Fourth Edition

Musculoskeletal and Sports Medicine for the Primary Care Practitioner

Fourth Edition

Musculoskeletal and Sports Medicine for the Primary Care Practitioner

Edited by

Richard B. Birrer
Professor of Medicine
Cornell University, New York, USA
eMD LLC
Locust Valley, New York, USA

Francis G. O'Connor
F. Edward Hebert School of Medicine
Uniformed Services University of the Health Sciences
Bethesda, Maryland, USA

Shawn F. Kane
F. Edward Hebert School of Medicine
Uniformed Services University of the Health Sciences
Bethesda, Maryland, USA

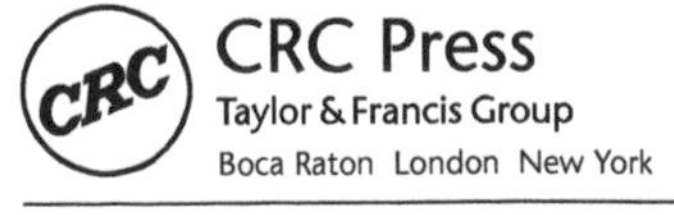

CRC Press is an imprint of the
Taylor & Francis Group, an **Informa** business

Disclaimer: The views expressed in this textbook are solely those of the authors and do not represent those of the Uniformed Services University of the Health Sciences or the Department of Defense.

CRC Press
Taylor & Francis Group
6000 Broken Sound Parkway NW, Suite 300
Boca Raton, FL 33487-2742

First issued in paperback 2020

ISBN-13: 978-1-4822-2011-7 (hbk)
ISBN-13: 978-0-367-78770-7 (pbk)

Visit the Taylor & Francis Web site at
http://www.taylorandfrancis.com

and the CRC Press Web site at
http://www.crcpress.com

Contents*

* Video links demonstrating important musculoskeletal maneuvers are available under the "Downloads" tab at http://www.crcpress.com/9781482220117.

SECTION IV Injury Management and Rehabilitation

SECTION V Regional Clinical Problems

Foreword

Now almost 25 years ago, Rich Birrer asked me to write the preface for the second edition of this textbook, then entitled *Sports Medicine for the Primary Care Physician*. The time was very different as sports medicine was just beginning to be recognized as an important domain of the primary care physician. The first three fellowship programs created to train primary care physicians in the discipline of sports medicine at the Cleveland Clinic, Michigan State University and University of California, Los Angeles (UCLA) had been in existence for five years, and additional fellowships were beginning to be developed at other institutions. The subspecialty of sports medicine had just been approved by the American Board of Medical Specialties (ABMS) with the American Boards of Emergency Medicine, Family Medicine, Internal Medicine, and Pediatrics, serving as the initial sponsoring boards of the subspecialty. The first certification examination in sports medicine would be given to 428 candidates in 1993, the same year that the second edition was eventually published. (It took what seemed like an eternity to get the second edition into press as the publisher changed three times!)

Of course, those of us who have been deeply involved in sports medicine know what subsequently has happened in the field since the second edition was published; interest in the discipline has exploded. The Accreditation Council for Graduate Medical Education (ACGME) would eventually adopt program requirements for accredited training in sports medicine and would begin the initial accreditation of fellowships in 1996. Twenty-seven fellowships sponsored by the specialty of family medicine were initially approved along with one internal medicine program, one emergency medicine program, and three programs in pediatrics. The American Board of Physical Medicine and Rehabilitation was approved by the ABMS to become the fifth sponsoring board for certification in sports medicine in 2006, and they began accrediting their first fellowship programs through the ACGME in 2008.

We now have over 150 accredited sports medicine fellowship programs across the specialties that sponsor the certificate and close to 3000 physicians who are board certified in sports medicine. Along with this increase in the number of primary care physicians who devote a significant amount of time to practicing sports medicine, a surprisingly large number of textbooks and journals have been published devoted to disseminating information about the clinical practice of sports medicine and cutting-edge research affecting this practice. So where does yet another textbook fit into this vast array of resources available to the practicing clinician?

To answer this question, it would be informative to note that the first edition of *Sports Medicine for the Primary Care Physician* found its origins in the Sports Medicine Committee of the Society of Teachers of Family Medicine that was created in 1980. This committee was chaired by Daniel Garfinkel, and he and its members had the foresight to develop a curriculum for family medicine residency training programs. Just as the first edition mirrored the curriculum created by that committee, the fourth edition draws from the suggested sports medicine curriculum created by the American Academy of Family Physicians (AAFP) for family medicine residency training programs. This is important as the new ACGME program requirements in family medicine mandate that residents must have at least 200 hours (or 2 months) devoted to the care of patients with a breadth of musculoskeletal problems, and a structured sports medicine experience must be provided.

So, the fourth edition is focused not exclusively on providing information to those with advanced sports medicine training, but rather on delivering information at the right level to medical students, residents, ancillary and mid-level providers, and clinicians who wish to expand their sports medicine knowledge base. Each chapter is written in an evidence-based fashion with emphasis on key clinical considerations and provision of appropriate clinical pearls. Each chapter ends with a Strength of Recommendation Taxonomy (SORT) table for the key clinical recommendations made in each chapter.

Of particular note is that the chapters that focus on orthopedic conditions are written using a symptom-oriented approach, and most importantly, they highlight the criteria that should lead to orthopedic referral by the primary care physician. This is critically important information that should assist residents and young clinicians with facilitating the appropriate referral of cases to their orthopedic colleagues.

The book concludes with an array of appendices that serve as useful resources for clinicians, and we should not overlook the links to the publisher's website that will host videos to demonstrate many important clinical features mentioned in the text.

In the preface to Birrer's second edition, I wrote as follows: "The family physician is confronted with the unique challenge of motivating his or her patients to become physically active. In so doing, it is necessary to provide appropriate education and counseling, as well as care for some of the maladies that may occur as a direct result of increased physical activity. This excellent text provides essential information which should allow family physicians to confidently practice Sports Medicine within the framework of their practices."

While much within the field has changed since I wrote those words in 1991, much has remained the same. Given the obesity epidemic in our country, the need for primary care physicians to actively engage their patients in the discussion about nutrition, physical activity, and wellness has never been greater. This latest edition of *Musculoskeletal and Sports Medicine For the Primary Care Practitioner* serves as a wonderful resource to help them do so.

James C. Puffer, MD
President and Chief Executive Officer
American Board of Family Medicine
Professor of Family and Community Medicine
College of Medicine
University of Kentucky
Lexington, Kentucky

Preface

> And is not bodily habit spoiled by rest and idleness but preserved for a long time by motion and exercise?
>
> **Plato, *Theaetetus***

Exercise in the natural form of work was a necessary and regular part of life before the Industrial Age. With the advent of work-saving machinery, people turned more and more to the "sedentary studious life."[1] Despite the clairvoyant exhortations of some of our nation's political leaders (Thomas Jefferson and Benjamin Franklin) and the world's medical giants (George Cheyne and Joseph Addison), the "pamper'd Race of Men" prospered.[2] Yet, the tempo of the past several decades has shown the wisdom and benefits of regular exercise. Serendipity has played a significant role in the observations that physically active individuals do not suffer proportionately from atherosclerosis, strokes, myocardial infarctions, and other chronically debilitating diseases as do their sedentary counterparts. Exercise research has begun to yield the secret successes of fitness training. Established health benefits of regular physical activity include a reduction of coronary heart disease, hypertension, non-insulin-dependent diabetes, colon cancer, anxiety, depression, and all-cause death rates; maintenance of appropriate body weight and functional capacity; and increased bone mineral content. The general sociocultural swing back to naturalism, homeopathy, holism, and self-help has embraced exercise and sports activities as a necessary component and has once again brought us full circle to our ancestors' philosophies.

Because the world of sports and recreational activity encompasses all ages and both genders, as well as the entire health spectrum, it is fitting that the primary care physician should be the frontline sports medicine specialist. It is this individual who first sees the injured athlete at home, on the field, or in the office. Very often, the physician recognizes the family or personal problem affecting a person's performance. Above all, it is the primary care physician who is best suited to integrate the patient's work, sport, family, and school environment so that maximum exercise potential and function under the safest health conditions can be realized.

The first edition of this book sprang from the Society of Teachers of Family Medicine sports medicine panel in 1980. This invigorating panel and its chairman, Daniel Garfinkel, MD, designed the sports medicine curriculum for the family practice programs of this country. The second edition moved to a problem-oriented, field-side format and became a practical authoritative guide for primary care physicians involved in the study and practice of sports medicine. The third edition brought further evolutionary changes, including several new chapters (complementary/alternative sports medicine options, the radiologic evaluation of the athlete, and a revised and streamlined medical illness section) and incorporated the growing science of evidence-based medicine. In addition, Francis G. O'Connor, MD, MPH, a recognized family physician who is a sports medicine authority and well-known educator, became the associate editor. This fourth edition specifically targets primary care providers who are increasingly called upon to deliver the majority of musculoskeletal and sports medicine evaluation and treatment in our current health-care system. The fourth edition focuses on an evidence-based approach with the identification of referral criteria where appropriate, clinical pearls' "call outs," and chapter-concluding Strength of Recommendation Tables (SORT). The editors, in addition, specifically developed a table of contents to reflect current educational requirements in primary care residency training. The majority of the authors have an active clinical practice in musculoskeletal and sports medicine or are well-respected experts in their specialty. We have included important video links that demonstrate important musculoskeletal maneuvers used in sports medicine. Finally, the fourth edition welcomes Shawn F. Kane, MD, as an assistant editor. Dr. Kane is a recognized leader in military sports and family medicine; he is a consultant to the surgeon general of the Army in family medicine, as well as a fellow in the American College of Sports Medicine, where he additionally serves as a section editor for one of their leading clinical journals.

Much work remains to be done in achieving the 2020 national objectives for physical fitness and exercise.[6] While the number of employer-sponsored fitness programs has significantly increased and the majority of primary care physicians include a careful exercise history as part of their initial examination of new patients, fewer than 50% of children aged 10 to 17 years regularly participate in appropriate physical activities, particularly cardiorespiratory fitness programs that can be carried into adulthood. Only 21% of adults aged 18 years and over are participating in vigorous physical exercise, and fewer than 8% of adults aged 65 years or older engage in appropriate physical activity (i.e., regular walking, swimming, or other aerobic activity). Only 5% of adults can accurately identify the variety and duration of exercise thought to promote cardiovascular fitness most effectively. Over 60% of adults and up to 17% of children are overweight or obese. These are profound challenges that must be addressed in the next decade through clinical practice and scholarly research. The message is clear: "Exercise is the easiest way to preserve health."[7] We are the medium. This textbook is one small effort in making the message happen. Read, learn, enjoy, and profit.

Video links demonstrating important musculoskeletal maneuvers are available under the "Downloads" tab at http://www.crcpress.com/9781482220117.

REFERENCES

1. Cheyne, G., Letter to Samuel Richardson, April 20, 1740.
2. Dryden, J., To John Driden of Chesterton, in *Fables, Ancient and Modern*, c. 1680.
3. Siwek, J., Gourlay, M.L., Slawson, D.C., Shaughnessy A.F., How to write an evidence-based clinical review article. *Am. Fam. Physician,* 65, 251–258, 2002.
4. Agency for Healthcare Research and Quality, Systems to rate the strength of scientific evidence. Summary, evidence report/technology assessment. Number 47. AHRQ pub. no. 02-E015, March 2002. Rockville, MD. Available at: www.ahrq.gov/clinic/epcsums/strengthsum.htm.
5. Clarke, M., Oxman, A.D., *Cochrane Reviewer's Handbook 4.0.* The Cochrane Collaboration, 2003. Available at: www.cochrane.org/resources/handbook/handbook.pdf.
6. U.S. Department of Health and Human Services, *Healthy People 2020: Leading Health Indicators: Nutrition, Physical Activity and Obesity.* U.S. Government Printing Office, Washington, DC, May 2014.
7. Mendez, C., *Book of Bodily Exercise*, 1553.

Acknowledgments

Special thanks to Barbara Norwitz, Kyle Meyer, Christine Selvan, Laurie Oknowsky, and the staff of Taylor & Francis (CRC Press) who enthusiastically and competently produced the textbook. Thanks also to our colleagues—the teachers, clinicians, and consultants who wrote these chapters, and to any of their illustrators, secretaries, and assistants.

Thanks also to our wives and families, who provided understanding and encouragement during the long hours of preparation and editing.

Editors

Richard B. Birrer, MD, is a graduate of Cornell University Medical College, New York, New York. He did his internship in family medicine at the Hunterdon Medical Center in Flemington, New Jersey, and completed his training at the State University of New York, Health Sciences Center of Brooklyn. As chief resident, he was the recipient of the Parke-Davis Teacher Development Award. He completed a master of public health degree from Harvard University and was a senior Fulbright scholar, introducing the principles and practice of family medicine in Egypt. He was chosen as a health exchange scientist to the former Union of Soviet Socialist Republics under the Fogarty program and is a Salzberg fellow. He holds a master's in medical management and is a certified physician executive. Currently, he is the CEO and president of eMD LLC and is a professor of medicine at Cornell. He is a diplomat and fellow in the specialties of family practice, sports medicine, geriatrics, emergency medicine, and medical management (certified physician executive). Dr. Birrer is the author of multiple peer-reviewed articles and monographs and 12 textbooks and serves on a number of editorial boards. He has run multiple marathons and has climbed the seven highest continental summits.

Francis G. O'Connor, MD, MPH, is currently professor and chair of the Department of Military and Emergency Medicine at the Uniformed Services University, Bethesda, Maryland and associate director for the Consortium on Health and Military Performance (CHAMP). He has been a leader in sports medicine education and research for the military for over 20 years. Dr. O'Connor has authored over 70 articles in scientific journals and numerous book chapters/technical reports/health promotion resources for the military. In addition, Dr. O'Connor is the editor of four texts on sports medicine, including the *Textbook of Running Medicine*, *Sports Medicine for the Primary Care Physician, 3rd Edition* and *ACSM's Sports Medicine: A Comprehensive Review*. He has been on the board of several leading organizations in sports medicine, including the American College of Sports Medicine, and the American Medical Athletic Association; he is a past president of the American Medical Society of Sports Medicine. A colonel in the United States Army, Dr. O'Connor is a graduate of the United States Military Academy at West Point.

Shawn F. Kane, MD, graduated from Gettysburg College, Gettysburg, Pennsylvania in 1991 and earned his medical degree from the F. Edward Hebert School of Medicine, Uniformed Services University of the Health Sciences, Bethesda, Maryland in 1995. He completed an internship and residency in family medicine at Womack Army Medical Center, Ft. Bragg, North Carolina. He completed a primary care sports medicine fellowship in 2004 at the National Capital Consortium/USUHS/DeWitt Army Community Hospital. Dr. Kane currently is the Deputy Chief of Staff Surgeon for the U.S. Army Special Operations Command (Airborne). He is an associate professor in the Department of Family Medicine and assistant professor in the Department of Military and Emergency Medicine at USUHS and serves as the consultant to the U.S. Army Surgeon General for Family Medicine. He is a fellow of the American College of Sports Medicine and the American Academy of Family Physicians. He has authored 25 peer-reviewed articles and textbook chapters.

Contributors

Alain Michael P. Abellada, MD
Blanchfield Army Community Hospital
Fort Campbell, Kentucky

William B. Adams, MD
Naval Medical Clinic
Quantico, Virginia

Venu Akuthota, MD
University of Colorado School of Medicine
Denver, Colorado

Jason B. Alisangco, DO
Dwight D. Eisenhower Army Medical Center
Fort Gordon, Georgia

Chad A. Asplund, MD, MPH, FACSM
Georgia Regents University
Augusta, Georgia

Selasi Attipoe, MS
Uniformed Services University of the Health Sciences
Bethesda, Maryland

Kenneth B. Batts, DO
Womack Army Medical Center
Fort Bragg, North Carolina

Blair A. Becker, MD
Group Health Family Medicine Residency
Seattle, Washington

Holly J. Benjamin, MD, FAAP, FACSM
University of Chicago
Chicago, Illinois

Erik Berger, MD
SCL Physicians
Lafayette, Colorado

Anthony I. Beutler, MD
Uniformed Services University of the Health Sciences
Bethesda, Maryland

Kenneth Bielak, MD
University of Tennessee Health Science Center
Memphis, Tennessee

Richard B. Birrer, MD, FAAFP, FACSM, FACP, FAGS, FACEP
Cornell University Medical College
New York, New York

and

eMD LLC
Locust Valley, New York

Daniel H. Blatz, MD
Spine and Sports Rehabilitation Center
Rehabilitation Institute of Chicago
Chicago, Illinois

and

Northwestern University
Evanston, Illinois

Barry P. Boden, MD
Uniformed Services University of the Health Sciences
Bethesda, Maryland

Ronald E. Bowers, Jr., DHSc, PA-C
Kettering College
Dayton, Ohio

Fred H. Brennan, Jr., DO, FAOASM, FAAFP, FACSM
University of New Hampshire
Durham, New Hampshire

and

157th Medical Group
Pease Air National Guard Base, New Hampshire

and

Seacoast Orthopedics and Sports Medicine
Somersworth, New Hampshire

David L. Brown, MD
Blanchfield Army Community Hospital
Fort Campbell, Kentucky

Linda L. Brown, MD
Blanchfield Army Community Hospital
Fort Campbell, Kentucky

Douglas J. Casa, PhD, ATC, FACSM, FNATA
University of Connecticut
Storrs, Connecticut

Evan Corey, MD
Cone Health System
Greensboro, North Carolina

Sarah De La Motte, PhD, MPH, ATC
Uniformed Services University of the Health Sciences
Bethesda, Maryland

B. Elizabeth Delasobera, MD
Georgetown University
and
MedStar Health
Washington, DC

Jesse DeLuca, DO
NCC/Fort Belvoir Primary Care Sports Medicine Fellowship
Fort Belvoir, Virginia

Arthur Jason De Luigi, DO
MedStar NRH
and
Georgetown University School of Medicine
Washington, DC

Patrick J. Depenbrock, MD
United States Army Special Operations Command
Fort Bragg, North Carolina

Patricia A. Deuster, PhD, MPH, FACSM
Uniformed Services University of the Health Sciences
Bethesda, Maryland

Kevin deWeber, MD
University of Washington
and
Clark College
Vancouver, Washington

Jay Dicharry, MPT, SCS
REP Lab, Rebound Physical Therapy
Bend, Oregon

Timothy Ryan Draper, DO
University of North Carolina
and
Sports Medicine Fellowship Cone Health System
Greensboro, North Carolina

Ted Epperly, MD
Family Medicine Residency of Idaho
Boise, Idaho

and

University of Washington
Seattle, Washington

Kenton H. Fibel, MD
Hospital for Special Surgery
New York, New York

Karl B. Fields, MD
University of North Carolina
and
Sports Medicine Fellowship Cone Health System
Greensboro, North Carolina

Jonathan T. Finnoff, DO
Mayo Clinic Sports Medicine Center
Minneapolis, Minnesota

and

Mayo Clinic School of Medicine
Rochester, Minnesota

Scott Flinn, MD
Blue Shield of California
Poway, California

Katherine Walker Foster, MD
The University of North Carolina at Chapel Hill
Chapel Hill, North Carolina

and

Cabarrus Family Medicine Residency Program
Concord, North Carolina

Jason Friedrich, MD
University of Colorado
Aurora, Colorado

Jennifer J. Gayagoy, MD
St. Joseph's Hospital Health Center
Syracuse, New York

and

MacNeal Hospital
Berwyn, Illinois

Melissa L. Givens, MD, MPH
Uniformed Services University of the Health Sciences
Bethesda, Maryland

Donald Lee Goss, PhD
U.S. Military Baylor University PT Sports Doctoral Fellowship
and
Keller Army Community Hospital
West Point, New York

Andrew J.M. Gregory, MD, FAAP, FACSM
Vanderbilt University School of Medicine
Nashville, Tennessee

Brian C. Halpern, MD, FAAFP
Hospital for Special Surgery
New York, New York

George D. Harris, MD, MS
West Virginia University-Eastern Division
and
University Healthcare Physicians Primary Care Division
Martinsburg, West Virginia

Mark D. Harris, MD, MPH
Fort Belvoir Community Hospital
Fort Belvoir, Virginia

and

Uniformed Services University of the Health Sciences
Bethesda, Maryland

Sally S. Harris, MD, MPH
Palo Alto Medical Foundation
Palo Alto, California

Bradley S. Havins, MD
Blanchfield Army Community Hospital
Fort Campbell, Kentucky

Robert Hayes, MD
University Park Family Medicine
South Bend, Indiana

Thomas Howard, MD, FACSM
Fairfax Family Practice
Fairfax, Virginia

Collin G. Hu, DO, EMT-E
Womack Family Medicine Residency Program
Fort Bragg, North Carolina

Yaowen Eliot Hu, MD
Herndon Family Medicine
Herndon, Virginia

Korin Hudson, MD
Georgetown University
and
MedStar Health
Washington, DC

Carrie A. Jaworski, MD
University of Chicago Pritzker School of Medicine
and
North Shore University Health System
Glenview, Illinois

Christopher E. Jonas, MD
Uniformed Services University of Health Sciences
Bethesda, Maryland

Wayne B. Jonas, MD
Samueli Institute
Alexandria, Virginia

Shawn F. Kane, MD, FAAFP, FACSM
United States Army Special Operations Command
Fort Bragg, North Carolina

and

F. Edward Hebert School of Medicine
Bethesda, Maryland

Osric S. King, MD
Hospital for Special Surgery
New York, New York

Jacqueline S. Lamme, MD
Naval Medical Center San Diego
San Diego, California

and

Uniformed Services University of Health Sciences
Bethesda, Maryland

Richard Levandowski, MD
Princeton Sports and Family Medicine
West Windsor Township, New Jersey

and

Rutgers Robert Wood Johnson Medical School
and
Rutgers New Jersey Medical School
Newark, New Jersey

David A. Levin, MD, FAAOS
The Orthopedic Center
A Division of the Centers for Advance Orthopedics
Bethesda, Maryland

Peter Lisman, PhD, ATC
Towson University
Towson, Maryland

Brian C. Lowell, MD
Family Medicine of Southwest Washington Residency
Vancouver, Washington

Christopher J. Lutrzykowski, MD
Dartmouth Medical School
Augusta, Maine

James H. Lynch, MD
Special Operations Command Africa
Stuttgart, Germany

and

Uniformed Services University of the Health Sciences
Bethesda, Maryland

Stephen W. Marshall, PhD
Gillings School of Global Public Health
and
University of North Carolina at Chapel Hill
Chapel Hill, North Carolina

Sean N. Martin, DO
Headquarters AFSOC
Eglin Air Force Base, Florida

Christopher D. Meyering, DO
1st Cavalry Division
Fort Hood, Texas

Sean W. Mulvaney, MD
Walter Reed National Military Medical Center
Bethesda, Maryland

Robert P. Nirschl, MD, MS
Nirschl Orthopedic Center
and
Virginia Sports Medicine Institute
Arlington, Virginia

Rochelle M. Nolte, MD
U.S. Public Health Service
San Diego, California

Nathaniel S. Nye, MD
Joint Base San Antonio
559th Trainee Health Squadron
Lackland, Texas

Francis G. O'Connor, MD, MPH, FACSM
Uniformed Services University of the Health Sciences
Bethesda, Maryland

Ralph P. Oriscello, MD
East Orange Veterans Administration Hospital
East Orange, New Jersey

Todd Palmer, MD
Family Medicine Residency of Idaho
Boise, Idaho

and

University of Washington
Seattle, Washington

Leigh E. Palubinskas, PT, DPT, OCS
Performance Physical Therapy
Stockbridge, Georgia

Andrea L. Pana, MD, MPH
Sports Medicine Physician
Austin, Texas

Michael J. Petrizzi, MD
VCU Sports Medicine Center & Hanover Family Physicians
and
Virginia Commonwealth University
Richmond, Virginia

Nicholas A. Piantanida, MD
Centura Health Physician Group
Colorado Springs, Colorado

Robert M. Barney Poole, PT, DPT, ATC
Performance Physical Therapy
Stockbridge, Georgia

and

Emory University
Atlanta, Georgia

Gayan P. Poovendran, MD
Meli Orthopedic Centers of Excellence
Fort Lauderdale, Florida

Scott W. Pyne, MD
United States Naval Academy
Annapolis, Maryland

and

Uniformed Services University of the Health Sciences
Bethesda, Maryland

Richard D. Quattrone, DO
Naval Health Clinic Hawaii
Pearl Harbor, Hawaii

Meghan F. Raleigh, MD, FAAFP
Fort Belvoir Community Hospital
Fort Belvoir, Virginia

Leslie H. Rassner, MD
Utah HealthCare Institute
Salt Lake City, Utah

Ulrich A. Rassner, MD
University of Utah School of Medicine
Salt Lake City, Utah

Mitchell J. Rauh, PhD, PT, MPH, FACSM
San Diego State University
San Diego, California

Brian V. Reamy, MD, FAAFP
Uniformed Services University of the Health Sciences
Bethesda, Maryland

Erika S. Reese, MD
Fort Belvoir Community Hospital
Fort Belvoir, Virginia

Scott Repa, DO
University of Chicago–North Shore
Glenview, Illinois

Jeffrey B. Roberts, MD, CAQSM
Bon Secours Sports Medicine
and
Virginia Commonwealth University
Richmond, Virginia

Sean C. Robinson, MD, CAQSM
Lewis and Clark College
and
Oregon Health & Science University
Portland, Oregon

David Rupp, MD, CAQSM
Marshall University School of Medicine
Huntington, West Virginia

R. Kent Sanders, MD
University of Utah School of Medicine
Salt Lake City, Utah

Christopher J. Sardon, MPH
Uniformed Services University of the Health Sciences
Bethesda, Maryland

Jonathan M. Scott, PhD, RD
Uniformed Services University of the Health Sciences
Bethesda, Maryland

Peter H. Seidenberg, MD, FAAFP, FACSM, RMSK
Pennsylvania State University
State College, Pennsylvania

Joel L. Shaw, MD
Grant Sports Medicine
MAX Sports Medicine
Columbus, Ohio

Ian Shrier, MD, PhD
Lady Davis Institute for Medical Research
and
McGill University
Montreal, Quebec, Canada

Lauren M. Simon, MD, MPH, FACSM
Loma Linda University
Loma Linda, California

and

University of California
Riverside, California

and

University of Redlands
Redlands, California

Marvin H. Sineath, Jr., MD
Family Medicine Residency
Nellis Air Force Base, Nevada

Michael A. Sirota, M.D.
San Diego Sports Medicine & Orthopedic Center
San Diego, California

Kristen L. Slappey, DO
Family Medicine Residency
Nellis Air Force Base, Nevada

Zachary Smith, DO
Cone Health System
Greensboro, North Carolina

Joshua S. Sole, MD
Texas Christian University
Arlington/Fort Worth, Texas

Mark B. Stephens, MD
Uniformed Services University of the Health Sciences
Bethesda, Maryland

Robert B. Stevens, DO
Oakland Family Medicine
Oakland, Maine

Steven D. Stovitz, MD, MS
University of Minnesota Medical School
Minneapolis, Minnesota

Jillian Sylvester, MD
Fort Belvoir Community Hospital
Fort Belvoir, Virginia

Michelle E. Szczepanik, MD
Carl R. Darnall Army Medical Center
Fort Hood, Texas

Rodney L. Thompson, MD
William Beaumont Army Medical Center
El Paso, Texas

James B. Tucker, MD
St Joseph's Hospital Health Center
and
Syracuse University
Syracuse, New York

Charles W. Webb, DO
Oregon Health & Science University
and
Portland State University
and
Lewis & Clark College
Portland, Oregon

Peter C. Wenger, MD
Rutgers New Jersey Medical School
Newark, New Jersey

Russell D. White, MD
University of Missouri–Kansas City
Kansas City, Missouri

and

Veterans Healthcare System of the Ozarks
Mount Vernon, Missouri

Robert Alan Whitehurst, DPT
Womack Army Medical Center
Fort Bragg, North Carolina

John H. Wilckens, MD
Johns Hopkins School of Medicine
Baltimore, Maryland

Robert P. Wilder, MD, FACSM
The University of Virginia
Charlottesville, Virginia

Scott E. Young, DO, FACEP
Madigan Army Medical Center
Joint Base Lewis-McChord
Tacoma, Washington

Section I

General Principles

1 Evidence-Based Medicine in Musculoskeletal and Sports Medicine

Steven D. Stovitz and Ian Shrier

CONTENTS

TABLE 1.1
Key Clinical Considerations

1. The modern evidence-based medicine (EBM) movement began in the early 1990s due to an increasing recognition that recommendations for diagnosing and treating illnesses were often based on personal opinions. Prior to EBM, there was not a strong emphasis that opinions be justified by peer-reviewed evidence.
2. Evidence-grading systems try to objectify the evaluation of both individual studies and bodies of evidence (multiple studies) on particular clinical questions.
3. EBM requires the integration of the best research evidence with our clinical expertize and our patient's unique values and circumstances.[11]

1.1 INTRODUCTION

This textbook aims to help primary care clinicians in their practice of musculoskeletal and sports medicine. With the intent of summarizing the highest quality evidence, authors of this chapter have been asked to present the information and conclude all chapters, when possible, in the form of a standardized evidence-grading system. Evidence-grading systems have been advocated by many in the evidence-based medicine (EBM) movement as an attempt to validate the quality of evidence as it pertains to particular clinical questions. The objective of this chapter is to review the purpose of the EBM movement with a focus on the rationale behind the evidence-grading systems. We will discuss the benefits and limitations of evidence-grading systems and also refer to controversies surrounding the proper role of evidence in the context of patient care (Table 1.1).

While the practice of medicine has always tried to incorporate evidence, the origin of the modern EBM movement dates back to the early 1990s.[1] At that time, there was an increasing recognition that recommendations for diagnosing and treating illnesses were often based on what was considered "expert-based medicine."[9] Expert-based medicine refers to opinions of experts or leaders in the field, without documentation of the rationale behind the opinions. Prior to the modern EBM movement, the medical community did not require these experts to explicitly explain or evaluate the evidence they used in making recommendations. Therefore, it was difficult to differentiate between recommendations that were based on either personal opinion (little rationale and likely biased) and/or studies with substantial flaws (high probability of large bias), from those recommendations based on sound science and rational decision making (least biased). The principles of EBM can be applied to examining disease etiology, diagnosis, and/or treatment. For the purposes of this chapter, we will focus on treatment evaluation EBM.

1.2 EVIDENCE-BASED MEDICINE (EBM) AND EVIDENCE-GRADING SYSTEMS

Figure 1.1 graphically displays a commonly used pyramid to assess evidence quality as it pertains to treatment. Additionally, a variety of organizations have developed grading systems for a body of evidence. One of the most detailed systems, shown in Table 1.2, comes from the multinational working group entitled, Grading of Recommendations, Assessment, Development and Evaluation (GRADE).[6] Leaders in the field of primary care medicine recognized that the emphasis on *evidence quality* often obscured the fact that the outcome of many studies was disease oriented rather than patient oriented. A disease-oriented outcome (e.g., increases in bone density) is not as important to the patient as a patient-oriented outcome (e.g., fewer hip fractures).

Clinical Pearl

The strength-of-recommendation taxonomy (SORT) system emphasizes patient-oriented outcomes (e.g., fewer hip fractures) over disease-oriented outcomes (e.g., increases in bone density).

TABLE 1.2
Grading of Recommendations Assessment, Development, and Evaluation (GRADE)

Code	Quality of Evidence	Definition
A	High	Further research is very unlikely to change our confidence in the estimate of effect. Several high-quality studies with consistent results In special cases: one large, high-quality multicenter trial
B	Moderate	Further research is likely to have an important impact on our confidence in the estimate of effect and may change the estimate. One high-quality study Several studies with some limitations
C	Low	Further research is very likely to have an important impact on our confidence in the estimate of effect and is likely to change the estimate. One or more studies with severe limitations
D	Very low	Any estimate of effect is very uncertain. Expert opinion No direct research evidence One or more studies with very severe limitations

Source: GRADE (Grading of Recommendations Assessment, Development and Evaluation) Working Group 2007. (Evidence-Based Medicine Working Group, *Journal of the American Medical Association*, 268, 2420, 1992.) Modified by the EBM Guidelines Editorial Team.

Consequently, in 2004, a number of leading journal editors in primary care medicine put forth a new grading system with further emphasis on patient-oriented outcomes, the SORT, see Table 1.3.[2]

Since this textbook is geared toward primary care providers, chapters will typically use the SORT system. The developers of GRADE also discuss how to operationalize the transition from "evidence" to "recommendations."[5] In doing so, GRADE attempts to keep the evidence "patient centered" by incorporating patient's values and preferences.[5]

1.3 ERRORS AND THE RELATIONSHIP OF STUDY DESIGN TO EVIDENCE QUALITY

The various evidence-grading systems have differences, but share a common goal; that is, to help the clinical-research community systematically evaluate a body of evidence in order to obtain the highest level of validity (i.e., "truth") when answering clinical questions. To understand the rationale behind the structure of these systems, it is important to recognize some general categories of errors.

1.3.1 Errors May Be Random or Systematic Events

Errors that cause evidence to stray from the truth are often divided into errors that are either random or systematic. One key distinguishing factor between random and systematic errors is that, within individual studies, random errors decrease when the studies are larger, whereas systematic errors do not. For a particular research question, random errors from individual studies are expected to cancel each other out when there are a higher number of studies. More studies on a topic can also potentially decrease systematic errors toward a particular research question. This assumes that multiple studies do not repeat the same systematic errors and that the errors from particular studies act in opposing directions. Repetition of research, although often discouraged by funding agencies, is crucial toward the goal of minimizing errors and obtaining the most valid evidence.[7]

Clinical Pearl

Research errors can be categorized into those that are either random or systematic. Random errors tend to decrease with an increase in study sample size. Systematic errors persist despite increases in study sample size.

Systematic errors are often thought of as "bias." The physician who reports results only on patients who return for follow-up visits after treatment is likely reporting on a biased sample (assuming that less than 100% of patients follow-up). Losses to follow-up are unlikely to be random events. It may be that patients who do worse are "lost to follow-up" as they did not like the manner in which they were treated. Conversely, for some problems, patients who do better may be lost to follow-up, as they did not see a need to return. Note that, within a particular study, systematic error (i.e., bias) does not decrease if there are more subjects.

An "expert" physician at a tertiary care medical center who randomizes his/her patients to either a new treatment or "usual care" may also be reporting results on a "biased" sample. Tertiary care medical centers likely see a disproportionate percentage of patients who have failed "usual care." Consequently, a new treatment under study may appear to be relatively superior at the tertiary care medical center. The clinician reader of the research who works with a less selective population may find that the new treatment is not as beneficial as the study results suggested. Note that some would not call this latter example "bias," but rather a problem of generalizability. For the purpose of the non-tertiary care clinician, whether one calls it bias or a problem of generalizability, the fact remains that research from a tertiary care center may have a systematic error when trying to apply the findings to one's own patients, and this error does not diminish as the number of subjects increases. Unfortunately, by definition, errors of generalizability are not well captured by standardized evidence-grading systems even though SORT and GRADE do make attempts to do so.

1.3.2 Study Design and Evidence Hierarchy

Clinicians do not have time to carefully analyze all possible studies on the problems they encounter during clinical care. They must rely on research summaries. The pyramid shown

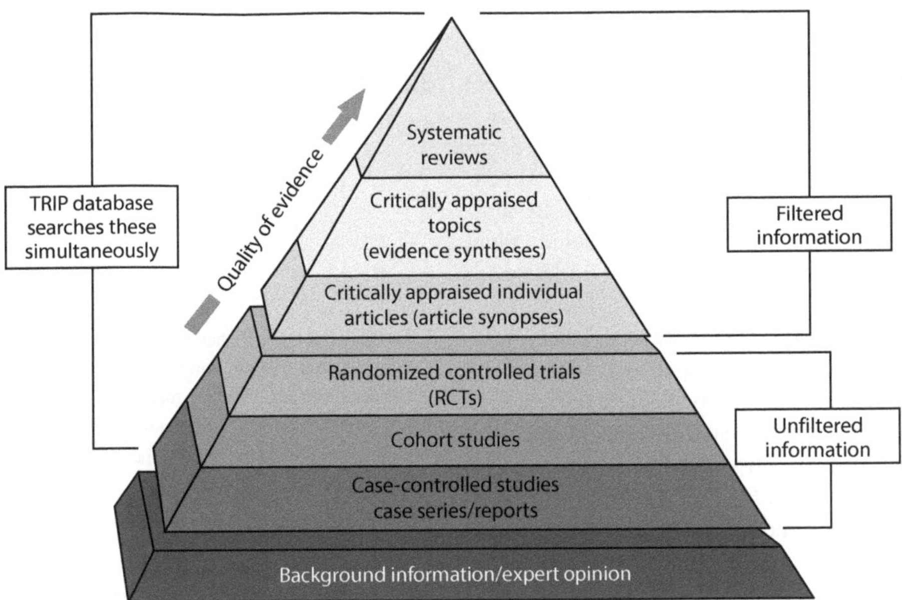

FIGURE 1.1 Evidence hierarchy. (From Evidence-based clinical practice resources: Pyramid, http://guides.library.yale.edu/content.php?pid=9786&sid=73113, accessed October 17, 2015.)

in Figure 1.1 places categories of evidence that are felt to be less valid (i.e., higher potential for bias) at the bottom of the pyramid and evidence that is felt to be more valid (i.e., least biased) at the top of the pyramid. Careful consideration of the categories quickly reveals that the pyramid, like other evidence hierarchy ranking systems, has the potential to garner false conclusions. Expert opinion based on years of experience might be closer to the truth than any singular study, regardless of the design. Although EBM was created, in part, to stop recommendations based solely on expert opinion, occasionally, experts are correct and studies may be wrong for a large variety of reasons.

For example, even a well-designed and well-conducted study may have random errors. Studies with no "statistically significant difference" may have low "power" (i.e., small sample size) and be misinterpreted as "no difference." However, absence of proof of a difference is not proof of absence of a difference, and a difference between treatments may, in fact, exist. Problems such as low power resulting in a lack of a statistically significant effect within a particular study can be overcome with well-conducted analyses of bodies of evidence, e.g., systematic reviews and/or meta-analyses. Other reasons for mistakes within studies include measurement error and flaws in the statistical analysis.

Although the evidence hierarchies, such as that shown in Figure 1.1, can have flaws, they are based on a strong rationale. While all studies have the potential for bias, some study designs are more likely to produce biased results. As stated here, a case series might be biased due to issues of follow-up. When evaluating treatment, the most obvious unbiased study is one that assesses two groups who have equal probability for the outcome (except for the treatment that is being applied) and are treated exactly the same throughout the study (except for the treatment). In other words, if no treatment was given, we would expect the results to be the same in both groups. This is the strength of a randomized controlled trial (RCT). Note that even a large well-conducted RCT on a clinician's exact question may not be applicable to the patient if the population in the study differed from the person in the clinic. A large observational cohort study may be the representative of your patient population (i.e., generalizable). However, important prognostic factors that are unknown to investigators may either (a) cause some patients to be more likely to suffer a bad outcome or (b) cause some patients to take treatment and others to not take treatment. If either occurs then there is bias because the two groups are not expected to have the same results if treatment did not occur. Statistical adjustment can minimize some of the effect of the differences between groups for prognostic factors but only if they are known, and measured.

An RCT is considered the study design with the least potential for bias, since, by its design, RCTs are expected to create two groups with equal prognosis (i.e., known and unknown variables are expected to be evenly distributed between the groups). However, RCTs with poor follow-up, or which treat patients and controls differently after randomization, may also be very biased. To improve our assessment of bias within and between study designs, more elaborate methods are currently being proposed,[13,14] but more work needs to be done before these tools become widely used and useful for the clinician.

1.4 ASSESSING A BODY OF EVIDENCE

The developers of SORT refer to the fact that evidence should be judged on quality (especially of individual studies), quantity (i.e., multiple studies), and consistency.[2] When judging evidence, in total, for the purpose of comparing treatments, the ultimate goal is to know the truth. Toward that goal, combining studies has obvious advantages.

As stated here, when evaluating multiple studies on a topic, random errors from individual studies will tend to cancel out each other. Combining studies can also minimize the effect of systematic error (bias) within any one study on the total body of evidence if the biases from individual studies occur in different directions (i.e., some make the treatment appear better and some make the treatment appear worse). In addition, when outcomes are rare, it may be hard for individual studies to capture treatment differences, even if differences actually exist.

Consequently, well-done systematic reviews and meta-analyses are felt to provide the highest quality evidence. The pyramid shown in Figure 1.1 specifically places evidence synthesis that comes from combining studies atop of even the best designed singular studies. The GRADE system emphasizes evidence consistency. In GRADE, the final summary takes the approach related to finding the truth and operationalizes it as whether future studies are likely or not likely to change a recommendation (Table 1.2). Obviously, if many well-conducted studies obtain similar results, one can be fairly confident that further research will not likely change the conclusions. According to GRADE, the quality of evidence is considered high (i.e., "A") when "Further research is very unlikely to change our confidence in the estimate of effect." The SORT system emphasizes quantity (i.e., multiple studies) and uses the word "consistent" to describe how multiple studies reaching a similar conclusion are valued higher than singular studies.

TABLE 1.3
Strength of Recommendation Taxonomy (SORT)

Code	Definition
A	Consistent, good-quality patient-oriented evidence[a]
B	Inconsistent or limited-quality patient-oriented evidence[a]
C	Consensus, disease-oriented evidence,[a] usual practice, expert opinion, or case series for studies of diagnosis, treatment, prevention, or screening

[a] Patient-oriented evidence measures outcomes that matter to patients: morbidity, mortality, symptom improvement, cost reduction, and quality of life. Disease-oriented evidence measures immediate, physiologic, or surrogate end points that may or may not reflect improvements in patient outcomes (e.g., blood pressure, blood chemistry, physiologic function, pathologic findings).

Clinical Pearl

EBM requires the integration of the best research evidence with our clinical expertise and our patient's unique values and circumstances.[11]

1.5 INTEGRATING EVIDENCE AND SHARED DECISION MAKING IN MUSCULOSKELETAL AND SPORTS MEDICINE

Evaluating the quality of evidence and integrating it into patient care are the foundation of EBM. However, many now apply the principles used to assess evidence quality, and infer that little further judgment is needed to apply the evidence in the practice of EBM. As summarized by Greenhalgh, this is an inappropriate and simplistic interpretation of EBM.[5] As stated by the founders of EBM on page one of their book, "Evidence-based medicine (EBM) requires the integration of the best research evidence with our clinical expertise and our patient's unique values and circumstances."[11] This message is unfortunately lost when the emphasis is solely on the relevant level of study designs within the pyramid of Figure 1.1. This does not mean we should ignore evidence. Rather, it means we must remember that evidence can only be understood in context, and value judgments are always required. For example, within GRADE, words like "unlikely" and "confidence" for Grade A evidence are not precise. Therefore, GRADE explicitly requires value judgments to be made. In fact, EBM was designed to help clinicians make judgments, not to replace clinician judgment. When this is kept in mind, it is a very powerful tool. When it is forgotten, it can lead to inappropriate care for both small and large numbers of patients.

As much of this textbook will suggest, one of the important roles of the physician is to empower the patient in decision making that affects their health. The physician's role is not merely to summarize the evidence for the patient. The goal of shared decision making is to make decisions in a manner consistent with the patient's wishes.[4,8,10] This process asks clinicians to translate, in an understandable manner, the available knowledge that might affect a patient's decision.[3,12] The SORT (Table 1.3) and GRADE (Table 1.2) systems are useful reminders that the patients' general health and well-being must remain our focus.

Due to a variety of reasons, patients may choose treatments that the evidence finds inferior. These reasons may include personal preferences ("I don't like creams, so I would rather take a pill"), or fears ("my uncle died during a similar operation"), or issues related to the baseline risk for the outcome ("why would I undergo surgery if there is a high likelihood that I will get better without surgery?"). In brief, high-quality evidence is better than low-quality evidence. However, we need to remember that when evidence, no matter how high the quality, suggests that a particular treatment is superior, this is within the context of what was chosen for the primary outcome and the value placed on particular adverse events; this does not necessarily signify that the particular treatment is the best for your patient who may place a different value on the possible outcomes and adverse events.

REFERENCES

1. Evidence-Based Medicine Working Group. Evidence-based medicine. A new approach to teaching the practice of medicine. *Journal of the American Medical Association*. 1992;268(17):2420–2425. Accessed August 18, 2014.

2. Ebell M, Siwek J, Weiss B et al. Strength of recommendation taxonomy (SORT): A patient-centered approach to grading evidence in the medical literature. *Journal of the American Board of Family Practice.* 2004;17(1):59–67. Accessed August 18, 2014.
3. Epstein R, Alper B, Quill T. Communicating evidence for participatory decision making. *Journal of the American Medical Association.* 2004;291(19):2359–2366.
4. Epstein RM, Street RL, Jr. Shared mind: Communication, decision making, and autonomy in serious illness. *Annals of Family Medicine.* 2011;9(5):454–461.
5. Greenhalgh T, Howick J, Maskrey N, Evidence Based Med Renaissance Group. ESSAY evidence based medicine: A movement in crisis? *BMJ: British Medical Journal.* 2014;348:g3725. Accessed August 14, 2014.
6. Guyatt GH, Oxman AD, Schuenemann HJ, Tugwell P, Knottnerus A. GRADE guidelines: A new series of articles in the journal of clinical epidemiology. *Journal of Clinical Epidemiology.* 2011;64(4):380–382. Accessed August 30, 2014.
7. Ioannidis JPA. Why science is not necessarily self-correcting. *Perspectives on Psychological Science.* 2012;7(6): 645–654. Accessed September 1, 2014.
8. Kon AA. The shared decision-making continuum. *Journal of the American Medical Association.* 2010;304(8):903–904.
9. Smith R, Rennie D. Evidence-based medicine—An oral history. *Journal of the American Medical Association.* 2014;311(4):365–367. Accessed August 8, 2014.
10. Stiggelbout AM, Van der Weijden T, De Wit MPT et al. Shared decision making: Really putting patients at the centre of healthcare. *BMJ: British Medical Journal.* 2012;344:e256.
11. Straus SE, Glasziou P, Richardson WS, Haynes RB. *Evidence-Based Medicine: How to Practice and Teach it,* 4th edn. Toronto, Ontario, Canada: Elsevier; 2011.
12. Straus SE, Tetroe JM, Graham ID. Knowledge translation is the use of knowledge in health care decision making. *Journal of Clinical Epidemiology.* 2011;64(1):6–10.
13. Thompson S, Ekelund U, Jebb S et al. A proposed method of bias adjustment for meta-analyses of published observational studies. *International Journal of Epidemiology.* 2011;40(3):765–777. Accessed September 9, 2014.
14. Turner RM, Spiegelhalter DJ, Smith GCS, Thompson SG. Bias modelling in evidence synthesis. *Journal of the Royal Statistical Society Series A: Statistics in Society.* 2009;172:21–47. Accessed September 1, 2014.

2 Epidemiology

Stephen W. Marshall and Mitchell J. Rauh

CONTENTS

2.1 INTRODUCTION

This chapter provides an introduction to the fundamentals of epidemiologic methods as applied to musculoskeletal and sports medicine. The number of people who participate in sport is large, with 470,000 collegiate athletes, 7.8 million high school athletes,[28,29] and an unknown number (undoubtedly in the tens of millions) of adults and children who play in club and recreational leagues. While involvement in organized sports bestows many health benefits and rewards, it also carries the risk of injury and other negative effects. Sports-related musculoskeletal injuries lead to chronic musculoskeletal problems and osteoarthritis,[20,21,34] limiting the ability to experience pain-free mobility or participate in fitness-enhancing activities later in life.[10]

The purpose of epidemiology in musculoskeletal and sports medicine is to identify the determinants of the prevalence and incidence of sports injury and related musculoskeletal conditions. For example, is the risk of injury greater in some sports than others? What environmental conditions increase the likelihood of heat-related conditions such as exertional heat illness? What preventive measures available are effective in preventing injuries and musculoskeletal conditions? The goal of epidemiology in sports medicine is to provide answers to these types of questions. A formal definition appears in the following box.

Clinical Pearl

Sports medicine epidemiology is the study of the distribution and determinants of injuries and disorders for the purpose of identifying and implementing measures to prevent their development.

2.2 STUDY DESIGNS

To understand and interpret data on sports injuries and musculoskeletal conditions, a basic understanding of study design is necessary. There are two basic types of study designs: descriptive and analytical. Descriptive studies (i.e., case series and cross sectional) are used primarily for understanding the scope of the problem and identifying trends. Analytical studies (i.e., case–control, case crossover, and prospective cohort) are used for assessing risk and identifying risk factors. Currently, most of the sports injury literature is descriptive epidemiology, but the number of analytical studies is increasing.

The research question to be answered should drive the choice of study design. Table 2.1 shows the general types of study designs that are used in epidemiology and the types of research questions that each design can be used to address. Each design has its strengths and limitations and are discussed in the remainder of this section.

TABLE 2.1
Types of Epidemiologic Study Designs

Study Design	Purpose(s)	Population
Case series	Assess the scope of a problem.	Injured persons.
Cross sectional	Determine the prevalence of a problem in a defined population.	All persons or a sample of persons in a defined area (school, county, state).
Case–control	Evaluate risk factors among injured and non-injured person. Assess effectiveness of an intervention.	Injured persons and representative controls (uninjured persons).
Case crossover	Evaluate time-related risk factors, usually among injured persons. Assess effectiveness of an intervention.	Events resulting in injury and representative control times in the same athletes.
Prospective cohort	Evaluate risk factors among injured and non-injured persons. Assess effectiveness of an intervention.	Defined cohort with assessment of exposure and prospective monitoring of injuries.
Randomized controlled trial	Assess effectiveness of an intervention.	Randomly assigned treatment and nontreatment subjects in a well-defined sample.

2.2.1 Case Series

The goal of a case series study is typically to collate information on a type of clinical event, its severity, the circumstances surrounding the event, and other elements to further describe the injured population. A case series can help the clinician/researcher generate ideas for further study. However, case series do not include uninjured people, and thus, this study design is unable to identify risk factors for prevention purposes.

2.2.2 Cross Sectional

Studies that are conducted on a sample of a target population provide valuable information on the prevalence (i.e., the percentage of the target population currently experiencing) of certain diseases, conditions, or even risk factors. A cross-sectional study on concussions, for example, can be conducted on a target population of high school athletes. If information is requested of all high school athletes (both injured and uninjured), then there is a denominator to use to calculate prevalence (see Section 2.3).

However, cross-sectional studies have limited ability to identify risk factors because all of the information on injuries/musculoskeletal conditions is collected at the same time. For example, athletes may over-recall or under-recall their injury/condition, particularly if disclosure is perceived to be associated with perceived incentives (e.g., exaggerating injuries due to bravado) or consequences (e.g., under-reporting injuries due to concern about being withheld from competition). Therefore, cross-sectional studies are a weak basis for the quantification of a causal relationship between the risk factor (not wearing ankle brace) and the outcome such as injury (high ankle sprains). Study designs that account of the temporal nature of cause and effect are better suited to assessing risk factors.

2.2.3 Case–control

One study design that is well suited to assessing risk factors is the case–control study. In this study design, cases (e.g., injured athletes from a clinic) and comparable controls (e.g., uninjured athletes from the clinic's source population) are selected, and the two groups are compared on possible risk factors. For example, one may be interested in studying female high school athletes who incurred or did not incur an anterior cruciate ligament (ACL) injury during a basketball or soccer game.[27] For each person with an ACL injury (a case), another soccer or basketball player without an ACL injury would be selected as a "control," typically from the same team or a comparable team at the same school. Potential risk factors that could be explored might include examining motor control strategies or anatomical/anthropometric differences between cases and controls.

There are many advantages of the case–control design. These studies are usually relatively cheap to conduct because there is no waiting time for an injury to occur. The downside of this efficiency is that the researchers have to find a way to document retrospectively the potential risk factors. Bias may result if recall of risk factors differs between cases and controls.

Note that subjects are recruited into a case–control study based on their outcome status, e.g., injured or noninjured. Therefore, the particular outcome (e.g., ACL injury) must be clearly defined, and unambiguous study entry rules must be operationalized, prior to conducting the study. Also, this design is only useful for studying risk factors that are not affected by injury, such as genomics, or anatomical characteristics. If the injury changes the risk factor, this design should not be used.[36] If the investigator is relying on self-reported data or risk factors, e.g., family history of ACL injury, then recall bias may occur if cases remember their risk factor data with greater clarity than controls (i.e., non-injured).

The most fundamental point concerning case–control studies is that controls serve as a sample from the population in which the cases occurred. The control and the case groups should come from the same core "source population." This simple rule is often ignored. The first step in designing a case–control study is to identify a source population to study, e.g., all basketball or soccer players in a geographical area. The next step is then to identify a means to find the cases in this population, e.g., by implementing a standardized case identification process in all local orthopedic clinics. The final step is to determine how a sample will be drawn from this population—for example, from team members or lists of league members. This sample will be the controls.

Clinical Pearl

In a case control study, the cases and controls must come from a common "source population."

2.2.4 Case Crossover

In certain situations, it is possible for a case to serve as his/her own control. In this type of study, it is possible to assess whether the injury was preceded by a trigger event that occurred immediately prior to the injury event. This design is useful to examining time-varying risk factors, e.g., climatic conditions, fatigue inducted by practice schedules, and time in menstrual cycle. The injured person would be assessed for deviations from his/her usual activity that may have triggered the injury or condition. Because each person serves as his/her own control, the problems of finding an appropriate control group are mitigated. For acute traumatic injuries (e.g., ACL rupture) or sudden-onset conditions (e.g., sudden cardiac arrest, or exertional heatstroke), this is a very strong design to use. The case-crossover design is also well suited for studying transient factors that have an immediate or near-immediate effect on injury, e.g., fatigue.

2.2.5 Prospective Cohort

One of the strongest study designs for assessing risk factors is the prospective cohort study. In this study design, a group of athletes are followed over time (usually a season). Potential risk factors are collected at baseline and, at follow-up, comparisons can be made to see if the injury rates differ between athletes with different initial exposures. For example, to study the effect of a particular type of helmet on the occurrence of concussions among college athletes, a prospective cohort study could follow two groups of athletes over the season: those who wore helmets made by vendor A and those who wore helmets made by vendor B. Then the rate of new concussions in each helmet group is compared, thus allowing some conclusions to be made about the efficacy of the new helmet in preventing or reducing concussion injuries. The key characteristic of this type of study is that the risk factor (helmet use) is identified prior to the injury (concussion).[4]

While the prospective cohort study is very powerful in its ability to identify potential risk factors, evaluate the performance of interventions and identify the incidence (new cases) of an injury; it may be expensive because of the prospective follow-up to capture incident injuries or conditions and it usually requires a larger sample size. Thus, for injuries or conditions with low incidence, case–control studies might be more feasible.

Clinical Pearl

The key feature and strength of the prospective cohort study, as compared to other observational epidemiological designs, is that the risk factor is identified prior to the injury.

2.2.6 Randomized Control Trial (RCT)

An RCT randomly assigns subjects to a "treatment" or "control" group. For example, to assess the benefits of wearing a knee brace as a primary prevention for knee sprains among college football players, randomly selected athletes would wear braces, while other athletes would wear no brace. In practice, it is often easier to randomize at the level of the team, or school, rather than to randomize individuals. Some interventions, such as a team-based dynamic warm-up program, can only be randomized at the level of the team. However, this "cluster-randomization" decreases the statistical power of the study.

A study by Gilchrist et al.,[11] which evaluated an ACL injury prevention program in female collegiate soccer players, illustrates the use of the RCT design in sports medicine. In this study, NCAA division I women's soccer teams were randomly assigned to a treatment or control group. The treatment group participated in a program that included stretching and strengthening activities three times a week during the season, while the control group continued performing only their usual activities. This study was able to document a reduction in ACL injuries occurring during practice and games throughout the 2002 season.[11]

However, RCTs can be difficult to carry out in practice. True random assignment is difficult to achieve, and compliance can become an issue. For studies assessing equipment, the athletes may stop using the intervention equipment unless they are closely monitored. The Gilchrist study used teams' certified athletic trainers (ATCs) to monitor compliance with the intervention program.[11] Note that, if the intervention is a training program or an item of equipment, it is often difficult or impossible to blind subjects and study staff as to which athletes are in the treatment or control group. Thus, double-blind RCTs are rare in observational sports medicine.

Selecting an appropriate control condition is an important aspect of the design of an RCT. The control group in an RCT could be a total placebo (e.g., a pill without any active ingredients), or a known treatment that is the usual standard of care. Note that the "control group" in an RCT serves a very different function from the "control group" in a case–control study. Controls in a case–control study are *selected* by the researchers based on their outcome status (e.g., uninjured). The controls in an RCT are *assigned* by the researchers to the "no-intervention condition." Thus, controls in case–control study are *uninjured*, whereas controls in an RCT are *unexposed*.

These study designs, with specific advantages and disadvantages, are summarized in Table 2.2. The pragmatic elements of time and resources (e.g., available funds) are often an important consideration in conducting a specific study. For example, case series studies often use records that are available for other

TABLE 2.2
Advantages and Disadvantages of Various Study Designs

Study Design	Advantages	Disadvantages
Case series	Easy to conduct. Can use existing records. Generates hypotheses for further study.	No control group so no comparisons can be made. Cannot provide incidence. Cannot provide risk factor data. Selective survival/recall.
Cross sectional	Inexpensive (data collected at one time). Many sampling techniques available. Can evaluate many exposures or outcomes. Can identify injury trends using repeated cross-sectional studies.	Cannot establish cause and effect. Cannot calculate incidence. Not good for rare injuries. Cannot study natural history of injuries.
Case–control	Well suited to unusual conditions (e.g., fatal cardiac arrest). Relatively quick and inexpensive. Existing records may be used to document past exposure. No risk to subjects because data are obtained after injury has occurred. Allows for the study of multiple potential risk factors.	Relies on recall or existing records for past exposures. Validation of exposure often impossible. Appropriate control group difficult to obtain. Not well suited to determining incidence or prevalence.
Case crossover	Same advantages as for case–control studies. Particularly appropriate for acute injuries or sudden-onset conditions. Useful for time-related risk factors (risk factors that change over time, e.g., heat and humidity).	Same disadvantages as for case–control studies. Time-related confounders.
Prospective cohort	Provides information on exposure prior to injury. Provides rates of progression and natural history of injury. Can study multiple outcomes. In sports medicine, often not more expensive than a case–control study.	May require long follow-up or large number of subjects. Less practical for rare injuries.
Randomized control trial	Same advantages of prospective cohort design. Intervention is assigned at random.	Those who consent to be in a randomized trial may be a highly selective subgroup of population. Compliance may be a problem.

purposes, which make data collection very time efficient. However, without a non-injured group, only limited inferences can be drawn. A cross-sectional study includes those with and without injury, but because all data are collected at present, it is not possible to look for associations within the sample. Case–control and case-crossover studies provide a comparison group, but the temporal sequence of the risk factor and the outcome (injury) may be harder to identify. The prospective cohort and the randomized clinical trial study designs are the most powerful studies from which to draw inferences about cause and effect (risk factors), but these are also the most difficult to conduct.

2.3 INCIDENCE AND PREVALENCE

Incidence and prevalence are fundamental concepts in epidemiology. However, these concepts are frequently misunderstood. The definitions are very simple and are summarized here.

Clinical Pearl

Incidence is the occurrence of **new** injury or conditions in a defined **population** at risk over a defined **time** period. **Prevalence** is the **proportion** of defined population that is **currently injured** or has the musculoskeletal condition of interest **at this moment in time.**

2.3.1 Prevalence

Prevalence is the proportion of currently injured athletes, both new and existing, in a sports population. For example, in a high school, the prevalence of injury would be the proportion of athletes who were currently injured on any given day. Note that prevalence is defined at a specific moment in time—it provides a "snapshot" of the *current status* of the athletes—who is or is not injured. Prevalence is sometimes referred to as the prevalence rate; however, prevalence is actually a proportion.

2.3.2 Incidence

Incidence measures the occurrence of *new injuries* in a defined population. Incidence is the pace at which the non-injured becomes injured. To measure incidence, one must define a subset of the population that is not currently injured (i.e., those that are injury free or do not have any prevalent injury), and then prospectively monitor this subgroup to determine how many of them become injured over time.

2.3.3 Relationship between Incidence and Prevalence

Figure 2.1 provides a simple model of the relationship between incidence and prevalence. In this diagram, a group of athletes—for example, all NCAA athletes at a college—have been divided into two groups: those who are currently

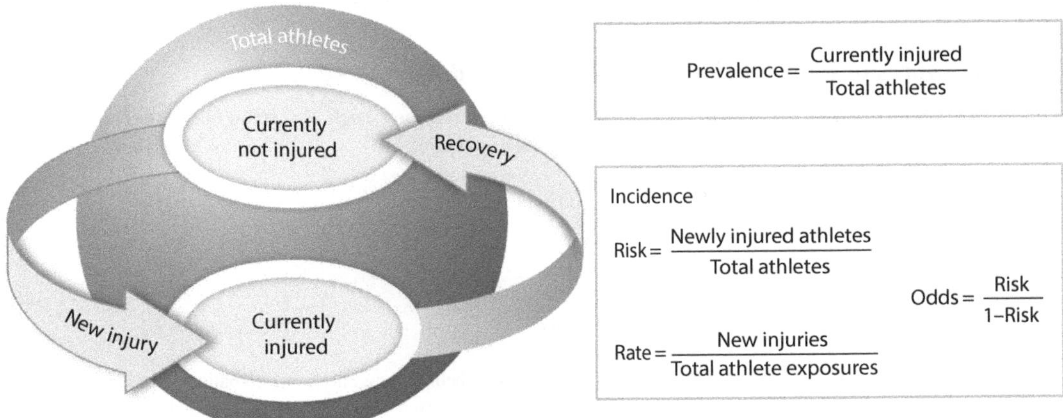

FIGURE 2.1 Relationship between prevalence and incidence. (Reprinted from Rauh, M.C. and Marshall, S.W., *Selected Topics in Sports Injuries and Rehabilitation*, pp. 730–772, Copyright 2010, with permission from Elsevier.)

free of injury (top circle) and those who are who are currently injured (bottom circle). The total number of NCAA athletes at the college is the sum of the two circles (all non-injured and all injured athletes).

Prevalence is defined by the size of the lower circle relative to the size of both circles combined. That is, it is the number currently injured (bottom circle) divided by the total number of athletes (size of both circles together). *Incidence* is defined by the pace at which athletes move from a non-injured state to an injured state. This is the "flow" from non-injured group (top circle) to the injured group (bottom circle), as indicated by the descending left hand arrow. As athletes heal, they leave the injured group (bottom circle) and return to the non-injured group (top circle).

Note that prevalence can be high even when incidence is low. This is because prevalence is a function of both incidence and healing time. Thus, if the average healing time is long, even very low incidence can lead to high prevalence.

2.4 INCIDENCE: RISKS, ODDS, AND RATES

These are three main measures of incidence:

- *Injury risk* (incidence proportion or cumulative incidence)—the proportion of athletes who are injured at least once over a defined interval of time (such as a season)
- *Injury odds*—this is the risk divided by 1 minus risk
- *Injury rate* (incidence rate or incidence density)—the number of new cases per unit of athlete time at risk

Note that the numerator for injury risk and injury odds is injured athletes, whereas the numerator for injury rate is injuries. Thus, athletes who have more than one injury during the monitoring period would contribute multiple events to the calculation of injury rate, but only once to the calculation of injury risk and odds.

Table 2.3 presents example calculations of injury risk, injury odds, and injury rate. The data (originally presented in Knowles et al., 2006)[18] are taken from two real high school teams enrolled in the North Carolina High School Athletic Injury Study: a football and a volleyball team. On the football team, 22 of the 36 athletes were injured. On the volleyball team, 5 of the 17 athletes were injured.

To compute the *risk* of injury in a football season, you divide the number of athletes injured during the season by the number of athletes on the team: 22/36 or 61%. When reporting an injury risk, you must always state the period of time that the risk applies to (one season, in this case), otherwise the statement is meaningless.

Clinical Pearl

Never report an injury risk without also specifying the time period. For example, "the risk of injury in football is 61%" is incorrect because the reader does not know if the risk applies to a season, a half-season, or just one game. The correct statement is "the risk of injury in a football *season* is 61%."

Injury odds is simply an injury risk divided by 1 minus risk. The odds of injury for the football season is 0.61/(1 – 0.61) or 1.57 to 1. Odds can sometimes be a useful surrogate for risk in some situations in which risk cannot be estimated directly (such as case–control studies). Other than that, odds has no direct use.

On the football team, there were 44 injuries and 3760 athlete-exposures during the follow-up period. Therefore, the *injury rate* per 1000 athlete-exposures was

$$\frac{44}{3860} \times 1000 = 11.3.$$

TABLE 2.3
Comparing Three Measures of Injury Incidence (Risk, Odds, and Rate)

	Football (1 Season for 1 High School Team)	Volleyball (1 Season for 1 High School Team)	Ratio Measure (Football vs. Volleyball)	Comment
Athletes	36	17		
Injuries	44	5		
Injured athletes	22	5		
Athlete-exposures	3860	741		
	$\frac{22}{36} = 61.1\%$	$\frac{5}{17} = 29.4\%$	**Risk ratio = 2.1**	
Injury risk	The average risk of being injured in a football season is 61%.	The average risk of being injured in a volleyball season is 29%.	Footballers have twice the risk of injury, per season, relative to volleyballers.	Useful for parents, athletes, administrators.
Injury odds	$\frac{0.611}{1-0.611} = 1.57:1$	$\frac{0.294}{1-0.294} = 0.42:1$	**Odds ratio = 3.7**	
	The average odds of being injured in a football season is 1.6 to 1 (about 3:2).	The average odds of being injured in a volleyball season is about 0.4 to 1 (about 1:2).	Footballers have nearly four times greater odds of injury, per season, relative to volleyballers.	Tracks close to the risk ratio if risk is 10% or less, otherwise useless.
Injury rate	$\frac{44}{3860} = 11.3$ per 1000 athlete-exposures	$\frac{5}{741} = 6.8$ per 1000 athlete-exposures	**Rate ratio = 1.7**	
	The average rate of injury on the football team is 11.3 per 1000 athlete-exposures.	The average rate of injury on the volleyball team is 6.8 per 1000 athlete-exposures.	Footballers have nearly the twice the rate of injury, per game or practice, relative to volleyballers.	Useful for scientists.

Source: Knowles, S.B. et al., *J. Athl. Train.*, 41(2), 201, 2006.

The choice of multiplier—1000—is arbitrary. Its purpose is simply to make the result more readable. Athletes who have multiple injuries are counted multiple times—once for each injury—in the numerator of the *injury rate.*

Most researchers prefer *injury rate* to *injury risk* because injury rate has the ability to account for differences between athletes in their denominator and allows the researcher to identify risk factors and compare sports in a manner that is scientifically more rigorous. Note that we divide the *injured athletes* by *total athletes* to determine injury risk and divide *injuries* by *athlete-exposures* to determine injury rate. Over the football season there were 44 injuries in the 36 injured athletes (12 athletes having a single injury, 4 athletes having two injuries, and 6 athletes having three injuries, and one unfortunate athlete having six injuries). All of these injuries are used for calculating the injury rate. Injury risk uses only the 22 "first injuries"—the first injury for each athlete during the follow-up period. Thus, the *injury rate* is also a more efficient use of the data than *injury risk.*

Clinical Pearl

Rates, risks, and *odds* are three different ways of measuring *incidence.*

Risk is NOT the same as a *rate*! When reporting a risk, you must indicate what length of time (e.g., a season) the risk applies to. Unfortunately, many sports medicine researchers incorrectly refer to risks as rates and vice versa.[18] In fact, the term "risk" is used far too loosely in sports medicine. The use of "risk" as a general synonym for "incidence" is highly unfortunate and should be severely curtailed. For example, if a surveillance study found that football had twice the injury rate of volleyball, people might say "the injury risk is twice as high in football." However, the fact that the *rate* is twice as high in football does not mean that the *risk* is twice as high in football. Watch out for this common error, and limit use of "risk" to situations in which the quantity measured is truly a risk.

2.5 MEASURING THE EFFECT OF A RISK FACTOR

Ultimately, we want to be able to identify risk factors and measure the effect of interventions. Ratio measures are often used to accomplish this. Table 2.3 includes some example calculations for the risk ratio, odds ratio, and rate ratio, under the hypothetical scenario that one might want to compare the injury incidence in football to the injury incidence in volleyball (volleyball is the "reference" category). To do this, one simply divides the risk (or odds or rate) in football by the risk (or odds or rate) in volleyball.

2.6 INJURY DEFINITION

To standardize data collection, an explicit and clear injury definition should be created and reported in every study. This states the criteria used to include an injury in the study. A wide range of injury definitions have been used. Most injury definitions involve either criteria for time lost from participation in the sport and/or criteria for clinical attention, such as requiring physician assessment. The North Carolina High School Athletic Injury Study, for example, defined an injury as "a result of participation in a high school sport that either limited the student's full participation in the sport the day following the injury or required medical attention by a health care professional (i.e., athletic, trainer, physician, nurse, emergency medical technician, emergency room personnel, or dentist)."[42]

Clinical Pearl

A clear injury definition should be reported in every study.

Note that the use of a standardized injury definition does NOT guarantee that reported incidence can be compared between different studies, since different populations have widely differing levels of access to health care. Most NCAA Division I teams, for example, have ready access to clinical services through the provision of ATCs, while many high schools and recreational club athletes have very limited access to on-site services.

Definitions that involve time lost from the sport may also mean different things in different populations. A sprained ankle may be a debilitating injury for a track athlete but might only be a mild inconvenience in crew (rowing). Furthermore, some overuse injuries, such as early-stage stress fractures, may cause considerable distress for the athlete without resulting in any time lost from the sport. There are also physiologic and psychological differences between athletes in pain thresholds and wide variations in clinical management of some injuries, such as concussions. All of these factors mean that one must be very careful when comparing reported incidence between different studies, or even when comparing two sports from the same study.

2.7 DENOMINATOR DATA

To compute incidence and prevalence, some measure of the population at risk, or denominator data, is needed. At a minimum, the denominator should at least quantify the number of athletes in the population under study. More detailed denominator data collection might involve measuring hours and minutes of participation for each athlete, but this may become exceedingly time consuming and expensive. Fortunately, denominator data can often be approximated (or estimated) from preexisting sources of information, such as team rosters and practice schedules.

The most common type of denominator used in computing injury rates is "athlete-exposure." Athlete-exposures are computed by summing up the total number of athletes who participated in every game and every practice during the monitoring or follow-up period. Athlete-exposures are often approximated using the scheduled number of games and practices, multiplied by the average number of athletes participating in each game and practice. The use of athlete-exposures is common in analytical studies that are trying to identify risk factors and in descriptive studies that compare rates between different sports.

Clinical Pearl

Athlete-exposure is the preferred denominator for studies that seek to identify risk factors or make comparisons of injury incidence across sports.

2.8 STATISTICAL METHODS

The choice of statistical method is mainly driven by the goals of the study and the study design. The statistical analysis should address the stated research questions and will depend on the study design. Table 2.4 lists some common statistical methods. A statistician/biostatistician should be consulted if there is any doubt about these factors.

Multivariable regression is an important tool in sports medicine epidemiology, since it allows the researcher to account for covariates (i.e., other factors) that potentially might confound an analysis. The solutions ("beta coefficients") produced by a regression model have useful interpretations: linear regression produces means, binomial regression produces risk ratios, logistic regression produces odds ratios, and Poisson regression produces rate ratios. A variant of Poisson regression named negative binomial regression may be used for injury rates with extra-Poisson variance. Finally, the Cox model (proportional hazards regression) is used if the outcome measure is a time-to-event variables (such as number of days from injury to full return-to-play).

A note of caution: regression models can give misleading results if variables are entered into the model without any understanding of the interrelationships between the variables in the model. Thus, it is wise to develop a written analysis plan and make sure that the regression models (and all statistics) directly address the aims of the study in a logical and coherent fashion. Be aware that the thoughtless and ill-considered inclusion of variables in a regression model can produce misleading and confusing results.

2.9 INJURY SURVEILLANCE

Injury surveillance systems are very important in sports medicine and serve a variety of functions. The data collected may be used to estimate the total burden of morbidity or mortality,

TABLE 2.4
Statistical Analyses Overview

Dependent Variable (Outcome Measure)	Independent Variable (Predictors or Risk Factors)	Typical Statistical Analysis	
		Non-model	Regression Model
Continuous[a] (e.g., BMI, VO_2Max)	Continuous (e.g., BMI, age, VO_2Max)	Correlation coefficient	Linear regression
	Categorical (e.g., sex, injury history, HIV+)	Student's *t*-test	ANOVA
Categorical (e.g., sex, injury history)	Continuous (e.g., BMI, age, VO_2Max)	Trend test	Logistic or binomial regression
	Categorical (e.g., sex, injury history, HIV+)	Chi-square test	Logistic or binomial regression
[a]Two types of continuous data that require special methods:			
Injury rate (continuous count)	Continuous or categorical	Chi-square test	Poisson/negative binomial regression
Time-to-injury (continuous survival time)	Continuous or categorical	Log-rank test	Proportional hazards (Cox) model

and/or to identify risk factors and high-risk groups in sport populations.[25] This information can also be used as a basis for safety decision making and for the allocation of health care and other resources. Finally, the data may serve as an outcome measure for research on injury prediction and form the basis for assessing the effectiveness of interventions aimed at injury prevention.[25]

Over the past three decades, a wide variety of injury surveillance systems have been developed to assess sport-related injury. Table 2.5 summarizes the major current injury surveillance systems in the United States. Some systems are based on the reporting of a specific injury type (e.g., fatalities and other catastrophic conditions), while others are specific athletic populations (e.g., high school or collegiate).

A sports injury surveillance system, to be useful, requires easy-to-use, uniform and unambiguous definitions of the variables. In addition, the system should also collect information in a form that is of relevance across a broad range of potential users of the data: sports participants themselves,

TABLE 2.5
Major Current Nationally Focused Sports Surveillance Systems in the United States

Surveillance System	Active Years	Data Collected	Source of Data	Current Website
Case registry				
National Center for Catastrophic Sports Injury Research[26]	Began in 1982/1983 academic year; ongoing; system expanded and updated in 2014. NCAA mandated catastrophic reporting for colleges and universities in 2014.	Any severe injury (fatality, permanent, or transient severe disability) incurred during any sport; focused on high school, college, and semi-pro/pro sports.	Coaches, athletic trainers, athletic directors, executive officers of state and national athletic organizations, parents and athletes can report an event for review and investigation.	nccsir.unc.edu sportinjuryreport.org
Cohort design				
NCAA Injury Surveillance System (ISS)[17]	Began by NCAA in 1982/1983 academic year; ongoing; moved to online platform in 2004/2005; NCAA contracted with the Datalys Center in 2009/2010.	Sport-related injuries, participation data (athletes and athlete-exposures).	Injuries reported by certified athletic trainers in NCAA colleges and universities.	datalyscenter.org
High School RIO™ Sports-Related Injury Surveillance Study[33]	Began in 2005/2006 academic year; ongoing.	Sport-related injuries and participation data (athlete-exposures).	Injuries reported by athletic trainers from 100 U.S. high schools (nationally representative) weekly via Internet-based surveillance system for nine sports. Expansion to all sports and a larger convenience sample of high schools began in 2008/2009.	www.ucdenver.edu/academics/colleges/PublicHealth/research/ResearchProjects/piper/projects/RIO/Pages/default.aspx

TABLE 2.6
Recommended Components of a Sports Injury Surveillance System

The sports activity the injured person was engaging in at the time of the injury (e.g., football, running).
The location where the injury was incurred (e.g., football field, basketball course, running surface).
The particular activity initiating the injury (e.g., pitching, tackling).
What went wrong? (e.g., collided with another player).
The level of supervision of the initiating activity (e.g., recreation vs. competition).
The nature of the injury (e.g., sprain, fracture, concussion).
The body region(s) injured (e.g., head, shoulder, knee).
The severity of the injury (e.g., number of participation days lost, emergency department visit).
The characteristics of the injured person (e.g., age, gender, race, etc.).
The places of the presentation and referral for treatment (hospital emergency room, physical therapist, athletic trainer).
Sports participation data (e.g., number of exposures, hours, or minutes spent in an activity, competition vs. training).
The use of sports injury countermeasures (e.g., modified rules, protective equipment).

Source: Finch, C.F., *Sports Med.*, 24(3), 157, 1997.

sport medicine physicians, other sports medicine professionals and researchers, coaches, trainers and sports administrators.[39] Some important components of sports injury systems, as recommended by Finch[6], are presented in Table 2.6.

2.10 PREVENTIVE INTERVENTIONS

The widespread reduction of sports injuries and other musculoskeletal conditions would have a major impact on quality of life through the maintenance and promotion of physical activity. Physical fitness level is a significant predictor of all-cause mortality, morbidity, and disease-specific morbidity (i.e., cardiovascular disease, diabetes, cancer).[3,16,31] Sports injuries, particularly knee injuries, result in an increased risk of osteoarthritis.[19] Thus, there is a significant public health impact associated with sports injuries and future development of osteoarthritis and other diseases associated with decreased levels of physical activity.

Clinical Pearl

Minimizing the occurrence of injury would help maintain the benefits of sport participation at all ages. Benefits of sport participation include good health, greater self-esteem, relaxation, competition, socialization, teamwork, fitness, and motor skill development.

Table 2.7 provides a list of interventions for selected sports, along the level of supporting evidence.[12] This is not intended to be a complete or authoritative list. Rather, it is intended to convey the large number of the interventions for which is substantial supporting evidence, and the wide diversity of interventions that have been studied and shown to be successful.

2.11 THE FOUR-STEP MODEL FOR INJURY PREVENTION

A four-stage approach for injury prevention has been proposed by van Mechelen et al.[38,39] (Figure 2.2). First, surveillance (see Section 2.9) is used to measure the extent or magnitude of injury in a given sport population and to determine the most common injuries. Descriptive epidemiologic tools, such as rates and rate ratios, are used to determine which sports have the highest injury incidence, quantify gender differences, explore the role of practice vs. competition setting. Typically, the body location, severity of injury, injury type, amount of time loss, risk of re-injury, and incidence of major or catastrophic injuries are quantified, if possible. Extensive reviews of descriptive epidemiology are available elsewhere.[32]

Second, the causes of injury or risk factors must be identified. Risk factors can be divided into modifiable and non-modifiable factors.[1,2,23] Modifiable risk factors are those that can be altered by injury prevention strategies to reduce injury rates.[5,24] Non-modifiable risk factors are those that cannot be altered, but still may affect the relationship between modifiable risk factors and injury. While non-modifiable risk factors, such as age, gender, and previous injury, may be of worthy consideration in studies of sport injury prediction and prevention, it may be more important to study factors that are potentially modifiable, such as physical training, flexibility, balance, proprioception, or psychological/social factors.[2,5]

Clinical Pearl

In terms of injury prevention, a higher priority should be placed on studying factors that are potentially modifiable (alterable) rather than non-modifiable (unalterable) factors.

Modifiable risk factors are often subdivided into those that are intrinsic to the athlete and those that are extrinsic. Potentially modifiable intrinsic factors include neuromuscular systems, anatomic and biomechanical factors, body composition, and psychosocial factors. Potentially modifiable extrinsic factors include exposure/setting, environment and climatic factors, personal equipment, and coaching experience and education.

The third step of the van Mechelen model is to introduce prevention measures that are likely to reduce future risk and/or severity of sports. Prevention measures (or interventions) should be based on information on the etiological factors and/or injury mechanisms as identified in the second step. Then, in step four, the effect of these prevention measures can be evaluated by repeating the first step, e.g., by time trend analysis of injury patterns.

TABLE 2.7
Examples of Injury Prevention Interventions in Selected Sports

Activity	Proven	Promising/Potential	Not Evaluated, Insufficient, or Conflicting Evidence
Baseball/softball	Breakaway bases Reduced impact balls Faceguards/protective eyewear	Batting helmets Pitch count	Chest protectors
Basketball	Protective eyewear Mouthguards	Ankle disk training Semi-rigid ankle stabilizers (esp. with h/o instability)	Preventive knee braces
Bicycling	Helmet use (Educational campaigns, laws, and subsidies all increase use)	Bike paths/lanes Retractable handlebars	Lighting on bike trails
Football	Helmets and other equipment Ankle braces rather than taping Minimizing cleat length Rule changes (no spearing, etc.) Playing field maintenance Preseason conditioning Cross training reduces overuse Coach training/experience	Limiting practices with contact	Preventive knee braces Body pads
General physical activity	Fitness/conditioning	Return to play guidelines Attention to training parameters	Pre-exercise stretching Coaching attitudes to injury prevention
Ice hockey	Helmet with full face shield down Rules: fair play, checking, high sticking	Enforcement of rules Discouraging fighting	Body pads
Inline skating/skateboarding	Wrist guards Knee/elbow pads	Helmets	
Playgrounds	Shock absorbing surfacing Height standards Maintenance standards		
Running/jogging	Altered training regimen	Shock absorbing insoles	Reflective clothing
Skiing/snowboarding	Training to avoid risk situations Binding adjustment Wristguards in snowboarding	Helmets	
Soccer	Anchored, padded goal posts Shin guards Movement and strength training		Head gear "fair head" rule

Source: Gilchrist, J. et al., Chapter 7: Interventions to prevent sports and recreation-related injury, in: Doll, L.S. et al. (eds)., *Handbook of Injury and Violence Prevention*, Springer, New York, 2007, p. 117.

2.12 THE HADDON MATRIX

A helpful framework for developing interventions is the Haddon Matrix. This matrix was developed in the 1970s by William Haddon, a pioneer in highway safety research.[13–15] Haddon observed that all injuries and musculoskeletal conditions arise from uncontrolled energy transfers, e.g., the uncontrolled exchange of kinetic energy that occurs when two players collide unintentionally on a sports field. Haddon pointed out that mechanisms for limiting and mitigating energy transfers were a unifying concept in injury epidemiology.[13,15] The Haddon Matrix[14] divides the chain of injury causation into three phases: prior to the injury event, during the injury event, and after the event. These form the rows of the Haddon Matrix. The columns are the levels at which intervention can occur: the host (the athlete), the energy that causes the injury (e.g., kinetic or thermal energy), and the environment (both physical and social). The concept of the Haddon Matrix is illustrated in Table 2.8 using the example of all sports injuries. In practice, detailed Haddon Matrices that are specific to the injuries or disorders of interest would be needed by intervention developers.

2.13 ADOPTION OF INTERVENTIONS

Unfortunately, many sports injury interventions are underutilized. Table 2.7 demonstrates that there are a large number of "proven" interventions. However, developing and testing an intervention should not be the end of the story. Research is

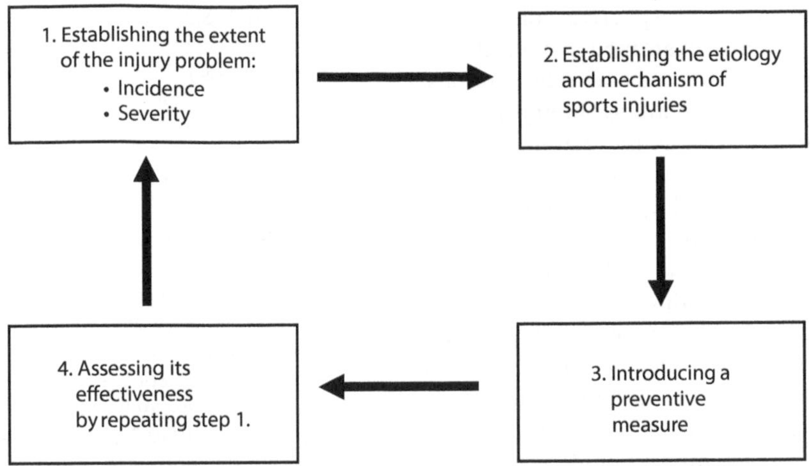

FIGURE 2.2 Four-step sequence of injury prevention. (With kind permission from Springer Science+Business Media: Sports Med., Incidence, severity, aetiology and prevention of sports injuries: A review of concepts, 14(2), 1992, 82–99, van Mechelen, W. et al.)

TABLE 2.8
Example Haddon Matrix for Sports Injury

	Host (Athlete)	Agent/Vehicle (Energy)	Physical Environment (Playing Field)	Social Environment (Team/Coach/School/Parents)
Pre-event (before the injury)	Appropriateness of the activity to the skills of the child.	Visibility of child (reflective materials).	Condition, design, maintenance, and lighting of playing surfaces.	Support for defined play areas (skateboard parks, playgrounds).
				Attitudes toward competition.
	Recognition of injury risk factors.			Restriction of dangerous play.
				Neuromuscular training programs.
Event (during the injury event)	Physical characteristics (joint laxity, physique).	Energy absorbing equipment and surfaces.	Surfacing (artificial or natural).	Monitoring of children by parents and others.
	Response time during the event.	Protective equipment appropriate to the activity.	Padding on goalposts and other surfaces near field of play.	Financial support for certified athletic trainers at all sporting events.
Post-event (after the injury)	Conditioning.	Reporting and replacing faulty equipment.	Ensure emergency medical personnel have access to environment.	Quick and appropriate response.
	Adherence to rehabilitation.			Access to appropriate clinicians trained in sports medicine.
	Parental management of rehabilitation compliance.			Evidence-informed return-to-play guidelines and institutional support for evidence-informed return-to-play decisions.

Sources: Weaver, N.L. et al., *Patient Educ. Couns.*, 46(3), 199, 2002; Marshall, S.W. et al., Sports and recreational injuries, in: Liller, K. (ed.), *Injury Prevention for Children and Adolescents*, 2nd edn., American Public Health Association, Washington, DC, 2012.

needed on adoption and implementation of interventions. For example, coach's attitudes and beliefs are influential to adoption of an intervention by players, but a favorable coach attitude does not guarantee adoption.[9,30] Implementation science is a well-developed field that describes the process of change through public health interventions.[7,8]

Of particular not, RE-AIM (Reach, Effectiveness, Adoption, Implementation, and Maintenance) is a model for describing the update of interventions that is particularly relevant to sports medicine.[7,30] There has been little translational research to date on how to generate more widespread use of proven sports injury interventions, and very little use of implementation science in sports medicine; there is a pressing need for more work in this area.[7,30]

2.14 SUMMARY

The epidemiology of sports injuries and musculoskeletal conditions is an important area. To date, most literature in this field has been descriptive epidemiology. There have been relatively few RCT, prospective cohort, and case–control studies that have examined potential risk factors or addressed the effectiveness of interventions. Nevertheless, there are many promising injury prevention efforts in many competitive and recreational sports. Studies of the effect of neuromuscular training and reduction of ACL injuries among high school and collegiate athletes highlight these efforts.[11,27] Future research needs to address the evolving nature of America's recreational patterns. For example, athletes are specializing and training year-round at an increasingly younger age; the effects of this "mono-sport" specialization on their risk of acute and overuse injuries remains unstudied. Likewise, numerous aspects of current clinical practices, such as preseason screening exams and guidelines for the rehabilitation of injured athletes for graduated return to play, remain under-researched. Finally, there is a need to greatly increase the use of currently proven interventions. Finding answers to these and other important questions will be pressing issues for current and future sports medicine epidemiologists.

REFERENCES

1. Bahr R, Holme I. Risk factors for sports injuries: A methodological approach. *British Journal of Sports Medicine.* 2003;37(5):384–392.
2. Bahr R, Krosshaug T. Understanding injury mechanisms: A key component of preventing injuries in sport. *British Journal of Sports Medicine.* 2005;39(6):324–329.
3. Blair SN, Kohl HW, Barlow CE et al. Changes in physical fitness and all-cause mortality. A prospective study of healthy and unhealthy men. *Journal of the American Medical Association.* 1995;273(14):1093–1098.
4. Collins M, Lovell MR, Iverson GL et al. Examining concussion rates and return to play in high school football players wearing newer helmet technology: A three-year prospective cohort study. *Neurosurgery.* 2006;58(2):275–286; discussion 275–286.
5. Emery CA. Injury prevention and future research. *Medicine and Sports Science.* 2005;48:179–200.
6. Finch, C.F. An overview of some definitional issues for sports injury surveillance. *Sports Medicine.* 1997;24(3):157–163.
7. Finch CF No longer lost in translation: The art and science of sports injury prevention implementation research. *British Journal of Sports Medicine.* 2011;45(16):1253–1257.
8. Finch CF, Donaldson A. A sports setting matrix for understanding the implementation context for community sport. *British Journal of Sports Medicine.* 2010;44(13):973–978.
9. Frank BS, Register-Mihalik J, Padua DA. High levels of coach intent to integrate a ACL injury prevention program into training does not translate to effective implementation. *Journal of Science and Medicine in Sports.* 2015;18(4): 400–406.
10. Garrick JG, Requa RK. Sports and fitness activities: The negative consequences. *Journal of American Academic Orthopedic Surgery.* 2003;11(6):439–443.
11. Gilchrist J, Mandelabum BR, Melancon H et al. A randomized controlled trial to prevent noncontact anterior cruciate ligament injury in female collegiate soccer players. *American Journal of Sports and Medicine.* 2008;36(8):1476–1483.
12. Gilchrist J, Saluja G, Marshall SW. Interventions to prevent sports and recreation-related injury. In: Doll LS, Mercy JA, Sleet DA (eds.). *Handbook of Injury and Violence Prevention.* New York: Springer; 2007.
13. Haddon W Jr. On the escape of tigers: An ecologic note. *American Journal of Public Health and the Nations Health.* 1970;60(12):2229–2234.
14. Haddon W Jr. A logical framework for categorizing highway safety phenomena and activity. *Journal of Trauma.* 1972;12(3):193–207.
15. Haddon W Jr. Energy damage and the ten countermeasure strategies. *Journal of Trauma.* 1973;13(4):321–331.
16. Jebb SA, Moore MS. Contribution of a sedentary lifestyle and inactivity to the etiology of overweight and obesity: Current evidence and research issues. *Medicine and Science in Sports and Exercise.* 1999;31(11 Suppl):S534–S541.
17. Kerr ZY, Dompier TP, Snook EM et al. National collegiate athletic association injury surveillance system: Review of methods for 2004–2005 through 2013–2014 data collection. *Journal of Athletic Training.* 2014;49(4):552–560.
18. Knowles SB, Marshall SW, Guskiewicz KM. Issues in estimating risks and rates in sports injury research. *Journal of Athletic Training.* 2006;41(2):207–215.
19. Koh J, Dietz J. Osteoarthritis in other joints (hip, elbow, foot, ankle, toes, wrist) after sports injuries. *Clinical Sports and Medicine.* 2005;24(1):57–70.
20. Lohmander LS, Englund PM, Dahl LL et al. The long-term consequence of anterior cruciate ligament and meniscus injuries: Osteoarthritis. *American Journal of Sports and Medicine.* 2007;35(10):1756–1769.
21. Lohmander LS, Ostenberg A, Englund M et al. High prevalence of knee osteoarthritis, pain, and functional limitations in female soccer players twelve years after anterior cruciate ligament injury. *Arthritis and Rheumatism.* 2004;50(10):3145–3152.
22. Marshall SW, Gilchrist J, Saluja G, Liller K. Sports and recreational injuries. In: Liller K (ed.). *Injury Prevention for Children and Adolescents*, 2nd edn. Washington, DC: American Public Health Association; 2012.
23. Meeuwisse WH. Predictability of sports injuries. What is the epidemiological evidence? *Sports and Medicine.* 1991;12(1):8–15.
24. Meeuwisse WH. Assessing causation in sport injury: A multifactorial model. *Clinical Journal of Sports and Medicine.* 1994;4(3):166–169.
25. Meeuwisse WH, Love EJ. Athletic injury reporting. Development of universal systems. *Sports and Medicine.* 1997;24(3):184–204.
26. Mueller FO, Cantu RC. *Football Fatalities and Catastrophic Injuries, 1931–2008.* Durham, NC: Carolina Academic Press; 2010.
27. Myer GD, Ford KR, Barber Foss KD, Liu C, Nick TG, Hewett TE. The relationship of hamstring and quadriceps strength to anterior cruciate ligament injury in female athletes. *Clinical Journal of Sports Medicine.* 2009;19(1):3–8.
28. National Collegiate Athletic Association. 1981-82–2013-14 NCAA sports sponsorship and participation rates report. NCAA Indianapolis, IN.
29. National Federation of State High School Association. 2013–2014 Participation Survey. Indianapolis, IN: NFHS.
30. O'Brien J, Finch CF. The implementation of musculoskeletal injury-prevention exercise programmes in team ball sports: A systematic review employing the RE-AIM framework. *Sports and Medicine.* 2014;44(9):1305–1318.

31. Paffenbarger RS Jr, Hyde RT, Wing AL et al. Changes in physical activity and other lifeway patterns influencing longevity. *Medicine and Science in Sports and Exercise.* 1994;26(7):857–865.
32. Rauh MC, Macera CA, Marshall SW. Epidemiology of sports injuries. In: Magee DJ, Manske RC, Zachazewski JE, Quillen WS (eds.). *Selected Topics in Sports Injuries and Rehabilitation.* St Louis, MI: Elsevier; 2010.
33. Rechel JA, Yard EE, Comstock RD. An epidemiologic comparison of high school sports injuries sustained in practice and competition. *Journal of Athletics and Training.* 2008;43(2):197–204.
34. Roos EM. Joint injury causes knee osteoarthritis in young adults. *Current Opinion in Rheumatology.* 2005;17(2):195–200.
35. Saunders N, Otago L, Romiti M et al. Coaches' perspectives on implementing an evidence-informed injury prevention programme in junior community netball. *British Journal of Sports and Medicine.* 2010;44(15):1128–1132.
36. Schootman M, Powell JW, Torner JC. Study designs and potential biases in sports injury research. The case-control study. *Sports and Medicine.* 1994;18(1):22–37.
37. van Mechelen W. Sports injury surveillance systems: 'One size fits all'? *Sports and Medicine.* 1997;24(3):164–168.
38. van Mechelen W, Hlobil H, Kemper HC. Incidence, severity, aetiology and prevention of sports injuries. A review of concepts. *Sports and Medicine.* 1992;14(2):82–99.
39. van Mechelen W, Hlobil H, Kemper HC. *How Can Sports Injuries be Prevented?* Oosterbeek, the Netherlands: National Institute for Sports Health Care (NISGZ); 1987.
40. von Porat A, Roos EM, Roos H. High prevalence of osteoarthritis 14 years after an anterior cruciate ligament tear in male soccer players: A study of radiographic and patient relevant outcomes. *Annals of the Rheumatic Disease.* 2004;63(3):269–273.
41. Weaver NL, Marshall SW, Miller MD. Preventing sports injuries: Opportunities for intervention in youth athletics. *Patient Educations and Counseling.* 2002;46(3):199–204.
42. Weaver NL, Mueller FO, Kalsbeek WD et al. The North Carolina High School Athletic Injury Study: Design and methodology. *Medicine and Science Sports and Exercise.* 1999;31(1):176–182.

3 Role of the Team Physician

Christopher J. Sardon, Anthony I. Beutler, and John H. Wilckens

CONTENTS

TABLE 3.1
Key Clinical Considerations

1. The most important responsibility of the team physician is the medical care of athletes at all ages and all levels of participation.
2. Team physicians should have core knowledge of injuries and illnesses typical in athletes and teams under their supervision.
3. The team physician should review the pre-participation examinations of all athletes under their care. The team physician has the responsibility to clear each athlete to participate at the start of the season and to clear injured athletes to return to play.
4. Successful team physicians deliver expert and ethical medical care and clearly communicate needed information to each member of the athlete's care team, without violating the patient's privacy and trust.

3.1 INTRODUCTION

Athletics play a significant role in our culture. But whether it is a young child joining their first soccer team, a weekend warrior trying to recreate their glory days on the basketball court, a master athlete running his or her first marathon, or a professional athlete playing in the Super Bowl, injuries are inevitable. The team physician has the responsibility to aid these athletes by preventing, identifying, and managing potential injuries during individual, team, and mass participation sporting events (Table 3.1).

3.2 WHAT IS A TEAM PHYSICIAN?

The American College of Sports Medicine published a Team Physician Consensus Statement in 2013 to define the role of the team physician:

> The team physician must have an unrestricted medical license and be a medical doctor (MD) or doctor of osteopathy (DO). He or she has the leadership role in the organization, management, and provision of medical care for individual, team, and mass participation sporting events. The most important responsibility of the team physician is the medical care of athletes at all ages and all levels of participation.
>
> The team physician should possess special proficiency in the prevention and care of musculoskeletal injuries and medical conditions encountered in sports. The team physician integrates medical expertise with medical consultants, certified and/or licensed athletic trainers, and other allied health care professionals (athletic care network). Aided by the athletic care network, the team physician also educates athletes, coaches, parents/guardians, and administrators. The team physician is ultimately responsible for the clearance to participate and the return-to-play (RTP) decision.[13]

Although doctors of any specialty can be a team physician, the majority are family medicine physicians and orthopedic surgeons. Without regard to the physician's particular medical specialty, the team physician should aid in the prevention of injuries, maximization of training and preparation for competitions, diagnosis, and treatment of sport-specific injuries and emergencies, and rehabilitation of injuries.

3.3 TIME REQUIREMENTS OF A TEAM PHYSICIAN

A team physician must have an office schedule that can accommodate athletes with urgent and time-sensitive medical needs. Most team physicians have designated training room time each week, at least one to two evenings, where they can evaluate new and follow-up existing injuries of team members. Training room time is an especially important setting in which to communicate with the athletic trainer on the rehabilitation progress of athletes' injuries.[4] An athlete's behavior and responses can vary widely, depending on the familiarity of the environment; therefore, training rooms should ideally be held in the athlete's "native environment," at a location convenient to the athletes and close to practice or training facilities.

Although knowledge and ability are certainly important, the most valuable asset to the team physician is trust. Trust is earned by connecting with the athletes, coaches, and school officials.

Team physicians do not routinely attend team practices. Although it is not necessary to attend all practices, occasional, brief appearances during practice will allow the physician to gain insight into the environment and conditions in which the athletes train, the team's training regimen, and interactions between coaches and players. A better appreciation of all these factors can prove invaluable in the physician's medical decision making. Additionally, brief appearances at practice help the physician build collegial relationships with coaches and players, establishing his or her role as a part of the team and distinguishing the physician from other officials, support staff, and media representatives who participate only in game-day activities.

The amount of time spent at the actual competition depends on the team physician's role and availability as well as on state laws and the regulations of the governing athletic association. Some laws mandate that a physician be in attendance for every game. Other laws allow nonphysician medical personnel, such as an athletic trainer, to cover an event with on-call physician backup.[5]

The clinician who is the team physician for an entire institution must decide whether to attend all the games for a few teams, or to attend a few games for every team. We recommend that team physicians attend at least part of one practice and at least one game for each team they supervise. Providing good "team medicine" is very difficult without observing the interactions and conditions of play and practice.

3.4 CORE KNOWLEDGE OF A TEAM PHYSICIAN

The team physician must have core knowledge of the typical injuries seen in athletes to ensure a strong understanding of the type of injuries specific to the sport(s) of the teams and/or the individuals under their care and supervision. The American College of Sports Medicine has issued consensus statements on multiple issues that are key to the knowledge base of the team physician. Among these wide-ranging issues are the following: injury/illness prevention, conditioning, nutrition, return-to-play decisions, concussions, master athletes, adolescent athletes, female athletes, sideline preparation, and mass participation events. Each of these issues is discussed in greater depth in subsequent chapters throughout the textbook. But highlights of these consensus documents, including specific pearls and responsibilities of the team physician, are presented in concise format in the following sections.

3.4.1 Injury/Illness Prevention

One of the most important roles of the team physician involves injury and/or illness prevention in recreational and professional athletes prior to athletic endeavors. The team physician's broad comprehension allows for the identification of both intrinsic (anatomy, prior injury, muscle weakness, inflexibility, etc.) and extrinsic (equipment, environment, etc.) risk factors. Understanding and mitigating these factors can allow the team physician to encourage specific protocols and programs in an attempt to minimize the occurrence of injuries or illnesses in sports.

3.4.2 Conditioning

The conditioning of athletes is an important concern for the team physician. A well-planned conditioning program can maximize an athlete's performance and minimize the risk for injury. The American College of Sports Medicine discusses the importance of the team physician being knowledgeable about general conditioning principles, status of conditioning during competition as well as pre- and postseason issues, and any available resources to maximize a conditioning program. The general principles of conditioning should first focus on progressive overload by starting at a lower level and gradually increasing the intensity and amount of exercise performed.[6] This approach is key in avoiding overuse injuries like stress fractures. Another important principle of conditioning is the concept of periodization. A periodization-training program fluctuates the intensity and quantity of exercise during a set time period, which has shown to be more effective when compared to low-volume, single set training.[6] Finally, a conditioning program should incorporate aerobic exercise, sport-specific training, and injury/illness prevention. It is essential for the team physician to recognize the different aspects required to design a conditioning program for preseason, in-season competition, and off-season. Based on the goals of the team or individual, the conditioning program will differ in order to reflect the needs of the specific sport the athlete has chosen for competition.

3.4.3 Nutrition

Nutrition plays a critical role in sports for a team physician to understand. Many athletes have the misconception that they need to take supplements in order to maximize their potential. Despite this common misconception, solid scientific evidence suggests that athletes can meet 100% of their dietary needs from a well-balanced nutrition plan combining carbohydrates, proteins, and fats.[14] Balance is critical to an effective nutrition plan. The team physician should recognize that an insufficient intake of energy can lead to muscle loss, fatigue, increased risk of injury/illness, and longer recovery times, whereas an overload of energy intake can lead to weight gain, fatigue, and poor performance.[14] The consensus statement from the American College of Sports Medicine suggests that 50%–70% of calories should be from carbohydrates, 10%–35% of calories from protein, and 20%–35% of calories from fats.[14] See Chapter 15, Sports Nutrition and the Athlete, for further discussion.

Clinical Pearl

As general rule, the athlete's calorie intake should be

50%–70% Carbohydrate
10%–35% Protein
20%–35% Fat

3.4.4 Return to Play

Making the decision on when to return a player to the playing field after an injury is a very important task of the team physician. The overall goal is to rehabilitate the athlete's injury and return the player to action without putting the athlete at an increased risk for further injury. In order to carry out this task, the team physician must first establish a return-to-play protocol. During this process, the team physician must evaluate the status of an athlete's injury (medical factors, psychological factors, and functional testing), the potential risk of returning to play, and any extrinsic factors that can negatively impact the athlete.[11] The treatment and rehabilitation process must focus on restoring sport-specific function of the injury, as well as identifying any equipment or orthotics required to return to play safely. Last, the team physician must understand the sports governing body and the federal, state, and local regulations related to returning an athlete to the playing field.

Determining which injured athletes may safely return to same-day competition can be especially problematic. The passions of game day, the adrenaline of the moment, and the complexities of an acute musculoskeletal examination can each complicate the decision of who is safe to return to play and who is not. In these situations, it can often be helpful for the team physician to remember that the goal is to win the war, not just the battle. In situations where the team is winning the battle with a lopsided score (or losing the battle by the same margin) athletes who might otherwise be safely returned to play will probably be better off waiting for the next struggle in the war.

One of the most controversial injuries for the team physician to assess and return to play is a concussion. A sports-related concussion is a rapidly evolving issue due to an increase in information about concussion complications. The team physician must stay up-to-date on the latest developments regarding the identification and treatment of concussions. The "golden rule" a team physician must abide by is that any athlete suspected of having a concussion must be removed from play and cannot return to play that same day.[9] It is the responsibility of the team physician to inform and educate players and coaches about the signs and symptoms of concussions as well as the necessity of the athlete to be evaluated by a health-care provider before returning to the playing field. See Chapter 31, Injury Management and Rehabilitation, for further discussion of return-to-play issues.

Clinical Pearl

There is no same-day return to play in any athlete suspected of a concussion, even if symptoms have resolved during the competition.

3.4.5 Psychological Issues

A commonly overlooked aspect of medicine is the psychological stress that an injured player experiences. Many athletes will have increased amounts of stress when they are injured, because exercise is often their method of stress relief. The role of stress is important to understand in an athlete, because it plays a role in injury development, injury rehabilitation, and return-to-play decisions.[1] It has been shown that athletes who experience high levels of stress, on or off the field, are at an increased risk of injury, because it alters their attention (narrowing of attention and general distraction) and increases muscle tension and coordination difficulties.[8] At the onset of injury, it is difficult to predict how an individual athlete is going to express his or her emotions. Since exercise is a common coping mechanism for athletes, they may react to an injury with sadness, feeling isolated from their team, irritated, unmotivated, angry, or depressed (IBID). By recognizing psychological stress, the team physician's role is to provide the injured athletes with support and medical care that they may need.

The psychological framework that an athlete is in during the rehabilitation period is a significant factor affecting the quality and speed of recovery. Some emotions that an athlete may experience during the rehabilitation period are loss of confidence, fear, and anxiety, which can all negatively impact the progression of the rehabilitation process. The American College of Sports Medicine states that goal-setting, positive self-statements, cognitive restructuring, and imagery/visualization can lead to a faster recovery and help to reduce stress.[8] In addition, it is important for the team physician to build trust with the injured athletes, educate them about the injury and the recovery process, and encourage them to use new coping skills to relieve stress.[8] Last, the psychological state of mind that an athlete is in affects their return to play considerably. Even though an athlete may be physically capable, he or she may not be mentally ready to return to the playing field. It is the team physician's role to identify the mental readiness of the player, because if a player returns to play before being mentally ready, there may be an increased risk of injury. The team physician's training in sports psychology can serve as a resource to players, coaches, and other professionals in identifying and fostering the proper psychological state in training, competing, and rehabilitating athletes.

3.4.6 Adolescent Athletes

A team physician must have a strong age-specific knowledge of an athlete and what specific injuries plague that age group. The adolescent athlete is a particular age group that warrants some special consideration, because they are still growing and developing physically, mentally, and emotionally.

Overtraining has become a significant cause of injury and illness in the adolescent population. These young athletes are increasingly playing year-round sports as they begin to specialize in a specific sport. As a result, this emphasis on specialization during the adolescent years has led to an increase in overuse injuries, and it is important for the team physician to recognize this correlation. A team physician can help prevent these types of injuries by making sure that pitch counts are being enforced, and proper conditioning programs are being implemented. In addition, they should educate players, coaches, and parents of recommendations by the American College of Sports Medicine that adolescents take off 1 month out of every 6 months, or 2 months out of every year in order to let their body rest and recover.[3]

Adolescent athletes are different from adult athletes in at least three key ways, each related to their capacities for growth. First, the growth plates of the adolescent athlete's immature skeletal system are the weakest link in the musculoskeletal chain and are frequently injured. Second, adolescent athletes have different nutritional requirements since they are both growing and performing. And finally, in addition to their musculoskeletal immaturity, adolescent athletes are emotionally and psychologically immature. This immaturity often affects their ability to interact with physicians and coaches and to really understand the instructions and warnings given them. When dealing with young athletes, the prudent team physician will remember that true understanding often lags behind the ability to simply repeat spoken words. Chapter 64, The Young Athlete, contains a more in-depth discussion of these and other issues related to young athletes.

3.4.7 Master Athletes

The other age group requiring special attention from the team physician is master athletes (over age 50). When dealing with master athletes, it is essential that the physician have the athlete identify the goals of their fitness and encourage them to tailor their exercise regimen to these goals. Athletes may need to be encouraged over time to adjust their mind-set from their last period of competitive athletics. A lot has physically changed from their early 20s: their mind-set needs to change, too.

Older athletes often exercise in order to maintain good health through an active lifestyle. Team physicians must consider the specific injuries and illnesses of the older population, and the fact that these athletes are likely on medications that can be dangerous in athletics. Additionally important are the physiological changes that come with age and the specific injuries and illnesses that affect the master athlete. As athletes continue to age, chronic conditions, such as coronary artery disease, diabetes mellitus, hypertension, and osteoarthritis, begin to limit their ability to exercise. In particular, athletes begin to see a decline in their cardiopulmonary capacity and their muscle strength.[10] Chronic medical conditions and age-dependent physiological changes of older athletes are fundamental for the team physician to understand, because it will alter the intensity, duration, and type of exercise that these athletes should be participating in. The American College of Sports Medicine recommends resistance training and regular aerobic exercise for older athletes in order to slow the decline of muscle strength and cardiopulmonary function.[10] See Chapter 66, The Older Athlete, for further discussion of these issues.

3.4.8 Female Athletes

Female athletes constitute another specific group of athletes requiring special attention from the team physician. Female athletes are at an increased risk of ACL tears, patellofemoral pain, and stress fractures when compared to their male counterparts.[4] Osteopenia and osteoporosis are additional concerns in female athletes, especially since the majority of their bone mineral content is obtained during the adolescent years. With this concept in mind, the team physician can address menstrual dysfunction, eating disorders, and other conditions that can have negative immediate and future consequences on the athlete's bone mineral content.

Disorders of eating are a significant problem seen in female athletes. In fact, female athletes are more likely to have an eating disorder as compared to nonathletes, especially in sports that place emphasis on aesthetics, endurance, and weight classifications.[4] It is of high importance that the team physician educates athletes, coaches, and parents of the signs, symptoms, and consequences of eating disorders as they can significantly damage the immediate and future health of an athlete. Pregnancy occurring in female athletes is another concern for the team physician. The team physician must educate female athletes that exercise during pregnancy is generally healthy and beneficial, but there are some recommended limitations to exercise as the pregnancy progresses. A more in-depth discussion of the female athlete is found in Chapter 65.

3.4.9 Pharmacology

The team physician must be an expert in sports-related pharmacology. In addition to being knowledgeable about the medications to treat injuries/illnesses and their implications for physical performance, a team physician must also have a strong knowledge base of the performance-enhancing substances and herbal remedies. Many athletes look to boost their performance thru supplements. "Although all manufacturers are required by the Food and Drug Administration to analyze the identity, purity, and strength of all their products' ingredients, they are not required to demonstrate the safety and efficacy of their products."[14] The team physician should continuously stay updated on the safety and efficacy of these products, the potential adverse effects, and the list of substances that are banned in athletics.

The team physician should also stay abreast of new developments in injury treatment technologies and pharmaceuticals (i.e., platelet-rich plasma injections, stem cell therapies, and other novel biologic agents). When advising athletes regarding new therapies, team physicians weigh safety, potential benefit, the presence or absence of proven treatment alternatives, and ethical concerns. In addition to their advice to individual athletes, team physicians often provide input to athletic trainers, coaches, and administrators regarding new therapies and treatments. Chapter 29, Medications and Substances, provides more information on medical treatment of athletes.

3.5 RESPONSIBILITIES OF THE TEAM PHYSICIAN

3.5.1 Medical Responsibilities

The medical responsibilities of the team physician start before the athletic season begins by assessing whether or not an athlete is fit to play. This is usually conducted through a pre-participation physical. Although it is not necessary for the team physician to conduct the physical, it is necessary for the team physician to review the documentation prior to allowing an athlete to compete. This assessment should be performed far enough in advance of the season so that there are no conflicts with participation for the player.

The primary responsibility of the team physician is to be available to provide medical care from the sideline of a game or event. The covering physician should ensure that sideline care is their sole assigned responsibility. He or she should not be simultaneously on call or distracted by other work-related or personal concerns. Competitions that have a high risk of injury, such as collision sports (i.e., football, basketball, soccer, rugby, etc.), ideally should be covered by a physician, while other health professionals may cover competitions with a lower risk of injury.

Seasoned team physicians understand that they must surrender some of their desire to be fans, so that they can concentrate more on the delivery of good health care than on the score. The conflict between the emotion of the game and the responsibility to care for its athletes is as old as the team physician role. Every team physician may adapt to this conflict differently. But it is essential that each team physician recognizes the conflict and takes personal steps to mitigate its interference with their professional role.

Recent changes in legislation, practice guidelines, and local practice patterns have made the relationship between team physician and athletic trainer more formal and precise. Team physicians should work with athletic trainers and other medical professionals to ensure that roles and responsibilities are mutually understood, agreed upon, and rehearsed before game-day arrives. Injured athletes are more likely to receive optimal care in an environment characterized by implicit trust, professional courtesy, and open communication between team physician, athletic trainer, and other professionals.

The covering physician should actively watch the competition and anticipate potential injuries. Once an injury occurs, the team physician must properly diagnose and treat the injured player while also determining whether the athlete should return to play, remain on the sideline, or be transferred to more definitive care. When evaluating the injured athlete on the sideline, the physician should make sure that the athlete is in a safe location, far enough back from the action of the field and preferably partially screened from the inquiring eyes of fans. In addition to caring for the athletes actively competing, the team physician must also be prepared to care for any spectators or officials who may need medical assistance.

Another important medical responsibility of the team physician is to help rehabilitate the injured athlete. Ranging from developing specific physical therapy plans to arranging for appropriate specialty care, this can be a difficult area for the team physician to coordinate because there are many moving parts to the rehabilitation process, especially if outside subspecialty care is required. Once the athlete is deemed ready to compete, the team physician makes the final decision to allow the athlete return to competition or not. The team physician should not delegate this important role and should actively seek to minimize influence on their professional judgment from coaches, parents, or the athletes themselves. When determining return to play, the context of the injury may vary based on the different positional requirements for each athlete. For instance, a sprain of the medical collateral knee ligament will affect a gridiron football lineman, a volleyball player, and a competitive rifle shooter very differently.

Building a rehabilitation plan for an injured athlete is an inherently collaborative process. The physician, athletic trainer, coach, athlete, parent/agent, and other interested parties must all be on the same page. In instances where consensus is elusive or where stakes are especially high, an MRI can often be an effective management tool. In some cases, a normal MRI exhibits magical healing properties and allows the athlete to return to normal, pain-free function. In other cases, the MRI functions to bring all members of a treatment team to a unified diagnosis—a common starting place on the athlete's road to recovery. As these two examples illustrate, even when the MRI provides no diagnostic benefit to the team physician, it can be extraordinarily helpful in facilitating the multidisciplinary team management of an injury.

3.5.2 Administrative Responsibilities

In addition to medical responsibilities, the team physician engages in important administrative responsibilities, such as emergency procedure and mass event preparation. The team physician must organize a health-care team so that there are health-care professionals available for the athletic practices

TABLE 3.2
Administrative Responsibilities

- Develop an agreement between medical team and organizing body
- Evaluate potential environmental and site risk factors and develop a hazardous conditions plan
- Organize medical team
- Develop protocols for acute medical care and return-to-play decisions
- Notify local police, fire department, and emergency medical facilities of event and location
- Follow OSHA and HIPAA precautions
- Prepare medical aid stations with appropriate supplies
- Maintain medical records
- Include staff that can provide basic first aid and CPR
- Provide fluids, food, shelter, and sanitation facilities for competitors, staff, and spectators
- Provide documentation of all injuries and illnesses

Sources: Herring, S.A. et al., *Med. Sci. Sports Med.*, 36(11), 2004, 2004; Herring, S.A. et al., *Med. Sci. Sports Med.*, 44(12), 2442, 2012.

and competitions. Table 3.2 illustrates some of the administrative responsibilities of the team physician, as suggested by the American College of Sports Medicine.

3.5.3 Communication

Communication is another significant responsibility of the team physician. Whether the focus is on injuries, rehabilitation, or return-to-play decisions, the team physician creates and maintains open lines of communication with coaches, players, administrators, and parents. The ability to communicate needed information clearly to each individual, without violating the patient's privacy and trust, is a valuable skill indeed.

Establishing open communication and developing good rapport with the athletes will allow the team physician to provide optimal care. Good team physicians will understand that patients—even athletes—always have the final say on what treatment they will and will not pursue. With this in mind, second opinions on diagnosis and recommended treatment options should be encouraged. If the second physician agrees with your original diagnosis, you will look smarter and your patient will be grateful to you. If the second physician finds something other than your original diagnosis, you may have another treatment option to help you provide better care for your athlete, and that athlete will be grateful to you. Allowing or encouraging second opinions builds transparency. In our experience, suggesting to an athlete that a second opinion could be obtained if desired often increases their confidence in that physician's transparency to a point where the athlete no longer feels that a second opinion is needed.

Last, a team physician may be called upon to discuss an injury with the media. However, the wise team physician will remember that his/her primary responsibility is to protect the athlete's personal information. If the patient wishes to release by Facebook, Twitter, etc., the details of their condition, that right is theirs. But a team physician is better off never discussing an individual athlete's condition with the media.

If a press conference is needed, our recommendation is to get the head athletic trainer and the head coach or manager together. After making sure the athlete's rights are protected, share the required information with the coach and have him give the press conference. If he or she states everything correctly, then you have communicated well! But even if he or she misstates the facts, you have avoided being on the hook, and it is much easier for a coach to medically correct themselves than for a medical professional to do the same. Remember that the press can and will take sentences out of context, confounding the issue even when information has been communicated correctly and appropriately.

3.6 LEGAL AND ETHICAL CONSIDERATIONS

Team physicians have an obligation to treat athletes in the same manner they would treat any patient under their care and supervision. The standard of care must be met in all patient encounters in order to avoid litigation for negligence. In addition, it is important for the team physician to obtain informed consent prior to procedures as well as to establish the guidelines and limitations with the organization for which team physician professional services are being provided. All care provided in all venues (clinic, training room, sideline, etc.) must be documented in the medical record. If care is undocumented, then it did not happen.

In sports, being second-guessed is just part of the game. Coaches are second-guessed after every game, management is second-guessed after every season, and as a team physician you can expect that your decisions will be second-guessed as well. You can also expect that coaches and other professionals will push this second-guessing as far as they think they can. You must establish your "line in the sand" that you will not cross. When you establish this line, expect people to walk right up to it and push you every time, for a while. While this can be uncomfortable at first, knowing beforehand that it will happen can empower you to take a stand, without taking offense. After holding your line for a while, most individuals will respect the line and not challenge it further, and some individuals will just continue pushing. But if you do not have a line, people will just keep pushing, and just keep walking, until they have walked right over you. Chapters 4 and 5 are dedicated to the Ethics and Legal Issues of the Team Physician.

3.7 SUMMARY

The team physician is a position of trust in the eyes of the coaches, the institution, the medical team, and most importantly, the athletes. A successful team physician will develop

TABLE 3.3
SORT: Key Recommendations for Practice

Clinical Recommendation	Evidence Rating	References
The Team Physician should review the pre-participation physicals of each athlete under his care. The Team Physician has the responsibility to clear each athlete under his/her care for the season's participation.	C	[11–13]
Clearing injured athletes to return to play is a key duty of the Team Physician.	C	[7,11,13]
Same-day return to play is not appropriate for any concussed athlete.	B	[2,9,13]
Team Physicians should adhere to the same standards of care, consent, and documentation whether athletes are seen in the training room or in a traditional clinic setting.	C	[13]

and adhere to their own philosophy and standards, based on proven guidelines such as those outlined here. While the team physician is not the most visible member of the athletic team, he or she does play a vital role to enhance the experience and the safety of all involved in sport (Table 3.3).

REFERENCES

1. Filbay SR, Ackerman IN, Russell TG, Macri EM, Crossley KM. Health-related quality of life after anterior cruciate ligament reconstruction: A systematic review. *American Journal of Sports Medicine.* May 2014;42(5):1247–1255.
2. Halstead ME, Walter KD. Sport-related concussion in children and adolescents. *Pediatrics.* 2010;126(3):597.
3. Herring SA, Bergfeld JA, Bernhardt DT et al. Selected issues for the adolescent athlete and the team physician: A consensus statement. *Medicine & Science in Sports Medicine.* November 2008;40(11):1997–2012.
4. Herring SA, Bergfeld JA, Boyajian-O'Neill LA et al. Female athlete issues for the team physician: A consensus statement. *Medicine & Science in Sports Medicine.* October 2003;35(10):1785–1793.
5. Herring SA, Bergfeld JA, Boyajian-O'Neill LA et al. Mass participation event management for the team physician: A consensus statement. *Medicine & Science in Sports Medicine.* November 2004;36(11):2004–2008.
6. Herring SA, Bergfeld JA, Boyd JL et al. The team physician and conditioning of athletes for sports: A consensus statement. *Medicine & Science in Sports Medicine.* October 2001;33(10):1789–1793.
7. Herring SA, Bernhardt DT, Boyajian-O'Neill LA et al. Selected issues in injury and illness prevention and the team physician: A consensus statement. *Medicine & Science in Sports Medicine.* November 2007;39(11):2058–2068.
8. Herring SA, Boyajian-O'Neill LA, Coppel DB et al. Psychological issues related to injury in athletes and the team physician: A consensus statement. *Medicine & Science in Sports Medicine.* November 2006;38(11):2030–2034.
9. Herring SA, Cantu RC, Guskiewicz KM et al. Concussion (mild traumatic brain injury) and the team physician: A consensus statement-2011 update. *Medicine & Science in Sports Medicine.* December 2011;43(12):2412–2422.
10. Herring SA, Kibler BW, Putukian M et al. Selected issues for the master athlete and the team physician: A consensus statement. *Medicine & Science in Sports Medicine.* April 2010;42(4):820–833.
11. Herring SA, Kibler BW, Putukian M et al. The team physician and the return-to-play decision: A consensus statement-2012 update. *Medicine & Science in Sports Medicine.* December 2012;44(12):2446–2448.
12. Herring SA, Kibler BW, Putukian M et al. Sideline preparedness for the team physician: A consensus statement-2012 update. *Medicine & Science in Sports Medicine.* December 2012;44(12):2442–2445.
13. Herring SA, Kibler BW, Putukian M et al. Team physician consensus statement: 2013 update. *Medicine & Science in Sports Medicine.* 2013;45(8):1618–1622.
14. Herring SA, Kibler BW, Putukian M et al. Selected issues for nutrition and the athlete: A team physician consensus statement. *Medicine & Science in Sports Medicine.* December 2013;45(12):2378–2386.

4 Ethical Considerations for the Sports Medicine Provider

Christopher E. Jonas and Ralph P. Oriscello

CONTENTS

TABLE 4.1
Key Clinical Considerations

1. The same principles that govern standard medical practice have application in sports medicine including *do no harm*, nonmaleficence, confidentiality, and informed consent.
2. The sports medical provider is to expend his or her best effort and judgment for the athlete patient so as to maintain or restore health and functional ability. The athlete's welfare must be the guide for all efforts.
3. It is never appropriate to give medications that would allow activity that would otherwise be impossible for an injured or ill athlete to perform.
4. Sports medical providers can never condone the use of nor participate in supplying prohibited substances. Sports medical providers must also ensure proper knowledge and education regarding supplements.
5. Sports medicine providers should have a basic understanding of genetic and other medical testing and its implications upon athlete participation. Expert consultation should be sought promptly if needed.
6. Return-to-play decisions can be challenging and must be governed solely by the health of the athlete, independent of conflicting motives or individuals.

4.1 INTRODUCTION

Ethics is the conformation to accepted professional standards of conduct. It would be extremely difficult, if not impossible, to write a prescription for ethical behavior. Almost instinctively, one knows if a thought or action is ethical or not. All primary care medical providers (physicians, nurse practitioners, and physician assistants) have anguished over conflicts between ethics and expediency. No one achieves ethical perfection, but most medical providers are good by nature and are guided by high ethical standards. Ethical considerations in the area of sports medicine are similar to those in medicine in general including basic principles and rules.[10] The main reason for insisting upon the highest ethical standards by medical providers involved in sports medicine is that sport is considered to reflect values generally considered to be important to society: character building, health promotion, the pursuit of competitive excellence, and enjoyment. This chapter introduces the principles of medical ethics as applied to the musculoskeletal primary care provider and discusses situations unique to sports medicine (Table 4.1).

4.2 PRINCIPLES OF ETHICAL DECISION MAKING IN SPORTS MEDICINE

Sports medicine shares common ethics with standard medical practice. *Do no harm* and nonmaleficence, principles prohibiting recommendations or actions detrimental to an athlete's short-term and long-term health, are considered with every action taken in the training room when tending to an injured athlete. Confidentiality, informed consent, and truthfulness are absolutely essential for the ethical management of any sports-related medical decision.[3] Finally, beneficence, the principle of performing acts or making recommendations only potentially beneficial to an athlete, is the premier principle. These taken together form the foundation of ethical decision making in sports medicine and will be elaborated upon further in this chapter.

Clinical Pearl

Confidentiality, informed consent, and truthfulness are absolutely essential for the ethical management of any sports-related medical decision.

4.3 CONFIDENTIALITY

Confidentiality in medicine should not be graded, more or less, depending upon the individual's public persona. In sports medicine, confidentiality is of the utmost importance; an ethical principle that is inviolate. Athletes are very public persons. Society wants to know the most intimate details of their lives, including medical evaluations and treatments. By being an athlete, amateur or professional, the patient does not forfeit his or her right to medical privacy. Inquiries made of the sports medical provider by the press or other interested persons should not be answered without the specific permission of the athlete. Even with permission, the medical provider must be extraordinarily sensitive about details revealed. If any sense of doubt exists about what to tell or what not to tell, it is best to keep the athlete's status in confidence. Despite claims regarding the public's right to know, the right of privacy remains with the patient. It must be remembered that the press is very resourceful in obtaining information. If inaccurate information finds its way into print, the medical provider may, with the athlete's permission, attempt to correct it.

Information released to coaches, parents, and, spouses most often should be appropriate information about the athlete's care, especially when prohibition or limitation of competition or practice is necessary. The medical provider's explanation of the benefits of disclosure will usually result in permission from the athlete to do so. In the absence of such permission, the medical provider must consider the welfare of the athlete, the importance of the information, and the potential for harm or embarrassment to the athlete that might arise from disclosure (or nondisclosure), before sharing or withholding information. No greater breach of confidentiality can occur when any health information is released to anyone remotely related to the athlete's career without forewarning the individual.

Clinical Pearl

Confidentiality should not be graded, more or less, depending upon the individual's public persona. By being an athlete, amateur or professional, the patient does not forfeit his or her right to medical privacy. Despite claims regarding the public's right to know, the right of privacy remains with the patient.

When medical providers are employed by or volunteer their services to a school, team, or similar entity, the expectations of both parties should be agreed upon at the outset, preferably in writing. Frank and open communications will usually forestall misunderstanding and conflict. In all cases, medical providers should strive to protect their autonomy in medical decision making so that they will be able to maintain their position as advocate for the athletes' welfare.

4.4 SPORTS MEDICINE PROVIDER RESPONSIBILITIES

General trust continues to exist between a medical provider and any private patient who is also an athlete, whether in high school or an amateur. While rare in high school and uncommon in college sports, there can be major distrust between professional athletes and team medical providers.[7] The medical provider always makes a decision in conjunction with the desires of his or her patient that is in the patient's best interest. Whether the decision is regarding eligibility to participate in an event or to undergo diagnostic or therapeutic intervention, the end result is the maintenance of good health with the least risk to the patient/athlete. Conflict is minimal to absent. While we live in an era of informed consent, confidentiality, and truthfulness, patient autonomy reigns. Nevertheless, many patients still rely upon their medical provider to lead them in the decision-making process. In the majority of cases, this works very well.

Sports medicine is little different ethically from other aspects of medical practice. It does contain unique traps that can cause a medical provider to stumble if unaware. Included in this chapter will be suggestions to make decision making by sports medical providers less difficult while still recognizing that rarely does one solution fit all and that more rarely is the medical provider's decision the only one under the circumstances. Exactness and infallibility, while desirable, are not traits of even the finest medical providers.[11,12]

The primary duty of the sports medical provider is to expend his or her best effort and judgment for the athlete patient so as to maintain or restore health and functional ability.[2,9] The athlete's welfare must be the guide for all efforts. The medical provider must seek out and try to know the athlete's goals and motivations. Importantly, the medical provider must have a genuine appreciation for the importance of athletics in human life. Dr. O'Donoghue, in his now classic text,[13] lists five precepts for the sports medical provider: accept athletics, avoid expediency, adopt the best methods, act promptly, and pursue perfection.

The ill or injured athlete must know the diagnosis, understand its implications, and participate in all therapeutic decisions. Despite the athlete's wishes, the medical provider cannot do less than seek the best possible outcome.[1] While all recommendations or forms of therapy have risks as well as benefits, knowledge and judgment can come only from experience. A medical degree does not ensure perfect decision making. Harm can come to the athlete patient from unnecessary or excessive restrictions as well as from failure to restrict activity when appropriate.

Periodically, the medical provider/patient relationship is strained by a difference of opinion. If negotiation between the two fails, even with accepted intermediaries (family, other consultants, financial, or religious advisors), the relationship may be terminated. The medical provider involved in making sports-oriented medical decisions must be well versed in current recommendations for eligibility and continued participation and not depend upon his limited personal experience or unscientific reasoning.[4,5,16] For the most part, patients themselves end the relationship with their medical providers if the answers they wish to hear are not forthcoming. Under this set of circumstances, ethical conduct is not breached with the patient acting unilaterally. Recognizing the wide range of opinions and individual fallibility, the patient can assert his right to another opinion.

A sports medical provider must develop a suitable level of skill and knowledge and then maintain it.[5] Primary care sports medical providers generally know their level of competence. This group can definitively care for about 85%–90% of athletic problems but must know when to refer for specialized consultation or therapy. The referring medical provider must know the consultant's ability, personality, and empathy for athletes in order to make a competent referral.[6,14] The primary care medical provider should not abandon the care of the referred athlete and must maintain surveillance over the referral/therapeutic process. The consultant may gain insights from the referring medical provider, and the athlete is then afforded the continuing support of his or her medical provider. Referring medical providers can always question the recommendations of consultants if they seem incongruent with their knowledge of the patient. The trust established between athlete and medical provider, more likely than not, allows for resolution and comfort with the decision-making process.

4.5 POTENTIAL FOR DIVIDED LOYALTIES

While rare at the high school level and uncommon at the college level, major distrust can exist among professional athletes and team medical providers.[7] The athletes feel that too many times the quality of their treatment is secondary to the doctor's obligation to team owners and coaches.[2] A salaried position can interfere with a traditional medical provider/patient relationship. To many, the role of the salaried medical provider leads to a conflict of interest. A conflict of interest for a medical provider exists when his or her objective professional duties are compromised by personal interests (e.g., the financial reward of being associated with a professional team or individual athlete, as well as the publicity and high visibility one gets from such a position). At any and all levels, it is an ethical breach for anything but the athlete's best health interest to be considered, recognizing that judgment errors in regard to too conservative or too liberal therapy can occur.

At times, there may seem to be confusion as to where the loyalty of the sports medical provider lies. The ultimate welfare of the athlete may seem in conflict with the wishes of parents or spouse, coaches or team management. The fact that an entity other than the athlete pays the medical provider is immaterial. The loyalty of the medical provider is to the medical provider/patient relationship. Decisions must be based solely on sound medical judgment. Reasonable third parties will understand this. If any party insists otherwise, medical providers should consider removing their services from that party. It is not infrequent for the wishes of the patient to conflict with what the medical provider believes are in the athlete's best interest. These situations are very delicate, require much effort in explanation, and may indicate the need for further consultation. If, after further consultation, the treating sports medical provider still feels uncomfortable with another recommendation, continued care of such an athlete patient may be difficult if not impossible. Reassignment to another medical provider should be strongly considered.[5]

At the highest level of sports, the unfavorable mix of high salaries and short careers makes for risky decision making by both the athlete and the medical provider. Coaches often encourage medical providers to rush players back to the playing fields to win games. Players themselves often desire to rush back too quickly.[17] Teammates are thrown into the mix by suggesting that nonplaying team members are malingering while collecting a substantial income. Under these circumstances, many medical providers play by the rules of the coaching staff. With a substantial number of complications from such behavior, as demonstrated by court-authorized awards to players in the millions of dollars and a current suit seeking $100,000,000 for a heat-related death, players are at the point of not trusting team medical providers. Salaried medical providers must make the effort to assure players that it is their utmost responsibility to protect each player, and any player who should not be on the playing field will not be there.[15]

Clinical Pearl

At any and all levels, it is an ethical breach for anything but the athlete's best health interest to be considered, recognizing that judgment errors in regard to too conservative or too liberal therapy can occur.

4.6 DRUG USE

Sports medicine and ethics have several unique aspects. A major one is drug use by athletes at all levels.[17,24] Therapeutic medications are an integral part of sports medicine practice. Used appropriately, they control pain and inflammation, speed recovery, and hasten return to function. The medical provider must understand each drug thoroughly, including its potential effects on the safety or effectiveness of an athlete's performance.

It is never appropriate to use narcotics or local anesthetics to permit activity that would otherwise be impossible. The use of medications that alter the sensorium or affect coordination must be restricted to times when performance and safety will not be affected. The use of agents that will artificially enhance performance, whether effective or not, is unethical.

The use of drugs, hormones, and blood transfusions invariably is in the public's mind when outstanding performances in any sport are recorded.[8] From baseball to cycling, any new record is suspect. The use of ergogenic substances to enhance performance is often aided by covert, if not overt, support and supply by unethical team medical providers. Because of this, the World Anti-Doping Agency has banned five classes of substances: stimulants (e.g., amphetamines), narcotics, anabolic agents (e.g., steroids), diuretics, and peptide hormones (e.g., erythropoietin, growth hormone).[18] Sports medical providers can neither condone the use nor participate in supplying any of these agents.[15,17] The medical provider must also provide careful guidance of athletes regarding supplements as these can contain banned substances. The downfall of the individual, the program, and the medical provider can be significant. Key to preventing this is knowledge and application of information by the sports medical provider.

Some appropriately used medications are banned at certain serum levels or types of competition. The sports medical provider must be familiar with these so that any drugs appropriately prescribed do not expose the athlete to potential disqualification. Lists of banned drugs are published by regulating bodies (e.g., U.S. Olympic Committee). Usually, when use of a drug to permit athletic performance is appropriate, as in the prevention of exercise-induced asthma, an effective, acceptable medication can be found.

Clinical Pearl

Sports physicians can neither condone the use nor participate in supplying any of banned substances. The physician must also provide careful guidance of athletes regarding supplements as these can contain banned substances.

Current available testing makes it impossible to catch all participants whose behavior includes unethical use of banned substances. Because of that, some favor lifting the ban on hormones, for instance, feeling that it would be preferable to have a free-for-all and allow unrestricted use. The major argument against such a philosophy is the need not to condone cheating along with the essence of sport itself.

4.7 GENETIC TESTING

Advances in genetic testing have raised new ethical concerns. Although these advances have the potential to improve the health and well-being and safe athletic participation of patients, they also have the potential to cause harm depending upon how they are used.[20] Genetic testing can also be used to predict or enhance performance but it can also be used to discriminate others. Sports medicine providers should be familiar with and have a basic understanding of genetic testing and its implications upon athlete participation. Expert consultation should be sought promptly if needed. Appropriate ordering, interpretation, and education of patient athletes are key for the sports medicine provider. As with standard medical practice, candid discussions of risks, benefits, and responsibility can help clarify questions and avoid unwanted outcomes.

4.8 RELATIONSHIPS WITH COLLEAGUES

Many problems can arise when serving as a team medical provider. Because team members may be receiving care from other medical providers, team medical providers must be sensitive to their relationships with colleagues. A team medical provider must never criticize the actions of another medical provider directly to the patient. Concerns regarding therapy should be discussed with the primary medical provider in private. Sports medical providers can often positively influence their colleagues' care of athletes by such positive input.

A fail-safe approach to handling playing restrictions imposed or removed by the athlete's primary medical provider is important. No playing restriction should ever be countermanded by the team medical provider, who should, however, always insist upon the final say in approving the athlete's return to play. Consultation between the team medical provider and the athlete's primary medical provider usually solves the problem and may provide an opportunity for education.

Sports medicine is a team effort involving medical providers plus representatives of many paramedical disciplines. Sports medical providers should be able to recognize where one or more of these can be helpful and should coordinate the services of all in the care of an athlete. In doing so, sports medical providers must insist that such assistants adhere to the same high ethical standards they practice. Unfortunately, athletic medicine has proved a fertile ground for quackery and unproved practices employed in the guise of improving performance. The sports medical provider has an ethical responsibility to expose these practices and protect athletes from being victimized by them.

Except for the most basic training room treatment, an athlete is best referred back to his primary medical provider for definitive therapy of any illness or injury with a detailed note describing the team medical provider's concern. Medical societies generally have rules about medical provider advertising, a troublesome area today even though it is permitted. Medical providers promoting themselves as experts in sports medicine have an obligation to provide true expertise in that area, the same as experts in any other field.

4.9 ETHICS AND THE RETURN-TO-PLAY DECISION

The sports medicine provider regularly makes return-to-play decisions, both during events and during the period of injury management.[19,20] Return-to-play decisions are unique to sports medicine and can be challenging.[19,22] The burden of responsibility can be great, as catastrophic outcomes can follow bad decisions.[19,20] Health-care professionals identify return-to-play decisions as one of the main ethical conflicts in sports medicine.[20,21] The athlete's goal is usually to return to play as soon as possible.[19,20] For professional athletes, financial concerns add pressure to return to play. The sports medicine provider's chief concern must be to evaluate and decide based solely upon the health of the athlete and should not be influenced by competition, coaches, or others.[22]

Clinical Pearl

Return-to-play decisions are unique to sports medicine and can be challenging. The sports medicine provider's chief concern must be to evaluate and decide based solely upon the health of the athlete and should not be influenced by competition, coaches, or others.

4.10 FEAR OF LEGAL ENTANGLEMENT

Finally, a question remains regarding ethics and the law when the risk of a life-threatening situation or a potentially permanently disabling condition is uncertain. The medical provider should be most cautious and recommend against participation. It would not be unreasonable to recognize that the athlete may legally challenge such a recommendation. When operating at the highest ethical level with support from the medical literature and the medical community, such an event should never alter a medical provider's role in the future evaluation of other athletes. They would be best served by such a medical provider.

TABLE 4.2
SORT: Key Recommendations for Practice

Clinical Recommendation	Evidence Rating	References
The sports medicine provider must adhere to basic principles of ethics including do no harm, beneficence, nonmaleficence, confidentiality, and informed consent.	C	[3,10,20]
The health of the patient athlete must be the ultimate motivation and goal of the sports medicine provider in all settings.	C	[1,2,9]
Sports medicine providers cannot condone, supply, encourage, or conceal the use of prohibited substances. The provider must also provide careful guidance of athletes regarding supplements.	C	[15,17,20]
Sports medicine providers must not give medications that would permit activity that would otherwise be impossible for an injured or ill patient athlete to perform.	C	[8,15,23]
Return-to-play decisions must be governed solely by the health and well-being of the patient athlete.	C	[19–21]

4.11 SUMMARY

Medical providers involved in sports medicine soon realize the awesomeness of the responsibility and the magnitude of potential problems. Athletes can only be allowed to participate if they are not a danger to themselves or others. Medical providers must be familiar with the many disease states that affect the ability of athletes to participate without endangering themselves and others. They must be familiar with the unethical means used to enhance performance.[8,17] They must be aware of resources available to construct an authoritative opinion.[1,3] They must be devoted to the principles of confidentiality, informed consent, and truthfulness. They must be aware that occasional decisions may require legal enforcement. Most of all, they must realize that no table of contents exists to refer to for every decision. A backbone, on occasion, is more important than an ethics primer (Table 4.2).[23]

REFERENCES

1. *American College of Sports Medicine: Code of Ethics*. Available at www.acsm.org/content/navigationmenu/memberservices/memberresource/codeofethics (accessed July 31, 2015).
2. Anderson L. Contractual obligations and the sharing of confidential information in sport. *Journal of Medical Ethics*. 2008;34:1–5.
3. Anderson L. Writing a new code of ethics for sports medical providers: Principles and challenges. *British Journal of Sports Medicine*. 2009;43:1079–1082.
4. Graham TP, Bricker JT, James FW, Strong WB. *26th Bethesda Conference*: Recommendations for determining eligibility for competition in athletes with cardiovascular abnormalities. *Journal of the American College of Cardiology*. 1994;24:845.
5. Capozzi JD. Ethics in practice: Terminating the medical provider-patient relationship. *Journal of Bone and Joint Surgery*. 2008;90:208–210.
6. Dunn WR. Ethics in sports medicine. *American Journal of Sports and Medicine*. 2007;35(5):840–844.
7. George T. Care by team doctors raises conflict issue. *New York Times (print)* Sect. 8 (col 5), July 28, 2002.
8. Holm S. Ethics in sports medicine. *BMJ: British Medical Journal*. 2009;339:1–4.
9. Howe WB. Primary care sports medicine: A partimer's perspective. *The Physician and Sports Medicine*. 1988;16:103.
10. Johnson R. The unique ethics of sports medicine. *Clinical Sports and Medicine*. 2004;23:175–182.
11. Maron B. Surviving competitive athletics with hypertrophic cardiomyopathy. *American Journal of Cardiology*. 1994;73:1098–1104.
12. Mitten MJ. *The Athlete and Heart Disease: Diagnosis, Evaluation & Management*. Philadelphia, PA: Lippincott Williams & Wilkins; 1999: p. 307.
13. O'Donoghue DH. *Treatment of Injuries to Athletes*, 4th edn. Philadelphia, PA: W.B. Saunders; 1984: p. 7.
14. Rizve AA, Thompson PD. Hypertrophic cardiomyopathy: Who plays and who sits. *Current Sports Medicine Report*. April 2002;1(2):93–99.
15. Salkeld LR. Ethics and the pitchside medical provider. *Journal of Medical Ethics*. 2008;34:456–457.

16. Simone G. A new professional code in sports medicine. *BMJ: British Medical Journal.* 2010;341:c4931.
17. Tucker AM. Ethics and the professional team medical provider. *Clinical Sports and Medicine.* 2004;23:227–241.
18. World Antidoping Agency. List of prohibited substances and methods. Available at http://list.wada-ama.org/prohibited-all-times/prohibited-substances/ (December 31, 2015).
19. Johnson R. The unique ethics of sports medicine. *Clinical Sports and Medicine.* 2004;23(2):175–182.
20. Testoni D. Sports medicine and ethics. *American Journal of Bioethics.* 2013;13(10):4–12.
21. Anderson LC, Gerrard DF. Ethical issues concerning New Zealand sports doctors. *Journal of Medical Ethics.* 2005;31(2):88–92.
22. Stovitz S, Satin, D. Professionalism and the ethics of the sideline physician. *Current Sports Medicine Reports.* 2006;5:120–124.
23. Vernec AR. Doping, ethics, and the sports physician. *American College of Sports Medicine.* 2013;12(5).
24. Williams, J. *World Medical Association Medical Ethics Manual. 2.* Ferney-Voltaire, France: World Medical Association; 2009: p. 23.

5 Legal Aspects of Sports Medicine*

Lauren M. Simon

CONTENTS

TABLE 5.1
Key Clinical Considerations

1. The sports medicine physician should perform careful cardiovascular examination in a quiet venue during the preparticipation physical evaluation in order to auscultate murmurs, rate, or rhythm abnormalities, which may indicate a concerning cardiovascular condition.
2. Team physicians need to safeguard the protected health information (PHI) of the athletes at all times and take special precautions to minimize unauthorized/inadvertent disclosure of PHI or exposure of athlete's injury while providing care at public athletic venues.
3. When traveling with a team, physicians need to be aware that many states do not have a legal method to allow team physicians from another state to care for their team in the state they are visiting without exposing them to risk of prosecution from practicing without a license there. They should confirm regulations with the medical board of that state before travel.
4. If a preparticipation evaluation concludes with restricted sports clearance, then the physician should discuss with the athlete/parent/guardian (and document the discussion) alternate sports or fitness activities that the athlete can safely participate in.
5. The evaluation of an athlete for return-to-play (RTP) postinjury or illness should include evaluation of the athlete's general health status, nature of illness/injury, participation risks to athlete or others, medical/musculoskeletal interventions to facilitate RTP, and psychological readiness.

5.1 INTRODUCTION

With the growth of participation in sports, the role of the sports medicine team and the legal aspects of sports medicine have also grown in importance. Although the legal aspects of sports medicine are constantly evolving, having a foundation of the basic legal principles involved in providing medical care to athletes of all ages is vital to the successful practice of sports medicine. That knowledge can also help promote the safety of the athlete and reduce fears about liability that otherwise may prevent some physicians from engaging in the practice of sports medicine. This chapter is designed to familiarize physicians and other primary care providers with basic legal issues affecting sports medicine including discussion of roles of the team physician, preparticipation physical evaluations (PPEs), return-to-play (RTP) decisions, liability, malpractice, insurance, contracts, traveling with the team, and privacy and confidentiality regulations (Table 5.1). The information provided in this chapter is not a substitute for advice from legal counsel.

5.2 ROLE OF THE TEAM PHYSICIAN

Although team physicians come from a variety of medical specialty backgrounds, they should practice sports medicine

* In the second edition, this chapter was authored by Emidio A. Bianco and Elmer J. Walker.

according to relevant standards of care for both emergency and nonemergency situations. They should keep updated on the treatment of individual athletes and teams.[4,9] Some physicians are hired by a school or team to provide medical services for a specific athletic contest or series of events, whereas others volunteer to provide those services *gratis* (without charge). A spectator at an athletic event who happens to be a physician may also aid an athlete in case of an emergency (see Section 5.7).

A team physician consensus statement, which outlines the qualifications, duties, and responsibilities of a team physician, has been developed and updated by a sports medicine project-based alliance of six major professional medical organizations: American Academy of Family Physicians, American Academy of Pediatrics, American College of Sports Medicine, American Medical Society for Sports Medicine, American Orthopaedic Society for Sports Medicine, and American Osteopathic Academy of Sports Medicine.[9] The consensus statement outlines major responsibilities of the team physician, which include preparation of preparticipation evaluations of athletes, treatment and management of injuries and illness, coordination of rehabilitation, RTP determinations, medical care coordination, documentation and education of athletes (parent/guardian), teams, athletic staff, and schools. Some of the education provided by team physicians includes the topics of injury prevention, minimizing injury and reinjury, protective equipment, conditioning guidelines, infection precautions, avoidance of banned substances, and nutrition. The team physician should be familiar with the injury patterns commonly seen in specific sports and psychological response to injury. It is also important for the team physician to be cognizant of the rules regarding the athletes' medical eligibility and to be vigilant when prescribing any medication for any potential impact on an athlete's ability and eligibility to play. Administrative duties of the team physician also include coordinating medical supplies needed for event coverage, developing chain of command, preparation, planning and practice of emergency action plans to handle medical emergencies, and involvement in decisions about athletes or teams playing in adverse environmental conditions/hazardous condition plans. Although the details of actual emergency situations vary, ideally a trial run should be performed to smooth out any apparent wrinkles in the emergency plan before an actual emergency arises.

5.3 TEAM PHYSICIAN AGREEMENT

Team physician responsibilities can vary depending on the sport, level of competition, sports governing body, school league, university, age of athlete, etc. In addition, the team physician may be treating the athlete in a variety of situations from the relative calm of the office to the intense pressure of an important game. In order for the team physician to be able to treat the athletes according to the standard of care, no matter what the situation, it is strongly suggested that prior to beginning to serve as a team physician, the physician should have a written letter of agreement or contract that delineates the team physician's duties roles and responsibilities such as practice and game coverage expectations, travel expectations, liability coverage, medical supply provision, athlete preparticipation decisions, and authority regarding RTP decisions.[9] The agreement should be between the physician and the team or governance organization for the team such as the school district, university, or sports league. The agreement should specify physician compensation or if the team physician is a volunteer (i.e., provides services without remuneration), which may be important in states that have legislation that offers some protection for volunteer team physicians. The agreement/contract should also specify the duties and responsibilities of the team with regard to the team physician.[4,6,28] Legal counsel can assist the team physician with preparation of an appropriate document.

5.4 SPORTS MEDICINE LIABILITY

Some physicians are hesitant to practice sports medicine because of the fear of being sued. If a sports medicine physician is sued for medical treatment given or failure to treat an athlete or any aspect thereof and if the case results in a trial, the key question will be, "Did the physician abide by the standard of care?" The standard of care in sports medicine is constantly evolving, and the plaintiff and the defense will bring in experts to testify on the issue. To be found liable for medical malpractice, a sports medicine physician must be found to have been negligent. For a litigant to prevail against the physician on a claim of medical malpractice, four elements of negligence must be considered: duty, breach, causation, and damages. The full scope of these elements is beyond this coverage but is summarized in the succeeding text.

The first element, *duty*, refers to whether the team physician has a physician–patient relationship, an obligation recognized by law that results in a duty to care for the athlete in question. Where such a relationship or duty exists, the physician must competently care for the athlete at the minimum skill level of other physicians who provide medical treatment for such an injury.

The second element, *breach*, reflects a failure to conform to the requisite standard of care (expected of a reasonably competent sports medicine physician in similar circumstances) for the athlete. Much of the testimony in medical malpractice cases consists of expert witnesses for the patient/plaintiff and the physician/defendant who attempt to demonstrate that the physician's diagnosis/treatment did or did not conform to the standard of care owed to the patient.

The third element, *causation*, is proven if the plaintiff demonstrates that the physician's breach of the duty of care (that is, the failure to provide the minimum skill level to the patient) resulted in (that is, had a sufficient causal connection to) the specific harm befalling the patient/athlete. A physician cannot be found negligent by causation unless the medical treatment (or failure to treat) fell below the standard of care and resulted in harm or injury to the patient. For example, if a team physician fails to diagnose a fractured fibula in a football player who returns to the game and subsequently dislocates his shoulder, causation has not been proven. This is because the treatment (or lack thereof) of the fibular injury did not directly cause the injury to the shoulder.

The fourth element of negligence is *damages*. To have a viable case against a physician, the patient/athlete must have sustained some quantifiable damages, whether they are physical, financial, or emotional costs.[4] This means that if the team physician renders medical treatment below the standard of care that proximately causes an injury but no damages result, a negligence claim should not hold up in court. A sports medicine physician who engages in care of athletes must possess a similar degree of skill, learning, and care compared to reasonably competent sports medicine physicians acting under similar circumstances. For example, a reasonably competent sports medicine physician should be aware that an athlete who sustains a head injury and is knocked unconscious should be assumed to have an associated cervical spine injury and an immediate circulation, airway, breathing (CAB), and appropriate neurological evaluation plus immobilization should be performed.[3,20] If a sports medicine physician does what a reasonably competent sports medicine physician would do under the same or similar circumstances, an athlete/plaintiff will be unlikely to prevail on a claim of negligence against the physician.

5.5 MEDICAL MALPRACTICE INSURANCE

It is essential that a team physician's malpractice insurance cover the scope of the physician's practice of sports medicine. Because many of the patients treated by team physicians (particularly in a school setting) are minors (who in certain circumstances can file lawsuits upon reaching the age of majority), careful consideration must be given to the type of insurance coverage selected by the team physician.

Malpractice insurance is a complicated issue; the full discussion of which is beyond what is covered here but, in summary, can be divided into two main types: *occurrence* and *claims-made* insurance. Occurrence insurance provides coverage for alleged malpractice events that occur during the policy period but which can be brought to court during or after the period of the policy. Because occurrence insurance covers the physician for the alleged events, even after the time period of the policy may have ended, it does not require tail coverage. In contrast, claims-made insurance provides coverage for alleged malpractice events that occur *and* were brought to court during the time that insurance policy was in effect. When a physician has claims-made insurance, it is recommended that the physician acquire tail coverage to ensure malpractice coverage in case a claim is filed at a later date.

Clinical Pearl

Before changing jobs, physicians should check the "tail" coverage on their malpractice insurance to protect them against malpractice claims initiated after they leave their current job.

Some malpractice carriers place restrictions that deny coverage for certain activities. If a physician's malpractice insurance does not cover sports medicine activities, he should obtain additional insurance coverage before participating in uncovered medical practice. It is important for the physician to be knowledgeable about potential exclusions on the malpractice policy, such as the practice of medicine outside the physical confines of an office or hospital that may preclude the physician from conducting examinations at a gymnasium or covering athletic events. Additionally, if a physician travels with a team, it is important to check the "territory" section of a malpractice policy to see if the locale to which the physician is traveling is within the scope of coverage of the insurance policy and see if the malpractice carrier will cover the physician in states in which they do not hold a license.

5.6 TRAVELING TEAM PHYSICIAN

It is possible that when a team physician accompanies a team out of state (where the team physician is not licensed to practice medicine) that the physician might be perceived as practicing medicine without a license. In order to avoid this problem, team physicians must become familiar with the laws governing the practice of medicine in other states. A good place to gather information or resources concerning another state's medicolegal policies is through that state's medical board. Some states allow physicians who are licensed in another state to practice medicine occasionally in their state, as long as the physician does not have an office in that state or purport to be licensed in the visiting state; others do not.[35] It is the responsibility of team physicians to know the laws of the state that they are visiting.

Viola et al. performed a survey of state licensing medical boards in the United States, which asked if they have laws or exemptions to allow a traveling team physician (from another state [home/primary state]) to practice medicine using their current home state license on their own team while traveling to that state (secondary state where they are not licensed). If response was not obtained, then their statutory language was searched. Of the 58 licensing boards in the United States, they received information on 54 (93% response rate). Their findings indicate that 18 states (33%) allow team physicians traveling with their team to the secondary state to practice medicine with their primary state license, but 36 states (67%) do not have a legal pathway to allow traveling team physicians to practice medicine in the secondary state without a license. Twenty-seven of those 36 states (50% of all states) actually have laws that require a license in the secondary state for the practice of medicine, and thus, traveling team physicians could be faced with criminal liability if practicing medicine there. Some states have specific exemptions for temporary practice such as Massachusetts for U.S. Olympic Committee events. It is important to note that, in general, Good Samaritan laws for medical personnel to respond in an emergency do not cover team physician activity. In addition to surveying state medical boards, the study also surveyed medical malpractice carriers and found that most of them would not cover the malpractice for the traveling team physician to secondary state.[35]

To address these issues, legislation has been introduced in the U.S. Congress in 2014 in the Senate (S.2220) and House of Representatives (H.R.3722) to provide licensure clarity and malpractice coverage for sports medicine professionals who travel outside their primary licensure state. The outcome of the proposed legislation is currently pending.

When traveling to other states, physicians should familiarize themselves with the protocols and standard of care for sports medicine providers in that domain. It is important to learn the emergency policies and procedures before the visiting athletes engage in sports activities to provide for their safety. It is also recommended that the local sports medicine providers be apprised of any special medical needs of traveling team members. Physicians repeatedly traveling with a university or professional teams often form informal relationships with physicians in the same sports leagues who can help inform them of local policies and provide for any special medical needs of their athletes. Some physicians meet at officially sanctioned league/organization medical meetings to discuss and exchange similar information to obtain specific information physicians should refer to the local medical board or legal counsel.

Physicians traveling with their teams must also be aware of travel restrictions on the contents of the sports medicine bag. For example, airline carriers restrict flammable substances such as ethylene glycol spray and some sprays used for athletic taping, as well as sharp objects that are frequent components of a physician's medical bag. For domestic travel, sports medicine physicians need to be aware of what medications can be legally carried across specific state lines and those that may be restricted such as narcotics.[30] Additionally, there are often restrictions on who may carry the prescription medication (the athlete to whom it was prescribed versus physician/sports medicine staff). There are often strict labeling requirements for the medication including patient name so the team physician may not be able to legally carry prescription medications (such as antibiotics) for general prescribing if a need arises. Internationally, some prescription medications such as narcotics may be illegal to carry into some foreign countries and may place the physician at risk of being accused of drug trafficking. The U.S. Embassy can provide such information before foreign travel. Depending on where the team travels internationally, a ready supply of emergency equipment that we have come to expect domestically, such as spine boards and external defibrillators, may not be available. Another aspect of traveling with teams domestically and abroad arises when the team comprises minors. Traveling team physicians should ensure that each player's parent or guardian has completed *written* treatment authorization forms in case the need for treatment arises and the parent or guardian cannot be reached.[30]

5.7 GOOD SAMARITAN

Many physicians volunteer their time to serve as team physicians and/or to perform PPEs. Other physicians fear legal liability so they do not volunteer their time. It is quite reasonable for prospective team physicians to question whether they are protected from a lawsuit under a Good Samaritan statute. Good Samaritan statutes were enacted to protect persons who offer medical assistance to those in need of treatment from liability[4] and exist in some form in all 50 states.

Unfortunately, it is not possible for a team physician to be totally protected from liability. Anyone can be sued; however, just because a case is filed does not mean it has any merit or will proceed to trial.[4,29] It is not uncommon for cases to be dismissed or verdicts to be found in favor of the physician in those instances where the doctor voluntarily came to the aid of another person in an emergency situation. In such cases, the Good Samaritan law has been successfully invoked as a defense.[4]

The parameters of Good Samaritan laws can vary from state to state. As a general rule, however, most state Good Samaritan statutes protect a particular class of persons (i.e., some states protect all persons rendering assistance, while other statutes specifically protect particular healthcare providers such as physicians and nurses) acting in good faith in an "emergency" setting, where the provider's assistance has conformed to the profession's conduct standards under the circumstances and where the assistance has been provided without compensation.[4,21] In other words, the Good Samaritan must rescue or aid with honest intentions (good faith) at an emergency scene (such as an automobile accident, sporting event, or other locations specified by statute, normally not in a hospital or office), performing the aid with the minimum standard of care (without negligence) and performing the aid gratuitously (for free). PPEs are not emergency activities so usually are not covered under Good Samaritan laws, but if a physician volunteers to perform PPEs at a nonprofit clinic, the physician may be covered under federal charitable immunity legislation such as The Volunteer Protection Act of 1997.

It is essential that team physicians know the parameters of the Good Samaritan law in each state where they will be rendering athletic coverage. Some states, in order to encourage the rendering of volunteer medical care by physicians, have passed Good Samaritan legislation that specifically protect from liability those physicians who volunteer as athletic team physicians and/or who render care at athletic events or in other emergency situations. But in other states, team physicians, even if uncompensated, are considered persons who have a duty to act and are not covered by the Good Samaritan laws.[21,29]

5.8 PREPARTICIPATION EVALUATION

Physicians are often asked to perform PPEs to certify if an athlete can participate in certain sports or activities (see Chapter 6). The goal in performing PPEs is to promote the health and safety of the athlete in training and competition. Many school systems and states require these evaluations.[2] It is important to be aware that although many physicians perform PPEs without charge, most state Good Samaritan statutes do not protect physicians from potential liability, such as failure to diagnose a medical condition or injury, as a PPE is not an emergency evaluation.[20,29] One area of the PPE that poses the greatest liability risk is failure to diagnose a cardiac abnormality, such as an arrhythmia or other anomaly, that can be associated with sudden cardiac death in an athlete. This is one reason why physicians must be in a setting during PPEs where they can adequately auscultate the heart. Unfortunately, many PPEs are conducted in mass settings that may be quite noisy.

One of the most publicized legal cases involving cardiac sudden death in an athlete surrounded the death of basketball star Hank Gathers.[14] The cardiac anomaly known as hypertrophic cardiomyopathy (HCM) has been associated with sudden death in athletes, such as Hank Gathers, and can be a significant challenge for sports physicians because HCM is often asymptomatic and thus not easily identified during a medical history and/or physical examination.[4] Another cardiac anomaly associated with sudden death in athletes is rupture of the aorta in an athlete with Marfan's disorder. Athletes may also have unknown cardiac electrical abnormalities, such as prolonged QT syndrome, which can also lead to sudden death or may develop cardiac arrhythmia from other abnormalities that present as sudden cardiac death. One example of this was 28-year-old American long-distance runner Ryan Shay who died during the U.S. Olympic marathon trials in 2007 in New York City and whose autopsy results indicated cardiac arrhythmia due to cardiac hypertrophy with patchy fibrosis of undetermined etiology.

An athlete who has a prior injury that was inadequately rehabilitated and is subsequently reinjured by participating in sports poses another source of liability for physicians. Athletes or their families have been known to sue sports medicine physicians, alleging negligent failure to discover latent injuries or physical defects.[20] The best protection from liability for latent injury or reinjury is for the physician to adhere to accepted sports medicine practices under the circumstances.

Clinical Pearl

Athletes need to be prepared to safely participate in their sport or can be liable for their own injuries.

Athletes and teams also have responsibility to disclose preexisting injury or illness to the sports medicine physician. Sometimes, athletes fail to disclose information about medical conditions or prior injuries on their history or, in the case of minors, they may have signed their history sheet without their parent's knowledge and input. A physician can be held liable if found negligent in determining fitness or giving sports clearance that subsequently results in a causal injury.

Being aware of the potential liability from performing PPEs, physicians should pay close attention to their selection of venue in which to perform those evaluations. Some of the venues include individual visits by athletes to the doctor's office; a location such as a gymnasium, where multiple athletes are seen individually at sequential stations where each examiner performs one section of the exam; or locker room *en masse* examinations. Although station-based rotations or locker room examinations allow a large number of athletes to be examined efficiently, drawbacks of these methods include noise and lack of privacy, which may preclude an adequate history taking and make it difficult to auscultate the heart and lungs effectively. In the station-based type of examination, someone must sign the ultimate clearance determination, and this raises the question as to whether a physician wants to assume potential liability from another provider's assessment, particularly the cardiovascular evaluation.

5.9 PREPARTICIPATION EVALUATION STANDARDS

In order to guide preparticipation clearance determinations, many professional medical organizations have issued recommendations that address common medical problems that athletes who desire preparticipation clearance may have and which may increase their risk if participating in certain sports.[6,16,27] The *Preparticipation Physical Evaluation* fourth edition published by the American Academy of Pediatrics and authored by six major professional medical associations contains expert opinion and evidence-based principles and practice for PPEs (see Appendix A).[2] One clearance consideration is the type of sport the athlete is requesting to play. Sports can be classified according to the degree of physical contact between players and the level of static and dynamic cardiovascular demand of the sport (see Appendix B).[2,16] The contact classification divides sports into three categories: contact/collision, limited contact, or noncontact. For example, football is considered a contact/collision sport, while baseball is a limited contact sport, and swimming is categorized as a noncontact sport. The dynamic (volume) and static (pressure) cardiovascular demands of specific sports are divided into low, moderate, and high categories achieved during competition.

For example, rowing is a high-static/high-dynamic cardiovascular demand sport, whereas golf is low-dynamic and low-static cardiovascular demand sport.[2,16] If an athlete is medically restricted from participating in a particular sport, these classifications may be helpful to determine which other sport(s) the athlete may participate in.

Another source for athletic clearance guidance can be found in the guidelines from the 36th Bethesda Conference, which are used for eligibility recommendations for athletes with cardiovascular abnormalities.[19] When evaluating adults for cardiovascular clearance, it is helpful to utilize the American College of Sports Medicine's *Guidelines for Exercise Testing and Prescription*[24] to ensure that appropriate risk screening for cardiovascular diseases is being conducted. Even using appropriate guidelines to help determine clearance, some athletes may incur serious injury or death before they reach standard age for screening or before they develop risks triggering cardiovascular screening, such as occurred with the sudden cardiac death of 33-year-old St. Louis Cardinal pitcher Darryl Kile who died in his sleep from a myocardial infarction in the summer of 2002.[13]

A physician who has completed the history and physical examination of a person desiring participation in sports should render conclusions about clearance or the need for specific evaluations before a clearance determination can be finalized. The physician should document the decision in writing and include discussion of decision-making points if an athlete is not given clearance. Sometimes, members of a school athletic staff or a sports organization may help to expedite any further evaluations that are needed, but physicians are limited by confidentiality as to what medical information they can divulge without the express consent of the adult athlete or the parent/guardian of a minor athlete.

5.10 PREPARTICIPATION EVALUATION: ATHLETIC CLEARANCE

After the PPE and appropriate follow-up evaluations when indicated (such as an echocardiogram) are performed, the clearance determination is made. According to the PPE monograph, the types of clearance assessments for sports participation are (1) cleared for all sports without restriction, (2) cleared for all sports without restriction with recommendations for further evaluation or treatment for (specific condition), and (3) not cleared. Not cleared is further divided into not cleared pending further evaluation, not cleared for any sports, or not cleared for certain sports.[2] The sports classifications are very useful for determining the sports in which an athlete is physically capable of participating and for counseling an athlete who may have a restricted clearance as to which sports to consider. Consideration of the findings of the PPE, the 36th Bethesda classifications, and the effect of various medical conditions on sports participation[27] can help physicians to determine which activities, if any, are safe for a particular athlete. For example, if an athlete has a medical condition that warrants restricted clearance for a contact/collision, high-dynamic sport such as soccer, that athlete might be cleared for a noncontact/low-dynamic/low-static sport such as golf.

Determining risk is essential when clearing athletes. For example, during the musculoskeletal assessment portion of the exam, the physician should carefully examine previous injury sites, as this is a frequent source of liability. Sport-specific evaluation should also be performed, such as examining a soccer goalkeeper for broken fingers or deformities or evaluating the shoulder range of motion and stability of a baseball pitcher's throwing arm. When evaluating minors, physicians should also assess the physical size of the athlete, which can be helpful when discussing risks of participation in sports where age cutoffs are used to divide athletes rather than weight.

Physicians should make clearance determinations based on the standard of care and in the best interests of the athlete. Decisions should be individualized, reasonable, and based on competent medical evidence. The physician should not be influenced by outside considerations such as a team official or recruiter. Even though physicians exercise their best medical judgment to make clearance determinations, some special situations require additional documentation, such as athletes with unpaired organs or cardiac abnormalities. An athlete with unpaired organs or cardiac abnormalities who wants to participate in any contact/collision or limited contact sports should be given a thorough explanation of the choice of sports and the inherent risks. For example, an athlete with only one eye who desires to play a racquet sport should wear sports-approved polycarbonate or CR-39 eye protection.[2]

The decision to exclude an athlete from participation in a particular sport, like the decision to permit an athlete to play a particular sport, can be fraught with unexpected legal repercussions. Some athletes use legal avenues to reverse a team physician's or school district's clearance determinations.[12] In *Pace v. Dryden Central School District*,[23] a 17-year-old male with a solitary kidney was prohibited by the school district physician from participating in the high school football and basketball interscholastic athletic programs. His parents filed a lawsuit to compel the school to permit him to play. As part of their case, the parents submitted evidence showing that the particular health risks involved with the selected sports had been discussed with the family and that the student's own physician as well as a urology specialist had attested that the student's participation in contact sports was, in the opinion of the physicians, "reasonably safe." The court reversed the school district's decision and permitted the student to play.[23] Most significantly, the court held that, by virtue of its legal challenge to the restriction, the family waived any future liability claim against the school district in the event that the athlete's kidney was injured. The import of this decision is that litigation is often inevitable whether an athlete is cleared or not cleared for participation in sports. Team physicians should always rely on the clearance guidelines when making their determinations even if they are subsequently challenged in court.[20,29] It is important to note that if a court overrules a physician's clearance decision and permits an athlete to play or if an athlete has been conditionally cleared after the athlete has signed a written waiver of risk, the team physician continues to have the responsibility to help the athlete participate in that sport as safely as possible. Thus, if an athlete with a significant arrhythmia is playing a particular sport, whether by court order or by the athlete's decision after waiving the risks of participation, the team physician must ensure that a defibrillator is within immediate reach and that people are present who are trained in its use.

Although athletes do not have a constitutionally protected right to participate in sports,[10] they need to be given due process under the law if they are excluded from participation due to medical reasons. Thus, constitutional problems can occur if a high-risk athlete is barred from play due to a medical condition.[5] Multiple laws prohibiting discrimination, arbitrary classifications, and disparate treatment can be applied to the athletic context.[5] These include the Federal Rehabilitation Act (FRA) of 1973, the Individuals with Disabilities Education Act of 1989, and the Americans with Disabilities Act of 1990.[31,32,34] Athletes have utilized these laws to challenge team physicians' decisions to exclude athletes from participation. For example, in *Lambert v. The West Virginia State Board of Education*,[12] a school district excluded a deaf student from participating in basketball. The student took the district to court and the court decided that the FRA and the Individuals with Disabilities Education Act barred such discrimination against the handicapped student. The court ruled that the student could participate in the sport by using the services of a signer.[12]

Not all physicians and institutions evaluate risk and determine clearance in a similar manner potentially resulting in different clearance determinations. In 1996 Knapp v. Northwestern University, an athlete who had suffered a cardiac arrest as a high school senior who was successfully resuscitated and later had an implantable defibrillator placed, was cleared by several cardiologists to play basketball. He obtained a scholarship to play basketball at Northwestern University but the university team physician did not clear him based on the 26th Bethesda guidelines of the time and the opinion of the university's consulting cardiologist.[15] Knapp sued Northwestern University citing the FRA of 1973. The courts upheld Northwestern's position and ruled that Northwestern University's decision was reasonable, based on accepted medical guidelines, and the FRA did not apply.[11] Another case involved a high school football player (Larkin) who passed out at practice and was found on evaluation for the syncope to have HCM. When he was subsequently restricted from playing football, he sued his high school and the Archdiocese of Cincinnati in order to be permitted to play. The court in *Larkin v. Archdiocese of Cincinnati*[13] ruled that schools have the power to enforce medical standards, even if that means barring some athletes from competition.[4,5,13]

The Americans with Disabilities Act has also been used to challenge potentially discriminating practices by sports leagues to inhibit the ability of an athlete with a physical impairment to compete. In *PGA Tour, Inc. v. Martin*,[25] the court ruled that denying the use of a golf cart to Casey Martin (a professional golfer with a circulatory disorder that impaired his ability to walk), per the policy of the time of the PGA Tour that all golfers must walk during tournament play, violated the Americans with Disabilities Act, and Martin's request for a waiver to the "walking rule" should have been granted.[25]

5.11 RISK RELEASES/WAIVERS OF LIABILITY

There are inherent risks of injury by participating in sports, which vary by factors such as type of sport, competitive level, and environmental conditions. One of the responsibilities of the sports medicine physician is to inform prospective athletes (or their parents or guardians) of the risks involved in participating in a specific sport. Schools and athletic organizations often have printed handouts that include sport-specific information. In cases in which athletes have increased risks participating in sports due to known medical conditions, physicians should carefully document those risks and the potential consequences of participation on the risk release sheet that the adult athlete or parent or guardian of a minor must sign.

The rationale for these waivers is to try to protect the school or athletic organization and its staff from being sued. The premise is that if an athlete (or parent or guardian) is aware of the dangers or inherent risks of a particular sport and chooses to participate in the sport anyway, then the adult athlete (or parents, if a minor) assumes the risk and the school district, team, athletic organization, or activity sponsor and physician are insulated from liability. Waivers and risk releases do not always protect the parties from liability. Some states do not accept some types of waivers of risk as legally binding. As with any contract, the courts are often used to determine whether a waiver is valid and binding. The courts consider whether the waiver was clearly written, specific, and not subject to different interpretations.[5] Additionally, if a physician is negligent regarding treatment of an injury that occurs in that sport, the waiver of risk in the decision to play does not absolve the physician or athletic personnel from liability regarding injury negligence.

Sports medicine physicians should be knowledgeable about the laws in the states where they are practicing because they differ in the legal interpretation of risk release waivers or contracts. The physician can also seek legal counsel. The safest approach is for physicians to be familiar with sports medicine consensus statements and guidelines and use their best medical judgment when determining whether a person should be cleared to play a particular sport.

5.12 RETURN-TO-PLAY DECISIONS

A major area that exposes a sports physician to potential liability from negligence is making RTP decisions after injury or illness. The sports physician is the one who must determine whether or not an injured athlete may safely resume participation in the sport. Even though there are often pressures from the athlete or coach to reduce the time an athlete is restricted from participating in the game, the team physician must never compromise the athlete's safety. The physician must inform the athlete of the potential short- and long-term risks of playing injured if the athlete is allowed to return to play. The standard of care to be used when making RTP decisions is to consider what a reasonably prudent physician would do under the same or similar circumstances.[4] The team physician can use consensus statements, such as The Team Physician

Consensus Statement and the Return-to-Play Decision: a Consensus Statement 2012, as resources for making RTP decisions. One of the most common RTP decisions concerns players with sport-related concussion. The consensus statement on concussion in sport: the Fourth International Conference on Concussion in Sport held in Zurich, November 2012 is one of the consensus statements that may be used when considering RTP issues in an athlete with sports-related concussion.

Prior to engaging in athletic coverage, it is helpful for the physician to clarify, in writing, the role of the team physician for making the ultimate RTP decisions. This can minimize the RTP conflicts that can invariably arise during the excitement of a game.

5.13 TREATMENT

In contrast to emergency treatment that may occur on the sidelines with or without informed consent (if adult athlete is unconscious or medically unable to consent), elective or nonemergency treatment requires informed consent from an adult athlete or from a parent or guardian if the athlete is a minor. In situations where a parent is unavailable, a permission-to-treat form signed by the parent may be used for basic treatment of a minor. Informed consent means giving the athlete sufficient information to make an informed decision about whether or not to accept medical advice. When an athlete allows himself to be treated by a team physician without objection, it is considered implied consent.[20] The elements of informed consent include explaining the nature of the medical condition or diagnosis and treatment, inherent risks of the condition or treatment, and the likelihood of success of the treatment, alternatives to the treatment, or risks of not accepting treatment. An example of informed consent would be to inform an athlete of options for treating a painful injury with an anti-inflammatory medication such as ibuprofen plus discussing potential risks that the drug can have on various organ systems and the likelihood that it will work versus other options for treatment or lack of treatment. The team physician should document informed consent discussion and his or her treatment given to the athlete.

Clinical Pearl

It is important for the team physician to perform a condition-specific, medical, physical, and psychosocial assessment for an ill or injured athlete to aid in treatment and RTP decisions.

5.14 CONFIDENTIALITY, PRIVACY, AND DISCLOSURE

Until the advent of the Health Insurance Portability and Accountability Act of 1996 (HIPAA), it was understood by the legal community that the communications between a doctor and patient were privileged unless the privilege was expressly waived by the patient. Sports physicians had a legal responsibility to protect an athlete's medical information, even about injuries, from athletic staff, teammates, and press unless given specific permission to release that information. Now, under the HIPAA, not only physicians but also health plans, covered schools can suffer significant civil and criminal penalties for failure to protect the confidentiality of the patient (athlete).[18,33] Health providers may only disclose specific patient information to other health providers solely for health-care treatment purposes. The Family Educational Rights and Privacy Act (FERPA) is the applicable law when information is considered part of the educational record and applies to entities such as public schools that receive specific government educational funds. FERPA has a similar intent to HIPAA and may apply to PPEs and school-based training room medical records. It also limits the information a physician may share with a school or university or that they in turn may share with the public. This presents a dilemma when an athlete sustains a severe injury in a nationally televised athletic contest and sports teams and the public want information about the athlete's condition and the injury.[18,33] Physicians must be very careful not to release any information without the express consent of their patients. Whether traveling between athletic venues and medical practice sites or information transfer within/between health systems, the sports medicine professionals and their staff must take precautions to protect the athletes' protected health information (PHI).

The HIPAA *Privacy Rule*, which has the greatest impact on the practice of sports medicine, creates national standards to protect an individual's personal health information, gives patients increased access to their medical records, and affects the way health information is shared (see Section 45 Code of Federal Regulations [CFR], Parts 160 and 164).[33] Sports medicine providers, schools, and sports teams need to confer with their legal counsel to determine how they will comply with HIPAA. The Privacy Rule protects "individually identifiable health information" held and transmitted in any form or media (electronic, paper, or oral) and that information is called protected health information.

Individually, identifiable health information is information including demographic data that relate to the individual's past, present, or future physical or mental health or condition; the provision of health care to the individual; or the past, present, or future payment for the provision of health care to the individual and that identifies the individual or for which there is a reasonable basis to believe it can be used to identify the individual.[33]

In addition to HIPAA and FERPA legislation, the Affordable Care Act of 2010 (including standards for patients' information privacy), the American Recovery and Reinvestment Act of 2014, including the Health Information Technology for Economics and Clinical Health Act (which expands the scope of existing HIPAA privacy and security rules for electronic PHI), and the updated HIPAA regulations of 2014 protect the use of PHI.

Some specific items from the HIPAA Privacy Rule that will be discussed here include the Notice of Privacy Practices (NPP) and the Authorization to Release PHI because they affect the practice of sports medicine and applicable consent procedures.

5.15 NOTICE OF PRIVACY PRACTICE

Health-care providers are mandated to make a good faith effort to get a *written* acknowledgement of receipt of the NPP from a patient. The NPP describes the uses and disclosures that may be made of a person's PHI. The HIPAA does not prescribe a specific form for the NPP or require that the patient sign the actual NPP form, so the patients can sign a separate sheet or cover sheet to acknowledge they have read the NPP. Emergency treatment situations are exempted from the good faith effort requirement. However, as soon as is reasonably practicable after the emergency situation, the good faith effort to obtain patient acknowledgment of receipt of the NPP applies (45 CFR 164.520[c][2][ii]).

5.16 AUTHORIZATION TO RELEASE INFORMATION

Health-care providers (including sports medicine providers) and other covered entities are required to obtain authorization for disclosure of PHI and for nonroutine uses of PHI to parties that are *not* part of the chain of health-care providers (e.g., the media, teammates, athletic directors).

According to the HIPAA, the list of required elements (Table 5.2) that must be present for authorization of the PHI to be valid includes the following.

TABLE 5.2
Requirements for Protected Health Information Disclosure

Description of the information to be used or disclosed.
Identification of the persons/class of persons authorized to use or disclose the protected health information (PHI).
Identification of the persons/class of persons to whom the "covered entity" is authorized to make use or disclosure of PHI.
Description of the purpose of each use or disclosure.
Expiration date or event.
Individual's (patient or representative) signature and date.
Description of a personal representative's authority to act for the individual if not signed by the individual.
Statement that the individual may revoke the authorization in writing (including statement on right to revoke and instructions on how to do so or reference to Notice of Privacy Practices if that notice already includes this information).
Statement that the treatment is not conditioned on obtaining signed authorization, which is prohibited by the HIPAA privacy rule.
Statement that PHI may be re-disclosed by the recipient.
The individual must be provided with a copy of the signed authorization form.

It is important to note that the patient (athlete) is supposed to grant permission in advance for *each* disclosure or nonroutine use of the PHI on a per incident (per injury) basis. This brings into question the validity of blanket and universal authorization forms. Also, in cases involving minors, state law supersedes the federal HIPAA so that sports medicine providers need to be aware of applicable state laws regarding disclosure of information about a minor to a parent. Even under HIPAA, treating physicians of any patient (including athletes) can use and disclose whatever information they deem necessary for the treatment of the patient to other members of the health-care treatment team (e.g., releasing information about an injured athlete to an emergency room physician who will be assuming treatment of the patient). However, what is limited is disclosure to other parties, such as the media, athletic staff, or other team members.

This is not an all-inclusive discussion of the HIPAA, and more information can be obtained by accessing the website www.hhs.gov/ocr/privacy/hipaa/understanding/summary/privacysummary.pdf (accessed July 5, 15).

Protecting athletes' PHI from the public is especially challenging due to multimedia coverage of sports. A study of English newspapers in the month of March 2010 found they were replete with athletes' medical details (5640 specific articles) yet only 10% of the newspaper citations clearly identified the source of the information.[26] Whether in print, audio, electronic or social media, etc., it is imperative that physicians do *not* release athletes' health or injury information without express consent from the athlete. Some universities and professional teams use athletes' waivers to allow the team to disclose some details about their injury/illness status.

Confidentiality rules also apply to the use of radiologic or medical images or case reports involving athletes (or other patients). Even with deidentified images, written consent with specific proposed use delineated should be obtained from the athlete (or legal guardian) in order to use those images or medical details in publications, presentations, or media. If the athlete is deceased, consent should be obtained from the family before use.

Clinical Pearl

Any nontreatment-related use of an athlete's radiologic images or case information requires written "disclosure" consent from the athlete even when the data are deidentified.

5.17 INFECTIOUS DISEASE

Potential confidentiality issues can occur when athletes who possess infectious diseases such as hepatitis B, human immunodeficiency virus (HIV), herpes simplex, and fungal infections choose to play sports in which potential transmission to other athletes could occur. The physician should inform the athlete about the transmission risks of the infection and should discuss with the athlete precautionary steps to be taken to prevent transmission.[1] Of note, the American Academy of Pediatrics Committee on Sports Medicine Guidelines recognizes that the chance of transmitting the HIV virus during sports is extremely low and recommends that HIV-positive athletes be permitted to participate in all sports.[1] Thus, even though a nominal risk exists in blood exposure with HIV-infected athletes who choose to participate in contact sports, physicians must maintain the confidentiality of these athletes and not disclose their HIV status to others (including the athletic staff) without the express consent of the athletes.

5.18 PRESCRIBING MEDICATION

Prescribing medication also raises confidentiality issues. At times, it is important to inform both the athlete and someone other than the athlete of the potential side effects that might occur from specific medications, but doing so may compromise an athlete's confidentiality. In those instances, the physician should explain why it would be helpful for someone other than the athlete to be alert for side effects and obtain the athlete's permission to give limited disclosure. Additionally, a physician can incur liability from prescribing a medication that will cause an athlete to be disqualified or restricted from participation if found on drug testing. The physician must be aware of all drug regulations and all medications that are on the banned list of sports governing bodies and organizations such as those published by the National Collegiate Athletic Association,[22] the U.S. Olympic Committee, and the World Anti-Doping Agency. For example, an uninformed physician may prescribe a diuretic medication for an athlete with hypertension, which violates the drug prohibitions of the sport(s) in which the athlete competes. If a question arises about the use of a medication that is not clear from any published list, or internet resource such as the Global Drug Reference online, www.Globaldro.com, the physician could contact the sports organization without identifying the athlete to clarify if a specific medication may be used.

5.19 DRUG TESTING

Illicit drug use by athletes also creates confidentiality issues. Drug testing has been implemented in many collegiate and professional sports and some high school athletic programs with the goal of maintaining competitive fairness. However, when an athlete discloses to the team physician that he or she is using performance-enhancing or illicit drugs, the team physician cannot disclose that information without the specific consent of the athlete. Due to the potential conflict of interest and risk of compromising the physician–patient relationship, it is advised that the physician who is involved in an institution's drug testing compliance be someone other than the team physician. If an athlete admits to the use of such drugs as anabolic steroids or cocaine, the team physician should take advantage of that opportunity to have an honest, balanced discussion regarding the risks and benefits of the particular drug with the athlete in an attempt to discourage its use.[29]

5.20 LEGISLATION AFFECTING CLINICAL CARE

Sometimes, legislation or legal settlements that affect the clinical practice of sports medicine have roots in the unfortunate morbidity or mortality that has occurred in sports. One example of this in the United States includes the development of the Korey Stringer Institute (KSI), which is dedicated to prevention of sudden death in sports via health and safety initiatives. The KSI has a special focus on prevention of exertional heatstroke and provides valuable information/resources on this issue. This institute arose from the 2009 settlement of a wrongful death lawsuit against the National Football League by Kelci Stringer (widow of football player Korey Stringer, a Minnesota Vikings lineman who died from exertional heatstroke sustained during training camp in 2001).[37]

Concussion legislation also began due to an untoward event. The first state to pass legislation on school-sponsored sport-related concussion was Washington State in 2009. The law is named the Zackery Lystedt Law[36] after a youth football player who sustained a head injury while playing football, which resulted in severe, persistent disabilities. Between 2009 and 2014, all 50 states and the District of Columbia have passed laws on concussion in youth sports, but the laws vary in their scope and details. The most complete laws include three components: the parent/student athlete signs a concussion information form, any student athlete suspected of having sustained a concussion is to be removed from play, and written medical clearance is required prior to returning to play. Physicians who treat athletes need to be aware of the specific concussion laws that apply where they practice.

5.21 RISK MANAGEMENT

Sports medicine litigation is on the increase. In order for the sports medicine physician to deter litigation or prevail if litigation occurs, it is important for sports medicine physicians to practice the "4Cs" of good risk management: *compassion*, *communication*, *competence*, and *charting*.[4] Compassion is exhibited by those physicians who foster good relationships with the athletes and athletic staff and perhaps, not coincidentally, are less likely to be sued even if a bad outcome occurs. Communication focuses on the exchange of information between the patient and the physician. Physicians who communicate effectively are those who give the athletes and parents (if the athlete is a minor) clear informed consent about the risks of sports and the risks and treatment options for certain conditions or injuries. Competence is found in physicians who stay knowledgeable about sports medicine and deliver the required standard of care to the patient athlete. The fourth component, charting, concerns the physician's duty to maintain complete medical records. Meticulously prepared medical records can save a physician untold grief if litigation ensues.

The team physician must ensure that an organized system for record retention and retrieval is in place. Each patient's file should, at a minimum, contain the preparticipation physical examination record.[29]

Although team physicians often practice medicine on the field instead of in an office, the need for specific medical records is not removed. If a physician renders sideline care without much time for detailed documentation, the physician (as well as any assisting athletic trainers) should use a notepad or electronic device to contemporaneously document the essential medical information. Then, as soon as feasible, the physician should complete the notes, make a copy, and place the document in the patient's file. The record should be typed or legibly written and signed by the physician and should contain the athlete's name, sport, date of event, assessment of injury or illness, immediate treatment, and further recommendations for treatment and rehabilitation.[4,29] The storage of that information must also be in compliance with HIPAA/FERPA regulations regarding storage of identifiable patient information.[33]

Medical records should be maintained by the team physician for extended periods of time, often beyond the time an athlete is participating on a particular team or organization. Physicians who care for minor athletes who may be able to sue for medical malpractice after they reach the age of maturity (depending on the laws of their state) should consult with an attorney before destroying any medical records.

While the "4Cs" of good risk management are useful for all physicians, two additional "Cs" can be added to the list for the team physician: contract and confidentiality. The *contract* should be between the team physician and the entity for which the physician is providing services. The team physician should insist upon a contract or letter of agreement that delineates what services he or she will provide the team and what services the team will provide (see Section 5.3). Finally, the contract or agreement should include a statement that the final decision on participation or RTP considerations is to be made by the team physician after providing informed consent to the athlete. Maintaining the *confidentiality* of the physician–athlete relationship and adhering to the HIPAA/FERPA rules are also paramount to good risk management.

5.22 SUMMARY

The sports medicine physician needs an understanding of basic legal principles that affect the practice of sports medicine. These principles build on the legal aspects of other medical practice such as medical competence, standards of care, informed consent, malpractice, licensure, liability, and confidentiality, but sports medicine legal issues have added complexities such as medical practice occurring on the sidelines and across state lines. To promote athlete safety, provide excellent care to athletes, and protect physician licensure, the sports medicine physician needs to be aware of the specific legal issues that apply to the practice of sports medicine (Table 5.3).

TABLE 5.3
SORT: Key Recommendations for Practice

Clinical Recommendation	Evidence Rating	References
Physicians caring for athletes should check each prescribed or recommended medication against the banned substance list for the sport(s), sport organization, or governing body to avoid adversely affecting the athlete's eligibility.	C	[2,6,9,22,30]
The team physician should have a written letter of agreement with the organization, team, or school that defines the duties, responsibilities of both parties, and the authority of the team physician for return-to-play decisions.	C	[4,6–9]
The team physician should coordinate the development and rehearsal of a venue-specific emergency action plan for practice and competition, which includes access to CPR, early defibrillation, local emergency medical services, organizational/institutional administrators, and safety personnel.	C	[7,9,30]
Physicians caring for athletes should conform to regulations to protect individually identifiable health information (e.g., HIPAA/The Family Educational Rights and Privacy Act) and comply with disclosure regulations relevant to care of the athlete.	C	[2,7–9, 20,28,33]
Sports medicine physicians should be familiar with major professional organizations' Team Physician Consensus Statements (e.g., sideline preparedness, return to play, concussion) to use as guides for common issues in sports medicine practice.	C	[7–9,17]

REFERENCES

1. American Academy of Pediatrics Committee on Sports Medicine and Fitness. The human immunodeficiency virus and other blood-borne pathogens in the athletic setting. *Pediatrics.* 1999;104:1400–1403.
2. Bernhardt D, Roberts W (eds.). *PPE Preparticipation Physical Evaluation*, 4th edn. Washington, DC: American Academy of Pediatrics; 2010.
3. Bianco EA, Walker EJ. Legal aspects of sports medicine. In: Birrer RB (ed.). *Sports Medicine for the Primary Care Physician*, 2nd edn. Boca Raton, FL: CRC Press; 1992, Chapter 4.
4. Gallup EM. *Law and the Team Physician.* Champaign, IL: Human Kinetics; 1995.
5. Greenberg, M.J. Benching of an athlete with medical problems may spur legal claims. *National Law of Journal.* 1993;15:29.

6. Herbert DL. *Legal Aspects of Sports Medicine*, 2nd edn. Canton, OH: PRC Publishing; 1995.
7. Herring S, Kibler W, Putukian M. Sideline preparedness for the team physician: A consensus statement-2012 update. *Medicine and Science Sports and Exercise*. 2012;44(12):2442–2445.
8. Herring S, Kibler W, Putukian M. The team physician and the return-to-play decision: A consensus statement-2012 update. *Medicine and Science Sports and Exercise*. 2012; 44(12):2446–2448.
9. Herring S, Kibler W, Putukian M. Team physician consensus statement: 2013 update. *Medicine and Science Sports and Exercise*. 2013;45:1618–1622.
10. *JM, JR v. Montana High School Association*, 875 P.2d 1026 (1994).
11. *Knapp v. Northwestern*. U.S. Court of Appeals for the Seventh Circuit No. 96-3450.
12. *Lambert v. The West Virginia State Board of Education*, 447 S.E. 2d 901 (1994).
13. *Larkin v. Archdiocese of Cincinnati*, c-1-90-619 S.D. Ohio (1990).
14. Lavelle M. A star basketball player's death rattles the college sports world and creates a nightmare of numerous legal battles. *National Law of Journal*. 1991;13:1.
15. Maron B, Mitten M, Quandt E, Zipes D. Competitive athletes with cardiovascular disease: The case of Nicholas Knapp. *New England Journal of Medicine*. 1998;339(22):1632–1635.
16. Maron B, Zipes, D. *36th Bethesda Conference*: Eligibility recommendations for competitive athletes with cardiovascular abnormalities. *Journal of the American College of Cardiology*. 2005;45(8):1317–1375.
17. McCrory P, Meeuwisse W, Aubry M. et al. Consensus statement on concussion in sport. *The 4th International Conference on Concussion in Sport* held in Zurich, November 2012. *British Journal of Sports Medicine*. 2013;47:250–258.
18. McLeod P. Injuries become a federal case. *The Los Angeles Times*, October 10, D1, 2002.
19. Mitten M, Maron B, Zipes D. Task Force 12: Legal aspects of the *36th Bethesda Conference* recommendations. *Journal of the American College of Cardiology*. 2005;45(8):1373–1375.
20 Mitten MJ. Emerging legal issues in sports medicine: A synthesis, summary, and analysis. *St. John's Law Review*. 2002;76(5):5–86.
21. Moore MA, Lee HP (eds.). *California Physician's Legal Handbook 1999*. San Francisco, CA: California Medical Association; 1999.
22. National Collegiate Athletic Association. *2013–14 NCAA Sports Medicine Handbook*, 24th edn. Indianapolis, IN: The National Collegiate Athletic Association, p. 122.
23. *Pace v. Dryden Central School District*, 574 N.Y.S. 2d 142 (1991).
24. Pescatello L. (ed.). *ACSM'S Guidelines for Exercise Testing and Prescription*, 9th edn. ACSM 2013. Philadelphia, PA: Lippincott Williams & Wilkins.
25. PGA Tour, Inc. v. Martin, 532 U.S. 661 (2001).
26. Ribbans B, Ribbans H, Nightingale C. Sports medicine, confidentiality and the press. *British Journal of Sports Medicine*. 2013;47:40–43.
27. Rice S. American Academy of Pediatrics Committee on Sports Medicine and Fitness. Medical conditions affecting sports participation. *Pediatrics*. 2008;121(4):841–848.
28. Rubin A. Legal issues in sports medicine. In O'Connor FG, Casa DJ, Davis RA, Pierre P St, Sallis RE, Wilder RP (eds.). *ACSM's Sports Medicine: A Comprehensive Review*. Philadelphia, PA: Lippincott Williams & Wilkins; 2013.
29. Simon LM. Medical–legal issues in pediatric sports medicine. In Birrer RB, Griesemer BA, Cataletto MB (eds.). *Pediatric Sports Medicine for Primary Care*. Philadelphia, PA: Lippincott Williams & Wilkins; 2002, Chapter 10.
30. Simon L, Rubin A. Traveling with the team. *Current Sports Medical Report*. 2008;7(3):138–143.
31. U.S. Congress. *Americans with Disabilities Act of 1990*, 42 U.S.C. §§ 12101 *et seq*. Washington, DC: U.S. Government Printing Office; 1990.
32. U.S. Congress. *Federal Rehabilitation Act of 1973*, Section 701 *et seq*. Washington, DC: U.S. Government Printing Office; 1973.
33. U.S. Congress. *Health Insurance Portability and Accountability Act of 1996*, Public Law 104-191 (42 U.S.C. 1301 et seq); Standards for Privacy of Individually Identifiable Health Information; Final Rule, 45 CFR Parts 160 and 164.
34. U.S. Congress. *Individuals with Disabilities Education Act of 1989*. Washington, DC: U.S. Government Printing Office; 1989.
35. Viola T, Carlson C, Trojan T et al. A survey of state medical licensing boards: Can the traveling team physician practice in your state? *British Journal of Sports Mediicne*. 2013;47:60–62.
36. Washington State Engrossed House Bill 1824, Chapter 475, Laws of 2009, 61st legislature, 2009 regular Session. Effective July 26, 2009, http://apps.leg.wa.gov/documents/billdocs/2009-10/pdf/bills/session%20law%202009/1824/sl/pdf (accessed August 10, 2014).
37. Weber D. Tragedy brings issues to light. *The Press Enterprise*, July 21, 2002, C1.

6 Preparticipation Examination

Jennifer J. Gayagoy, Katherine Walker Foster, and James B. Tucker

CONTENTS

TABLE 6.1
Key Clinical Considerations

1. The preparticipation examination (PPE) is an important aspect of athletic competition and is meant to assess general fitness, identify medical conditions that may limit participation, predispose injury to self and/or other athletes, and identify high-risk behaviors in order to provide further education and counseling.
2. The PPE should ideally be performed approximately 5–6 weeks before the start of the season by the athlete's PCP who knows the athlete well.
3. A focused cardiac history (including family history) and physical examination should be included in every PPE due to carefully evaluate the athlete for conditions that may predispose to sudden cardiac death.
4. Musculoskeletal findings during the PPE are the most common cause of restriction and/or delayed participation of the athlete.
5. Determining clearance of the athlete can be difficult and is often individualized. Consensus guidelines have been developed to aid PCPs, sports medicine physicians, and specialists in making the appropriate decision to ensure safety in sport.

6.1 INTRODUCTION

The preparticipation examination (PPE) is an important aspect of recreational and athletic competition. Its purpose is to identify athletes with medical conditions that limit participation or predispose to injury, to assess physical maturity and physical fitness, to assess general health and identify health-risk behaviors, and to meet legal and insurance requirements.[12,25,57,58,65,89,90] It was not designed to prevent participation and rarely does it do so. The largest study documenting the administration of the PPE evaluated 2739 athletes and resulted in disqualification of only 1.9% from participation in sports.[91] Another study of 596 athletes resulted in only a 0.2% clearance failure rate (Table 6.1).[42]

Although the PPE has been routinely performed for over 40 years, its effectiveness in screening and preventing injury or sudden death in the athletic population remains uncertain.[6,7] Many institutions use their own screening tools and evaluation forms making the lack of standardization difficult to collect objective data.[6,18,73] However, the PPE is still widely recommended by many medical organizations. The PPE provides an opportunity for the primary care provider (PCP) to facilitate general health care, update immunizations, identify chronic health conditions, and provide counsel for high-risk behaviors. It does not attempt to replace an athlete's routine health maintenance examination, but for most athletes, it is their only interaction with a health-care provider, making its implementation even more necessary.[6,37,105]

This chapter intends to provide the PCP with updated general consensus recommendations for the performance of the PPE and guidelines for clearance of the athlete for sports participation. A more standardized approach to the PPE will allow for improved data collection and provide evidence-based groundwork for future recommendations.[6,18,73]

6.2 ADMINISTRATION OF THE PPE

The PPE should be completed approximately 5–6 weeks prior to the beginning of the sports season in order to allow adequate time for rehabilitation and to order further diagnostic tests if necessary before final decisions for clearance can be made.[12,40,57,58,90,85] State regulations determine which healthcare providers are allowed to perform the PPE.[6,88,96,97] Many states allow the exams to be done by nonphysicians, such as physician assistants and nurse practitioners.[30] The ultimate responsibility for the PPE and decision for clearance, however, should be assigned to the physician and any problems beyond the comfort level of the evaluator should be referred to the appropriate specialist.[6,88,96,97]

Clinical Pearl

Although many states allow the PPE to be performed by nonphysicians, the final decision for clearance is the ultimate responsibility of the overseeing physician.

The two main formats of the examination are group setting/coordinated medical team and individual evaluation by the athlete's PCP. The locker room–based examination is considered inappropriate and is no longer recommended.[6] Advantages and disadvantages exist for each. Group setting is usually more efficient, as it involves various health professionals, possibly decreasing the time for referrals and obtaining clearance. The stations usually consist of vital signs, vision screening, medical, orthopedic, and occasionally cardiology. Physical therapists, nutritionists, and athletic trainers may also be available to advise on proper rehabilitation. The history and physical examination should be done by a single provider who will then coordinate care with additional providers if needed. Advantages include familiarity with sports medicine, on-site consultation, decreased referral time, and earlier clearance. Disadvantages include having a large enough space, noise, lack of a personalized approach, possible incomplete or inaccurate health history, poor communication with the athlete's PCP and parent or guardian, and difficulty in obtaining privacy or confidentiality.[6,12,18,25,57,58,65,89,90]

The most common and ideal approach is to have the PPE performed at the athlete's PCP's office; this format is recommended by most medical societies. Advantages include continuity of care; familiarity with the athlete's personal and family history; ease of arranging follow-up; ease of keeping record of referrals, tests, and treatments; and privacy and more honest disclosure of high-risk behaviors or mental health concerns. Disadvantages of the office-based setting are lack of knowledge in how physical findings may affect risk for participation, time, and cost. Some athletes do not have access to a PCP, making an individual exam difficult. Communication among the athlete's PCP, coach, and athletic trainer is sometimes poor, making coordination of care difficult.[6,12,18,25,40,57,58,65,73,89,90]

Guidelines regarding appropriate screening intervals have not been established. Many authorities believe that a complete exam at the least should be performed with each entry into a higher level of competition (e.g., middle school to high school, high school to college), with interim histories and limited physical examinations completed in between.[12,18,40,85,90] There is no evidence supporting the assumption that increased frequency of the PPE leads to decreased injuries or death. Due to the significant physical and psychological growth that occurs from middle school to college, however, consensus recommendations propose that a comprehensive PPE be performed every 2 years in younger athletes and every 2–3 years in older athletes with annual interim updates. Interim examinations should focus on any injuries and/or medical problems that have occurred since the prior comprehensive.[6,64,105]

6.3 HISTORY

The history section is the most important component of the PPE. Studies have reported that history alone can detect anywhere between 65% and 88% of medical and/or orthopedic conditions that could potentially affect athletic participation.[17,31,42,83,84] The PCP should inquire about chronic medical illnesses, surgical history, family history, allergies, consumption of energy drinks, any supplements the athlete may be taking in hopes to improve performance and current medications, including both prescription and over-the-counter. Review of medications provides additional information on medical conditions that may have been omitted or forgotten on the history form and discuss risks for disqualification. Many common over-the-counter cold preparations and supplements (which are not regulated by the Food and Drug Administration) contain banned substances.[6,18,73,101,103] A comprehensive list of substances prohibited by the National Collegiate Athletic Association (NCAA) and World Anti-Doping Agency can be found online. Any chronic medical conditions identified, such as diabetes, asthma, and seizures, should be assessed for present control.

Clinical Pearl

The most important aspect of the PPE is the athlete's history. Obtaining a thorough medical history allows identification of approximately 68%–85% of medical and/or orthopedic conditions that could affect participation.

Answers to questionnaires often differ between the athlete and their parent or guardian.[16] Ideally, the parent or guardian will fill the questionnaire first and the athlete second to obtain as much information as possible and respect the athlete's privacy. Questions pertaining to sensitive issues such as body image and high-risk behaviors have been removed from the history section and are now placed as "PCP reminders" at the top of the physical examination portion of the PPE form to guide discussion in a private setting.

The American Academy of Pediatrics in conjunction with multiple expert medical societies has created a history and physical examination document that can direct the PCP in conducting an appropriate and thorough PPE (see Appendix A).[6] The PPE begins with measuring vitals (blood pressure, height, weight, and calculating BMI) and visual acuity and performing a systems-based approach physical examination as outlined in the following.

6.4 HEENT

Many times the head and neck, eye, ear, nose, and throat (HEENT) portion of the exam is deemphasized. Any differences in pupil size (anisocoria) at baseline should be documented. Such information can help prevent unnecessary evaluation if the athlete sustains a head injury.[73] The PCP should also examine visual acuity with and without corrective lenses.[27] Any difference between the eyes of two lines or greater in the visual acuity examination chart warrants referral for further evaluation. An athlete whose best corrected vision is worse than 20/40 in one eye and it is determined that the loss of the better eye would result in a significant change in lifestyle is deemed "functionally one-eyed." An athlete should have corrected vision of 20/40 or better if engaging in collision and contact sports. Protective eyewear approved by the American Society for Testing and Materials must be worn by all "functionally one-eyed" athletes participating in sports that are high risk for eye injuries, such as basketball, baseball, and field hockey. Such athletes are not cleared to participate in sports in which eye protection cannot be effectively worn such as boxing, wrestling, and full-contact martial arts. Examination of the ears is important in those participating in water and contact sports. Perforated tympanic membranes in a swimmer or diver should prompt the PCP to advise use of protective ear plugs. Any damage noted to the auricular cartilage in wrestlers and rugby players warrants the use of ear protection. If nasal septum deviation is noted, a referral to an otolaryngologist should be placed.[6,73,77,106] Examination of the mouth may show evidence of bulimic activity (i.e., parotid gland enlargement, gingival atrophy, and decreased tooth enamel) and/or tobacco use (i.e., leukoplakia) and may help tip off the examiner to delve into these topics. A high, arched palate may be a clue to a patient with Marfan's syndrome. Additional criteria are discussed in the musculoskeletal section. Palpation of the neck may reveal adenopathy suggestive of malignancy or infection.[6]

6.5 CARDIAC

The cardiac history and physical exam are most critical and require extra attention because of the severity of the consequences if abnormalities are overlooked. Sudden cardiac death (SCD) among high school athletes is estimated to occur at a frequency of 1/100,000 to 1/300,000 per year.[4,30,46,47,49,51,85,89] These numbers are even higher among older athletes. The most common cause of SCD among high school athletes is hypertrophic cardiomyopathy. In athletes over the age of 35, atherosclerotic disease accounts for the majority of deaths. The next most common cause of SCD in young athletes is congenital coronary artery anomalies. Other causes include ruptured aorta from Marfan's syndrome, aortic stenosis, myocarditis, dilated cardiomyopathy, arrhythmogenic right ventricular dysplasia, ion channelopathies (long QT syndrome [LQTS], catecholaminergic polymorphic ventricular tachycardia [CPVT], and Brugada syndrome), mitral valve prolapse, and intramural coronary arteries.[4,6,30,46,47,49]

Clinical Pearl

The most common cause of SCD among high school athletes is hypertrophic cardiomyopathy. The most common cause of SCD among athletes greater than 35 years of age is atherosclerotic disease.

While most authorities agree that cardiac screening is appropriate prior to participation in sports for young athletes, the recommendations vary. The 2007 American Heart Association (AHA) recommendations include a focused history and physical examination, whereas the European Society of Cardiology recommends an electrocardiogram (EKG) in addition to a history and physical examination.[37] A positive response to any of the 12 questions recommended by the AHA may require further cardiovascular evaluation (Table 53.2).

While an EKG can improve the sensitivity of detecting cardiac abnormalities that may predispose to a sudden cardiac arrest, it does lack specificity. Proponents of adding the EKG to cardiac screening cite the improved sensitivity and decreased rates of SCD. In Italy, since the introduction of a mandatory screening program that included routine EKGs for athletes between the ages of 12 and 35 participating in sports, the incidence of SCD dropped considerably. Opponents often argue against it due to the increased cost, low incidence of SCD, difficulty in training health-care providers to accurately interpret the EKGs, and the large number of athletes that may be excluded from sports unnecessarily. It is estimated that it would cost up to $3.4 billion to save one life and 600–1700 athletes would need to be restricted from sports to save one life.[11,52,71,867–40] Fortunately, continued research and developments, such as the European and Seattle criteria, have been made to help PCPs distinguish normal athletic physiologic adaptations and pathologic cardiac abnormalities (see Table 53.3).[20] Further research and education in this area may change the cardiac screening recommendations in the future.

Questions regarding the cardiac history are very important, as it carries the highest risk for sudden death on the athletic field. A number of personal historical questions need to be addressed, including a history of exertional chest pain/discomfort, unexplained syncope or near syncope, excessive fatigue with exercise, prior recognition of a heart murmur, or a history of elevated blood pressure. A history of irregular heartbeats or palpitations related to exercise is also important. Many cardiac abnormalities can be familial, and therefore, a thorough family history is important. It should address specific known cardiac conditions such as hypertrophic cardiomyopathy, Marfan's syndrome, arrhythmogenic right ventricular dysplasia, LQTS, Brugada syndrome, and CPVT, as well as a family history of SCD before the age of 50 years. A family history of unexplained syncope, unexplained drowning or near drowning, unexplained MVA, unexplained seizure disorder, or sudden infant death syndrome can be a trigger to consider an ion channel disorder such as LQTS or CPVT. Arrhythmias, conduction abnormalities, anomalous coronary arteries, and valvular disease may result in symptoms of fatigue, lightheadedness, dizziness, or syncope.[4,30,40,46,47,49,51,57,58,85,86,89,90] Syncope during exercise is a much more ominous and worrisome finding than syncope after exercise (see Chapter 53 for further discussion).[46]

Clinical Pearl

Syncope *during* exercise is worrisome and much more likely related to an underlying life-threatening medical condition, whereas syncope *after* exercise is likely related to exercise-associated collapse, a benign condition related to the abrupt cessation of skeletal muscle contraction and reflex vasodilation.

Older individuals require a more in-depth cardiac examination if they plan on engaging in regular strenuous exercise or competitive sports competition. Maron et al.[52] make the following recommendations for older athletes. Men over the age of 40–45 and women over the age of 50–55 with one or more risk factors for coronary artery disease should undergo exercise stress testing. These risk factors include hypercholesterolemia or dyslipidemia, systemic hypertension, current or recent cigarette smoking, diabetes mellitus (DM), or history of myocardial infarction or SCD in a first-degree relative less than 60 years old. All athletes 65 years of age and older and all athletes with symptoms of coronary disease should undergo an exercise test. Athletes younger than 65 who are asymptomatic and without cardiac risk factors do not need to undergo exercise stress testing. An EKG is recommended for all masters athletes >40 years old. Echocardiography should be performed on all patients if the history or physical is suggestive of valvular heart disease, hypertrophic cardiomyopathy, arrhythmogenic right ventricular cardiomyopathy, or prior myocardial infarction.[49] The American College of Sports Medicine has different guidelines for older athletes that are more stringent and rely on risk stratification and moderate versus. strenuous exercise (see Table 53.4 and Figure 53.1).[24] Other guidelines are not as aggressive. The ACC/AHA reports little evidence to support routine screening in asymptomatic men older than 45 and women greater than 55 preparing to begin a vigorous exercise program (Class IIb), unless the patient has diabetes (Class IIa).[28] If cardiac abnormalities are identified in both older and younger athletes, the guidelines from the 36th Bethesda Conference[103] are an excellent reference regarding recommendations for participation for various cardiac problems. All recommendations are level C (consensus/expert opinion).[48]

The cardiac exam is the single most important aspect of the physical exam because undetected cardiac abnormalities can lead to sudden death. The examiner should listen in a quiet area with the patient in both standing and supine positions. A murmur that is louder with a Valsalva maneuver or with a position that decreases venous return should be further investigated, as such a finding is associated with hypertrophic cardiomyopathy. Any diastolic murmur and any murmur that is higher than a grade 3/6 should also be further evaluated. Femoral and brachial arteries should be palpated to rule out coarctation of the aorta. The patient should also be evaluated for signs of Marfan's syndrome, as this syndrome is associated with aortic rupture and SCD. The physical exam findings include an unusually tall person with a wide arm span, kyphoscoliosis, high-arched palate, pectus excavatum or carinatum, mitral valve prolapse, aortic insufficiency murmur, long slender fingers, myopia, and displaced lenses.[4,40,46,47,49,51,85,89,90]

Clinical Pearl

The heart exam should be performed in a quiet room and auscultation performed with the athlete in both supine and standing positions. Any murmur louder with Valsalva maneuver or a position that decreases venous return or any murmur greater than grade 3/6 warrants further evaluation.

Blood pressure readings should be taken preferably in a quiet, relaxed setting with an appropriate-sized cuff. If it is initially elevated, the reading should be taken again after a few minutes. If it is elevated a second time, the athlete should lie down and rest for 10–15 minutes. Unfortunately, this is sometimes difficult to do, especially in a mass screening type of examination format. The Fourth Report on the Diagnosis, Evaluation and Treatment of High Blood Pressure in Children and Adolescents has established blood pressure normative data based on gender, height, and age and can be used to stage hypertension. Stage 1 hypertension is defined as a blood pressure value (measured on three separate occasions) between the 95th and 99th percentile +5 mmHg of age-, gender-, and height-based norms, and stage 2 is defined as a blood pressure above the 99th percentile + 5 mmHg. For adults, stage 1 is defined as a blood pressure between 140 and 159 over 90 and 99 and stage 2 is defined as a blood pressure of 160/100 or greater. Athletes found to have stage 2 hypertension or findings of end-organ damage should not be allowed to participate in sports until the blood pressure is further evaluated, treated, and controlled.[6,68]

6.6 PULMONARY

Exercise-induced asthma (EIA) and exercise-induced bronchospasm (EIB) are the most common pulmonary conditions affecting athletic performance in young athletes and can be discovered by asking questions pertaining to wheezing, shortness of breath, chest tightness, and/or coughing during exercise. The athlete may also admit to nonspecific complaints such as feeling out of shape, excess fatigue, chest or abdominal pain, or headaches.[95,101] Positive answers to the aforementioned screening questions should lead to further peak flow testing with measurements taken before and after exercise. A decrease in peak flow/FEV1 of 10%–15% is suggestive of EIA/EIB. Those with a known history of EIA/EIB should be asked questions to determine severity and current level of control such as frequency of beta-agonist use, number of missed practices or games, and number of doctor visits, urgent care/emergency room visits, and/or hospitalizations over the past year. The use of beta-agonist medication twice a week, nighttime symptoms, and difficulty in sleeping more than once per month indicates poor control and may require the addition of an inhaled corticosteroid.[60,66] This can prove to be an invaluable diagnosis because appropriately diagnosed athletes can be optimally treated to perform at their best. These athletes should be advised to have a rescue inhaler available at all times.[18] The lung exam is normal in most cases. Even those with EIA will usually have a normal exam at rest. Participation is allowed for all sports if the asthma is well controlled. Only athletes with severe asthma will need restrictions on activity.

Another common pulmonary condition diagnosed in athletes is vocal cord dysfunction (VCD). These athletes may describe the feeling of "trouble getting air in" or describe stridor after the start of physical activity. Due to symptoms also being associated with exertion, these athletes may be misdiagnosed and treated for EIA/EIB. Suspicion for VCD should rise for those with equivocal pulmonary function testing and failure of symptom improvement with beta-agonist use. Diagnosis is made with inspiratory–expiratory flow loop testing or laryngoscopy. Referral to a speech pathologist should be placed so that the athlete may learn proper breathing techniques to control symptoms. Triggers or risk factors include allergic rhinitis, reflux disease, anxiety, and poorly controlled asthma.[6,73]

Clinical Pearl

In most athletes with EIA/EIB and/or VCD, the pulmonary exam will be normal at rest. Therefore, a good history is key to guide diagnosis, treatment, and decision for participation in sport.

A less common abnormality is primary spontaneous pneumothorax. Those who have undergone only conservative management should be counseled on the risks of recurrence if they are involved in strenuous or contact sports. Athletes who have undergone thoracotomy or other invasive procedures should be allowed to return to all sports in 2–4 weeks. In either case, if a pneumothorax does recur, the athlete should be advised not to participate in contact sports.[62]

6.7 ABDOMEN

The abdominal exam should be done with the athlete in a supine position. Auscultation should be performed before palpation to avoid palpation-induced cessation of bowel sounds.[9] All four quadrants should be palpated to identify any masses, hernias, or organomegaly. An enlarged liver and/or spleen should prompt further evaluation for acuity versus chronicity and etiology determined. Acute hepatomegaly may indicate infection or malignant disease. An acutely enlarged liver or spleen is a contraindication to collision/contact or limited-contact sports. An enlarged liver beyond the body protection of the rib cage is at risk for injury. Infectious mononucleosis can cause acute splenomegaly and puts the athlete at risk for splenic rupture. Because splenic rupture can occur in the absence of trauma (with the greatest risk being within 3 weeks of illness onset), athletes should be restricted from all forms of sports-related activity for approximately 4–5 weeks. Another important finding that should not be missed in young female athletes is the presence of a gravid uterus.[6,80]

6.8 NEUROLOGIC

6.8.1 Concussion

> Concussion is a brain injury and is defined as a complex pathophysiologic process affecting the brain induced by biomechanical forces.[55]

Concussion is easily the most topical medical condition in athletics today. The Centers for Disease Control and Prevention (CDC) reports about 175,000 concussions in children and adolescents related to athletics and recreational activities are seen annually in emergency rooms.[29] Obviously, the number is much higher as PCPs probably see the majority of such injuries. Some estimates go as high as 3.8 million per year.[32] Multiple reviews in the lay press have examined sports-related concussion: among them, *Sports Illustrated*,[92,93] *The New Yorker*,[100] *the New York Daily News*,[98] *The New York Times*,[99] *Los Angeles Times*,[44] *Scientific American*,[87] *ESPN The Magazine*,[23] *USA Hockey Magazine*,[102] and *National Geographic*.[67]

Over the past decade, international conferences on concussion in sport have redefined the definition/diagnosis,[3,54–56] and return to participation guidelines have been standardized to some degree.[3,32,54–57] The potential for long-term affects has been established, but the exact risk and patterns are unknown. Between 2000 and 2010, there was more research and more scholarly articles published regarding concussions—both clinical and basic sciences—than in the previous five decades combined. Yet, there is still far more unknown than is known. While neurocognitive testing has become a part of the assessment armamentarium, it is far from the complete answer. While it provides some objective data, it can only be used in concert with the clinical picture. Comparing baseline neurocognitive data to postconcussion testing gives us numbers, but the implications of those numbers are really not established.

We all completely agree that sustaining a concussion is not good. Most agree that sustaining multiple concussions is worse because of an increased risk of depression and cognitive impairment in later life. This risk is probably geometric rather than simply additive. We all completely agree that an athlete should not be returned to participation until all concussion symptoms have cleared. Reasons for this consensus, however, vary and include the increased risk of another concussion, worsening/prolonging the initial concussion, and potential death from a very rare condition called second impact syndrome (SIS). There is significant controversy as to whether SIS even exists.[8,14,53]

Clinical Pearl

Any athlete diagnosed with a concussion should not be cleared for return to play until all concussion symptoms have resolved. Return to full participation requires a stepwise approach involving a gradual increase in physical activity.

It is imperative for the PCP performing a PPE to obtain as thorough a past history of concussions/head trauma as possible. Parents, athletes, and treating PCPs must be queried. Information sought must include the severity and frequency of occurrence, symptoms and duration of symptoms, imaging studies if done, neurocognitive testing if done, limitations on participation invoked, and as complete contemporaneous medical records of each event as are obtainable.

This may help to identify those individuals at greater risk for recurrent injury. The many guidelines regarding return-to-play criteria following concussions all agree that an athlete should not be allowed to return to play if still symptomatic from a concussion. All PCPs should be familiar with guidelines for continued participation in contact/collision sports after repeated concussions. Guidelines evolved through the Vienna,[3] Prague,[54] Zurich,[56] and Zurich[55] conferences and most recently the AMSSM position statement on concussion in sport have for the most part replaced those proposed by Cantu,[13] the Colorado Medical Society,[81] and the American Academy of Neurology[75]. Concussion management is detailed in Chapter 40, Head.

6.8.2 Others

It is rare in this day and age that seizure disorders cannot be controlled with a single medication or combination of medications. Medications should be chosen to maximize control of seizures and to minimize side effects. Seizures precipitated by exercise or hyperventilation may be challenging to control in an athlete. Obviously, participation in water sports requires awareness of risk and implementation of the buddy system. Participation in certain sports such as archery, riflery, and motor sports requires individualization, consultation, and caution. While athletes with posttraumatic and postinfectious seizures are theoretically and logically more at risk to seize secondary head trauma in contact sports, participation should not be arbitrarily limited, but each situation should be individualized.[26,33,85]

Burners/stingers or pinched nerves are neurologic complications that should be addressed and recorded. They usually are the result of stretching or compression of the cervical nerve roots or brachial plexus. In athletes with a history of recurrent burners or stingers, the examiner should inquire about transient quadriplegia. This is a rare problem that presents as burning pain, numbness or tingling, and weakness or paralysis of all four extremities. If an athlete has recurrent burner/stingers or transient quadriplegia, further workup should be performed to rule out a structural abnormality. If such an abnormality exists, competition in contact/collision sports should be restricted.[57,89]

Migraine headaches are rarely a reason for limitation or restriction from participation in sports. The most important challenge is control, and either prophylactic or "rescue" medications may be used individually or in combination to minimize the frequency, intensity, and duration of symptoms. Athletes with migraine headaches should be approached individually depending on triggers, frequency, and intensity of symptoms. Vascular headaches precipitated by exertion, dehydration, or contact are infrequent but may be problematic in treatment.

6.9 MUSCULOSKELETAL

Musculoskeletal findings are one of the most common reasons for the restriction of activity or delayed clearance in athletes. The majority of musculoskeletal injuries can be detected by history alone. The athlete should wear appropriate clothing that allows full inspection and range of motion. In the asymptomatic athlete with no history of prior injuries, a quick general screening examination is all that is required with the addition of a detailed joint-specific examination reserved for any positive findings (i.e., swelling, tenderness, decreased strength, or range of motion) (see Table 6.2).

An athlete with current complaints or a history of injury should prompt the examiner to ask questions regarding prior evaluation, casting and/or bracing, surgery, number of missed practices or games, mechanism of injury, training schedule at the time of injury, and rehabilitation.[18,73,101] A history of injury puts the athlete at increased risk for reinjury especially if not adequately rehabilitated.[16,37,41] Any joint previously injured requires a more detailed joint-specific examination. Unresolved symptoms or concerning findings on examination require further evaluation and possible referral.

TABLE 6.2
General Musculoskeletal Screening Examination

Instruction	Observation
Stand facing the examiner.	Trunk symmetry, general habitus
Look at the ceiling, floor, and over the shoulders, and touch the ear to the shoulder.	Cervical spine range of motion
Shrug shoulders (against resistance).	Trapezius strength
Abduct shoulders to 90° (resistance at 90°).	Deltoid strength
Do full internal and external rotation of the arms.	Shoulder range of motion, glenohumeral joint
Flex and extend the elbows.	Elbow range of motion
Put the arms at the sides, elbows at 90° flexed; pronate and supinate the wrists.	Elbow and wrist range of motion
Spread fingers; make a fist.	Hand and finger range of motion and strength
Tighten (contract) quadriceps; relax quadriceps.	Alignment, symmetry, knee and/or ankle effusions
"Duck walk" away and toward examiner (4 steps).	Hip, knee, and ankle range of motion, strength, balance
Stand facing away from the examiner.	Trunk symmetry, scoliosis
Keep knees straight, and touch toes.	Scoliosis, range of motion, hamstring flexibility
Raise upon toes and then heels.	Calf symmetry, strength, balance

Sources: Adapted from and a combination of Conley, K.M. et al., *J. Athl. Train.*, 49(1), 102, 2014; Bernhardt, D.T. et al., *PPE Preparticipation Physical Evaluation*, 4th edn., American Academy of Family Physicians, American Academy of Pediatrics, American College of Sports Medicine, American Medical Society for Sports Medicine, American Orthopaedic Society for Sports Medicine, and American Osteopathic Academy of Sports Medicine, 2010.

Clinical Pearl

Musculoskeletal findings during the PPE are the most common cause of delayed clearance and/or restriction of activity in athletes. Any concerning finding (i.e., instability, impaired function) requires further evaluation and rehabilitation.

Another variation of the musculoskeletal exam is to do a sports-specific examination. Sports-specific examinations focus on joints under continuous repetitive stress and therefore at higher risk of injury.[10] For example, an examiner may spend more time on the shoulder exam of baseball players and swimmers in order to maximize strength and conditioning programs. Joint-specific and sports-specific exams are more time-consuming than the general screening exam. The sports-specific examination is usually done by sports medicine physicians, as it requires more in-depth knowledge of individual sports.[21,25,40,57,63,85,89,90]

In general, clearance is denied to an athlete with a musculoskeletal injury who has persistent effusion or edema, ligament instability, loss of functional ability, strength that is less than 85%–90% of the unaffected side, and significantly decreased range of motion. Any of the aforementioned findings requires further treatment and rehabilitation. The athlete may be able to participate if the activity does not directly affect the area of injury or if the use of protective padding and/or bracing allows the athlete to compete safely without the risk of worsening the injury.[6,18,89] Referral to a specialist is warranted when the examining PCP is unsure of the clearance guidelines for particular musculoskeletal disorders.

Included in the PPE history and physical examination forms are screening questions and findings that may suggest Marfan's syndrome. Any history of a family member diagnosed with Marfan's syndrome along with musculoskeletal examination findings such as pectus carinatum or excavatum, arm span-to-height ratio >1.05, pes planus, scoliosis, and reduced elbow extension requires further evaluation before clearance can be granted.[6]

6.10 DERMATOLOGIC

The dermatologic examination is essential for athletes who participate in sports that involve mats and/or close skin-to-skin contact such as wrestling and rugby since active infection prohibits participation.[73,101] The PCP should inquire about the history and current presence of certain skin infections, such as tinea, herpes simplex, impetigo, boils, scabies, and molluscum contagiosum. When an athlete is contagious, participation in sports that involve mats as well as contact/collision sports or limited-contact sports should not be allowed.[40,57,59,63,85,89] Return to play should not be granted until the athlete has been adequately treated and is no longer contagious in order to minimize the risk of transmission. Herpes gladiatorum is epidemic in wrestlers; therefore, some athletes and teams have incorporated the use of prophylactic antiviral medication (i.e., acyclovir) to prevent recurrence and outbreaks.[2,73] Community-acquired methicillin-resistant *Staphylococcus* is a growing problem within the athletic population and should be suspected in any skin infection not responding to standard antibiotics and all abscesses. The athlete should be advised to avoid sharing personal items such as towels, razors, and helmets. Open wounds should be cleaned and covered for practice and play with a nonpermeable occlusive dressing as per standard precautions recommended by the CDC. Any open wound or skin infection that cannot be protected warrants exclusion from participation (see Chapter 55, Dermatology, for further discussion).[6,73]

6.11 GENITOURINARY

The genitourinary exam is typically performed with the male athlete standing. In male athletes, the contents of the scrotum should be palpated to determine the presence of two descended testicles, their size (a smaller size may be a sign of steroid use), and shape (contour irregularities are suspicious of cancer).[6,73,106] A single testicle is not a contraindication to athletic participation, but a protective cup should be worn. The athlete and parents must be informed of the risks of injury or loss to the remaining testicle.[40,57,62,85,89] An undescended or irregular testicle requires referral to a urologist for further evaluation.

A history of a solitary or horseshoe kidney does not automatically disqualify an athlete from participation. Again, referral to a urologist or nephrologist is recommended and eligibility determined on an individual basis. A discussion about the risk (albeit low) of loss of the remaining kidney, including the need for transplantation and/dialysis, should be included in the decision process for return to play. The use of a "flak" or shock-absorbing jacket may be recommended for moderate-contact sports;[58,89] however, its use has not been proven to reduce the risk of injury.[6,73,82]

Evaluation for a hernia should be performed in the athlete who complains of groin pain. Asymptomatic athletes do not need to be screened; however, any incidental finding on physical exam should be documented. The presence of a hernia does not prohibit participation from play. The athlete should be educated about signs and symptoms of strangulation such as increased pain, unresolved swelling, nausea, and/or vomiting.[15,82]

Clinical Pearl

Although not a contraindication for participation, due to the serious consequences of injury to the athlete with a single testicle (infertility) or kidney (dialysis), a thorough discussion of these risks should be undertaken between the physician, the athlete, and their parent/guardian if the athlete chooses to participate in sports.

The female genitourinary examination is not a standard part of the PPE.

6.12 ENDOCRINE

Athletes with a history of type 1 or type 2 DM should be routinely screened for signs and symptoms of complications including cardiovascular disease (hypertension), peripheral vascular disease, retinopathy, nephropathy, neuropathy (autonomic and peripheral), foot conditions (sensation and ankle reflexes), and gastrointestinal problems (gastroparesis). In athletes with retinopathy, strenuous activity can cause retinal detachment or vitreous hemorrhage. Therefore, the American Diabetes Association recommends against participation in activities that cause a significant rise in blood pressure such as weight lifting or high-impact sports such as jogging. Autonomic disturbances may increase the risk of postural hypotension and impair thermoregulation predisposing the athlete to heat injury. Gastroparesis can lead to electrolyte disturbances and hinder attempts at appropriate rehydration. Referral may be warranted so that the athlete in conjunction with a certified endocrinologist may create an individualized diabetes management plan including appropriate dietary and blood glucose monitoring regimens to ensure safe participation.[10,34]

6.13 MENTAL HEALTH

For many adolescent athletes, the PPE is their only interaction with a clinician.[6,18,73,106] Therefore, time should be taken to ask questions and screen for sensitive topics such as signs or symptoms of anxiety, depression, distortions in body image, disordered eating, and high-risk behaviors. The new PPE forms have removed these screening questions from the history portion and have instead placed "PCP reminders" at the top of the physical examination form (Appendix A). Depending on the severity of the condition, the presence of depression, anxiety, substance abuse, and/or disordered eating does not warrant disqualification. The athlete should be encouraged to seek help and utilize mental health services within the community. The possibility of improved sports performance as symptoms become better controlled should be emphasized.[73,106]

6.14 HEAT ILLNESS

A prior episode of heat-related illness increases the athlete's risk for future recurrence. Other risk factors include sickle-cell trait, obesity, and poor prior conditioning.[38] The PCP should also inquire about medications such as diuretics, antihistamines, amphetamines, selective serotonin reuptake inhibitors, and ergogenic aids such as ephedra and creatine that may predispose to dehydration and disrupt thermoregulation. Younger athletes are at an even greater risk for heat illness due to decreased ability to produce sweat, longer time needed to acclimate, delayed thirst response, and increased body-surface-area-to-mass ratio leading to increased heat gain from the environment.[1,22,101] Coaches, trainers, and athletes at risk need to be educated about the signs and symptoms of heat illness and prevention strategies such as ensuring proper acclimatization and allowing adequate time for rehydration. Assessments for clearance need to be done on an individual basis if there is a history of heat illness. A restriction to cooler environments might be warranted in certain cases.[11,85,89]

6.15 SPECIAL CONSIDERATIONS FOR THE FEMALE ATHLETE

The female athlete population is a special one that requires additional screening. Female athletes are at increased risk for noncontact anterior cruciate ligament injuries, recurrent dislocation of the patella, patellofemoral pain syndrome, and adolescent idiopathic scoliosis.[45] The female athlete is also at risk of exhibiting a pattern of low energy availability, menstrual dysfunction, and altered bone mineral density referred to as the "female athlete triad." The definition has been broadened over the years to encourage earlier detection before serious clinical manifestations such as amenorrhea and/or osteoporosis occur.[69] Many female athletes are positive for 1 or 2 of the triad's components making screening during the PPE important to allow early intervention if needed. It is a common problem encountered among women athletes and seen in higher frequency in sports where appearance is important or thinness is an advantage such as gymnastics and distance running. Female college athletes in aesthetic sports versus endurance and team sports experience more muscle and bone injuries.[5] Therefore, any complaints of unresolved musculoskeletal pain require further evaluation to exclude an occult fracture and/or tendinopathy. The examiner should inquire about age at menarche, frequency of menstrual periods, history of stress fractures, and eating patterns. If index of suspicion for an eating disorder is high, questions about laxative use, diuretic use, and complaints of a chronic sore throat (from purging) may provide additional information. Athletes with amenorrhea or oligomenorrhea require further evaluation for other etiologies before attributing the cause to the female athlete triad. For athletes who screen positive for the triad, the International Olympic Committee has guidelines for further evaluation.[74] The benefit of hormonal therapy for amenorrheic athletes has been unconvincing. The use of oral contraceptives has not been shown to reverse low bone mineral density, and evidence in reduction of fractures has been inconclusive.[43,104] Low energy bioavailability is the main contributing factor to the female athlete triad; therefore, athletes should be educated on proper nutrition and adequate caloric intake.[72] Current recommended daily intake for calcium in adolescents and young adults is 1300 mg/day. For vitamin D, 400 IU for children and adolescents and 1000–2000 IU for young adults are advised.[35] Athletes with hypermenorrhea are at increased risk of iron-deficiency anemia and should be screened for signs and symptoms due to the potential adverse effect on athletic performance. Iron supplementation may be warranted; however, it may take 2–3 months until the anemia is corrected.[6]

Clinical Pearl

The *female athlete triad* is a pattern of low energy availability, menstrual dysfunction, and altered bone mineral density seen more commonly in sports where appearance and thinness are considered advantageous. Screening all athletes during the PPE allows for early intervention and education.

On physical exam, the clinician may look for parotid gland enlargement, erosion of dental enamel, yellow skin discoloration, dry mucous membranes, lanugo, and Russell's sign. However, in most female athletes who are suffering from an eating disorder, the physical examination is completely normal. While the presence of eating disorders is rarely cause for disqualification (unless there is evidence of impaired health status and/or athletic performance), recognizing them can aid in getting the athlete the appropriate counseling. Left untreated, eating disorders can lead to osteoporosis, poor cold tolerance, bradycardia, electrolyte abnormalities, gastrointestinal problems, acid–base disorders, cardiac abnormalities, infertility, organ failure, and even death.[6,35,58,79,85,89]

It is important to note that although the triad has been classically described in females, it can occur in male athletes who also participate in sports that focus on leanness or achieving a particular weight class.[72]

6.16 ROUTINE SCREENING TESTS

Present consensus recommends against the use of routine laboratory or other screening tests in determining clearance in the asymptomatic athlete.[6] If, however, the history or physical examination raises concerns, then further tests should be ordered. For example, a female with a history of heavy menstrual flow, poor eating habits, and fatigue should have her hematocrit checked and perhaps iron studies evaluated. A person with a family history of sickle-cell disease or personal history of sickle-cell trait should also have a complete blood count with peripheral smear or confirmatory testing performed if no records are on file.[18] Sickle-cell trait was earlier believed to be a benign condition. There have been recent case reports, however, of sudden death in athletes performing prolonged strenuous activity within a hot, humid, and/or high altitude environment, leading to dehydration, sickling of cells, and vasoocclusion.[39,76,82] Athletes positive for sickle-cell trait should be advised to maintain adequate hydration at all times, abstain from diuretics, and avoid overexertion in hot, humid weather.[39] Urinalysis should be performed if the athlete provides a history of hematuria, dysuria, or kidney disease. The debate on obtaining routine screening EKGs and/or echocardiograms in order to prevent SCD is controversial and ongoing. A fasting lipid profile should be performed on those with a family history of premature coronary artery disease to evaluate for familial types of hyperlipidemia.[6,90]

Although the use of routine screening tests is not supported, the athlete and PCP may be subject to requirements of their respective sports governing body. For example, in 2010, the NCAA mandated testing for sickle-cell trait in all division I and II athletes regardless of personal and/or family history unless a waiver of exemption is signed. Certain boxing organizations require screening for human immunodeficiency virus (HIV) even though routine screening for HIV and hepatitis is not currently recommended due to the low risk of transmission during sports.[6]

6.17 CLEARANCE

Determining clearance for an athlete is a difficult task for PCPs. The purpose of the PPE is not to restrict play but to ensure safe participation of the athlete. The decision for clearance is multifactorial, taking into account the desires of the athlete, the desires of the parent or guardian, the specific sport, availability of protective equipment, and the risk of injury or death to the athlete, teammates, and other competitors.[18,73] Clearance falls into four categories: (1) clearance without restriction; (2) clearance with recommendations for further evaluation and treatment; (3) not cleared, restricted until completion of further testing/consultations; and (4) complete restriction from certain or all sports.[6] Determining clearance is not always a straightforward decision for evaluating PCP. Judgment should take into account the amount of contact/risk of collision (see Table 6.3) and the level of intensity (see Table 6.4) of the sport the athlete wishes to participate.

Current guidelines for the clearance of cardiac abnormalities as described in the 36th Bethesda Conference guidelines and general clearance guidelines endorsed by multiple medical societies are two excellent resources.[6,48] Clearance is typically determined on an individual basis and for very difficult cases may require a coordinated consensus among multiple medical specialists before a final decision is made.

TABLE 6.3
Classification of Sports by Contact

Contact/Collision	Limited Contact	Noncontact
Basketball	Baseball	Archery
Boxing[a]	Bicycling	Badminton
Diving	Cheerleading	Body building
Field hockey	Canoeing/kayaking (white water)	Canoeing/kayaking (flat water)
Football	Fencing	Crew/rowing
Flag	Field (high jump, pole vault)	Curling
Tackle	Floor hockey	Dancing
Ice hockey	Gymnastics	Field (discus, javelin, shot put)
Lacrosse	Handball	Golf
Martial arts	Horseback riding	Orienteering
Rodeo	Racquetball	Power lifting
Rugby	Skating (ice, inline, roller)	Race walking
Ski jumping	Skiing (cross-country, downhill, water)	Riflery
Soccer	Softball	Rope jumping
Team handball	Squash	Running
Water polo	Ultimate Frisbee	Sailing
Wrestling	Volleyball	Scuba diving
	Windsurfing/surfing	Strength training
		Swimming
		Table tennis
		Tennis
		Track
		Weight lifting

Source: From American Academy of Pediatrics Committee on Sports Medicine and Fitness, *Pediatrics*, 94(5), 757, 1994. With permission.

[a] Participation not recommended by the American Academy of Pediatrics; the American Academy of Family Physicians, American Medical Society for Sports Medicine, American Orthopaedic Society for Sports Medicine, and American Osteopathic Academy of Sports Medicine have no stand against boxing.

TABLE 6.4
Classification of Sports by Strenuousness

High-to-Moderate Intensity			Low Intensity
High-to-Moderate Dynamic and Static Demands	**High-to-Moderate Dynamic and Low Static Demands**	**High-to-Moderate Static and Low Dynamic Demands**	**Low Dynamic and Low Static Demands**
Boxing[a]	Badminton	Archery	Bowling
Crew rowing	Baseball	Auto racing	Cricket
Cross-country skiing	Basketball	Diving	Curling
Cycling	Field hockey	Equestrian	Golf
Downhill skiing	Lacrosse	Field events (jumping)	Riflery
Fencing	Orienteering	Field events (throwing)	
Football	Ping pong	Gymnastics	
Ice hockey	Race walking	Karate or judo	
Rugby	Racquetball	Motorcycling	
Running (sprint)	Soccer	Rodeoing	
Speed skating	Squash	Sailing	
Water polo	Swimming	Ski jumping	
Wrestling	Tennis	Water skiing	
	Volleyball	Weight lifting	

Source: From American Academy of Pediatrics Committee on Sports Medicine and Fitness, *Pediatrics*, 94(5), 757, 1994. With permission.

[a] Participation not recommended by the American Academy of Pediatrics; the American Academy of Family Physicians, American Medical Society for Sports Medicine, American Orthopaedic Society for Sports Medicine, and American Osteopathic Academy of Sports Medicine have no stand against boxing.

Occasionally, an athlete or an athlete's parents will disagree with the PCP's recommendation to deny clearance. Under the Rehabilitation Act of 1973 and the Americans with Disabilities Act of 1990, the athlete may have the right to participate against medical advice. If the athlete does decide to participate, an exculpatory waiver should be signed by the athlete and/or parent(s)/guardian(s) that indicates awareness of the risks of participation and prohibits bringing suit against the PCP in the event of injury. Unfortunately, the validity of this type of waiver varies from state to state, so it may not completely protect the PCP from legal action. An alternative to the exculpatory waiver, suggested by some legal experts, is to have the parent or guardian and athlete write, in their own words and in their own handwriting, a signed letter indicating their understanding of the risks of continued participation and that they understand the risks they are taking. Having such a letter would make it difficult to convince a jury that the parents or guardian and athlete did not understand the risks involved in comparison with understanding the written material on a standard waiver form.[6,36,61]

TABLE 6.5
SORT: Key Recommendations for Practice

Clinical Recommendation	Evidence Rating	References
The PPE should be completed approximately 5–6 weeks prior to the beginning of the sports season to allow adequate time for rehabilitation and order further diagnostic tests if necessary before final decisions for clearance can be made.	C	[12,40,57,58,85,90]
Ideally, a comprehensive PPE should be performed every 2 years in younger athletes and every 2–3 years in older athletes with annual interim updates focusing on any new injuries and/or medical problems.	C	[6,64,105]
A focused personal and familial cardiac history and physical examination should be included in every PPE with positive findings guiding the need for further evaluation. If any cardiac abnormalities are identified, recommendations for participation for participation can be found in the 36th Bethesda Conference report guidelines.	C	[48]
Any athlete diagnosed with a concussion should not be allowed to return to play until all symptoms of a concussion have cleared. Further consensus guidelines for treatment and clearance of the athlete who has suffered multiple concussions and/or has prolonged complicated symptoms are per the 4th International Conference on Concussion in Sport, held in Zurich in 2013, and/or the AMSSM position statements.	C	[3, 54–56]
Routine laboratory or other screening tests are not recommended in determining the clearance of the asymptomatic athlete. Further testing should only be guided by the athlete's history or any abnormal physical findings.	C	[6]

6.18 CONCLUSION

The PPE is important to help ensure safety in athletic participation. It is not intended to and rarely does it result in disqualification of athletes from competition. The exam should be scheduled at least 5–6 weeks prior to the beginning of the sports season, allowing adequate time for further evaluation of identified abnormalities. The authors favor individual exams by qualified primary care or sports medicine physicians. Whenever doubt arises as to whether an athlete should be allowed to compete in a particular sport, it is recommended to refer to appropriate resources/specialists to aid in the decision process. Because many athletes use this exam as their only interaction with health-care professionals, it should be used as an opportunity to establish trust and foster a PCP–patient relationship (Table 6.5).

REFERENCES

1. American Academy of Pediatrics Committee on Sports Medicine and Fitness. Climatic heat stress and the exercising child and adolescent. *Pediatrics.* 2000;106(1 Pt 1):158–159.
2. Anderson BJ. The effectiveness of valacyclovir in preventing reactivation of herpes gladiatorum in wrestlers. *Clinical Journal of Sports Medicine.* 1999;9(2):86–90.
3. Aubry M, Cantu R, Dvorak J et al. Summary and agreement statement of the first International Conference on Concussion in Sport, Vienna 2001. *British Journal of Sports Medicine.* 2002;32:6–7.
4. Basilico FC. Cardiovascular disease in athletes. *American Journal of Sports Medicine.* 1999;27(1):108–121.
5. Beals KA, Manore, MM. Disorders of the female *athlete triad* among collegiate athletes. *International Journal of Sport Nutrition and Exercise Metabolism.* 2002;12(3):281–293.
6. Bernhardt DT, Roberts WO (eds.). *PPE Preparticipation Physical Evaluation*, 4th edn., American Academy of Family Physicians, American Academy of Pediatrics, American College of Sports Medicine, American Medical Society for Sports Medicine, American Orthopaedic Society for Sports Medicine, and American Osteopathic Academy of Sports Medicine, 2010.
7. Best TM. The preparticipation evaluation: An opportunity for change and consensus. *Clinical Journal of Sports Medicine.* 2004;14:107–108.
8. Bey T, Ostick B. Second impact syndrome. *The Western Journal of Emergency Medicine.* 2009;10(1):6–10.
9. Bickley LS, Szilagyi PG. *Bates' Guide to Physical Examination and History Taking*, 8th edn. Philadelphia, PA: Lippincott Williams & Wilkins; 2003.
10. Birrer RB, Sedaghat VD. Exercise and diabetes: Optimizing performance in patients who have type 1 diabetes. *Physician and Sportsmedicine.* 2003;31(5):29–41.
11. Borjesson M, Dellborg M. Is there evidence for mandating electrocardiogram as part of the pre-participation examination? *Physician and Sportsmedicine.* 2011;21:13–17.
12. Bratton RL, Agerter DC. Preparticipation sports examinations: Efficient risk assessment in children and adolescents. *Postgraduate Medicine.* 1995;98(2):123–126, 129–132.
13. Cantu RC. Posttraumatic retrograde and anterograde amnesia: Pathophysiology and implications in grading and safe return to play. *Journal of Athletic Training.* 2001;36(3):244–248.
14. Cantu RC. Second-impact syndrome. *Clinical Sports Medicine.* 1998;17(1):37–44.
15. Carek PJ, Mainous A. III. The preparticipation physical examination in athletics: A systematic review of current recommendations. *BMJ: British Medical Journal.* 2003;1327: E170–E173.
16. Carek PJ, Futrell M, Hueston WJ. The preparticipation physical examination history: Who has the correct answers? *Clinical Journal of Sports Medicine.* 1999;9(3):124–128.

17. Chun J, Haney S, DiFiori J. The relative contributions of the history and physical examination in the preparticipation evaluation of collegiate student-athletes. *Clinical Journal of Sports Medicine.* 2006;16(5):437–438.
18. Conley KM, Bolin DJ, Carek PJ et al. National Athletic Trainers' Association Position Statement: Preparticipation physical examinations and disqualifying conditions. *Journal of Athletic Training.* 2014;49(1):102–120.
19. De Paepe A, Devereux RB, Dietz HC et al. Revised diagnostic criteria for the Marfan Syndrome. *American Journal of Medical Genetics.* 1996;62:417–426.
20. Drezner JA, Ackerman MJ, Anderson J et al. Electrocardiographic interpretation in athletes: The "Seattle criteria. *British Journal of Sports Medicine.* 2013;47:122–124.
21. Dyment PG. The sports physical. *Adolescent Medicine.* 1991;2(1):1–12.
22. Eberman LE, Cleary CM. Preparticipation physical exam to identify at-risk athletes for exertional heat illness. *Athletic Therapy Today.* 2009;14(4):4–7.
23. ESPN The Magazine December 12, 2013. Leonard Marshall leads concussion charge against NFL.
24. Expert Panel on Detection, Evaluation, and Treatment of High Blood Cholesterol in Adults, Summary of the second report of the National Cholesterol Education Program (NCEP) expert panel on detection, evaluation, and treatment of high blood cholesterol in adults (Adult Treatment Panel II). *Journal of the American Medical Association.* 1993;269:3015–3023.
25. Feinstein RA. Preparticipation physical examinations: Critical controversies. *Adolescent Medicine.* 1997;8(1):149–158.
26. Fountain N, May A. Epilepsy in athletes. *Clinical Sports Medicine.* July 2003;22(3):605–616,x-x1.
27. Fuller CM, McNulty CM, Spring DA et al. Prospective screening of 5,615 high school athletes for risk of sudden cardiac death. *Medicine and Science Sports and Exercise.* 1997;29(9):1131–1138.
28. Gibbons RJ, Balady GJ, Bricker JT et al. ACC/AHA 2002 guideline update for exercise testings: Summary article. A report of the American College of Cardiology/American Heart Association Task Force on Practice Guidelines (Committee to Update the 1997 Exercise Testing Guidelines). *Journal of the American College of Cardiology.* 2002;40(8):1531.
29. Gilchrist J, Thomas KE, Xu L et al. Nonfatal sports and recreation related traumatic brain injuries among children and adolescents treated in emergency departments in the United States 2001–2009. *MMWR.* 2011;60(39):1337–1342.
30. Glover DW, Maron BJ. Profile of preparticipation cardiovascular screening for high school athletes. *Journal of the American Medical Association.* 1998;279:1817–1819.
31. Goldberg, B., Saraniti, A. et al. Preparticipation sports assessment: An objective evaluation. *Pediatrics.* 1980;66(5):736–745.
32. Harmon K, Drezner JA, Gammons M et al. American Medical Society for Sports Medicine position statement: Concussion in sports. *British Journal of Sports Medicine.* 2013;47(1):15–26.
33. Howard G, Radloff M, Sevier T. Epilepsy and sports participation. *Clinical Sports Medicine Report.* February 2004;3(1):15–19.
34. Jimenez CC, Corcoran MH, Crawley JT et al. National Athletic Trainer's Association position statement: Management of the athlete with type I diabetes mellitus. *Journal of Athletic Training.* 2007;42(4):536–545.
35. Johnson MD. Tailoring the preparticipation exam to female athletes. *Physician and Sportsmedicine.* 1992;20:61–72.
36. Jones C. College athletes: Illness or injury and the decision to return to play. *Buffalo Law Review.* 1992;40:113–115.
37. Joy EA, Paisley TS, Price R et al. Optimizing the collegiate preparticipation physical evaluation. *Clinical Journal of Sports Medicine.* 2004;14(3):183–187.
38. Kark JA, Posey DM, Schumacher HR et al. Sickle cell trait as a risk factor for sudden death in physical training. *New England Journal of Medicine.* 1987;31(13):781–787.
39. Kerle KK, Nishimura KD. Exertional collapse and sudden death associated with sickle cell trait. *American Family Physician.* 1996;54(1):237–240.
40. Krowchuk DP. The preparticipation athletic examination: A closer look. *Pediatric Annals.* 1997;26(1):37–49.
41. Kurowski K, Chandra S. The preparticipation athletic evaluation. *American Family Physician.* 2000;61(9):2683–2690.
42. Lively MW. Preparticipation physical examinations: A collegiate experience. *Clinical Journal of Sports Medicine.* 1999;9(1):3–8.
43. Lopez LM, Grimes DA, Schulz KF et al. Steroidal contraceptives: Effect on bone fractures in women. *Cochrane Database System Review.* 2006;4:CD006033.
44. *Los Angeles Times*, February 17, 2014. Football helmets and concussion: A new study opens new questions.
45. Loud KJ, Micheli LJ. Common athletic injuries in adolescent girls. *Current Opinion in Pediatrics.* 2001;13(4):317–322.
46. Luckstead EF. Cardiovascular evaluation of the young athlete. *Adolescent Medicine.* 1998;9(3):441–455.
47. Lyznicki JM, Nielsen NH, Schneider JF. Cardiovascular screening of student athletes. *American Family Physician.* 2000;62(4):765–774.
48. Maron BJ, Zipes DP. Journal of the American College of Cardiology 36th Bethesda Conference Eligibility Recommendations for Competitive Athletes with Cardiovascular Abnormalities. *Journal of the American College of Cardiology.* 2005;45.
49. Maron BJ, Thompson PD, Puffer JC et al. Recommendations for preparticipation screening and the assessment of cardiovascular disease in masters athletes: An advisory for healthcare professionals from the working groups of the World Heart Federation, the International Federation of Sports Medicine, and the American Heart Association Committee on Exercise, Cardiac Rehabilitation, and Prevention. *Circulation.* 2001;103(2):327–334.
50. Maron BJ, Thompson PD, Puffer JC et al. Cardiovascular preparticipation screening of competitive athletes: A statement for health professionals from the Sudden Death Committee (Clinical Cardiology) and Congenital Cardiac Defects Committee (Cardiovascular Disease in the Young), American Heart Association. *Circulation.* 1996;94850–94856.
51. Maron BJ. Risk profiles and cardiovascular preparticipation screening of competitive athletes. *Cardiology Clinic.* 1997;15:473–483.
52. Maron BJ, Thompson PD, Ackerman MJ et al. Recommendations and considerations related to preparticipation screening for cardiovascular abnormalities in competitive athletes; 2007 update: A Scientific Statement from the American Heart Association Council on Nutrition, Physical Activity, and Metabolism: Endorsed by the American College of Cardiology Foundation. *Circulation.* 2007;115:1643–1655.
53. McCrory P. Does second impact syndrome exist? *Clinical Journal of Sports Medicine.* 2001;11(3):144–149.
54. McCrory P, Johnston K, Meeuwisse W et al. Summary and agreement statement of the 2nd International Conference on Concussion in Sport, Prague 2004. *British Journal of Sports Medicine.* 2005;39:196–204.

55. McCrory P, Meeuwisse W, Aubry M et al. The 4th International Conference on Concussion in Sport held in Zurich, November 2012. *British Journal of Sports Medicine.* 2013;47:250–258.
56. McCrory P, Meeuwisse W, Johnston K et al. Consensus Statement on Concussion in Sport: The 3rd International Conference on Concussion in Sport held in Zurich, November 2008. *British Journal of Sports Medicine.* 2009;43:i76–i84.
57. Metzl JD. Pediatric and adolescent sports injuries: The adolescent preparticipation physical examination: Is it helpful? *Clinical Sports Medicine.* 2000;19:577–592.
58. Metzl JD. Preparticipation examination of the adolescent athlete, part 1. *Pediatric Review.* 2001;22(6):199–204.
59. Metzl JD. Preparticipation examination of the adolescent athlete, part 2. *Pediatric Review.* 2001;22(7):227–239.
60. Miller MG, Weiler JM, Baker R et al. National Athletic Trainers' Association position statement: Management of asthma in athletes. *Journal of Athletic and Training.* 2005; 40(3):224–245.
61. Mitten MJ. Team physicians and competitive athletes: Allocating legal responsibility for athletic injuries. *University of Pittsburg Law Review.* 1993;55(1):129–169.
62. Moeller JL. Contraindications to athletic participation: Cardiac, respiratory, and central nervous system conditions. *Physician and Sportsmedicine.* 1996;24:47–58.
63. Moeller JL. Contraindications to athletic participation: Spinal, systemic dermatologic, paired-organ, and other issues. *Physician and Sportsmedicine.* 1996;24:59–75.
64. Montalto NJ. Implementing the guidelines for adolescent preventive services. *American Family Physician.* 1998; 57(9):2181–2190.
65. Myers A, Sickles T. Preparticipation sports examination. *Primary Care.* 1998;25(1):225–236.
66. National Asthma Education and Prevention Program. Expert panel report 3 (EPR 3): Guidelines for the diagnosis and management of asthma-summary report 2007. *Journal of Allergy and Clinical Immunology.* 2007;120(5 suppl):S94–S138.
67. National Geographic, February 2011. *The Big Idea: Brain Trauma.*
68. National High Blood Pressure Education Program Working Group on High Blood Pressure in Children and Adolescents. The fourth report of the diagnosis, evaluation, and treatment of high blood pressure in children and adolescents. *Pediatrics.* 2004;114(2 suppl 4th report):555–576.
69. Nattiv A, Agostini R, Drinkwater B et al. The female athlete triad. The inter-relatedness of disordered eating, amenorrhea, and osteoporosis. *Clinical Sports Medicine.* 1994; 13:405–418.
70. O'Connor FG, Oriscello RG, Levine BD. Exercise-related syncope in the young athlete: Reassurance, restriction or referral. *American Family Physician.* 1999;60:2001–2008.
71. Patel A, Lantos JD. Can we prevent sudden cardiac death in young athletes: The debate about preparticipation sports screening. *Acta Paediatrica.* 2011;100:1297–1301.
72. Payne JM, Kirchner JT. Should you suspect the female athlete triad? *Journal of Family Practice.* 2014;63(3):187–192.
73. Peterson AR, Bernhardt DT. The preparticipation sports evaluation. *Pediatric Review.* 2011;32(5):e53–e65.
74. Position stand on the female athlete triad. The International Olympic Committee Web site. Available at: http://www.olympic.org/Documents/Reports/EN/en_report_917.pdf.
75. Practice parameter—The management of concussion in sports (summary statement): report of the Quality Standards Subcommittee. *Neurology.* 1997;48:581–585.
76. Pretzlaff RK. Death of an adolescent athlete with sickle cell trait caused by exertional heat stroke. *Pediatric Critical Care Medicine.* 2002;3(3):308–310.
77. Protective eyewear for young athletes. *Pediatrics.* 2004; 113:619–622.
78. Psooy K. Sports and the solitary kidney: How to counsel parents. *Canadian Journal of Urology.* 2006;13(3):3120–3126.
79. Putukian M. The female athlete triad. *Current Opinion in Orthopaedics.* 2001;12:132–141.
80. Putukian M., O'Connor FG, Stricker P. Mononucleosis and athletic participation: An evidence-based subject review. *Clinical Journal of Sports Medicine.* 2008;18(4):309–315.
81. Report of the Sports Medicine Committee: Guidelines for the Management of Concussion in Sport. Colorado Medical Society 1990 (revised May 1991).
82. Rice SG, the American Academy of Pediatrics Council on Sports Medicine and Fitness. Medical conditions affecting sports participation. *Pediatrics.* 2008;121:841–848.
83. Risser WL, Hoffman HM, Bellah GG. Frequency of preparticipation sports examinations in secondary school athletes: Are the University Interscholastic League guidelines appropriate? *Textile Medicine.* 1985;81(7):35–39.
84. Risser WL, Hoffman HM, Bellah GG et al. A cost-benefit analysis of preparticipation sports examinations of adolescent athletes. *Journal of School Health.* 1985;55(7):270–273.
85. Sahoo S, Fountain N. Epilepsy in football players and other land-based contact or collision sport athletes: When can they participate and is there an increased risk? *Current Sports Medicine Reports.* October 2004;3(5):284–288.
86. Schmeid C, Borjesson M. Sudden cardiac death in athletes. *Journal of Internal Medicine.* 2014;275:93–103.
87. *Scientific American*, September 2, 2008. Concussions exact toll on football players long after they retire.
88. Sideline preparedness for the team physician: A consensus statement. *Medicine and Science Sports and Exercise.* 2001;33(5):846–849.
89. Smith DM. Preparticipation physical examinations. *Sports Medicine and Arthroscopy Review.* 1995;3:84–94.
90. Smith DM, Kovan JR, Rich BS, Tanner SM. *Preparticipation Physical Examination*, 2nd edn. Minneapolis, MN: American Academy of Family Physicians, American Academy of Pediatrics, American Medical Society for Sports Medicine, American Orthopaedic Society for Sports Medicine, and American Osteopathic Academy of Sports Medicine; 1997.
91. Smith J, Laskowski ER. The preparticipation physical examination: Mayo Clinic experience with 2739 examinations. *Mayo Clinic Proceedings.* 1998;73(5):419–429.
92. *Sports Illustrated*, November 1, 2011. Concussions.
93. *Sports Illustrated*, October 2, 2013. Adapted from the League of Denial: The NFL, Concussions, and the battle for Truth.
94. Standing Committee on the Scientific Evaluation of Dietary References Intakes, Food and Nutrition Board, Institute of Medicine. *Dietary Reference Intakes for Calcium, Phosphorus, Magnesium, Vitamin D and Fluoride.* Washington, DC: The National Academies Press; 1997.
95. Storms WW. Review of exercise-induced asthma. *Medicine and Science Sports and Exercise.* 2003;35(9):1464–1470.
96. Team physician consensus statement. *American Journal of Sports Medicine.* 2000;28(3):440–441.
97. Team physician consensus statement. *Medicine and Science Sports and Exercise.* 2000;32(4):877–878.
98. *The New York Daily News*, January 19, 2014. President Obama says he wouldn't let his son play pro football.

99. *The New York Times*, May 21, 2014. Brain changes in college football players raise new concerns.
100. *The New Yorker*, January 31, 2011. Football and the Concussion Crisis.
101. Tucker A, Grady M. Role of the adolescent preparticipation physical examination. *Physical Medicine and Rehabilittion of Clinical North America*. 2008;19:217–234.
102. *USA Hockey Magazine*, January 2011. Time out for concussion.
103. Van Thuyne W, Van Eenoo P, Delbeke FT. Nutritional supplements: Prevalence of use and contamination with doping agents. *Nutrition Research Review*. 2006;19(1):147–158.
104. Warren MP, Brooks-Gunn J, Fox RP et al. Persistent osteopenia in ballet dancers with amenorrhea and delayed menarche despite hormone therapy: A longitudinal study. *Fertility and Sterility*. 2003;80(2):398–404.
105. Wingfield K, Matheson GO, Meeuwisse WH. Preparticipation evaluation: An evidence-based review. *Clinical Journal of Sports Medicine*. 2004;14(3):109–122.
106. Womack M.D. Give your sports physicals a performance boost. *Journal of Family Practice*. 2010;59(8):437–444.

7 Physical Activity Counseling and Exercise Prescription*

Mark B. Stephens

CONTENTS

TABLE 7.1
Key Clinical Considerations

1. Inadequate physical activity is one of the three leading actual causes of death in the United States.
2. There is insufficient evidence to recommend routine physical activity counseling in the office setting.
3. Low-risk patients do not need formal exercise testing before beginning a physical activity program.
4. Intermediate- to high-risk patients benefit from formal exercise testing and individualized exercise prescription as part of a comprehensive exercise program.
5. Exercise prescriptions are simple and cost-effective. They are based on the principles of frequency, intensity, type, and time.

7.1 INTRODUCTION

Physical inactivity is a leading contributor to overall mortality in the United States.[19] Fewer than half of all American adults meet recommended physical activity levels of 150 minutes of moderate-to-vigorous physical activity per week.[1,15] As a result of this pandemic of physical inactivity, nearly 70% of adult Americans are currently classified as being overweight or obese.[16] The role of physical inactivity in health and disease remains a major focus of *Healthy People 2020*,[17] an ongoing initiative designed to promote wellness and prevent disease in the general population (Table 7.1).

Clinical Pearl

Physical activity is the most cost-effective prescription available for a multitude of chronic diseases from heart disease to diabetes.

The disease burden associated with inadequate physical inactivity has been well documented. Diabetes,[2] coronary artery disease,[24] hyperlipidemia,[18] hypertension,[25] and certain cancers[9] have all been associated with physical inactivity. Age, social class, and previous experience also impact an individual's attitude, motivation, and response to physical activity.[6] These are important factors to consider when providing individual patients with advice about physical activity. A formal exercise prescription also considers other health behaviors such as tobacco use and dietary habits. Physical activity counseling can be brief and easily conducted in the

* The opinions contained herein are those of the authors. They are not official policy of the Uniformed Services University, the Department of the Navy, or the Department of Defense.

office setting. Behavioral counseling within primary care settings to promote physical activity has a small impact on health outcomes.[20] An exercise prescription, on the other hand, refers to a formal, written document based on history, physical examination, clinical exercise testing, and specific patient goals. The exercise prescription is designed to provide patients with specific information regarding the frequency, intensity, type, and duration of physical activity with specific objectives in mind.

7.2 HISTORY

A formal exercise prescription is based on three core elements. A thorough and accurate clinical history is first and foremost. In addition to inquiring about the patient's general medical history, primary care providers should also explore social, cultural, familial, environmental, and personal factors that impact an individual exercise prescription. For instance, it is normal for adults to become less active as they age. Many others "complain" that they are too busy to exercise (see Table 7.2).[13] Minority populations, individuals from low-income families, and adults with physical disabilities are less likely to engage in regular physical activity.[23]

Adults who spend significant amounts of time watching the television or using a computer are also less physically active and at increased risk for diabetes, heart disease, and all-cause mortality.[11] All of these factors contribute to the contextual framework upon which a holistic exercise prescription is based.

7.3 MEDICAL HISTORY

A thorough medical history is foundational for any exercise prescription. All medical diagnoses that might impact a patient's ability to exercise should be explored and appropriately documented. Specifically, any prior history of coronary artery disease, hypertension, diabetes, hyperlipidemia, peripheral vascular disease, asthma, chronic obstructive pulmonary disease, cancer, or musculoskeletal disease should be elicited and documented. The medical history forms the basis for determining if further evaluation is indicated prior to initiating a new physical activity program.[16]

7.4 ACTIVITY HISTORY

In addition to a general medical history, it is important to determine each patient's experiential base of exercise and physical activity. Patients should describe physical activity related to their lifestyle or occupation as well. It is also important to ask patients to describe current television, computer, and video viewing habits. Does the individual have experience with formal activity programs? Have they participated in sports or recreational activities? A prior history of musculoskeletal injury is the leading risk factor for subsequent injury. This information is helpful in targeting recommendations for injury prevention. Patients should describe their current pattern of exercise. Based on current guidelines, adults should obtain at least 150 minutes of moderate physical activity on a weekly basis.[3] Patients should be asked to explicitly define individual goals. Are they interested in losing weight, improving cardiovascular endurance, improving muscular strength, decreasing cardiovascular risk, or improving their overall health?

7.5 PHYSICAL EXAMINATION

The physical examination is the second cornerstone upon which formal exercise prescriptions are based. The physical examination should be conducted in a standard fashion.

TABLE 7.2
Overcoming Activity Barriers

Roadblock	Strategy for Overcoming Roadblock
I am usually too tired to exercise.	Regular activity actually improves your energy level.
The weather is too bad.	Many activities can be done in the comfort of your home, no matter what the weather.
I can't afford a health club.	You do not need a health club to be physically active; walk around the mall, use public facilities, and find others to join you in an activity group.
Exercise is boring.	Try listening to music or exercising with a friend or family member.
I get sore when I exercise.	Slight muscle soreness after physical activity is common when just starting out; limit this by starting slowly, building up gradually, and stretching before and after each activity.
I do not enjoy exercise.	Don't "exercise." Try becoming physically active through any hobby or enjoyable activity that gets you moving.
I'm afraid of getting hurt.	Make sure you wear proper clothing and footwear; do not exercise on uneven terrain or push yourself beyond your limits.
I'm not any good at exercise.	You do not have to be good at exercise to walk. Start low and go slow; as you develop confidence and establish a pattern of activity, try new things.
I do not have time.	Thirty minutes a day is equivalent to a half-hour television show; can you give up one show per day?

Source: Adapted from Patrick, K. et al., *Sportmedicine*, 22, 45, 1994.

Blood pressure, height, and weight should be recorded to calculate body mass index (BMI):

$$\text{BMI} = \text{Weight (kg)/height (m)}^2$$

For adults, a BMI of 20–24.9 is considered normal. An adult with a BMI between 25 and 29.9 is considered overweight. Individuals with a BMI of greater than 30 are considered to be obese. Particular attention should be directed to the cardiopulmonary, musculoskeletal, and neurological systems during the examination. The purpose of the physical exam is to screen for conditions that would merit further evaluation prior to beginning an exercise program.[3] The cardiopulmonary exam should include documentation of pulses (rate and rhythm); auscultation for murmurs, rubs, gallops, and clicks; auscultation of lung fields; and peripheral pulses. The musculoskeletal examination should focus on the range of motion of all major joints as well as the presence of pain and/or swelling. The abdominal examination should focus on the presence of organomegaly, tenderness, bruits, or masses. An extremity examination should be performed to rule out edema. If areas of concern are identified, further evaluation is appropriate prior to initiating a new exercise program.[3]

Clinical Pearl

Low-risk patients do not need a formal exercise test before beginning a program of regular activity.

Who needs clinical exercise testing prior to beginning a program of physical activity? Clinical exercise testing is the third cornerstone upon which formal exercise prescription is based. An accurate decision regarding the need for clinical exercise testing requires information from the history and physical examination. Several useful clinical tools are also available to assist clinicians when confronted with the question of who needs clinical exercise testing prior to beginning a program of regular physical activity.

One approach, endorsed by the American College of Sports Medicine, is based on the concept of clinical risk stratification.[3] Using information from the patients' past medical history and physical examination, individuals are categorized into three categories: low, moderate, and high risk (see Table 7.3).

Patients who are at low risk do not need a formal clinical exercise test before beginning a program of regular physical activity. For these patients, physical activity counseling is sufficient. Those who are an moderate risk require clinical exercise testing only if they plan to only engage in activities that are vigorous in intensity. All high-risk patients should have clinical exercise testing performed before beginning a program of regular exercise (see Table 7.4). The clinical exercise test provides important diagnostic and therapeutic information (e.g., maximum heart rate [MHR] and/or an estimation of maximal oxygen consumption) that can be used to tailor an individualized exercise prescription (see Chapter 22).

TABLE 7.3
Risk Stratification[a]

Risk Category	Description
Low risk	Men under the age of 45 and women under the age of 55 who are asymptomatic and have a maximum of one clinical risk factor
Moderate risk	Men over the age of 45 and women over the age of 55 or individuals who have two or more clinical risk factors
High risk	Individuals who are either symptomatic or who have known cardiopulmonary disease

Source: Adapted from American College of Sports Medicine, *ACSM's Guidelines for Exercise Testing and Prescription*, 9th edn., Lippincott Williams & Wilkins, Philadelphia, PA, 2013.

[a] Symptoms include exertional chest pain, exertional dyspnea, exertional syncope, palpitations, orthopnea, paroxysmal dyspnea, peripheral edema, palpitations, and claudication.

7.6 PHYSICAL ACTIVITY GUIDELINES: WHAT'S RECOMMENDED?

The health benefits of physical activity are well recognized. Physically active individuals have lower rates of all-cause mortality,[8] improved psychological well-being,[22] lower rates of cardiovascular morbidity,[24] and a reduced risk of developing diabetes,[2] hypertension,[25] and certain cancers.[9] Additionally, physical activity promotes bone, joint, and muscular health, enhances work performance capability, and is associated with improved self-esteem.

It is recommended for all Americans to accumulate 150 minutes of moderate-intensity physical activity on a weekly basis.[1] This guideline is important in that it suggests that the benefits of physical activity can be accumulated in relatively short bouts throughout the course of the day, as opposed to single daily "training" sessions. Multiple bouts of physical activity, as short as 8–10 minutes, can be accumulated throughout the day with "lifestyle activities" such as stair climbing, brisk walking, housework, and yard work. Short bouts of activity have a cumulative health benefit.[4] Recent data also indicate that standing at work or taking frequent walking breaks provides health benefit.[7]

Health-related gains can be realized with mild-to-moderate levels of activity, particularly in previously sedentary individuals. Moderate-to-vigorous levels of physical activity, however, are still recommended for individuals who wish to achieve higher levels of cardiovascular conditioning. In short, any level of physical activity is beneficial for health, but more does appear to be better. Current guidelines also recommend that activities promoting muscular strength and flexibility also be included to improve balance, strength, and coordination.[10,12]

Recognizing the importance of physical activity in combating chronic disease, the U.S. Department of Health and Human Services has made physical activity one of the leading health indicators by which the nation's health will be

TABLE 7.4
Clinical Exercise Testing

Indications for Exercise Testing	Contraindications to Exercise Testing
Evaluation of patients with suspected coronary artery disease	Absolute contraindications
Typical angina pectoris	Recent myocardial infarction
Atypical angina pectoris	Unstable angina
Evaluation of patients with known coronary artery disease	Acute myocarditis/pericarditis
Following myocardial infarction	Acute systemic infection
Following therapeutic intervention	Symptomatic heart failure
Screening of healthy, asymptomatic patients	Symptomatic aortic stenosis
Individuals in high-risk occupations (pilots, firefighters, law enforcement officers, mass transit operators, etc.)	Relative contraindications
Men over age 40 and women over age 50 who are sedentary and plan to start a vigorous exercise program	Severe hypertension (uncontrolled)
Individuals who are identified as being at risk based on multiple cardiac risk factors or concurrent chronic diseases	Persistent arrhythmias (poorly controlled)
Evaluation of exercise capacity in patients with valvular heart disease (excluding severe aortic stenosis)	Obstructive cardiomyopathy
Evaluation of patients with cardiac rhythm disorders	Uncontrolled diabetes or thyroid disease
Evaluation of exercise-induced arrhythmia and response to treatment	Systemic neuromuscular, musculoskeletal, or rheumatologic disease that limits the patient's ability to exercise
Evaluation of rate-adaptive pacemaker setting	Heart block (second- or third-degree atrioventricular block)
	Stenotic valvular heart disease
	Undifferentiated electrolyte abnormalities (hypokalemia, hypomagnesemia, etc.)

Sources: Adapted from American College of Sports Medicine, *ACSM's Guidelines for Exercise Testing and Prescription*, 9th edn., Lippincott Williams & Wilkins, Philadelphia, PA, 2013; Gibbons, R.J. et al., *Circulation*, 106(14), 1883, 2002.

measured over the next decade. The specific goals of *Healthy People 2020* are to reduce the burden of chronic disease and to improve health, fitness, and quality of life by increasing daily physical activity.[17] The following points can be summarized from current guidelines[1,8]:

- All individuals should engage in at least 30 minutes of physical activity of moderate intensity on 5 days each week.
- Additional health benefits can be achieved by increasing the time spent in moderate-intensity activity or by increasing the intensity of the activity.
- Activities that promote muscular strength (resistance training) should be performed at least twice a week.
- Previously inactive men over age 45, women over age 55, and people at high risk for coronary artery disease should consult a physician prior to beginning a new exercise program, especially if they plan to incorporate *vigorous* physical activity into their routine.

7.7 PUTTING THE GUIDELINES TO WORK: THE EXERCISE PRESCRIPTION

General physical activity guidelines provide a solid foundation for activity counseling and can be easily incorporated into a routine office visit. An exercise prescription is more involved and can be considered analogous to any other medical prescription.[4] It takes time to give patients clear instructions, about medication and about physical activity. Much like counseling patients about how to properly take medications, an exercise prescription should address the frequency, intensity, type, and time (duration) of exercise each patient is to perform. These components of the exercise prescription are easily remembered as the frequency, intensity, type, and time *(FITT) principle* for exercise prescription (see Table 7.5 and Figure 7.1).

TABLE 7.5
Components of an Exercise Prescription: The "Frequency, Intensity, Type, and Time" Principle

Frequency
Intensity
Type of activity
  Resistance training
  Cardiovascular training
    Flexibility
Time (duration of activity)

7.8 FREQUENCY

All patients should strive to be physically active every day. This is particularly true for patients who are most interested in improving their overall general health. Although improvements in cardiorespiratory conditioning are possible in previously sedentary individuals who exercise only once or twice a week, programs with such limited activity are ineffective at increasing endurance and cardiovascular conditioning and are often abandoned. Individuals interested in improving cardiovascular endurance should engage in physical activity five times per week.

Name: Date:

Age: Gender:

Medications:

Type of physical activity:

Frequency:

Duration:

Intensity: Training heart range:

Maximum heart rate:

Special instructions:

Precautions:

Risk factors to work on:

Reevaluation date:

(Doctor's signature)

(Patient's signature)

(Guardian's signature, if applicable)

FIGURE 7.1 Suggested exercise prescription form.

7.9 INTENSITY

Exercise intensity is the central component of the exercise prescription. Intensity represents the strength of the training stimulus. In general, the benefits of physical activity follow a typical dose–response curve. Previously sedentary patients and others who are interested in health-related physical fitness should always begin at low intensities, typically 40%–50% of their maximum aerobic capacity (VO_{2max}). Patients interested in improving cardiovascular endurance should exercise at between 50% and 85% of VO_{2max}. VO_{2max} represents the maximum amounts of oxygen that an individual can breathe in, transport to metabolically active tissues, and use for productive work during maximal exertion (see Chapter 27, Maximal Aerobic Capacity). VO_{2max} can be measured directly during clinical exercise testing or estimated using several simple tools such as target heart rates, ratings of perceived exertion (RPE), or the talk test (discussed in Section 7.13). The intensity of activity must also be specifically tailored to the patient's goals.

7.10 TARGET HEART RATE

At moderate levels of exercise, a linear relationship exists between heart rate and VO_{2max}. This facilitates the ability to provide simple exercise prescriptions based on an individual's resting heart rate (RHR). To do this, the patient must be comfortable taking his or her own pulse. If individuals have a difficult time finding their pulse, commercial heart rate monitors are also available. The most common areas for a pulse check during exercise are the distal radial artery and the carotid artery. Patients should be instructed to count the number of pulsations in 15 seconds and multiply this number by four to determine their heart rate in beats per minute (bpm). MHR can be either measured directly during clinical exercise testing or calculated based on the patients' age:

$$\text{MHR} = 220 - \text{Patient age}$$

For the exercise prescription, patients should be instructed to keep their heart rate within the target zone for the duration of their training session. The most common target heart rate range (THRR) is between 40% and 80% of maximal heart rate. Patients who are new to their exercise prescription should exercise toward the lower portion of the target zone. The target zone is an attractive clinical tool because it can be easily modified if patients are on cardioactive medications. The target zone can also be adjusted as patients become more conditioned with continued exercise.

7.11 HEART RATE RESERVE

A modification of the THRR is the heart rate reserve (HRR). This formula compensates for individual differences in RHR. The HRR is calculated by subtracting the patient's RHR from his or her age-predicted MHR (220 – age):

$$\text{HRR} = \text{MHR} - \text{RHR}$$

$$\text{HRR} = ([220 - \text{Age}] - \text{RHR})$$

The THRR is calculated by multiplying the desired training intensity (typically 40%–80%) by the HRR and then adding the RHR:

$$\text{THRR} = ([\text{MHR} - \text{RHR}] \times \%\ \text{Training heart rate}) + \text{RHR}$$

$$\text{THRR} = ([\text{HRR}] \times \text{Training intensity}) + \text{RHR}$$

For example, a 45-year-old male has an RHR of 85 bpm. His calculated maximal heart rate is 220 bpm – 45 bpm = 175 bpm. His HRR is 175 bpm – 85 bpm = 90 bpm. He plans exercise at 40%–60% of his maximal capacity. Using the HRR formula, his target heart rate range is 121–139 bpm. Note that this rate is slightly higher than if it were based on the age-predictable MHR. The target heart rate range is a useful concept that patients can use to monitor exercise intensity.

7.12 RATING OF PERCEIVED EXERTION

For patients who are not interested in using the target heart rate or are uncomfortable taking their pulse, self-RPE are another useful tool for prescribing activity intensity (see Table 7.6). Similar to the association between heart rate and VO_{2max}, scales of perceived exertion are also based upon a relatively linear association between heart rate and the level of perceived physical exertion.[5] Scales of perceived exertion are very useful for assessing exercise intensity, particularly for individuals on medications that slow the heart rate (e.g., beta blockers, certain calcium channel blockers) or patients with abnormal cardiac rhythms (e.g., atrial fibrillation, atrial flutter).

For example, using the original scale of 6–20, it is easy to teach patients the concepts of rest (scale = 6) and maximal exertion (scale = 20). Based upon these anchors, patients can grade their exercise intensity in a relatively linear fashion from light to moderate to difficult. The relative perception of intensity of each patient is a reproducible level that can be used reliably for exercise prescription. The concept of perceived exertion is easiest to reinforce during the clinical exercise test but can be taught to anyone. Extending the example for the 45-year-old male with an MHR of 175, his maximum level of exertion (HR = 175) would correspond to an RPE of 20. His target zone (40%–60% of maximal capacity—HR of 121–139 bpm) would correspond to an RPE of 10–14. Patients who prefer can use the modified Borg scale, which rates exertion on a scale from 0 (rest) to 10 (maximal exertion).[5]

TABLE 7.6
Borg Scale of Perceived Exertion

Traditional Borg RPE Scale		Modified Borg RPE Scale	
6		0	Nothing
7	Very, very light	0.5	Extremely weak
8		1	Very weak
9	Very light	2	Weak
10		3	Moderate
11	Fairly light	4	
12		5	Strong
13	Somewhat hard	6	
14		7	Very strong
15	Hard	8	
16		9	
17	Very hard	10	Very, very strong (maximal)
18		11	
19	Very, very hard	12	Absolute maximum

Source: Borg, G.A., *Borg's Perceived Exertion and Pain Scale*, Human Kinetics, Champaign, IL, 1998. With permission.

7.13 TALK TEST

The talk test allows patients to exercise to a level where they are comfortable carrying out a conversation without undue breathlessness. The talk test allows patients to stay below their ventilatory threshold (the intensity of exercise at which respiratory rate markedly increases to buffer lactic acid that accumulates within vigorously exercising muscle). For example, patients who are exercising at a moderate intensity should be able to engage in conversation with an exercise partner without stopping or slowing down to catch their breath. A useful variation of the talk test is the talk–sing test. Using this variant, patients are instructed to exercise at an intensity where they can comfortably talk but would be unable to sing. Here again, the principle is to ensure that patients exercise at an adequate intensity without exceeding the ventilatory threshold.

Clinical Pearl

The "talk test" is a simple way to monitor exercise intensity. Have patients exercise at a level where they are able to hold a conversation (but would be unable to sing).

7.14 TYPE (CHOICE OF ACTIVITY)

When writing an exercise prescription, the type of physical activity should be based on each individual's interests as well as his or her current level of fitness. It is important to recommend a variety of activities to maintain patient interest and discourage boredom. Activities should employ large-muscle groups that are used in continuous and rhythmic motion. By far, the most common physical activity is walking. Walking is an excellent way to begin an exercise prescription. Walking requires no specialized equipment or exercise facilities. Walking can also be used as both a fitness activity and a lifestyle activity. Examples of fitness activities include traditional sports and recreational activities such as swimming, running, basketball, tennis, or bicycling. Lifestyle activities include walking, yardwork, housework, and stair climbing. Both types of activity can be used to provide an adequate exercise stimulus. The choice of activity depends on each patient's goals and preferences. Depending on availability, accessibility, and affordability, patients can also use specialized facilities such as gymnasiums, pools, and fitness centers to increase variety in their exercise program (see Table 7.7). Yoga is a holistic activity that is gaining in popularity to improve balance, flexibility, strength, and wellness.[14,21]

TABLE 7.7
Approximate Energy Expenditure for Common Physical Activities

Energy	Recreation	Occupation
1.5–2 MET mL/kg/min[a]	Standing	Shaving/dressing/showering
4–7 mL O_2/min/kg	Card playing	Desk work
2–2.5 kcal/min	Sewing/knitting	Electric typing/writing
	Flying, motorcycling	Auto driving
	Walking (1–2 mph/1.6–3.2 kph)	Dusting/light house work
	Model ship building	Calculator machine operation
	Bed exercise	Watch repair
		Light assembly work
		Hammering
2–3 MET	Golf (powercart)	Car washing
7–11 mL O_2/min/kg	Bowling, billiards	Auto repair
2.5–4 kcal/min	Darts, piano playing	Kneading dough
	Fishing (standing, sitting), croquet	Manual typing
	Power boating, shuffleboard	Ironing/tailoring
	Skeet shooting, light woodworking	Bartending
	Walking (2–3 mph/3.2–4.8 kph)	Heavy level work, dredge
	Cycling (5 mph/8 kph)	Riding power lawn mower
	Shopping	Television, radio repair
	Kayaking, rowing, canoeing (2.5 mph/4 kph)	Crane operator
	Horseback riding (walk)	Upholstering
	Horseshoe pitching	Using hand tools
		Cleaning/scrubbing/waxing
		Washing/polishing/sanding
Aerobic Threshold		
3–4 MET	Calisthenics (light)	Janitorial work
11–14 mL O_2/min/kg	Fly fishing	Brick laying/plastering
4–5 kcal/min	Archery	Twisting cables/pulling on wires
	Badminton (doubles)/tennis (triples)	Raking leaves
	Sailing (small boat)	Machine assembly
	Ice boating	Hitching trailers
	Horseback riding (trot)	Cranking up dollies
	Badminton (social doubles)	Mopping/hanging wash
	Softball (noncompetitive)	Window cleaning
	Music (energetic)	Light plumbing
	Golf (pulling bag cart)	Welding (moderate)
	Volleyball (six-man noncompetitive)	Plowing, tractor
	Walking (3–3.5 mph/5–5.8 kph)	Trailer-truck driving
	Cycling (6 mph/10 kph)	Light lawn mower pushing
		Wheelbarrow (100 lb or 45 kg); assembly line work (light or medium, parts appearing at an approximate rate of 500/day or more; lifting a 45 lb/20 kg part every 5 min or so)
		Stocking shelves, packing or unpacking light or medium objects
4–5 MET	Table tennis	Heavy machine repair (farm, airplane, plumbing)
14–18 mL O_2/min/kg	Golf (carrying bag)	Using power saw on hardwood
5–6 kcal/min	Dancing (social)	Pushing a power mower/cart/dolly
	Tennis (doubles)	Gardening/hoeing
	Badminton (singles)	Baling hay
	Calisthenics (moderate)	Carpentry (light)
	Swimming (light)	Painting
	Tetherball	Masonry
	Baseball (noncompetitive)	Paperhanging

(Continued)

TABLE 7.7 (*Continued*)
Approximate Energy Expenditure for Common Physical Activities

Energy	Recreation	Occupation
	Walking (3.5–4 mph/5.8–6.4 kph)	Interior repair/remodeling
	Cycling (6.5–8 mph/10.4–12.8 kph)	Stair climbing (slow)
	Kayaking, rowing, canoeing (3 mph/4.8 kph)	Putting in a sidewalk
		Carrying trays/dishes
		Gas station mechanic
		Military marching
		Lifting and carrying 20–44 lb/9–20 kg
		General heavy industrial labor
		Walking from room to room
		Pumping tire
		Plowing with a horse
5–6 MET	Weight training (light to moderate)	Garden digging
18–21 mL O_2/min/kg	Hunting (small game)	Shoveling light earth
6–7 kcal/min	Fishing (wading)	Stair climbing (moderate)
	Softball (competitive)	Exterior remodeling or construction
	Horseback riding (posting at a trot)	
	Soccer (noncompetitive)	
	Walking (4 mph/6.4 kph)	
	Ice/roller skating (9 mph/15 kph)	
	Cycling (8–8.5 mph/12.8–13.6 kph)	
	Kayaking, rowing, canoeing (4 mph/6.4 kph)	
6–7 MET	Backpacking (5 lb/2.2 kg)	Shoveling 10 lb or 4.5 kg 10×/min
21–25 mL O_2/min/kg	Tennis (singles)	Snow shoveling
7–8 kcal/min	Scuba diving (warm water)	Mowing lawn (push mower)
	Downhill skiing (light)	Splitting wood
	Water volleyball	Using pneumatic tools
	Ski touring (2.5 mph/4 kph)	Carrying/lifting 45–64 lb/20–29 kg
	Calisthenics (heavy)	Spading
	Water skiing	
	Cycling (9 mph/14.4 kph)	
	Badminton (competitive)	
	Walking (5 mph/8 kph)	
	Cross-country hiking	
	Dancing (rumba, square)	
	Swimming (moderate)	
7–8 MET	Horseback riding (gallop)	Stair climbing (fast)
25–28 mL O_2/min/kg	Snowshoeing (3 mph/4.8 kph)	Ditch digging
8–10 kcal/min	Sledding/tobogganing	Hand saw/ax on hardwood
	Ice hockey	Carrying or lifting 65–84 lb/30–38 kg
	Touch/flag football	Laying railroad track
	Paddle ball	Carrying 20 lb/9 kg up stairs
	Swimming (fast)	
	Mountain climbing	
	Basketball (nongame)	
	Walking (6 mph/9.6 kph)	
	Cycling (12 mph/19 kph)	
	Kayaking, rowing, canoeing (5 mph/8 kph)	
	Jogging (5 mph/8 kph)	
	Downhill skiing (vigorous)	
	Aerobic dance	
8–9 MET	Light sparring (boxing, martial arts)	Carrying/lifting 85–100 lb/39–45 kg
28–32 mL O_2/min/kg	Fencing	Shoveling 14 lb or 6 kg/10×/min

(*Continued*)

TABLE 7.7 (*Continued*)
Approximate Energy Expenditure for Common Physical Activities

Energy	Recreation	Occupation
10–11 kcal/min	Scuba diving (cold water)	Tending furnace
	Handball (social)	Using a pick
	Endurance motorcycling	Using bar, sledgehammer
	Basketball (vigorous)	Climbing a ladder or stairs
	Soccer (competitive)	Moving or pushing desks, file cabinets
	Squash (social)	Stocking furniture; also pushing against heavy spring tension
	Running (5.5 mph/9 kph)	
	Cycling (13 mph/21 kph)	
	Ski touring (4 mph/6.5 kph) in loose snow	
	Backpacking (30 lb/14 kg)	
	Rope jumping (60–80/minute)	
	Weight training (heavy)	
10+ MET	Basketball (competitive)	Shoveling 16 lb or 7 kg 10×/min
32+ mL O_2/min/kg	Hunting (big game)	Heavy labor
11+ kcal/min	Heavy sparring (boxing, martial arts)	Ax chopping (heavy)
	Ski touring (5+ mph/8+ kph)	
	Running, 6 mph = 10 MET	
	Running, 7 mph = 11.5 MET	
	Running, 8 mph = 13.5 MET	
	Running, 9 mph = 15 MET	
	Running, 10 mph = 17 MET	
	Cycling, 14 mph = 10 MET	
	Cycling, 15 mph = 11.5 MET	
	Cycling, 16 mph = 12.5 MET	
	Swimming 850 yd/18–20 minutes = 10 MET	
	Swimming (crawl) 950 yd/20–22 minutes = 11 MET	
	Swimming 1000 yd/20–22 minutes = 12 MET	
	Paddle ball or racquetball (competitive)	
	Rope jumping (120–140/minute)	
	Snowshoeing	
	Judo	
	Squash (competitive)	
	Handball (competitive)	
	Gymnastics	
	Spaceball	
	Trampolining	
	Wrestling	
	Backpacking (heavy)	

[a] MET, metabolic equivalent. 1 MET = 3.5 mL O_2/kg/min.

7.15 TIME (LENGTH OF ACTIVITY SESSIONS)

The goal for every individual is 30–60 minutes of physical activity each and every day. Short, intermittent bouts of low-intensity exercise can be accumulated throughout the day and are useful for improving overall health.[10] Individuals who are interested in developing cardiorespiratory fitness or increasing their VO_{2max}, however, must exercise at progressively greater intensities for increasingly longer periods of time. Individuals who are just beginning an exercise program can be safely instructed to limit their initial activity sessions to 10–15 minutes. This helps reduce the risk of injury and assists patients with acclimation to an increasingly active lifestyle. Once patients are comfortable with this routine, they should be instructed to gradually increase their activity sessions to the recommended 30–60 minutes. A common strategy is to have patients perform an initial warm-up period of 5–10 minutes. During the warm-up, patients should engage in light calisthenics and stretching activities in preparation for more strenuous activity. The actual training or activity session follows the warm-up and should be 20–40 minutes in length depending on the patient's level of interest and ability. Following the activity session, patients should spend an additional 5–10 minutes performing cooldown activities. While this traditional paradigm has never been shown

TABLE 7.8
SORT: Key Recommendations for Practice

Clinical Recommendation	Evidence Rating	References
Patients should aim for 150 minutes of moderate-to-vigorous activity on a weekly basis.	A	[1]
Routine behavioral counseling to promote physical activity has not been shown to have a significant impact on health outcomes.	B	[20]
Low-risk patients need no formal exercise testing prior to beginning a program of physical activity.	C	[3]
Intermediate- to high-risk patients benefit from formal exercise testing in conjunction with an exercise prescription as part of a comprehensive physical activity program.	C	[3]

to augment patient compliance or reduce the rate of musculoskeletal injury, it is familiar to many patients and can add variety to the exercise routine. To avoid injury, patients should be instructed to gradually increase the frequency, duration, and intensity of their exercise sessions over a period of several months.

7.16 SUMMARY

When writing an exercise prescription, physicians must always consider each patient's specific goals and objectives. Physical activity has an unparalleled impact on health and disease. Exercise is arguably the most powerful (and important) prescription in a physician's arsenal. Physical activity should be a routine part of everyone's lifestyle. Prescribing regular physical activity has a profound impact on the ability of patients to live better and healthier lives. No other medical prescription can make such a claim (Table 7.8).

REFERENCES

1. U.S. Department of Health and Human Services. Physical activity guidelines for Americans. http://www.health.gov/paguidelines/ (accessed June 23, 2015).
2. American Diabetes Association, Standards of medical care in diabetes—2013. *Diabetes Care.* 2013;36(Suppl. 1):S1–S114.
3. American College of Sports Medicine. *ACSM's Guidelines for Exercise Testing and Prescription*, 9th edn. Philadelphia, PA: Lippincott Williams & Wilkins; 2013.
4. Blair SN, Cheng Y, Holder JS. Is physical activity or physical fitness more important in defining health benefits? *Medicine and Science Sports and Exercise.* 2001;33(6 Suppl.), S379–S399, discussion S419–S320.
5. Borg GA. *Borg's Perceived Exertion and Pain Scales.* Champaign, IL: Human Kinetics; 1998.
6. Charansonney OL, Vanhees L, Cohen-Solal A. Physical activity: From epidemiological evidence to individualized patient management. *International Journal of Cardiology.* 2014;170(3):350–357.
7. Dunstan DW, Howard B, Healy GN, Owen N. Too much sitting—A health hazard. *Diabetes Research and Clinical Practise.* 2012;97(3):368–376.
8. Erlichman J, Kerbey AL, James WP. Physical activity and its impact on health outcomes. Paper 1. The impact of physical activity on cardiovascular disease and all-cause mortality: An historical perspective. *Obesity Review.* 2002;3(4):257–271.
9. Friedenreich CM, Orenstein MR. Physical activity and cancer prevention: Etiologic evidence and biological mechanisms. *Journal of Nutrition.* 2002;132(11 Suppl.):3456S–3464S.
10. Garber CE, Blissmer B, Deschenes MR et al. Quantity and quality of exercise for developing and maintaining cardiorespiratory, musculoskeletal and neuromotor fitness in apparently healthy adults: Guidance for prescribing exercise. *Medicine and Science Sport and Exercise.* 2011;3(7): 1334–1359.
11. Grontved A, Hu FB. Television viewing and risk of type 2 diabetes, cardiovascular disease and all cause mortality: A meta-analysis. *Journal of the American Medical Association.* 2011;305:2448–2455.
12. Haskell WL, Lee IM, Pate RR et al., Physical activity and public health: Updated recommendation for adults from the American College of Sports Medicine and the American Heart Association. *Circulation.* 2007;116:1081–1093.
13. Hebert ET, Caughy MO, Shuval K. Primary care providers perceptions of physical activity counseling in a clinical setting: A systematic review. *British Journal of Sports Medicine.* 2012;46(9):625–631.
14. Howe TE, Rochester L, Jackson A et al. Exercise for improving balance in older people. *Cochrane Database System Review.* November 9, 2011;(11):CD004963.
15. Centers for Disease Control. Division of Nutrition, Obesity and Physical Activity. http://www.cdc.gov/physicalactivity/data/facts.html (accessed June 23, 2015).
16. Centers for Disease Control. Division of Nutrition, Obesity and Physical Activity. http://www.cdc.gov/nchs/fastats/obesity-overweight.htm (accessed June 23, 2015).
17. U.S. Department of Health and Human Services. http://www.healthypeople.gov/2020/default (accessed June 23, 2015).
18. Kraus WE, Houmard JA, Duscha BD et al., Effects of the amount and intensity of exercise on plasma lipoproteins. *New England Journal of Medicine.* 2001;347(19):1483–1492.
19. Mokdad A, Marks JS, Stroup DF, Gerberding J. Actual causes of death in the United States, 2000. *Journal of the American Medical Association.* 2004;291:1238–1245.
20. Moyer VA, US Preventive Services Task Force, Behavioral counseling interventions to promote a healthful diet and physical activity for cardiovascular disease prevention in adults: US Preventive Services Task Force recommendation statement. *Annals of Internal Medicine.* 2012;157(5):367–371.
21. Patel NK, Newstead AH, Ferrer RL. The effects of yoga on physical functioning and health related quality of life in older adults: A systematic review and meta-analysis. *Journal of Alternative Complement Medicine.* 2012;18(10):902–917.
22. Penedo FJ, Dahn JR. Exercise and well-being: A review of mental and physical health benefits associated with physical activity. *Current Opinion in Psychiatry.* 2005;18(2):189–193.

23. Stahl T, Rutten A, Nutbeam D et al. The importance of the social environment for physically active lifestyle: Results from an international study. *Social Science and Medicine.* 2001;52(1):1–10.
24. Tanasescu M, Leitzmann MF, Rimm EB et al., Exercise type and intensity in relation to coronary heart disease in men. *Journal of the American Medical Association.* 2002;288(16):1994–2000.
25. Whelton PK, He J, Appel LJ. et al., Primary prevention of hypertension: Clinical and public health advisory from the National High Blood Pressure Education Program. *Journal of the American Medical Association.* 2002;288(15):466–471.
26. Patrick K, Sallis JF, Long B et al. *A new tool for encouraging activity: Project PACE. The Physician and Sportsmedicine.* 1994;22:45–55.
27. Gibbons RJ, Balady GJ, Bricker JT et al. ACC/AHA practice guidelines. ACC/AHA 2002 guideline update for exercise testing: Summary article; A report of the American College of Cardiology/American Heart Association task force on practice guidelines (committee to update the 1997 Exercise Testing Guidelines). *Circulation.* 2002;106(14):1883–1892.

SUGGESTED READINGS

American College of Sports Medicine, *ACSM's Guideline for Exercise Testing and Prescription*, Pescatello, L.S. (ed.), 9th edn., Lippincott Williams & Wilkins, Philadelphia, PA, 2013.

Jonas, S. and Phillips, E.M. (eds.), *ACSM's Exercise is Medicine: A Clinician's Guide to Exercise Prescription*, Lippincott Williams & Wilkins, Philadelphia, PA, 2009.

U.S. Department of Health and Human Services, The Surgeon General's Vision for a Healthy and Fit Nation, U.S. Department of Health and Human Services, Office of the Surgeon General, Rockville, MD, January 2010.

U.S. Department of Health and Human Services, Public Health Service, Centers for Disease Control and Prevention, National Center for Chronic Disease Prevention and Health Promotion, Division of Nutrition and Physical Activity, *Promoting Physical Activity: A Guide for Community Action*, 2nd edn., Human Kinetics, Champaign, IL, 2010.

Section II

Fundamentals

8 Bone

Nathaniel S. Nye

CONTENTS

TABLE 8.1
Key Clinical Considerations

1. Bones are vital not only to physiologic life but to all aspects of human performance. Bones have important roles in weight bearing, human locomotion, enabling respiration, protecting vital organs, serum calcium homeostasis, hearing, and harboring hematopoietic cells.
2. A finely controlled interplay between osteoblasts (deposit bone material) and osteoclasts (resorb bone) is essential for proper bone formation, remodeling, fracture healing, and maintenance of serum calcium levels. Conditions affecting this balance result in bone diseases such as osteoporosis, osteomalacia, and Paget's disease of bone.
3. The 206 bones in the adult human skeleton can be classified into long, short, flat, irregular, and sesamoid bone types. Each type of bone conveys specific structural, physiologic, and biomechanical advantages.
4. Many bones elongate at the growth plate, or physis, until they close in mid- to late adolescence. An open physis is vulnerable to injury. Fractures involving the physis are described by the Salter–Harris classification, and some types impart risk for disordered growth.
5. Peak bone mass is reached around age 18 (females) to 20 (males) and is an important modifiable risk factor for osteoporosis later in life. Bone mass can be maintained through a healthy diet, regular weight-bearing exercise, and avoidance of smoking and certain drugs.

8.1 INTRODUCTION

Although bones are widely viewed in American society as a symbol of death, living bone tissue is incredibly dynamic and versatile. Indeed, the bone is arguably the single most essential adaptation to terrestrial life.[31] Its important roles include serving as a framework and support for the body in bearing its own weight against gravity, providing levers to translate muscular contraction into locomotion, protecting vital organs and structures from trauma, providing both a reservoir and sink for serum calcium homeostasis (without which, cells cannot function), harboring an important hematopoietic cell machinery, and even in translating sound waves into nerve signals for hearing. In short, all human performance from hitting a baseball to performing a violin solo to flying a fighter jet depends intimately upon bone and calcium fulfilling their vital roles (Table 8.1).

8.2 BASIC OSTEOLOGY

Understanding the bone must begin with a knowledge of its component cells, proteins, and minerals. The most important cells in the bone are the osteoclasts and osteoblasts, which form an intimately linked pair in the formation and remodeling of the bone. Osteoclasts are related to macrophages and function in the resorption of the bone. Osteoblasts (of mesenchymal stem cell origin) function in deposition of new bone matrix.[19] Working together through an intricate pattern of intercellular communication under local and systemic hormonal control, osteoblasts and osteoclasts execute the critical ongoing process of bone remodeling.[29] Both the structural integrity of the bone and serum calcium balance depend on this process occurring correctly. Several common disorders of bone remodeling are discussed in the succeeding text. Other important cells in the bone include osteocytes, fibroblasts, chondrocytes, and lining cells; a summary of bone cells and their corresponding functions is listed in Table 8.2.

Clinical Pearl

Osteoblasts deposit new bone matrix, while osteoclasts resorb bone. These cells work together to develop and maintain healthy bone structure and heal fractures.

TABLE 8.2
Bone Histology

Cell	Depiction (Figure 8.1)	Functions
Osteoblast	1	Responds to local cytokines and systemic hormones in the process of remodeling, deposits organic bone matrix, and creates a calcium-rich extracellular fluid.
Osteoclast	2	Resorbs old bone tissue in preparation for osteoblastic activity, driven by hormonal influence; plays a critical role in serum calcium homeostasis.
Osteocyte	3	Osteoblasts that become surrounded by bone matrix mature into osteocytes, to remain in place to nourish and maintain healthy bone microarchitecture.
Fibroblast	4	Synthesizes and repairs collagen fibers.
Chondrocyte	Not depicted	Synthesizes cartilage at the physes, resulting in linear growth, as well as at joint surfaces.
Lining cell	5	Osteoblasts remaining on the surface of mineralized bone after remodeling is complete become quiescent and form a protecting/nourishing layer.

8.3 BONE MATRIX

The formation of new bone begins as osteoblasts secrete an organic matrix called osteoid. Osteoid is composed of type I collagen fibers (90% osteoid weight) and other proteins such as osteocalcin (strongly binds calcium) and is surrounded by an aqueous gel of glycosaminoglycans.

When mineralized, this organic matrix gives tensile and compressive strength to the bone; it is analogous to civil engineers adding iron rebar or fiberglass to cement. Osteoblasts, through the action of alkaline phosphatase, secrete high concentrations of Ca^{2+} and $(PO_4)^-$ ions. In turn, the osteoid matrix attracts these ions, which precipitate around the collagen fibers as crystals of hydroxyapatite, $Ca_{10}(PO_4)_6(OH)_2$. Hydroxyapatite confers bone its hardness and rigidity.[30]

8.4 BONE ARCHITECTURE AND REMODELING

Lamellar bone refers to an organized, ring-like pattern of bone mineralization organized around a central canal (Haversian canal, containing nutrient blood supply) (see Figure 8.1). While lamellar bone provides excellent strength, its formation is slow. On the other hand, woven bone is a more haphazard pattern of bone mineralization, with the advantage that it can be formed much more rapidly than lamellar bone. Not surprisingly, the new bone formed at a fracture site is woven bone. In healthy bones, woven bone is formed in locations of bone growth or healing and is gradually replaced by lamellar bone. However, when osteoblast/osteoclast regulation is impaired, as in Paget's disease of bone, excessive amounts of woven bone are formed without regard to the normal stimuli of bone stresses and hormonal influences.[7] This results in more brittle bones.

Clinical Pearl

Dysregulation of osteoblast/osteoclast activity in Paget's disease of bone leads to brittle bones with excessive woven bone tissue. Prevalence in the United States is estimated at 1%–2% of the general population, but incidence has decreased in recent years. Risk factors include northern European ancestry and age >65.

All bones display one or a combination of two macroscopic architectural patterns (see Figure 8.1):

- Cortical (compact) bone, forming the dense outer layer
- Cancellous (trabecular or spongy) bone, forming strong inner struts

Each bone is subjected to unique forces depending on anatomic position and the activity level of the individual. Through the constantly ongoing process of remodeling, osteoblasts and osteoclasts respond to these forces to produce a precisely tuned arrangement of trabeculae within a cortical shell that is optimally adapted to withstand the forces. On the other hand, factors that impair osteoblast/osteoclast activity (e.g., advanced age, sedentary lifestyle, smoking) may result in weaker bones or delayed bone healing.

8.5 BONE ANATOMY

The 206 bones in the adult human body can be categorized into five types:

- Long bones (e.g., humerus, femur, metacarpals)
- Short bones (e.g., carpals of hand, tarsals of foot)
- Flat bones (e.g., plates of skull)
- Irregular bones (e.g., vertebrae, sphenoid, ethmoid)
- Sesamoid bones (e.g., patella, pisiform, sesamoids of thumb and great toe)

Each type of bone conveys specific structural, physiologic, and biomechanical advantages. Indeed, each surface of each individual bone, as well as the orientation of one bone in relation to its neighboring bones, is specially adapted to suit necessary purposes of locomotion (femur, tibia, humerus), hand dexterity (pronating/supinating surfaces of radius/ulna, carpals of wrist), supporting the weight of the body against gravity (pelvis, spine), protecting or housing vital organs (skull, ribs), enabling respiration (ribs), providing resonating chambers for vocal communication (sinuses of maxilla,

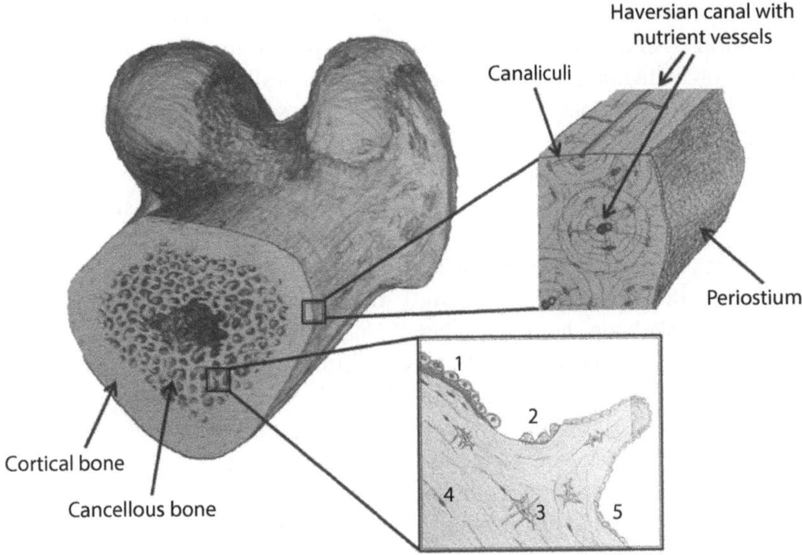

FIGURE 8.1 Internal bone architecture. A sectioned distal femur is shown to demonstrate macroscopic and microscopic internal bone architecture. Macroscopically, cortical bone provides a very strong, dense outer layer, while trabecular bone adds structural integrity to resist loads while contributing little additional weight. Microscopically, the osteon or "Haversian system" is shown, with canaliculi emanating from a central Haversian canal, which provides blood and nutrients to neighboring osteocytes. Finally, important bone cell types are represented (1, Osteoblast; 2, Osteoclast; 3, Osteocyte; 4, Fibroblast; 5, Lining cell; see also Table 8.1).

ethmoids, etc.), transmitting sound waves into nerve impulses (inner ear ossicles), and so forth.

Noting the predominance of long bones in the skeleton, it is important to recognize their special anatomic patterns (some of which apply variably to other types of bone) (see Figure 8.2).

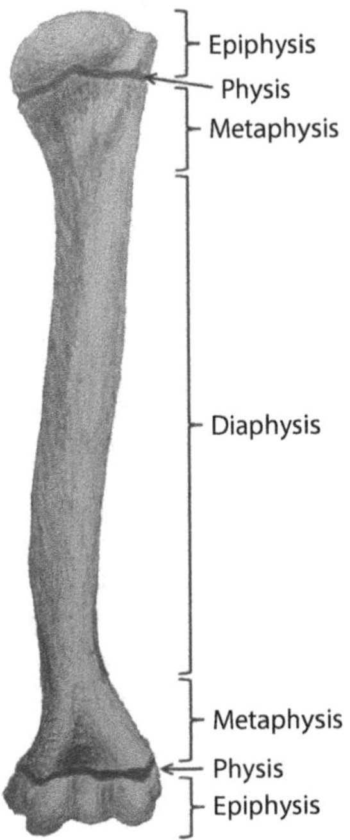

FIGURE 8.2 Long bone morphology. The humerus displays common anatomical elements seen among all long bones. The epiphysis is the primary articulating part of the bone beyond the physis. The physis is a growth center whereby the bone elongates. The metaphysis is a transitional "conical" segment between the physis and the roughly tubular bone shaft, termed the diaphysis.

- *Physis*: the "growth plate." Physes typically exist near one or both ends of a long bone. Linear growth (elongation) of the bone occurs at this site until the physis closes. Physis closure occurs at various times depending on sex and anatomic location. Open physes are generally the weakest part of a bone and are susceptible to fracture.
- *Epiphysis*: the terminal portion of the bone beyond the physis (may be proximal or distal), typically where an articulation occurs. It consists of mostly trabecular bone.
- *Metaphysis*: the transitional zone between the bone's "shaft" (diaphysis, see in the following text) and the physis.
- *Diaphysis*: the "shaft" of the bone, typically providing the bulk of the bone's lever arm capability. It comprises mostly a thick, cortical cylinder filled with marrow or fat.

8.6 BONE FORMATION

Most bones in the human body are formed by a remarkable process called endochondral ossification, wherein a cartilage anlage (or bone template) develops from mesenchymal tissue and then gradually becomes ossified through several ossification centers. In the fetus and neonate, multiple, anatomically predictable ossification centers develop within these bone templates as blood vessels, osteoblasts, osteoclasts, and bone marrow cells invade the cartilage. Ossification extends peripherally from these centers. This process enables a bone to develop hardness through much of its structure while preserving an actively proliferating cartilaginous center for linear growth (the physis). The biochemical and cellular pathways responsible for endochondral ossification are extremely complex; multiple cytokines, growth factors, and hormones (including growth hormone, thyroid hormone, insulin-like growth factors, and the locally secreted Indian hedgehog, parathyroid hormone (PTH)-related peptide, and fibroblast growth factors) must work in harmony to execute normal skeletal growth and maturation.[18]

Some bones develop without a cartilage anlage through a process called intramembranous ossification. The main example is almost the entire craniofacial skeleton; however, other examples include the clavicle and parts of the scapula. Here, condensations of preosteogenic mesenchymal stem cells form a nidus and begin to expand within a tissue layer, followed by differentiation into osteoblasts. The osteoblasts secrete osteoid, which ossifies directly, without need for a cartilage template. Seen on microscopy, the bone expands centripetally as finger-like bone columns extend outward adjacent to proliferating vascular sinuses. This process is less well understood than endochondral ossification, but it is known to depend critically on angiogenesis.[26,36]

8.7 SKELETAL MATURATION AND PHYSIS CLOSURE

As a healthy child ages, the bones grow under hormonal influences. Linear growth occurs relatively rapidly at the physes, while circumferential growth occurs more slowly along all contours of a bone. Osteoblasts lining the outer surfaces of bones slowly lay down the bone just underneath the tough, fibrous periosteum, thereby adding thickness to the bone. Within the cancellous portion of the bone, osteoclasts resorb some bone to balance this circumferential growth, thereby ensuring that cortical bone does not become too thick. Around the time of puberty, physes will begin to narrow and then close; in other words, the cartilaginous growth center will ossify, fusing the metaphysis to the epiphysis. Timing of physis closure varies between one bone and another and even between two ends of a bone. However, the overall pattern of physis closure is highly predictable and has been carefully studied. In general, physes will close approximately 2–3 years earlier in girls than in boys. Until the physes close, they remain the weakest part of the bone and are vulnerable to injury. Fractures involving the physis are commonly described by the Salter–Harris classification scheme. Displacement of fracture fragments involving the physis may result in a bony bridge or "bar" across the growth plate, leading to bone angulation or growth arrest.[5]

8.8 BONE HOMEOSTASIS

The structural strength and thickness of bone depend primarily on hormonal influences, genetic factors, and load-bearing stresses applied to the bone. Analogous to muscle, bone tissue will undergo hypertrophy in response to increased load stress. Individuals who exercise regularly will generally have a higher bone mineral density than those who are sedentary. To illustrate this principle from a clinical standpoint, the mantra "abnormal stress on a normal bone, or normal stress on an abnormal bone" is instructive. While most exercise results in healthy bone remodeling and increased bone strength, excessive exercise may result in cumulative stress above the capacity of the bone's cellular repair machinery (osteoblasts and osteoclasts) to remodel. Uncorrected, this situation will eventually lead to stress fractures. On the other hand, in an individual with osteoporosis, a simple activity such as walking may result in a pathologic fracture of the lower extremity (normal stress on abnormal bone).

Clinical Pearl

Stress fractures result from abnormal stresses on a normal bone. Pathologic fractures, such as in patients with osteoporosis, result from normal stresses on an abnormal bone. However, the underlying process is similar (bone damage exceeding rate of healing).

Additionally, hormones are important drivers of bone structure. During and after puberty, growth and sex hormone levels increase greatly, causing bones to grow both linearly and in thickness. Most females reach 90% of their peak bone mass by the age of 18, while males on average reach 90% of their peak bone mass at the age of 20.[24] Peak bone mass is one of the most important determinants of osteoporosis risk in later life.[20] After the age of 25–30, bone mineral density tends to slowly decline as individuals reach older age. This decline can be minimized through continued exercise and a healthy diet (specifically, adequate levels of protein, calcium, vitamin D, and vitamin C are essential); however, genetic and environmental factors (certain medications such as systemic corticosteroids, medroxyprogesterone, and proton pump inhibitors as well as cigarette smoking may increase risk for osteoporosis) are also very important. In women, the loss of ovarian estrogen supply at the time of menopause leads to a higher risk of bone mineral loss and development of osteopenia or osteoporosis.

Clinical application: When the pituitary gland fails to produce adequate growth hormone, global skeletal growth deficiency ensues in a condition called pituitary dwarfism. Bodily proportions remain relatively unchanged, but the individual is very small unless treated with supplemental human growth hormone. By contrast, achondroplasia (a genetic disorder of growth plate regulation) causes accelerated physeal closure, resulting in disproportionately short limbs with a relatively normal trunk.

In addition to growth hormone and sex hormones, PTH is a critical factor in maintaining bone homeostasis. PTH is released by the parathyroid glands in response to hypocalcemia. It upregulates osteoclast activity that increases serum calcium levels by mobilizing calcium ions from the inorganic matrix of bone. PTH also acts on the kidneys to increase the renal absorption of calcium, decrease the absorption of phosphate, and increase the synthesis of 1,25$(OH)_2$-vitamin D. The primary role of 1,25$(OH)_2$-vitamin D is to increase intestinal absorption of calcium. Vitamin D precursors are derived both from the diet (as cholecalciferol and ergocalciferol) and through UV radiation to the skin and subsequently converted to 1,25$(OH)_2$-vitamin D (the active form) in the kidney under the influence of PTH.[31]

Clinical application: A group of related metabolic disorders are known to cause decreased calcification of otherwise normal organic bone matrix. These include rickets, osteomalacia, and renal osteodystrophy. Rickets may be caused by inadequate stores of either calcium or phosphate (termed hypocalcemic and hypophosphatemic rickets). Historically, hypocalcemic rickets was much more common than it is today due to supplementation of vitamin D for infants. With their rapid skeletal development, infants have particularly high demand for calcium and vitamin D. Infants depending solely upon breast milk for nutrition without supplementation of vitamin D, particularly those with dark skin, limited sunlight exposure, or mothers with a vegetarian diet, are at high risk for rickets. Affected infants present around 15–18 months with muscle weakness, delayed walking, bowed limbs, carpopedal spasms, and diffuse limb pain. The American Academy of Pediatrics recommends a total daily intake of 400 IU vitamin D daily for all infants beginning within the first few days of life.[35] Achieving this intake requires supplementation in all breastfed infants, and in formula-fed infants receiving less than 1 L of formula per day. Conversely, osteomalacia is analogous to rickets in adults. Osteomalacia results from vitamin D and/or dietary calcium deficiency, which causes a secondary hyperparathyroidism as the body attempts to maintain serum calcium levels. This disorder is particularly common in elderly patients who are bound to beds or wheelchairs (e.g., many nursing home residents) who often have poor appetites and low sunlight exposure. Those affected present with diffuse, aching bone pain, fatigue, and possibly pathologic fractures. Renal osteodystrophy occurs in adults with chronic renal failure, due to impaired ability to excrete phosphate as well as synthesize 1,25$(OH)_2$-vitamin D. This results in low serum calcium and a secondary hyperparathyroidism, causing increased osteoclast activity. In all of these conditions, the essential building blocks for hydroxyapatite are deficient, and much of the osteoid created by osteoblasts never mineralizes, resulting in weak, painful, brittle bones.[4,23]

Clinical Pearl

Vitamin D deficiency is a popular and debated topic. In February 2013, the USPSTF issued recommendations regarding vitamin D and calcium supplementation to prevent fractures in adults. In short, there was insufficient evidence to support supplementation with >400 IU vitamin D3 and >1000 mg calcium for fracture prevention in community-dwelling adults of any age and either gender. Adequate evidence shows that lower doses are ineffective for fracture prevention in postmenopausal women. There is limited evidence that 700–800 IU vitamin D3 daily may reduce risk for falls in older adults.

8.9 VARIABILITY IN BONE ANATOMY

The anatomy of the normal human skeleton, while remarkably consistent, does display a broad spectrum of variability from one person to the next. These variations in skeletal structure may be asymptomatic and purely incidental radiographic findings or they may create significant pain syndromes or predispose to certain injury patterns. It is important to consider variations in structure of normal bones, such as hooked or flat acromial morphology or pectus deformities, and "accessory bones" or bones that are present in some individuals but absent in most. Table 8.3 discusses many of the most common bony variants and clinical implications.

Clinical application: In certain conditions, nonbone tissue may ossify abnormally. This is called heterotopic ossification. For example, myositis ossificans may occur at the site of a large intramuscular hematoma (often the result of trauma in sports or motor vehicle accidents) or sometimes postoperatively. The hematoma transforms into clot, followed by fibrosis, and eventually ossification may occur as collagenous fibers attract calcium and phosphate ions. This condition is followed radiographically until the lesion stabilizes, usually around 6–12 months, and then excised if symptomatic.[16,33] In ankylosing spondylitis, heterotopic ossification occurs due to autoinflammation in and around many joints, ligaments, and tendons throughout the body but predominantly involves the spine.

8.10 SUMMARY

The bone is a dynamic, living tissue that imparts tremendous capabilities to the human body. An important network of cells work under local and systemic hormonal influences to create and remodel bones that are very specifically adapted to the demands placed upon each bone. The human skeleton develops and matures in a very predictable pattern, with linear growth occurring at the physes until they close around the second decade of life. A wide variety of genetic, nutritional, metabolic, and environmental disorders lead to bone diseases. By helping patients maintain an active lifestyle, a balanced diet, and avoid unhealthy behaviors, these diseases can potentially be prevented (Table 8.4).

TABLE 8.3
Common Variants of Skeletal Anatomy

Skeletal Variant	Description	Prevalence	Clinical Relevance
Bipartite patella	Incomplete bony union of the ossification centers of patella, usually a superolateral isolated fragment[15]	2%[15]	May be mistaken for acute patellar fracture; may become symptomatic and painful, particularly with trauma or overuse; more common in males than in females by ratio 9:1.[15]
Bipartite hallux sesamoid	Incomplete bony union of ossification centers of hallux sesamoids	2.7%–33.5%[8,21]	Clinically irrelevant unless painful, as they may become with overuse (e.g., long-distance runners); must be distinguished from a fracture.[21]
Fabella	Accessory sesamoid within proximal portion of medial head of gastrocnemius	10%–20%[11]	Common incidental finding on knee radiographs; may be mistaken for a loose body within the knee or an osteophyte.[37]
Tarsal coalition	Fusion of two or more tarsal bones; calcaneonavicular most common, followed by talocalcaneal[37]	<1%[34]	Depending on which joint is involved, the motion of the ankle and midfoot becomes limited. Common cause of painful pes planus, usually in older children or adolescents.[34] Usually congenital but may be acquired posttrauma or postsurgery.
Accessory navicular	Type 1: sesamoid within distal tibialis posterior tendon. Type 2: Incomplete bony union of the ossification centers of navicular[17,21]	4%–21%[21]	Type 1: almost always asymptomatic. Type 2: tibialis posterior tendon inserts onto accessory ossicle when present and may become partially avulsed and osteonecrotic causing medial foot pain (usually in middle-aged women).[21]
Os trigonum	Incomplete bony union of the ossification centers of posterior talus	2.5%–14%[12]	Repeated ankle plantar flexion (i.e., ballet dancing) may cause painful compression and bony impingement of os trigonum or tenosynovitis of the flexor hallucis longus as it courses adjacent to os trigonum.[14]
Os acromiale	Incomplete bony union of the ossification centers of acromion	8.2%[9]	Usually an incidental finding on radiographs. May become locally tender or cause impingement syndrome. Associated with rotator cuff tear.
"Hooked" acromion	Bigliani acromion classification: Type 1: Flat Type 2: Curved Type 3: Hooked[13]	Type 1: 17%–26% Type 2: 43%–56% Type 3: 18%–40%[13,25]	Relationship of acromial type to rotator cuff tears and impingement is controversial. Using Bigliani classification, early studies found positive correlation[3] but recent studies found no correlation.[2,22] Other acromial measurements have been proposed with varying predictive value.[2,22] No difference in outcomes of surgical rotator cuff repair with or without acromioplasty.[1,28]
Transitional lumbosacral vertebrae	Usually partial fusion of L5–S1, transverse processes articulate with sacrum	7%–36%[10]	Sacralization of L5 associated with the protection of the L5-S1 disc but increased stress and degeneration of L4–L5 disc.[10]
Cervical rib	Accessory rib, usually at C7 vertebra	<1%[27]	May lead to compression of brachial plexus or subclavian artery/vein, causing thoracic outlet syndrome or upper extremity deep vein thrombosis.[6]

TABLE 8.4
SORT: Key Recommendations for Practice

Clinical Recommendation	Evidence Rating	References
Exercise, physical therapy, and home hazard assessment decrease fall risk in older adults.	B	[32]
All women aged ≥ 65 years should be screened for osteoporosis.	A	[32]
All men aged ≥ 70 years should be screened for osteoporosis.	C	[32]
To prevent vitamin D deficiency and rickets, recommend total daily vitamin D intake of 400 IU per day for infants and children through adolescence.	B	[4,35]
Daily vitamin D supplementation (at least 700–800 IU), with or without calcium, decreases fall risk in persons aged 60 years and older.	B	[4]

REFERENCES

1. Abrams GD, Gupta AK, Hussey KE et al. Arthroscopic repair of full-thickness rotator cuff tears with and without acromioplasty: Randomized prospective trial with 2-year follow-up. *American Journal of Sports Medicine.* April 2014;42(6):1296–1303.
2. Balke M, Schmidt C, Dedy N, Banerjee M, Bouillon B, Liem D. Correlation of acromial morphology with impingement syndrome and rotator cuff tears. *Acta Orthopaedica.* April 2013;84(2):178–183.
3. Bigliani LU, Ticker JB, Flatow EL, Soslowsky LJ, Mow VC. The relationship of acromial architecture to rotator cuff disease. *Clinical Sports Medicine.* October 1991;10(4):823–838.
4. Bordelon P, Ghetu MV, Langan RC. Recognition and management of vitamin D deficiency. *American Family Physician.* October 15, 2009;80(8):841–846.
5. Brown JH, DeLuca SA. Growth plate injuries: Salter-Harris classification. *American Family Physician.* October 1992;46(4):1180–1184.
6. Chang KZ, Likes K, Davis K, Demos J, Freischlag JA. The significance of cervical ribs in thoracic outlet syndrome. *Journal of Vascular Surgery.* March 2013;57(3):771–775.
7. Corral-Gudino L, Borao-Cengotita-Bengoa M, Del Pino-Montes J, Ralston S. Epidemiology of Paget's disease of bone: A systematic review and meta-analysis of secular changes. *Bone.* August 2013;55(2):347–352.
8. Coskun N, Yuksel M, Cevener M, et al. Incidence of accessory ossicles and sesamoid bones in the feet: A radiographic study of the Turkish subjects. *Surg Radiol Anat.* January 2009;31(1):19–24.
9. Edelson JG, Zuckerman J, Hershkovitz I. Os acromiale: Anatomy and surgical implications. *Journal of Bone Joint Surgery British.* July 1993;75(4):551–555.
10. Farshad-Amacker NA, Herzog RJ, Hughes AP, Aichmair A, Farshad M. Associations between lumbosacral transitional anatomy types and degeneration at the transitional and adjacent segments. *The Spine Journal* June 2015;15(6):1210–1216.
11. Lateral radiograph of the knee. http://www.wheelessonline.com/ortho/lateral_radiograph_of_the_knee. 2012. Accessed June 28, 2015.
12. Os trigonum/posterior talar impingement. http://www.wheelessonline.com/ortho/os_trigonum_posterior_talar_impingement. 2012. Accessed June 28, 2015.
13. X-ray findings in rotator cuff tears/impingement syndrome. http://www.wheelessonline.com/ortho/x_ray_findings_in_rotator_cuff_tears_impingement_syndrome. 2012. Accessed June 28, 2015.
14. Iovane A, Midiri M, Finazzo M, Carcione A, De Maria M, Lagalla R. Os Trigonum Tarsi Syndrome. Role of magnetic resonance. *Radiology Medicine.* January–February 2000;99(1–2):36–40.
15. Kavanagh EC, Zoga A, Omar I, Ford S, Schweitzer M, Eustace S. Mri findings in Bipartite Patella. *Skeletal Radiology.* March 2007;36(3):209–214.
16. Larson CM, Almekinders LC, Karas SG, Garrett WE. Evaluating and managing muscle contusions and myositis ossificans. *Physician and Sportsmedicine.* February 2002;30(2):41–50.
17. Lawson JP, Ogden JA, Sella E, Barwick KW. The painful accessory navicular. *Skeletal Radiology.* 1984;12(4):250–262.
18. Mackie EJ, Ahmed YA, Tatarczuch L, Chen KS, Mirams M. Endochondral ossification: How cartilage is converted into bone in the developing skeleton. *International Journal of Biochemistry and Cell Biology.* 2008;40(1):46–62.
19. Matsuo K, Irie N. Osteoclast-osteoblast communication. *Archives of Biochemistry and Biophysics.* May 15, 2008; 473(2):201–209.
20. McGuigan FE, Murray L, Gallagher A et al. Genetic and environmental determinants of peak bone mass in young men and women. *Journal of Bone and Mineral Research.* July 2002;17(7):1273–1279.
21. Mellado JM, Ramos A, Salvado E, Camins A, Danus M, Sauri A. Accessory ossicles and sesamoid bones of the ankle and foot: Imaging findings, clinical significance and differential diagnosis. *European Radiology.* December 2003;13 Suppl 6:L164–177.
22. Moor BK, Wieser K, Slankamenac K, Gerber C, Bouaicha S. Relationship of individual scapular anatomy and degenerative rotator cuff tears. *Journal of Shoulder and Elbow Surgery.* April 2014;23(4):536–541.
23. Moyer VA, LeFevre ML, Siu AL. Vitamin D and calcium supplementation to prevent fractures in adults. *Annals of Internal Medicine.* December 17, 2013;159(12):856–857.
24. National Institutes of Health. Osteoporosis and Related Bone Diseases National Resource Center. http://www.niams.nih.gov/Health_Info/Bone/Osteoporosis/bone_mass.asp. Accessed April 26, 2014.
25. Paraskevas G, Tzaveas A, Papaziogas B, Kitsoulis P, Natsis K, Spanidou S. Morphological parameters of the acromion. *Folia Morphology (Warsz).* November 2008;67(4):255–260.
26. Percival CJ, Richtsmeier JT. Angiogenesis and intramembranous osteogenesis. *Developmental Dynamics.* August 2013;242(8):909–922.
27. Sanders RJ, Hammond SL. Management of cervical ribs and anomalous first ribs causing neurogenic thoracic outlet syndrome. *Journal of Vascular Surgery.* July 2002;36(1):51–56.
28. Shin SJ, Oh JH, Chung SW, Song MH. The efficacy of acromioplasty in the arthroscopic repair of small- to medium-sized rotator cuff tears without acromial spur: Prospective comparative study. *Arthroscopy.* May 2012;28(5):628–635.
29. Sims NA, Gooi JH. Bone remodeling: Multiple cellular interactions required for coupling of bone formation and resorption. *Seminars in Cell and Developmental Biology.* October 2008;19(5):444–451.
30. Stevens AL, Lowe JS. Bone. In Andreoli TE (ed.). *Human Histology*, 3rd edn.; 2005. Philadelphia, PA: Saunders Elsevier.

31. Stewart AF. Normal physiology of bone and mineral homeostasis. In Stevens A (ed.). *Andreoli and Carpenter's Cecil Essentials of Medicine*, 7th edn.; 2007. Philadelphia, PA: Elsevier, pp. 749–760.
32. Sweet MG, Sweet JM, Jeremiah MP, Galazka SS. Diagnosis and treatment of osteoporosis. *American Family Physician.* February 1, 2009;79(3):193–200.
33. Trojian TH. Muscle contusion (thigh). *Clinical Sports and Medicine.* April 2013;32(2):317–324.
34. Vincent KA. Tarsal coalition and painful flatfoot. *Journal of the American Academy of Orthopedic Surgery.* September–October 1998;6(5):274–281.
35. Wagner CL, Greer FR. American Academy of Pediatrics Section on B, American Academy of Pediatrics Committee on N. Prevention of rickets and vitamin D deficiency in infants, children, and adolescents. *Pediatrics.* November 2008;122(5):1142–1152.
36. Yang Y. Skeletal morphogenesis during embryonic development. *Critical Reviews in Eukaryotic Gene Expression.* 2009;19(3):197–218.
37. Yochum TR, Rowe LJ. *Essentials of Skeletal Radiology*, 3rd edn.; 2005. Philadelphia, PA: Lippincott Williams & Wilkins.

9 Cartilage

Richard D. Quattrone

CONTENTS

TABLE 9.1
Key Clinical Considerations

1. Physical exam of the cartilage is joint specific versus cartilage specific and should include evaluation of alignment, range of motion, swelling, effusion, stability, strength, and neurovascular status.[20]
2. Weight-bearing radiographs provide a more accurate estimate of joint space narrowing, which can allude to the presence and degree of cartilage thinning in load-bearing joints.[35]
3. Magnetic resonance imaging is considered the gold standard to evaluate the articular cartilage.[32]
4. Arthroscopic evaluation remains the most accurate way to assess location, depth, size, shape, and stability of chondral or osteochondral defect of the articular surface.[20]
5. The Modified International Cartilage Repair Society classification system can be used to describe lesions both arthroscopically and using advanced radiologic imaging techniques.[14]
6. Meta-analyses of randomized placebo-controlled trials in knee OA patients have demonstrated the efficacy of oral chondroitin sulfate to relieve OA joint pain.[37,41,45]
7. Persistent loss of mechanical function, mechanical locking, catching, or laxity despite maximizing nonsurgical management should be considered for surgical intervention.[20]

9.1 INTRODUCTION

Cartilage problems and osteoarthritis (OA) are extremely common. It is vital that the primary care provider understand the basics of the anatomy and physiology of cartilage in order to better inform the patient of realistic diagnostic and treatment options available to them. The apophyseal articular cartilage and its role in decreasing friction and distributing loads across major diarthrodial joints such as the hips and knees will be the focus of this chapter in addition to the discussion on the properties of meniscal fibrocartilage. Injury to diarthrodial articular cartilage is very common affecting approximately 900,000 Americans annually and results in over 200,000 surgical procedures (Table 9.1).[17]

9.2 ANATOMY AND PHYSIOLOGY OF THE CARTILAGE

Cartilage is a unique flexible connective tissue produced from embryonic mesenchymal stem cells that can differentiate into chondroblasts. Chondroblasts in turn secrete an extracellular matrix composed of collagen fibers, proteoglycan-rich ground substance, and elastin fibers. These three components further combine with exogenous glycosaminoglycan substrates such as chondroitin sulfate (CS) to form a resilient cartilaginous matrix. Chondroblasts that get trapped in the extracellular matrix cavities, or *lacunae*, are referred to as chondrocytes. The cartilage matrix is avascular and relies on diffusion to supply the chondrocytes and therefore grows and repairs more slowly than most other connective tissue.

There are three main types of cartilage: elastic cartilage, fibrocartilage and articular, or *hyaline* cartilage. Elastic cartilage is found in the external ear pinna, epiglottis, and larynx. The fibrocartilage functions at the site of tendon and ligament insertion to bone and is additionally found in intervertebral discs, interarticular menisci, and circumferential labrum joint capsules. Fibrocartilage additionally constitutes the healing tissue of articular cartilage when produced from associated subchondral bone.

In the skeletally immature, the articular cartilage has a stem cell population that functions at the physis, or growth plate, and is crucial to bone formation.[13] The ribs, nose, larynx, and trachea are all composed of mature articular cartilage. The articular cartilage, however, has a more predominant role within diarthrodial joints.

The articular cartilage is an avascular layered matrix composed of 65%–80% water, 10%–20% predominantly type II collagen, 10%–15% proteoglycans, and 5% chondrocytes.[20] Type II collagen forms the framework of articular cartilage and provides overall tensile strength. Proteoglycans are responsible for compressive strength, forming a porous structure that traps water. The high water content allows deformation of the cartilage surface in response to stress by shifting in and out of the cartilage matrix.[13] Water also provides nutrition and oxygen to the chondrocytes, allowing them to synthesize proteoglycans and collagen. A physiologic tidemark exists at the demarcation between the deep articular cartilage layer and the underlying calcified layer. An avascular articular cartilage that sustains a superficial laceration that does not cross the tidemark will cause chondrocytes to proliferate but not heal. Deep lacerations that cross the tidemark into the vascular subchondral bone, however, may heal with fibrocartilage.[13,15,18] The articular cartilage stiffens with age due to a relative increase in protein content compared to water content. This occurs as aging chondrocytes become larger and fail to reproduce resulting in the production of shortened CS chains. Shortened CS chains produce proteoglycan complexes with decreased mass and thus less water absorptive ability.[13]

Clinical Pearl

Deep lacerations extending across the avascular articular cartilage into the vascular subchondral bone may *heal* with less durable fibrocartilage, forming the basis for several surgical reparative techniques.

The fibrocartilage is primarily composed of type I collagen and is not as durable as the articular cartilage.[20] It can be produced by subchondral undifferentiated marrow mesenchymal stem cells that can differentiate into cells capable of producing a fibrocartilage matrix that can *fill in* articular cartilage defects in diarthrodial joints. The meniscal fibrocartilage, however, is supplied by an extensive paramedical microvascular plexus, which runs circumferentially and extends to supply 10%–30% of the peripheral meniscus.[33] The remainder of the periphery remains avascular, which influences surgical repair considerations.

9.3 HISTORY AND PHYSICAL EXAM

Articular cartilage injury can be caused by an acute injury that results in a focal chondral or osteochondral injury, or from chronic subacute injuries or conditions that result in degenerative lesions. Damage can occur in isolation or in association with other intra-articular injuries.[20] Details of the onset and mechanism of joint injury, prior history of injury or surgery, provocative and palliative activities, effusion, instability, or mechanical symptoms will aid in a thorough work-up.

Clinical Pearl

Joint-specific physical examination should focus on the disruption of joint mechanical properties.

Physical exam of a cartilage is joint specific versus cartilage specific and should include evaluation of alignment, range of motion, swelling, effusion, stability, strength, and neurovascular status. Particular attention is required to evaluate for disruption of mechanical properties of the joint to include crepitus, catching, locking, or grinding that can occur from articular irregularities.[20]

9.4 DIAGNOSTIC PROCEDURES AND IMAGING

Plain radiographs are used to rule out fractures, identify osteochondral lesions, identify intra-articular loose bodies, assess limb alignment, and detect degenerative changes. Typical radiographic evaluation of articular surfaces should include a minimum of both posterior–anterior and 45° lateral views. Weight-bearing joints should be viewed posteriorly–anteriorly to better assess joint space narrowing (JSN).[35] Often addition of joint-specific views is required to better assess subchondral sclerosis, osteophytes, and cysts, allowing grading of chondral injury. Damage to cartilage is difficult to be directly assessed by radiograph since the hyaline articular cartilage does not contain calcium and is therefore not visualized.[1]

Computed tomography may be used to assess lesions associated with osseous involvement.

Magnetic resonance imaging (MRI) is considered the gold standard to evaluate articular cartilage and identify subchondral edema and can be useful in the assessment of ligaments and menisci but can underestimate the degree of cartilage abnormalities seen during arthroscopy.[32]

Arthroscopic evaluation remains the most accurate way to asses for location, depth, size, shape, and stability of chondral or osteochondral defect of the articular surface.[20]

The Modified International Cartilage Repair Society (ICRS) classification system can be used to describe lesions both arthroscopically and by advanced radiologic imaging tchniques[14] (see Table 9.2).

Clinical Pearl

- Articular cartilage appears gray on both T1- and T2-weighted images.
- Fibrocartilage appears dark on both T1- and T2-weighted images.

TABLE 9.2
Modified International Cartilage Repair Society (ICRS) Classification System for Chondral Injury

Grade of Injury	Modified ICRS System
Grade 0	Normal cartilage
Grade I	Superficial fissuring
Grade II	< ½ cartilage depth
Grade III	> ½ cartilage depth up to subchondral plate
Grade IV	Through subchondral plate, exposing subchondral bone

Source: Mainil-Varlet, P. et al., *J. Bone Joint Surg. Am. Vol.*, 85-A(Suppl 2), 45, 2003.

9.5 COMMON CARTILAGE PATHOLOGIC CONDITIONS

9.5.1 Focal Chondral Defects

Localized full thickness loss of articular cartilage with exposed subchondral bone, most often occurring in the hip. Typically, this is a result of a direct blow to the greater trochanter with a transfer of forces from the femoral head to the acetabulum, or from shear and/or rotational forces in the knee most commonly involving the medial femoral condyle.[49]

9.5.2 Apophyseal Injuries

Several areas of traction apophyses can occur whose muscle attaches to bone. They are typically present in the hip and pelvis in the skeletally immature with the ischial tuberosity being the most commonly involved region. This is often seen in avid adolescent runners and most often respond to conservative treatment[49] (see Table 9.3).

9.5.3 Femoroacetabular Impingement

Femoroacetabular impingement (FAI) is a condition in which abnormal contact exists between the femoral head–neck junction and the acetabulum that results in injury to the articular cartilage and labrum of the hip. The location of the pathology determines one of two types of deformity. A Cam-type femoral deformity is a *pistol grip* deformity of the femoral neck, which decreases the head–neck offset leading to an abutment of this region with the normal acetabulum. Conversely, a pincer-type acetabular deformity is created by increased acetabular retroversion leading to the abutment of the normal femoral head–neck junction on the acetabular rim.[49] Correction of structural abnormalities is increasingly becoming the standard treatment for FAI. Recent studies have shown that acetabular labral preservation and repair appear to provide superior results when compared to debridement alone.[21]

Clinical Pearl

Two types of FAI deformities are as follows:

1. Cam-type femoral neck deformity
2. Pincer-type acetabular deformity

9.5.4 Osteochondroses

Plural of osteochondrosis, these are a group of articular and nonarticular cartilage disease processes in children and adolescents (see Table 9.4).

9.5.5 Osteoarthritis

OA is a degenerative disease of the articular cartilage that occurs as a result of an age-related decrease in proteoglycan content.[39] With less water-absorptive proteoglycan present, there is a resultant decreased matrix water content allowing collagen to become more susceptible to degradation and degeneration.[39,50] Diagnosis is confirmed by radiologic evidence of JSN, subchondral sclerosis (increased bone formation around the joint), subchondral cyst formation, and the presence of osteophytes.[3]

TABLE 9.3
Traction Apophysis of the Hip

Traction Apophysis	Muscle Attachments
Iliac crest	Internal and external obliques
Anterior superior iliac crest (ASIS)	Sartorius and tensor fascia lata
Anterior inferior iliac crest (AIIS)	Rectus femoris
Ischial tuberosity	Hamstrings
Greater trochanter	Abductors
Lesser trochanter	Iliopsoas

Source: Reprinted from Netter's Sports Medicine, Turman, K.A.H.J. and Miller, M.D., in: *Netter's Sports Medicine*, Madden, C.C.P.M. and Young, C.C., eds., 2010, pp. 438–444, Saunders/Elsevier, Philadelphia, PA, with permission from Elsevier.

Clinical Pearl

Classic radiologic signs of OA are as follows:

1. JSN
2. Subchondral sclerosis
3. Subchondral cysts
4. Osteophytes

9.6 TREATMENT CONSIDERATIONS AND PROGNOSIS

Initial conservative treatment of articular cartilage injuries include activity modification, nonsteroidal anti-inflammatory drugs (NSAIDS), supplemental oral glucosamine and CS, corticosteroid injections, and consideration of viscosupplementaiton.[19] Those who exhibit persistent loss of mechanical function, mechanical locking, catching, or laxity despite nonsurgical management should be considered for surgical intervention.[20] The knee is the most common area for cartilage restoration, though ankle and knee problems may also be treated.

Meniscal fibrocartilage arthroscopic surgical repair has become one of the most common orthopedic surgical procedures in the United States[24] with nonoperative treatment management directed only toward less active patients with minor symptoms.

9.6.1 Chondroitin Sulfate

CS belongs to the glycosaminoglycan family and is a major component of articular cartilage. On OA joint tissues, CS has been shown to modify the chondrocyte death process, to improve the anabolic/catabolic balance of the extracellular

TABLE 9.4
Osteochondroses

Disorder	Location Affected	Presentation	Course and Treatment
Freiberg's infraction	Second metatarsal head	• Commonly seen in skeletally immature females. • Caused by direct or repetitive microtrauma.	• Self-limited • Conservative treatment
Kohler's disease	Tarsal navicular	• Typically seen in childhood. • Idiopathic osteonecrosis.	• Self-limited • Conservative treatment
Panner's disease	Elbow	• Results from a lateral compression overuse injury. • Formation occurs when an avascular segment develops followed by subsequent revascularization over time.	• Self-limited • Conservative treatment
Kienbock's disease	Lunate	• Vascular necrosis and collapse as a result of overuse and repetitive compressive loading of the wrist and ulnar negative variance.	• Surgical intervention required
Osgood–Schlatter disease	Patellar tendon insertion at the tibial tuberosity	• A traction apophysis in the skeletally immature.	• Self-limited • Conservative treatment
Sinding–Larsen–Johansson syndrome	Patellar tendon origin at the inferior pole of the patella	• A traction apophysis in the skeletally immature.	• Self-limited • Conservative treatment
Sever's disease	Achilles tendon insertion on the calcaneal tuberosity	• Skeletally immature patients during a period of rapid growth. • Occurs as a consequence of traction on the calcaneal apophysis from the gastrocsoleus complex.	• Self-limited • Conservative treatment
Osteochondritis dissecans	Can occur anywhere, commonly on the lateral aspect of the medial femoral condyle or talar dome	• More common in children and teenagers. • Result of direct trauma creating a localized separation of subchondral bone form overlying the articular cartilage, which then becomes lodged within the joint.	• Surgical intervention often required

Source: Reprinted from Netter's Sports Medicine, Turman, K.A.H.J. and Miller, M.D., in: *Netter's Sports Medicine*, Madden, C.C.P.M. and Young, C.C., eds., 2010, pp. 438–444, Saunders/Elsevier, Philadelphia, PA, with permission from Elsevier.

cartilage matrix, to reduce some proinflammatory and catabolic factors, and to reduce the resorptive properties of subchondral bone osteoblasts.[8,40] Moreover, meta-analyses of randomized placebo-controlled trials in knee OA patients have demonstrated the efficacy of CS to relieve OA joint pain.[37,41,45] CS at a dose of 800 mg orally once daily has been shown to slow significantly the rate of JSN over a period of 2 years in patients with symptomatic radiographic knee OA.[28,31,36,42]

Clinical Pearl

Eight hundred milligrams of CS orally once daily may slow JSN.

9.6.2 Arthroscopic Debridement and Lavage

Considered the first-line surgical intervention in a patient with symptomatic articular cartilage injury,[20] arthroscopic debridement and lavage allows for diagnostic direct visualization of the chondral injury and the remainder of the joint. As a therapeutic intervention, arthroscopic debridement and lavage provides for removal of degenerative debris, loose nonviable chondral fragments, and lavage of associated inflammatory cytokines,[2] which has shown to give at minimum a 50%–70% short-term benefit.[2,23] This can be of particular benefit with in-season athletes with a priority of rapid recovery and return to play. Over time however, the therapeutic benefits diminish while the diagnostic information obtained can continue to be used to guide future treatment decisions.[11,29,30,46,48]

9.6.3 Fragmentation Fixation

There are several variables that must be accounted for when choosing fragmentation fixation as a therapeutic intervention for successful articular cartilage osteochondritis dissecans (OCD) repair. The size, shape, location, condition, and adequacy of subchondral bone attached to the OCD all must be taken into consideration.[20] Arthroscopically, the defect and the fragment are prepped by debriding the fibrocartilage at the base of the lesion, microfracturing of the base to promote bleeding, and reduction of the fragment anatomically into the bed followed by rigid compression fixation by one of several techniques. Success has been reported in patients up to 90% depending on the fixation method used.[1,2]

9.6.4 Marrow-Stimulation Techniques

Mesenchymal progenator stem cell can be delivered to the articular cartilage defect bed and can subsequently aid in the formation of fibrocartilage-like repair tissue from these cells. There are a number of marrow-stimulation techniques that may be employed. Ultimately, the penetration of the calcified cartilage layer into the subchondral bone by arthroscopic drilling, abrasion, or microfracture allows for the migration of mesenchymal stem cells to the articular surface.[20] The resultant fibrocartilage repair tissue is less durable than the original articular cartilage, and therefore, best results are achieved in small defects with low demand placed on them physically by the patient.[1,2]

9.6.5 Osteochondral Autograph

The use of articular cartilage and bone plugs from load-sparing donor sites to areas of symptomatic chondral defect is known as an osteochondral autograft. Transplant of multiple viable hyaline cartilage plugs can be performed in a single arthroscopic operation and allow for a relatively brief period of rehabilitation.[1,22,34] Outcomes have been promising showing greater than 90% good to excellent results.[26,27] Limitations, however, include availability of low-contact harvest areas, potential damage to donor sites, and the potential for donor plug incongruity resulting in uneven articular surfaces. This may cause mechanical obstacles to the proper functioning of the joint postoperatively.

9.6.6 Osteochondral Allograft

Osteochondral allograft from a fresh cadaveric source of intact viable articular cartilage and associated subchondral bone is placed into an articular cartilage defect. This technique provides the ability to replace large defects in a single procedure without potential to create donor-site morbidity. As with any allograft there is the potential risk of immunologic rejection, incomplete graft incorporation, and potential disease transmission.[6,9,16] Despite the relative expense of the procedure and frequent requirement to perform this as an open surgical procedure versus arthroscopically, successful outcome rates of 91% at 5 years and 84% at 10 years have been documented.[1,5,51]

9.6.7 Autologous Chondrocyte Implantation

Use of autologous chondrocytes avoids the risk of immunologic rejection and disease transmission and has the ability to fill large articular cartilage defects with hyaline-like cartilage rather than fibrocartilage. The procedure, however, is demanding and quite expensive, requiring a two-stage procedure during which chondrocytes are harvested, cultured in the lab for expansion of the chondrocyte cell line, and transplanted beneath a periosteal or collagen matrix patch.[20] Studies have demonstrated varied results, but some studies have documented up to a 92% success rate in patients 10–20 years after surgery.[44]

9.6.8 Meniscal Operative Repair

The determinants of successful outcomes of a torn meniscal repair include location and configuration of the tear, patient age, chronicity, and underlying condition of the joint.[33,43] Classic criteria for meniscal repair include complete vertical tear >10 mm in length, location within the peripheral 10%–30% of the meniscus (or within 3–4 mm of the vascular meniscosynovial junction), and displacement of no more than 3–5 mm on arthroscopic probing.[25,33] Partial meniscectomy is indicated for complete, oblique, radial, horizontal, degenerative, or complex tears[33] with the goal of removing nonfunctional tissue, maximizing meniscal preservation, and creating a stable configuration of the remaining tissue.[43]

TABLE 9.5
SORT: Key Recommendations for Practice

Clinical Recommendation	Evidence Rating	References
Acetabular labral preservation and repair in FAI provides superior results when compared to debridement alone.	A	[21]
Early treatment of fibrocartilage meniscal peripheral tears is improved with surgical repair performed within the first 4 months from the time of injury.	A	[25]
CS at a dose of 800 mg orally once daily can significantly slow the rate of joint space narrowing over a period of 2 years in patients with symptomatic radiographic knee OA.	A	[28,31,36,42]
In knee OA, corticosteroids have better short-term response rate and equal to hyaluronic acid in the intermediate four to eight weeks range, but is inferior to hyaluronic acid after eight weeks from the time of injection.	A	[7]
Arthroscopic debridement and lavage provides good short-term improvement in symptomatic articular cartilage injury.	A	[2,23]
Autologous chondrocyte implantation has shown good improvement in the long term 10–20 years after surgery.	B	[1,5,51]

9.6.9 Intra-Articular Injections

The use of corticosteroids or hyaluronic acid supplementation for treating OA is commonly used to allow symptomatic relief of pain. Intra-articular corticosteroids typically provide 4–8 weeks of short-term relief, particularly in the knee.[4,47] Repeat injections are possible in the same joint but limited to four injections annulally.[12] Viscosupplementation with intra-articular hyaluronic acid injections is widely used for OA of the knee despite debate of early studies. Subsequent trials have shown treatment effectiveness lasting up to 4 months of pain reduction, though cost remains the biggest drawback (Table 9.5).[10]

REFERENCES

1. Articular Cartilage Restoration. American Academy of Orthopaedic Surgeons OrthoInfo. http://orthoinfo.aaos.org/topic.cfm?topic=a00422. Accessed April 20, 2014.
2. Alford JW, Cole BJ. Cartilage restoration, part 2: Techniques, outcomes, and future directions. *The American Journal of Sports Medicine.* March 2005;33(3):443–460.
3. Altman RD. Osteoarthritis: Joint Disorders. Merck Sharp & Dohme Corp; 2013. http://www.merckmanuals.com/professional/musculoskeletal-and-connective-tissue-disorders/joint-disorders/osteoarthritis-oa?qt=&sc=&alt=. Accessed April 16, 2014.
4. Arroll B, Goodyear-Smith F. Corticosteroid injections for osteoarthritis of the knee: Meta-analysis. *BMJ: British Medical Journal.* April 10, 2004;328(7444):869.
5. Aubin PP, Cheah HK, Davis AM, Gross AE. Long-term followup of fresh femoral osteochondral allografts for posttraumatic knee defects. *Clinical Orthopaedics and Related Research.* October 2001(391 Suppl):S318–S327.
6. Bakay A, Csonge L, Papp G, Fekete L. Osteochondral resurfacing of the knee joint with allograft. Clinical analysis of 33 cases. *International Orthopaedics.* 1998;22(5):277–281.
7. Bannuru RR, Natov NS, Obadan IE, Price LL, Schmid CH, McAlindon TE. Therapeutic trajectory of hyaluronic acid versus corticosteroids in the treatment of knee osteoarthritis: A systematic review and meta-analysis. *Arthritis and Rheumatism.* December 15, 2009;61(12):1704–1711.
8. Bassleer CT, Combal JP, Bougaret S, Malaise M. Effects of chondroitin sulfate and interleukin-1 beta on human articular chondrocytes cultivated in clusters. *Osteoarthritis and cartilage/OARS, Osteoarthritis Research Society.* May 1998;6(3):196–204.
9. Beaver RJ, Mahomed M, Backstein D, Davis A, Zukor DJ, Gross AE. Fresh osteochondral allografts for posttraumatic defects in the knee. A survivorship analysis. *The Journal of Bone and Joint Surgery. British Volume.* January 1992;74(1):105–110.
10. Bellamy N, Campbell J, Robinson V, Gee T, Bourne R, Wells G. Viscosupplementation for the treatment of osteoarthritis of the knee. *The Cochrane Database of Systematic Reviews.* 2006(2):CD005321.
11. Bernard J, Lemon M, Patterson MH. Arthroscopic washout of the knee—A 5-year survival analysis. *The Knee.* June 2004;11(3):233–235.
12. Bettencourt RB, Linder MM. Arthrocentesis and therapeutic joint injection: An overview for the primary care physician. *Primary Care.* December 2010;37(4):691–702, v.
13. Brinker MR. Joints. In: Miller MD, Brinker, Mark R. (eds.). *Review of Orthopaedics*, 3rd edn. Philadelphia, PA: Saunders; 2000: pp. 40–60.
14. Brittberg M. Evaluation of cartilage injuries adn cartilage repair. *Osteologie.* 2000(9):17–25.
15. Buckwalter JA RL, Hunziker EB. Articular cartilage: composition and structure. In: Woo SLBJ (ed.). *Injury and Repair of the Musckuloskeletal Soft Tissues.* Park Ridge, IL: American Academy of Orthopeaedic Surgeons; 1988: pp. 405–425.
16. Chu CR, Convery FR, Akeson WH, Meyers M, Amiel D. Articular cartilage transplantation. Clinical results in the knee. *Clinical Orthopaedics and Related Research.* March 1999(360):159–168.
17. Cole BJ FR, Levy AS, Zaslav KR. Management of a 37-year old man with recurrent knee pain. *Journal of Clinical Outcomes Manage.* 1999;6(6):46–57.
18. Curl WW, Krome J, Gordon ES, Rushing J, Smith BP, Poehling GG. Cartilage injuries: A review of 31,516 knee arthroscopies. *Arthroscopy: The Journal of Arthroscopic & Related Surgery: Official Publication of the Arthroscopy Association of North America and the International Arthroscopy Association.* August 1997;13(4):456–460.
19. Daher RJ, Chahine NO, Greenberg AS, Sgaglione NA, Grande DA. New methods to diagnose and treat cartilage degeneration. *Nature Reviews: Rheumatology.* November 2009; 5(11):599–607.
20. Dhawan AKV, Cole BJ. Articular Cartilage Injury. In: O'Connor FG (ed.). *ACSM's Sports Medicine: A Comprehensive Review.* Philadelphia, PA: Wolters Kluwer Health/Lippincott Williams & Wilkins; 2013: pp. 30–38.
21. Fayad TE, Khan MA, Haddad FS. Femoroacetabular impingement: An arthroscopic solution. *The Bone & Joint Journal.* November 2013;95-B(11 Suppl A):26–30.
22. Feczko P, Hangody L, Varga J et al. Experimental results of donor site filling for autologous osteochondral mosaicplasty. *Arthroscopy: The Journal of Arthroscopic & Related Surgery: Official Publication of the Arthroscopy Association of North America and the International Arthroscopy Association.* September 2003;19(7):755–761.
23. Friedman MJ, Berasi CC, Fox JM, Del Pizzo W, Snyder SJ, Ferkel RD. Preliminary results with abrasion arthroplasty in the osteoarthritic knee. *Clinical Orthopaedics and Related Research.* January–February 1984(182):200–205.
24. Greis PE, Bardana DD, Holmstrom MC, Burks RT. Meniscal injury: I. Basic science and evaluation. *The Journal of the American Academy of Orthopaedic Surgeons.* May–June 2002;10(3):168–176.
25. Greis PE, Holmstrom MC, Bardana DD, Burks RT. Meniscal injury: II. Management. *The Journal of the American Academy of Orthopaedic Surgeons.* May–June 2002;10(3):177–187.
26. Hangody L, Feczko P, Bartha L, Bodo G, Kish G. Mosaicplasty for the treatment of articular defects of the knee and ankle. *Clinical Orthopaedics and Related Research.* October 2001(391 Suppl):S328–336.
27. Hangody L, Kish G, Karpati Z, Udvarhelyi I, Szigeti I, Bely M. Mosaicplasty for the treatment of articular cartilage defects: Application in clinical practice. *Orthopedics.* July 1998;21(7):751–756.
28. Hochberg MC, Zhan M, Langenberg P. The rate of decline of joint space width in patients with osteoarthritis of the knee: A systematic review and meta-analysis of randomized placebo-controlled trials of chondroitin sulfate. *Current Medical Research and Opinion.* November 2008;24(11):3029–3035.

29. Hubbard MJ. Arthroscopic surgery for chondral flaps in the knee. *The Journal of Bone and Joint Surgery: British volume.* November 1987;69(5):794–796.
30. Jackson RW. Meniscal and articular cartilage injury in sport. *Journal of the Royal College of Surgeons of Edinburgh.* 1989;34(6 Suppl):S15–S17.
31. Kahan A, Uebelhart D, De Vathaire F, Delmas PD, Reginster JY. Long-term effects of chondroitins 4 and 6 sulfate on knee osteoarthritis: The study on osteoarthritis progression prevention, a two-year, randomized, double-blind, placebo-controlled trial. *Arthritis and Rheumatism.* February 2009;60(2):524–533.
32. Khanna AJ, Cosgarea AJ, Mont MA et al. Magnetic resonance imaging of the knee. Current techniques and spectrum of disease. *The Journal of Bone and Joint Surgery. American volume.* 2001;83-A (Suppl 2 Pt 2):128–141.
33. Klimkiewicz JJ, Shaffer B. Meniscal surgery 2002 update: Indications and techniques for resection, repair, regeneration, and replacement. *Arthroscopy: the Journal of Arthroscopic & Related Surgery: Official Publication of the Arthroscopy Association of North America and the International Arthroscopy Association.* November–December 2002;18(9 Suppl 2):14–25.
34. LaPrade RF, Botker JC. Donor-site morbidity after osteochondral autograft transfer procedures. *Arthroscopy: The Journal of Arthroscopic & Related Surgery: Official Publication of the Arthroscopy Association of North America and the International Arthroscopy Association.* September 2004;20(7):e69–e73.
35. Leach RE, Gregg T, Siber FJ. Weight-bearing radiography in osteoarthritis of the knee. *Radiology.* November 1970;97(2):265–268.
36. Lee YH, Woo JH, Choi SJ, Ji JD, Song GG. Effect of glucosamine or chondroitin sulfate on the osteoarthritis progression: A meta-analysis. *Rheumatology International.* January 2010;30(3):357–363.
37. Leeb BF, Schweitzer H, Montag K, Smolen JS. A metaanalysis of chondroitin sulfate in the treatment of osteoarthritis. *The Journal of Rheumatology.* January 2000;27(1):205–211.
38. Mainil-Varlet P, Aigner T, Brittberg M et al. Histological assessment of cartilage repair: A report by the Histology Endpoint Committee of the International Cartilage Repair Society (ICRS). *The Journal of Bone and Joint Surgery: American volume.* 2003;85-A(Suppl 2):45–57.
39. Maroudas AI. Balance between swelling pressure and collagen tension in normal and degenerate cartilage. *Nature.* April 29, 1976;260(5554):808–809.
40. Martel-Pelletier J, Kwan Tat S, Pelletier JP. Effects of chondroitin sulfate in the pathophysiology of the osteoarthritic joint: A narrative review. *Osteoarthritis and Cartilage/ OARS, Osteoarthritis Research Society.* June 2010;18(Suppl 1): S7–S11.
41. McAlindon TE, LaValley MP, Gulin JP, Felson DT. Glucosamine and chondroitin for treatment of osteoarthritis: A systematic quality assessment and meta-analysis. *Journal of the American Medical Association.* March 15, 2000;283(11):1469–1475.
42. Michel BA, Stucki G, Frey D, et al. Chondroitins 4 and 6 sulfate in osteoarthritis of the knee: A randomized, controlled trial. *Arthritis and Rheumatism.* March 2005;52(3):779–786.
43. O'Connor FG. *ACSM's Sports Medicine: A Comprehensive Review.* Philadelphia, PA: Wolters Kluwer Health/Lippincott Williams & Wilkins; 2013.
44. Peterson L, Vasiliadis HS, Brittberg M, Lindahl A. Autologous chondrocyte implantation: A long-term follow-up. *The American Journal of Sports Medicine.* June 2010;38(6):1117–1124.
45. Richy F, Bruyere O, Ethgen O, Cucherat M, Henrotin Y, Reginster JY. Structural and symptomatic efficacy of glucosamine and chondroitin in knee osteoarthritis: A comprehensive meta-analysis. *Archives of Internal Medicine.* July 14, 2003;163(13):1514–1522.
46. Sprague NF, 3rd. Arthroscopic debridement for degenerative knee joint disease. *Clinical Orthopaedics and Related Research.* October 1981(160):118–123.
47. Stephens MB, Beutler AI, O'Connor FG. Musculoskeletal injections: A review of the evidence. *American Family Physician.* October 15, 2008;78(8):971–976.
48. Timoney JM, Kneisl JS, Barrack RL, Alexander AH. Arthroscopy update #6. Arthroscopy in the osteoarthritic knee. Long-term follow-up. *Orthopaedic Review.* April 1990;19(4):371–373, 376–379.
49. Turman KAHJ, Miller MD. Netter's sports medicine. In: Madden CCPM, Young CC (eds.). *Netter's Sports Medicine.* Philadelphia, PA: Saunders/Elsevier; 2010: pp. 438–444.
50. Venn M, Maroudas A. Chemical composition and swelling of normal and osteoarthrotic femoral head cartilage. I. Chemical composition. *Annals of the Rheumatic Diseases.* April 1977;36(2):121–129.
51. Bugbee WD. Fresh osteochondral allografting. *Operative Techniques in Sport Medicine.* 2000;8(2):158–162.

10 Muscle Injury

Michelle E. Szczepanik and Christopher D. Meyering

CONTENTS

TABLE 10.1
Key Clinical Considerations

1. Type I myofibers are slow-twitch, have numerous mitochondria, use oxidative metabolism for energy, and are fatigue-resistant.
2. Type II myofibers are fast-twitch, utilize glycogen stores for brief-duration intensity activity, have a higher velocity and force of contraction, and are susceptible to fatigue.
3. The greatest chance of injury to a muscle occurs at the myotendinous junction during an eccentric contraction.
4. The most common muscle injury in athletics is a muscle strain.
5. Biarticular muscles span two joints and are more susceptible to a strain injury.
6. Muscle strains are graded and typically do not require surgery.
7. Treatment principles involve NSAIDs and RICE in the first 72 hours following injury.
8. Delayed-onset muscle soreness most commonly occurs in fast-twitch muscle fibers and after performing eccentric muscle exercises.
9. Muscle contusions can result in myositis ossificans in some instances.

10.1 INTRODUCTION

Injury to muscles in sports is a relatively common occurrence regardless of the type of activity and level of participation. Even though most muscular injuries are self-limiting, they can drastically affect athletic performance making prevention and treatment extremely important in the athlete's care. Remembering how muscles are composed and the differences in types and function helps clinicians understand how muscles become damaged and how to best repair them (Table 10.1).

All muscle injuries will follow a typical pattern of repair from the initial injury to recovery. There are generally accepted guidelines for muscle injury management regardless of the type of injury. In addition to a discussion on general treatment guidelines, we will also review the specific types of injuries and patterns such as muscle strain, the most frequently encountered muscle injury, as well as contusions, cramps, and delayed-onset muscle soreness (DOMS).

10.2 MUSCLE PHYSIOLOGY

Each muscle is made up of multiple muscle bundles called fascicles that in turn contain the basic unit of muscle, the muscle fiber. Each muscle fiber contains many myofibrils that are made up of a number of sarcomeres, the functional unit of muscle. Within the sarcomere, there are I bands that are attached to Z lines and composed of thin actin filaments, and there are H bands that are made up of thick myosin filaments that slide over the I bands during a contraction[22] (see Figure 10.1).

Every action of movement involves several steps for a muscle fiber to contract. The first step consists of a nerve impulse traveling along the length of the nerve to the skeletal muscle ending at the motor end plate, a special synapse between the muscle and nerve. That stimulus in turn results in the release of acetylcholine by the presynaptic axons into the synaptic clefts. Acetylcholine binds to acetylcholine receptors on the postjunctional folds of the myofibers and causes depolarization of the muscle cell. With depolarization, the electrical impulse passes into the interior of the cell causing the release of calcium from the sarcoplasmic reticulum. Calcium then binds to troponin on the thin filaments that change the position of the tropomyosin. The position change of the tropomyosin exposes the actin filament on the I band leading to an interaction of the myosin, or thick

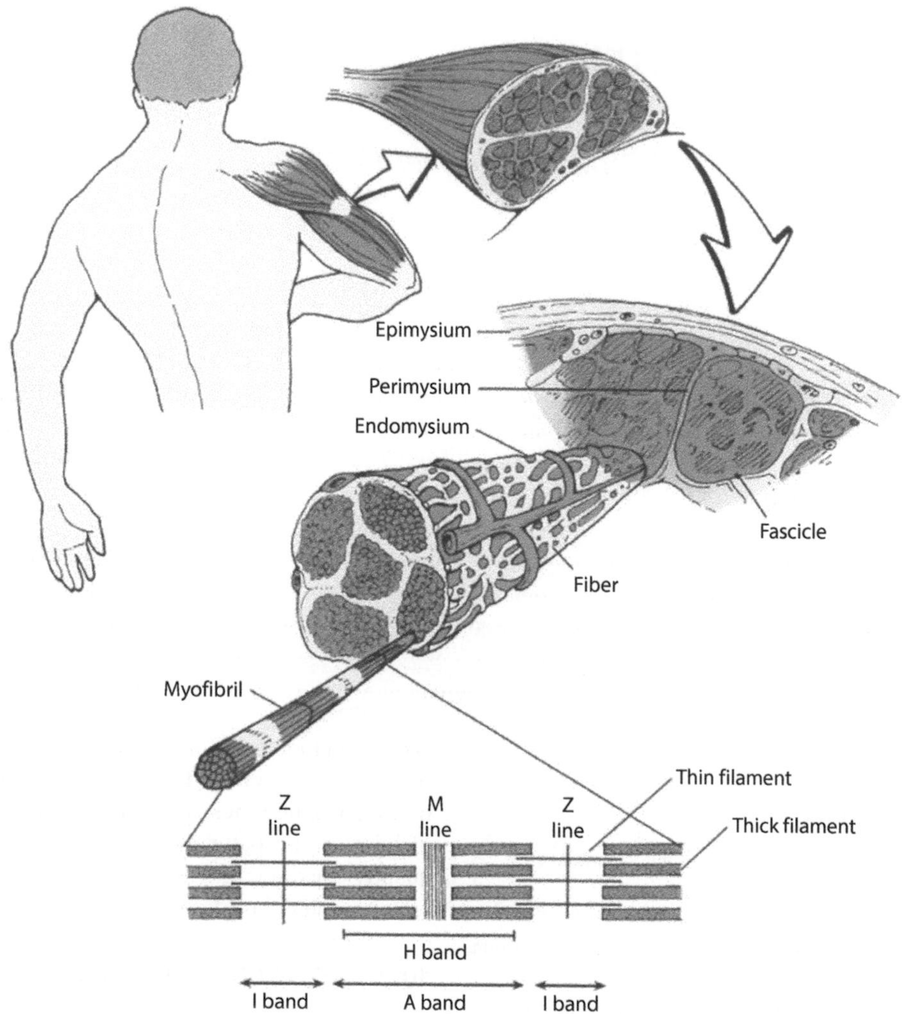

FIGURE 10.1 Skeletal muscle architecture. (Reprinted from *Fundamentals of Orthopaedics: Review of Orthopaedics*, 1st edn., Brinker, M.R. and Miller, M.D., 1999, Philadelphia, PA, with permission from Elsevier.)

filaments in the H band, and the filaments then slide past each other to shorten the muscle fiber.[2,15] All of the filament interaction process is driven by the breakdown of adenosine triphosphate (ATP).

10.3 MUSCLE COMPOSITION

The complex of a muscle fiber and motor neuron is called a motor unit. There are differing numbers of muscle fibers in a motor unit as well as varying numbers of motor units per skeletal muscle depending on the function of the particular muscle. As an example, if fine motor control is the primary function, then there will be fewer numbers of muscle fibers in the motor unit. Conversely, if the muscle is meant for strength and larger movements like the quadriceps, then there are many muscle fibers contained in the motor unit.[2,15]

Muscles come in different shapes and sizes based upon in their function within the body. Biarticular muscles like the biceps femoris or the rectus femoris span two joints making them more susceptible to a strain injury.[2,9] Uniarticular muscles, on the other hand, cross a single joint, are typically located close to bone, and have a responsibility in postural maintenance.[9] There are also muscles with long tendons like the plantaris or muscles with long muscle bellies like the sartorius. There are unipennate muscles that have fibers aligned in a linear fashion versus bipennate muscles that insert at an angle thereby increasing muscle fiber density and contractile muscle forces as well.[12]

Clinical Pearl

Biarticular muscles span two joints and are more susceptible to a strain injury.

10.4 MUSCLE CONTRACTION

There are three different types of muscle contraction: isometric, isotonic, and isokinetic. In isometric contractions, the muscle contracts but does not change its length such as pushing against an immoveable object or holding a weight in a steady position. In contrast, both isotonic and isokinetic contractions involve changing muscle length throughout the range of motion. In isotonic, the muscle tension is constant throughout the range of motion. In isokinetic, the muscle maximally contracts at a constant velocity over the full range of motion. Both isotonic and isokinetic have two phases of contraction as well: concentric and eccentric. Concentric contraction is when the muscle shortens while contracting as in performing a bicep curl. Eccentric contraction is when the muscle lengthens while contracting as when lowering the weight from a bicep curl. The greatest chance of injury to a muscle occurs during an eccentric contraction.[2,13,14,22]

Clinical Pearl

The greatest chance of injury to a muscle occurs during an eccentric contraction.

10.5 NUMBER/TYPES OF MUSCLE

Muscle fibers can also be classified as type I or type II based on their physiologic properties. Type I myofibers are called slow-twitch fibers because they have a slow contraction time and they generate less force than type II fibers. They have numerous mitochondria and intracellular lipids for oxidative metabolism which means they resist fatigue and are used for sustained, low-level activity. Type II myofibers are fast-twitch fibers that generate a higher velocity and force of contraction than type I, but they are less efficient and therefore are susceptible to fatigue. Type II muscle fibers are specialized for anaerobic metabolism and utilize glycogen stores for brief-duration intense activity.[2,9,15]

Clinical Pearl

Type I myofibers are slow-twitch, have numerous mitochondria, use oxidative metabolism for energy, and are fatigue-resistant.

Type II muscle fibers may be further divided into type IIa, which are oxidative glycolytic, and type IIb, which are glycolytic. Type IIa fibers have some aerobic capacity and have some fatigue resistance but generate less power than type IIb. Type IIb fibers generate the most force but fatigue the quickest. Although muscles are composed of a mixture of type I and type II muscle fibers, training can change the balance of muscle fiber types in a given muscle based on demands.[15]

Clinical Pearl

Type II myofibers are fast-twitch, utilize glycogen stores for brief-duration intensity activity, have a higher velocity and force of contraction, and are susceptible to fatigue.

10.6 MUSCLE INJURY

Whether injury occurs to a muscle by strain, contusion, or other modality, the same injury and repair process occur. This three-step process of repair following the injury includes the reparative phase, muscle degeneration, and fibrosis development. Healing results in connective tissue scar formation at the site of muscle injury.

The reparative process of muscle injury involves degeneration of muscle tissue, hemorrhage, and inflammation. This stage occurs in the first few days following injury and involves inflammatory cells such as neutrophils, macrophages, and fibroblasts. Neutrophils present at the injury site trigger the release of cytokines resulting in the formation of oxygen free radicals that induce local inflammation. Macrophages phagocytose the injured tissue and are followed by fibroblasts that proliferate and generate new collagen.[18]

The second phase of muscle regeneration involves vascularization of the injured area with capillary infiltration and begins about a week after the injury; this phase takes a few weeks before it is complete. The last stage of fibrosis development starts about 2–3 weeks after the injury and is characterized by collagen formation at the site of injury.[2,9,15,18] Newly formed fibers are aligned based upon the stressors on the tissue.

On the periphery of the muscle fibers are satellite cells that function as a stem cell in response to mechanical or chemical insults. When a muscle is injured, satellite cells are activated through various growth factors and differentiate into myoblasts. These myoblasts will then fuse together into multinucleated muscle fibers and function to replace the damaged muscle tissue.[2,9,15,18]

10.7 GENERAL TREATMENT PRINCIPLES FOR MUSCLE INJURY

Few well-designed studies exist regarding the treatment of muscle injuries although there are several generally accepted management principles. Understanding the previously mentioned phases of muscle regeneration helps guide the provider with not only what treatments to use but also what treatments may potentially cause harm or interference with healing. The exact time to full recovery may vary with each athlete, but the steps to return to activity typically follow the same pattern.

Treatment in the first few days after injury involves a short course of NSAIDs and utilizing the RICE principle: relative rest to prevent continued pain and injury, ice to decrease pain, compression to prevent large hematoma formation, and elevation of the affected area to decrease the amount of swelling. A brief period of immobility, usually 72 hours or less, assists with decreasing the size of swelling and hematoma formation. Although the early use of NSAIDs seems to help with earlier return to activity, there is debate concerning the overall benefits as the inhibition of chemotaxis may affect the recurrence of injury.[11,18] NSAID use after the acute phase of injury is considered a hindrance to recovery.[18,23]

Following the initial period of immobility of about 3 days, early mobilization appears to induce a more rapid and concentrated capillary ingrowth to the injured area and more parallel orientation of muscle fiber regeneration when compared to immobilization.[18] The end benefit is a decreased rate of repeat injury. The underlying concept is preventing the injured muscle from overstretching and this can be done if the patient remains in the painless range of motion.

Return to sports-specific training is considered once the injured muscle can be stretched without pain to the same limit as the contralateral muscle and basic activities are also pain-free.[18] Steadily increasing the amount and intensity of activity helps prevent repeat injury. There are some studies to suggest that strengthening with eccentric exercises reduces the rate of reinjury.[4,5,10,13,27]

10.8 MUSCLE STRAIN

The most common muscle injury in sports is a muscle strain, which is a tear of the muscle sustained mostly commonly during an eccentric load. This can occur during sprinting, starting or stopping with running, cutting or quick change in direction, and jumping.[10,13] An athlete may feel a "pop" followed by pain and weakness of the affected muscle.[2,9] Risk factors for muscle strain include a previous muscle injury, muscle strength imbalance, muscle tightness or poor flexibility, improper warm-up, muscle fatigue, or overuse.[2,10,11]

At a cellular level, there is disruption of the myofibers, usually at the myotendinous junction, resulting in hemorrhage and inflammation. This injury is most often seen in biarthrodial muscles (cross two joints) such as the rectus femoris, biceps femoris, and gastrocnemius or in a muscle such as the adductor longus that has a complex architecture.[2] Most injuries occur at the myotendinous junction; however, any disruption of the muscle–tendon unit can be categorized as a strain.

Clinical Pearl

Most strain injuries occur at the myotendinous junction.

Muscle strains are classified into three grades. A grade I muscle strain is the mildest injury that consists of pain and partial disruption of muscle fibers but no loss of strength. Grade II is also a tear of some but not all muscle fibers; however, there is associated loss of strength and reduced movement due to pain. Grade III is the most severe with complete disruption of the muscle–tendon unit and loss of function[2,11,12] (see Table 10.2).

On clinical exam, there will be tenderness to palpation at the site of the muscle strain. With complete disruption as in a grade III strain, a defect may be palpable.[2,9] Ultrasound may be used to evaluate the degree of the strain; however, clinical exam is most important when determining the grade. MRI is usually not needed for the diagnosis.

TABLE 10.2
Classification of Muscle Strains

Grade I	Some disruption of muscle fibers and pain but no loss of strength.
Grade II	A tear of some but not all muscle fibers; however, there is associated loss of strength and reduced movement due to pain.
Grade III	Complete disruption of the muscle–tendon unit with loss of function.

Source: Bruckner, P. et al., eds, *Bruckner and Khan's Clinical Sports Medicine*, 4th edn., McGraw Hill Australia Pty Ltd, Sydney, New South Wales, Australia, 2012.

Treatment is directed at controlling the initial inflammatory response and preventing further tissue damage. Ice, compression, and short-term immobilization may help control the pain and inflammation. Other modalities such as therapeutic ultrasound and cryotherapy may be used although their exact mechanism in speeding recovery is not known.[18] After the initial period of immobilization, gentle range of motion exercises that avoid aggressive stretching are essential to limit adhesions and speed recovery. Surgery is usually not needed for a muscle strain except in some instances of complete avulsion of the muscle–tendon complex.[9] NSAID use continues to be debated regarding potential for delayed or incomplete healing. The general consensus is that a short course of NSAIDs may reduce inflammation and potentially speed functional recovery following an acute strain; however, prolonged use is not recommended.[24,25,26]

Once the injured muscle can be stretched to the same degree as the contralateral side, can go through basic movements without pain, and has returned strength, gradual return to play may be considered.[18] Scar formation following a strain may make the muscle more susceptible to future injury; therefore, strengthening following a muscle strain is essential in order to prevent reinjury. Multiple studies have shown a decrease in the recurrence of muscle strains with eccentric strengthening techniques.[4,5,10,13,27]

10.9 DELAYED-ONSET MUSCLE SORENESS

DOMS is classified as skeletal muscle pain that occurs 24–72 hours after unfamiliar physical activity. It most commonly occurs in the fast-type muscle fibers and after performing eccentric exercises.[3,6,9,20] At the cellular level, there is cytoskeletal disruption that creates an influx of intracellular calcium; this influx then induces myoprotein degeneration and the resultant inflammatory process stimulates nociceptors causing pain.[3,20,28]

Clinical Pearl

DOMS most commonly occurs in type II muscle fibers after eccentric exercises.

Pain and soreness intensity vary with DOMS and a patient will typically experience tenderness of the muscles, decreased joint range of motion, decreased muscle strength due to pain, and decreased force-generating capability of the muscle fibers. Although muscle enzyme serum levels may be elevated, no permanent muscle damage occurs and pain normally resolves within 5–7 days.

Over time, adaptation occurs and less soreness is generated with subsequent workouts. Treatment for DOMS consists of stopping the offending exercise, stretching the affected muscles, and performing gentle range of motion activities.[25] NSAIDs may be beneficial in the acute phase although their benefit may decline if used more than 72 hours after injury.[18,23]

10.10 MUSCLE CONTUSION

Most often seen in the lower extremity, muscle contusions are caused by contact from a direct force like a blunt object or another player.[1,11] Within hours following the trauma to the muscle, edema, inflammation, and hematoma formation develop. Symptoms include pain, swelling at site of impact, loss of range of motion if located near a joint, and sometimes a palpable mass. Diagnosis is often clinical but associated fracture may need to be ruled out.

Treatment is similar to the general treatment principles described previously with initial therapy involving RICE and less than 72 hours of immobilization with the muscle in a lengthened position, followed by early mobilization in a pain-free range. Prolonged immobilization appears to cause more muscle atrophy and slower restoration of the contused muscle with a delay in return of muscle activity.[16,17,19,29] Although corticosteroids and NSAIDs reduce inflammation, there is debate concerning delayed muscle regeneration and subsequent decreased tensile properties with their use.[8] Scar formation with a muscle contusion seems to be less than following a muscle strain.

10.11 MYOSITIS OSSIFICANS

Myositis ossificans is a rare complication, which involves heterotopic bone formation resulting from the hematoma after muscle contusion. In a study done at the U.S. Military Academy, researchers found that about 9% of muscle contusions resulted in myositis ossificans.[16,29] Although the etiology is unclear, there is an increased incidence in individuals with a higher degree of muscle contusion and those subjected to repetitive trauma.[7]

Symptoms include tenderness and swelling as seen with a muscle contusion, but there is also an increase in pain and warmth at the area plus a firm mass often palpable on exam. By about 1 month, abnormal bone formation can be seen on x-ray.[17] This heterotopic bone formation may remodel or absorb over the ensuing 3–12 months. Uncommonly, a mature bone persists and a patient has continued pain, swelling, weakness, or even loss of motion. In these instances, surgical intervention may be warranted; however, the ectopic bone should not be excised until osteoblastic activity has subsided and the ectopic bone has fully matured without an increased uptake on bone scan, typically 12–24 months.[9,18,21]

10.12 MUSCLE CRAMPS

A muscle cramp is the result of a painful, spasmodic, involuntary contraction of skeletal muscle that happens during or immediately after exercise.[30] The source of this abnormal muscle behavior seems to come from the nerve that supplies that muscle and these fatigue-induced alterations lead to muscle cramping.[9] Typically, the vulnerable muscle will be in a shortened position and twitch, often referred to as the "cramp-prone state." If activity continues, then cramping ensues, and the patient will experience a painful, hard, contracted muscle.[31]

The most common places for muscle cramping to occur are the lower extremity muscles like the gastrocnemius, quadriceps, or hamstrings although cramping can involve nearly any muscle in the body. Hydration status or metabolic abnormalities are often blamed for muscle cramping; however, dehydration and electrolyte imbalances are seldom the culprit. Rather, studies suggest that intrinsic risk factors such as a previous history of cramping or performance at an increased level of intensity or duration of exercise and extrinsic factors such as heat and humidity play a more important role.[31]

TABLE 10.3
SORT: Key Recommendations for Practice

Clinical Recommendation	Evidence Rating	References
There is a decrease in the recurrence of muscle strains with eccentric strengthening techniques.	B	[4,5,10,13,27]
The greatest chance of injury to a muscle occurs during an eccentric contraction.	A	[2,13,14,22]
NSAID use after the acute phase of injury is considered a hindrance to recovery.	B	[18,23]
Early use of NSAIDs may help with earlier return to activity, but the inhibition of chemotaxis needed for repair may affect the recurrence of injury.	B	[11,18]
After immobilization for 3 days, early mobilization appears to improve capillary ingrowth to the injured area and more parallel orientation of regenerated muscle fiber when compared to immobilization resulting in fewer repeat injuries.	B	[17,18]
Immobilization past 72 hours appears to cause more muscle atrophy and slower restoration of the contused muscle with a delay in return of muscle activity.	A	[16,17,19,29]

Treatment involves stopping the offending activity and passive stretch of the cramping muscle.[11,31] Fluids and electrolyte replacement continue to be used in the treatment of muscle cramps even though their role in this condition is controversial. Although a previous history of cramping in a muscle appears to be a risk factor for future episodes, frequent cramping or cramping in a muscle that is not exercising should prompt a work-up for a metabolic or endocrinologic abnormality (Table 10.3).

REFERENCES

1. Anderson JE. The satellite cell as a companion in skeletal muscle plasticity: Currency, conveyance, clue, connector and colander. *Journal of Experimental Biology.* 2006;209(Pt 12):2276–2292.
2. Armfield DR, Kim DH, Towers JD, Bradley JP, Robertson DD. Sports-related muscle injury in the lower extremity. *Clinical Sports and Medicine.* 2006;25(4):803–842.
3. Armstrong RB. Mechanisms of exercise-induced delayed onset muscular soreness: A brief review. *Medicne and Science Sports and Exercise.* 1984;16(6):529–538.
4. Arnason A, Andersen TE, Holme I, Engebretsen L, Bahr R. Prevention of hamstring strains in elite soccer: An intervention study. *Scandinavian Journal of Medical Science Sports.* 2008;18(1):40–48.
5. Askling C, Karlsson J, Thorstensson A. Hamstring injury occurrence in elite soccer players after preseason strength training with eccentric overload. *Scandinavian Journal of Medical Science Sports.* 2003;13(4):244–250.
6. Balnave CD, Thompson MW. Effect of training on eccentric exercise-induced muscle damage. *Journal of Applied Physiology.* 1993;75(4):1545–1551.
7. Beiner JM, Jokl P. Muscle contusion injuries: Current treatment options. *Journal of American Academy Orthopeadic Surgery.* 2001;9(4):227–237.
8. Beiner JM, Jokl P, Cholewicki J, Panjabi MM. The effect of anabolic steroids and corticosteroids on healing of muscle contusion injury. *American Journal of Sports Medicine.* 1999;27(1):2–9.
9. Best TM. Soft-tissue injuries and muscle tears. *Clinical Sports and Medicine.* 1997;16(3):419–434.
10. Brooks JHM, Fuller CW, Kemp SPT, Reddin DB. Incidence, risk and prevention of hamstring muscle injuries in professional rugby union. *American Journal of Sports Medicine.* 2006;34(8): 1297–1306.
11. Bruckner P, Bahr R, Blair S, Cook J, Crossley K, McConnell J, McCrory P, Noakes T, Khan K (eds.) *Bruckner and Khan's Clinical Sports Medicine*, 4th edn. Sydney, South Wales, Australia: McGraw Hill Australia Pty Ltd; 2012.
12. Carrilero LP, Hamming M, Nelson BJ, Taylor DC. Muscle and tendon injury and repair. In: O'Connor FG, Casa DJ, Davis BA, St. Pierre P, Sallis RE, Wilder RP (eds). *ACSM's Sports Medicine: A Comprehensive Review.* Philadelphia, PA: Lippincott Williams & Wilkins; 2013.
13. Crosier JL, Ganteaume S, Binet J, Genty M, Ferret JF. Strength imbalances and prevention of hamstring muscle injury in professional soccer players: A prospective study. *American Journal of Sports Medicine.* 2008;36(8): 1469–1475.
14. Garrett WE Jr, Nilcolaou PK, Ribbeck BM, Glisson RR, Seaber AV. The effect of muscle architecture on the biomechanical failure properties of skeletal muscle under passive extension. *American Journal of Sports Medicine.* 1988;16(1):7–12.
15. Huard J, Li Y, Fu FH. Muscle injuries and repair: Current trends in research. *Journal of Bone and Joint Surgery American.* 2002;84-A(5):822–832.
16. Jackson DW, Feagin JA. Quadriceps contusions in young athletes. Relation of severity of injury to treatment and prognosis. *Bone and Joint Surgery American.* 1973;55(1):95–105.
17. Jarvinen M. Healing of a crush injury in rat striated muscle. Part 2. A histological study of the effect of early mobilization and immobilization on the repair process. *Acta Pathologica et Microbiologica Scandinavica (A).* 1975;83(3):269–282.
18. Jarvinen TA, Jarvinen TL, Kaariainen M, Kalimo H, Jarvinen M. Muscle injuries: Biology and treatment. *American Journal of Sports Medicine.* 2005;33(5):745–764.
19. Lehto M, Duance VC, Restall D. Collagen and fibronectin in a healing skeletal muscle injury. An immunohistological study of the effects of physical activity on the repair of injured gastrocnemius muscle in the rat. *Journal of Bone and Joint Surgery British.* 1985;67(5)820–828.
20. Lieber RL, Friden J. Morphologic and mechanical basis of delayed onset muscle soreness. *Journal of the American Academy of Orthopaedic Surgery.* 2002;10(1):67–73.
21. McCarty EC, Walsh WM, Hald RD, Peter LE, Mellion MB. Musculoskeletal injuries in sports. In: Madden CC, Putukian M, Young CC, McCarthy EC (eds.) *Netter's Sports Medicine.* Philadelphia, PA: Saunders-Elsevier; 2010.
22. Miller MD, Thompson SR, Hart J (eds.) *Review of Orthopaedics*, 6th edn. Philadelphia, PA: Saunders, 2012.
23. Mishra DK, Friden J, Schmitz MC, Lieber RL. Anti-inflammatory medication after muscle injury. A treatment resulting in short-term improvement but subsequent loss of muscle function. *Journal of Bone and Joint Surgery American.* 1995;77(10):1510–1519.
24. Nikolaou PK, Macdonald BL, Glisson RR, Seaber AV, Garrett WE Jr. Biological and histological evaluation of muscle after controlled strain injury. *American Journal of Sports and Medicine.* 1987;15(1):9–14.
25. Noonan TJ, Garrett WE Jr. Muscle strain injury: Diagnosis and treatment. *Journal of American Academy of Orthopaedic Surgery.* 1999;7(4):262–269.
26. Obremsky WT, Seaber AV, Ribbeck BM, Garrett WE Jr. Biomechanical and histologic assessment of a controlled muscle strain injury treated with piroxicam. *American Journal of Sports and Medicine.* 1994;22(4):558–561.
27. Petersen J, Holmich P. Evidence based prevention of hamstring injuries in sports. *British Journal of Sports and Medicine.* 2005;39(6):319–323.
28. Proske U, Morgan DL. Muscle damage from eccentric exercise: Mechanism, mechanical signs, adaptation and clinical applications. *Journal of Physiology.* 2001;537(Pt 2):333–345.
29. Ryan JB, Wheeler JH, Hopkinson WJ, Arciero RA, Kolakowski KR. Quadriceps contusions. West Point update. *American Journal of Sports and Medicine.* 1991;19(3):299–304.
30. Schwellnus MP, Derman EW, Noakes TD. Aetiology of skeletal muscle 'cramps' during exercise: A novel hypothesis. *Journal of Sports Science.* 1997;15(3):277–285.
31. Schwellnus MP, Drew N, Collins M. Muscle cramping in athletes—Risk factors, clinical assessment, and management. *Clinical Sports and Medicine.* 2008;27(1):183–194.

11 Ligaments

Blair A. Becker

CONTENTS

TABLE 11.1
Key Clinical Considerations

1. Ligament injuries range from sprain (mild) to complete rupture (severe).
2. Injuries can be graded by the amount of pain, joint opening, and the presence or absence of an end point.
3. Examine all surrounding joint structures when a ligament injury is suspected.
4. MRI is the imaging modality of choice for suspected ligament pathology.
5. Dynamic ultrasound is useful for assessing superficial ligaments.
6. Healing progresses from hematoma, to collagen proliferation, and then to remodeling.
7. Need for operative management is determined by the location of ligament and degree of injury.

11.1 PHYSIOLOGY

Ligaments connect directly to bone and resist deforming stresses placed across joints. Their main role is to ensure the dynamic stability of joints. Ligaments are made up of collagen, which is the most prevalent protein in the human body (Table 11.1).

There are a variety of unique collagen types, but of particular relevance to the musculoskeletal system, type I collagen is present in ligament, tendon, and bone. Type I collagen is composed mainly of fibrils, which provide it with considerable tensile strength.[15] Type III and type V collagens also play a role in ligament structure, with type III forming a healing matrix around injured ligament tissue.[2]

Collagen architecture of ligaments reflects the tensile stresses that these tissues face. Type I collagen tends to be oriented parallel to the force it most commonly encounters. Tendons typically transmit a unidirectional long-axis vector, and their collagen fibrils are correspondingly longitudinal. Ligaments, on the other hand, have a more dynamic array of fibrils mirroring the multiple force vectors they encounter during activity.[5]

Three ligaments that have inspired a good deal of research in athletes are the anterior cruciate ligament (ACL) of the knee, the medial collateral ligament (MCL) of the knee, and the ulnar collateral ligament (UCL) of the elbow. What all of these structures have in common is the function of maintaining joint stability during the complex movement patterns of sport. They are dynamic tissues that are capable of resisting numerous deforming forces, which allows competitors to perform incredible feats of athleticism while preserving joint congruity. All biologic tissues have a limit, however, and ligaments are no different. When a ligament encounters a force that overwhelms its load threshold, the tissue will have some degree of failure. Ligament injuries constitute a spectrum of stretch injury, ranging from a mild stretch insult (sprain) with minimal resultant joint instability to a complete tear (rupture) with the potential for significant instability and even joint dislocation.

11.2 ANATOMY

Perhaps the most studied ligament in the body, the MCL, spans the medial knee joint with roughly 80 mm of ligament tissue. Proximally, it attaches to the medial femoral condyle, and distally, it attaches to the medial metaphysis of the tibia. It resists valgus stress to the knee. Much of what we know about the interface of ligament and bone is a result of studies conducted on MCL bony attachments.

The MCL inserts onto bone in both a direct and an indirect fashion. The proximal attachment of the MCL is an example of direct insertion, consisting of a fibrocartilage transition from ligament to bone. The distal attachment of the MCL, conversely, inserts indirectly onto the tibia. An indirect attachment consists of both superficial fibers inserting onto periosteum and deep fibers inserting onto bone.[20]

The ACL is situated within the knee joint, attaching at the lateral femoral condyle and running to the medial tibial plateau. It resists both anterior translation and internal rotation of the tibia, as it relates to the femur.

A good example of the dynamic nature of ligaments, the UCL complex of the elbow is made up of multiple unique structures. This complex includes an anterior oblique ligament (AOL), which spans from the medial epicondyle of the humerus to the proximal ulna. The AOL is the strongest component in the UCL complex and serves as the primary restraint against valgus stress at 90° of elbow flexion. This is important to overhead athletes, who are often placing maximal valgus stress on the elbow in this position while throwing or serving.[12]

11.3 EPIDEMIOLOGY

Knee injuries are common in an active population, and many of these are ligament injuries. More than 90% of ligamentous knee injuries occur at the ACL and MCL and are typically found in athletes.[17] The incidence of MCL injury is 0.24 per 1000 in the United States and is considered the most common ligamentous knee injury, with males being more commonly injured.[6] The prevalence of ACL injury is 1 in 3000 in the United States, with women being disproportionately affected.[13]

11.4 PATHOLOGY

Ligaments are injured when they encounter a deforming force that exceeds their ability to prevent joint displacement. The MCL serves to protect the knee against valgus stress and, to a lesser extent, external rotation and internal rotation. It has served as the basis of numerous studies due to its ability to spontaneously heal after injury.

The MCL contains distinct superficial and deep components that demonstrate how the ligament is able to counter multiple unique stresses applied to the knee during activity.[16] This again demonstrates the complex architecture of collagen fibers in ligament tissue, designed to resist multiple vectors of stress.

The superficial MCL serves as the foremost check to valgus stress and external rotation, with the deep MCL also providing some stability. The superficial and deep MCLs have a more equal role when it comes to resisting the force of internal rotation.[6] Injuries occur when the ability of the MCL to resist these forces is overwhelmed. Though noncontact mechanisms of injury can occur with the MCL, it is most often injured by the excessive valgus stress of a lateral blow or forced external rotation of the foot with a flexed knee.

The ACL is also commonly injured. One study found that more than 70% of patients who presented with a traumatic hemarthrosis had a partial or complete ACL tear.[3] More than two-thirds of ACL injuries occur without any trauma to the knee, but rather with landing from a jump or pivoting or cutting in such a way that exceeds the load threshold of the ligament.[13] Early attempts at primary repair of the torn segments did not result in ligament healing. Histologic evaluation of ruptured ACLs demonstrates no evidence of cross bridging between the ligament remnants. In fact, a synovial layer forms at the surface of the ligament fragments that seems to inhibit the healing process observed in other ligaments, like the MCL.[18] To reestablish ACL function, it must be reconstructed from a grafted tendon or ligament.

Clinical Pearl

Maintain an index of suspicion for an intra-articular ligament tear in an athlete with hemarthrosis.

Another ligament that is unlikely to spontaneously heal after rupture is the UCL of the elbow. It is often injured in throwing athletes such as baseball pitchers and football quarterbacks, but also overhead athletes such as volleyball and tennis players.

During the late cocking phase of a baseball pitch, the elbow undergoes extreme torque, about 65 Newtons (N). College pitchers will routinely generate 82 N of torque at their elbow.[10] The load threshold of the UCL has been determined to be only 34 N. This shows not only the significant load the UCL routinely resists in throwing athletes but also the valgus support provided by bony and muscular structures of the elbow.[9] With this degree of repetitive loading to the UCL ligament, it is not hard to imagine how it can break down over time and even rupture.

11.5 LIGAMENT HEALING

Much of what we know about the ligament healing process comes from the MCL, due to the ligament's consistent diameter and inherent healing properties.[19] Phases of ligament healing are not dissimilar to those seen in fracture healing. An inflammatory phase is marked by hematoma formation. A reparative phase follows a few weeks later with a fibroblast-constructed matrix of proteoglycans and mostly type III collagen. The matrix is gradually replaced by type I collagen over the next 6 weeks. The remodeling phase then commences, with collagen aligning in response to physiologic stress. The maturation seen in the remodeling phase can last years after an injury. Significant remodeling is known to occur for at least 2½ years after an injury.[11]

As we have seen, collagen fibril architecture reflects joint stresses. Not surprisingly then, weight bearing plays an essential role in ligament repair. One study showed that 9 weeks of immobilization led to replacement of typical ligamentous collagen with newer and weaker cross-linking collagen that is less capable of withstanding the dynamic stresses encountered during joint loading.[1] Early mobilization plays an essential role in improved functional outcome after ligament injury. Following ligament injury, immobilization leads to a loss in size, stiffness, and strength of collagen fibrils. Conversely, normal activity improves all three parameters. Exercise training can similarly aid in functional healing of ligament, but too much training can have a deleterious effect on collagen fibrils.[19]

Growth factors also seem to influence the strength of healing ligament tissue. In an animal study, injured ACLs treated with transforming growth factor-β1 withstood higher maximum loads and showed superior stiffness when compared to untreated groups.[14] Additional growth factors seem to encourage collagen synthesis. Another study took ACL remnants procured during reconstruction surgery and exposed one group to autologous platelet-rich plasma (PRP) and another to platelet-poor plasma. The PRP used was found to contain much higher levels of not only transforming growth factor-β1 but also epidermal growth factor and vascular endothelial growth factor. The ACLs in the PRP group showed a significantly higher rate of collagen proliferation than the platelet-poor plasma group.[7]

11.6 HISTORY AND PHYSICAL

Patients will often present after a ligament injury complaining of a sudden onset of pain to the affected ligament or associated joint. The history can alternatively suggest a more chronic course, such as a thrower describing a period of elbow soreness or decreased velocity with a progressive UCL injury. Investigating the mechanism of injury is vital. For example, if the sideline practitioner observes a football player sustaining a lateral blow to the knee, he or she will likely consider an acute MCL injury in his or her differential.

Ask about activity level, e.g., how often a pitcher is throwing or if they play multiple positions on multiple teams. The patient will sometimes describe a "pop," which can suggest a ligament rupture rather than a sprain or partial tear. Asking about and examining for an effusion can be helpful to differentiate between intra- or extra-articular ligament etiologies.

Clinical Pearl

Using pitch counts for youth throwers is vital to preventing UCL injury.[21]

When approaching the exam for a suspected ligament injury, recall that the level of force required to damage a ligament can also injure nearby structures. A skier may describe catching an edge of their ski and externally rotating their tibia with a flexed knee. You are right to suspect an MCL injury, but there may be a concomitant ACL injury as well. In the knee, all key structures should be examined, even if one suspects an isolated MCL injury.

When examining the affected ligament, begin with inspection and palpation. In the case of the MCL, complete rupture occurs most commonly at the proximal attachment. Palpating for the point of maximal tenderness can thus be helpful in distinguishing the degree of injury. For the UCL of the elbow, start posterior to the medial epicondyle and palpate distally.

TABLE 11.2
AMA Guidelines for Grading Medial Collateral Ligament or Lateral Collateral Ligament Complex Injuries of the Knee

Grade	Description
I	0–5 mm joint line opening
II	5–10 mm joint line opening
III	>10 mm opening; no firm end point

TABLE 11.3
Degree of Ligament Injury

	Pain and Inflammation	Instability on Exam	Endpoint
First degree (sprain)	Yes	No	Yes
Second degree (partial tear)	Yes	Yes	Yes
Third degree (complete tear)	Yes	Yes	No

Next, consider the ligament's function. This should help recall exam maneuvers designed to replicate the dynamic stress to which a given ligament is exposed. Among other tests, the ACL is examined with the Lachman and anterior drawer maneuvers, the MCL is tested with valgus stress (Table 11.2), and the UCL is likewise tested with valgus stress. An uninjured ligament should resist these forces without pain or increased laxity, when compared to the unaffected side. Care should also be taken to assess neurovascular status of the affected extremity.

As Table 11.2 indicates, ligament injuries are often graded I–III, based on objective joint opening. It is also helpful to describe the degree of ligament injury (Table 11.3), which is separate from grading the injury. While injury grade is purely objective, degree is a more inclusive, clinically oriented scale that can help guide treatment.

11.7 DIAGNOSTICS

Mild ligament injuries can often be diagnosed clinically and have excellent healing potential with conservative treatment. More severe injuries, or injuries to ligaments that will not heal with conservative treatment such as an ACL or UCL rupture, typically require advanced imaging to guide management.

T2-weighted MRI provides the best imaging of ligaments. It can reveal the entire spectrum of ligament injury, ranging from the increased signal intensity of a first-degree sprain to the complete rupture of a third-degree tear. In the right hands, musculoskeletal ultrasound can also be diagnostic for injuries of extra-articular ligaments and has the added advantage of providing dynamic views while stressing a given ligament, e.g., the UCL of the elbow.

As a general rule, if a second- or third-degree MCL injury is suspected, an MRI is warranted to rule out associated damage to the cruciate ligaments, meniscus, or chondral surfaces. If any one of the Ottawa knee rules is met, then x-rays should be obtained.[6] MR arthrogram is helpful in suspected acute tears of the UCL, as the mechanism often involves tearing of the joint capsule, which becomes evident with extra-articular contrast extravasation.[12]

11.8 TREATMENT CONSIDERATIONS

Treatment of ligament injuries can be nonoperative or operative, but the goal remains the same: reestablishing a ligament's tensile strength in order to restore normal joint function and stability. Due to the inherent healing potential of the MCL, conservative treatment is typically appropriate. Even an isolated complete tear of the MCL is often treated without surgery. Treatment consists of rest, ice, compression, elevation, and bracing. Isolated third-degree tears may require an initial 1–2 weeks of nonweight bearing to ensure ligament healing.

Recall that the heavily studied MCL is known to heal well, as long as the ruptured segments are in close proximity to one another. The one exception to this rule is a third-degree injury with associated bony avulsion or concomitant cruciate rupture. Though it remains controversial, many advocate surgically repairing these injuries. Surgery is also indicated for patients who fail to achieve ligament healing with conservative therapy and continue to demonstrate valgus instability.

When the ligament is able to resist valgus stress on exam and the patient is pain free, a gradual return to play program can be initiated. A study showed that the average time to return for football players with first-degree injury is about 10 days. In a second-degree injury, average return is about 3 weeks.[6]

Though it was once the accepted standard to repair the ruptured ACL by suturing its remnants together, surgeons quickly learned that this technique did not result in ligament healing. Eventually, techniques for ACL reconstruction using auto- or allograft were introduced. This landmark surgical advancement for athletes of all ages transformed the ACL rupture from a career-ending injury to a season-ending one. If an athlete wishes to continue activities that involve jumping, cutting, pivoting, and rapid deceleration, then reconstruction is indicated.

The goal of ACL reconstruction is to reestablish the stabilizing force of native ligament as closely as possible, namely, resisting anterior tibial translation and internal rotation. A reconstructed ACL's stabilizing function will prevent future joint displacement.[8] Without ligament reconstruction, an active patient can expect ongoing joint instability, which may lead to meniscal tears, chondral injury, and potentially early osteoarthritis.[3] A recent systematic review of long-term outcomes showed that patients treated with surgical reconstruction for ACL rupture had fewer later meniscus injuries, fewer knee surgeries, and were more active when compared with patients who elected to not have surgery.[4]

Surgical reconstruction involves removal of the ACL remnants, creating tibial and femoral tunnels at the native ligament's former bony attachments and then spanning the two locations with a graft. The graft is harvested from the patient's own semitendinosus–gracilis tendons, bone–patellar tendon–bone, or a cadaver ACL.

It is important to note that even with reconstruction, a history of ACL rupture is likely to lead to posttraumatic osteoarthritis within two decades. With an associated meniscal tear at the time of injury, the likelihood of developing osteoarthritis approaches 80%. Despite attempts to restore physiologic function of the native ACL, joint kinematics and kinetics are not returned to their preinjury levels. This has raised questions about the complex factors that affect ligament function, such as geometric position, proprioception, and neuromuscular control. It seems clear that regardless of the graft type utilized, anterior tibial translation and internal rotation after surgery are still more lax, when compared to the uninjured side.[13]

The treatment of UCL injuries lands somewhere between the nonoperative approach to MCL injury and the surgical approach to ACL rupture. Partial tears of the UCL are generally allowed an 8–12-week period of rest from all throwing. The athlete is given NSAIDs and provided rehabilitative exercises with a gradual return to throwing program when he or she is pain free. If there is a failure of conservative management or a complete rupture, surgical treatment is indicated.

Similar to ACL ruptures, the UCL rupture was once seen as a career-ending injury. Outcomes with primary surgical repair of the ligament were poor. With the advent of reconstructive surgery, however, throwers were able to successfully return to high-level throwing after about a year. Graft choice includes palmaris longus, hamstring, and toe extensor, among others. Today, a good number of successful Major League Baseball pitchers have undergone UCL reconstruction.

11.9 FUTURE DIRECTIONS

Researchers continue to investigate avenues for improving ligament healing. From aiding primary ligament healing to

TABLE 11.4
SORT: Key Recommendations for Practice

Clinical Recommendation	Evidence Rating	References
Use Ottawa knee rules to determine need for x-ray when MCL is injured.	A	[6]
Check MRI for greater than or equal to second-degree MCL injury.	B	[6]
MRI arthrogram is the study of choice for acute UCL injury.	B	[12]
Patients who undergo ACL reconstruction have improved function and fewer subsequent meniscal tears and surgeries.	A	[4]
Prescribe 8–12 weeks of rest, followed by progressive throwing program for partial UCL tear.	B	[12]

augmenting surgical repair, there may be a future role for growth factors, gene therapy, and even biologic scaffolds (Table 11.4).

REFERENCES

1. Akeson WH, Amiel D, Mechanic GL et al., Collagen cross-linking alterations in joint contractures: Changes in the reducible cross-links in periarticular connective tissue collagen after nine weeks of immobilization. *Connective Tissue Research.* 1977;5:15–19.
2. Birk DE, Mayne R. Localization of collagen types I, III and V during tendon development. Changes in about 70% of a ligament is made up of water. collagen types I and III are correlated with changes in fibril diameter. *European Journal of Cell Biology.* 1997;72:352–361.
3. Butler DL. Anterior cruciate ligament: Its normal response and replacement. *Journal of Orthopedic Research.* 1989; 7:910–921.
4. Chalmers PN, Mall NA, Moric M et al. Does ACL reconstruction alter natural history. *The Journal of Bone and Joint Surgery.* 2014;96:292–300.
5. Cooper RR. Misol S. Tendon and ligament insertion: A light and electron microscopic study. *Journal of Bone & Joint Surgery.* 1970;52:1–20.
6. Duffy PS, Miyamotos RG. Management of medial collateral ligament injuries in the knee: An update and review. *The Physician and Sports Medicine.* 2010;38:48–54.
7. Fallouh L, Nakagawa K, Sasho T et al. Effects of autologous platelet-rich plasma on cell viability and collagen synthesis in injured human anterior cruciate ligament. *Journal of Bone and Joint Surgery.* 2010;18:2909–2916.
8. Finsterbush A, Frankl U, Matam Y. Secondary damage to the knee after isolated injury of the anterior cruciate ligament. *American Journal of Sports Medicine.* 1990;15:225–229.
9. Fleisig GS, Andrews JR, Dillman CJ et al. Kinetics of baseball pitching with implications about injury mechanisms. *American Journal of Sports Medicine.* 1995;23:233–239.
10. Fleisig GS, Kingsley DS, Loftice JW et al. Kinetic comparison among the fastball, curveball, change-up, and slider in collegiate baseball pitchers. *American Journal of Sports Medicine.* 2006;34:423–430.
11. Frank C, Schachar N, Dittrich D. Natural history of healing in the repaired medial collateral ligament. *Journal of Orthopedic Research.* 1983;2:179–188.
12. Hariri S, Safran MR. Ulnar collateral ligament injury in the overhead athlete. *Clinical Sports Medicine.* 2010;29:619–644.
13. Kiapour AM, Murray MM. Basic science of anterior cruciate ligament injury and repair. *Bone and Joint Research.* 2014;3:20–31.
14. Kondo E, Yasuda K, Yamanaka M et al. Effects of administration of exogenous growth factors on biomechanical properties of the elongation-type anterior cruciate ligament injury with partial laceration. *American Journal of Sports Medicine.* 2005;33:188–196.
15. Liu SH, Yang R, Al-Shaikh R et al. Collagen in tendon, ligament, and bone healing. *Clinical Orthopaedics and Related Research.* 1995;318:265–278.
16. Miyamoto RG, Bosco JA, Sherman OH. Treatment of medial collateral ligament injuries. *Journal of the American Academy of Orthopedic Surgery.* 2009;17:152–161.
17. Miyasaka KC, Daniel DM, Stone ML et al. The incidence of knee ligament injuries in the general population. *American Journal of Knee Surgery.* 1991;4:3–8.
18. Murray MM, Martin SD, Martin TL et al. Histological changes in the human anterior cruciate ligament after rupture. *Journal of Bone and Joint Surgery.* 2000;82A:1387–1397.
19. Woo SL, Abramowitch SD, Kilger R et al. Biomechanics of knee ligaments: Injury, healing, and repair. *Journal of Biomechanics.* 2006;39:1–20.
20. Woo SL, Inoue M, McGurk-Burleson E et al. Treatment of the medial collateral ligament injury II: Structure and function of canine knees in response to differing treatment regimens. *American Journal of Sports Medicine.* 1987;15:22–29.
21. Andrews, J.R., Fleisig, G.S., Preventing Baseball Injuries, n.d., STOPsportsinjuries.org. Accessed June 28, 2015.

12 Nerve Injury

Yaowen Eliot Hu and Thomas Howard

CONTENTS

TABLE 12.1
Key Clinical Considerations

1. The most common nerve injury in athletics is the "stinger" or "burner."
2. Nerve injury starts with Wallerian degeneration 24–36 hours after injury.
3. The most common upper extremity nerve involved in injuries is the ulnar nerve.
4. Special provocative maneuvers such as Phalen's sign and direct irritation of the nerve with Tinel's sign may be helpful in identifying nerve injury but is not pathognomonic and the physical exam is often normal.
5. At 3–4 weeks of injury, EMG is the most helpful in localizing the lesion.
6. Avulsion-type injuries have the worst prognosis and compression-type injuries have the best prognosis for recovery.

12.1 INTRODUCTION

Musculoskeletal complaints are among the most common encounters seen by primary care providers (PCPs), with pain being a principal chief complaint. As nearly all pain is transmitted from the peripheral to the central nervous system for interpretation by the brain through nerves, it is critical that the PCP understand the anatomy and function of working nervous system pathways. The nerve represents a unique bundle of axons that through a complex electrochemical process facilitates both voluntary and involuntary action. As the nerve anatomically extends throughout the axial and appendicular skeleton, and in many cases is quite superficial, this tissue is vulnerable and can be injured through both overuse and acute trauma. In addition, nerve tissue can be injured by neoplastic, infectious, autoimmune, and idiopathic etiologies. Therefore, the PCP must carefully evaluate the patient's complaint to identify the pain generator in order to facilitate appropriate treatment. An adequate history and physical exam are essential in distinguishing nerve injuries and are pivotal in localizing the lesion. Advanced imaging and ancillary testing may also assist in accurate diagnosis when properly employed and interpreted. Since some nerve injuries require urgent surgical referral for treatment, it is important to recognize and diagnose various nerve injuries in a timely manner to avoid significant long-term disability, especially in older patients with severe pain and brachial plexus injuries.[11] This chapter reviews the anatomy and function of the peripheral nerve, identifies common pathologic terminology, and concludes with an introduction to evaluation and management. Detailed assessment and management of specific nerve injuries are discussed in the appropriate musculoskeletal chapter (Table 12.1).

12.2 ANATOMY OF NERVES

Nerves are generated from collections of neurons, which consist of a central cell body with outward projections known as axons. Axons arise from the cell body and propagate electrical signals known as action potentials downstream with the help of voltage-gated sodium and calcium channels distributed along the length of the axon. Axons also help with the transport of nutrients within the cell and may be wrapped with myelin, a substance produced by Schwann cells. The myelin is layered to form a sheath around the axon to provide insulation for faster and more efficient action potential conduction. The individual axon is surrounded by connective tissue known as the endoneurium. Multiple axons form a bundle of fibers and are surrounded by a layer of connective tissue called the perineurium. These axonal bundles are further grouped together and surrounded by loose connective tissue known as the epineurium.[15]

Nerves are classified as central and peripheral depending on their location. Central nerves involve signaling in the brain and spinal cord, while peripheral nerves involve the nerve roots, ganglia, and all of the other nerves to the rest of the body. Efferent nerves send signal from the central nervous system to the rest of the body, while afferent

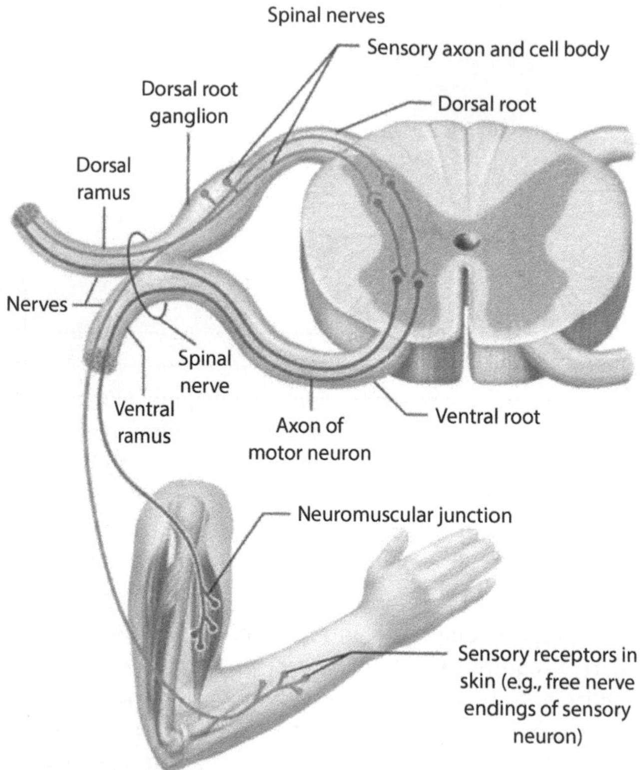

FIGURE 12.1 Nervous system: Spinal nerves and plexuses. (From www.antranik.org, accessed October 17, 2015. With permission.)

nerves receive signals back from the periphery. Efferent motor neurons are located in the anterior horn of the spinal cord and afferent sensory neurons are located in the dorsal root ganglion outside of the spinal cord. Nerves exit the spinal cord and connect to peripheral nerves to innervate the organs of the body (see Figure 12.1). Some nerves are organized into clusters close to the spinal cord known as ganglia prior to innervating the rest of the body, while others directly connect to peripheral nerves. As nerves traverse through the body, they may lie superficial to, between, or through muscles. With concurrent limb movement, nerves glide and may have tether points at their origin, destination, and between floats, causing symptoms of nerve entrapment or compression. Thus, it is important to distinguish between spinal cord, nerve root, and peripheral nerve symptoms to identify the points of entrapment or compression.

12.3 PHYSIOLOGY AND FUNCTION

The peripheral nervous system consists of the nerves outside of the brain and spinal cord (central nervous system) and its function is to connect the central nervous system to the limbs and organs. Peripheral nerves may be purely sensory, purely motor, or a combination of both. Electrical impulses known as action potentials are propagated down the axon to relay electrical and chemical information to other nerves, organs, and muscle across synapses and neuromuscular junctions.[15] Once the action potential reaches the synaptic terminal between nerves, neurotransmitters are released into the synapse and bind to receptors on the downstream nerve. Another action potential is generated and the process repeated until the desired function is achieved.

12.4 PATHOLOGY OF NERVES

Nerve injuries occur in musculoskeletal medicine with both overuse and trauma. Injury may happen with recreation or during occupation. Specific mechanisms include stretching, traction, compression, laceration, or ischemia[2] and may occur at the spinal cord, nerve root, the ganglia, or the individual nerve. With recreation, the sports involved are usually throwing sports such as softball or baseball, racquet sports such as tennis, and sports where nerves are prone to overuse or compression such as volleyball and cycling.[17] The patient's occupation may also contribute to repetitive compression from lifting and poor ergonomic posturing, leading to carpal tunnel syndrome, the most common overuse nerve entrapment in primary care. Most traumatic peripheral nerve injuries involve the upper extremity. The most common nerve involved with trauma is the ulnar nerve[2] and the most common traumatic nerve injury encountered is the "stinger" or "burner."[10]

Clinical Pearl

Nerve injury starts with Wallerian degeneration 24–36 hours after the event.

With nerve injury, there is damage to the nerve itself and its surrounding connective tissue. Nerve injury starts with Wallerian degeneration and is followed by axon regeneration and nerve reinnervation. Wallerian degeneration involves axonal degeneration distal to the injury and starts 24–36 hours after injury. Axon regeneration typically occurs at a rate of 1 mm/day and the entire recovery process may take up to 12 months to complete.[3,15] Dependent upon the location of the injury, there exists specific terminology: Myelopathy refers to injury of the spinal cord, while radiculopathy refers to injury of the nerve root and neuropathy involves injury of the peripheral nerve.

12.5 SEDDON AND SUNDERLAND CLASSIFICATION OF NERVE INJURY

Nerve injuries are classified via the Seddon or the Sunderland classification systems to delineate the treatment options and prognoses associated with different injuries. In the Seddon classification system, complete axonotmesis and neurotmesis cannot be differentiated with electrodiagnostic studies since the difference between the two involves the damage in the supporting connective tissue.[13] On the other hand, the Sunderland classification system organizes the injury based on the neural anatomy[16] (see Tables 12.2 and 12.3).

TABLE 12.2
Seddon Classification of Nerve Injury

Neurapraxia	There is injury to the myelin alone with conduction block and conduction velocity slowing along the affected nerve segment on electrodiagnostic studies.
Axonotmesis	There is axonal injury with Wallerian degeneration and conduction loss at the affected nerve segment on electrodiagnostic studies. Later, there will be decreased or absent evoked potential amplitudes distal to the injury site on electrodiagnostic studies.
Neurotmesis	There is complete disruption of the nerve with axonal injury, Wallerian degeneration, and supporting connective tissue damage. There is conduction loss at the affected nerve segment on electrodiagnostic studies. There is a poor prognosis of recovery and needs surgical intervention for treatment.

Source: Adapted from Seddon, H.J., *Brain*, 66, 237, 1943.

TABLE 12.3
Sunderland Classification of Nerve Injury

Class 1	There is injury to myelin alone and is the equivalent of neurapraxia in the Seddon system. There is excellent prognosis for recovery.
Class 2	There is axonotmesis with axonal injury and intact endoneurium, perineurium, and epineurium. There is good prognosis for recovery, but this depends on the percentage of axonal injury and the distance of the injury from the muscle.
Class 3	There is axonotmesis with endoneurium injury and sparing of the perineurium and epineurium. There is poor prognosis for recovery and surgery may be needed.
Class 4	There is axonotmesis with endoneurium and perineurium injury with sparing of the epineurium. There is poor prognosis for recovery and surgery is required.
Class 5	There is neurotmesis with complete transection of the nerve. There is poor prognosis for recovery and surgery is required.

Source: Adapted from Sunderland, S., *Nerves and Nerve Injuries*, 2nd edn., Churchill Livingston, London, U.K., 1978.

12.6 HISTORY AND PHYSICAL EXAM

Clinical Pearl

Neurotmesis is the complete transection of a nerve with disruption of the surrounding connective tissue and surgical treatment is required.

The history and physical examination is core to the diagnosis and management of injury to the peripheral nerve. A careful history must be taken with nerve injuries, and important areas to cover include past medical history such as diabetes, hypertension, thyroid disorders, and other psychiatric disorders. Past surgical history, medications, family history, and social history are also important aspects to cover as nerve injuries may have many potential causes. The mechanism of injury, description of symptoms, duration of symptoms, and distribution of symptoms are helpful in the evaluation of acute versus chronic injuries and overuse versus traumatic injuries. Assessing whether the patient is right- or left-handed is useful in establishing baselines in strength testing during physical examination. Nerve injuries often present with numbness, tingling, burning, or electrical sensations in the distribution of the nerve or dermatome. They may also present with poorly localized pain, paresthesia, weakness, and loss of reflexes. Allodynia is an important finding on physical exam where the patient exhibits hypersensitivity or pain along the distribution of the nerve with light touch.

One of the most important aspects in the history and physical examination involves localization of the pathologic lesion to the spinal cord, nerve root, or peripheral nerve. With myelopathy, symptoms depend on the level of the lesion, and the patient may present with upper motor neuron signs including spasticity, weakness, hyperreflexia, and reappearance of early reflexes (i.e., Babinski reflex) that have already disappeared. Because of the central location of the pathologic lesion, there may also be unilateral or bilateral symptoms involving multiple spinal levels, gastrointestinal and genitourinary symptoms, and sexual dysfunction. In radiculopathy, the pathologic lesion is localized to the nerve root, and there may be unilateral weakness, decreased reflexes, altered sensations, and pain radiating from along the spine to the peripheral distribution of the nerve root and its corresponding nerves. Special provocative maneuvers for nerve root and peripheral nerve entrapment (Phalen's sign, Spurling's test, etc.) or direct irritation of the nerve (Tinel's sign) may reproduce the patient's symptoms but are not pathognomonic. Weakness of individual muscles and altered sensation with two-point pinprick discrimination testing may be useful in localizing the lesion. However, the patient may have a completely normal physical exam, and having the patient repeat the offending motion to reproduce symptoms may help with diagnosis.[2,4,10]

Clinical Pearl

Special provocative tests such as Phalen's sign are helpful in diagnosing nerve entrapments but are not pathognomonic.

12.7 DIAGNOSTIC TESTING

X-rays are usually not helpful in evaluating nerve injuries unless there are bony pathologies contributing to compression or ischemia of the nerve. Ultrasound and MRI may be helpful in identifying the sites of compression and entrapment. Nerves that are entrapped may appear to be enlarged and may be surrounded by fluid signal on ultrasound or MRI. Dynamic ultrasound and dynamic MRI evaluation may reveal subluxation or dislocation of the nerve from its normal anatomic position. Diagnostic lidocaine injections at potential points of compression or entrapment, especially under ultrasound guidance for needle placement, may also assist in identifying and confirming the pathology that is creating the patient's symptoms.

Electrodiagnostic testing with electromyography (EMG) and nerve conduction studies (NCSs) are necessary in determining the location, severity, and prognosis of the nerve injury (see Chapter 21, Electrodiagnostic Testing). If the date of injury is less than 7 days, NCS is useful in localizing the injury and identifying conduction block versus axonotmesis. If the date of injury is within 1–2 weeks, electrodiagnostic studies are helpful in distinguishing between complete and incomplete lesions and may be beneficial in differentiating axonotmesis and neurotmesis from neurapraxia. If the date of injury is within 3–4 weeks, EMG is able to characterize the lesion with the best yield. At 3–4 months after injury, electrodiagnostic studies detect reinnervation of muscles.[1,12]

Clinical Pearl

At 3–4 weeks after injury, EMG will yield the most information in localizing the lesion.

12.8 TREATMENT OPTIONS AND PROGNOSIS

Treatment of nerve injuries depends on the diagnosis and the timing, location, and severity of the lesion. There may be nonsurgical and surgical treatment options for a variety of nerve injuries. Initial nonsurgical treatment includes pain control with options including nonsteroidal anti-inflammatories, anticonvulsants, and antidepressants along with physical therapy and splinting to preserve function and range of motion. Anti-inflammatory medications are used to decrease inflammation and swelling around the nerve. Gabapentin is an anticonvulsant that interacts with voltage-sensitive calcium channels to increase release of GABA, an inhibitory neurotransmitter, thereby decreasing the excitability of the downstream axon. Pregabalin is another anticonvulsant that is commonly used because it decreases the secretion of substance P, a pain-generating neurotransmitter. Antidepressants such as amitriptyline and duloxetine inhibit the reuptake of serotonin and norepinephrine, outcompeting substance P for its receptor to decrease pain. Furthermore, it is important to allow for passive range of motion of the affected limb. Nerve glides and physical therapy to reduce compression, traction, and stretching may be needed for improvement.

Pain refractory to initial medications and physical therapy interventions may require topical anesthetics, transcutaneous electrical nerve stimulators, or peripheral nerve blocks in severe cases. Desensitization techniques may be helpful in complex regional pain syndrome or symptoms of hypersensitivity and allodynia.[2,6,8] Incomplete nerve lesions are typically treated conservatively with monitoring for electrodiagnostic recovery.[2] Surgical release and decompression of the nerve may ultimately be needed if the patient fails all avenues of conservative nonsurgical therapy.

Surgery within 72 hours of the injury is indicated in nerve transection, laceration, or compression from a hematoma or aneurysm. If the injury was a blunt transection or an avulsion of the nerve, then surgery should be performed within several weeks of the injury to repair the nerve. Delayed surgery 3–6 months from the injury should be performed in cases where the degree of nerve damage is uncertain. Reinnervation of the muscle must be performed within 12–18 months of the injury because of the potential for irreversible damage to the denervated muscle.[2,12]

Prognosis depends on the mechanism, severity, and type of nerve injury. Avulsion injuries have the worst prognosis when compared with compression injuries. Neurapraxia usually has excellent prognosis for recovery, while axonotmesis and neurotmesis have variable outcomes depending on the number of axons involved. Comparison of the degree of axonal loss to the contralateral side is helpful in evaluation of prognosis as an amplitude difference of 50% on EMG is indicative of significant axonal loss. For motor recovery, if the affected side's amplitude on electrodiagnostic studies is 0%–10% that of the contralateral side, then the prognosis is poor. But the prognosis is good if the affected side's amplitude is 10%–30% that of the contralateral side, and the prognosis is excellent if the affected side's amplitude is >30% that of the contralateral side (Table 12.4).[12,14]

TABLE 12.4
SORT: Key Recommendations for Practice

Clinical Recommendation	Evidence Rating	References
Substantial long-term disability was found in patients after nerve injury with higher pain scores, older age, and brachial plexus injury.	B	[11]
Successful response to carpal tunnel surgery may be predicted by positive response to injection.	B	[7]
A positive Tinel's sign has a 44%–75% sensitivity and a 48%–100% specificity for the diagnosis of cubital tunnel syndrome.	C	[4]
A positive Tinel's sign has a 42%–73% sensitivity, 85%–100% specificity, and an 89%–100% positive predictive value for the diagnosis of carpal tunnel syndrome.	A	[9]
A positive Phalen's sign has a 91% sensitivity, 85%–95% specificity, and a 91%–92% positive predictive value for the diagnosis of carpal tunnel syndrome.	A	[9]
A positive Flick sign has 93% sensitivity and 96% specificity in ruling in carpal tunnel syndrome.	C	[5]

REFERENCES

1. Aldridge JW, Bruno RJ, Strauch RJ et al. Nerve entrapment in athletes. *Clinical Sports and Medicine*. 2001;20(1):95–122.
2. Campbell WW. Evaluation and management of peripheral nerve injury. *Clinical Neurophysiology*. 2008;199(9): 1951–1965.
3. Coleman MP, Freeman MR. Wallerian degeneration, Wld(s), and NMNAT. *Annual Review of Neuroscience*. June 2010; 33(1):245–267.
4. Cummines CA, Schneider DS. Peripheral nerve injuries in baseball players. *Neurological Clinic*. 2008;26:195–215.
5. D'Arcy CA, McGee S. The rational clinical examination: Does this patient have carpal tunnel syndrome? *Journal of the American Medical Association*. 2000;283(23):3110–3117.
6. Dworkin RH, Backonja M, Rowbothan MC et al. Advances in neuropathic pain: Diagnosis mechanisms and treatment recommendations. *Archives of Neurology*. 2003;60(11): 1524–1534.
7. Edgell SE, McCabe SJ, Breidenbach WC et al. Predicting the outcome of carpal tunnel release. *Journal of Hand Surgery (Am.)*. 2003;28(2):255–261.
8. Kingery WS. A critical review of controlled clinical trials for peripheral neuropathic pain and complex regional pain syndromes. *Pain*. 1997;73(2):123–139.
9. Kotevoglu N, Gulbahce-Saglam S. Ultrasound imaging in the diagnosis of carpal tunnel syndrome and its relevance to clinical evaluation. *Joint Bone Spine*. 2005;72(2):142–145.
10. Krivickas LS, Wilbourn AJ. Peripheral nerve injuries in athletes: A case series of over 200 injuries. *Seminars in Neurology*. 2000;20(2):225–232.
11. Novak CB, Anastakis DJ, Beaton DE et al. Patient-reported outcome after peripheral nerve injury. *Journal of Hand Surgery*. 2009;34(2):281–287.
12. Robinson LR. AAEM Minimonograph 28: Traumatic injury to peripheral nerves. *Muscle Nerve*. 2000;23:863–873.
13. Seddon HJ. Three types of nerve injury. *Brain*. 1943; 66:237–288.
14. Sillman JS, Niparko JK, Lee SS et al. Prognostic value of evoked and standard electromyography in acute facial paralysis. *Otolaryngology Head and Neck Surgery*. 1992;107(3):377–381.
15. Snell RS. *Clinical Neuroanatomy,* 7th edn. Philadelphia, PA: Lippincott Williams & Wilkins; 2009.
16. Sunderland S. *Nerves and Nerve Injuries*, 2nd edn. London, U.K.: Churchill Livingston; 1978.
17. Toth, C. Peripheral nerve injuries attributable to sport and recreation. *Neurology Clinical*. 2008;26(1):89–113.

13 Bursae

Korin Hudson and B. Elizabeth Delasobera

CONTENTS

TABLE 13.1
Key Clinical Considerations

1. There are approximately 160 bursae in the human body. Bursae function to reduce friction between adjacent structures in the musculoskeletal system such as in areas where tendons pass over or between bones, between overlapping muscles, or between bones and skin. Bursal pathology should be considered when patients present with symptoms in these areas.
2. While bursitis accounts for less than 1% of primary care visits, it is commonly seen in athletes, particularly runners, and in workers who are required to do a significant amount of lifting and/or kneeling.
3. The diagnosis of bursitis is largely clinical, and the etiology can often be ascertained from history and physical exam alone. Evaluation of bursal fluid may aid in diagnosis.
4. Most cases of septic bursitis respond to drainage and oral antibiotics. Intravenous antibiotics are only required for severe cases or in patients with accompanying systemic symptoms. Surgical management is rarely needed and is generally reserved for patients with refractory or recurrent bursitis.

13.1 INTRODUCTION

Bursae (singular: bursa; the term derived from the Latin for "purse") are small, closed sacs, lined with a synovial membrane, which secretes synovial fluid. Bursae are generally found in areas of the musculoskeletal system that are subject to friction, such as where a tendon passes over a bone, between bones, between overlapping muscles, or between bones and skin. Deep bursae are located in the fascia, whereas superficial bursae are located in the subcutaneous tissue. These fluid-filled bursae function to decrease friction between skin, tendons, and bones (Table 13.1).

13.2 ANATOMICAL CONSIDERATIONS

There are approximately 160 discrete bursae in the human body. Most true bursae form during embryonic development, though some, such as the olecranon bursa, may develop later in life.[1] Adventitial bursae also form later in life in response to repeated trauma, constant pressure, or friction. While anatomic/true bursae are lined with epithelial cells and contain synovial cells that secrete lubricating fluid rich in collagen and proteoglycans, adventitial bursae lack endothelial cells and do not secrete or contain synovial fluid. Most of the bursae described in this chapter are anatomic/true bursae. Examples of adventitial bursae include those that form over a bunion or over an osteochondroma.

13.3 PHYSIOLOGIC CONSIDERATIONS

The primary pathologic condition that affects the bursae is bursitis. Though the term denotes an inflammatory condition, bursitis may have any one of many etiologies including infection, trauma, hemorrhage, or a range of inflammatory conditions including autoimmune disorders, conditions that lead to crystal deposition, or overuse injuries.

13.3.1 Septic Bursitis or Infectious Bursitis

Septic bursitis or *infectious bursitis* is most common in superficial bursae due to direct introduction of microorganisms from the skin, either through trauma or via contiguous spread from overlying cellulitis. The olecranon bursa is a common location for infectious bursitis for this reason. An infection of deep bursae is rare, accounting for only about 10% of all septic bursitis.[2] A septic bursitis in a deep bursa is most likely either due to hematogenous spread from a distant infection or due to direct spread from a septic joint. Aspiration of the bursa in cases of suspected bursitis may yield cloudy fluid or frank pus. Gram stain and culture of this fluid can be used to direct therapy.

13.3.2 Traumatic bursitis

Traumatic bursitis, as the name implies, results from direct trauma to the area. This either may be a single acute traumatic injury or may be due to repetitive microtrauma. The latter is more common and leads to a chronic inflammatory process described in the following. Acute traumatic bursitis may have both hemorrhagic and acute inflammatory components. Aspiration of the bursa (which should be reserved for patients in whom there is no concern for infection and who have symptoms so severe that they are causing significant pain or are limiting function) may show blood and/or serous fluid. Management of traumatic bursitis is found in Section 13.8.

13.3.3 Inflammatory bursitis

Inflammatory bursitis may also have a number of etiologies. The inflammatory cascade may be initiated by repetitive microtrauma, systemic rheumatologic or autoimmune conditions, or hypermobility syndromes in which unstable joints can lead to tendinosis, frequent sprains, and bursitis. The pathophysiology of the inflammatory cascade that follows is described in Section 13.5. If aspirated, synovial fluid may provide clues to the etiology.

13.3.4 Hemorrhagic bursitis

Hemorrhagic bursitis can mimic inflammatory bursitis because blood can cause some degree of inflammation and can present with physical findings similar to infectious or inflammatory processes (see physical exam findings in Section 13.6). When not associated with trauma, hemorrhagic bursitis is most often seen with patients who are predisposed to bleeding, such as patients who are on systemic anticoagulant medications (e.g., heparin, enoxaparin, warfarin, or newer agents such as fondaparinux, rivaroxaban, or dalteparin) or those who have inherent bleeding disorders such as Von Willebrand's disease and hemophilia.

13.4 EPIDEMIOLOGY

While bursitis accounts for approximately 0.4% of all visits to primary care clinics, the incidence is higher in athletes, occurring in up to 10% of runners.[2] Superficial septic bursitis occurs more frequently in men (85% of cases) compared to women (15%) and is often seen in workers whose job requires frequent lifting or kneeling.[3] Morbidity associated with bursitis is most often related to pain and decreased range of motion, which may affect function and ability to perform in sports- or job-specific movements. Mortality associated with bursitis is very low, and almost all patients can be treated in the outpatient setting.

13.5 PATHOLOGY

As aforementioned, bursitis is most often caused by infection or inflammation, or rarely from bleeding or trauma. The pathophysiology of the reaction within the bursa and the fluid that accumulates depends on the etiology.

Septic bursitis, as described earlier, occurs when bacteria are introduced into the bursal sac, leading to increased production of synovial fluid and proliferation of white blood cells (WBCs). The most common organism associated with all infectious bursitis is *Staphylococcus aureus*, which accounts for about 80% of the cases.[4] The second most common organisms involved are *Streptococcus* species, though many other organisms may be implicated and polymicrobial infections are not uncommon.[5]

In cases of inflammatory bursitis, the synovial lining becomes thickened and produces excessive fluid, which leads to localized swelling and pain. There are three phases or types of inflammatory bursitis: acute, recurrent, and chronic. In the acute subtype, local inflammation occurs, synovial fluid accumulates, and the bursal sac becomes swollen and thickened, which leads to localized tenderness and pain with movement. In the chronic subtype, long-standing or repeated inflammation leads to a situation in which the lining of the bursal sac is replaced by granulation tissue and later by fibrous tissue. This long-standing inflammatory process leads to chronic, continuous pain and may cause weakening of the nearby ligaments and tendons. Ultimately, these chronic changes may lead to tendon rupture. The recurrent subtype occurs when there are relapses of acute inflammatory bursitis, with periods in between in which the patient is asymptomatic. In such cases, each episode presents more like an acute episode, though over time, frequent and recurrent episodes may lead to chronic changes.

Clinical Pearl

INFECTIOUS AGENTS

S. aureus is responsible for 80% of cases of septic bursitis.

The most commonly affected bursae in the upper extremity are the subacromial, the subscapular, and the olecranon bursae. The subacromial bursa lies on the surface of the supraspinatus tendon, separating it from the overlying coracoacromial arch and the deltoid muscle. Its location here, overlying the tendons of the rotator cuff, predisposes the subacromial bursa to repetitive microtrauma and inflammation. The subscapular bursa is found between the anterior surface of the scapula and the posterior chest wall. Inflammation in the subscapular bursa occurs as a result of abnormal bony architecture or scapular dyskinesis.

The olecranon bursa is composed of two different structures; one lies between the triceps tendon and the posterior joint capsule of the elbow, while the other is more superficial, lying between the insertion of the distal triceps tendon and the skin. As noted earlier, the location of the superficial bursa at the olecranon makes it particularly susceptible to acute trauma (direct blow), chronic microtrauma (so-called student's elbow due to leaning onto one's elbows on a desk), or infection. The majority of cases of olecranon bursitis are noninfectious with septic bursitis accounting for only approximately 20% of acute cases.[6]

The most commonly affected bursae in the lower extremity are the ischial/gluteal, the iliopsoas, the trochanteric, the bursae around the knee (prepatellar, infrapatellar, and popliteal), and the bursae around the Achilles. The ischial/gluteal bursa lies deep to gluteus maximus and over the ischial tuberosity. This bursa often becomes inflamed in patients who have sedentary occupations and spend a great deal of time sitting. The iliopsoas or iliopectineal bursa is the largest in the body and is found between the iliopsoas and the lesser trochanter, extending superiorly beneath the iliacus. The iliopsoas bursa can become irritated especially in runners and in patients with rheumatologic disease or osteoarthritis. The trochanteric bursa has both a superficial and deep component, with the superficial lying between the tensor fascia lata and the skin and the deep lying between the tensor fascia lata and the greater trochanter. Trochanteric bursitis has typically been described in overweight women who complain of hip and lateral thigh pain that is worse at night and with activity. However, recent improved diagnosis through use of bedside ultrasound (US) (see Section 13.7) demonstrates that perhaps much of what was once thought to be trochanteric bursitis in fact represents other muscular or tendon pathology in the area, most frequently tendinopathy or tears of the gluteus medius or gluteus minimus.

In the knee, the prepatellar bursa lies anteriorly over the patella, just deep to the skin. Similar to the olecranon bursa, the prepatellar bursa is susceptible to direct trauma, chronic microtrauma (such as in laborers with so-called housemaid's knee), or infection due to superficial soft tissue infections. The infrapatellar bursa has two components, one superficial and one deep to the patellar tendon. The popliteal bursa lies in the posterior aspect of the knee joint and is anatomically located where a Baker's cyst may form, at the junction of the semimembranosus and the medial head of the gastrocnemius. In one study, 37% of patients undergoing knee arthroscopy had an identifiable popliteal bursa communicating with the posteromedial compartment of the knee joint.[7] Patients with popliteal bursitis or Baker's cyst often complain of pain with walking, jumping, or squatting.

In the Achilles region, there are two bursae at the insertion of the Achilles on the calcaneus, one is superficial, between the tendon and the skin, while the other is deep, located between the tendon and the calcaneus. Retrocalcaneal bursitis is frequently seen in patients who report acute pain and swelling associated with wearing new shoes, which cause friction in the area. In athletes, retrocalcaneal bursitis may accompany Achilles tendinopathy. In more chronic cases, a "pump bump" may develop in this area, with evidence of the thickened tissue beneath.

13.6 HISTORY AND PHYSICAL EXAM

Many patients presenting with bursitis-related pain will report a history of repetitive movements (e.g., frequent kneeling, repetitive lifting, or from sports with repetitive motions, such as running). These patients may report limited range of motion due to swelling and/or pain, and they may have significant limitations in their sports-specific or work-related activities. In severe cases, activities of daily living (sitting, climbing stairs, sleeping on one side, dressing and other overhead activities, etc.) may cause exacerbation of symptoms as well. Upon questioning, they may report a history of systemic inflammatory disease such as rheumatoid arthritis, lupus, or gout. Furthermore, it is important to ask about any history of direct trauma, systemic symptoms such as fevers, or any history consistent with coagulopathy.

On physical exam, the clinician will often identify localized tenderness, edema, erythema, palpable warmth, and/or decreased active range of motion in the area of the affected bursa. Passive range of motion is often preserved. Not surprisingly, erythema and edema are more often seen with superficial bursitis and both are often very localized and well demarcated as the inflammation is confined to the bursa itself. The symptoms of bursitis are often reproduced by the movement of the joint and/or tendon that is associated with the affected bursa. Chronic bursitis may lead to weakening and tenderness of the tendon itself.

Cutaneous temperature may also be helpful when there is concern for septic bursitis. Smith et al. measured a significant difference in skin temperature between the skin overlying the infected bursa and the contralateral/unaffected side. Overall, average surface temperature difference between affected and unaffected extremities was 0.7°C (1.26°F) in aseptic cases compared to 3.7°C (6.66°F) in septic cases. Using a surface temperature probe, a measured temperature difference (≥ 2.2°C or 3.96°F) was 100% sensitive and 94% specific for a septic process.[8] Clinically, a surface temperature probe may be used; however, even a palpable difference in temperature may increase the suspicion for an infectious etiology.

Clinical Pearl

EVALUATION OF SKIN TEMPERATURE

The skin overlying septic bursitis is always warmer than the contralateral side (100% sensitive).

13.7 DIAGNOSTICS/IMAGING

Routine lab work is generally not helpful in making a diagnosis unless systemic or rheumatic disease is suspected. In these cases, a rheumatologic panel (anti-CCP, ANA, ESR, CRP, RF, uric acid, etc.) may be useful. Aspiration of the bursa may be useful to evaluate the presence of crystals or bacteria. If the etiology is unclear, any aspirated fluid should be sent for uric acid–level determination; identification of crystals; and cell count with differential, gram stain, and culture; protein and glucose are rarely helpful but can be sent if there is enough fluid. Nontraditional synovial markers such as fluid lactate level have also been described in the diagnosis of septic arthritis and may prove helpful in the future for making the early diagnosis of septic bursitis as well.

In the acute setting, cell count is the test that often yields the fastest results and may be used to make a preliminary diagnosis and guide initial therapy. Aseptic or inflammatory bursitis has white cell counts (WBC) less than 1000/μL, with a predominance of mononuclear cells. A WBC count of 10,000–20,000/μL or higher usually signifies an infectious etiology. For cases between 1,000 and 10,000/μL, the WBC differential can be helpful, as a predominance of mononuclear cells tends to indicate inflammatory processes, while an increased proportion of polynuclear cells is indicative of an infectious etiology. Gram stains of bursal fluid are unfortunately only positive in 50%–60% of samples that later yielded positive cultures, so the gram stain cannot be relied upon exclusively.[6] However, the bursal fluid culture will provide the definitive diagnosis, and the culture and sensitivities should be used to guide definitive antibiotic therapy in cases of septic bursitis.

Clinical Pearl

UTILITY OF RADIOGRAPHS

Bursitis is generally a clinical, not a radiographic, diagnosis.

In general, plain radiographs usually are not helpful. However, x-rays may be useful for identifying osteophytes or other underlying bony pathology, which can exacerbate tendinopathy and bursal inflammation. In severe or chronic cases of bursitis, x-rays may also show joint effusions, bony erosion, and/or crystal deposition. Bone scintigraphy is neither sensitive nor specific for bursitis, but may be performed in cases where the diagnosis is unclear, in order to evaluate other causes of pain. Magnetic resonance imaging (MRI) and computed tomography scanning are usually not necessary as the diagnosis may be made clinically, though these scans may reveal bursitis in cases where the entire joint is being imaged for another reason. Bird et al. used an MRI to assess 24 patients with clinical findings consistent with greater trochanteric bursitis (i.e., lateral hip pain and tenderness over the greater trochanter) and found that only two patients who had clinical signs consistent with trochanteric bursitis had evidence of bursal distension on MRI.[9]

Of all radiologic studies, US may be the most useful for many reasons. When diagnosis is unclear, US may aid in the evaluation for other etiologies for pain. US can also be used to look for fluid or increased blood flow (using Doppler flow studies), which can be signs of inflammation, infection, or trauma. Furthermore, US can also identify adjacent and associated pathologies such as tendinopathy in cases of chronic symptoms. In cases in which a bursa is overlying a tendon, bursal edema, as seen on US, is often a sign of associated tendinopathy, a finding that may help guide treatment and rehabilitation strategies. Finally, US can be used as an adjunct for procedures, such as aspiration and injection. One of the best arguments in favor of the use of US is that it is widely available in many clinic settings and can help make the diagnosis, in the office, in a single visit.

Table 13.2 reviews the strength of recommendations for various evaluation methods for bursitis.

13.8 TREATMENT CONSIDERATIONS

The focus of treatment should be tailored based on the specific etiology. For overuse or inflammatory etiologies, conservative therapies aimed at reducing inflammation are first-line treatments. These include recommendations for rest, cold therapy, elevation, nonsteroidal anti-inflammatory drugs, and physical therapy. Aspiration is also often part of the treatment strategy, especially for acute and/or traumatic bursitis. However, this should be limited to patients with acute or severe symptoms that are significantly affecting their range of motion and functional abilities. Chronic inflammatory conditions, including gouty bursitis, may respond only temporarily to aspiration and reaccumulation of fluid often occurs. A light compression dressing and/or intrabursal steroid injection may help prevent this. However, caution must be taken when injecting steroids especially if an infectious etiology is part of the differential diagnosis. Physical therapy may be helpful in patients with severe or ongoing symptoms. Other possible treatment modalities include therapeutic US and steroid iontophoresis; however, there is little evidence to suggest that these modalities provide significant benefit in most cases.

For cases of suspected septic bursitis, empiric antibiotic therapy should be initiated while gram stain and culture results are pending. Superficial septic bursitis may be treated with oral therapy in the outpatient setting with therapy directed at common skin flora. Coverage for *S. aureus* should be ensured, and coverage for methicillin-resistant *S. aureus* should be considered in high-risk populations.[10,11] However, those with evidence of deep bursitis, septic joint, or systemic symptoms may require hospital admission for intravenous antibiotics. For traumatic or hemorrhagic bursitis, aspiration followed by rest, ice, and physical therapy can be useful.

Clinical Pearl

TREATMENT OF SEPTIC BURSITIS

Most cases of septic bursitis respond to drainage and oral antibiotics.

Intravenous antibiotics are required for severe cases and/or patients with systemic symptoms.

Surgery is rarely needed and is reserved for refractory or recurrent cases.

Surgical washout and excision of bursal tissue may be required for chronic or frequently recurring cases or in cases of septic bursitis that has not responded appropriately to antibiotics. However, surgical treatment is most often considered a "last resort" after all other treatment options have been exhausted. Most patients will respond well to conservative management. Those who fail standard therapy or those who have signs of tendon or ligamentous injury should be referred to an orthopedic surgeon for further evaluation. In a recent review article, the described rates of surgery were lower in cases of septic bursitis due to *S. aureus* (8%) compared to 18% in cases where other bacteria were implicated.[6]

There are no set return-to-play (or return to work) guidelines for bursitis. Management and return to activity will depend on the etiology, location, limitations of movement or sport-specific activity, and the response to treatment. Once the patients have normal range of motion (passive and active) and normal strength and have passed functional testing without pain, they will be able to return to their job/sport. However, all patients should be aware that bursitis may be exacerbated or recur with the repetitive motions involved in sports and activity, particularly if the initial onset was insidious and due to chronic repetitive motions. Activity modification and/or protective equipment may be helpful in facilitating healing and return to work/activity while minimizing recurrence of symptoms. For cases such as "housemaid's knee" and prepatellar bursitis that is often seen in construction workers who kneel while performing tasks such as laying carpet or tile, protective knee pads can be used to help distribute the force and minimize the repetitive trauma to the area.

TABLE 13.2
SORT: Key Recommendations for Practice

Clinical Recommendation	Evidence Rating	References
Twenty percent of olecranon bursitis is septic bursitis.	C	[6]
In the evaluation of bursal fluid, the following occurs: • WBC count >10,000 WBC/μL is consistent with septic bursitis. • WBC count <1000 WBC/μL is consistent with aseptic bursitis. • When WBC count >1,000/μL and <10,000/μL, cell type can help with the diagnosis where a predominance of polynuclear cells is indicative of septic bursitis.	B	[6]
Temperature difference between skin overlying affected bursa compared to contralateral side of >2.2°C predicts septic bursitis with 100% sensitivity and 94% specificity.	B	[7]

13.9 CONCLUSION

Bursitis is a common condition seen both in primary care and in sports medicine clinics. The astute clinician should be able to recognize this condition based on the relevant history and physical exam findings and will be able to guide initial evaluation and management accordingly. The vast majority of patients will respond to conservative management and can be managed in the outpatient setting (Table 13.2).

REFERENCES

1. Chen J, Alk D, Evantov I, Wientroub S. Development of the olecranon bursa: An anatomic cadaver study. *Acta Orthopaedica Scandinavia*. 1987;58(4):408–409.
2. Lohr K, Gonsalves A, Root L, Talbot-Stern JK. Bursitis; Medscape on-line reference, http://emedicine.medscape.com/article/2145588-overview (accessed April 21, 2014).
3. Le Manac'h AP, Ha C, Descatha K, Imbernon E, Roquelaure Y. Prevalence of knee bursitis in the workforce. *Occupational Medicine (London)*. 2012;62(8):658–660.
4. Cea-Pereiro JC, Garcia-Meijide J, Mera-Verela A, Gomez-Reino JJ. A comparison between septic bursitis caused by Staphylococcus aureus and those caused by other organisms. *Clinical Rheumatology*. 2001;20(1):10–14.
5. Torralba KD, Quismorio FP Jr. Soft tissue infections. *Rheumatic Disease Clinics of North Americal*. 2009;35(1):45–46.
6. Aaron D, Patel A, Kayiaros S, Calfee R. Four common types of bursitis: Diagnosis and management. *Journal of the Academy of Orthopaedic Surgery*. 2011;19(6):359–367.
7. Johnson LL, van Dyk GE, Bays BM, Gully SM. The popliteal bursa (Baker's cyst): An arthroscopic perspective and the epidemiology. *Arthroscopy*. 1997;13(1):66–72.
8. Smith DL, McAfee JH, Lucas LM, Kusum LK, Romney DM. Septic and nonseptic olecranon bursitis: Utility of the surface temperature probe in the early differentiation of septic and nonseptic cases. *Archives of Internal Medicine*. 1989;149(7):1581–1585.
9. Bird PA, Oakley SP, Shnier R, Kirkham BW. Prospective evaluation of magnetic resonance imaging and physical examination findings in patients with greater trochanteric pain syndrome. *Arthritis Rheumatoid*. 2001;44(9):2138–2145.
10. Hamann F, Dulon M, Nienhaus A. MRSA as an occupational disease: A case series. *International Archives of Occupational and Environmental Health*. 2011;84(3):259–266.
11. Hanrahan J. Recent developments in *Septic Bursitis. Current Infectious Disease Report*. 2013;15(5):421–425.

14 Exercise Physiology

Joshua S. Sole and Jonathan T. Finnoff

CONTENTS

TABLE 14.1
Key Clinical Considerations

1. Resistance training results in muscle cell hypertrophy not hyperplasia and occurs after 6–8 weeks of training. Initial strength gains prior to 6–8 weeks are attributed to neural factors. Resistance exercise can result in an improved aerobic exercise but the converse has not been demonstrated. Resistance training also increases bone mineral density, ligament, and tendon strength (increased collagen content), and anaerobic energy stores (glycogen, ATP, phosphocreatine).
2. There are three main stretching techniques: proprioceptive neuromuscular facilitation (PNF), ballistic stretching, and static stretching. The most effective stretching technique is PNF. Ballistic and static stretching have similar efficacy, but ballistic stretching has a higher risk of injury.
3. Individual lactate (anaerobic) threshold is trainable. Although lactate is the prime energy source for glycolysis, lactate accumulation has not been shown to cause the subjective "muscle burn" from exercise.
4. Exercise has profound effects on multiple organ systems including but not excluded to the cardiovascular, respiratory, endocrine, immune, neurologic, and musculoskeletal systems.
5. Physiologic changes with aging are of clinical importance, especially when counseling and treating the masters-/senior-level athlete. Additionally, regular exercise is beneficial as an adjuvant treatment to many chronic disease states including but not limited to hypertension, peripheral vascular disease, osteoarthritis, chronic obstructive pulmonary disease, chronic pain, depression, osteoporosis, and obesity.
6. Weight loss requires negative caloric balance (more calories expended than consumed). Dieting alone is superior for weight loss than exercise alone, but individuals are more likely to maintain weight loss if they participate in regular physical activity/exercise. Furthermore, regular exercise modifies multiple cardiovascular disease–risk factors in the obese patient.

14.1 MUSCLE MICROANATOMY AND PHYSIOLOGY

Muscle cells (myofibers) are multinucleated cells that contain sarcomeres, which are the smallest functional unit of skeletal muscle contraction. Sarcomeres extend from Z-line (disk) to Z-line (disk) (Figure 14.1).[7,8,12] The contractile elements (myofibrils) of the sarcomere are myosin (thick filament) and actin (thin filament). Actin has a double helical structure and contains myosin-binding sites where the globular head of myosin filaments binds during muscle contraction. In the resting state, the myosin-binding sites on the actin filaments are covered by a protein called tropomyosin, thus preventing myosin from binding to actin. Another protein, named troponin, is bound to tropomyosin. The role of the troponin–tropomyosin protein complex in muscle contraction will be discussed later. Key considerations for this chapter are contained in Table 14.1.

Actin attaches to the Z-lines at the end of each sarcomere, while myosin attaches to the M-lines in the center of the sarcomeres.[12] The A (dark) band includes the region where actin and myosin overlap. The I (light) band only contains actin. The H zone contains only myosin. During muscle contraction, the H zone and I band shorten.[7,12]

The process of muscle contraction begins when an alpha-motor neuron depolarizes, releasing acetylcholine (Ach) into the neuromuscular junction, which binds to receptors on the muscle cell membrane (sarcolemma), causing the muscle cell to depolarize. Depolarization is rapidly transmitted into the interior of the muscle cell via the transverse tubules, which signals the sarcoplasmic reticulum to release calcium (Ca^{++}) inside the muscle cell (Figure 14.1). The Ca^{++} binds to troponin causing a shift in the tropomyosin position, uncovering the actin filament's myosin-binding sites. A myosin head, with an attached adenosine triphosphate (ATP) molecule, then binds to the actin filament. When this occurs, the ATP is hydrolyzed to adenosine diphosphate (ADP) by the enzyme ATPase. This chemical reaction releases energy, which is used to flex the myosin head, which slides the actin filament across the myosin filament (sliding-filament theory), causing muscle contraction. The ADP is released from the myosin filament, allowing a new ATP molecule to attach to the myosin head, and the

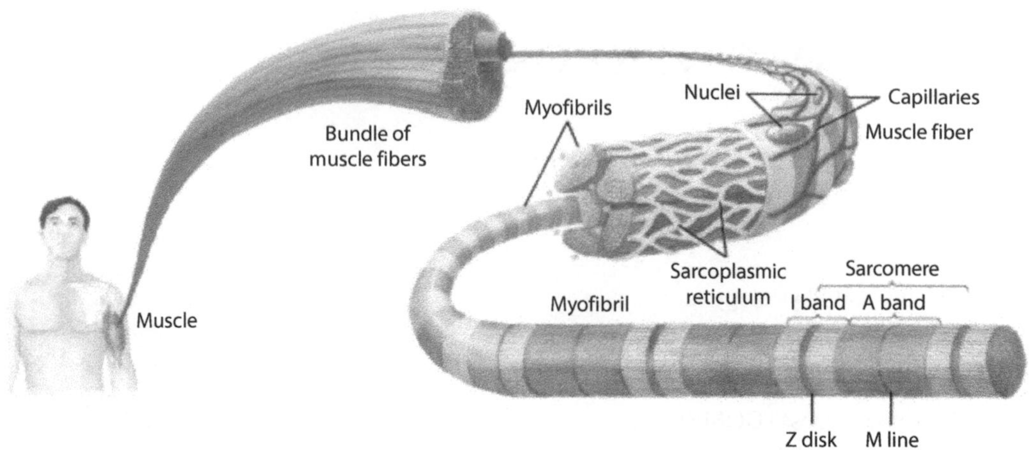

FIGURE 14.1 Basic skeletal muscle anatomy. (Reprinted with permission from http://crescentok.com/staff/jaskew/isr/anatomy/anatomy1/unit9.htm.)

myosin detaches from the actin. The ATP is again converted to ADP, and the energy from this reaction allows the myosin head to return to its original position in preparation for another contraction. Thus, two ATPs are required for each contraction cycle.[7,12]

A motor unit is made up of a single alpha motor neuron and all the muscle cells it innervates. The number of muscle cells per motor unit varies from tens to thousands. Smaller motor units are involved in fine motor movements, while large motor units are involved in gross motor activities. When a motor unit is activated, all of the muscle cells it innervates contract. This is called the "all or none law."[7,8,12]

Muscles have special sensory organs called muscle spindles, which are innervated by gamma motor neurons. Muscle spindles are intrafusal muscle fibers that sense and respond to muscle position and movement. Rapid stretching of the muscle is sensed by the muscle spindles, and they signal the muscle to contract and resist the rapid stretch (e.g., patellar tendon reflex). Golgi tendon organs are located inside of the tendons. When excessive muscle force is sensed by the golgi tendon organ, it causes the muscle to relax, which protects the muscle from tearing.[12]

Muscles have three connective tissue layers including the endomysium, perimysium, and epimysium. Each muscle cell is surrounded by the endomysium, which is continuous with the muscle cell membrane (sarcolemma). Multiple muscle cells are bundled into fascicles, which are surrounded by the perimysium. The epimysium surrounds the entire muscle. At either end of the muscle, the endomysium, perimysium, and epimysium connect to the muscle's tendon, which in turn connects to the periosteum of bone.[7]

There are two primary muscle fiber types in humans: Type I (slow twitch-oxidative) and Type II (fast twitch-glycolytic). They are delineated by their expression of different myosin heavy chains. Type II muscle fibers are further subdivided into Type IIa (fast twitch-oxidative glycolytic) and Type IIx (fast twitch-glycolytic). While some muscles are predominantly composed of one fiber type, nearly all muscles have a mixture of both fiber types. However, each motor unit is composed of a single fiber type. The characteristics of each muscle fiber type are listed in Table 14.2.[12]

Muscle recruitment behaves according to the Henneman size principle. According to this principle, motor units with Type I muscle fibers are recruited first followed by motor units with Type II fibers.[7]

14.2 METABOLIC PATHWAYS IN EXERCISE

The energy for muscle contraction is supplied by three metabolic pathways (energy systems).[7] The first pathway is the ATP–phosphocreatinine system. In this pathway, phosphocreatinine donates a phosphate to regenerate ATP from ADP within the muscle. This process is driven by the enzyme creatinine kinase. This enables rapid replenishment of ATP during short, high-intensity exercises lasting up to 30 seconds in duration. It takes about 3 minutes of rest to replenish the phosphocreatinine supply.[7,8]

The second metabolic pathway is the anaerobic (glycolytic) system, which metabolizes glucose to pyruvate via glycolysis. No oxygen is required for glycolysis, and the two or three ATP molecules are produced depending on whether the initial substrate is glucose (2 ATP) or glycogen (3 ATP). The rate-limiting enzyme of glycolysis is phosphofructokinase. In the presence of oxygen, pyruvate enters the aerobic metabolic system. Otherwise, it is reversibly converted to lactate. This is the primary energy system for sustained maximal exercise lasting between 1 and 3 minutes.[7,8]

The third metabolic pathway (aerobic or oxidative pathway) involves the metabolism of pyruvate through a process known as oxidative phosphorylation. This process takes place in the mitochondria. Oxidative phosphorylation has two parts: the Kreb's cycle and electron transport chain. In the presence of oxygen, pyruvate is converted to acetyl coenzyme A (acetyl CoA), which is metabolized in the Kreb's cycle and electron transport chain to produce 36 ATP molecules. The by-product on this process is carbon dioxide (Kreb's cycle) and water (electron transport chain). Thus, the net ATP produced from glycolysis and oxidative

TABLE 14.2
Characteristics of Skeletal Muscle Fiber Types

Characteristic	Type I	Type IIa	Type IIx
Contraction speed	Slow	Fast	Fast
Force production	Low	Intermediate	High
Endurance	High	Intermediate/low	Low
Glycolytic capacity	Low	High	High
Myosin ATPase activity	Low	Intermediate	Intermediate
Aerobic enzymes	High	Intermediate/low	Low
Anaerobic enzymes	Low	High	High
Fatigability	Low	Intermediate/high	High
Capillary density	High	Intermediate	Low
Fiber size	Small	Intermediate	Large
Mitochondria	High	Intermediate	Low
ATPase activity	Low	High	High
Myoglobin content	High	Low	Low
Glycogen content	Low	Intermediate	High
Triglyceride content	High	Intermediate	Low
Color	Red	White	White
Myosin heavy chain (MHC)	MHCIβ	MHCIIa	MHCIIb
ATP/ADP	Low	Intermediate	High

Sources: Howatson, G. and van Someren, K.A., *Sports Med.*, 38(6), 483, 2008; Pate, R.R. et al., *Journal of the American Medical Association*, 273(5), 402, 1995.

phosphorylation is 38 ATP if glucose is the initial substrate and 39 ATP if glycogen is the starting substrate. Aerobic metabolism serves as the primary energy pathway for exercise lasting greater than 3 minutes.[7,8]

Fat can also be metabolized via the aerobic pathway via β-oxidation. This begins with the breakdown of triglycerides into glycerol and three fatty acids. The fatty acids are converted into acetyl CoA, which then enter the Kreb's cycle and electron transport chain. The net energy production from free fatty acid metabolism is far greater than for glucose metabolism. For instance, 129 ATP molecules are produced from the metabolism of one palmitic acid molecule, the most common saturated fatty acid found in animals, plants, and microorganisms.[7,8]

14.3 EXERCISE CONCEPTS

Endurance or aerobic exercise involves the repetitive contraction of large muscle groups over time, whereas anaerobic exercise involves higher-intensity, short-duration activities. The anatomic and physiologic adaptations to aerobic and anaerobic exercises are listed in Table 14.3.

Regular aerobic exercise training results in preferential metabolism of fat, sometimes referred to as "glycogen sparing," which also reduces lactate production during exercise. Furthermore, because of the increase in aerobic enzymes, less pyruvate is converted to lactate.[7]

Oxygen uptake (VO_2) is defined as the amount of oxygen consumed by the body to produce the energy necessary for a given activity. Maximal oxygen uptake ($VO_{2\,max}$) is the amount of oxygen used during maximal exercise and is a commonly used measurement for aerobic fitness (see Section 14.7). The best way to determine $VO_{2\,max}$ is by performing an incremental exercise test to failure. $VO_{2\,max}$ has been achieved during the exercise test when an increase in the amount of work no longer results in an increase in VO_2.[31] Simple in-office clinical and field tests that can be used to estimate $VO_{2\,max}$ include the 1–2 mile run, 12 minute run, 3 minute step test, shuttle runs, and submaximal cycle ergometry.[12]

Resistance exercise training is used to improve muscle strength, endurance, and power (how fast strength/force can be applied).[12] Resistance exercise causes more hypertrophy than endurance exercise. Muscle hypertrophy is secondary to an increased number of sarcomeres per muscle cell (no more muscle cells [hyperplasia]) and predominantly occurs in Type II muscle fibers, although some hypertrophy also takes place in Type I fibers. It takes approximately 6–8 weeks of resistance training to induce muscle hypertrophy.[7,12] Strength gains prior to 6 weeks are due to improved neuromuscular recruitment patterns and suppression of inhibitory reflexes.[7,12] Resistance training can also improve aerobic exercise performance. However, aerobic training does not appear to augment the strength gains acquired from resistance training.[7]

Clinical Pearl

Initial strength gains from resistance exercise are due to neural factors. Gains from muscle cell hypertrophy take 1.5–2 months to develop. Resistance training only results in muscle hypertrophy and has never been shown to cause muscle cell hyperplasia in humans.

TABLE 14.3
Anatomic and Physiologic Adaptations to Aerobic and Anaerobic Exercise

Adaptation	Aerobic	Anaerobic
Muscular capillary density	↑↑	↓
Mitochondrial number and size	↑↑	↓
Oxidative (aerobic) enzymes	↑↑	↑
Glycolytic (anaerobic) enzymes	—	↑↑
Fatty acid transportation across sarcolemma	↑↑	—
Fat metabolism	↑↑	—
Glucose/glycogen metabolism	↓	—
Arterial oxygen extraction/arteriovenous oxygen difference	↑↑	—
Lactate production	↓	↓
Lactate-buffering capacity	—	↑↑
Type IIx to Type IIa fiber-type conversion	↑↑	—
Muscle hypertrophy	—	—
Improved aerobic exercise performance	↑↑	↑
Increased bone mineral density	—	↑↑
Increased connective tissue content	—	↑↑

Source: Howatson, G. and van Someren, K.A., *Sports Med.*, 38(6), 483, 2008.

Metabolic energy equivalents (MET) are the standard unit used to measure exercise intensity. One MET (resting metabolic rate) is equal to 1 kcal/kg/h or 3.5 mL of O_2/kg/min. Table 14.4 depicts how many METs are required for specific activities.

Another commonly used scale for exercise intensity is the Borg Rating of Perceived Exertion (RPE) (Table 14.5). This is a subjective scale and does not require any objective measurements.

14.4 LACTATE KINETICS

During rest and low activity, serum lactate levels are between 0.8 and 1.5 mmol/L and generally remain constant.[8,12] As exercise intensity increases, there is a point where metabolism shifts from predominantly aerobic to anaerobic metabolism and lactate begins to accumulate. This point is

TABLE 14.4
Physical Activity and Metabolic Equivalents

Physical Activity	MET
Light-Intensity Activities <3	
Sleeping	0.9
Watching television	1.0
Writing, desk work, typing	1.8
Walking, 1.7 mph (2.7 km/h), level ground, strolling, very slow	2.3
Walking, 2.5 mph (4 km/h)	2.9
Moderate-Intensity Activities 3–6	
Bicycling, stationary, 50 W, very light effort	3.0
Walking 3.0 mph (4.8 km/h)	3.3
Calisthenics, home exercise, light or moderate effort, general	3.5
Walking 3.4 mph (5.5 km/h)	3.6
Bicycling, <10 mph (16 km/h), leisure, to work or for pleasure	4.0
Stationary bicycling (100 W) light effort	5.5
Vigorous-Intensity Activities >6	
Jogging, general	7.0
Calisthenics (e.g., push-ups, sit-ups, pull-up, jumping jacks), heavy, vigorous effort	8.0
Running or jogging, in place	8.0
Jumping rope	10.0

Sources: American College of Sports Medicine et al., *ACSM's Guidelines for Exercise Testing and Prescription*, 8th edn., Philadelphia, PA, Lippincott Williams & Wilkins, 2010; Andersen, R.E., *Phys. Sportsmed.*, 27(10), 41, 1999; Borg, G.A., *Med. Sci. Sports Exerc.*, 14(5), 377, 1982.

TABLE 14.5
Borg Rating of Perceived Exertion (RPE) Scale

RPE	Description
6	No exertion at all
7	Extremely light
8	
9	Very light
10	
11	Light
12	
13	Somewhat hard
14	
15	Hard (heavy)
16	
17	
18	
19	Extremely hard
20	Maximal exertion

Sources: Cuccurullo, S. *Physical Medicine and Rehabilitation Board Review*, 2nd edn., New York, Demos Medical Publishing, 2010; Dunn, A.L. et al., *Med. Sci. Sports Exerc.*, 33(6 Suppl), S587, discussion 609, 2001.

called the lactate (anaerobic) threshold and usually occurs when the serum lactate concentration is 4 mmol/L. Lactate threshold is often reported as a percentage of $VO_{2\,max}$ and is trainable (i.e., can occur at a higher percentage of $VO_{2\,max}$ following consistent training). In untrained people, the lactate threshold may be 50%–60% of the $VO_{2\,max}$, but it trained individuals that this threshold may be closer to 80%–90% of $VO_{2\,max}$.[7] Lactate threshold as a percentage of $VO_{2\,max}$ is considered one of the best measures of aerobic fitness. Muscle cells release lactate into the circulation during exercise, where it is converted to glucose via gluconeogenesis and serves as an energy source in the heart and non-exercising muscles. Lactate does not appear to cause the "muscle burn" associated with exercise.[7,12]

Clinical Pearl

Lactate accumulation and release from muscle cells during exercise has not been shown to correlate with the subjective "muscle burn" during exercise activity.

14.5 DELAYED ONSET MUSCLE SORENESS (DOMS)

Delayed onset muscle soreness (DOMS) can be seen in elite or novice athletes after novel eccentric exercises or resistance training.[6,12] Symptoms are temporary and can include pain, tenderness, stiffness, and decreased muscle force production. Following a novel eccentric or resistance exercise, there is disruption of the sarcomere's Z-lines termed "Z-line streaming." Release of calcium activates proteolytic enzymes that degrade the damaged sarcomeres. Neutrophils are attracted to the site of injury within a few hours and monocytes within 6–12 hours. Monocytes differentiate into macrophages and phagocytose the damaged tissue. Prostaglandin E2 and histamine are released causing sensitization of nociceptive nerves, edema, and hyperthermia. Oxygen-free radicals are produced, which cause further cell damage. Pain typically presents 6–12 hours following exercise or activity and peaks 2–3 postexercise and typically resolves within a week.[6,7]

Performing a single bout of eccentric exercise prevents DOMS from the same type of exercise for approximately 6 weeks (termed repeated bout effect).[7] Many symptomatic treatments have been used for DOMS including nonsteroidal anti-inflammatories (NSAIDs), acetaminophen, massage, physical modalities (e.g., electrical stimulation, cryotherapy, heat), and rest. However, the most effective treatment appears to be light exercise starting 1–2 days after the onset of DOMS and progressing over 1–2 weeks back to normal levels.[6]

Clinical Pearl

The most effective means of preventing DOMS is the repeated bout effect. This involves a single bout of eccentric exercise to prevent the development of DOMS from the same exercise for around 6 weeks.

14.6 FLEXIBILITY AND STRETCHING TECHNIQUES

There are three main categories of stretching techniques: static, ballistic, and proprioceptive neuromuscular facilitation (PNF). Static stretching typically involves holding a muscle in a stretched position for 30–60 seconds. Static stretching is relatively easy to perform and results in minimal activation of the muscle spindles.[7] Static stretching prior to exercise may have a deleterious effect on exercise performance. Ballistic stretching utilizes a "bouncing" motion to facilitate muscle stretch. This activates muscle spindle fibers resulting in reflexogenic contraction of the muscle being stretched. Ballistic stretching has been shown to be as effective as static stretching, but is known to be more painful and to have a higher injury predisposition. PNF stretching involves contracting the muscle being stretched (agonist) or the antagonist muscle to facilitate the stretch through inhibitory (antagonist) and facilitatory (agonist) reflexes.[7] PNF has been shown to be more effective than static or ballistic stretching, which are considered equal in efficacy to each other.[7]

Clinical Pearl

Effectiveness of stretching techniques: PNF > Static stretching = Ballistic stretching.

14.7 EXERCISE AND THE CARDIOVASCULAR SYSTEM

With increased exercise intensity, there is a linear increase in heart rate (HR). Stroke volume (SV) increases initially, but eventually plateaus. Increases in cardiac output (CO) with lower intensity exercise are due to a combination of increased HR and SV. However, increased CO during higher intensity exercise is almost completely secondary to increases in HR.

Clinical Pearl(s)

$$CO = HR \times SV$$

$a\text{-}VO_2$ = Arteriovenous oxygen content difference

Fick equation: $VO_2 = CO \times (a\text{-}VO_2)$

There is a linear relationship between CO and VO_2.[7] This is based on the Fick equation (see Clinical Pearl). Thus, cardiac output is a vital determinant of aerobic capacity.[7,12] During prolonged aerobic exercise, there is a gradual increase in HR and gradual decrease in SV at any given workload. This phenomenon, termed "cardiac drift," is secondary to a greater percentage of blood being shunted to the skin for heat dissipation and reduced blood volume secondary to sweating during aerobic exercise.[7]

Long-term aerobic exercise training results in various anatomic and physiologic adaptations to the cardiovascular system. There is increased stroke volume at rest and at maximum exercise capacity. Resting HR decreases due to increased vagal tone. The left ventricular (LV) wall thickness, internal diameter, and overall size increase (eccentric cardiac hypertrophy). Moreover, total blood volume increases. This is initially secondary to increased plasma volume, but eventually results from an increase in both plasma volume and red blood cell quantity. However, since the increase plasma volume is larger than red blood cell volume, a "pseudoanemia" occurs.

Long-term resistance training increases LV wall thickness and mass, but does not increase the LV internal diameter.[7]

14.8 EXERCISE AND THE RESPIRATORY SYSTEM

The total volume of air moved into and out of the lungs each minute is called the minute ventilation (MV). MV is equal to the tidal volume times the respiratory rate. At rest, MV is around 5–7 L/min, but during exercise it can increase as high as 60–180 L/min, depending on one's health status. With exercise, MV has an initial rapid increase, followed by a plateau, then a gradual increase until steady state is achieved. The initial increase in MV is due to an increase in tidal volume. With increased exercise intensity, the increase in MV is primarily due to an increase in respiratory rate. There is a linear relationship between submaximal VO_2 and MV.[7]

14.9 PHYSIOLOGIC CHANGES WITH AGING

Tables 14.6 and 14.7 summarize many physiologic changes that occur with aging and training. These changes need to be taken into consideration when working with the aging population.

TABLE 14.6
Physiologic Changes in Aging

System	Physiologic Change	Effect/Amount of Change
Cardiovascular	↓ Maximum heart rate	10 beats/min/decade
	↓ Blood vessel compliance	↑ blood pressure 10–40 mmHg
	↓ Restring stroke volume	
	↓ Maximum cardiac output	30% by 85 years of age
	↓ Maximum cardiac output	20%–30% by the age of 65
Respiratory	↑ Residual volume	30%–50% by the age of 70
	↓ Vital capacity	40%–50% by the age of 70
Metabolic	↓ $VO_{2\,max}$	9% per decade
Neurologic	↓ Nerve conduction velocity	1%–15% by the age of 60
	↓ Proprioception	↑ falls 35%–40% by the age of 60
Musculoskeletal	↑ Bone loss (35–55 years old)	1% per year
	↑ Bone loss (>55 years old)	3%–5% per year
	↓ Muscle strength	20% by the age of 65
	↓ Flexibility	

Sources: Howatson, G. and van Someren, K.A., *Sports Med.*, 38(6), 483, 2008; Moy, C.S. et al., *Am. J. Epidemiol.*, 137(1), 74, 1993.

TABLE 14.7
SORT: Key Recommendations for Practice

Clinical Recommendation	Evidence Rating	References
Initial strength gains from resistance exercise are due to neural factors. Gains from muscle cell hypertrophy take months to develop.	A	[7,12]
Resistance training only result in muscle cell hypertrophy (increase in cell size) not hyperplasia (increase in cell number).	A	[7]
Resistance training can improve aerobic exercise performance, but aerobic exercise does not enhance strength gains from resistance training.	A	[7]
The buildup of lactic acid (lactate) does not appear to cause the subjective "muscle burn" during exercise.	A	[7,8,12]
Proprioceptive neuromuscular facilitation (PNF) is more effective than static or ballistic stretching. Static and ballistic stretching are equal in effectiveness.	A	[7]
There are predictable physiologic effects of aging that affect performance and exercise tolerance, involving many body systems, that need to be accounted for in the master's/senior athlete.	A	[7,8]

REFERENCES

1. American College of Sports Medicine, W. R. Thompson, N. F. Gordon, and L. S. Pescatello. *ACSM's Guidelines for Exercise Testing and Prescription*, 8th edn. Philadelphia, PA: Lippincott Williams & Wilkins; 2010.
2. Andersen RE. Exercise, an active lifestyle, and obesity: Making the exercise prescription work. *The Physician and Sportsmedicine.* October 1999;27(10):41–50.
3. Borg GA. Psychophysical bases of perceived exertion. *Medicine and Science in Sports and Exercise.* 1982;14(5):377–381.
4. Cuccurullo S. *Physical Medicine and Rehabilitation Board Review*, 2nd edn. New York: Demos Medical Publishing; 2010.
5. Dunn AL, Trivedi MH, O'Neal HA. Physical activity dose-response effects on outcomes of depression and anxiety. *Medicine and Science in Sports and Exercise.* June 2001; 33(6 Suppl):S587–S597; discussion 609–610.
6. Durstine JL, American College of Sports Medicine. *ACSM's Exercise Management for Persons with Chronic Diseases and Disabilities*, 3rd edn. Champaign, IL: Human Kinetics; 2009.
7. Howatson G, van Someren KA. The prevention and treatment of exercise-induced muscle damage. *Sports Medicine.* 2008;38(6):483–503.
8. Miller WC. How effective are traditional dietary and exercise interventions for weight loss?. *Medicine and Science in Sports and Exercise.* August 1999;31(8):1129–1134.
9. Moy CS, Songer TJ, LaPorte RE, Dorman JS, Kriska AM, Orchard TJ, Becker DJ, Drash AL. Insulin-dependent diabetes mellitus, physical activity, and death. *American Journal of Epidemiology.* January 1, 1993;137(1):74–81.
10. North TC, McCullagh P, Tran ZV. Effect of exercise on depression. *Exercise and Sport Sciences Reviews.* 1990; 18:379–415.
11. O'Connor F.G. *ACSM's Sports Medicine: A Comprehensive Review.* Philadelphia, PA: Wolters Kluwer Health/Lippincott Williams & Wilkins; 2013.
12. Pate RR, Pratt M, Blair SN et al. Physical activity and public health. A recommendation from the centers for disease control and prevention and the american college of sports medicine. *Journal of the American Medical Association.* February 1, 1995;273(5):402–407.

15 Sports Nutrition and the Athlete

Jonathan M. Scott and Patricia A. Deuster

CONTENTS

TABLE 15.1
Key Clinical Considerations

1. An athlete's nutritional requirements may differ vastly from those of the general population. Typically, athletes have increased calorie, carbohydrate, and protein needs compared to the general population.
2. Through a well-rounded, calorically appropriate diet, an athlete can meet his or her nutrient needs through food alone and does not require dietary supplements.
3. Dietary supplements are not regulated as strictly as drugs.
4. Athletes' fuel and macronutrient needs differ depending on the type of sport, such as endurance, strength/power, and intermittent high intensity.
5. The concept of nutrient timing, although studied for years, has recently gained attention as researchers aim to determine when the optimal combination of nutrients should be consumed before, during, and after an activity, based on the type of athletic event.

15.1 INTRODUCTION TO SPORTS NUTRITION

The energetic, biomechanical, physiological, and psychological demands imposed by exercise are substantial. Appropriate nutritional habits and selected nutritional interventions can enhance performance, delay muscle fatigue, accelerate recovery, enhance uptake of important nutrients, and achieve individual performance goals. This chapter provides key information on nutritional considerations for optimizing performance for able-bodied athletes by describing energy sources, pathways, and needs; presents current knowledge with regard to nutrient timing; and reviews various nutritional topics, including hydration, vitamins, minerals, and dietary supplements (Table 15.1).

15.2 ENERGY PATHWAYS

Adenosine triphosphate (ATP) is the cellular currency responsible for providing energy to cells. The dominant metabolic pathways for generating/regenerating ATP are the creatine phosphate shuttle, glycolysis, the tricarboxylic acid (TCA) cycle, electron transport chain, and beta-oxidation (lipid/free fatty acids as substrate). The TCA cycle, electron transport chain, and beta-oxidation represent aerobic pathways,[2] whereas the creatine phosphate shuttle and glycolysis can generate ATP in the absence of oxygen (anaerobically). Aerobic metabolism dominates at rest, but the initiation of exercise invokes anaerobic pathways followed by a highly regulated interplay between anaerobic and aerobic pathways. The predominant substrates used to produce ATP by the body are carbohydrates (CHO: glycogen, blood glucose, and blood, muscle, and liver lactate) and lipids (free fatty acids). Amino acids from protein comprise less than 8% of total energy metabolism and are not a primary fuel at any time, except during starvation or when other fuel sources are unavailable.

Exercise intensity dictates the capacity and dominance of the various pathways to generate ATP, which affects the relative contributions of CHO and free fatty acids as energy sources.[28] The crossover point depends on energy intensity and occurs at the point where an individual switches from a predominant reliance on free fatty acids (low intensity) to CHO as the main source of energy (high intensity). Figure 15.1 presents an overview of the relative contribution of fats and CHO as substrates at rest and as a function of exercise intensity. At rest and during exercise of moderate intensity (i.e., the subject is able to speak while exercising or approximately 45%–65% VO_2 max), free fatty acids dominate; however, as exercise intensity increases, CHO becomes the primary substrate. Consequently, CHO is the preferred energy source for competitive-level endurance running, cycling, swimming, and other high-intensity activities.

It is important to remember that men and women are different in their use of energy sources. Healthy active men utilize CHO at significantly higher rates and oxidize lipids at lower rates than women both at rest and during moderate-intensity endurance exercise.[11] The high estrogen levels in women

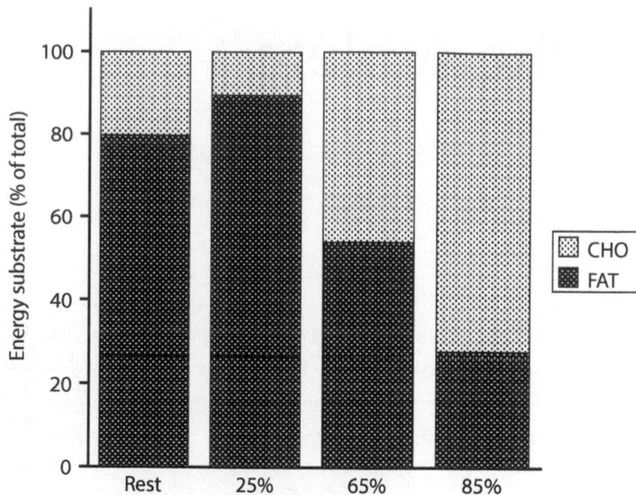

FIGURE 15.1 The relative contributions of fat and carbohydrate to energy at rest and during exercise at 25%, 65%, and 85% of maximal aerobic capacity. (Adapted from Romijn, J.A. et al., *J. Appl. Physiol.*, 88(5), 1707, 2000. Copyright 2000 by the American Physical Society.)

during the luteal phase of the menstrual cycle enhance muscle glycogen storage compared to the early follicular phase.[21] Likewise, reliance on muscle glycogen during exercise is lowest in women during the luteal as compared to the follicular phase because of higher estrogen levels.[21]

15.3 ENERGY BALANCE

Calorie (kcal) is the basic unit used to measure heat energy. Energy balance represents the equilibrium between kcal intake and kcal output (expenditure). Maintaining energy balance is a critical aspect for optimizing performance in active populations, where energy expenditure can be very high. Being able to estimate an individual's total energy expenditure (TEE) over a 24 hour period provides the foundation to develop appropriate nutritional recommendations to maintain energy balance. The three major contributors to TEE are resting energy expenditure (REE), physical activity, and energy for digesting foods, also known as the "thermic effect of food." REE, the amount of energy required just to maintain life, can be easily estimated. Although not 100% accurate, such estimates are useful. The most accurate equations for estimating REE are as follows[9]:

$$\text{Men} = 9.99 \times \text{Weight (kg)} + 6.25 \times \text{Height (cm)} - 4.92 \times \text{Age (years)} + 5$$

$$\text{Women} = 9.99\ \text{Weight (kg)} + 6.25 \times \text{Height (cm)} - 4.92 \times \text{Age (years)} - 161$$

Once REE has been estimated, a factor applied to account for physical activity yields TEE (Black 1996). Table 15.2 lists recommended physical activity level (PAL) factors (Black 1996), which range from 1.3–2.4 depending on exercise intensity and the number of hours spent training on a weekly basis. Although not exact, this estimate does provide a baseline that can be used to guide energy intake and energy balance. Environmental extremes such as heat, cold, and altitude can increase TEE by an additional 15%–25%.[5,6,31] By monitoring energy intake and changes in body weight, a more accurate assessment of TEE can be determined.

TABLE 15.2
Suggested Ranges for Physical Activity Factors Based on Activity

Level of Physical Activity	PAL
Sedentary	1.0–1.39
Low active	1.4–1.59
Active	1.6–1.89
Very active	1.9–2.4

Clinical Pearl

Energy needs can increase by as much as 15%–25% when a person is exposed to extreme conditions such as cold, heat, and/or altitude.

15.4 NUTRIENTS

Nutrients are substances found in food that provide calories, promote growth and repair of tissues, and help regulate metabolism. Six broad categories of nutrients include carbohydrates, proteins, fats, water, vitamins, and minerals.

15.4.1 Carbohydrates

Carbohydrates, found in a variety of foods from cereals and grains to fruits, vegetables, and dairy (Table 15.3), are necessary to maintain blood glucose levels during exercise and replete muscle glycogen; glucose is also a primary source of energy for the brain. Total CHO intake is sport specific, depends on TEE, and is determined by the setting (preexercise, during exercise, and postexercise), duration, intensity, and type of activity.

15.4.2 Protein

Dietary protein requirements can be met by making wise choices from among animal and/or plant sources. Athletes do not need protein powders or amino acid supplements when they make appropriate food selections.[26] Table 15.4 provides a list of select protein sources. To meet protein needs, all of the essential amino acids (EAA) must be provided in the diet, including leucine, isoleucine, valine, histidine, lysine, methionine, phenylalanine, threonine, and tryptophan. Most plant

TABLE 15.3
Carbohydrate Content of Select Foods

Food	Serving Size	Carbs (g)
Fruit, dried	¼–½ cup	60
Baked potato	1 large	50
Fruit yogurt	1 cup	50
Rice, cooked	1 cup	45
Granola, low fat	½ cup	45
Frozen yogurt	1 cup	44
Spaghetti, cooked	1 cup	40
Sports Bar	2–2.4 oz	40–60
Pancake	3″–4″	35
Regular soda	12 oz	35–45
Bagel	1 mini	31
Raisin bran	¾ cup	30
Oatmeal, instant	1 packet	30
Beans, peas, lentils	1 cup	30–45
Ramen noodles	½ package	25
English muffin	1	25
Banana	1 medium	25
Fruit juice	8 oz	25–30
Pita	1 small	21
Apple	1 medium	20
Tortilla, corn or flour	5″–6″	15
Waffle	1	15
Popcorn	3 cup popped	15
Bread, sliced	1 slice	15
Orange	1 medium	15
Corn	½ cup	15
Honey, jam, maple syrup	1 tablespoon	15
Gatorade	8 oz	14
Milk, whole, 2%, skim	8 oz	12
Graham crackers	2 squares	10
Saltines	5	10
Carrot	1 medium	10
Salad greens	2 cups raw	5
Green beans, broccoli	½ cup	5

sources are not complete proteins, in that they do not provide all of the EAA needed to make protein, so it is important to select combinations of foods to ensure adequate EAA intake. Examples of such complementary proteins include grains with legumes (beans and tortillas; lentils and rice) or grains with dairy (pasta and cheese). Animal sources of protein such as chicken or fish contain all of the EAA.

15.4.3 Fats

Fats (specifically fatty acids and triglycerides) are the major form of stored energy and an important energy substrate at rest, during exercise, in cold environments, at altitude, and during starvation. Stored fat serves essential functions such as insulating the body, protecting organs, and as a key component of cell membranes. Total fat intake (saturated, trans, monounsaturated, and polyunsaturated) is sport specific and based on TEE. Fats are found in many foods, notably nuts, seeds, dairy and animal protein, and fish, to name a few (Table 15.5).

TABLE 15.4
Protein Content of Select Foods

Food	Serving Size	Protein (g)
Tuna (canned)	1 can (6 oz)	40
White meat chicken	3 oz cooked	26
White meat turkey	3 oz cooked	26
95% lean ground beef	3 oz cooked	25
Pork tenderloin	3 oz cooked	24
Salmon	3 oz cooked	22
Greek yogurt	6 oz	17
Cottage cheese	½ cup	14
Tofu (firm)	4 oz	10
Milk or regular yogurt	1 cup (8 oz)	8
Beans/legumes[a]	½ cup	8
Almonds (most nuts)[a]	¼ cup	7
Egg	1 large	7
Egg whites	¼ cup	7
Hard cheese	1 oz	7
Peanut butter[a]	2 tablespoons	7
American cheese	1 slice (0.75 oz)	6
Bread[a]	1 slice	2
Cold cereal[a]	1 cup	2
Vegetables[a]	½ cup	2
Rice, noodles, pasta[a]	½ cup	2
Fruit[a]	1 piece	<1

[a] Not a complete protein source because this food does not contain all the essential amino acids needed to make protein.

TABLE 15.5
Fat Content of Select Foods

Food	Serving Size	Fat (g)
Almonds, raw	¼ cup (~24 nuts)	18
Avocado	½ medium	15
Coconut oil	1 tablespoon	13.5
Olive oil	1 tablespoon	13.5
Butter	1 tablespoon	12
Mayonnaise	1 tablespoon	11
Salad dressing, ranch-type	1 tablespoon	8
Bacon	2 slices	6
Olives, black	6 medium	3
Cream, half-and-half	1 tablespoon	1.5

15.4.4 Hydration

Water, an essential nutrient, is the most abundant component of the human body. It constitutes approximately 50%–70% of body weight. Select functions of water include participation in digestion and absorption of nutrients, excretion of waste products, maintenance of blood circulation, and regulation of body temperature. Fluid requirements can vary greatly depending on diet and health status, exercise intensity and duration, and environmental conditions.[29] The Institute of Medicine in 2005 established daily adequate intake values: 3.7 L/day or ~4 quarts/day for men and 2.7 L/day or ~2.9 quarts/day for women. Requirements are higher for physically active people and may exceed 10 L/day or 10.6 quarts/day.[22] Overall fluid balance is compromised by exercise mainly through sweat losses and ventilation.[20,29] Sweat rates have been reported to vary from 0.3–3.5 L/h, depending on age, type of activity, physical fitness, acclimation status, clothing, and of course, environmental conditions.[29] Because of large differences among individuals, each person needs to determine his or her own propensity for sweating to more accurately estimate fluid losses and requirements across a variety of environmental conditions.

15.4.4.1 Dehydration

Sweat losses are the primary source of fluid losses during exercise, and dehydration occurs when a person fails to replace lost fluids with water or other fluid-replacement beverages. Dehydration results in reduced central blood volume, skin blood flow, and stroke volume and elevated heart rate.[29] Fluid losses can occur at higher altitudes, in the cold, in the heat, and even under conditions of low physical activity and are greater especially during exercise of long duration.[20,26,29] A ~2%–3% loss of body weight due to dehydration can impair performance and mood and predispose an individual to heat illness.[29] A greater loss of fluid can be life threatening.[30]

15.4.4.2 Electrolyte Balance

Electrolyte (i.e., sodium, potassium, chloride) and other mineral (e.g., calcium, zinc, iron) losses from sweating can be substantial, depending on training status, dietary intake, genetics, sweat rate, and prior heat exposure. Excessive losses can lead to severe medical problems.[3,17] Sodium losses can range in concentrations from 230–1610 mg/L and rates of 70–5100 mg/h; higher values are noted in heavy sweaters, those unaccustomed to working in the heat and those consuming a high-sodium diet.[29,33] Potassium losses can range in concentrations from 120–600 mg/L and rates from 40–2000 mg/h.[29,33]

Electrolytes lost through sweating can be replaced through foods and fluid-replacement beverages. Dried fruits are good food choices for potassium, and pretzels and pickles are good sources of sodium. For example, a small box of raisins provides 322 mg of potassium; a snack of 10 small, plain, salted hard pretzels (60 g) provides about 814 mg of sodium; and one small dill or kosher cucumber pickle provides about 569 mg of sodium. Adding only ½ teaspoon of table salt to food provides 1200 mg of sodium. The current published adequate daily dietary intake of sodium is 1500 mg for young adults, which is only slightly more than ½ teaspoon of table salt, but this may not be adequate for active populations.[22]

15.4.4.3 Fluid Ingestion and Timing

Fluids should be ingested before, during, and after exercise, depending on intensity, duration, and environmental concerns. The American College of Sports Medicine's position stand on fluid replacement provides multiple recommendations with regard to the timing and composition of prospective fluids.[29] In particular, it is essential to be well hydrated prior to exercise. Adequate hydration can be achieved by consuming 400–600 mL (14–22 oz) of fluid at least 4 hours prior to exercise.[26,29] Fluid ingestion needs can also be determined according to body weight: approximately 5–7 mL/kg (2–3 mL/lb) should be adequate to fully hydrate an individual prior to exercise.[26] In addition, fluids containing sodium (20–50 mEq/L or 460–1150 mg/L) or small amounts of sodium-containing foods at snacks or meals will help to offset sweat losses, enhance palatability, stimulate thirst, and promote fluid absorption to ensure adequate hydration status before exercise.[16,17] Hydrating at least 4 hours prior to exercise typically allows sufficient time to excrete any excess fluid as urine before starting an event. The only anion recommended for all fluid replacement beverages—before, during, and after—is chloride in the form of sodium chloride due to its high concentration in the plasma and role in optimizing fluid absorption.[7]

The recommended sodium intake during exercise is different from that for preexercise intake. The recommended range for sodium in commercial fluid replacement beverages for use during exercise is 10–35 mEq/L (230–800 mg/L).[1] Very-high-sodium concentrations (≥50 mEq/L or 1150 mg/L) decrease drink palatability,[1,34] which could compromise overall fluid intake. With regard to potassium, the recommended amount during exercise is 2–10 mEq/L (78–390 mg/L). Magnesium and calcium are sometimes included, but the amounts are typically low. Importantly, loss of electrolytes cannot be estimated from changes in body weight.[1,4,29] Endurance exercise longer than 1 hour is served well by coingestion of CHO and electrolytes. In particular, beverages containing 6%–8% (60–80 g/L) CHO (glucose, sucrose, fructose, glucose polymers, and the like) with electrolytes are recommended during prolonged exercise to optimize hydration.[1,4,17,25,26,29,34]

In addition, fluids should be replaced during exercise at a rate that will prevent losing more than 2% body weight.[17,26,29] Because it is usually impossible to obtain body weight during competition, the practical recommendation is to consume up to 350 mL (12 oz) of fluid every 20 minutes of exercise, depending on the environmental conditions and whether the activity lasts more than 1 hour.[8] Total fluid volume should not exceed 1 L/h. However, an individual should monitor his or her own fluid losses because general recommendations do not account for individual differences or for environmental conditions.

After exercise, fluid losses need to be replaced. Restoration of hydration status can be accomplished by consuming regular foods and beverages.[4,29] However, when dehydration equates to a 2%–4% loss of body weight, the person needs

TABLE 15.6
Practical Approaches for Monitoring Hydration Status with Clinical Cutoffs

Characteristic	Validity	Euhydration Cutoff
Urine specific gravity	Chronic	<1.020
Urine osmolality	Chronic	<700 mOsmol/kg
Loss of body weight	Acute and chronic	<1%

to be intentional about fluid ingestion. If actual changes in body weight are known, then the following can be applied: a 1 kg decrease in body weight requires ingesting between 1.25–1.5 L of fluid—and a 1 lb decrease requires 2.4–2.9 cups or 0.6–0.75 quarts—to fully restore fluid balance.[4,29] The fluid should contain sodium at a concentration of approximately 20–50 mEq/L (460–1150 mg/L) to stimulate thirst and fluid retention and promote a more rapid and complete recovery.[1,4,29]

15.4.4.4 Monitoring Hydration

Hydration status is best monitored by changes in body weight. Obtaining body weight first thing in the morning over several days is best for establishing a body weight that reflects a well-hydrated state or euhydration.[29] Nude weight should be recorded both before and after physical activity to estimate fluids lost through sweating. Of course, this requires that a scale be accessible. Urine specific gravity (USG) should be obtained when possible and can be measured in the field using a refractometer. USG <1.020 (UOsmol ≤ 700 mOsmol/kg) is considered to reflect euhydration[29] see Table 15.6 for a list of practical approaches for monitoring hydration status with clinical cutoffs. Alternatively, inspecting urine color offers a subjective method to assess hydration status: Pale yellow, almost-clear urine suggests adequate hydration. Conversely, dark yellow or smelly urine often indicates dehydration. However, urine may be neon yellow or not pale, regardless of hydration status, if the athlete is taking a B-vitamin supplement, particularly one high in riboflavin;[3,7,22,29] p. 432; p. 423).

15.4.5 Vitamins/Minerals

Vitamins and minerals serve important roles in active populations, as they are involved in pathways that produce energy, hemoglobin, bone growth and remodeling, and recovery from injury. In addition, they help protect against excessive oxidative stress. Athletes who consume a balanced, calorically appropriate diet typically do not need supplements, as any increased need above the recommended daily value of any single vitamin or mineral can be met through dietary intake. For those who actually have a deficiency, supplementation may be necessary to bring intake up to appropriate levels.

Clinical Pearl

Athletes who consume a balanced diet with sufficient energy will meet their recommended daily values for vitamins and minerals.

15.5 DIETARY SUPPLEMENTS

The use of dietary supplements has become increasingly popular among athletes to enhance performance. Consumers of dietary supplements should be aware that although the Food and Drug Administration (FDA) regulates dietary supplements, the regulations are not as strict as they are for drugs. Consequently, some unsafe and contaminated products end up on the market. FDA has noted four "high-risk" dietary supplement categories: bodybuilding, weight-loss, sexual-enhancement, and diabetes products; these products are more likely than vitamin and mineral supplements to contain unsafe and contaminated ingredients. In addition, many "high-risk" supplements may not conform to the labeling regulations required by FDA and may contain illegal (e.g., analogues of drugs, amphetamines) or controlled (e.g., steroids) substances. Such ingredients may be intentionally left off the label, as they would not meet the definition of a dietary supplement. Thus, consumers should be careful when purchasing dietary supplements. Supplements displaying seals from third-party verification/certification programs are better choices because they (1) are unlikely to contain contaminants, (2) likely to have ingredients present in the amounts listed on the supplement facts panel, and (3) likely to have accurate labels. See Figure 15.2 for sample seals of third-party certification/verification programs. Consumers should also be aware that (1) concentrations and combinations of ingredients are arbitrarily created by manufacturers with little to no scientific research

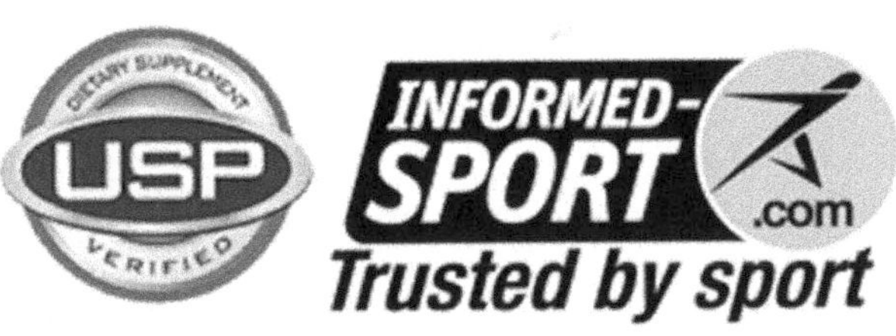

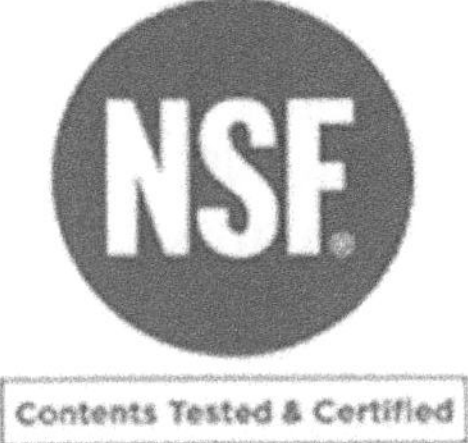

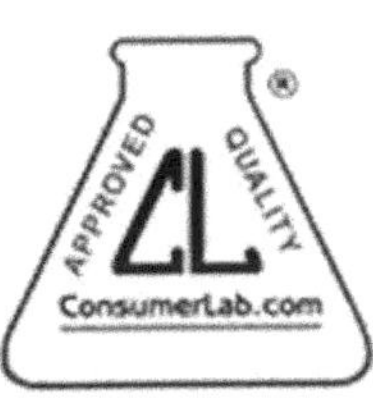

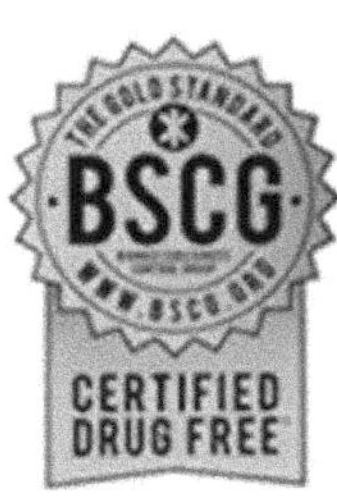

FIGURE 15.2 Examples of logos/seals from organizations that third-party verify/certify dietary supplements.

to support their recommendations and (2) using any dietary supplement, especially those from the high-risk categories, increases the probability of experiencing an adverse event. Adverse events associated with dietary supplements can range from very mild physical discomfort to severe, life-threatening incidents. Health-care providers should report adverse events and should educate patients on how to report adverse events through Natural Medicines MedWatch (https://naturalmedicines.therapeuticresearch.com/tools/natural-medwatch.aspx). As such, athletes should proceed with caution when considering and using dietary supplements. Primary care providers should query their patients about supplement use and discuss general safety issues with all patients.

Clinical Pearl

High-risk categories of dietary supplements include bodybuilding, weight-loss, sexual-enhancement, and diabetes products.

Clinical Pearl

Report adverse events through Natural Medicines MedWatch: https://naturalmedicines.therapeuticresearch.com/tools/natural-medwatch.aspx.

15.6 BODY COMPOSITION

The term "body composition" generally refers to a body's proportional makeup of fat-free mass and fat mass, expressed as a percentage of body fat. Fat-free mass can be further divided into lean mass (muscle mass), bone mineral content, and body water. Several different methods are available for assessing body composition: dual-energy x-ray absorptiometry, hydrostatic weighing, air-displacement plethysmography, bioelectrical-impedance analysis, and skinfold measurements. Each has its own inherent limitations. No standardized definition of ideal body composition exists; reference values for body composition use normative data, based on gender and sport (female soccer player, male swimmer or cyclist) or sport-specific positions (football linemen, linebackers, or skill positions) across a continuum.[10,19,27,35]

15.7 NUTRITIONAL RECOMMENDATIONS FOR SPECIFIC ATHLETIC POPULATIONS

Athletes have higher energy needs and subsequently greater carbohydrate, protein, and fat requirements compared to the general population. Specific recommendations for athletes are dependent upon frequency, intensity, duration, and the type of activity performed. Generally, athletes can be grouped into three main categories based on the type of activity including endurance, strength /power, and intermittent high intensity.

15.7.1 ENDURANCE

Endurance athletes rely on aerobic metabolism as their primary energy system. Consequently, endurance athletes have higher carbohydrate and lower protein needs compared to strength/power athletes and intermittent high-intensity athletes. Examples of endurance activities include road cycling, long-distance swimming, and marathon running.

15.7.1.1 Energy Needs

A typical PAL for an endurance athlete is 1.8–2.2, depending on weekly mileage. For someone whose primary activity is exercising 30 minutes, 5 days a week, at light to moderate intensity (cycling, walking, swimming, jogging), a PAL of 1.6–1.79 could be used. The PAL for someone exercising 60 minutes, 5 days a week at a moderate to strenuous intensity might be in the range of 1.8–2.4. For example, a 35-year-old female, 60 kg (132 lb) and 165 cm (65″), running 40 miles/week or cycling 100 miles/week, would have an REE of 1298 kcal/day, a PAL factor of 1.8 would yield an initial TEE estimate of 2336 kcal/day. Depending on energy intake data, her PAL could be adjusted up or down and TEE revised accordingly.

15.7.1.2 Carbohydrate

Carbohydrate needs of endurance athletes range from 6–10 g/kg body weight/day (2.7–4.5 g/lb body weight/day), depending on energy needs. This equates to approximately 360–600 g/day for a 60 kg (132 lb) athlete.[26] Stated differently, the percentage of kcals in an athlete's diet derived from CHO will likely range between 55%–70%. For example, a 60 kg athlete who requires 2350 kcal/day should consume 1293–1645 kcal from CHO, which equates to 325–410 g of CHO/day.

15.7.1.2 Protein

Daily protein needs of endurance athletes are 1.2–1.4 g/kg body weight/day (0.55–0.64 g/lb body weight/day).[26] This equates to a protein intake of 72–84 g/day for a 60 kg (132 lb) athlete, which translates to 288–336 kcal, or 12.3%–14.3% of a total energy requirement of 2350 kcal.

15.7.1.3 Fat

Generally, fat needs of endurance athletes are 20%–35% of the total kcals, with 10% or less of these coming from saturated fat and the balance from mono- and polyunsaturated fats. Trans fat intake should be less than 1% of total kcals each day. When energy intakes are high (>4000 kcal/day), fat intake may approach 35% or higher to ensure adequate kcal intake. Thus, a 60 kg (132 lb) athlete who consumes 2350 kcal/day would consume no more than 91 g of fat (823 kcal), with only 26 g from saturated and 65 g from unsaturated fats emphasizing fatty fish, nuts, seeds, canola oil, and olive oil. Some endurance athletes in training decrease their intake of fat to only 20%–25% of total energy in order to consume adequate amounts of CHO without going over their energy allowances, but intakes less than 20% of fat are not recommended under any circumstances.[26]

15.7.2 Strength/Power

Strength/power athletes rely on anaerobic metabolism as their primary energy system. Consequently, strength/power athletes have higher protein and lower carbohydrate needs compared to endurance and intermittent high-intensity athletes. Examples of strength/power activities include Olympic weight lifting, throwing (shot put, hammer, discus), and football linemen.

15.7.2.1 Energy

A typical PAL for strength/power athletes is 1.8–2.2, depending on duration and intensity of training. If an athlete spends <5–7 hours/week training, a PAL of 1.6–1.79 would be used, whereas someone training 8–14 h/week (moderate to strenuous exercise) would use 1.8–2.4. For example, if a 25-year-old male Olympic weight lifter, 100 kg (220 lb) and 183 cm (72″), was training 10 h/week, his REE would be approximately 2024 kcal/day. A PAL factor of 2.0 yields an initial TEE estimate of 4048 kcal/day.

15.7.2.2 Carbohydrate

Carbohydrate needs of strength/power athletes range from 4–6 g/kg body weight/day (1.8–3.2 g/lb body weight/day), depending on overall energy needs. This equates to approximately 400–600 g/day for a 100 kg (220 lb) athlete.[26] Stated differently, the percentage of kcal in the diet derived from CHO should be in the range of 50%–60%. For example, a 100 kg athlete who requires 4050 kcal/day should consume 1600–2400 kcal from CHO, which equates to 400–600 g of CHO/day.

15.7.2.3 Protein

Daily protein needs of strength/power athletes are 1.2–1.8 g/kg body weight/day (0.55–0.82 g/lb body weight/day),[26] which equates to a protein intake of 120–180 g/day for a 100 kg (220 lb) athlete. Overall, this would be 480–720 kcal, or 11.9%–17.8% of total energy needs of 4050 kcal.

15.7.2.4 Fat

Fat needs and intake recommendations of strength/power athletes are generally similar to those of endurance athletes. A 100 kg (220 lb) strength/power athlete who consumes 4050 kcal/day would obtain no more than 158 g from fat (1418 kcal), with only 45 g of saturated fat and 113 g of unsaturated fat. Some strength/power athletes in training increase their intake of fat to >35% of total energy as an adjunct to consuming excess protein, which can limit CHO intakes. However, intakes of fat >35% are not recommended.[26]

15.7.3 Intermittent High Intensity

Intermittent high-intensity athletes rely on both aerobic and anaerobic metabolism for energy. Consequently, intermittent high-intensity athletes have carbohydrate and protein needs in between endurance and strength/power athletes. Examples of intermittent high-intensity activities include team sports such as basketball, soccer, and volleyball.

15.7.3.1 Energy

A typical PAL for intermittent high-intensity athletes is 1.8–2.2, depending on hours spent training. For someone who spends <5–7 h/week (moderate to strenuous exercise), a PAL of 1.6–1.79 is appropriate, whereas someone training 10–20 h/week would use 1.8–2.4. For example, if a 28-year-old male soccer player, 85 kg (187 lb) and 178 cm (70″), was training 14 h/week, his REE would be estimated as 1828 kcal/day, and a PAL factor of 2.1 would yield an initial TEE estimate of 3838 kcal/day.

15.7.3.2 Carbohydrate

Carbohydrate needs of intermittent high-intensity athletes range from 6–8 g/kg body weight/day (2.7–3.6 g/lb body weight/day), depending on energy needs. This equates to approximately 510–680 g/day for an 85 kg (187 lb).[26] In other words, the percentage of kcal in the diet derived from CHO would range 55%–65%. For example, an 85 kg athlete who needs 3850 kcal/day should consume 2120–2500 kcal from CHO, which equates to 530–625 g of CHO/day.

15.7.3.3 Protein

Daily protein needs of intermittent high-intensity athletes are 1.2–1.6 g/kg body weight/day (0.55–0.73 g/lb body weight/day),[26] which equates to a protein intake of 102–136 g/day for an 85 kg (187 lb) athlete. Overall, this is 408–544 kcal or 10.6%–14.1% of total energy of 3850 kcal.

15.7.3.4 Fat

Fat needs and intake recommendations of intermittent high-intensity athletes are 20%–35%, similar to those of both endurance and strength/power athletes. Fat intakes can approach 35% or higher when energy intakes are high (>4000 kcal/day) to ensure adequate energy intake. As an example, an 85 kg (187 lb) athlete who requires

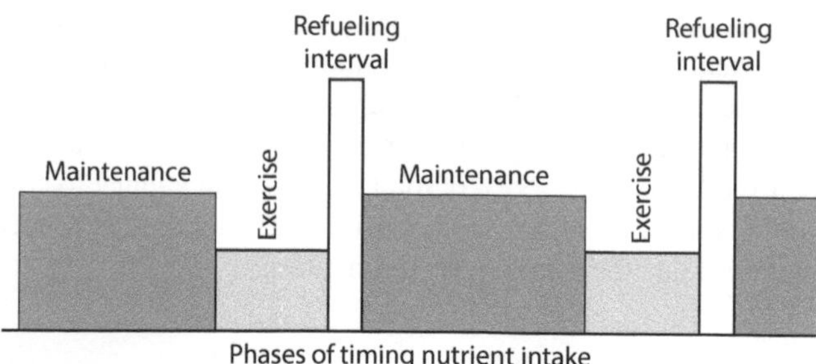

FIGURE 15.3 The three major phases for nutrient timing: maintenance and growth, exercise, and the refueling interval for recovery. Heights of bars are indicative of protein and carbohydrate balance—exercise indicates the breakdown of energy stores, the refueling interval reflects rebuilding energy stores, and maintenance displays homeostasis.

3850 kcal/day would consume no more than 150 g of fat (1348 kcal), with approximately 43 g from saturated and 107 g from unsaturated fats.

15.8 NUTRIENT TIMING

The goals of training are to optimize physiologic and molecular adaptations specific to one's sport. These training goals can be most effectively achieved when appropriate nutritional strategies are implemented before, during, and after training. "Nutrient timing" is the term originally coined by Drs. John Ivy and Robert Portman[13] to indicate that *when* food is consumed is as important as *what* food is consumed. The three phases of nutrient timing are (1) during exercise, (2) the refueling interval (RFI) immediately after exercise (recovery), and (3) the time between exercise sessions (maintenance and growth) (Figure 15.3).

Various strategies have been developed to maintain adequate energy stores, enhance recovery, stimulate muscle protein synthesis, maximize glycogen repletion, and minimize/protect against training injuries (Rodriguez et al., 2009). Nutrient timing, combined with adequate rest and recovery periods, is an important component of all training programs, regardless of sport. However, another consideration for competition is familiarity: foods and fluids consumed before and during but not after exercise should be the same as those used in training, to minimize possible gastric distress from unaccustomed foods.

15.8.1 Preexercise Meal/Snack

The optimal content and timing of a preexercise meal/snack have not been agreed upon. However, consuming a meal or snack providing 200–300 g of CHO 3–4 h before heavy training or competition will allow sufficient time for the food to be digested and for gastric emptying to occur. Consuming up to 25 g of protein before exercise may be important for those primarily engaged in strength/power training with regard to maximizing protein synthesis.[14] If a larger meal is desired, more time should be allowed for digestion. Table 15.7 provides a list of suggested preexercise foods.

TABLE 15.7
Suggested Foods for Preexercise Meal/Snack

Type of Food	kcal	CHO (g)	Fat (g)	Protein (g)
2 slices whole-wheat bread w/2 oz turkey, lettuce, and 1 medium orange	289	40	4	23
1 baked potato w/plain yogurt	197	41	1	7
8 oz low-fat yogurt w/fruit	250	47	3	11
½ cup low-fat granola w/½ cup skim milk	233	46	3	8
Bagel w/2 tbsp low-fat cream cheese	330	55	6	13
8 oz low-fat chocolate milk and 1 medium apple	253	51	3	9

Clinical Pearl

For a preexercise meal/snack, focus on carbohydrates, but include some protein and limit fat. Experiment with various foods to find what works best for you.

15.8.2 During Exercise

During exercise energy stores are being used to provide substrate to the working muscles, and muscle protein breakdown is higher than at rest. Consuming small amounts of CHO at regular intervals can minimize metabolic distress and enhance athletic performance, particularly if the exercise duration is greater than 1 hour.[4] During exercise lasting longer than 1 hour, ingesting CHO in a fluid can also help sustain hydration. Studies have shown that ingesting 0.7 g CHO/kg body weight (approximately 30–60 g CHO/hour or 7–20 g CHO every 15–20 minutes) can extend endurance performance.[14] When the exercise duration is greater than 3 hours, CHO intakes of up to 110 g/h may be needed, depending on the intensity of the exercise.[32] For ultraendurance events, athletes commonly ingest both solid foods and liquid foods to meet CHO needs.

Clinical Pearl

For exercise lasting less than 60 minutes, water is adequate; for longer than 60 minutes, consider a carbohydrate-electrolyte sports drink.

An athlete should try various foods during training to determine which are most suitable for competition. The amount of CHO and fluid required and/or tolerated by any individual athlete will be determined by the exercise intensity, duration, environmental conditions, and mode of exercise (running vs. soccer game vs. lifting competition). The athlete will have to do trial runs to determine his or her optimal fuel sources. Consuming protein during events confers no discernable benefit.[18]

15.8.3 Recovery: Refueling Interval

After exercise, the metabolic environment within the body needs to transition from a state of breakdown to rebuilding in order to promote recovery and restore what was depleted during the exercise phase. This is the "refueling interval" or RFI. Release of insulin, an important hormone for inhibiting muscle protein breakdown, can be stimulated by ingestion of both CHO and certain amino acids.[15] Thus, the goal of the RFI is to replenish glycogen stores and facilitate muscle protein synthesis. To enhance muscle glycogen synthesis following prolonged, strenuous exercise (over 60 minutes), start with a snack of approximately 50 g of CHO within 60 minutes after the activity, followed by approximately 1.0–1.5 g/kg body weight (0.5–0.7 g/lb) CHO (as liquid, gel, or solid food) at 2 hour intervals for up to 6 hours.[4,14]

Although somewhat controversial, it is generally believed that ingesting some protein (12–25 g) with CHO during recovery can increase muscle protein synthesis and improve nitrogen balance better than consuming CHO without protein.[12,26] Consuming foods with EAA—especially leucine—will promote the postexercise muscle protein synthesis needed for building and repairing muscle tissue.[23,24,26] For example, foods containing leucine include eggs, dairy, and chicken. Without appropriate refueling after a strenuous competition or hard training session, performance may be compromised, especially if a second workout is completed the same day or in less than 24 hours.

Clinical Pearl

If you are participating in multiple workouts each day (two-a-days) or have less than 24 hours between workouts, consuming a combination of carbohydrates and protein postwork is likely beneficial.

15.9 SUMMARY

Able-bodied athletes have unique nutrition requirements compared to the general population. Nutrition requirements include increased calorie, carbohydrate, protein, and fat needs.

TABLE 15.8
SORT: Key Recommendations for Practice

Clinical Recommendation	Evidence Rating	References
Athletes need to consume adequate calories based on gender and sport requirements to maintain weight and health and maximize training adaptation.	A	[26]
Carbohydrate needs range from 4–10 g/kg body weight depending on sport.	A	[26]
Protein intakes above 1.8 g/kg body weight do not confer additional benefits.	A	[26]
Total fat intake should comprise 20%–35% of total calories with saturated fat limited to no more than 10% of total calories.	A	[26]
Additional vitamin and/or mineral supplementation is not required for athletes who consume adequate calories from a variety of food sources unless a deficiency exists.	A	[26]
Weight loss of greater than ~2%–3% due to dehydration may decrease performance.	B	[26,29]
Nutrient timing related to pre-, during, and postactivity fueling may enhance performance during activity and facilitate faster recovery.	A	[26]

Unless a specific deficiency exists, athletes can meet all nutritional requirements through appropriate and deliberate food and beverage selections. Optimal performance requires the correct timing and combination of foods, and proper sports nutrition can be the difference between good and great athletes (Table 15.8).

REFERENCES

1. Baker LB, Jeukendrup AE. Optimal composition of fluid-replacement beverages. *Comprehensive Physiology.* 2014; 4(2):575–620.
2. Beneke R, Boning, D. The limits of human performance. *Essays Biochemistry.* 2008;44:11–25.

3. Bergeron MF. Exertional heat cramps: Recovery and return to play. *Journal of Sports Rehabilitation.* 2007; 16(3):190–196.
4. Burke L. Fasting and recovery from exercise. *British Journal of Sports Medicine.* 2010;44(7):502–508.
5. Burstein R, Coward AW, Askew WE, Carmel K, Irving C, Shpilberg O, Epstein Y. Energy expenditure variations in soldiers performing military activities under cold and hot climate conditions. *Military Medicine.* 1996;161(12):750–754.
6. Butterfield GE, Gates J, Fleming S, Brooks GA, Sutton JR, Reeves JT. Increased energy intake minimizes weight loss in men at high altitude. *Journal of Applied Physiology.* 1992;*(1985)* 72(5):1741–1748.
7. Committee on Military Nutrition Research, Food and Nutrition Board, & Institute of Medicine (Eds.). *Fluid Replacement and Heat Stress.* Washington, DC: The National Academies Press; 1994.
8. Convertino VA, Armstrong LE, Coyle EF, Mack GW, Sawka MN, Senay LC Jr, Sherman WM. American College of Sports Medicine position stand. Exercise and fluid replacement. *Medicine and Science Sports and Exercise.* 1996;28(1):i–vii.
9. Frankenfield D, Roth-Yousey L, Compher C. Comparison of predictive equations for resting metabolic rate in healthy nonobese and obese adults: A systematic review. *Journal of American Dietetic Association.* 2005;105(5):775–789..
10. Goncalves EM, Matias CN, Santos DA, Sardinha LB, Silva AM. Assessment of total body water and its compartments in elite judo athletes: Comparison of bioelectrical impedance spectroscopy with dilution techniques. *Journal of Sports Science.* 2014;33(6):634–640.
11. Hamadeh MJ, Devries MC, Tarnopolsky MA. Estrogen supplementation reduces whole body leucine and carbohydrate oxidation and increases lipid oxidation in men during endurance exercise. *Journal of Clinical Endocrinology Metabolism.* 2005;90(6):3592–3599.
12. Howarth KR, Phillips SM, MacDonald MJ, Richards D, Moreau NA, Gibala MJ. Effect of glycogen availability on human skeletal muscle protein turnover during exercise and recovery. *Journal of Applied Physiology.* 2010; 109(2):431–438.
13. Ivy J, Portman R. *Nutrient Timing: The Future of Sports Nutrition.* Laguna Beach, CA: Basic Health Publications, Inc; 2004.
14. Kerksick C, Harvey T, Stout J, Campbell B, Wilborn C, Kreider R, Antonio J. International Society of Sports Nutrition position stand: Nutrient timing. *Journal of International Society Sports Nutrition.* 2008;5:17.
15. Martinez-Lagunas V, Ding Z, Bernard JR, Wang B, Ivy JL. Added protein maintains efficacy of a low-carbohydrate sports drink. *Journal of Strength and Conditioning Research.* 2010;24(1):48–59.
16. Maughan RJ, Leiper JB, Shirreffs SM. Restoration of fluid balance after exercise-induced dehydration: Effects of food and fluid intake. *European Journal of Applied Physiology and Occupational Physiology.* 1996;73(3–4):317–325.
17. Maughan RJ, Shirreffs SM. Development of hydration strategies to optimize performance for athletes in high-intensity sports and in sports with repeated intense efforts. *Scandinavian Journal of Medical Science and Sports.* 2010;20(Suppl. 2):59–69.
18. McLellan TM, Pasiakos SM, Lieberman HR. Effects of protein in combination with carbohydrate supplements on acute or repeat endurance exercise performance: A systematic review. *Sports Medicine.* 2014;44(4):535–550.
19. Melvin MN, Smith-Ryan AE, Wingfield HL, Ryan ED, Trexler ET, Roelofs EJ. Muscle characteristics and body composition of NCAA division I football players. *Journal of Strength and Conditioning Research.* 2014; 28(12):3320–3329.
20. Montain SJ. Hydration recommendations for sport 2008. *Current Sports Medicine Reports.* 2008;7(4):187–192.
21. Oosthuyse T, Bosch AN. The effect of the menstrual cycle on exercise metabolism: Implications for exercise performance in eumenorrhoeic women. *Sports Medicine.* 2010; 40(3):207–227.
22. Panel on Dietary Reference Intakes for Electrolytes and Water, Standing Committee on the Scientific Evaluation of Dietary Reference Intakes, & Institute of Medicine (Eds.). *Dietary Reference Intakes: Water, Potassium, Sodium, Chloride, and Sulfate.* Washington, DC: The National Academies Press; 2005.
23. Pasiakos SM, McClung HL, McClung JP, Margolis LM, Andersen NE, Cloutier GJ, Young AJ. Leucine-enriched essential amino acid supplementation during moderate steady state exercise enhances postexercise muscle protein synthesis. *Americal Journal of Clinical Nutrition.* 2011; 94(3):809–818.
24. Pasiakos SM, McClung JP. Supplemental dietary leucine and the skeletal muscle anabolic response to essential amino acids. *Nutrition Review.* 2011;69(9):550–557.
25. Ray ML, Bryan MW, Ruden TM, Baier SM, Sharp RL, King DS. Effect of sodium in a rehydration beverage when consumed as a fluid or meal. *Journal of Applied Physiology.*1998;(1985), 85(4):1329–1336.
26. Rodriguez NR, Di Marco NM, Langley S. American College of Sports Medicine position stand. Nutrition and athletic performance. *Medicine and Science Sports and Exercise.* 2009;41(3):709–731.
27. Roelofs EJ, Smith-Ryan AE, Melvin MN, Wingfield HL, Trexler ET, Walker N. Muscle size, quality, and body composition: Characteristics of division I cross-country runners. *Journal of Strength and Conditioning Research.* 2014; 29(2):290–296.
28. Romijn JA, Coyle EF, Sidossis LS, Rosenblatt J, Wolfe RR. Substrate metabolism during different exercise intensities in endurance-trained women. *Journal of Applied Physiology.* 2000;88(5):1707–1714.
29. Sawka MN, Burke LM, Eichner ER, Maughan RJ, Montain SJ, Stachenfeld NS. American College of Sports Medicine position stand. Exercise and fluid replacement. *Medicine and Science Sports and Exercise.* 2007;39(2):377–390.
30. Sawka MN, Greenleaf JE. Current concepts concerning thirst, dehydration, and fluid replacement: Overview. *Medicine Science and Sports and Exercise.* 1992;24(6):643–644.
31. Schoeller DA. Recent advances from application of doubly labeled water to measurement of human energy expenditure. *Journal of Nutrition.* 1999;129(10):1765–1768.
32. Stellingwerff T, Cox GR. Systematic review: Carbohydrate supplementation on exercise performance or capacity of varying durations. *Applied Physiology and Nutrition Metabolism.* 2014;39(9):998–1011.

33. Taylor NA, Machado-Moreira CA. Regional variations in transepidermal water loss, eccrine sweat gland density, sweat secretion rates and electrolyte composition in resting and exercising humans. *Extreme Physiology and Medicine.* 2013;2(1):4.
34. Wemple RD, Morocco TS, Mack GW. Influence of sodium replacement on fluid ingestion following exercise-induced dehydration. *Internaitonal Journal of Sports Nutrition.* 1997;7(2):104–116.
35. Zapolska J, Witczak K, Manczuk A, Ostrowska L. Assessment of nutrition, supplementation and body composition parameters on the example of professional volleyball players. *Rocz Panstw Zakl Hig.* 2014;65(3):235–242.

16 Human Growth and Development

Daniel H. Blatz and Arthur Jason De Luigi

CONTENTS

TABLE 16.1
Key Clinical Considerations

1. Activity levels among the youth in the United States have been decreasing over recent decades. This is a concerning trend as there are many benefits to physical activity and youth sports. For each individual, the risks and benefits of any activity must be weighed.
2. The rate and milestones of growth and development vary for each individual. Common milestones can be used as a rough guide to monitor progress.
3. In order to determine an individual's readiness for all types of activities and sports, their physical, cognitive, and psychosocial development needs to be understood.
4. Early sport specialization, focusing on a single sport or discipline from a very early age, is becoming more and more common in the United States. However, most people do not understand that there may be risks associated with this trend.
5. The clinician is a valuable resource for each child/adolescent/athlete, as well as their parents and coaches, when issues arise related to their growth and development, their entry into youth sports, and/or their progression through the various stages of their life and activities in which they want to participate.

16.1 INTRODUCTION

In this chapter, the authors will discuss human growth and development from birth through adolescence. It is designed to offer a general outline of the typical motor, cognitive, and psychosocial maturation that occurs between infancy and adulthood. The chapter covers growth and development during infancy; however the main focus will be on childhood and adolescence (Table 16.1).

Whether a young person is ready or not for a specific sport or level of play largely depends on their individual rate of maturation. Therefore, chronological age is not a perfect indicator of readiness for a certain level of sport and sports development. However, age can be used as an approximate guide to discuss the various stages of growth and development. In addition to this, the authors will discuss the benefits of youth sports, the idea of sport readiness, sport specialization, and some of the factors that contribute to both success and failure in youth sports.

16.2 BENEFITS OF YOUTH SPORTS

Organized youth sports are a common setting for regular physical activity among kids, especially in the wealthier, *developed* countries of the world, like the United States. They are highly popular for youths and their families, with approximately 45 million child and adolescent participants in the United States and 75% of American families with school-aged children having at least one child participating in organized sports.[57] However, when you look at levels of physical activity among youths, there has been a steady decline in the number of hours devoted to physical activity. Some of this has been attributed to reduction in school time dedicated to physical activity (gym, recess, after-school programs, etc.), reduction in the number of kids walking to and from school, and increase in screen time (e.g., computer, smartphone, video games).[37,47,49,57] On average, youths 8–18 years old spend 7.5 hours/day sitting in front of a screen.[37,47] The Center for Disease Control (CDC) 2011 Youth Risk Behavior Surveillance System found that only 29% of students in grades 9–12 took part in 60 minutes of physical activity each day, which is the CDC's recommendation for children aged 6–17 years.[17] In addition to a decline in levels of physical activity, the average American now consumes more calories, more fat, and more sugar than in previous generations.[47,57]

The benefits of youth sports are copious. Organized sports have been shown to improve caloric expenditure and decrease snacking, decrease time spent in front of screens, and provide an arena for the development of motor, cognitive, and social skills.[49,57,71] The CDC reported a direct correlation between students who took part in high levels of physical activity and improved academics, decreased diabetes and cardiac disease, better weight control, and decreased psychological disorders.[86] Athletes have an increased likelihood of eating fruits and vegetables and a decreased likelihood of smoking tobacco, partaking in illicit drugs, and carrying a weapon.[57,65] Additionally, physically active girls have a decreased likelihood of developing breast cancer, osteoporosis, and obesity; a decreased rate of teenage pregnancy, depression, and suicide; and an increased likelihood of improved self-confidence and

TABLE 16.2
Kids Who Play Youth Sports Are

Less Likely To	More Likely To
• Break the law and go to prison	• Have better scores on national tests
• Join a gang	• Graduate from high school
• Abuse alcohol/drugs	• Get a job and maintain employment
• Cut class	• Become directors and managers in their jobs
• Have discipline problems in school	• Become leaders in politics and business
• Drop out of school	• Participate in charities
• Become a welfare recipient	

Source: Adapted from Kids Play USA Foundation website, available at http://kidsplayusafoundation.org/benefits-of-youth-sports.

body image.[57,82,84,88] Overall, teens who take part in sports are generally happier and less anxious, have better self-esteem, and have a reduced risk of suicidal behavior[54,84] (see Tables 16.2 and 16.3).

Clinical Pearl

Benefits of youth sports are profound and widespread and extend to positive effects on overall health, as well as physical, cognitive, and psychosocial well-being.

Participating in physical activity and youth sports is not without its risks. With increased activity and participation, there is an increase in sports-related injuries. A total of 2.6 million emergency room visits a year for those aged 5–24 years, a 70%–80% attrition rate from organized sports by the time a person is 15 years old, and programs overemphasizing winning are some of the problems encountered in youth sport.[57] Despite the latter, the authors believe that the benefits significantly outweigh the risks. And with better understanding of the stages of growth and development, sport readiness, and risks of sport specialization, the authors believe that the benefits will continue to outweigh risks by an even greater margin.

16.3 STAGES OF DEVELOPMENT

16.3.1 Infancy and Toddlerhood (0–24 Months)

Infants and toddlers typically follow a sequential path of acquisition of skills that cannot be sped up by early training.[11,13,68] Early in life, infants have certain primary (primitive) motor reflexes. These eventually diminish as other responses take their place. The ages at which infants typically start walking vary widely from 6 to 18 months. However, the ability of a child to walk at an early age does not mean the child will perform other motor skills early as well. Typical milestones for motor skills and reflexes in the infant and toddler can be seen in Table 16.4.[16]

TABLE 16.3
Benefits of Youth Sports

Physical and Psychological

- Increased energy expenditure
- Reduced body fat
- Reduced risk for obesity
- Stronger musculoskeletal system
- Increased participation in physical activity later in life
- Increased self-esteem
- Lower levels of depression
- Lower levels of suicidal ideation and attempts
- Lower levels of problem behaviors (aggression, delinquency)

Academic Performance

- Higher grade point averages (GPA) than non-athletes
- Increase in GPA as the number of sports teams increases
- Miss less school and more likely to go to college

Youth Athletes Report

- Eating more fruits and vegetables
- Smoking less
- Less television time
- Higher satisfaction with their body weight

Sports Can Provide

- Opportunities to make friends
- Positive role models
- Travel opportunities

Source: Adapted from the National Youth Sports Health and Safety Institute website, available at http://nyshsi.org/wp-content/uploads/2012/08/Benefits-of-Youth-Sports1.pdf.

TABLE 16.4
Typical Milestones of Infancy and Toddlerhood

Stage	Physical/Motor Milestones
By the age of 6 months	Rolls over in both directions, supports weight on legs when standing, begins to sit unsupported, and may crawl backward
By the age of 12 months	Gets to sitting position on his or her own, pulls to stand, cruises, may take a few steps without holding on, and may stand alone
By the age of 18 months	Walks alone, pulls toys while walking, can help undress, drinks from cup, and eats with spoon
By the age of 24 months	Stands on tiptoe, kicks ball, begins to run, walks up and down stairs holding on, climbs onto and down from furniture without help, throws ball overhand, and makes or copies straight lines and circles

Source: Adapted from the CDC Milestone Moments, available at http://www.cdc.gov/ncbddd/actearly/pdf/parents_pdfs/milestonemomentseng508.pdf.

By the time a toddler reaches the age of 2, they should be able to perform pretend play and parallel play. They can follow simple one-step or two-step commands and can listen for short periods of time. They also imitate adults, especially parents.[68]

This age is too young for sport participation to occur. However, there are some early intervention programs, such as swimming lessons, which many parents introduce their kids to before the age of 2. These have not been unequivocally proven to enhance swimming skills.[2] However, early water-survival skills training has not been shown to increase the risk of drowning and may be protective against drowning.[2,12] The American Academy of Pediatrics (AAP) continues to support swimming lessons after the age of 4 but has relaxed their 2000 position against water-survival skills prior to the age of 4.[2]

16.3.2 Early Childhood/Preschool Years (2–6 Years)

16.3.2.1 Physical Growth and Motor Skills

Compared to toddlerhood and infancy, the rate of physical growth in early childhood slows down considerably. Children's legs lose their typical bowlegged anatomy that is seen in infancy and toddlerhood. Their stride length increases as their legs straighten and lengthen. During this stage, significant advances are notable in neuromotor control. In part, this has to do with the incredible rate of synaptogenesis and myelination that is occurring from birth into early childhood. These processes occur through adolescence but the large increase in the brain's size, from 25% of adult size at birth to 90% of adult size by the age of 5, is largely due to myelination.[18] This enables motor nerves to improve firing rate and synchrony resulting in improved coordination of movement. It is during this time that children often learn to ride a bike and catch a ball.[11,33,60,68] They also improve their fine motor control of hands and fingers allowing them to manipulate small objects.[11,33,60,68] Typical milestones achieved during early childhood can be seen in Table 16.5.[16]

TABLE 16.5
Typical Milestones of Early Childhood

Stage	Physical/Motor Milestones
By the age of 3	Climbs well, runs easily, pedals a tricycle, and walks up and down stairs one foot on each step
By the age of 4	Hops and stands on one foot up to 2 seconds, pours, cuts with supervision, mashes food, and catches a bounced ball most of time
By the age of 5	Stands on one foot for 10 seconds or longer, hops, may be able to skip, somersault, use a fork and spoon and sometimes a knife, use toilet on his or her own, swings, and climbs
By the age of 6	Runs fast and steadily rarely falling, jumps backward on one foot, and sequences of motor movements in an organized manner

Source: Adapted from the CDC Milestone Moments, available at http://www.cdc.gov/ncbddd/actearly/pdf/parents_pdfs/milestonemomentseng508.pdf.

As children practice these motor skills, they become more refined and efficient.[33,68,89] Toward the end of early childhood, by the age of 5 and 6, children have much improved strength, endurance, balance, and coordination compared to toddlerhood and the beginning of early childhood. Further improvements in strength can be achieved with regular exercise and by physiologic adaptations in neural priming.

16.3.2.2 Cognitive Development

In this age group, kids tend to learn by imitation of others and by trial and error.[33,70] They have short attention spans that last no longer than 15 minutes, as well as poor selective attention. They can remember and recall very basic information. They are able to follow simple rules but often need the aid of reminders and visual aids.

16.3.2.3 Psychosocial Development

Early childhood is marked by egocentric tendencies. They have difficulty in seeing events and views from any other perspective than their own and have a hard time with not always being *first*.[68–70] They greatly desire to have their needs met immediately. This is the time when children just begin cooperative play. But they have yet to gain the ability to compare their abilities and performance with that of other kids.[31,33,66,68,80]

16.3.3 Late Childhood/Elementary School Years (6–11 Years)

16.3.3.1 Physical Growth and Motor Skills

The adult walking pattern is typically established during this period, due to the maturation and synergy of the physiologic, neurologic, and musculoskeletal systems.[4,68] This maturation in gait improves overall stability and efficiency in mobility.[4,68] In addition, mature patterns of fundamental skills are achieved during this time period (see Table 16.6).

TABLE 16.6
Fundamental and Transitional Motor Skills

Fundamental Motor Skills	Transitional Motor Skills
Catch	Catching overhead
Kick	Kicking on the run
Run	Running and throwing
Vertical jump	Jumping and striking
Overhand throw	Basketball layup
Ball bounce	Dribbling basketball on run
Leap	Leaping for various distances
Dodge	Dodging and leaping, roll dodge
Punt	Punting on the run
Forehand strike	Forehand strike while leaping
Two-hand sidearm strike	Hitting baseball vs. bunting baseball, slap shot in hockey vs. pass in hockey

Physical growth becomes steady during this stage of development. At this time, the physique of boys and girls is very similar, more so than what we find in later development.[27,48,68,79,80] However, there are gender differences in certain motor tasks. In general, girls tend to have better balance and learn to catch objects, as well as hop and skip, earlier than boys. In general, boys tend to have more explosive power in vertical jump, running, and throwing. Boys also typically learn to hit objects (e.g., as in baseball), kick, and throw more efficiently and accurately earlier than girls.[68,75,76] It is during this time that the transition from tee-ball to baseball with pitching can occur. As kids grow during this stage, more and more advanced tasks can be accomplished with more grace and efficiency. In addition, anaerobic and aerobic capacities increase steadily during late childhood. However, compared to adolescents, they are still very limited in this regard.

By the age of 11, most children have a mastery of all fundamental motor skills such as running, overhand throwing, kicking, and catching.[11,21,33,27,36,68,80] Additionally, they have already begun to work on transitional skills, the ones that require a combination of fundamental skills or are a variation of a fundamental skill.[71] Examples include throwing on the run, a basketball layup, and throwing long distances (see Table 16.6).

16.3.3.2 Cognitive Development

Prior to the cognitive improvements in adolescence, children in this stage of development have difficulty in thinking about consequences of actions and futuristic thinking. They typically are only concerned with the present situation and may not be able to differentiate the many varying outcomes of an action, rather seeing things only in black and white.[3,14,31,68–70] Therefore, parents and coaches will likely find discussions regarding future consequences fruitless. They also may still have some magical thinking and believe that they can perform the same actions that their sports idols can.[31,32,68,69]

Their attention spans, especially in the early part of this time period, are short. Therefore, instruction times should be kept on the short side, rules should be relatively flexible, and there should be a focus on simple activities that emphasize fundamental skills and the simpler transitional skills. Avoiding overly competitive situations is important as well.

Their memory continues to develop throughout this stage and there can be significant improvement in the ability to follow directions and rules. They also start to understand the reasoning behind the rules of the game or sport, and their judgment improves.[21,23,24,31,68] As attention and reasoning improves, coaches and parents may be able to gradually introduce more complex strategies and play combinations.

16.3.3.3 Psychosocial Development

During this stage, they often learn to like being part of a team. They begin to see the differences between their abilities and those of others.[25,66,68,80] Body image awareness begins as well.[1,68–70] In addition, they can recognize the kids that are popular and those that are not. They often enjoy comparisons between each other when it comes to athletic ability. Because of their lack of futuristic thinking, all young athletes in this stage, including the ones at opposite ends of the spectrum of ability, may have trouble realizing that their ability can change over time. Because of this, the more advanced kids may lack motivation to practice and improve their skills.[25,66,68,80,83] Conversely, the poorer performing kids may become discouraged and may lack the enthusiasm to continue to work on their skills to become better. Therefore, it is very important for coaches and parents to find activities that build confidence in all the participating young athletes. Differences in attention from coaches and other players due to athletic ability can be either positive or negative influences and may promote both positive and negative social adaptation. Thus, the focus should be on trying hard, putting in the effort, and less so on the outcome. If kids are praised for their effort and attempt of a challenging task as opposed to praise only for success (or winning), then they will learn to take on and relish the challenge and not just the success. If the opposite occurs, then kids may decide to take on lesser challenges to ensure success (and thus congratulatory praise from coaches, parents, etc.). This has the potential to minimize or halt their physical, cognitive, and social development.[59]

With regard to the increase in sport specialization, during this growth period it is believed that early diversification in sport and other activities may be important. An individual with a well-rounded sports regimen will more likely have positive psychosocial development and social adaptation and identity development down the road then an individual participating in one specialized sport.

16.3.4 Peripuberty and Early Adolescence (12–15 Years)

16.3.4.1 Physical Growth and Motor Skills

Peripuberty and early adolescence is characterized by rapid changes in physical growth and motor skills. The timing of these changes the timing of these changes depends on the onset of puberty and varies significantly from individual to individual. There is wide variability among boys and among girls with regard to rates of physical growth, motor skills development, and overall performance. In general, girls experience physical changes earlier than boys due to the earlier onset of puberty. Girls' growth spurts typically occur at a younger age, and thus, they are temporarily heavier and taller than boys. It is at this time that girls and boys can typically compete evenly.

During this period, the increases in muscle mass, overall strength, and cardiopulmonary endurance are greater than in any other period.[33,45,61,68,72,80] As opposed to prepubertal strength gains that are typically due to neural adaptations, postpubertal strength gains occur due to neural adaptations plus the addition of muscle hypertrophy. In general, boys can show dramatic increases in the performance of activities that require muscle strength such as jumping and sprinting, whereas girls tend to have more of a gradual increase and earlier plateau in performance of these activities.[33,55,56,68,80] In general, boys continue to improve in motor performance throughout early adolescence, whereas girls often do not demonstrate the same level of increased improvement after this age.[10,55,68,72,80] In boys, speed has been shown to be maximized before peak height velocity, while strength and power is maximized after peak height velocity; no clear pattern like this has been observed in girls.[10,53,55,68,72,80] Girls accumulate a greater amount of fat mass than boys during this time period. Boys who reach maturity early tend to be stronger and taller and have more muscle mass than late-maturing boys, whereas girls who reach maturity early tend to have wider shoulders and hips than later maturing girls.

Despite many of the gains seen in early adolescence, there can be temporary losses in coordination and balance. This is due to the rapidly growing musculoskeletal system and the time it takes to adapt to their changing body habitus. There can also be a loss of flexibility and increase in overuse injuries, especially apophyseal and physeal injuries. This is largely due to the disparity between the rate of growth between bone and soft tissues.

Clinical Pearl

Individual rates of growth and development vary widely. Therefore, chronological age is not a perfect indicator of the stage of development. However, it can be used as a general guideline of the various levels of development and when assessing sport readiness.

When discussing growth and development, it is important to mention that puberty is the time of menarche. If menses is delayed or absent during this period, this may be a sign of the female athlete triad and negative energy balance. Therefore, it is important that the sports medicine physician take into consideration these potential adverse effects and make appropriate inquiries into the general health of the adolescent female athlete.

16.3.4.2 Cognitive Development

Early adolescence is marked by improvements in inductive and deductive reasoning. In early adolescence, onset and advancement of abstract thinking, analytical capabilities, and problem solving occurs.[1,5,23,25,35,68–70] They can understand the theories and concepts of each sport and how it is played. They also have the ability to learn, remember, and apply complex strategies related to a given sport or activity.

Problems can arise with applying rules from one situation to the next as they progress in their development.[22,68] In addition, as intellectual abilities grow and reasoning skills advance, some adolescents will begin to argue and dispute concepts with coaches, parents, and other adults. They begin to test their boundaries and show their growing intellect.

16.3.4.3 Psychosocial Development

Early adolescence marks a heightened preoccupation with body image. Minor changes and alterations can be considered major concerns. Comparisons between an individual and his or her peers are very common, potentially causing feelings of inferiority or superiority. Young people in this stage of development also still need approval from their peers. Thus, they may push the limits of their boundaries, get into trouble, and stand up to authority figures in order to gain acceptance. Despite the common need for peer acceptance, family support and approval are very important during this period of development.[68–70] Sport participation provides a chance for adolescents to express themselves and develop independence.[50,61,68] It is important for adolescents to develop a sense of identity. It is at this time that individuals start to view themselves as a baseball player or tennis player, for example. Success in life and the activities that one attempts can lead to confidence and positive psychosocial maturation, whereas failure has the potential to lead to role confusion and a poorer sense of self and personal identity.[30] Of note, bullying often occurs during this stage with potentially deleterious effects. It can be difficult for adolescents to depersonalize comments from peers, coaches, parents, and other adults. Negative comments regarding a particular skill or activity can leave adolescents believing the commentator does not like them personally. Coaches and adults must choose carefully the comments and phrases they use to show support. As previously mentioned in the childhood section, it is best to use phrases that promote the effort, the attempt, and putting in the work rather than just the achievement or success.[59] It cannot be understated that family and friends play an important role in an individual's development of their own identity.[68–70]

16.3.5 Late Adolescence (15–18 Years)

16.3.5.1 Physical Growth and Motor Skills

As adolescence progresses, there is continued enhancement of strength, agility, coordination, power, and speed. However, it occurs at a slower rate than in early adolescence. Late-maturing boys and girls tend to catch up to those who reached maturity earlier. Specialization of gross motor skills also continues during this stage and will continue to develop long after adolescence. Girls at this age tend to be better at activities where balance is essential. By the end of this stage, full physical maturity is reached.

Specialization of skills can be enhanced by environmental factors such as increased practice of specific skills or a particular sport. However, there is evidence that the enhancement of sport-specific skills due to sport specialization can come at a cost (see Section 16.5). Cross-training has its benefits and can serve as a type of periodization in training. There is evidence that children and adolescents who specialize in one sport are more likely to develop overuse injuries, such as apophysitis, physeal injuries, and stress fractures, at a greater rate than adolescents who vary sport from season to season.[42] Often, sport specialization goes hand in hand with intense training and potentially overtraining. Due to these concerns, the AAP recommends that parents and pediatricians watch out for signs and symptoms of overtraining, such as decline in performance, weight loss, and sleep changes. By the age of 15, 75% of kids drop out of organized sports.[36] Ensuring enjoyment is a key aspect of maintaining sport participation and its many benefits presented earlier.

16.3.5.2 Cognitive Development

Abstract thinking continues to improve into late adolescence and beyond. They can begin to use creativity to apply strategies to various sports and activities.[68,73,90] They have a better understanding of the consequences of their actions.[1,33,40,68,70] They are able to analyze their actions, such as whether or not they played well, by comparing their recent performance with past performance, including personal bests and instances of above or below average play. They are able to assess strengths and weaknesses, determine what they need to change for the next activity or event, formulate a new strategy or game plan, and implement that game plan.[68,73,85,90] Adolescents can do this on their own; however, input from coaches, parents, and other knowledgeable individuals is valued.

As adolescence continues, more realistic goals are envisioned. Decision making becomes much more future oriented (as opposed to the *here and now* of early adolescence). Ideally, if development is proceeding well, personal values are much more clear and defined at this time.[1,31,40,68–70] By this stage, most adolescents are intellectually equipped for all competitive sports and specialization. However, enjoyment is still a major guiding principle for sport participation.

16.3.5.3 Psychosocial Development

Increasing levels of independence from parents and other authority figures is sought during this stage of development. Peers are relied on heavily as opposing viewpoints to parents. They also, consciously and unconsciously, use nonparental adults as role models, whether those people be coaches, professional athletes, or celebrities. Sports and physical acumen are often used to impress their peers and idols. Risk taking continues as a means to impress others.

As adolescence progresses and maturation continues, if they are well adjusted and healthy, a clearer sense of self and personal values has developed. They are better able to deal with peer pressures and pressure from parents and coaches and society in general. They are hopefully more secure with their body and gender role. They also tend to have a clearer idea of the role they wish sports to play in their lives, whether it be a primary and passionate focus, a tool to make and maintain friends, or just one of a number of activities that they take part in.[9,26,40,66–68]

16.4 READINESS FOR SPORTS

Sport readiness is the result of a process in which the young person acquires necessary physical, motor, cognitive, and psychosocial abilities,[71] thereby meeting the demands of a given sport or activity.[71] It is not always easy to know when an individual is ready for a particular sport or level within a certain sport. As previously mentioned, a mastery of fundamental skills is a prerequisite for most sports. These fundamental skills should be the focus of early training and youth sports. For example, the ability to balance on one leg is needed if one is going to be able to kick a soccer ball. Sports often require transitional skills, those that are a combination of fundamental skills (e.g., running and kicking as in kicking a soccer ball on the run) or more advanced fundamental skills with varying degrees of performance (e.g., throwing a ball in the strike zone or from center field to home plate; see Table 16.6).

Clinical Pearl

Sport readiness is the result of a process in which the child acquires necessary physical, motor, cognitive, and psychosocial abilities, thereby meeting the demands of a given sport or activity.

So how can one tell if a young person is ready for a particular sport? Observation during informal play is a good tool to use to assess motor skills. This may be done best in noncompetitive surroundings when the young person is unaware and the focus is on having fun. Regarding cognitive development, a young person has to be able to understand and attend to the basic rules of the particular sport before they can be expected to succeed in that sport. Therefore, they need to be able to follow basic instructions, learn over time, and learn with trial and error. Socially, kids have to show that they are able to interact with their peers and coaches in a positive way, be able to accept some level of feedback regarding their performance, and adapt to varying surroundings and situations. When coaches and parents have a better understanding about sport readiness and stages of growth and development, their interactions with the youth athlete can become more positive and constructive. Athletes playing under coaches who were instructed in coach effectiveness training report an enhanced sporting experience.[7,57,77,78] Via positive reinforcement and better teaching skills, player satisfaction, motivation, compliance, self-esteem, and attrition rates were all improved by coaches with this training.[7,57,78]

Clinical Pearl

Assessing sport readiness requires

- Understanding of the fundamental and transitional skills a sport requires
- Observation of the athlete to assess the presence of the necessary skills
- Inquiry to determine if the cognitive skills required to learn and play a sport are present
- Assessment of the level of psychosocial development present that will ensure success in potentially psychologically and socially challenging situations

As stated previously, chronological age is only a rough estimate of an individual's physical and motor, cognitive, and psychosocial development. Each person develops at their own rate. Development can be facilitated and hindered by positive and negative experiences, respectively. Placing a young person in a situation that does not provide enough of a challenge can slow development and hinder progress. Placing a young person in a situation that is overwhelming to them, whether it be because they are outsized physically, do not have the cognitive skills to follow strategy, or lack the psychosocial maturation to feel comfortable in their surroundings, may cause them to stop enjoying the sport. It cannot be overemphasized that enjoyment of the sport is one of the keys to success in any sport, and this can be maximized by fully understanding the idea of sport readiness.

So what specific activities may be best for a particular stage of growth and development? In general, the fundamental skills and balance are still limited in early childhood (2–6 years). Therefore, informal and simple activities are appropriate, such as running, swimming, throwing, and catching.[20] In middle childhood (6–12 years), balance is much improved and adult walking and running styles have been obtained. Most of the fundamental skills have been achieved and transitional skills are being forged. Therefore, more advanced activities and entry-level sports are appropriate, such as running, swimming, soccer, baseball, tennis, gymnastics, and martial arts.[20] Early adolescence includes the growth spurt of puberty. Mastery and refinement of fundamental and transitional motor skills is occurring. However, there can be minor setbacks in balance and coordination due to the changing body habitus. Despite this, entry-level sports that are a little more advanced, such as football, basketball, hockey, volleyball, and field hockey, are appropriate because of their overall advancing development.[20]

16.5 SPORT SPECIALIZATION

Sport specialization is considered "intensive, year-round training in a single sport at the exclusion of other sports."[20] In recent times, the move toward sport specialization has been driven by increased importance placed on competitive success with goals such as travel team selection, college and university scholarships, national and Olympic team selection, and the hope to play sports professionally. Due to these lofty goals and increasing competition, common thinking among lay people is that sport specialization at earlier and earlier ages is the only means to achieve these ends. However, a recent study published in 2013 reviewed all the studies that looked into age of sport specialization and outcome with regard to the achievement of elite status in athletics.[42] This review found 11 studies that compared age of specialization, early diversification, and outcome. Overall, for most sports, early sport diversification (i.e., taking part in numerous sports and waiting until adolescence to specialize) improves chances of achieving success in a certain sport.[42] Nine of eleven studies showed evidence that compared to near-elite athletes and non-international athletes, elite athletes and international team athletes were more likely to have begun intense training or sport specialization after the age of 12 and had early sport diversification.[42] This goes against the commonly held belief that the earlier one begins specialized training in a particular sport, the better the chance of elite-level success. The authors of that 2013 study noted that "early diversification provides the young athlete with valuable physical, cognitive, and psychosocial environments and promotes motivation."[42] It was also noted that "early diversification followed by specialization may lead to more enjoyment, fewer injuries, and longer participation, contributing to the chances of success."[42] However, there are certain *early entry sports*, such as gymnastics, swimming, and figure skating, where there is some evidence that chance of success is increased with early specialization.[20] In these *early entry sports*, the age at which elite level is often achieved comes well before full physical maturity, thus the need for early specialization.

In the American Medical Society for Sports Medicine position statement on overuse injuries and burnout in youth sports, one of their recommendations is "early sport specialization may not lead to long-term success in sports and may increase risk for overuse injury and burnout."[20] Of great concern is the idea that sport specialization done too early puts undue physical and emotional stress on the young athlete. This can lead to overuse injuries such as stress fractures, osteochondritis dissecans, and apophyseal and physeal injuries, among many others. Some statistics support this increased injury pattern.[20]

Clinical Pearl

Early sport specialization may be detrimental to the achievement of elite-level status, as compared to early diversification and sport specialization taking place after the onset of adolescence.

Specific shoulder and elbow injuries in the adolescent athlete will vary from sport to sport. Athletes involved in overhead sports, such as baseball and tennis, most commonly experience these upper extremity injuries.[19] Athletes who specialized only in tennis are 1.5 times more likely to report an injury.[42,43] In adolescent elite national tennis players, specifically boys 16–18 years old and girls 16 years old, over 20%–45% of all injuries were located in the upper extremity.[19,74] Of these athletes, 25%–30% had previous or current shoulder pain, while 22%–25% had previous or current elbow pain.[19,74]

It is estimated that over 2.5 million youth athletes competed in Little League Baseball in 2009.[19,52] Lyman et al. noted that 26%–35% of youth baseball pitchers experienced a shoulder and/or elbow injury during the course of a season.[19,52] Similarly, 30% of pitchers experienced shoulder pain and 25% experienced elbow pain after a specific game.[19,51] Potential risk factors for subsequent injury will depend upon the exact sport. In the throwing athlete, risk factors have included the number of pitches thrown in a game, the type of pitches, and the number of months pitched in a year.[19,44] These findings have led to recommendations including limiting the pitch count to less than 80 throws/game, limiting the use of curve balls and sliders, and pitching for less than 8 months in a year to avoid injury.[19,64] Baseball pitchers who pitched greater than 8 months per year have a greater likelihood of needing shoulder or elbow surgery.[42,64] Pitchers aged 9–14 years with more than 100 innings in a year are 3.5 times more likely to have an injury.[29,42] Other studies have started looking at the differences in pitching kinematics and kinetics in adolescent throwers compared to adults to identify biomechanical factors that may contribute to overuse and fatigue.[19,28,62,63] Earlier studies of adolescent pitchers suggested an increase in physeal width of the dominant shoulder regardless of symptoms. As the athlete matures, skeletal changes occur.

The intense training inherent with sport specialization can lead to early withdrawal or burnout from a sport that at one time afforded them great joy.[6,8,15,38,39,41,42,46,58,81,87] Burnout is described as departure from sport because of an athlete's perception that it is not possible for them to meet both the physical and psychological demands required.[20,34] Swimmers who specialized early had decreased time on the national team and withdrew from swimming earlier than those who specialized later.[8,42] The focus, especially in the early stages of growth and development, should be on fun, as well as fundamental and transitional skill development ahead of competition and outcome (i.e., winning).[20] The AAP recommends no sport specialization before the age of 10. Much of the evidence points to the fact that early specialization before the onset of adolescence and puberty could actually reduce the likelihood of achieving elite-level status in the sport and that early diversification and specialization after the onset of adolescence may be the most beneficial and give the greatest likelihood of success.[6,8,15,38,39,41,42,46,58,81,87] Certainly, more research is required. However, the evidence available presents an interesting counterpoint to the idea of early sport specialization.

16.6 CONCLUSION

Physical activity during youth and youth sports has been shown to be of great benefit for the physical and psychological health and well-being of its participants. It is important that doctors taking care of these young athletes are aware of the typical stages and patterns of growth and development so that the positive benefits of sport participation are maximized. Doctors can be a great resource for parents and coaches when it comes to understanding physical, cognitive, and psychosocial growth and development. Assessment of sport readiness is an important process because of the potential risks and benefits with placement of young athletes in sports and events that are not suitable to their skill level or maturity. Early sport specialization has become more widespread, and it has the potential to lead to increased rate of overuse injuries, early withdrawal from sport, and loss of enjoyment (Table 16.7).

TABLE 16.7
SORT: Key Recommendations for Practice

Clinical Recommendation	Level of Evidence	References
Benefits of youth sports are profound and widespread, and extend to positive effects on overall health, as well as physical, cognitive, and psychosocial well-being.	A	[49,54,57,65,71,84,86,88]
Individual rates of growth and development vary widely. Therefore chronological age is not a perfect indicator of the stage of development. However it can be used as a general guideline of the various levels of development and when assessing sport readiness.	B	[11,13,16,68]
Sport readiness is the result of a process in which the young person acquires necessary physical, motor, cognitive, and psychosocial abilities thereby meeting the demands of a given sport or activity.	B	[71]
Assessing sport readiness is not always easy. It requires • Understanding of the fundamental and transitional skills a sport requires, • Observation of the athlete to assess the presence of the necessary skills, • Inquiry to determine if the cognitive skills required to learn and play a sport are present, and • Assessment of the level of psychosocial development present that will ensure success in potentially psychologically and socially challenging situations.	B	[71]
Early sport specialization may be detrimental to the achievement of elite level status, as compared to early diversification with sport specialization taking place after the onset of adolescence.	B	[6,8,15,20,38,39,41,42,46,58,81,87]
Early sport specialization has the potential to contribute to injury, withdrawal from sport and/or burnout, and loss of enjoyment in a sport that once provided great joy.	B	[6,8,15,20,38,39,41,42,46,58,81,87]

REFERENCES

1. Abe JA, Izard CE. A longitudinal study of emotion, expression and personality relations in early development. *Journal of Personality and Social Psychology.* 1996;77:566–577.
2. American Academy of Pediatrics Committee on Injury, Violence and Poison Prevention. Policy statement—Prevention of drowning. *Pediatrics.* 2010;126(1):1–10.
3. American Academy of Pediatrics Committee on Psychosocial Aspects of Child and Family Health. *Guidelines for Health Supervision III.* Elk Grove Village, IL: American Academy of Pediatrics; 1997.
4. American Academy of Pediatrics Committee on Sports Medicine and Fitness. Intensive training and sports specialization in young athletes. *Pediatrics.* 2000;106:154–157.
5. American Academy of Pediatrics Committee on Sports Medicine and Fitness. Participation in boxing by children, adolescents, and young adults. *Pediatrics.* 1997;99:134–135.
6. Baker J, Côté J, Abernathy B. Sport-specific practice and the development of expert decision-making in team ball sports. *Journal of Applied Sports Psychology.* 2003;15:12–25.
7. Barnett NP, Smoll FL, Smith RE. Effects of enhancing coach-athlete relationships on youth sport attrition. *Sports Psychology.* 1992;6:111–127.
8. Barynina II, Vaitsekhovskii SM. The aftermath of early sports specialization for highly qualified swimmers. *Fitness Sports Revolution International.* 1992;27:132–133.
9. Begel D. The psychologic development of the athlete. In: Begel D, Burton RW, eds. *Sport Psychiatry: Theory and Practice.* New York: WW Norton; 2000: pp. 3–21.
10. Beunen G, Malina RM. Growth and physical performance relative to timing of the adolescent spurt. *Exercise and Sports Science Review.* 1988;16:503–540.
11. Branta C, Haubensticker J, Seefeldt V. Age changes in motor skills during childhood and adolescence. *Exercise and Sports Science Review.* 1984;12:467–520.
12. Brenner R, Teneja G, Haynie D et al. The association between swimming lessons and drowning in childhood: A case-control study. *Archives of Pediatrics and Adolescent Medicine.* 2009;163(3):203–210.
13. Burgess-Milliron MJ, Murphy SB. Biomechanical considerations of youth sports injuries. In: Bar-or O, ed. *The Child and Adolescent Athlete.* Oxford, U.K.: Blackwell Science; 1996: pp. 173–188.
14. Capute AJ, Accardo PJ. A neurodevelopmental perspective on the continuum of developmental disabilities. In: Capute AJ, Accardo PJ, eds. *Developmental Disabilities in Infancy and Childhood*, 2nd edn. Baltimore, MD: Paul H Brooks Publishing; 1996:pp. 1–24.
15. Carlson R. The socialization of elite tennis players in Sweden: An analysis of the players' backgrounds and development. *Sociol Sports Journal.* 1998;5:241–256.
16. Center for Disease Control. Milestone moments. Available at: http://www.cdc.gov/ncbddd/actearly/pdf/parents_pdfs/milestonemomentseng508.pdf. Accessed April 10, 2014.
17. Centers for Disease Control and Prevention. Youth risk behavior surveillance—United States, 2011. *MMWR.* 2012;61:1–168.
18. Colby JB, O'Hare ED, Bramen JE, Sowell ER. Structural brain development birth through adolescence. In Rubenstein J, Rakic P, eds. *Neural Circuit Development and Function in the Brain.* Amsterdam, the Netherlands: Academic Press/Elsevier; 2013; pp. 207–230.
19. De Luigi AJ. Common injuries of the throwing athlete. Available at http://diamondskillsbaseball.com/wp-content/uploads/2014/04/Common-Injuries-in-the-Adolescent-Throwing-Athlete.pdf. Accessed April 19, 2014.
20. DiFiori JP, Benjamin HJ, Brenner J et al. Overuse injuries and burnout in youth sports: A position statement from the american medical society for sports medicine. *Clinical Journal of Sports Medicine.* 2014;24:3–20.
21. Dixon SD, Stein MT, eds. *Encounters with Children: Pediatric Behavior and Development*, 3rd edn. Philadelphia, PA: Mosby; 2000.
22. Elkind D. *The Hurried Child: Growing Up Too Fast, Too Soon.* Reading, MA: Addison-Wesley; 1988.
23. Erickson E. *Childhood and Society.* New York: WW Norton and Co., Inc.; 1963.
24. Erickson E. *Identity, Youth and Crisis.* New York: WW Norton and Co., Inc.; 1968.
25. Ewing MW, Seefeldt VS, Brown TP. *Role of Sport in the Education and Health of American Children and Youth.* East Lansing, MI: Michigan State University Institute for the Study of Youth Sports; 1996.
26. Farrell EG. Sports medicine: Psychologic aspects. In: Greydanus DE, Wolraich ML, eds. *Behavioral Pediatrics.* New York: Springer-Verlag; 1992: pp. 425–434.
27. Feldman H, Bauer RE. Developmental-behavioral pediatrics. In: Zitelli BJ, Davis HW, eds. *Atlas of Pediatric Physical Diagnosis*, 3rd edn. St. Louis, MO: Mosby-Wolfe; 1997: pp. 47–74.
28. Fleisig G, Chu Y, Weber A, Andrews J. Variability in baseball pitching biomechanics among various levels of competition. *Sports Biomechanics.* March 2009;8(1):10–21.
29. Fleisig GS, Andrews JR, Cutter GR et al. Risk of serious injury for young baseball pitchers: A 10-year prospective study. *American Journal of Sports Medicine.* 2011;39(2):253–257.
30. Forbes Oste H. The art of social strategy. Erickson's psychosocial development adapted for social optimisation strategies. Available from: http://forbesoste.com/tag/erik-erikson/ Accessed April 20, 2014.
31. Gemelli R. *Normal Child and Adolescent Development.* Washington, DC: American Psychiatric Press; 1996.
32. Gesell A, Ilg FL, Ames LB. *The Child from Five to Ten.* New York: Harper and Row Publishers; 1946.
33. Gomez JE. Growth and maturation. In: Sullivan AJ, Anderson SJ, eds. *Care of the Young Athlete.* Park Ridge, IL: American Academy of Orthopaedic Surgeons and American Academy of Pediatrics; 2000: pp. 25–32.
34. Gould D. Intensive sport participation and the prepubescent athlete: Competitive stress and burnout. In: Cahill BR, Pearl AJ, eds. *Intensive Participation in Children's Sports.* Champaign, IL: Human Kinetics; 1993: pp. 19–38.
35. Greydanus DE, Pratt HD. Psychosocial considerations for the adolescent athlete: Lessons learned from the US Asian. *Journal of Pediatric Practice.* 2000;3:19–29.
36. Harris S. Readiness to participate in sports. In: Sullivan JA, Anderson SJ, eds. *Care of the Young Athlete.* Rosemont, IL: American Academy of Orthopaedic Surgeons and American Academy of Pediatrics; 2000: pp. 19–24.
37. Hedstrom R, Gould D. *Research in Youth Sports: Critical Issues Status, White Paper Summaries of the Existing Literature.* East Lansing, MI: Institute for the Study of Youth Sports, Michigan State University; 2004.
38. Helsen WF, Starkes JL, Hodges NJ. Team sports and the theory of deliberate practice. *Journal of Sport and Exercise Psychology.* 1998;20:12–34.

39. Hodges NJ, Starkes JL. Wrestling with the nature of expertise: A sport specific test of Ericsson, Krampe, and Tesch-Romer's (1993) theory of "deliberate practice. *International Journal of Sport Psychology*. 1996;27:400–424.
40. Hoffman AD. Adolescent growth and development. In: Hoffman AD, Greydanus DE, eds. *Adolescent Medicine*, 3rd edn. Stamford, CT: Appleton and Lange; 1997: pp. 11–22.
41. Hume PA, Hopkins WG, Robinson DM, Robinson SM, Hollings SC. Predictors of attainment in rhythmic sportive gymnastics. *Journal of Sports and Medcine Physical Fitness*. 1994;33(4):367–377.
42. Jayanthi N, Pinkham C, Dugas L, Patrick B, LaBella C. Sports specialization in young athletes: Evidence-based recommendations. *Sports Health*. 2013;5(9):251–257.
43. Jayanthi NA, Dechert A, Durazo R, Luke A. Training and specialization risks in junior elite tennis players. *Journal of Medical Science Tennis*. 2011;16(1):14–20.
44. Kocher MS, Walters PM, Micheli LJ. Upper extremity injuries in the paediatric athlete. *Sports Medicine*. August 2000;30(2):117–135.
45. Kreipe RE. Normal somatic adolescent growth and development. In: McAnarney ER, Kreipe RE, Orr DP, Comerci GD, eds. *Textbook of Adolescent Medicine*. Philadelphia, PA: WB Saunders; 1994: pp. 44–67.
46. Law M, Côté J, Ericsson KA. Characteristics of expert development in rhythmic gymnastics: A retrospective study. *International Journal of Exercise and Sport Psychology*. 2007;5:82–103.
47. LetsMove.org. Learn the facts. Available from: http://www.letsmove.gov/learn-facts/epidemic-childhood-obesity. Accessed April 25, 2014.
48. Levine MD. Neurodevelopmental dysfunction in the school age child. In Behrman RE, Liegman RM, Jensen HB, eds. *Nelson Textbook of Pediatrics*, 16th edn. Philadelphia, PA: WB Saunders; 2000: pp. 94–100.
49. Loprinzi PD, Cardinal BJ, Loprinzi KL, Lee H. Benefits and environmental determinants of physical activity in children and adolescents. *Obesity Facts*. 2012;5:597–610.
50. Luckstead EF, Greydanus DE. *Medical Care of the Adolescent Athlete*. Los Angeles, CA: Practice Management Information Corporation; 1993.
51. Lyman S, Fleisig GS, Andrews JR et al. Effect of pitch type, pitch count, and pitching mechanics on risk of elbow and shoulder pain in youth baseball pitchers. *American Journal of Sports Medicine*. 2002;30:463–468.
52. Lyman S, Fleisig GS, Waterbor JW et al. Longitudinal study of elbow and shoulder pain in youth baseball pitchers. *Medicine and Science Sports and Exercise*. 2001;33:1803–1810.
53. Malina RM, Bouchard C eds. *Growth, Maturation, and Physical Activity*. Champaign, IL: Human Kinetics; 1991.
54. Malina RM, Cumming SP. Current status and issues in youth sports. In: Malina RM, Clark MA, eds. *Youth Sports: Perspectives for a New Century*. Monterey, CA: Coaches Choice; 2003.
55. Malina RM. Physical growth and biologic maturation of young athletes. *Exercise Sport Science Review*. 1994;22:389–433.
56. Marshall WA, Tanner JM. Variation in the pattern of pubertal changes in girls. *Archives of Disease in Childhood*. 1969;44:291–303.
57. Merkel DL. Youth sport: Positive and negative impact on young athletes. *Journal of Sports Medicine*. 2013;4:151–160.
58. Moesch K, Elbe AM, Hauge ML, Wikman JM. Late specialization: The key to success in centimeters, grams, or seconds (cgs) sports. *Scandinavian Journal of Medical Science Sports*. 2011;21(6):e282–e290.
59. National Education Association. The praise paradox: Are we smothering kids in kind words? Available from: http://www.nea.org/home/42298.htm. Accessed April 12, 2014.
60. Needleman RD. Growth and development. In: Behrman RE, Kliegman RM, Jensen HB, eds. *Nelson Textbook of Pediatrics*, 16th edn. Philadelphia, PA: WB Saunders; 2000: pp. 23–65.
61. Nelson MA. Developmental skills and children's sports. *Physician and Sportsmedicine*. 1991;19:67–79.
62. Nissen CW, Westwell M, Ounpus S, Patel M, Tate JP, Pierz K, Burns JP, Bicos J. Adolescent baseball pitching technique: A detailed three-dimensional biomechanical analysis. *Medicine and Science Sports and Exercise*. August 2007;39(8):1347–1357.
63. Nissen CW, Westwell M, Ounpuu S, Patel M, Solomito M, Tate J. A biomechanical comparison of the fastball and curveball in adolescent baseball pitchers. *American Journal of Sports Medicine*. August 2009;37(8):1492–1498.
64. Olsen SJ 2nd, Fleisig GS, Dun S, Loftice J, Andrew JR. Risk factors for shoulder and elbow injuries in adolescent baseball pitchers. *American Journal of Sports Medicine*. June 2006;34(6):905–912.
65. Pate RR, Trost SG, Levin S, Dowda M. Sports participation and health-related behaviors among US youth. *Archives of Pediatric and Adolescent Medicine*. 2000;154:904–911.
66. Patel DR, Greydanus DE, Pratt HD. Youth sports: More than sprains and strains. *Contemporary Pediatrics*. 2000;18:45.
67. Patel DR, Pratt HD, Greydanus DE. Adolescent growth, development, and psychosocial aspects of sports participation: An overview. *Adolescent Medicine State of the Art Review*. 1998; 9:425–440.
68. Patel DR, Pratt HD, Greydanus DE. Pediatric neurodevelopment and sports participation When are children ready to play sports? *Pediatric Clinical North America*. 2002;49:505–531.
69. Piaget J, Inhelder B. *The Psychology of the Child*. New York: Basic Books; 1969.
70. Piaget J. Intellectual evaluation from adolescence to adulthood. *Human Development*. 1972;15(1):1–12.
71. Purcell LK. Sport readiness in children and youth. *Paediatric and Child Health*. 2005;10:343–344.
72. Roemmich JN, Rogol AD. Physiology of growth and development. Its relationship to performance in the young athlete. *Clinical and Sports Medicine*. 1995;14:483–502.
73. Ryckman RM, Hamel J. Perceived physical ability differences in the sport participation motives of young athletes. *International Journal of Sports and Psychology*. 1993;24:270–283.
74. Safran MR, Hutchinson MR, Moss R et al. A comparison of injuries in elite boys and girls tennis players. *Transactions of the 9th Annual Meeting of the Society of Tennis Medicine and Science*, March 1999. Indian Wells, CA.
75. Seefeldt V, Haunbenstricker J. Patterns, phases or stages: An analytical model for the study of developmental movement. In: Kelso JAS, Clark JE, eds. *The Development of Movement Control and Coordination*. New York: John Wiley & Sons; 1982: pp. 309–318.
76. Seefeldt V. The concept of readiness applied to motor skills acquisition. In: Magill RA, Ash MJ, Smoll FL, eds. *Children in Sports*, 2nd edn. Champaign, IL: Human Kinetics; 1982: pp. 31–37.
77. Smith RE, Smoll FL, Barnett NP. Reduction of children's sport performance anxiety through social support and stress-reduction training for coaches. *Journal of Applied Developmental Psychology*. 1995;16:125–142.

78. Smith RE, Smoll FL, Curtis B. Coach effectiveness training: A cognitive-behavioral approach to enhancing relationship skills in youth sport coaches. *Journal of Sport Psychology.* 1997;1:59–75.
79. Smoll FL, Schultz RW. Quantifying gender differences in physical performance: A developmental perspective. *Development Psychology.* 1990;26:360–369.
80. Smoll FL, Smith RE, eds. *Children and Youth in Sport: A Biopsychosocial Perspective.* Madison, WI: Brown and Benchmark, Inc.; 1996.
81. Soberlak P, Côté J. The developmental activities of elite ice hockey players. *Journal of Applied Sports Psychology.* 2003;15:41–49.
82. Staurowsky EJ, DeSousa MJ, Ducher G et al. *Her Life Depends On It II: Sport, Physical Activity, and the Health and Well-Being of American Girls and Women.* East Meadow, NY: Women's Sports Foundation; 2009.
83. Stryer BK, Tofler IR, Lapchick R. A developmental overview of child and youth sports in society. *Child Adolescent Psychiatric Clinical North America.* 1998;7:697–724.
84. Taliaferro LA, Rienzo B, Miller MD et al. High school youth and suicide risk: Exploring protection afforded through physical activity and sport participation. *Journal of School Health.* 2008;78:545–553.
85. Tofler IR, Stryer BK, Micheli LJ et al. Physical and emotional problems of elite female gymnasts. *New England Journal of Medicine.* 1996;335:281.
86. Ullrich-French S, McDonough MH, Smith AL. Social connection and psychological outcomes in a physical activity-based youth development setting. *Research Quarterly for Exercise and Sport.* 2012;83:431–441.
87. Wall M, Côté J. Developmental activities that lead to dropout and investment in sport. *Physical Education and Sports Pedagogy.* 2007;12:77–87.
88. Women's Sports and Fitness Facts and Statistics Women's Sports Foundation 3/26/09. Benefits of sport: The universal truths Available from:http://www.womenssportsfoundation.org/home/she-network/health/benefits-of-sport-the-universal-truths. Accessed April 25, 2014.
89. Yan JH, Thomas JR, Thomas KT. Children's age moderates the effect of practice variability: A quantitative review. *Research Quarterly for Exercise and Sport.* 1998;69:210–215.
90. Zimmerman BJ, Kitsantas A. Developmental regulations in self-regulation shifting from process goals to outcome goals. *Journal of Educational Psychology.* 1997;89:29–36.

Section III

Clinical Assessment

17 History and Physical Exam

Anthony I. Beutler and Bradley S. Havins

CONTENTS

TABLE 17.1
Key Clinical Considerations

1. The presenting area of injury may not always be the underlying source of the patient's problem.
2. A thorough history is the "key witness" in building a correct differential diagnosis for musculoskeletal injury.
3. The mistake of treating only the injured victim and ignoring the underlying culprit is the most common treatment error made by primary care physicians treating musculoskeletal injuries.
4. Extrinsic factors are common and the most easily correctable "culprits" underlying overuse injuries.
5. Physical exam is a key contributor to the overall, comprehensive, pathoanatomical treatment plan.

17.1 INTRODUCTION

Sustaining injuries is an unfortunate part of sports participation. A majority of injured patients will seek care with their primary care physician. When caring for sports-related injuries, the physician's task is to quickly and accurately diagnose injuries, institute effective therapies, and get the athlete back to sport as quickly and safely as possible. In the case of acute injuries, this can be a fairly simple process. For example, most acute fractures have a clear mechanism of injury and can be easily diagnosed by a combination of history, physical exam, and plain film radiography. After reduction as needed, immobilization for a prescribed duration, and proper rehabilitation, the structural healing is complete and the athlete is generally ready to return to play (Table 17.1).

In contrast to acute injuries, many chronic/overuse injuries do not respond predictably to rest, ice, compression, and elevation (RICE) and relative rest. All too commonly an athlete will self-treat with over-the-counter analgesics, rest for a while, use some ice, and buy a compressive brace to assist with the injury. Yet when they attempt to return to play, they find their pain returns, and they continue to perform below their desired level of excellence. An athlete in this situation is caught in the overuse injury cycle, which can be extremely frustrating.

In addition to being frustrating to the athlete, the overuse injury cycle can be perplexing for the treating physician. Physicians will face tough questions from athletes such as the following: "Why does my plantar fasciitis come back even after I take a break from running?" "Why is my shoulder impingement not gone after a couple weeks of rest?" "If my Achilles tendinosis is back again, will I ever be able to run pain-free again?" These are all questions that primary care physicians will face, and the intent of this chapter is to give you the tools to answer these questions, to correctly diagnose the problem, and to understand why the "injured" area may not always be the underlying source of the patient's problem.

Clinical Pearl

The presenting area of injury may not always be the underlying source of the patient's problem.

To help frame this concept, we will use the victim and culprit model. For our purposes, the victims will be the injured tissues (bone, muscle, tendon, etc.), and the culprits will be the underlying factors that contributed to that injury. Using the example of a Colles fracture, the victim would be the distal radius. In this acute injury, the culprit could be as straightforward as a fall on an outstretched hand. In the case of an overuse injury, however, the culprit is often not as easy to identify.

17.2 VICTIMS? CULPRITS? WHEN DID I BECOME A DETECTIVE?

No, you have not joined the police force, but to identify the culprit (or in other words, the underlying pathology behind an overuse injury), you may have to think like one. In police work, identification of the victim is easy. The victim is usually the one filing the complaint, or in a crime scene, they might be the one outlined in chalk. Detectives do not get paid the big bucks from identifying the victim. The real question detectives need to answer is "who did it?" and perhaps as importantly, why? The same is true with physicians. Many primary care physicians are well-trained at victim identification. They correctly identify what tissue structure has been injured. But the successful sports medicine physician must do more than just victim identification. Finding and apprehending the correct offending culprit distinguishes the truly excellent physician from the mediocre one. But before you can apprehend the culprit, you do first need to make sure that you have correctly identified the right victim.

17.2.1 Victim Identification

A thorough history is the "key witness" to correctly diagnosing a musculoskeletal injury. History combined with a thorough physical exam nearly always provide enough "evidence" that laboratory and radiological tests are merely used to confirm the diagnosis. The correct diagnosis always starts with a good history. An experienced sports medicine physician will be guided toward a diagnosis based on key historical points: "It hurts when I do this; it does not hurt when I do that." Or "My shoulder feels like it slips out of place when I open my sunroof." Based on historical clues, a differential diagnosis is formulated and physical examination is performed based on this differential. While it may be possible to correctly diagnose simple conditions (i.e., a lateral ankle sprain) on exam findings alone, even the most complete examination of more complex joint regions (like the hip or shoulder) is unlikely to yield a precise diagnosis without a careful and skillful history.

Clinical Pearl

A thorough history is the "key witness" in building a correct differential diagnosis for musculoskeletal injury.

Past injury history, surgical history, and medical history are of key importance to the sports medicine physician. The best predictor of future injury is a history of past injury. Injured areas are naturally predisposed to repeat injury. Additionally, efforts to rehabilitate, brace, or compensate for previously injured tissues may cause predictable increases in forces affecting surrounding tissues. Past surgical history for musculoskeletal injury is an obvious predictor of future injury, but non-orthopedic surgery can also predispose to future musculoskeletal injury (i.e., abdominal surgery leading to core muscle weakness, leading to patellofemoral pain on return to running). Past medical history is often and mistakenly overlooked in musculoskeletal diagnosis. Common medical conditions predispose to a variety injuries (i.e., diabetes and thyroid disease predispose to adhesive capsulitis of the shoulder). Yesterday's history is often a key culprit contributing to the demise of today's victim.

17.3 SPORTS MEDICINE PHYSICAL EXAMINATION

The sports medicine physical examination has six core components that will be briefly discussed here.[1] When performing physical examination, the skilled sports physician will remember to compare an injured limb with the often "normal" contralateral side and will remember that a complete examination requires interrogation of the joint proximal to and the joint distal to the presenting region. The six core components of physical examination are frequently performed and reported in the following sections.

17.3.1 Inspection

Inspection starts when the patient enters the room. Inspecting the gait of a patient with a lower extremity or running injury is mandatory. Observing a patient with shoulder pain as they remove their jacket is also useful. Look at the way the patient is positioned at rest. This is usually the position of comfort for the patient and can indicate which movements are particularly painful. Carefully check for changes in skin color or character. Note any deformities as well as muscle bulk or atrophy. Unless you are secretly Superman, you cannot do this through the patient's clothes. Proper patient exposure begins at inspection and should be maintained throughout the physical maneuver process.

17.3.2 Palpation

Palpate bony prominences, any palpable ligaments, and if possible find the point of maximal tenderness. Specific attention should be paid to tenderness to palpation occurring over bones versus over surrounding soft tissue. Be cognizant that palpation may be painful for the patient, but don't be shy about doing your job. Finding the most tender spot on palpation is often the most important part of the physical exam. If a point of tenderness is found, remember to ask the patient if this recreates the same pain they experience with their activity.

17.3.3 Range of Motion

Range should be tested in all planes of motion that correspond to each specific joint. Active range of motion (motion initiated by the patient) should be attempted first, since if active range of motion is full, then testing passive range of motion is usually not required. However, if deficits in active range of motion are observed, passive testing (the examiner attempts to move the patient's joint) should be documented. Be sure to note if the range of motion is painful or pain free. In cases where pain significantly affects passive motion, targeted injections of local anesthetic are useful to distinguish motion deficits due to pain-induced guarding from true mechanical blocks that physically impede motion.

17.3.4 Strength

Assessing muscular strength is key to the sports medicine evaluation. The standard X/5 strength assessment is used but is often less helpful in the sports medicine context as it lacks the granularity needed for fine distinctions. Clinicians should look for relative weakness compared to the contralateral extremity. When testing strength, physicians should endeavor to compare the point at which a patient's strength fails, or "breaks," from side to side. This "breaking" can be difficult to assess in strong athletes as their muscle mass and strength can mask important clinical findings. Strength is traditionally assessed by having the patient fire the tested muscle (i.e., flex the bicep), and then the examiner attempts to fight against the maximally activated muscle (i.e., pull the elbow into extension).

17.3.5 Neurovascular

A neurovascular exam is obviously of extreme importance in acute trauma and can also yield tremendous benefits in cases of chronic, overuse injury. Typically, light touch sensation is sufficient for the diagnosis of most musculoskeletal conditions. When assessing sensation of the hand, two-point discrimination is the most useful sensation exam. In spinal injuries, sensation, reflexes, and myotonal strength testing are key to determining injury severity as well as localizing the injury. Documentation of pulses is essential in establishing the neurovascular status of injured tissues.

17.3.6 Special Tests

Special tests are the glitzy, glamorous, Hollywood stars of the physical exam. They offer the allure of making a dazzling diagnosis with a single deft maneuver. And it certainly doesn't hurt than many special tests are named for famous orthopedic surgeons! Unfortunately, special tests usually aren't really all that "special." The sensitivity and specificity of many special tests are frankly more suspect than scintillating (Table 17.2) Three important rules of thumb apply to all special tests: First, be wary of new special tests. Initial studies often report nearly perfect sensitivity and specificity. However, subsequent studies in primary care patient populations typically show much less predictive value (see Thessaly test for meniscus tears). Second, the more special tests exist for a given injury, the worse those tests generally will be at predicting that injury (i.e., shoulder labrum). So because of rules 1 and 2, rule 3 is that special tests should be interpreted in the context of the full history and physical examination. Special tests are body region and joint specific, and the decision of whether or not to perform a specific special test depends on the patient's history and other aspects of their physical exam. Specific special tests will be discussed later in their respective chapters.

TABLE 17.2
Predictive Characteristics of Common Special Tests

Test Name	Sensitivity (%)	Specificity (%)
Lachman test	63	55
Ankle anterior drawer test	58	100
Syndesmosis squeeze test	30	93
Thompson test	96	93
Dynamic labral shear (crank test)	89	30
Empty can (pain)	78	40
Empty can (weakness)	87	43
Hawkins–Kennedy	74	50
Neer	68	30
Relocation test	44	54

Sources: Covey, C.J. and Mulder, M.D., *J. Fam. Pract.*, 62, 466, September 2013; Hegedus, E.J. et al., *Br. J. Sports Med.*, 46, 964, 2012; Lareau, C.R. et al., *J. Am. Acad. Orthop. Surg.*, 22, 372, June 2014; Ostrowski, J.A., *J. Athl. Train.*, 41, 120, 2006.

17.4 LABS/RADS AND THE DIFFERENTIAL DIAGNOSIS

Once the history and physical are complete, the diagnosis (or victim) should be apparent within a relatively limited differential diagnosis. Radiology studies and laboratory analysis are then used to corroborate the diagnosis or pinpoint the diagnosis within the differential. It is essential that radiological studies be used to confirm a suspected diagnosis rather than as a substitute for an adequate history and physical exam. Magnetic resonance imaging (MRI) offers amazing tissue resolution, but cannot take the place of history and physical exam. An incredibly high number of normal, pain-free adults have pathologic findings on MRI, making reliance on MRI alone exceptionally high risk for unnecessary procedures and iatrogenic complications. Additionally, there are many diagnoses that do not show up well (or at all) on MRI (i.e., iliotibial band syndrome). Just getting an MRI and then treating those findings is not good medicine. A better choice is to read this book, take a careful history, learn proper physical exam techniques, and use radiology and laboratory studies to confirm your suspicions when indicated with imaging.

17.5 MAKING A "PATHOANATOMIC" DIAGNOSIS

The anatomic victim and its pathology should be identified in the diagnosis. Diagnoses such as runner's knee, shin splints, or ankle sprain should be avoided as they only describe a region of pain or dysfunction, not the underlying pathologic part or process. Diagnoses such as patellar tendinopathy, anterior exertional compartment syndrome, or grade II anterior talofibular ligament sprain are preferred because they describe the underlying pathologic process and a precise location.

Now that the anatomic victim has been identified, the final step in a "pathoanatomic" diagnosis is identifying the underlying pathologic process along the kinetic chain of injury. The pathoanatomic diagnoses listed in the preceding text (i.e., patellar tendinopathy) are correct in their anatomic location of the injury, but they offer little insight into the true culprit's identity. The adept sports medicine physician must be able to recognize the anatomic injury, and in the case of overuse injuries, identify the underlying and often subclinical pathologic processes that lead to the injury along the entire kinetic chain. This investigation and the correction of the pathologic chain is typically an advanced and difficult task, even for experienced sports medicine physicians.

17.6 FINDING THE CULPRIT: "WHO DONE IT?"

In the setting of acute trauma, the culprit is easy to apprehend. The patient was doing fine until an acute traumatic episode occurred; for example, they fell on an out stretched hand, smashed their finger with a hammer, or hit their leg against a soccer goal. But in the case of an overuse injury, the underlying pathologic process is more difficult to unravel because the mechanism of injury may be less clear, and the symptoms of injury are more vague. Overuse injuries often result from cumulative subclinical trauma, or they might result from an acute event that would not have caused injury if not for a background of chronic dysfunction. Complicating the issue further is that for most common victims, there are multiple potential culprits.

Potential culprits in overuse injuries can be placed into two groups, intrinsic and extrinsic factors. Intrinsic factors include factors inherent in the athlete themselves, including any biomechanical or structural anomalies. One example of an intrinsic abnormality would be a leg length discrepancy, which can alter dynamic pelvic stabilization and lead to an overuse injury in the lower kinetic chain. On the other hand, extrinsic factors are external to the athlete. These include improper training, ill-fitting equipment, and ill-advised changes in training regimen (too much, too heavy, too soon, too fast). Extrinsic factors are the most common and most easily correctable etiologies of overuse injuries.

Clinical Pearl

Extrinsic risk factors like equipment or training errors are common and the most easily correctible "culprits" for musculoskeletal injury.

When searching for the culprit of a particular injury, the net should be cast broadly. Consider both intrinsic and extrinsic factors, especially those that are subclinical, like previous surgeries and current/previous training patterns. The physical exam should include the function of at least the joints proximal and distal to the painful region and often may include the entire kinetic chain. Complex athletic movements are rarely isolated to a single joint, and an evaluation of all of the "moving parts" should be undertaken to ensure that all areas of dysfunction are identified. Just as in real life, your musculoskeletal detective work may uncover more than one culprit! To start you on the path to being a super sleuth, Table 17.3 contains a list of "usual suspects": typical intrinsic and extrinsic culprits for common sports conditions.

17.7 TREATING THE VICTIM: WHAT'S WRONG WITH THAT?

Identifying and treating the right culprit(s) is critical to establishing the optimal treatment plan to return the injured athlete to sport. Imagine a patient showing up at your emergency room having been shot in the leg by an angry neighbor. You would of course treat the injured victim by cleaning and

TABLE 17.3
Usual Suspects: Common Victims and Culprits for Common Injuries

Victim	Intrinsic Factors	Extrinsic Factors
Plantar fasciitis	Tight heel chords, pes planus/cavus, weak foot and calf muscles	Training error, improper footwear
Achilles tendinopathy	Weak gastrocnemius/soleus, pronation errors	Training error, excessive hill running, fluoroquinolone antibiotic use, improper footwear
Patellofemoral pain syndrome	Weak quad/core muscles, tight quads/hamstrings/hip flexors, pes cavus/planus, musculoskeletal malalignment, obesity	Training error, improper footwear
Trochanteric pain syndrome (bursitis)	Weak core musculature, tight tensor fasciae latae	Training error, improper footwear
Rotator cuff syndrome	Rotator cuff weakness,[a] core muscle weakness, quadriceps weakness, glenohumeral internal rotation deficit, poor throwing mechanics, subacromial bone spurs	Training errors

[a] Notice that for rotator cuff syndrome the victim is the rotator cuff and the most common culprit is rotator cuff weakness. When both victim and culprit are the same, this is musculoskeletal (MSK) suicide!

bandaging the wound. But would you discharge the person from the ER without making sure that the offending neighbor had also been "treated" (apprehended!) by the police? Of course not! But all too often injured athletes receive care directed only at their symptomatic victim injury, while the offending culprit behind the injury goes completely unrecognized and untreated. This mistake of treating only the injured victim is the most common treatment error made by primary care physicians in treating musculoskeletal injuries. Victim-based treatment alone will lead to a cycle of repeated treatment failure and repeat injury as the same old culprit (or maybe new culprits from detraining and disuse) repeatedly stresses the victimized tissue. Using a pathoanatomic diagnosis and a rehabilitation plan allows the savvy sports medicine physician to not only heal victimized tissues but also correct underlying pathologic culprits and successfully, safely, and succinctly return the athlete to practice and play.

Clinical Pearl

Only treating the injured "victim" and ignoring the underlying "culprit" is the most common treatment error made by primary care physicians caring for musculoskeletal injuries.

The concept of victims and culprits can even be helpful in recovering from acute injuries if we change the paradigm slightly. For acute injuries, the primary offending culprit is usually easy to identify: the hammer that struck the thumb, the 260 lb lineman who hit the knee, the bucking bronco that threw the cowboy, and the ground that eventually caught his shoulder. And while these primary culprits are certainly real and often entertaining, identifying them may or may not significantly improve our patient's chances of returning safely to sport. Instead, the savvy sports medicine practitioner will address the secondary culprits or "culprits for reinjury" in acutely injured athletes. Acute injuries invariably lead to decreases in strength, range of motion, and proprioception (i.e., balance or sense of position in space). Any of these deficits will increase the athlete's risk for reinjury when they return to play, so it behooves both patient and physician to address these culprits for reinjury in the rehabilitation plan.

17.8 PUTTING IT ALL TOGETHER

Let's walk through a case to put the concepts from this chapter together. Consider the case of David, a 39-year-old recreational runner with 6 weeks of right greater than left heel pain. His pain started to bother him occasionally after long runs and on his first couple steps in the morning. It has progressed slowly over the past couple of weeks to being nearly constant with any walking or running activity, but excruciating with the first step in the morning, or the first steps of running. He has had to stop running because he was limping so badly that his knee began to bother him. He has no past surgical or past medical history and takes no prescription medications. Before coming to see you, he tried not running for 10 days, purchasing new running shoes, taking enough ibuprofen to give an elephant an ulcer, self-applied kinesiology tape, and he even bought cushioned heel pads with bioelectromagnetical healing properties. None of these has helped his pain, which he describes as being a dull toothache-like pain at rest, and then becoming more sharp when he steps on the heel. His pain began as he began to ramp up training for his first marathon.

Our differential diagnosis would include plantar fasciitis, Achilles tendinopathy, stress fracture, and nerve entrapment. On physical exam:

Inspection—Normal appearing heel without erythema, swelling, or deformity.
Palpation—Maximum tender to palpation over the plantar aspect of the medial calcaneal tubercle. No tenderness to palpation along the Achilles body, Achilles insertion, base of the fifth metatarsal, lateral/medial calcaneus, or lateral/medial ankle.
Range of motion—Full active range of motion without any exacerbation of pain; however, the patient does lack 15 degrees of dorsiflexion at the ankles bilaterally to passive motion.
Strength—Foot and ankle strength 5/5 and equal bilaterally.
Neurovascular—Intact sensation to light touch throughout with 2+ dorsalis pedis and posterior tibial pulses bilaterally.
Special tests—Thompson squeeze, anterior drawer, talar tilt, and Tinnel's test of the tarsal tunnel are all negative.

Since this is a chronic, overuse injury, further lab testing or radiographs are not indicated at this time.

Based on our differential and confirmed by physical exam, we would diagnose this patient with plantar fasciitis, which is what they patient thought he had. So why is he not getting better despite all his attempts at self-treatment?

Notice that most of the treatments tried by the patient (rest, NSAIDs, heel pads) are victim based: they attempt to address and heal the injured victim, the plantar fascia in this case. But we know this is insufficient. To properly treat plantar fasciitis, we need to find and address the culprits in addition to bandaging the victim. A quick glance at Table 17.3 indicates that common intrinsic culprits for plantar fasciitis include tight heel cords, weakness of foot/calf musculature, and pes planus/cavus, while common extrinsic factors include training error and improper shoe wear. Reexamining our history and physical examination, we see that the symptoms started while training for a marathon, which makes training error a very likely culprit. Similarly, we see on physical exam that the patient did have tight heel cords with deficits in ankle dorsiflexion.

Armed with this information, we can devise the following pathoanatomical treatment plan:

1. Stop running for now. It's not always necessary to stop running completely for plantar fascia pain, but when your gait is altered by pain, you're causing more problems by continuing to run. David should be able to bike, swim, or even elliptical without increasing his plantar fascia pain, and he can continue to train for his marathon using these modalities.[6]
2. David can continue any victim-oriented treatments he finds useful. I'd recommend ice and plantar fascia stretching, especially before getting out of bed in the morning.
3. Begin Achilles stretches (gastrocnemius and soleus) and plantar fascia stretches immediately.[6,7]
4. Consider towel drag exercises or other similar exercises to strengthen foot and calf intrinsic muscles.
5. As pain subsides over next 4–6 weeks, educate patient on proper return to running program and proper run training. In general, patients should increase their volume of running no more than 10% per week, with rest days in between running days.[7]

17.9 CONCLUSION

Physical exam is a key component of the overall concept of a comprehensive pathoanatomical treatment plan. Following the steps outlined in this chapter will allow physicians to utilize all components of the patient examination to return their injured athletes to sport more quickly, safely, and efficaciously by focusing treatment efforts not only on injured victim tissues but also on the likely intrinsic and extrinsic culprits that underlie the patient's injuries.

Clinical Pearl

Physical exam is one key contributor to a successful, comprehensive, and pathoanatomical treatment plan.

REFERENCES

1. Bickley LS, Szilagyi PG. *Bates' Guide to Physical Examination and History Taking*. Lippincott Williams & Wilkins, Philadelphia, PA; 2003.
2. Covey CJ, Mulder MD. Plantar fasciitis: How best to treat? *Journal of Family Practice*. September 2013;62(9):466–471.
3. Hegedus EJ, Goode AP, Cook CE et al. Which physical examination tests provide clinicians with the most value when examining the shoulder? Update of a systematic review with meta-analysis of individual tests. *British Journal of Sports Medicine*. 2012;46(14):964–978.
4. Lareau CR, Sawyer GA, Wang JH, DiGiovanni CW. Plantar and medial heel pain: diagnosis and management. *Journal of American Academy of Orthopaedic Surgery*. June 2014;22(6):372–380.
5. Ostrowski JA. Accuracy of 3 diagnostic tests for anterior cruciate ligament tears. *Journal of Athletic Training*. 2006;41(1):120–121.
6. Schmidt HG, Rikers RMJP. How expertise develops in medicine: Knowledge encapsulation and illness script formation. *Medical Education*. 2007;41:1133–1139.
7. Schwieterman B, Haas D, Columber K, Knupp D, Cook C. Diagnostic accuracy of physical examination tests of the ankle/foot complex: A systematic review. *International Journal of Sports Physical Therapy*. 2013;8(4):416–426.

18 Sports Medicine Radiology for the Primary Care Provider

Leslie H. Rassner, R. Kent Sanders, and Ulrich A. Rassner

CONTENTS

TABLE 18.1
Key Clinical Considerations

1. Sports medicine imaging should answer a diagnostic question and influence medical management.
2. Plain film radiography is the backbone of musculoskeletal (MSK) imaging and remains the initial imaging study for the majority of sports injuries.
3. CT scans are first-line imaging methods in the emergent management of moderate to severe head, spine, and abdominal injuries. CT scans are used to visualize complex fractures for preoperative planning or adjustment of treatment plan.
4. MRI is the test of choice for muscle, tendon, ligamentous, and cartilage injury as well as spine injury with neurologic deficits. MRI can define the location and extent of bone stress injuries and stress fractures.
5. Nuclear medicine scans can be used with great sensitivity to detect osteomyelitis, stress fractures, or avascular necrosis, but lack specificity to distinguish between bone turnover processes.
6. In the hands of a skilled provider, ultrasound may offer immediate office evaluation for MSK injuries as well as targeted in-office MSK injections.
7. Health-care providers should inform patients about radiation risks and ensure exposure is as low as reasonably achievable without sacrificing quality of care.
8. The most targeted radiologic exam can be performed when a diagnostic question and pertinent history are communicated to the radiologist.

18.1 INTRODUCTION

This chapter focuses on a division of musculoskeletal (MSK) imaging—radiology specifically for sports medicine providers. Before utilizing sports medicine imaging, the provider should combine knowledge of anatomy, clinical history, and physical exam to arrive at a specific diagnostic question. Ideally, radiologic imaging should confirm the provider's pathoanatomic diagnosis and influence medical management.[8] With the advances in imaging, real but distracting normal incidental developmental variants and asymptomatic degenerative changes can be detected.[24] Therefore, a radiologic search should be focused to ensure that imaging results will be relevant[8] (Table 18.1).

Communicating the diagnostic question and pertinent history to the radiologist is critical for imaging protocol selection and focusing the radiologic report. Modalities such as computed tomography (CT) and magnetic resonance imaging (MRI) may require IV or intra-articular contrast, joint-specific coils, and selection of specific sequences and planes of imaging. The most specific study might not be performed when key pieces of clinical information are not communicated. For example, an MRI of the entire foot for "foot pain" will generally lack the resolution to adequately diagnose a plantar plate injury that a targeted small field of view study of the forefoot or single metatarsophalangeal (MTP) joint could evaluate. The targeted study would only be performed if the *specific* clinical question regarding a particular injury were shared *prior to the scheduling and protocoling of the study.* In this example, the targeted exam would require not only a specific protocol but also a specific coil type and probably be performed on the highest field strength magnet available. In Figure 18.1, the higher field strength and spatial resolution of a 3T MRI demonstrates a meniscal tear inadequately visualized on a 0.7T MRI of the same knee. Anatomical nomenclature, localizing descriptors, and references to anatomic position all help to enhance communication and result in the most pertinent radiologic report.

Necessary elements of the history include mechanism of injury, timing, prior surgery, hand dominance and occupation, or sport when relevant. Sports medicine providers should be cautioned that allowing ancillary staff to order imaging with vague clinical history such as "pain" degrades this essential communication and might result in wasted time, expense, delayed diagnosis, or misdiagnosis.

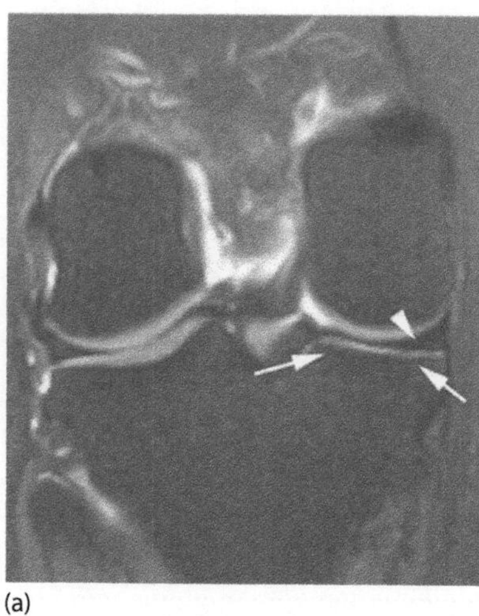
(a)

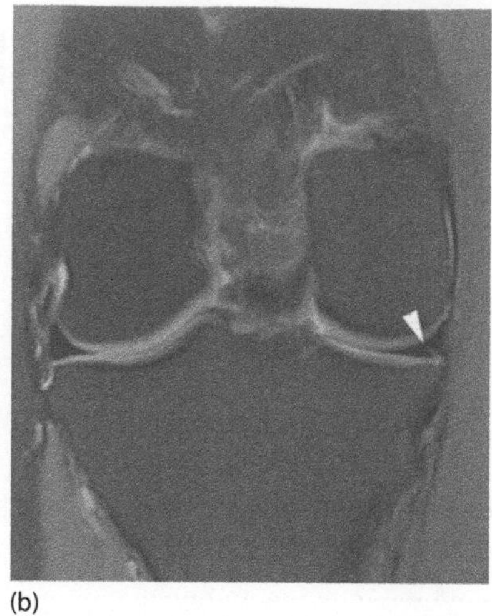
(b)

FIGURE 18.1 (a) Low field strength 0.7 Tesla (T) coronal proton density image of a right knee. Arrows indicate subtle linear truncation artifact from the bone–cartilage interface of the medial tibial plateau displaced inferiorly in the phase-encoding direction. Arrowhead shows a linear bright signal feature in the medial meniscus that appears similar to the truncation artifact. (b) 3T coronal proton density image of the same knee. Higher field strength allows for larger matrix and therefore finer spatial resolution. The truncation artifact is eliminated and an undersurface oblique meniscal tear is unequivocally demonstrated.

It is important for primary care sports medicine providers to know their surgical subspecialists. Obtaining the x-ray views and advanced imaging studies the specialists use avoids repeat imaging costs and potential radiation exposure. When possible, order imaging where specialists have electronic access to images or make certain patients know to bring CDs to specialty consultation appointments.

Remember that other biological processes, such as infection, tumor, and metabolic and rheumatologic/autoimmune disease, are commonly encountered on imaging and may clinically mimic sports injuries' physical presentations (Figure 18.2). Sports medicine providers are legally responsible to local radiology standard of care when reading and billing for in-office radiograph interpretation. In urban settings, the liability for such interpretations is higher as this would be equivalent to an MSK fellowship-trained radiologist.

18.2 IMAGING MODALITY OVERVIEW

18.2.1 Radiography

The term "x-ray" defines both images (radiographs) and the high-energy electromagnetic photons used to produce them. When x-rays pass through a patient, they are attenuated in different amounts depending on the linear attenuation coefficient (related to density) of the tissues they pass through. A film cassette or digital detector measures the x-rays exiting the patient, generating a negative. Denser tissues block more x-rays and therefore appear lighter on the image. Thus on radiographs, bone is white; fat, muscle, and joint effusions are varying shades of gray; while air is black.

Radiography is the backbone of MSK imaging and remains the initial imaging study for the majority of sports injuries.[8] The capabilities of plain radiographs are wide-ranging but heavily predicate on standard positioning, appropriate exposure, and image quality. Common well-visualized osseous pathology includes fracture, osteoarthritic changes, and joint space loss. Visible soft tissue pathology includes effusions, infection, some tumors, and radio-opaque foreign body implantation. Radiographs can be highly specific. Stress views allow the demonstration or exclusion of mechanical instability from ligamentous injury, shown in Figure 18.3.

Radiography is a first-line imaging technique because of its cost to diagnostic value and wide availability. A negative study might not exclude injury, but a positive one may be the end of the evaluation and thus minimize cost. In the setting of trauma, radiographs allow for cost-effective screening of the joint above and below the area of concern. When initial radiographs are normal but suspicion for nondisplaced fracture remains high, a patient may be treated as injured and repeat imaging performed in 7–10 days can look for periosteal reaction or a clear fracture line and/or fracture displacement (Figure 18.4).[8] In an outpatient setting, radiographs may be easily obtained without prior insurance authorization and in some cases may be required before an insurance company will authorize advanced imaging such as CT and MRI.

Radiography comes with few limitations and patient restrictions. Fractures may only be seen if they are in the plane, or direction, of the x-ray beam. Two views are required at a minimum and multiple views may be required to adequately assess for injury. The primary restrictions occur in pregnancy, with shielding of the abdomen recommended when possible. Pregnant patients considered for radiographs should be evaluated for risk versus benefit of the study. Risk varies inversely to maturation of the pregnancy, with the highest risk being in the first trimester. With appropriate shielding, extremity

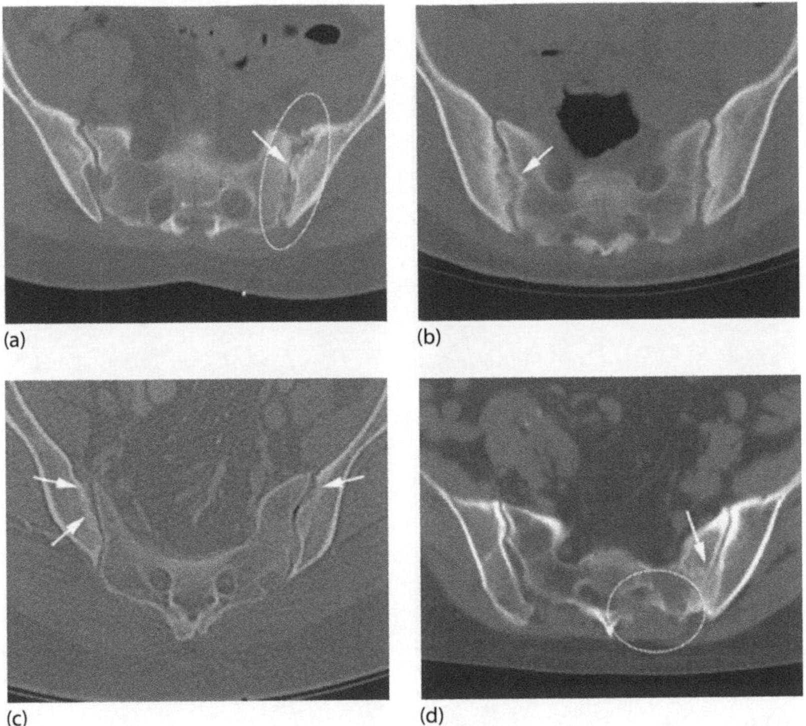

FIGURE 18.2 Axial CT images through the superior SI joints showing pathologies with similar appearances. (a) Unilateral left staphylococcus septic arthropathy (oval) with nonuniform sacral and iliac side bone destruction and severe narrowing of the remaining joint space (arrow). (b) Bilateral mildly asymmetrical ankylosing spondylitis–related erosive sacroiliitis. More extensive disease on the right includes sacral erosions (arrow). (c) Bilateral asymmetrical iliac-sided subarticular resorption (arrows) in renal osteodystrophy/secondary hyperparathyroidism. (d) Focal reactive sclerosis and SI joint ankylosis (arrow) in response to indolent lytic chordoma (oval) destroying the left sacrum.

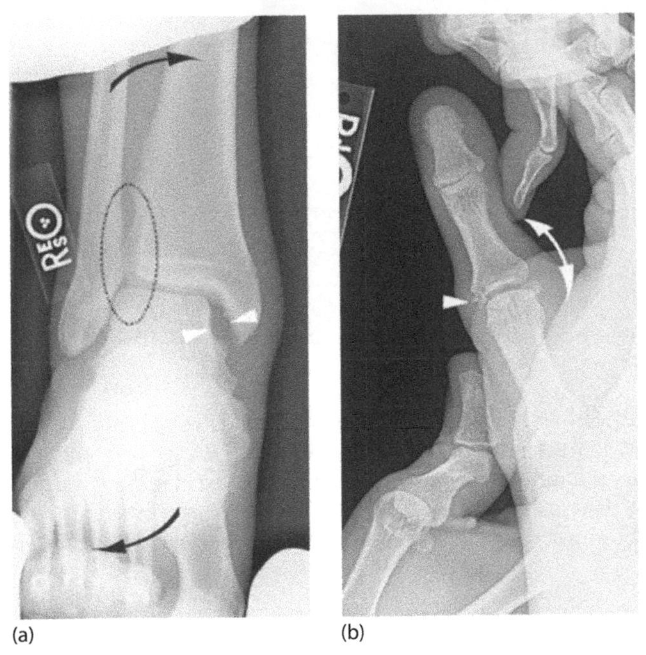

FIGURE 18.3 (a) Valgus stress view of a right ankle with abnormal widening of the medial mortise gutter (white arrowheads) and tibiofibular syndesmosis (oval) confirming deltoid and tibiofibular ligament injuries, respectively. Curved black arrows indicate direction of applied stress. (b) Reverse gamekeeper's fracture at the first phalangeal insertion of the radial collateral ligament (arrowhead). Tensile stress (curved double-headed arrow) is applied to the more critical ulnar collateral ligament that is found to be intact.

radiology carries a negligible radiation risk. For torso imaging, alternate imaging such as MRI or ultrasound may be considered where clinically relevant.

18.2.2 Computed Tomography

CT scans utilize x-rays sent through the patient to a detector while the x-ray tube and detector rotate around the patient. As a result, CT scans collect data from many hundreds of positions to form a reconstructed cross-sectional image. Advancements have led to faster, more efficient scanning, with less radiation exposure.[8] Still CT radiation doses remain higher than radiography for the same body part.

In sports injuries, the utility of CT comes from its wide availability, and capability to visualize complex anatomy, bone, and hemorrhage well. CT scans are first-line imaging methods in the emergent management of acute head and spine injuries, with ER protocols skipping cervical spine (C-spine) plain films in cases of severe trauma.[3,12] In sports injuries resulting from blunt abdominal trauma, body CT may be indicated to look for internal organ injury. CT is capable of revealing fine bony structure due to the high contrast of bone. Three-dimensional computer reconstructions allow definitive visualization of complex fractures critical for preoperative planning or adjustment of the treatment plan (Figure 18.5). In MSK radiology, CT scans are usually noncontrast unless there is concern for tumor or infection.

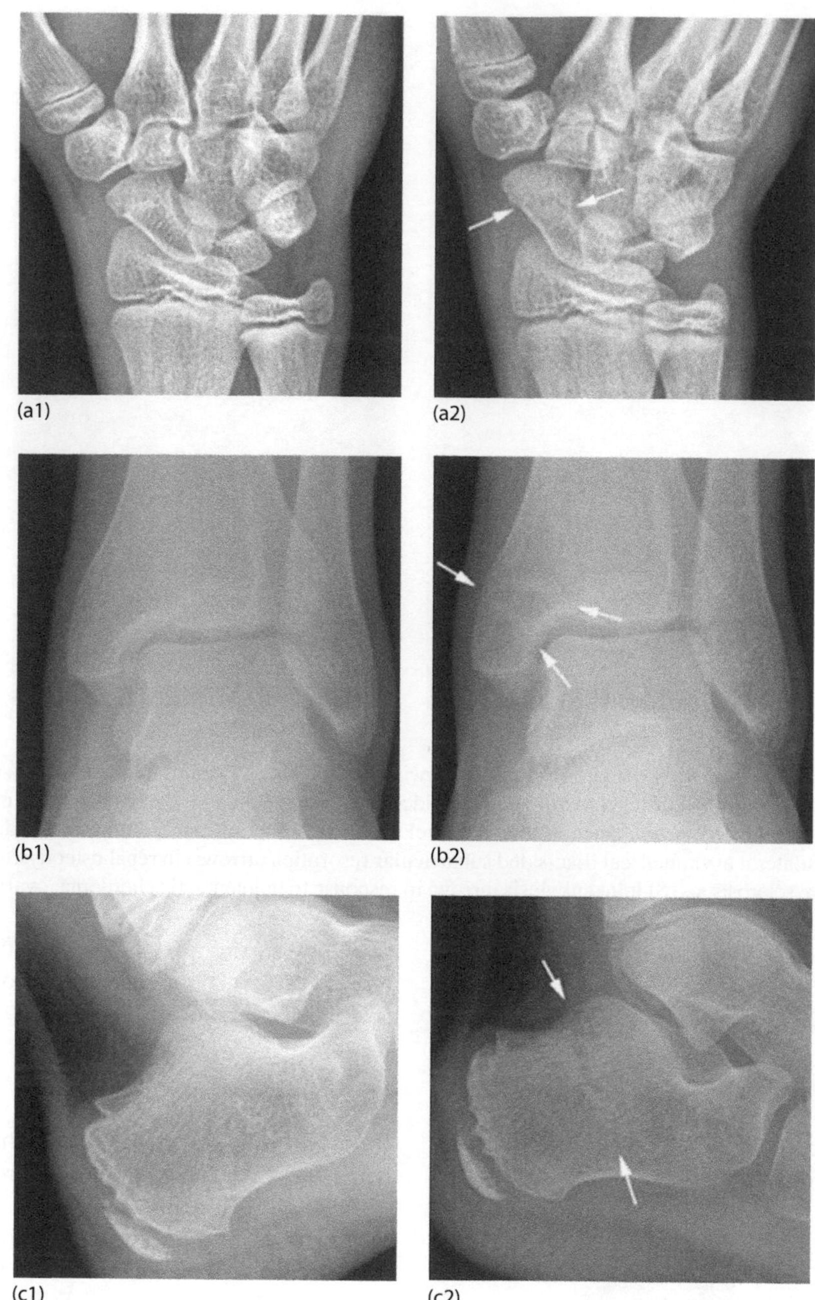

FIGURE 18.4 (1) Initial occult injuries and (2) follow-up radiographs of various fractures. (a1) 14-year-old male (YOM) with fall on an outstretched hand injury resulting in a nondisplaced oblique scaphoid waist fracture revealed as a linear lucency 9 days later during the resorptive phase of healing (arrows in a2). (b1) 22 YOM with running injury resulting in a nondisplaced transverse medial malleolus fracture revealed as transverse sclerotic bands in the delayed phase of healing 30 days later (arrows in b2). (c1) 10 YOM injured from unspecified fall. Nondisplaced calcaneal fracture revealed as a coronal linear lucency with surrounding sclerosis in the intermediate phase of healing 14 days later (arrows in c2).

CT scans come with several limitations. Artifacts caused by motion and metal can obscure pathology. CT scans have good spatial resolution (ability to depict small anatomic detail) but are inferior to MRI in soft tissue contrast (distinction of different soft tissue structures). For example, ligamentous injury is often difficult to diagnose on CT due to the low intrinsic contrast (differential absorption) of unenhanced soft tissue. CT comes with the risks of ionizing radiation, with doses higher than for plain films. As with radiography, pregnant patients considered for CT scanning should be evaluated for risk versus benefit of the study. For central imaging, alternate imaging such as MRI or ultrasound may be considered where clinically relevant.

18.2.3 Magnetic Resonance Imaging

MRI technique utilizes the magnetic moment of hydrogen nuclei found abundantly throughout the body, predominantly

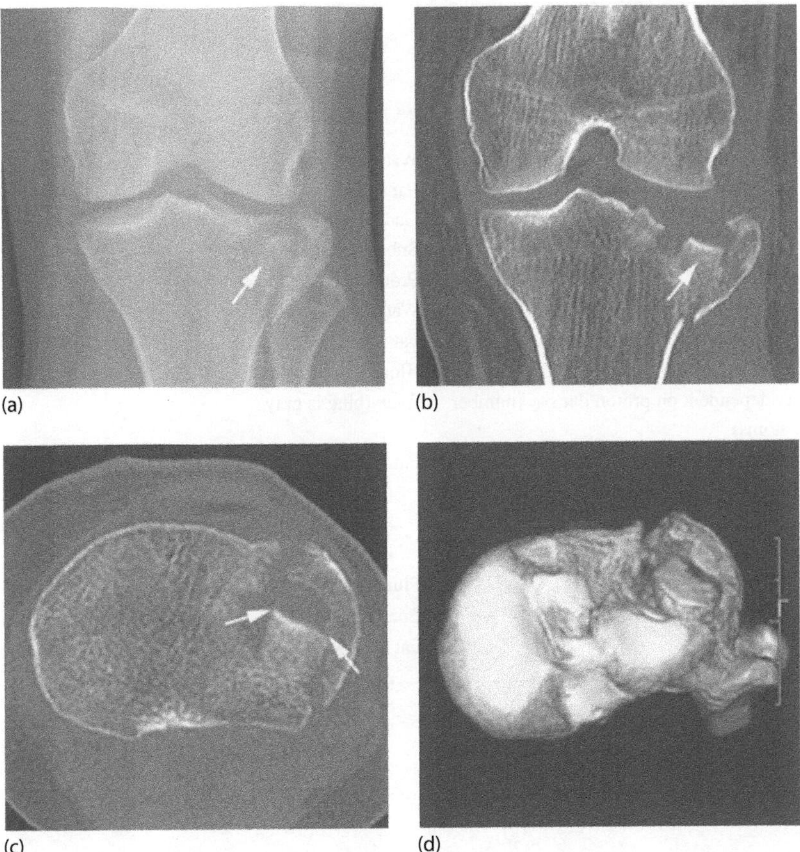

FIGURE 18.5 Lateral split/depression fracture of the tibial plateau. (a) AP radiograph makes the diagnosis while showing a depressed fragment of uncertain size and orientation. (b) Coronal CT image shows a centimeter-wide depressed fragment that appears oriented correctly to the cartilage side up. (c) Axial CT image shows a coronal–oblique cross section of the depressed fragment subchondral plate indicating obliquity. The injury is proved to be restricted to the lateral compartment. (d) The surface-volume rendering with the femur removed gives a virtual operative view of the joint, best depicting the 3D orientation of the depressed fragment as well as the degree of articular destruction of the anterior two-thirds of the lateral plateau.

in water and fat. When a patient is placed in the scanner's strong magnetic field, the patient becomes magnetized in the direction of the scanner field. Radio-frequency waves (radio waves) are sent into the patient and interact with hydrogen atoms, which turns the magnetization of the patient 90°. The decay and recovery of magnetization as well as the proton density can be measured via sequencing protocols (Table 18.2) to produce computer-generated cross-sectional images (Figure 18.6). The most commonly used MRI contrast agents are gadolinium based and make areas where contrast goes brighter on T1-weighted images. Thus, gadolinium-based IV contrast brightens the blood vessels and vascularized tissues, while arthrographic contrast brightens the joint space. In order to detect the magnetization of tissues and form MR images, coils for specific body parts are used. The use of optimized coils for specific body parts maximizes spatial resolution and signal-to-noise ratio, producing the highest image quality, as demonstrated in Figure 18.7.

MRI has revolutionized sports injury diagnosis and treatment. MRI has assumed a dominant role in imaging every major joint in the body.[8] Superior soft tissue characterization makes MRI the test of choice for muscle, tendon, ligamentous, and cartilage injury, as well as spine injury with neurologic deficits.[8] Contrasted MRI is used almost exclusively for the evaluation of tumors and infection, both in and out of the bone. MRI is exquisitely sensitivity to bone edema and trabecular microfracture, making it superior for the diagnosis of nondisplaced fractures, stress or insufficiency fractures, and stress reactions. Additionally, MRI comes with the great advantage of not using ionizing radiation.

The limitations of MRI include limited availability, cost, artifacts from motion and metal, and restrictions with certain implants. Patients may have difficulty in tolerating an MRI due to claustrophobia or prolonged imaging times of typically 20–45 minutes per body part.

Some MSK findings are highly dependent on MRI field strength, protocol, surface coils, and radiologist interpretation. Not all imaging centers may have a complete assortment of specialized joint coils, scanners above 1.5 T magnet strength, or MSK fellowship-trained radiologist staff. As a general rule, the smaller the structure being investigated, the more important the spatial resolution and signal-to-noise performance of the magnet and the receiver coil is in detecting the abnormality. Doubling of the magnet strength from 1.5T to 3.0T results in theory in a twofold increase in signal-to-noise performance. In reality, the signal-to-noise benefit will be less due to the

TABLE 18.2
MRI Sequences

Sequence	Descriptions	Tissue Brightness	Unique Clinical Features
T1	Signal dependent on differences in the recovery of longitudinal magnetization	Water is dark. Fat is bright. Gadolinium enhancement is bright. Subacute blood is bright. Proteinaceous fluid can be bright.	Normal fatty adult bone marrow is bright. Fractures and marrow replacement are dark.
T2	Signal dependent on the decay of transverse magnetization	Water is bright. Fat is bright. Blood can be bright or dark.	Many pathologies have edema and are bright on T2.
Proton density	Signal intensity dependent on proton density (number of hydrogen atoms)	Everything is gray.	
Fat saturation	Suppression of fat signal utilizing resonance frequency differences between fat and water.	Fat is dark.	Can be applied to any image sequence. Commonly used with gadolinium-enhanced T1-weighted images. Sensitive to field distortion (metal).
STIR		Fluid is bright. Edema is bright. Fat is dark.	Exquisitely sensitive to fluid/edema. Not as sensitive to field distortions. Not specific for fat.

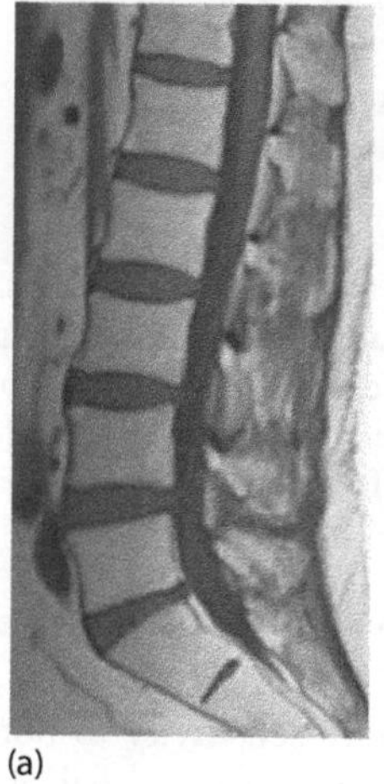
(a)

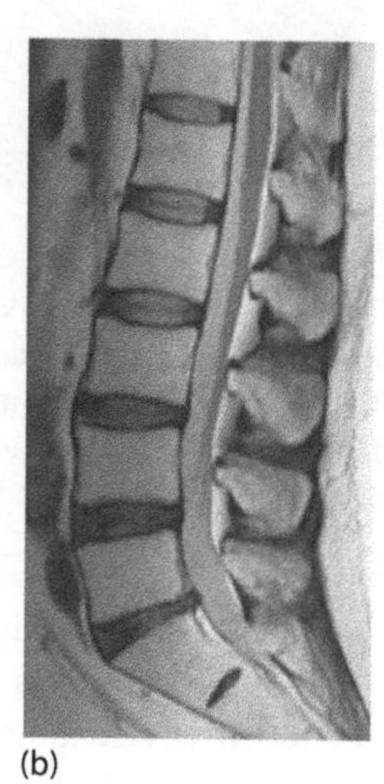
(b)

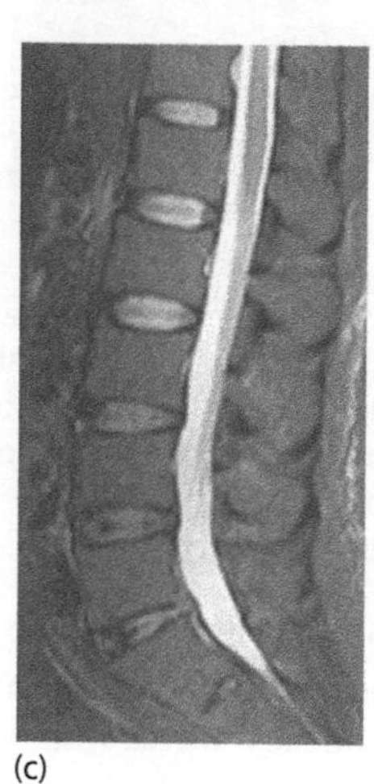
(c)

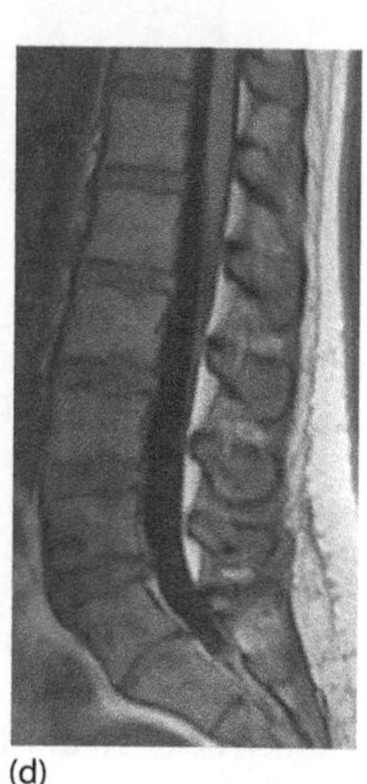
(d)

FIGURE 18.6 Typical noncontrast MR sequences for spine imaging represented here with a lumbar spine study of the same individual with fatty bone marrow in images (a–c) and a different individual with red marrow reconversion in D. (a) Fast spin echo (FSE) T1 without fat saturation: fatty marrow, epidural fat, and subcutaneous fat are bright, while CSF is darker than spinal cord and discs. (b) FSE T2 without fat saturation: fat remains bright and bright CSF nicely outlines the spinal cord and cauda equina. There is increased disc signal revealing internal anatomy of the nucleus pulposus and annular ligaments. (c) Short tau inversion recovery (STIR): a very fluid-sensitive sequence where fat is dark and CSF is very bright. The difference in fluid signal intensity between the superior three and the inferior three discs signals early disc degeneration with alteration of the glycosaminoglycan chemistry of the latter. (d) T1 inversion recovery without fat saturation: has the advantage over T1-FSE in that fluid signal is much darker making the chord and caudal equina more visible. The marrow signal is darker than in A from increased myeloid tissue that, since it contains microscopic fat, is still brighter than the disc or muscle.

effects of electronic noise and other sequence parameters, such as receiver bandwidth and various acceleration techniques. Additionally, with the use of surface coils, the signal strength will depend on the distance of the tissue from the coil. Coil designs that fit closely to the appendage or joint and have multiple channels/detectors result in the highest-resolution images. For most MSK studies, a 3T magnet with appropriate surface coil yields superior results to 1.5T. With large field of view imaging, such as lumbar and thoracic spine or whole pelvis imaging, the resolution advantage may not be as apparent and, for most types of cases involving larger body parts, not diagnostically significant. The amount of signal loss and image distortion from retained metal/hardware does double with doubling of the field strength. Therefore, if hardware is in close proximity to the structure of interest, imaging at 1.5T or less is recommended. Newer titanium alloy hardware generates far less artifact than older stainless steel, cobalt, or chrome alloys. Additionally, with various metal artifact suppression

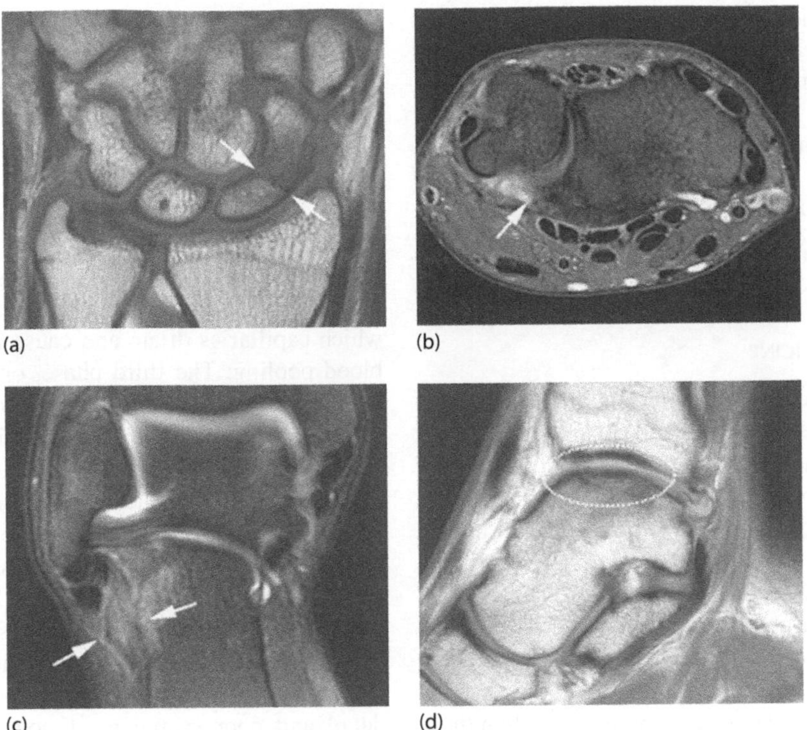

FIGURE 18.7 (a) 3T coronal T1 without fat saturation of the wrist showing a nondisplaced and radiographically occult scaphoid waist fracture (arrows). (b) 3T axial proton density with fat saturation of the wrist showing volar distal radial ulnar ligament tear (arrow). (c) 3T coronal T2 with fat saturation of the ankle showing calcaneal insertion calcaneofibular ligament tear (arrows). (d) 3T sagittal proton density without fat saturation of the ankle showing impacted talar dome osteochondral fracture (oval).

techniques, structures located from 0.5 to 1 cm are routinely resolved. As the amount of artifact will vary from each magnet and coil combination as well as with each individual piece of hardware, it is advisable to attempt MRI 1.5T before concluding that MRI cannot be performed (Figure 18.8).

MRI's strong magnetic field, gradient fields, and radiofrequency pulses can all interact with medical devices and ferromagnetic materials. Certain medical devices may malfunction and consequently have scan restrictions or may be contraindicated. The majority of pacemakers are rated unsafe for MRI; however, several newer devices are approved for MRI. Artificial cardiac valves usually can be scanned in 1.5 T MRI, but 3.0 T or greater MRI requires clearance by radiologist. Currently, all vascular stents are MRI safe; nevertheless, some stents have scan restrictions. Metal foreign bodies, body piercings, and jewelry can migrate, heat up, or torque. Tattoos and cosmetics containing metallic dyes can heat up or smear at edges if recently placed. The ordering clinician

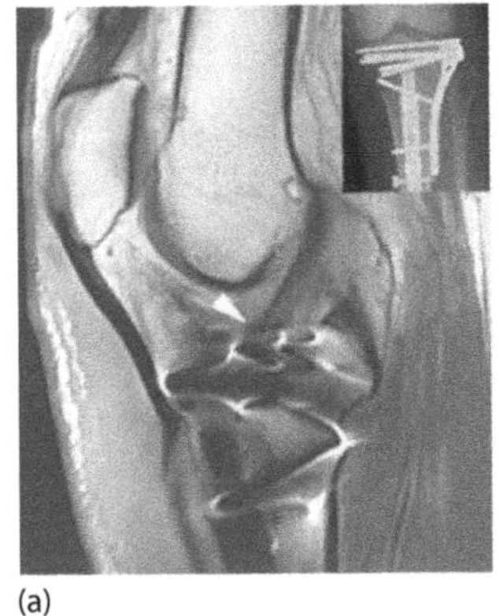

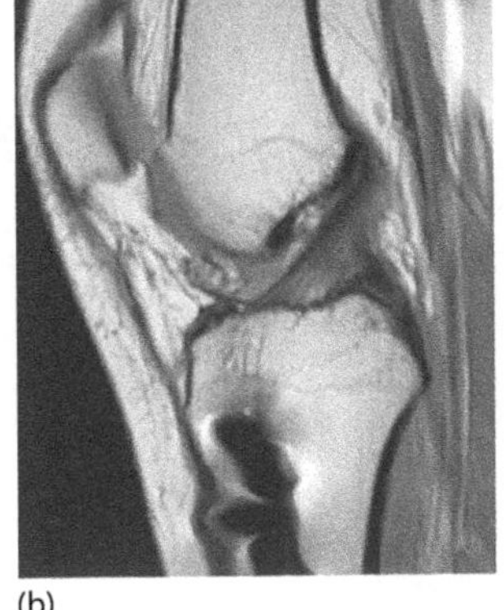

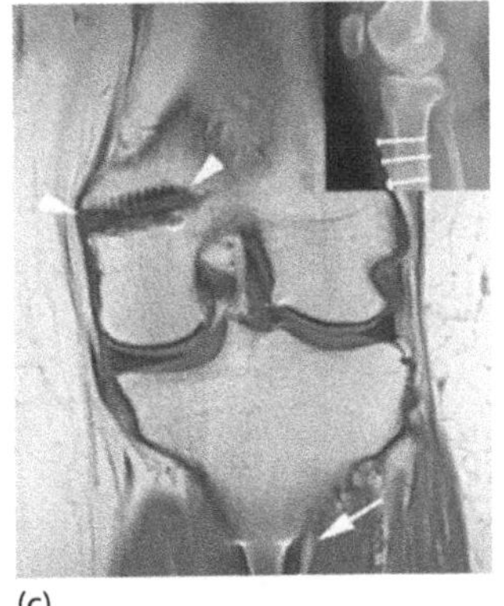

FIGURE 18.8 (a) 1.5T sagittal proton density without fat saturation of knee with intramedullary (IM) nail and lateral plate with subarticular screws (see inset) where metal artifact obscures the tibial plateau and meniscus. The ACL insertion remains visible however (arrowhead). (b) 1.5T sagittal proton density of knee with IM nail only. The tibial plateau and menisci are not obscured. (c) 3T coronal T1 without fat saturation of knee with bioabsorbable anchor in the medial femoral epicondyle (arrowheads) and anterior tibial screws (arrow at the bottom, inset). Joint visualization is unaffected.

and patient should provide as much information as possible about any medical devices and ferromagnetic materials, and the radiologist will ultimately determine if a scan can be performed safely.

MRI can be performed in any trimester of pregnancy; however, contrast is not routinely given due to the potential negative effects of gadolinium (a heavy metal) crossing the placenta, entering the fetal circulation, and affecting fetal development.

18.2.4 Nuclear Medicine

In nuclear medicine, radioactive materials are either given alone or linked to a molecule or cell and accumulate in areas of biological activity. Radioactivity emitted from the sites of biological activity can be measured with a gamma camera producing a 2D image from a certain projection (akin to a radiograph) or tomographically with a single-photon emission computed tomography (SPECT) scanner, which takes measurements from many directions and can reconstruct cross-sectional images (akin to a CT scanner). Nuclear medicine imaging studies are generally more organ or tissue specific (e.g., lung scan, heart scan, bone scan, brain scan) than those in conventional imaging, which focus on a particular section of the body (e.g., head, chest, abdomen, pelvis, spine, joints).

In sports medicine radiology, the two principal nuclear medicine techniques utilized are traditional bone scan and SPECT scans. Bone scans and SPECT scans use gamma ray–emitting radiopharmaceuticals (most commonly containing technetium 99m) to display increased areas of osteoblast activity, which correspond to areas of increased bone turnover. Initial dynamic images are acquired over the area of concern and then followed afterward by static images obtained over longer periods of time. The whole body or a part, like the feet or pelvis, can be imaged in a single delayed phase (typical for whole-body bone scan for cancer metastases) or in three phases—arterial, equilibrium, and delayed (typical in stress fracture evaluation). In three-phase scans, the first phase, or flow phase, consists of serial 2–5 second images obtained during injection of the radiopharmaceutical and demonstrates perfusion to a lesion. The second phase, or the blood-pool image, is obtained within 5 minutes after injection and demonstrates relative vascularity as in areas of inflammation, in which capillaries dilate and cause increased blood flow and blood pooling. The third phase, or bone image, is obtained about 3 hours after injection and demonstrates relative bone turnover associated with a lesion (Figure 18.9).

Bone and SPECT scans can be used to detect infection or osteomyelitis, stress fractures, or ischemia or avascular necrosis. Nuclear medicine scans are very sensitive for fractures and can well differentiate between shin splint or medial tibial stress syndrome and stress fracture. Myositis ossificans is best excised when bone formation slows, making follow-up bone scan useful in timing surgical excision.

While bone scans are limited by their lack of anatomical detail and poor spatial resolution, SPECT scans overcome this limitation by their reconstruction of cross-sectional images. Thus, SPECT scans can more precisely localize the location of increased activity, such as the facet joint versus vertebral body. Further improvement in activity localization can be achieved by merging SPECT images to CT images, as demonstrated in Figure 18.10. In spine imaging, SPECT has the advantage of potentially localizing a pain source in a patient with multiple levels and areas of degenerative changes. SPECT scans are sensitive to the very earliest development of pars stress fractures in athletes.

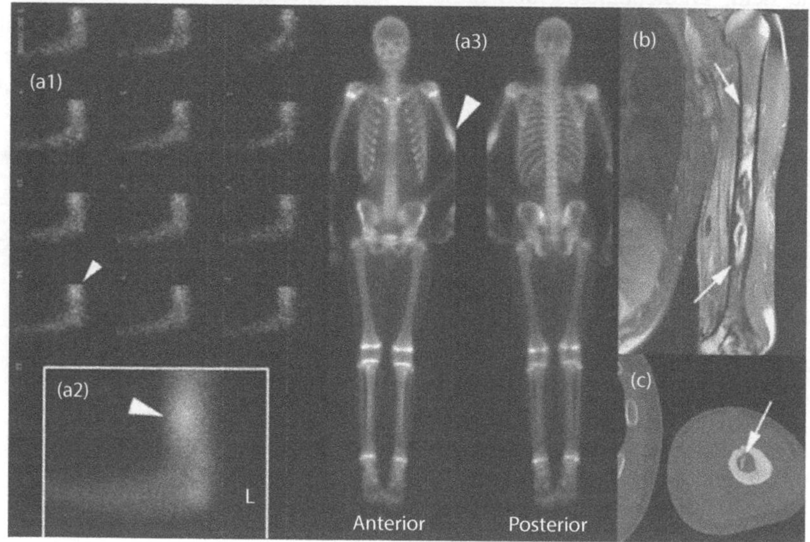

FIGURE 18.9 (a1–a3) Triple phase Tc99m methylene diphosphonate (MDP) bone scan with 5 seconds/frame infusion series of the affected left upper extremity (a1), blood pool phase in the lateral projection (a2), and the whole body delayed phase images in the anterior and posterior projection (a3). There is increased uptake in all three phases with strong localization in the left humerus (arrowheads). (b) Post-contrast T1 fat saturated MRI of the left humerus reveals a long segment Brodie's abscess (arrows). (c) Axial CT scan shows an intramedullary sequestrum (arrow).

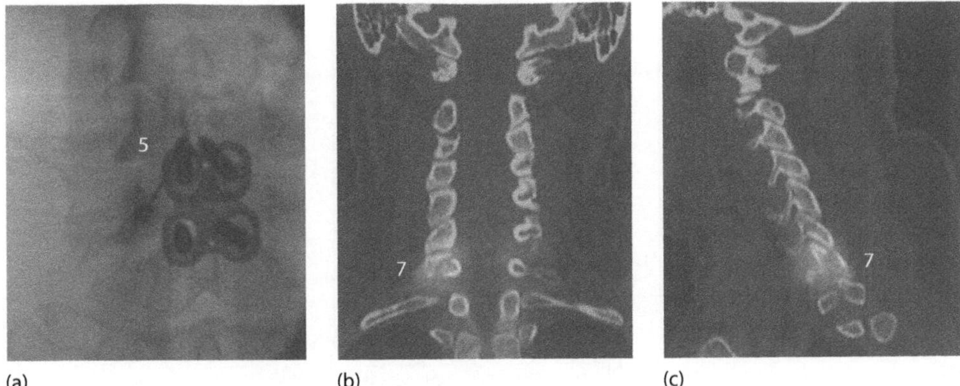

FIGURE 18.10 (a) 50 YOF with prior C6/C7 anterior cervical discectomy and fusion and neck pain that failed to respond to epidural steroid injection. (b) Coronal and (c) sagittal SPECT–CT 4 months later reveals an occult fracture of the C7 facet.

Nuclear medicine studies are limited by their expense, prolonged imaging times, and use of ionizing radiation, with radiation doses from a bone scan being similar to doses from a lumbar spine CT. Due to a lack of specificity, nuclear medicine imaging may not distinguish between bone-turnover processes, such as osteomyelitis from osteoarthritis. Nuclear imaging studies may remain positive for up to a year after clinical healing of a fracture, making them subject to potential false positives. Certain tumors with little osteoblast activity, such as multiple myeloma and lytic malignant metastasis, may not reliably be seen on bone scans. The risks versus benefits must be weighed before imaging children. Pregnant women may not undergo bone and SPECT scans, as there is no benefit worth the risk to the developing fetus.

18.2.5 Ultrasound

In medical ultrasound, sound waves are sent into the patient and reflected at interfaces of tissues with different acoustic impedance (tissue density and sound velocity). It allows real-time examination of moving structures. Spatial resolution can be high but depends on frequencies used. The higher the frequency, the higher the spatial resolution, but the shorter the depth that structures can be visualized.

Ultrasound has many capabilities including real-time dynamic evaluation of muscles and tendons, including stress views where relevant. Ultrasound can provide a focused evaluation of small joints, such as looking for synovitis of the hands and wrists. It can define masses and localize foreign bodies. For many common sports injuries, radiologic-guided injections have been shown to have superior outcomes over "blind" office injections.[27] Ultrasound is extremely safe and does not utilize ionizing radiation.

Ultrasound is heavily dependent on operator proficiency and proximity of the structure of interest to the probe.[2] Ultrasound has limited resolution for deep structures and is less effective in patients with a large body habitus. Ultrasound does not penetrate bone or air.

The initial purchase of ultrasound equipment and provider training can be expensive, but in the hands of a skilled operator, it can provide relatively inexpensive and fast on-field evaluation for MSK injury as well as targeted in-office MSK injections.

18.3 PEDIATRIC CONSIDERATIONS

Anatomic variations between children and adults result in different injuries from similar mechanisms of injury. For example, a fall on an outstretched hand (FOOSH) injury, depicted in Figure 18.11, will generally result in specific types of fractures in different age groups.

In skeletally immature children, the epiphysis is more susceptible to injury than the muscles, tendons, and ligaments.[22] The Salter–Harris classification system is the most widely used method of describing epiphyseal fractures and risk of growth arrest and angular deformity (Figure 18.12). When reviewing pediatric radiographs, subperiosteal hemorrhage at physis can be helpful in finding nondisplaced injuries (Figure 18.13).

Pediatric cortical bone is less mineralized and more fibrovascular than adult cortical bone with a thickened and less brittle periosteum. Therefore, pediatric bones bend more prior to fracturing resulting in "greenstick" fractures with incomplete separation of a diaphyseal bone on the tensile side and plastic deformity with or without cortical delamination and buckling on the compression side (Figure 18.14).

Additionally, children have a higher incidence of pure chondral injuries without fracture because rapidly growing epiphyseal bone has less robust bonding to the subchondral bone plate. Thus, any injury with normal x-rays but potential for a significant chondral injury requires advanced imaging with MRI. Children can have huge knee cartilage injuries with effusion but otherwise normal plain films, as seen in Figure 18.15.

Children heal rapidly. In 7–10 days, plain film reimaging will often confirm or exclude fractures based on the presence or absence of periosteal reaction or fracture remodeling.

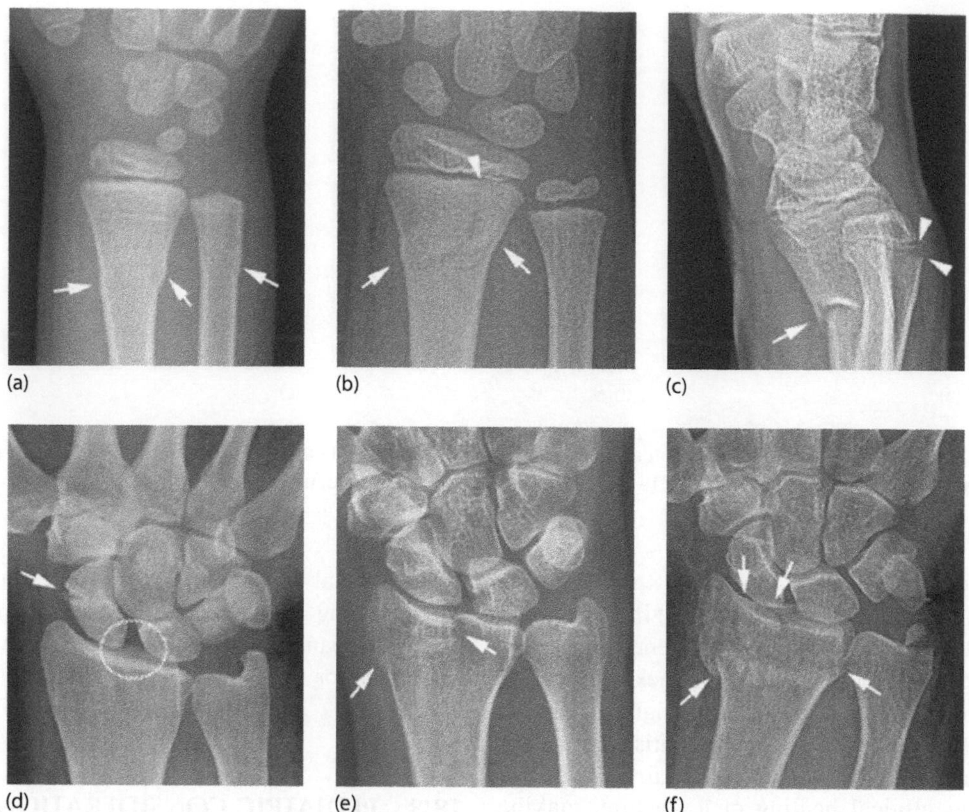

FIGURE 18.11 Changes in FOOSH fracture morphologies with aging. (a) Both-bone metadiaphyseal buckle fractures (arrows) at the age of 4. (b) Minimal cortical buckling (arrows) with oblique linear fracture (arrowhead) at the age of 8. (c) Lateral view showing an incomplete palmar transverse radial fracture (arrow) and Salter–Harris II fracture of the dorsal ulna (arrowheads) at the age of 14. (d) Minimally displaced scaphoid waist fracture (arrow) and scapholunate ligament tear and widened interval (oval) at the age of 23. (e) Minimally impacted oblique radial styloid fracture (arrows) at the age of 54. (f) Comminuted impacted intra-articular fracture (arrows) at the age of 67.

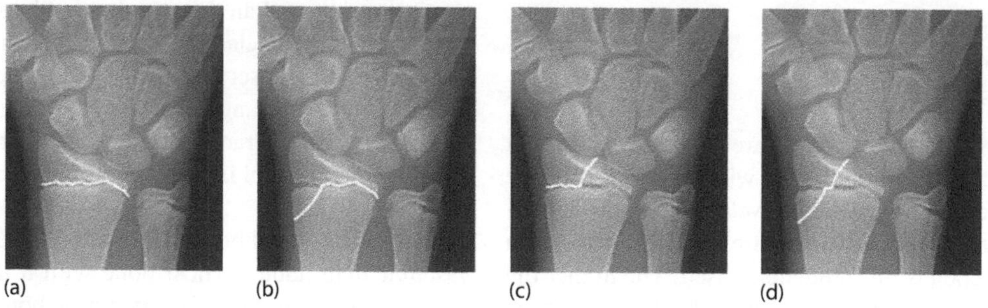

FIGURE 18.12 Salter–Harris classification applied to distal radius fractures. (a) Physeal only. (b) Physeal with metaphyseal extension. (c) Physeal with epiphyseal extension. (d) Oblique epiphyseal, transphyseal, and metaphyseal. Type V, not pictured here, is a compression fracture of the growth plate, resulting in a decrease in the perceived space between the epiphysis and diaphysis on x-ray.

Therefore, children may be splinted for presumptive injury until repeat films are obtained (Figure 18.4).

Secondary ossification centers appear in highly reliable patterns, and knowledge of their anatomy and timing of appearance is crucial for pediatric radiograph interpretation. Identifying avulsed and displaced ossification centers is extremely important, as treatment requires internal fixation. The elbow with its six ossification centers serves as a prime example (Table 18.3). An epicondylar fracture could be mistaken for a normal ossification center, or an avulsed and displaced medial epicondylar fracture could be missed (Figure 18.16). Contralateral films may be utilized for comparison.

18.4 RADIATION RISK

Ionizing radiation (x-ray and gamma ray) is composed of high-energy photons that are capable of damaging DNA

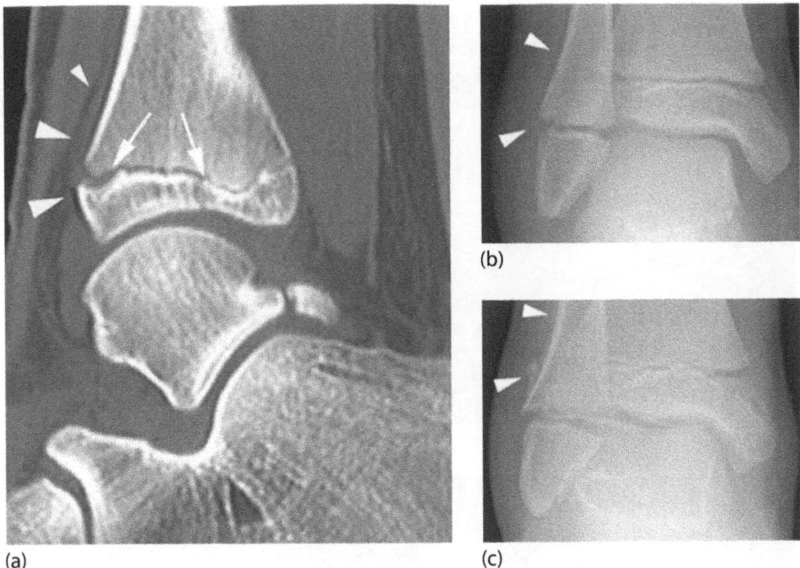

FIGURE 18.13 (a) Sagittal CT image of the ankle with Salter–Harris III fracture of the tibia (arrows) showing anterior subperiosteal hematoma and periosteal elevation (arrowheads). (b) AP ankle radiograph of different cases showing acute subperiosteal hemorrhage centered on fibular physis (arrowheads). (c) 14-day follow-up study shows periosteal new bone deposition (arrowheads).

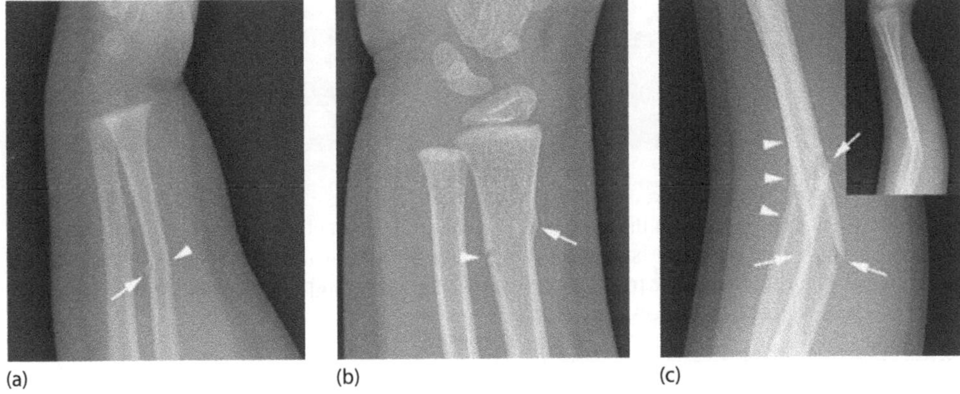

FIGURE 18.14 (a) Lateral oblique radiograph of forearm showing a diaphyseal buckle fracture of the radius with dorsal cortical delamination on the compression side (arrow) and plastic deformity on the tensile side (arrowhead) in a 1.5-year old. (b) Lateral oblique radiograph of the wrist showing metadiaphyseal buckle fracture with cortical delamination on the compression side (arrow) and cortical failure on the tensile side (arrowhead) in a 4-year old. (c) Lateral forearm radiograph (inset) showing a middiaphyseal both-bone fracture with tensile fracture of the volar cortices and bent fracture of the dorsal radius (arrows) and unfractured plastic deformity of the dorsal ulna (arrowheads) forming the greenstick deformity in an 11-year old.

and generating caustic free radicals. Experimental and epidemiological evidence has linked exposure to low-dose, ionizing radiation with the development of solid cancers and leukemia.[9] As a result, individuals at risk for repeated radiation exposure, such as healthcare and nuclear industry workers, are typically monitored and restricted to effective doses of 100 millisieverts (mSv) every 5 years (i.e., 20 mSv/year) with a maximum of 50 mSv allowed in any given year.[9] In some individuals, cumulative effective radiation doses from medical imaging can exceed recommended maximum exposures. Therefore, health-care providers should recognize and inform patients about cumulative risks of radiation and ensure exposure is *as low as reasonably achievable* (ALARA) without sacrificing quality of care.[9]

The range of doses provided by common MSK imaging is outlined in Table 18.3. Standard radiographic examinations have average effective doses that vary by over a factor of 1000 (0.01–10 mSv). CT examinations tend to be in a more narrow range but have relatively high average effective doses (approximately 2–20 mSv), and average effective doses for interventional procedures usually range from 5 to 70 mSv. Average effective dose for most nuclear medicine procedures varies between 0.3 and 20 mSv. These doses can be compared with the average annual effective dose from background radiation of about 3 mSv (Table 18.4).

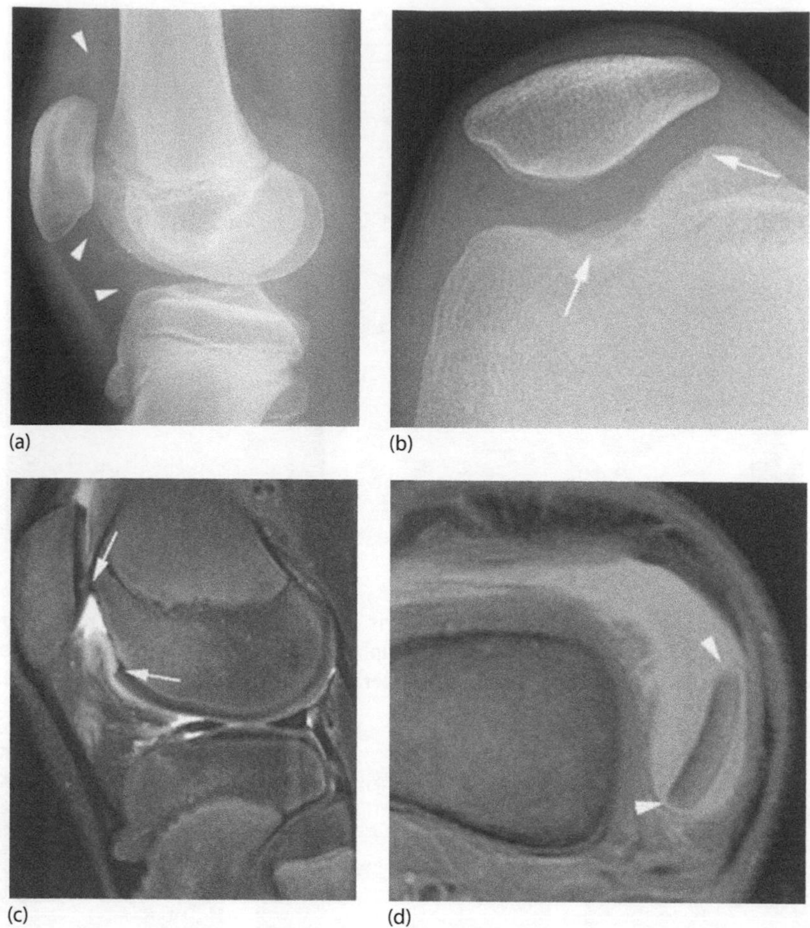

FIGURE 18.15 13 YOM with "soccer injury" to the left knee. (a) Lateral radiograph at the time of injury shows a small joint effusion (arrowheads). (b) Sunrise view shows subchondral bone plate irregularity (arrows) while joint space is preserved. (c) Sagittal T2 with fat saturation MRI shows a missing large section of the trochlear cartilage (arrows). Axial proton density with fat saturation MRI shows exfoliated slab of cartilage in the lateral suprapatellar recess (arrowheads).

TABLE 18.3
Ossification Centers of the Elbow

Order of Appearance of the Elbow Ossification Centers

- Capitellum—1 year
- Radial head—5 years
- Internal (medial) epicondyle—7 years
- Trochlea—10 years
- Olecranon—10 years
- Lateral epicondyle—11 years

Note: The order of "I" and "T" is most important to remember—the trochlea ossification center should not appear before the internal (medial) epicondyle ossification center.

18.5 HEAD AND SPINE SPORTS MEDICINE IMAGING

18.5.1 Head and Facial Trauma

Radiographs are rarely done for head or facial trauma but have been largely replaced by more sensitive CT scans. The substantial force necessary to cause a skull fracture typically justifies a CT scan to look for intracranial pathology. If plain films are desired to evaluate for a nasal fracture, a nasal bone series should be ordered. Temporomandibular joint (TMJ) radiographs are used for localized pain, arthritis, fracture, or dysplasia. Additionally, MRI dedicated to the TMJ can well visualize TMJ articular pathology.

In acute traumatic brain injury (TBI), CT scans are used to evaluate for hemorrhage, significant contusions, fractures, and stroke. In a sports medicine setting, strokes are typically a rare, secondary infarction due to a vascular injury.[34] CT or MRI angiography is utilized if vascular injury with dissection is suspected.

MRI is generally reserved for a TBI that fails to improve over time or acutely when axonal injury or ischemia due to traumatic vessel injury is of urgent concern. While MRI sensitivity equals CT in detecting acute intracranial pathology, MRI surpasses CT in detecting more subtle abnormalities, such as cerebral edema, hemosiderin deposition (older mild hemorrhage), and minor cerebral contusion.[34] In children and adolescents, MRI may be considered first-line imaging technique in an outpatient setting as it avoids the radiation

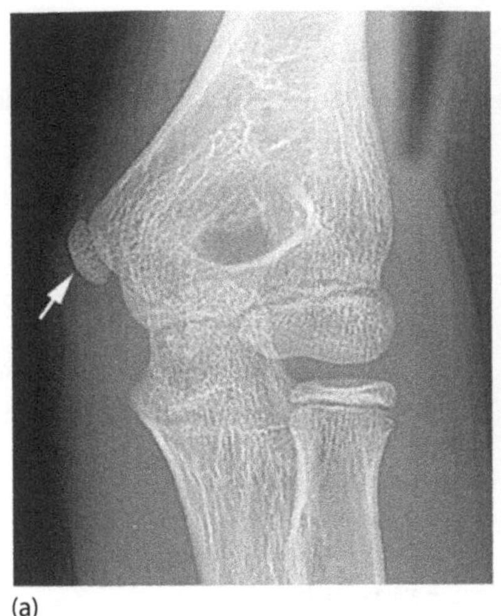
(a)

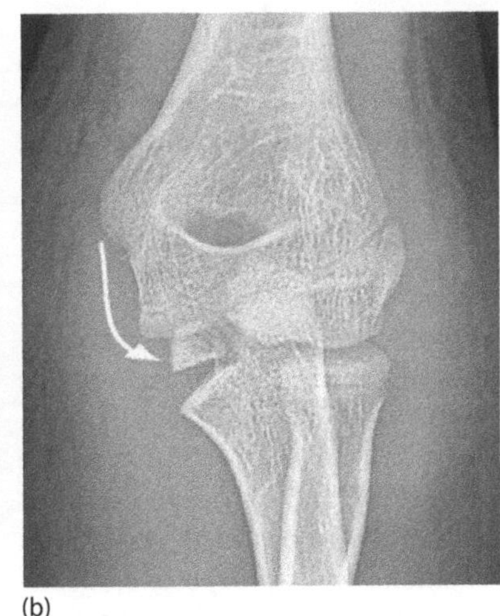
(b)

FIGURE 18.16 (a) AP radiograph of normal elbow in an 11-year old. Arrow indicates medial epicondyle apophyseal ossification center. (b) AP radiograph showing avulsed and displaced medial epicondyle apophyseal ossification center (curved arrow) in a 12-year old.

TABLE 18.4
Adult Effective Doses for Various Common Sports Medicine Imaging Procedures

Procedure	Average Effective Dose (mSv)	Values Reports in Literature (mSv)
Radiographs		
Cervical spine	0.2	0.07–0.3
Thoracic spine	1.0	0.6–1.4
Lumbar spine	1.5	0.5–1.8
PA and lateral chest	0.1	0.05–0.24
Abdomen	0.7	0.04–1.1
Pelvis	0.6	0.2–1.2
Hip	0.7	0.18–2.71
Shoulder	0.01	Not available
Knee	0.005	Not available
Other extremities	0.001	0.0002–0.1
Dual x-ray absorptiometry (without CT)	0.001	0.001–0.035
CT		
Head	2	0.9–4.0
Neck	3	Not available
Chest	7	4.0–18.0
Chest for pulmonary embolism	15	13–40
Abdomen	8	3.5–25
Pelvis	6	3.3–10
Spine	6	1.5–10
Nuclear medicine		
Bone (technetium 99 m)	6.3[a]	Not available

Source: Mettler, F.A. et al., *Radiology*, 248, 254, 2008.
[a] Actual effective dose (mSv), not "average effective dose."

exposure that accompanies CT scanning. In sports medicine, MRI of the brain is usually without contrast, unless there is concern for contrast-enhancing pathology such as meningitis, cerebritis, encephalitis, vasculitis, or tumor.

18.5.2 Concussion and Traumatic Brain Injury

A single concussion or repeated TBI may result in chronic neuropathologic changes and long-term associated disabilities.[30] Therefore, the accurate diagnosis of an initial concussion and measurement of return to preinjury brain function before return to sport is central to contemporary concussion management. Current diagnostic CT and MRI imaging are inconclusive in the diagnosis of concussion or measurement of return to baseline brain function.[5] Several neuroimaging techniques are emerging with potential for future use in concussion management, including diffusion tensor imaging (DTI), functional MRI (fMRI), and positron-emission tomography (PET) scans.[37]

DTI, a subtype of diffusion-weighted imaging (DWI), is a form of MRI based upon the diffusion of water molecules within an image element, or voxel. While DWI is applicable when isotropic water movement dominates the tissue of interest, DTI can give additional information in tissues with non-isotropic water movement and demonstrate injury to white matter tracts in the brain or muscle fibers. Abnormalities in the usually linear diffusion of water suggest postinjury disruption of white matter tracks that correlate with neuropsychological and cognitive impairments. Studies are ongoing to further establish a role of DTI in the diagnosis and management of concussion.[34,37]

fMRI evaluates brain function based on changes in brain capillary bed blood flow.[34] In particular, the blood-oxygen-ation-level-dependent technique reveals regional shifts in oxyhemoglobin and deoxyhemoglobin in the context of task-specific activity (Valerio and Illes, 2013). Research suggests that concussed brains "compensate" for disrupted areas by activating different ones, possibly reflecting chronic changes in brain networks.

PET imaging is being developed to detect changes in brain metabolism following a TBI. Brain cells take up deoxyglucose (DG) in proportion to glucose, but instead of being fully metabolized, DG is phosphorylated, becoming trapped in the brain cells with a slow clearance rate. The radioactive isotope 18F can be attached to DG, forming FDG, detectible in an FDG–PET scan. FDG–PET scans have shown promise in detecting changes in glucose uptake and utilization in the brain after an injury.[5]

18.5.3 Cervical Spine

In awake and alert patients, the National Emergency X-Radiography Utilization Study (NEXUS) criteria may be utilized when deciding whether to obtain radiological clearance of the C-spine. The decision instrument consists of five clinical findings from the history and physical examination (Table 18.5). The presence of any one of these findings requires radiographic evaluation. In a prospective, observational study, the decision instrument had a sensitivity of 99.6%, an NPV of 99.9%, a specificity of 12.9%, and a PPV of 2.7% for the identification of clinically significant C-spine injuries.[13] In an obtunded patient, CT or MRI can be used for C-spine clearance.

Radiographs for traumatic C-spine injury require three views, a cross-table lateral, an anteroposterior (AP), and an open-mouth odontoid. Radiographs must be reviewed systematically (Table 18.6 and Figure 18.17). Malalignment from spasm and straightening or mild kyphosis associated with C-collar and backboard immobilization should not be mistaken for occult fracture. Commonly, patients from low-velocity motor vehicle accidents (MVAs) will have increased spasm and splinting 48 hours after injury.

Oblique films can be helpful in patients with degenerative spine disease (such as facet arthritis and uncovertebral arthrosis) and radiculopathy. They may also be used for MVA patients where CT is not available. Pathology that is well visualized includes bony foraminal stenosis and facet fracture or malalignment (Figure 18.18).

In the setting of a chronic injury and with an alert, cooperative patient, dynamic flexion–extension radiographs can reveal cervical instability. In acute trauma, they would not be done due to the risk of neurologic injury. The study is aborted if it elicits pain or paresthesias. Flexion–extension radiographs can expose undetected ligament disruption when initial films are normal, but suspicion persists. They are positive when there is a widening greater than 3.5 mm of predental space from rupture of the transverse ligament, which holds C-1 against the dens (odontoid) of C-2, or more than 3 mm listhesis of any vertebra (Figure 18.19).[18,24]

CT is indicated when radiographs are normal but suspicion for fracture is high. High-speed MVAs with frontal impact patients directly undergo CT, skipping radiographs (Table 18.7: Hanson criteria).[3,8,12] CT is appropriate when x-rays are not normal but not definitive, such as with minimal listhesis, poor visualization, malsegmentation obscuring anatomy, or more than 2 mm of listhesis. All fractures found on radiography should undergo CT for further definition and evaluation for displacement. C-spine fractures are usually more involved than seen on x-ray. CT is usually noncontrast for traumatic injuries.

MRI is performed for injury with neurologic symptoms or impairment to evaluate cord or nerve root injuries. Additionally, MRI evaluates ligamentous, joint, and disc structures in patients with findings of instability or radiculopathy.[2,8]

TABLE 18.5
NEXUS Clinical Criteria

1. Tenderness at the posterior midline of the cervical spine
2. Focal neurologic deficit
3. Decreased level of alertness
4. Evidence of intoxication
5. Clinically apparent pain that might distract the patient from the pain of a cervical spine injury

The presence of any one of these findings is considered to be clinical evidence that a patient is at increased risk for cervical spine injury and requires radiographic evaluation.

Sources: Coris, E.E. et al., *Sports Med. Arthros. Rev.*, 17, 2, 2009; Hoffman, J.R. et al., *N. Engl. J. Med.*, 343, 94, 2009.

TABLE 18.6
Cervical Spine X-Ray Interpretation

ABCs
- A (i): appropriateness (correct patient)
- A (ii): adequacy of film?
  - C1 to top of T1, penetration
- A (iii): alignment (five lines), presence of lordosis
- Bones
- Connective tissue—prevertebral soft tissue, predental gap, intervertebral disc spaces

Lateral view

Alignment (five lines)
- Anterior vertebral bodies
- Posterior vertebral bodies
- Facet joints
- Base of the spinous processes
- Tip of the spinous processes

Soft tissue space—r/o occult fracture
- Choose your rules
- 6 at 2 and 2 at 6
  - 6 mm at C2 and 2 cm at C6

  or
- C1–C3 < 7 mm and C4–C7 = 14–22 mm

AP view
- Spinous processes

Odontoid view
- C1–C2 articulation.
- Lateral masses should line up. Displaced equals burst injury of the cervical ring.
- Usually axial load, with fragments displaced down the slope of the articular surface.

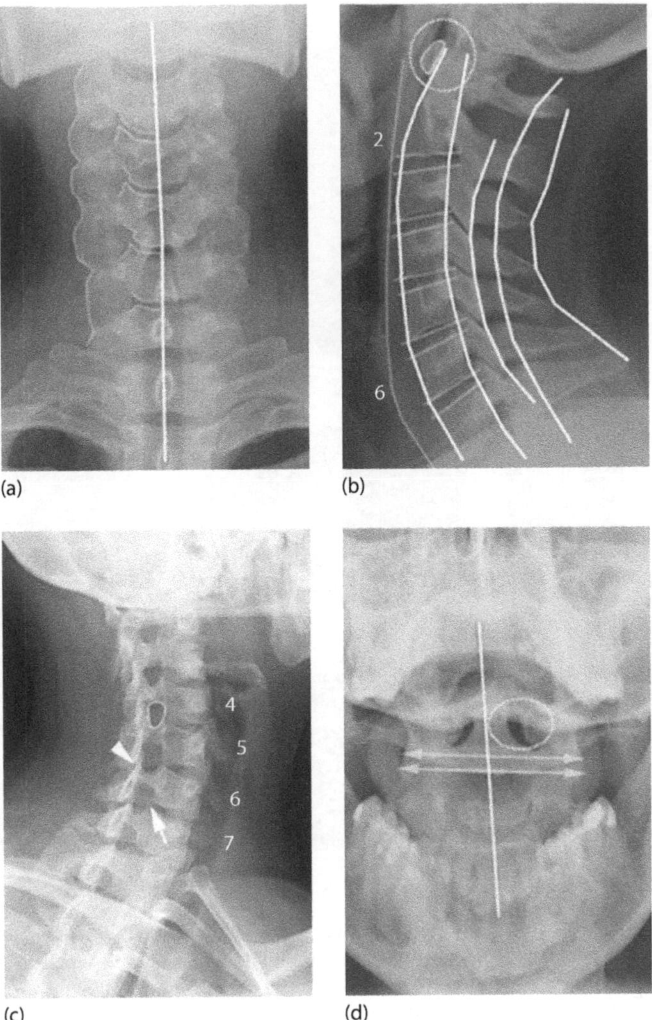

FIGURE 18.17 Normal C-spine radiographs in a 30-year-old female. (a) An AP frontal image shows less than 5° lateral curvature with normal alignment of spinous processes (vertical line). There is no facet arthropathy or malalignment (undulating outline to the left of the image) or facet arthropathy (normal uncovertebral joints outlined to the left of the midline). (b) The lateral radiograph shows normal sagittal alignment with normal lordosis and smooth transition of the boney spinal lines (white lines form anterior to posterior: anterior vertebral body line, posterior vertebral body line, spinolaminar/dorsal laminar line). The disc spaces are preserved (outlined in gray). The prevertebral soft tissues are normal in contour and thickness as demonstrated by the location of the posterior airway (gray line at the left), which in adults should be no thicker than 6 mm at C2 and 22 cm at C6. The atlanto-odontoid joint is normally aligned (circle) with the joint space in adults never being more than 3 mm wide as measured form the anterior cortex of the dens to the posterior cortex of the C1 arch (outlined). (c) An oblique radiograph showing the right lateral foramina (outlined at C4/C5). The foramina should appear as a smooth vertically oriented oval rather than as a "figure eight" with wasting from encroachment by osteophytes from the facet joints dorsally (arrowhead at C5/C6) and uncovertebral joints ventrally (arrow at C6/C7). (d) The open-mouth odontoid view is used primarily to assess the relationship of the C1 arch to the shoulders of C2 and the base of the dens. Seeing the tip of the dens is less critical. The transverse width of C1 should match C2 (double-headed arrows) with no more than 2 mm lateral displacement. The lateral dens spaces (oval) should be symmetrical within a millimeter in a properly positioned film where the sagittal incisor line falls over the middle third of the dens (vertical white line). The lateral dens space will widen to the ipsilateral side of chin displacement when there is head rotation.

CT angiograms are performed if mechanism of injury and history are concerning for vascular injury. Conventional angiography is generally for intervention only rather than solely diagnostic. Concerning injuries include high energy with fractures through a foramen or facet, or a skull-based fracture. Vascular dissections are not unusual in setting of high-energy trauma even without fracture. Of note, chiropractic cervical manipulations have been associated with vertebral artery dissections.[8,11,19,26,29]

18.5.3.1 Special and Pediatric Considerations

Certain developmental anomalies of the craniocervical spine such as vertebral segmentation and fusion abnormalities, os odontoideum and ligamentous instability, and developmental

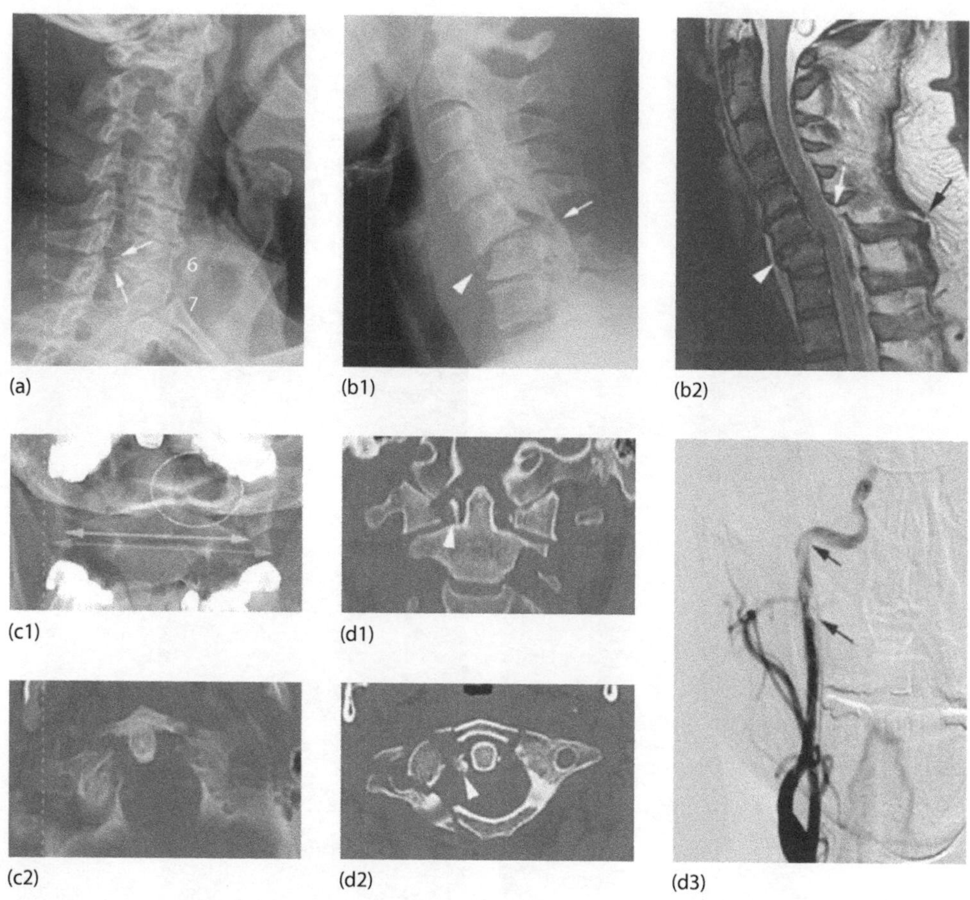

FIGURE 18.18 (a) Right anterior oblique C-spine radiograph showing bony lateral foraminal stenosis at C6/C7 from prominent uncovertebral spurs and degenerative disc disease (DDD). (b1) Lateral radiograph showing perched facets at C5/C6 (arrow) and flexion tear drop fracture at C6 (arrowhead) following MVA deceleration flexion injury. (b2) Sagittal non-fat-saturated T2 MR image from a similar case showing the same fracture (arrowhead) and dorsal distraction ligamentum flavum (white arrow) and supraspinous and nuchal ligament (black arrow) tears. (c1) Open-mouth odontoid view showing marked widening of the lateral dens space (oval) and widening of the transverse c1 arch diameter (longer double-headed arrow) compared to the shoulders of c2 (shorter double-headed arrow) in a c1 burst fracture. (c2) Axial CT image of the same case showing anterior displacement of dens and anterior c1 arch fragment. (d1, d2) Coronal and axial CT images, respectively, of different c1 burst fractures with similar widening of c1 arch and displaced transverse ligament tubercle (arrowheads). (d3) Conventional angiogram of the same case showing internal carotid artery dissection with filling defect (arrows) associated with the c1 fracture.

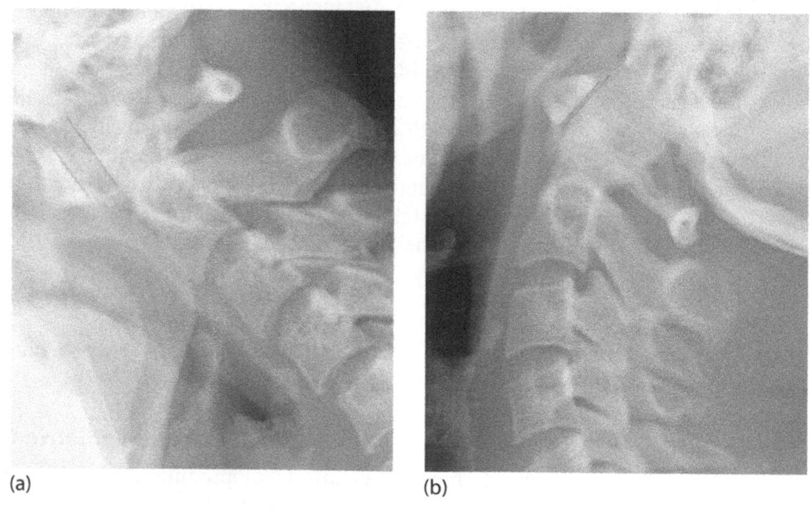

FIGURE 18.19 (a) Flexion and (b) extension images of atlantoaxial instability show widening of the atlanto-odontoid space to nearly 6 mm during flexion that reduces completely during extension (method of measuring joint space width is highlighted).

TABLE 18.7
Hanson Criteria

Clinical Decision Rule to Select High-Risk Patients to Undergo Helical CT of the Cervical Spine: Six Injury Mechanisms or Clinical Parameters
Injury mechanism parameters based on the initial report of emergency transportation personnel, patient, or witnesses
1. High-speed (≥ 35 mph [56 kmph] combined impact) motor vehicle accident
2. Crash with death at scene of motor vehicle accident
3. Fall from height (≥10 ft [3 m])
Clinical parameters based on primary patient survey
4. Significant closed head injury (or intracranial hemorrhage seen on CT)
5. Neurologic symptoms or signs referred to the cervical spine
6. Pelvic or multiple extremity fractures
The presence of any one parameter places the patient in the high-risk category (>5% risk of cervical spine fracture) and indicates that the patient should undergo helical CT.
It is assumed that CT of the head will be performed contemporaneously.

Source: Hanson, J.A. et al., *Am. J. Roentgenol.*, 174, 713, 2000.

spinal canal stenosis in the setting of neuropraxias have been demonstrated to place the cord at an increased risk of injury and may serve as an absolute contraindication to participation in contact sports. Evaluation by conventional radiographs with addition of flexion and extension views in the lateral projection is often sufficient for diagnosis.[2,8] The Torg ratio, defined as AP diameter of the spinal canal/vertebral body, may be measured to help stratify the risk of a neuropraxic event (Figure 18.20 Torg ratios).[8,16] Smaller Torg ratios are associated with an increased risk of recurrent spinal cord neuropraxia.[8,35] However, the Torg ratio is not always predictive and should not be used alone to determine return to contact sports.[7,16,27] Persistent neurological symptoms and intermittent cervical symptoms without a correlative conventional radiographic abnormality should be further evaluated with C-spine MRI. Occasionally, CT of the craniocervical junction is necessary to fully evaluate skeletal segmentation abnormalities.[2]

Up to 15% of individuals with Down's syndrome have a malalignment of the cervical vertebrae C-1 and C-2 in the neck known as atlantoaxial instability. Previously, it was believed that screening x-rays could predict Down's syndrome athletes at risk of spinal cord injury; however, research has not correlated radiographic instability, or lack thereof, with risk for spinal cord injury.[2,22] Nonetheless, Special Olympics–accredited programs do require athletes with Down's syndrome participating in certain "high-risk" physical activities complete a medical exam including flexion–extension C-spine radiographs. A case of atlantoaxial instability is demonstrated in Figure 18.21.

Pediatric pseudosubluxation is normal mobility of C-2 on C-3 in flexion in children and adolescents sometimes mistaken for pathologic motion. It is normal in children less than 8 years old, but may be seen in adolescents up to age 16. Pseudosubluxation can be distinguished from pathologic injury by a lack of anterior swelling and by the presence only on flexion views with resolution on extension views. Pseudosubluxation occurs due to relatively increased ligamentous laxity, the more horizontal nature of the facet joint, and the fulcrum of motion being greatest at C2–C3 (compared with C5–C6 in adults).[33,9,40]

18.5.4 Thoracic Spine

Radiographs of the thoracic spine include two upright views, AP and lateral. Due to the AP orientation of the thoracic facet joints, oblique views are useless. T1–T10 are stabilized by the ribs and the orientation of the facets, resulting in 60%–70% of thoracolumbar injuries occurring in the relatively less-stabilized T12–L2 region.

Fractures concerning for instability warrant CT imaging. Signs of potentially unstable fractures include two- or three-column injury, widening of the disc space, or widening of the interspinous distance (when the spinous processes are splayed apart). Compression fractures with greater than a 50% loss of height on radiography may actually be burst fractures. MRI is indicated for neurologic complaints or persistent pain with a significant mechanism of injury and negative plain films. MRI may reveal occult fracture with bone marrow edema and hemorrhage and define associated ligamentous injuries that may be braced to facilitate healing (Figure 18.22).

18.5.4.1 Special and Pediatric Considerations

In scoliosis evaluations, initial films include full-length upright posteroanterior (PA) and lateral (Figure 18.23 scoliosis measurements). A curvature of 10° or less is considered normal. Comparison films for rate of progression consist of a single full-length PA view. Referral or interval reimaging can be considered for curvatures greater than 20°. Consider bracing for curvature between 25° and 40° if patient is still growing. Surgery referral is indicated for curvature greater than 50°, since these curves are at higher risk for progression even after completion of growth.[9,40] Painful scoliosis is a red flag for the spectrum of osteoblastoma and osteoid osteoma malignancies, as well as pedicle/pars stress fractures. The malignancies present as a single curve with pain on the spastic side and are well visualized on MRI (Figure 18.24).

Scheuermann's disease, or Scheuermann's kyphosis, is a condition in which the kyphosis in the upper spine is increased due to anterior wedging of the thoracic spine (Figure 18.25 Scheuermann's). Scheuermann's presents midthoracic to thoracolumbar junction pain in adolescents and premature degenerative spine disease in young adults.[25,9] The criteria for diagnosis include thoracic kyphosis >45° (25°–40° being normal), wedging >5° of three adjacent vertebrae, and thoracolumbar kyphosis >30° (thoracolumbar spine is normally straight).[21,36,39,40] Treatment is usually physical therapy, but bracing until sexual maturity may prevent further progression.[23,34,38]

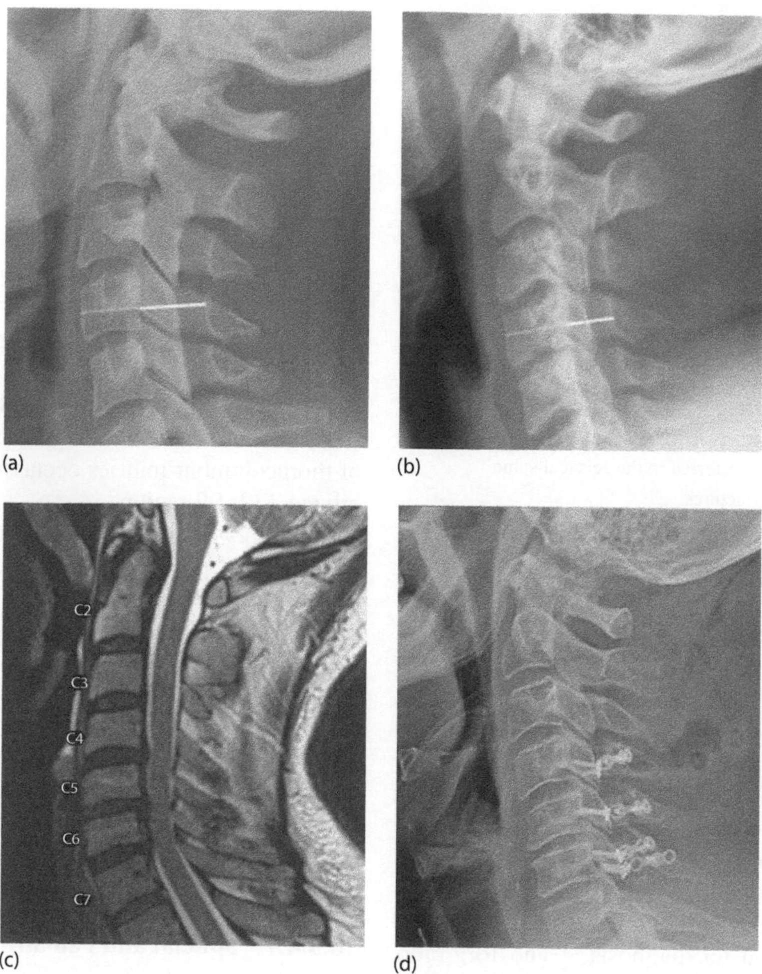

FIGURE 18.20 (a) Lateral C-spine radiograph of a normal 30 YOF with generous spinal canal and Torg ratio of 1.07. (b) 24 YOM with congenital spinal stenosis and Torg ratio of 0.7. Lines depict midbody location to obtain measurement, with C5 and C6 generally being the narrowest. (c) Sagittal non-fat-saturated T2 images showing severe multilevel spinal stenosis with chord compression as a result of mild multilevel DDD superimposed on congenital stenosis in a 45 YOM who presented with a C-spine "stinger" from minor trauma. (d) As his DDD was mild and there was no associated instability, he subsequently underwent dorsal decompression with a C4–C6 "open door" laminoplasty procedure.

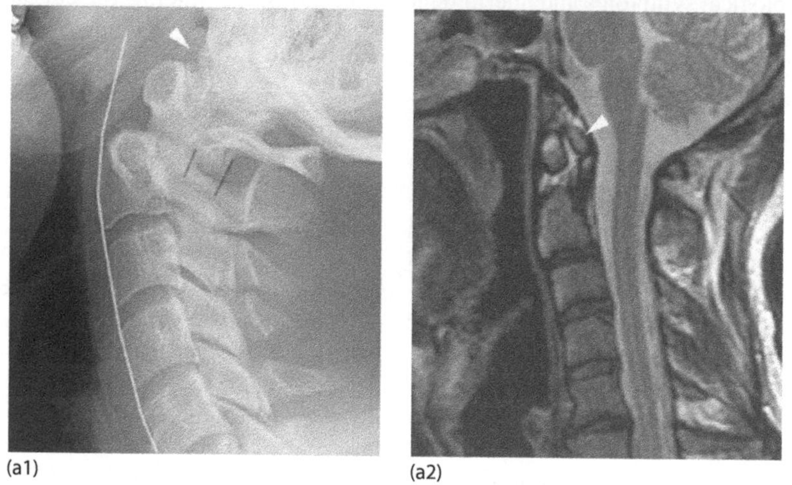

FIGURE 18.21 (a1) Lateral radiograph of a different case where there is gross atlantoaxial instability as shown by the marked posterior displacement of the hypertrophic anterior arch of C1 relative to the anterior spinal line. There is marked posterior lateral mass subluxation (method of measuring subluxation is highlighted). (a2) Sagittal T2 without fat saturation MR image shows an os odontoideum variant in which the lateral dental ossification centers remain in the anterior arch of C1 while the apical ossification center remains tethered between the basion and remaining C2 vertebral body (arrowhead in a1 and a2).

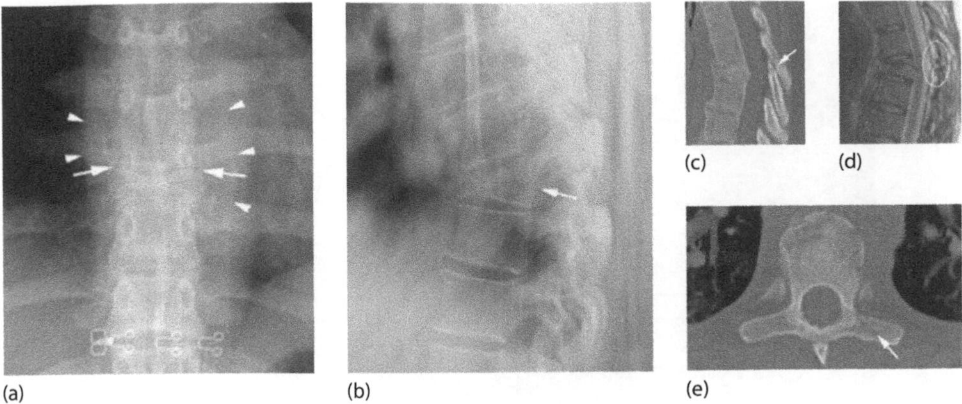

FIGURE 18.22 (a) An AP trauma portable radiograph of the T-spine shows a transverse fracture through the T7 vertebra (arrows) with paraspinal soft tissue swelling/bleeding (arrowheads). (b) The lateral radiograph confirms greater than 50% anterior wedging with posterior cortical buckling (arrow) and focal kyphosis. (c) A reconstructed sagittal CT image shows a transverse fracture in the lamina confirming posterior column extension of a mixed flexion/distraction injury. (d) A sagittal non-fat-saturated T2 MR image shows an intact dorsal thecal sac and ligamentum flavum (oval). (e) Axial CT image shows the severe comminution of the anterior vertebra and extension of the laminar fracture into the transverse process (arrow).

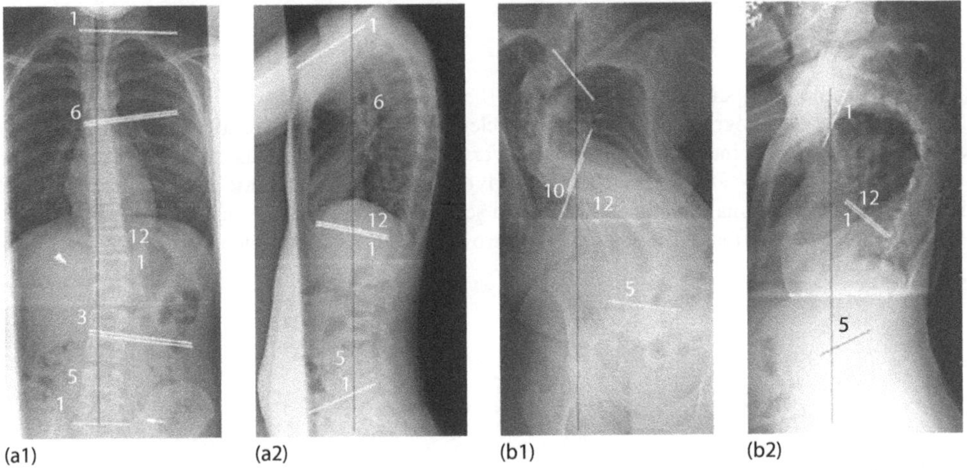

FIGURE 18.23 (a1) Standing AP scoliosis film of a mildly affected 14 YOM with a transitional right L1 rib (arrowhead) and lumbarized S1 vertebra bearing a transverse process on the right and an assimilation joint on the left (arrow). Cobb angle lines (white) are placed at the curvature transition points, in this case at T6 and L3, revealing the maximum degree of angular deformity. There is an 8° curvature of the convex-right T1–T6, 15° curvature of the convex-left T6–L3, and 6° curvature of the convex-right L3–S1. The lumbarized S1 vertebra is the last mobile segment in this case. As the total convex-right and convex-left curvatures are nearly equal (14° vs. 15°), the scoliosis is considered compensated, and the C7 plumb line (vertical black line) falls near the center of S1 reflecting no significant displacement of the coronal balance. (a2) The standing lateral shows 42° of thoracic kyphosis and 35° of lumbar lordosis with a normally located thoracolumbar transition at T12/L1. The sagittal plumb line falls at the anterior edge of S1 indicating a minimal amount of sagittal positive imbalance. (b1 and b2) This scoliosis series in a 65 YOF with postpolio spasticity and scoliosis illustrates the difficulty in evaluating severe deformities in osteopenic spines with 2D radiography. Note severe deformity of the chest wall that limits ventilatory effectiveness of the lungs and represents a significant source of morbidly in these patients (thoracic lateral curve 113°, lumbar lateral curve 77°, thoracic kyphosis 110°, lumbar lordosis 70°).

18.5.5 Lumbar Spine

A discussion of low back pain imaging should begin with the central question of when to image. The American College of Physicians/American Pain Society 2007 low back pain clinical guidelines provide an excellent evidence-based algorithm. Key recommendations include the following: (1) clinicians should not routinely obtain imaging or other diagnostic tests in patients with nonspecific low back pain and (2) clinicians should perform diagnostic imaging and testing for patients

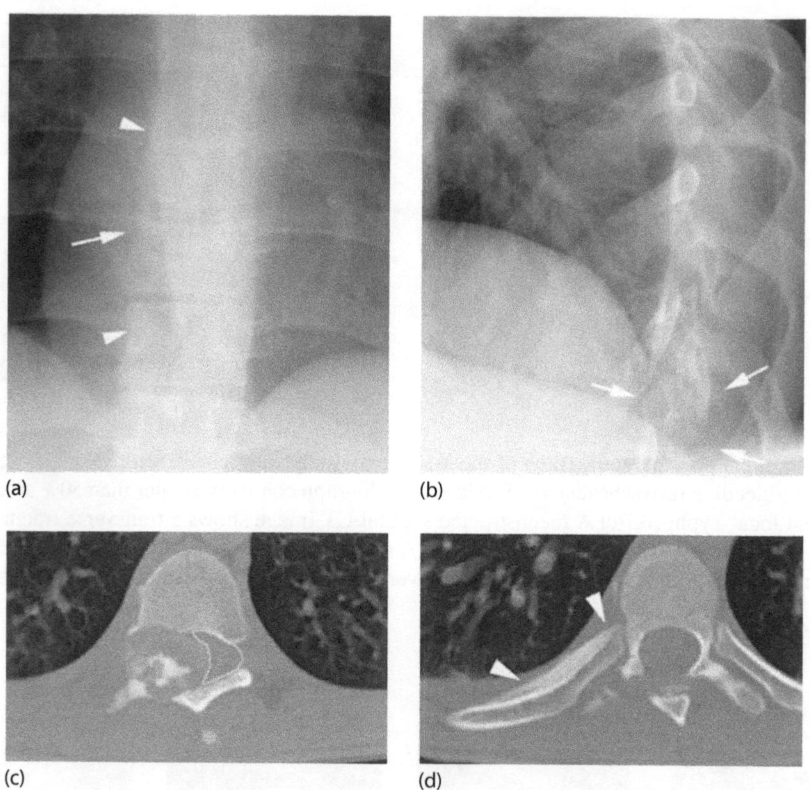

FIGURE 18.24 (a) Frontal radiograph showing subtle loss of the right T9 pedicle (arrow). Arrowheads indicate normal adjacent pedicle rings. (b) Close-up of lateral radiograph shows abnormal sclerosis in the T9/T10 lateral foramen and facets at the bottom margin of the image. In the absence of a specific indication/history of lower T-spine pain/symptoms, such "corner of the film" finding could be easily overlooked. (c) The follow-up CT scan reveals an expansile lytic and centrally sclerotic mass centered in the dorsal pedicle of the affected vertebra. Expansion into the spinal canal has resulted in severe stenosis. Outline indicates residual canal. (d) shows reactive sclerosis and periosteal new bone deposition of the adjacent rib (arrows) often seen in osteoid osteoma-like osteoblastomas that produce prostaglandin.

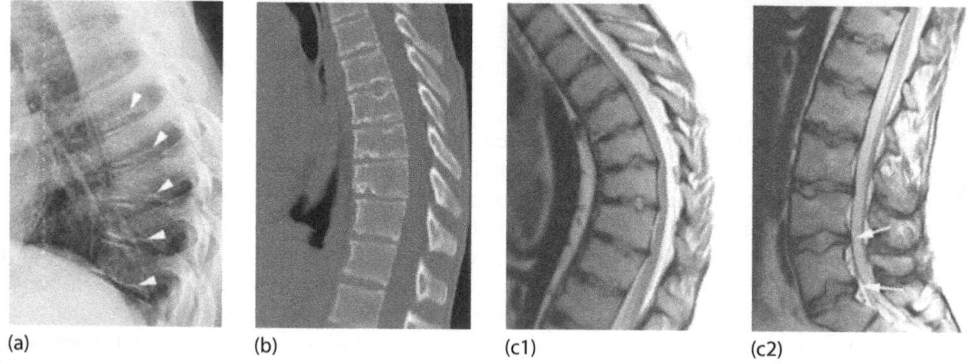

FIGURE 18.25 (a) Lateral T-spine radiograph of a symptomatic 24 YOM showing multilevel contiguous Schmorl's nodes (arrowheads) with mild wedging and kyphosis. (b) Sagittal reconstruction from trauma CT scan in a 22 YOM better showing multilevel midthoracic Schmorl's nodes and mild wedging. c1 and c2 show sagittal non-fat-saturated T2 MR images of the thoracic and lumbar spine, respectively, in severely affected 24 YOM. Thoracic kyphosis measures 64° in the supine position. Arrows in c2 show typical premature DDD.

with low back pain when severe or progressive neurologic deficits are present or when serious underlying conditions are suspected on the basis of history and physical examination.[6,34]

Initial radiographs for low back pain include an upright AP and lateral (Figure 18.26). In the past, lumbosacral spot views were performed centered on L5 to eliminate potential overread of disc space narrowing from beam diversion on a standard lateral. Currently, this view is not routinely done due to high radiation exposure. Oblique views of the lumbar spine are also discouraged due to radiation exposure and a lack of

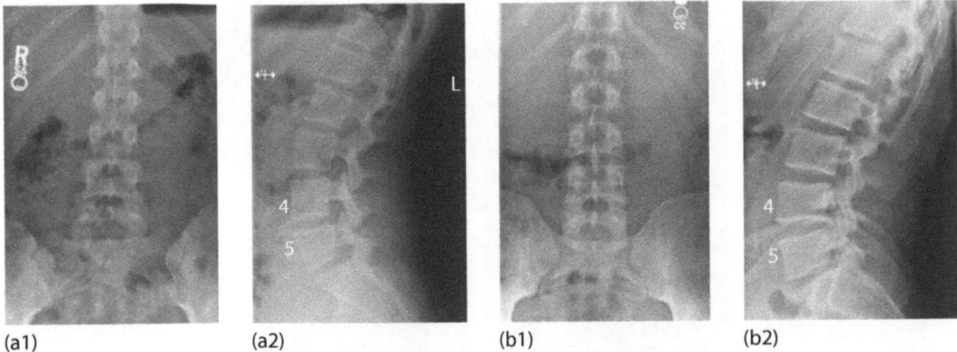

FIGURE 18.26 Upright AP and lateral L-spine films in normal gracile female (a1–a2) and robust male (b1–b2). Note that the vertebral bodies in the gracile form are taller than wide, while the opposite is true of the robust form. Both spines show remarkable left/right symmetry with normal alignment, segmentation, and distinct thoracolumbar and lumbosacral transitions. There is no dorsal dysraphism and the disc spaces are preserved without end plate spurring or listhesis. Note that the L4/L5 disc space is normally the widest. The lateral foramina are relatively larger in the gracile form, but neither shows any arthritic encroachment from the facets or posterior end plates.

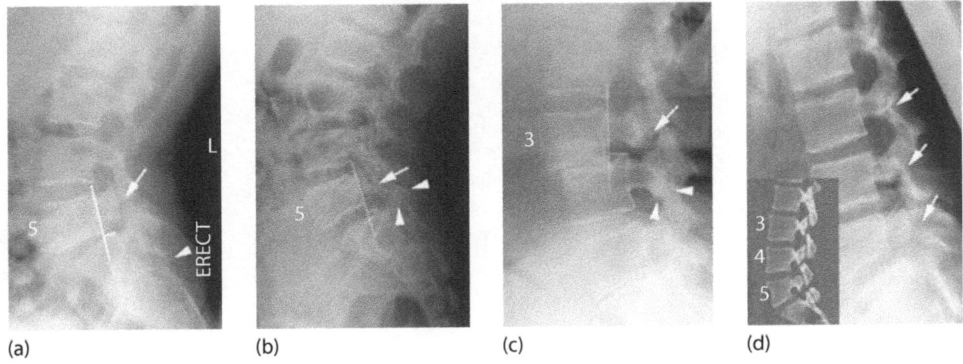

FIGURE 18.27 (a) Upright lateral L-spine radiograph of typical chronic bilateral pars defects (arrow) at L5 in a 37 YOM. Lines depict method for measuring the degree of L5 anterolisthesis. The arrowhead indicates an abnormal and hypoplastic S1/S2 facet joint that has occurred in conjunction with partial lumbarization of S1. (b) Lateral radiograph of an L5 pars defect (arrow) in a 14 YOM with dorsally dysraphic L5 vertebra and entire sacrum. The arrowheads indicate the splayed and hypoplastic L5 inferior facets. (c) Pars defects can occur at any level and may be seen higher in the hyperlordotic lumbar spine. In (c), arrow indicates a widely separated L3 pars defect. Arrowheads indicate severe reactive sclerosis/stress reaction of the L4 pars interarticularis without visible fracture. (d) shows multiple contiguous pars defects (arrows) in a 20 YOM college cheerleader. A preoperative CT (inset sagittal image) shows in better detail where bilateral fractures are.

true sensitivity for revealing pars defects. A pars defect will only be seen on oblique films when the fracture is perpendicular to the pars, but CT studies have demonstrated the majority of the lyses lie close to the coronal plane.[20,30] Lateral flexion films are the most sensitive radiographs for pars defects (Figure 18.27). Flexion/extension radiographs can reveal instability and pedicle fractures.

As with the cervical and thoracic spine imaging, CT can further define known vertebral fractures and determine if instability requiring bracing or surgery is present. MRI is indicated for neurologic complaints or persistent pain with a significant mechanism of injury and negative plain films. MRI may reveal occult fracture with bone marrow edema and hemorrhage and define associated ligamentous injuries. Severe or progressive neurologic deficits, including suspected cauda equina syndrome, warrant MRI. MRI is usually required prior to referral for interventional pain injections, but may not be necessary in certain clinical situations with straightforward history, physical exam, and radiographs with a compelling reason to circumvent MRI (Figure 18.28).

SPECT–CT and PET–CT may be used in patients with suspected or known spondylolysis or diffuse spondylosis. In a patient with multiple potential lumbar pathologies, SPECT and PET–CT can localize the most likely source of pain to direct management interventional pain injections or surgical decision making. Nuclear imaging remains the most sensitive for initial pars stress injuries in athletes, and a positive scan may result in early activity modification or bracing. Serial nuclear imaging of a spondylolysis may demonstrate resolving metabolic activity representing healing, and thus guide return to sport.

18.5.5.1 Special and Pediatric Considerations

Tethered spinal cord syndrome (also known as an occult spinal dysraphism sequence) is a neurological disorder caused

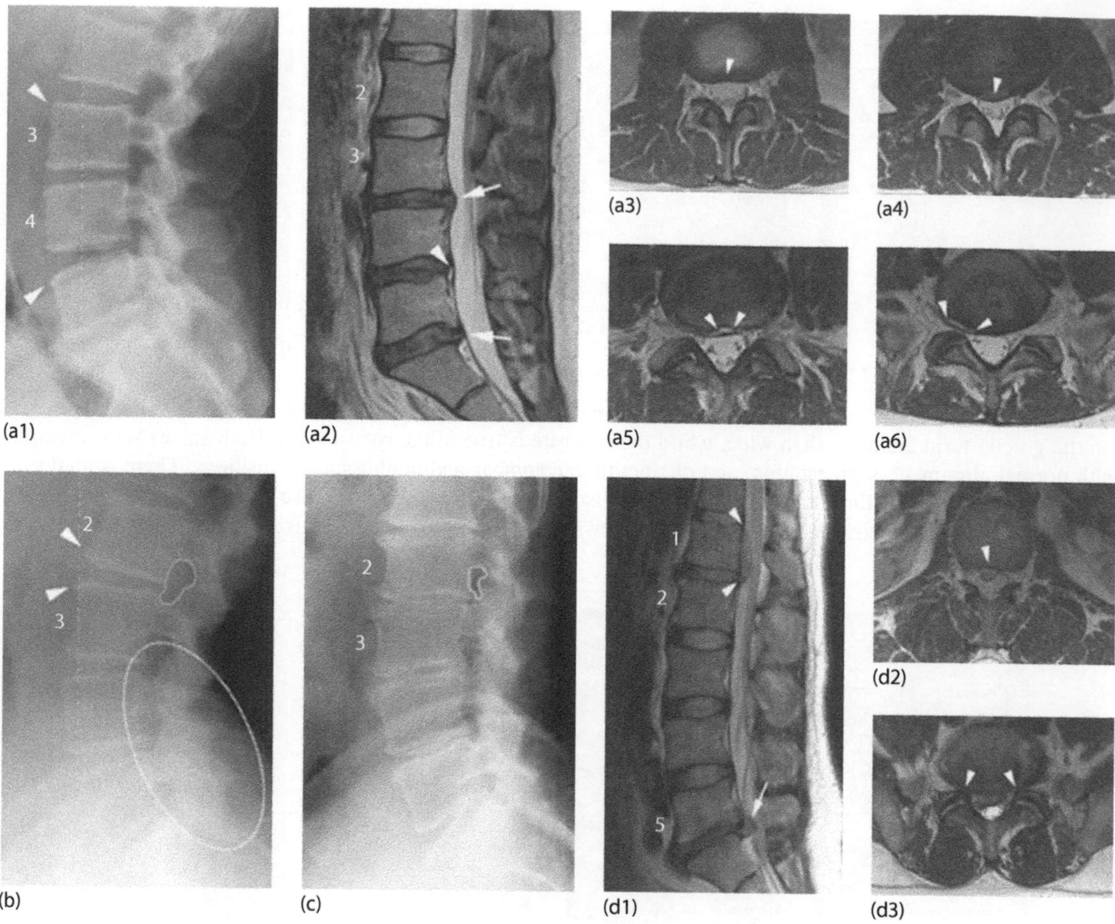

FIGURE 18.28 (a1) Upright lateral L-spine radiograph of mild/early lumbar DDD in which there is mild disc space narrowing at L3/L4 and L5/S1 and minimal end plate spurring (arrowheads). (a2) Sagittal non-fat-saturated T2 MR image of the same case showing darker fluid signal, when compared to the normal L2/L3 disc, in the degenerating inferior three discs. Arrows show abnormal midline posterior bulging. There is a central annular tear and small inferiorly directed disc extrusion at L4/L5 (arrowhead). Images a3 through a6 depict relevant axial disc features in the same case: (a3) normal disc anterior concavity at L2/L3, (a4) small central protrusion at L3/L4, (a5) small disc extrusion under posterior longitudinal ligament at L4/L5, and (a6) right subarticular zone (lateral recess) and foraminal annular tear at L5/S1. (b) Upright lateral L-spine radiograph of moderate DDD with greater end plate spurring (arrowheads) and moderate/severe inferior lumbar facet arthropathy (oval). (c) Severe multilevel DDD and facet arthropathy. Compare narrowed lateral foramen outlined at L2/L3 with normal foramen outlined in (b). d1 is a sagittal non-fat-saturated T2 MR image showing widely separated spinal stenosis due to two large disc extrusions at L1/L2 (arrowheads) and L5/S1 (arrow). (d2) The longer superior extrusion is transversely narrow and indents the thecal sac without nerve root compression. (d3) The broader inferior disc extrusion results in moderate spinal stenosis with compression of the transiting S1 nerve roots and posterior displacement of the remaining sacral nerve roots. There is an underlying disc bulge that extends into the lateral foramina contributing to foraminal stenosis (arrowheads).

by tissue attachments that limit the movement of the spinal cord within the spinal column (Figure 18.29). The condition is closely linked to spina bifida, and as such presentation in childhood may be with the cutaneous stigmata of dysraphism (hairy patch, dimple, subcutaneous lipoma). There may be associated foot and spinal deformities, leg weakness, low back pain, scoliosis, and incontinence. The condition may go undiagnosed until adulthood, with the development of sensory and motor problems and loss of bowel and bladder control. Imaging features are of a low conus medullaris (below L2) and thickened filum terminale (>2 mm). Untreated, tethered cord syndrome has a progressive course. Surgical release, in selected patients, can dramatically improve function.

The vertebral column is affected by a variety of variant anatomy of the body and/or neural arch as well as accessory ossicles. Vertebral body variants include hemivertebra, block vertebra, and butterfly vertebra. Neural arch variants include symmetrical and asymmetrical dorsal dysraphisms, absent or unfused spinous process, and absent or hypoplastic facets and/or pedicles (Figures 18.29 and 18.30). Morphologic boundary shifts can confuse the spinal segmentation boundaries resulting in transitional morphologies, absent vertebra, or supernumerary vertebra. Vertebral anomalies are noteworthy as they can cause pain and/or can occur with numerous syndromic as well as nonsyndromic conditions.

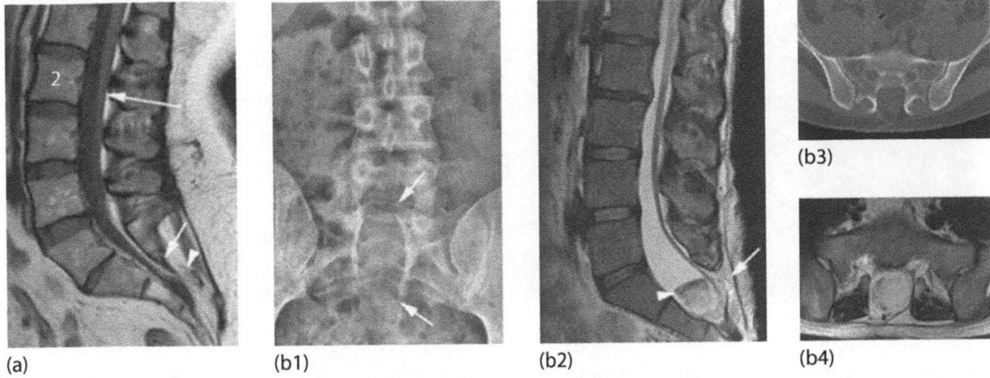

FIGURE 18.29 (a) Sagittal non-fat-saturated T1 MR image of a mild tethered chord with low conus at the inferior L2 level (long arrow), sacral dorsal dysraphism extending to the superior S2 lamina (short arrow), and mild dural ectasia adjacent a fatty dorsal plaque and filum terminale adhesion. (b1) AP upright L-spine radiograph showing a large sacral dysraphism with meningomyelocele (arrows). (b2) Sagittal non-fat-saturated T2 MR image of the same case showing dorsal fat (arrow) and neural placode (arrowhead). (b3) Axial CT image of the dorsal sacral defect with laterally projecting lamina. (b4) Axial non-fat-saturated T2 MR image showing meningomyelocele between multifidus muscles. (Courtesy of Dr. Lubdha Shah.)

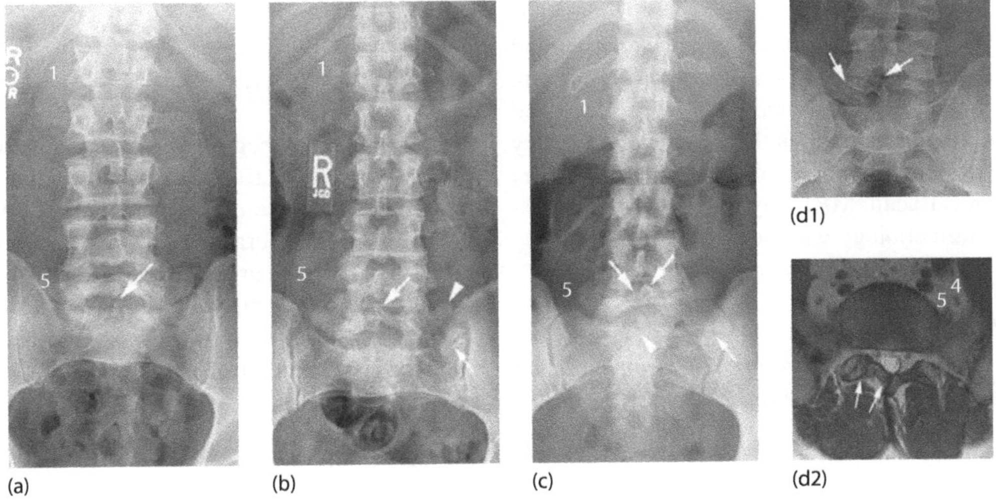

FIGURE 18.30 (a) Upright AP L-spine radiograph of a normally segmented spine with symmetrical dorsal dysraphism at L5 including an unfused spinous process ossification center centrally. The entire sacrum is dysraphic and may be associated with sacral dimple, pilonidal cyst, or tethered chord spectrum. Floating ossification centers can also be symptomatic from impingement/pseudoarthrosis. (b) A case of asymmetrical bypassing dysraphism (large arrow) with asymmetrical lumbarization of S1. The small arrow indicates a sacral transverse process to which attaches an "iliolumbar ligament." On the left, there is an assimilation joint (small arrow). (c) A case of similar appearance of left-sided hemisacralization of L5 (thoracic radiography confirms 12 ribs on the right). There is a small but otherwise normal rib outlined on the right at T12, while on the left, there is an unfused laterally projecting transverse process with a terminal ossification center typical of bone derived from the quadratus lumborum sclerotome. There is a normal transverse process on the right at L5, while on the left, there is assimilation joint (small arrow) from the development of the alar ossification center. On the left, T12 is lumbarized and L5 is sacralized. The large arrows at L5 and arrowhead at S1 show bifid spinous processes from minor dysraphism. (d1) Coned-down frontal view of another sacralized L5 vertebra with a floating laminar segment on the right due to a pars defect and midline bypassing dysraphism (arrows). (d2) Axial non-fat-saturated T2 MR image located just below the L5/S1 lateral foramen showing the floating hypoplastic right laminar segment (arrows). Note hypoplastic asymmetrical facets. The main contributions to the forming sciatic nerve in front of the sacral ala are from L4 laterally to L5 medially accounting for most of the peroneal and tibial nerves, respectively. Normally, this is L5 and S1, but in the sacralization of L5, the major spinal nerve contributions to the named lower extremity nerves originate from one level higher.[17,28]

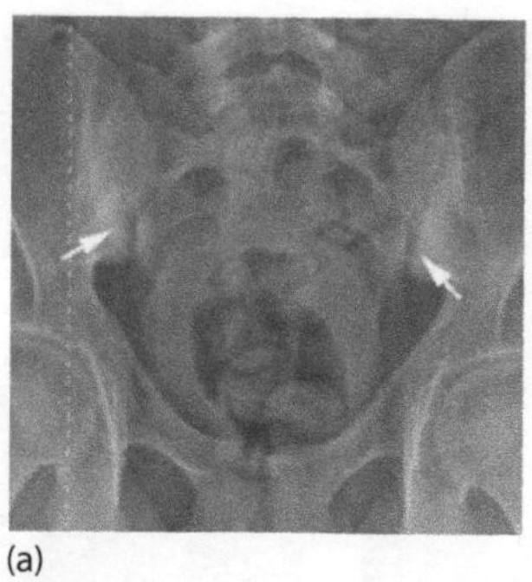

(a)

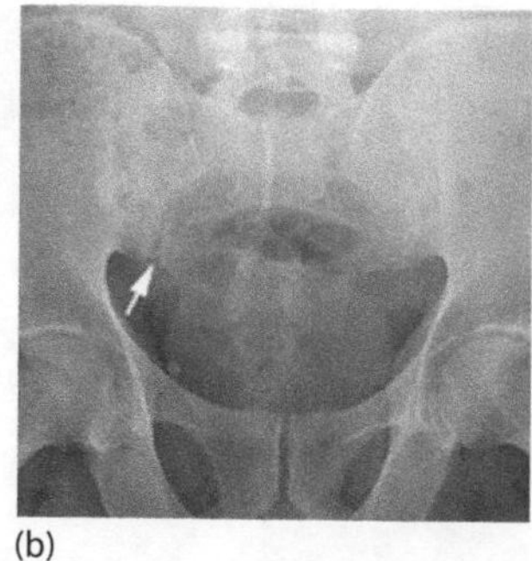

(b)

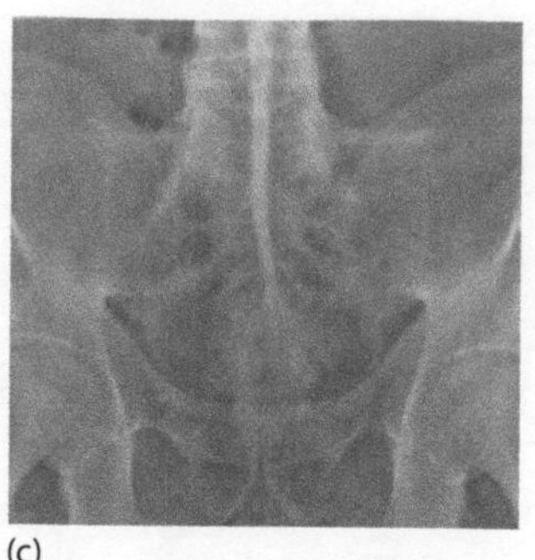

(c)

FIGURE 18.31 Images (a–c) are frontal pelvis radiographs showing the evolution of ankylosing spondylitis–related sacroiliitis. (a) In early disease, there is bilateral mildly asymmetrical sacroiliitis with iliac-sided erosions (arrows) and marked sclerosis but no appreciable ankylosis. (b) In the intermediate advanced stage, there is residual sclerosis with partial ankylosis on the right (arrow) and complete ankylosis on the left. Remnants of the SI joints are still visible as ill-defined broad lucencies. (c) In the final stage, the SI joints have been completely remodeled, and there are continuous trabecular arcades extending from the acetabula to the sacrum. The iliosacral, iliolumbar, interspinous, and supraspinous ligaments are ossified in the classic "bamboo" spine.

18.5.6 SI Joint

The imaging of the sacroiliac (SI) joints begins with a single view weight-bearing PA pelvis including acetabular joints. Pathologies visualized on radiographs may include inflammatory spondyloarthropathies, segmentation anomalies, joint erosions from infections (typically staphylococcal and gonococcal), and pelvic asymmetry secondary to leg length or ligamentous laxity from multiparity (Figures 18.2 and 18.31). CT scans may distinguish between inflammatory versus mechanical conditions. Rheumatologic erosions are well visualized on CT scan. MRI may be ordered for persistent pain of uncertain etiology with negative x-rays.

18.5.7 Sacrococcyx

Radiographs of the sacrococcyx are two views including an AP and a lateral, looking for mechanical instability, arthritis, or fracture. "Sitting fractures" typically present as a fall onto the buttocks on ice and are seen on lateral view as a transverse fracture with kyphosis, or folding, of sacrum (Figure 18.32). CT scans are generally not done. MRI may be ordered for persistent coccydynia of uncertain etiology with negative x-rays.

18.6 EXTREMITY IMAGING

Extremity imaging begins with radiographs. Ottawa knee and ankle rules may be utilized to assist in deciding when to order radiographs in the setting of acute injury (Ottawa Table 18.8 and Figure 18.33). Fractures are imaged with CT for additional detail when surgical or medical management will be impacted. MRI is employed for suspected injury, as it will visualize both bone and soft tissue abnormalities.

Arthrograms are utilized for suspected labral tears in the shoulders and hips. Arthrograms are also used in the wrist

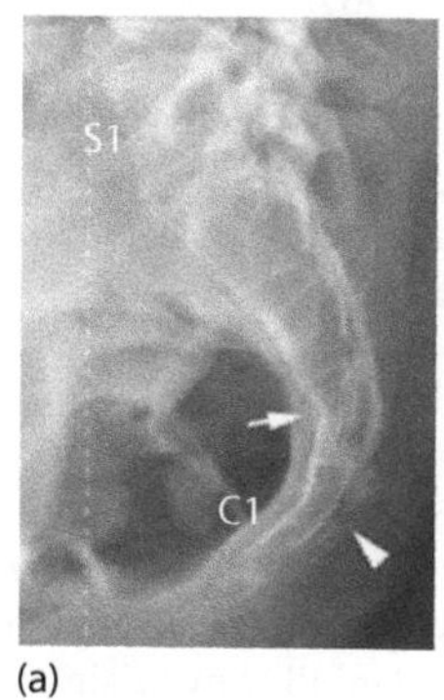

(a)

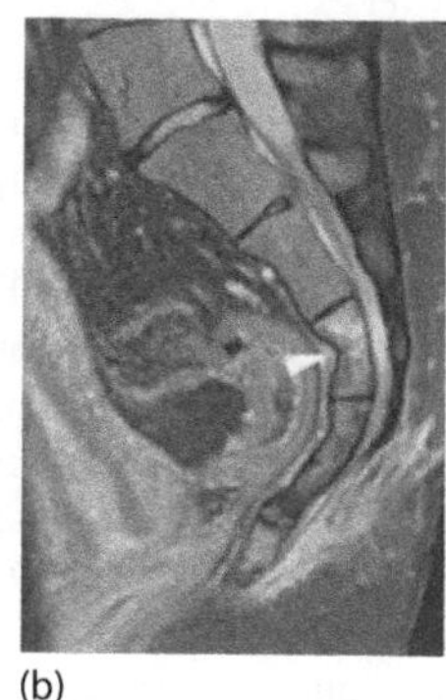

(b)

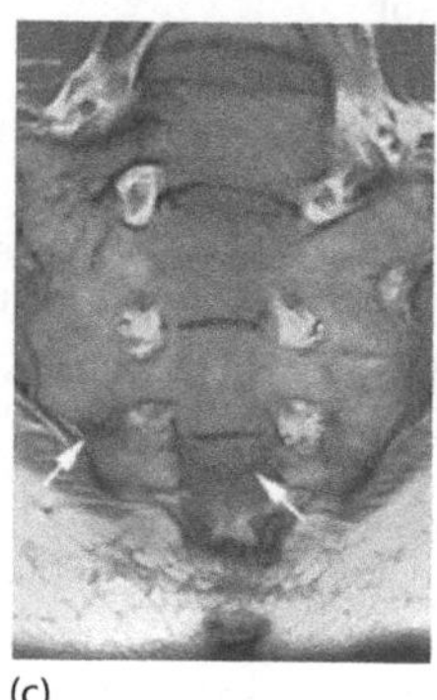

(c)

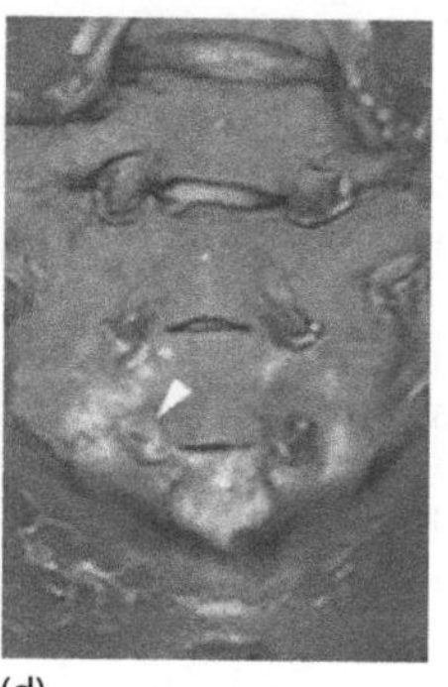

(d)

FIGURE 18.32 (a) A coned-down lateral view of the sacrum shows anterior cortical buckling (arrow) with minimal kyphosis at a transverse fracture of the superior S4 vertebra. S1 is lumbarized with a fully formed disc and failed separation/sacralization of C1 (the coccyx). The C1 cornu remains unfused to S5 (arrowhead). (b) Sagittal fat-saturated proton density MR image shows edema at the site of cortical buckling (arrowhead). Note the contusion edema in the subcutaneous tissues posterior to the inferior sacrum. (c) Coronal oblique non-fat-saturated T1 MR image shows low-signal fracture lines (arrows) partially obscured by bone edema that is dark on T1. (d) Coronal oblique fat-saturated T2 MR image shows bright edema outlining the fracture with edema/hemorrhage surrounding the S4 nerve in the arcuate foramen (arrowhead).

TABLE 18.8
Ottawa Knee Rules

Knee x-ray indications after acute knee injury
• Aged 55 years or over
• Tenderness at the head of the fibula
• Isolated tenderness of the patella
• Inability to flex knee to 90°
• Inability to bear weight (defined as an inability to take four steps, i.e., two steps on each leg, regardless of limping) immediately and at presentation
Exclusion criteria for the Ottawa rules are age <18 years, isolated superficial skin injuries, injuries more than 7 days old, recent injuries being reevaluated, and patients with altered levels of consciousness, paraplegia, or multiple injuries.

Source: Byrnes, K.R. et al., *Front. Neuroenerg.*, 5, 13, 2014; Coris, E.E. et al., *Neurosurg. Focus*, 31, E7, 2011; Yao, K. and Haque, T. *Aust. Fam. Phys.*, 41, 223, 2012.
Note: Sensitivity 100%, specificity 36%.

for suspected cartilage and ligament injuries. Some believe a 3 T or higher MRI does not require arthrogram to distinguish labral, cartilage, and ligament pathology. Consultation with your imaging center's radiology staff is advised for their recommendations based on the magnet strength, available coils, and joint-specific protocols.

IV contrast is reserved for evaluations suspicious for tumor and infection.

18.7 TUMORS

An extensive discussion of MSK tumors is beyond the scope of this chapter. Sports medicine providers should be aware that tumors might present as painful masses and pathologic fractures. Common benign lesions that may be encountered on radiography include bone islands, nonossifying fibroma (NOF)/fibrous cortical defect (FCD), osseous lipomas, and small, uncomplicated enchondromas/physeal rests (Figure 18.34: common benign lesions, bone island, NOF, osseous lipoma, enchondroma). Common tumor mimics include myositis ossificans and periosteal contusion (Figure 18.35: tumor mimics, myositis ossificans and periosteal contusion). Unless the sports medicine physician is certain that a radiographic lesion is benign and without complications, an MSK radiologist or orthopedic oncologist should be consulted.

18.8 STRESS (OVERUSE) FRACTURE IMAGING

Depending on location, stress fractures may be at higher risk for delayed union, nonunion, or completed fracture with displacement (Table 18.9). Any stress fracture with an intra-articular component is also considered high risk. In general, higher-risk stress fractures mandate more immediate radiologic imaging to confirm a clinical diagnosis and, in some cases, localize the fracture. For example, a femoral neck stress fracture localized to the compression side (without fracture line on radiographs) may be treated with a non-weight-bearing protocol, while if localized to the tension side, it could require

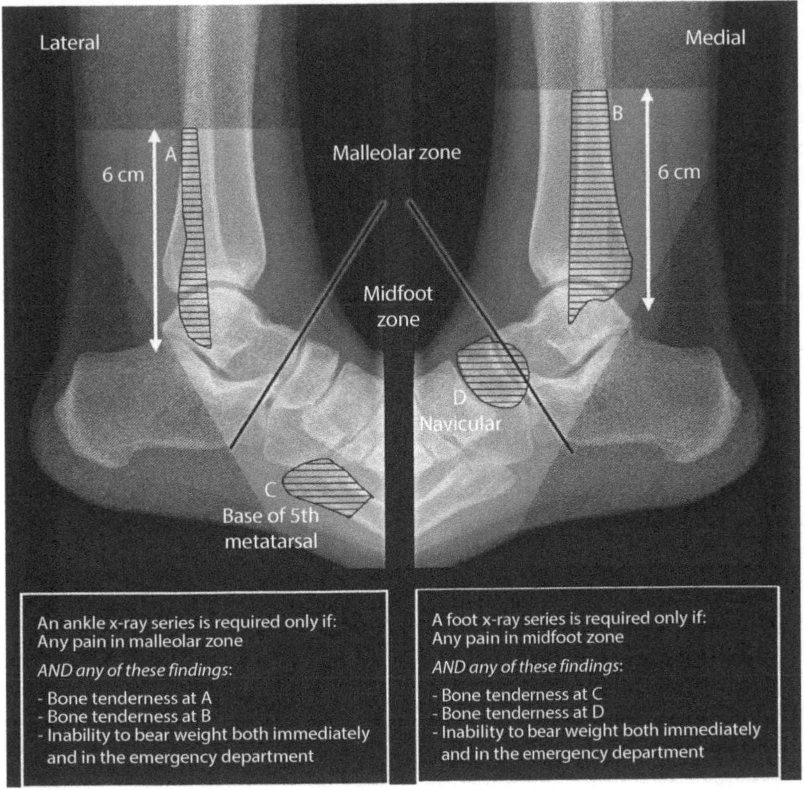

FIGURE 18.33 Ottawa ankle rules.

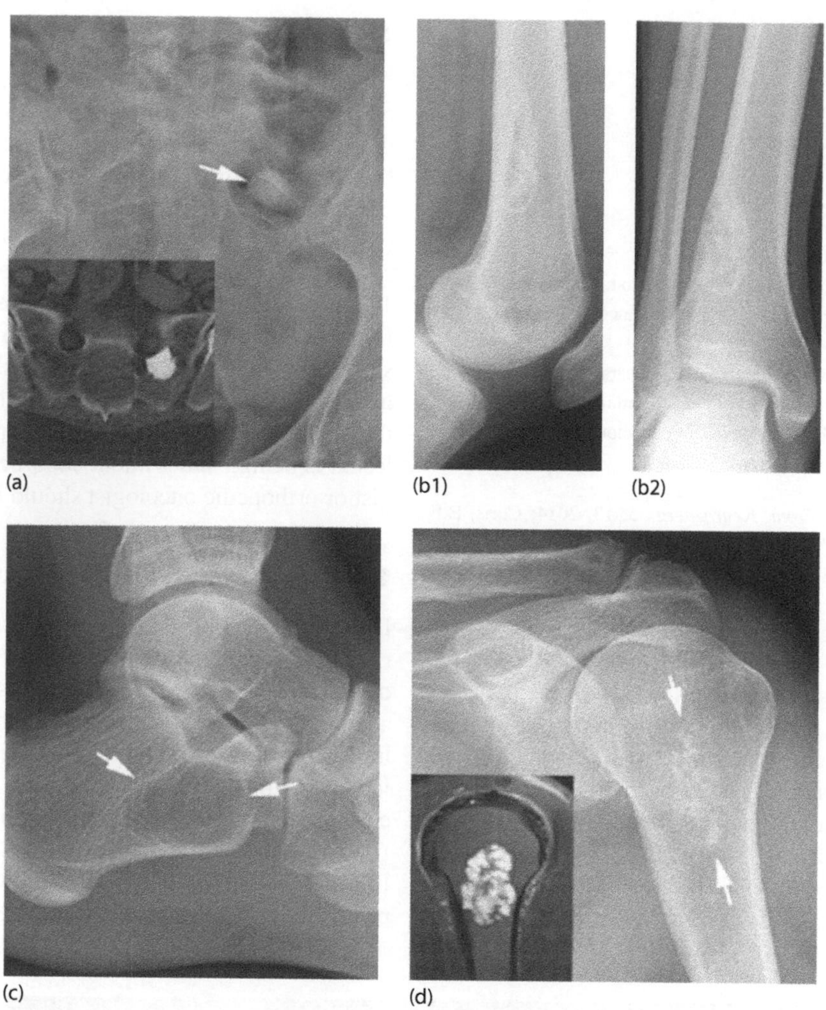

FIGURE 18.34 (a) Giant bone island (osteoma): AP radiograph of the pelvis shows a uniformly dense 2 cm mass with radiating spiculated margins (arrow) in a 65 YOF with prior history of breast cancer without metastasis. The surrounding lucency is bowel gas in sigmoid colon. Because of oncologic concerns, she underwent extensive additional workup including a CT (inset), which confirms an "ivory dense" lesion with spiculations extending into the adjacent normal trabecular arcades. (b) NOF: (b1) Lateral radiograph of the distal femur showing a well-circumscribed and peripherally sclerotic but otherwise lucent endosteal mass eccentrically located in the posterior metadiaphysis. (b2) AP radiograph of the ankle showing a nearly identical but slightly more sclerotic lesion. Despite the name, NOFs progressively ossify and become more sclerotic with age. (c) Intraosseous lipoma: Lateral radiograph of the ankle showing a typical calcaneal lipoma. Arrows show splaying of the trabecular arcades around the periphery of the lesion. (d) Enchondroma: AP radiograph of the shoulder revealing immature calcifications of an intramedullary metaphyseal enchondroma (arrows). Only a few calcifications approximate the classic "rings and arcs" of a chondroid matrix. MR is the preferred modality to further evaluate suspected chondroid lesions, particularly if they are painful. The inset shows a sagittal fat-saturated T2 MR image in which the hyaline lobules are clearly visible and show no aggressive features or fractures.

surgical fixation (Figure 18.36).[1,34,37] Stress fractures occur on a continuum, both physiologically and clinically, from early stress reactions developing into stress fractures with a distinct fracture line visible on imaging. Early radiologic diagnosis of stress reactions may be of value in some clinical situations for guiding and enforcing activity modifications to prevent progression to a complete stress fracture.[10,34]

Findings on radiographs are usually seen after 2–8 weeks of symptoms. In the early stages, the sensitivity of radiography may be as low as 10% and rise to 3%–70% at follow-up after at least 2 weeks. In early stress fractures, the most common radiographic sign is a region of focal periosteal bone formation, often subtle in nature. The gray cortex sign (a cortical area of decreased density) is also an early sign of stress fracture. Additional radiographic abnormalities may include osteopenia, endosteal reaction, ill-defined cortical margin, and, in severe cases, a discrete partial or complete fracture.[10,37] Stress fractures in cancellous bone, such as the calcaneus, usually appear as a linear band of sclerosis perpendicular to the trabeculae[5,31] (Figure 18.37).

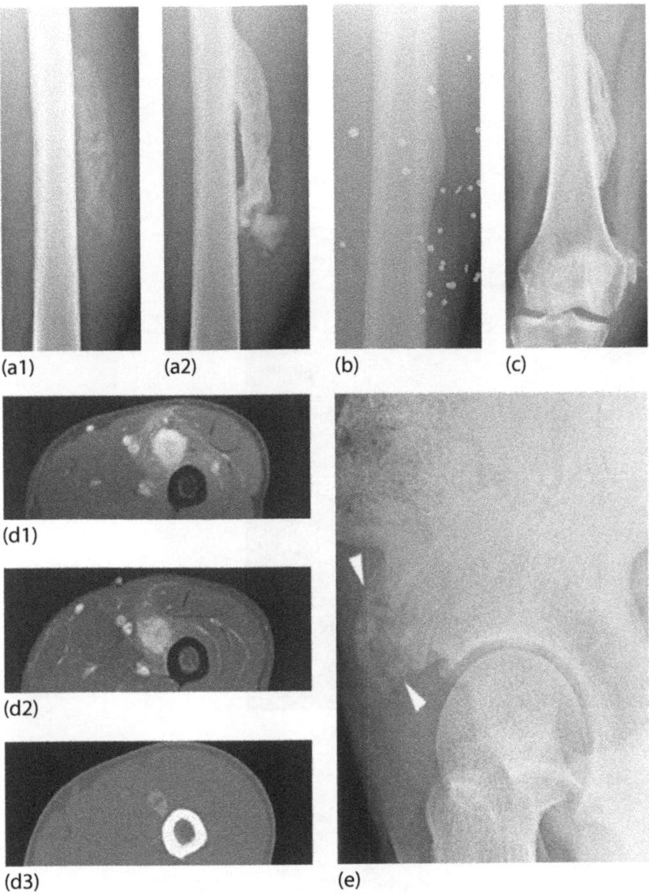

FIGURE 18.35 (a1) Lateral radiograph of the femur shows immature ossification in the vastus intermedius muscle that presented as a painful hard mass following a weight-lifting injury 2 months previously. Two years later, the myositis ossificans is fully mature with a well-established cortex and fatty medullary cavity. (b1) AP radiograph of the left midfemur shows fusiform periosteal new bone as a result of a healed periosteal/cortical contusion and shotgun wound. (c) AP radiograph of distal right femur showing focal myositis ossificans, more proximal periostitis, and MCL ossification from old medial thigh blunt trauma. (d1) Axial post-contrast fat-saturated T1 MR image showing an enhancing mass deep in the enhancing vastus medialis muscle and adjacent periosteal enhancement in a middle-aged farrier who presented with a painful palpable thigh mass but no specific injury. (d2) The follow-up MR image 2 months later shows a slight decrease in size and enhancement of the mass with progressive atrophy of the surrounding muscle. CT confirms the peripheral ossification pattern typical of myositis ossificans (d3). (e) Anterior oblique radiograph of the right anterior pelvis shows a classic hypertrophic tug lesion of the anterior inferior iliac spine apophysis (arrowheads) in a 13 YOM football player.

Nuclear medicine imaging is a more sensitive but less specific method for imaging stress fractures and can provide the diagnosis as early as 2–8 days after the onset of symptoms. There is the possibility of increased uptake in nonpainful sites, indicating subclinical accelerated remodeling. Pathological

TABLE 18.9
Critical and Less Critical Stress Fractures

High risk
Femoral neck
Anterior midtibia
Navicular
Body of talus
Proximal second metatarsal
Sesamoids
Pars interarticularis
Medium risk
Pelvis
Femoral shaft
Posterior or medial tibia
Medial malleolus
Proximal fifth metatarsal diaphysis
Low risk
Fibula/lateral malleolus
Calcaneus
Cuboid
Cuneiform
Distal metatarsals 2, 3, 4, and 5
At-risk fractures require early recognition, early and aggressive treatment, and both baseline and follow-up imaging to confirm union.

Source: Adapted from Baxter, D.E., *The Foot and Ankle in Sport*, Mosby, St Louis, 1994.

conditions such as infections and inflammatory disorders, tumors, arthropathies, or bone infarctions can also result in a positive bone scan Fredericson.[10,13] Patients are also subjected to prolonged imaging times and exposure to radiation.

CT scan is useful in differentiating conditions that mimic stress fractures on bone scan, such as osteoid osteoma, osteomyelitis with Brodie abscess, and various malignancies (as can MRI).[10] SPECT–CT scans are used to localize stress fractures in the spine, pelvis, and sacrum.

MRI provides the most comprehensive evaluation of stress injuries due to its sensitivity for stress fracture pathology, ability to precisely define the location and extent of bony injury, and its superior ability to diagnose other soft tissue injuries that present similarly to stress fractures. MRI is able to demonstrate a spectrum of bone injury from cortical or medullary edema to the presence of a distinct fracture line. MRI also has the advantage of lack of exposure to ionizing radiation and significantly less imaging time than a three-phase bone scan. Of note, asymptomatic bone marrow edema patterns or stress reactions may be present in relatively asymptomatic subjects, typically in the lower extremities of runners. The clinical relevance of these findings has been debated and underscores the importance of correlating MRI findings with clinical findings before making therapeutic decisions[10,31] (Table 18.10).

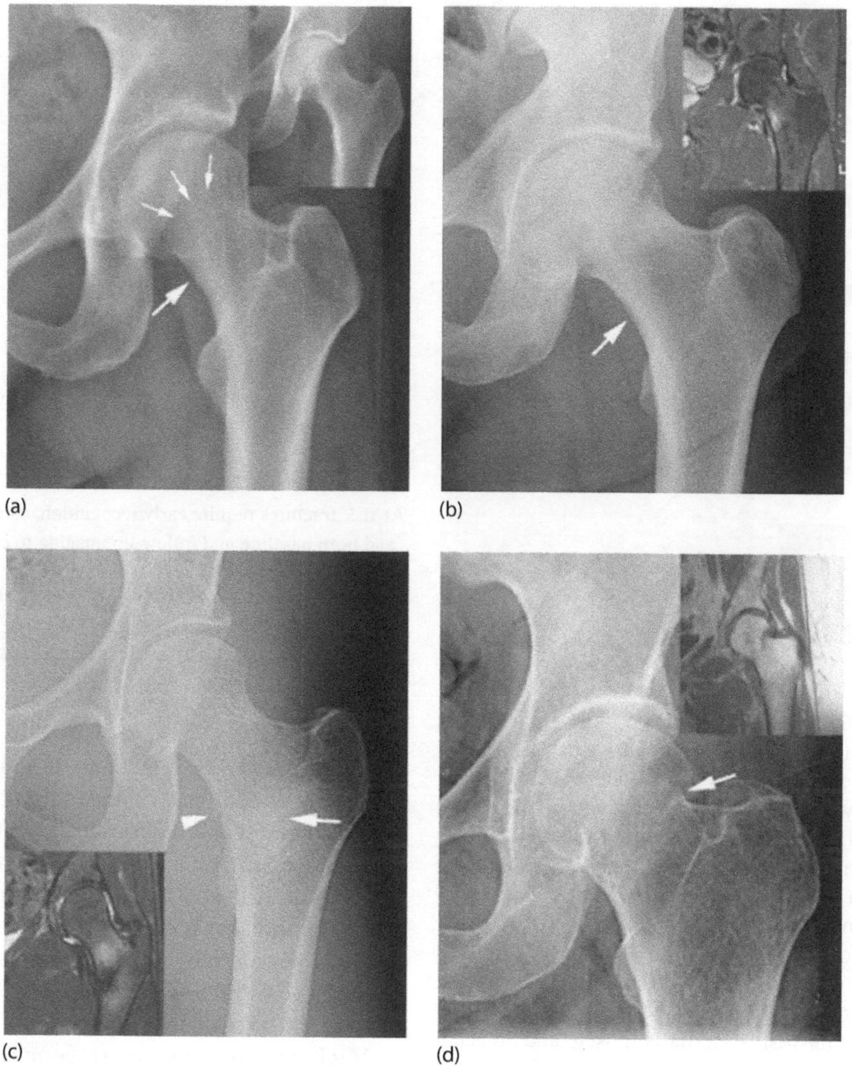

FIGURE 18.36 (a) AP hip radiograph showing successfully compensated femoral neck stress reaction with thickened inferior femoral neck cortex (large arrow) and primary compressive trabecular arcade (small arrows) in a 30 YOF runner. Compare to the inserted image of a normal femoral neck in a similar aged female. (b) Uncompensated stress reaction in which osteolysis is outpacing the blastic response and focal cortical osteopenia without transversely oriented fracturing is evident at the maximum stress riser of the inferior cervical cortex (arrow) in a 50 YOM runner. The inserted coronal postcontrast fat-saturated T1 MR image shows an enhancement parallel to the cortex in the region of active bone remodeling. A fracture is imminent. (c) Compressive failure of the femoral neck with a healing fracture (arrow) surrounded by extensive reactive sclerosis and callus at the basicervical femoral neck (arrowhead) in a 32 YOF runner. The inserted coronal TI MR image shows the dark low-signal fracture surrounded by bright marrow edema. (d) Osteopenic hip with tensile failure and valgus impaction along the subcapital superior femoral neck (arrow) in a 65 YOF. The inserted coronal non-fat-saturated T1 MR image shows the low-signal dark fracture propagating from superior to inferior.

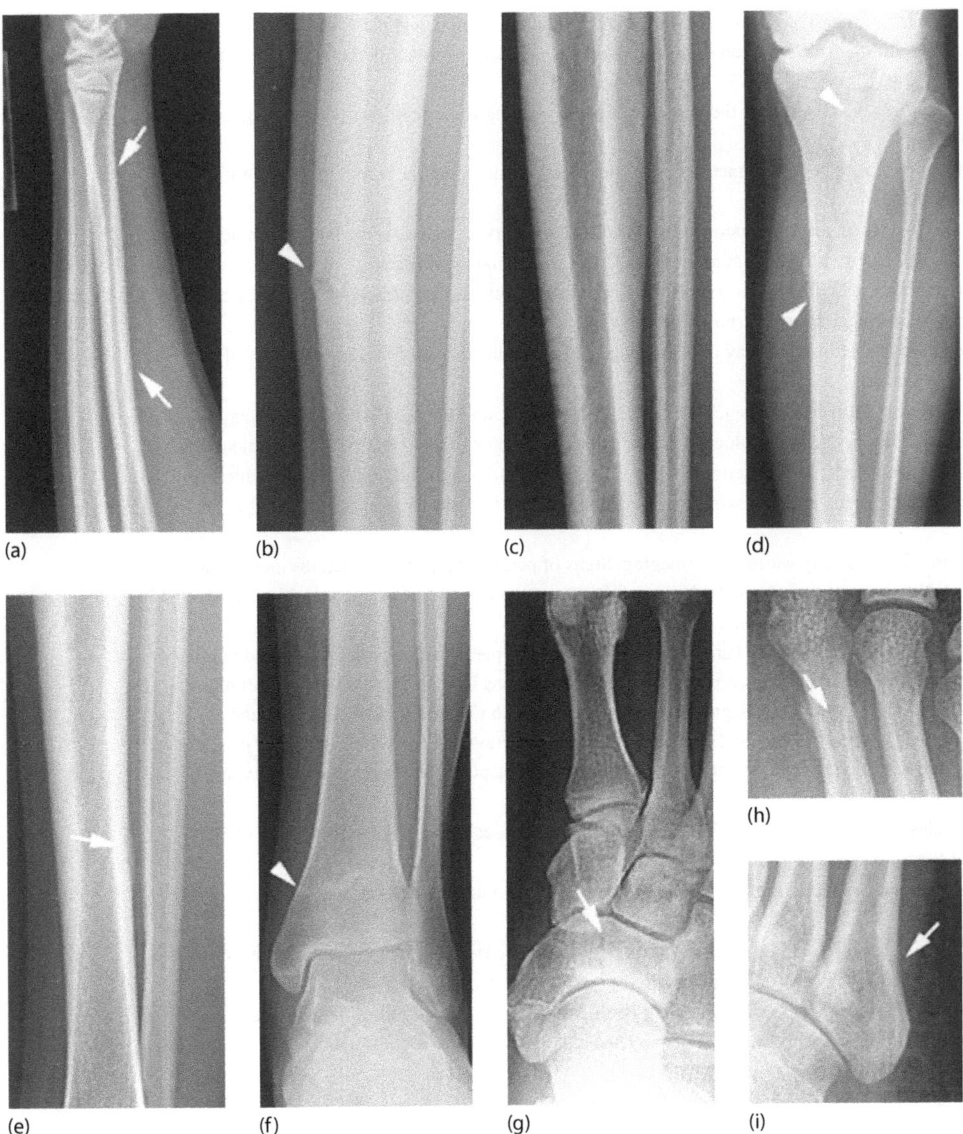

FIGURE 18.37 (a) Lateral radiograph of the forearm showing diaphyseal stress reaction with fusiform cortical thickening and narrowing of the medullary cavity (arrows) in 14 YOF cheerleader with forearm aching pain. (b) Lateral leg radiograph of the leg showing a typical chronic anterior cortical stress fracture (arrowhead) of the tibial middiaphysis in a running athlete. (c) Close-up of lateral leg radiograph with high-contrast windowing showing innumerable evolving anterior cortical tibial stress fractures sustained during aggressive triathlon training. (d) AP leg radiograph showing a healing vertical posterior cortical stress fracture of the tibia (arrowheads). (e) Lateral radiograph of the distal leg showing a healing posterior cortical stress fracture in young running athlete (arrow). (f) AP ankle radiograph showing a sclerotic transverse tibial metaphyseal stress fracture in an osteopenic female runner. (g) AP foot radiograph showing an incomplete navicular stress fracture (arrow) in a collegiate basketball player with bilateral lesions. (h) AP foot radiograph showing a healing distal second metatarsal stress fracture in a runner. (i) Oblique foot radiograph showing an early fifth metatarsal base fracture (arrow) in a hiker.

TABLE 18.10
SORT: Key Recommendations for Practice

Clinical Recommendation	Evidence Rating	References
Before utilizing sports medicine imaging, the provider should arrive at a specific diagnostic question and imaging results should influence clinical management.	C	[8,24]
Providers should remember that other biological processes, such as infection, tumor, and metabolic and rheumatologic/autoimmune disease, are commonly encountered on imaging and may clinically mimic sports injuries' physical presentations.	C	
Providers should utilize radiographs first line in the majority of MSK imaging because of their cost to diagnostic value and wide availability.	C	[8,24]
Providers should use CT to visualize complex fractures requiring additional imaging for preoperative planning or adjustment of treatment plan.	C	[8,14]
MRI is the test of choice for muscle, tendon, ligamentous, and cartilage injury as well as spine injury with neurologic deficits. Additionally, MRI comes with the great advantage of not using ionizing radiation.	C	[8,24]
Nuclear medicine scans can be used with great sensitivity to detect osteomyelitis, stress fractures, or avascular necrosis, but does lack specificity to distinguish bone turnover processes.	C	[10,31]
In the hands of a skilled provider, ultrasound may offer immediate office evaluation for MSK injuries as well as targeted in-office MSK injections.	C	[2,27]
In awake and alert patients, the National Emergency X-Radiography Utilization Study (NEXUS) criteria may be utilized when deciding whether to obtain radiological clearance of the C-spine (Table 18.5: NEXUS Clinical Criteria).	A	[4,13,14]
Providers should utilize Hanson's criteria to determine when CT scans should be utilized first line in the emergent management of acute head and spine injuries, skipping C-spine plain films in cases of severe trauma (Table 18.7: Hanson Criteria).	A	[12]
Spine fractures concerning for instability warrant CT imaging. Signs of potentially unstable fractures include two- or three-column injury, widening of the disc space, widening of the interspinous distance, or compression fractures with greater than a 50% loss of height on radiography.	C	[14]
The American College of Physicians/American Pain Society 2007 low back pain clinical guidelines should be used to determine when to image patients with low back pain. Key recommendations include the following: (1) clinicians should not routinely obtain imaging or other diagnostic tests in patients with nonspecific low back pain and (2) clinicians should perform diagnostic imaging and testing for patients with low back pain when severe or progressive neurologic deficits are present or when serious underlying conditions are suspected on the basis of history and physical examination.	A	[6]
Ottawa knee and ankle rules may be utilized to assist in deciding when to order radiographs in the setting of acute injury (Table 18.8 and Figure 18.30).	A	[8,32,41]
Higher-risk stress fractures mandate more immediate radiologic imaging to confirm a clinical diagnosis and, in some cases, localize the fracture.	C	[1,10,15,31]
Health-care providers should recognize and inform patients about cumulative risks of radiation and ensure exposure is *as low as reasonably achievable* (ALARA) without sacrificing quality of care.	C	[9]
When a provider communicates the diagnostic question and pertinent history to the radiologist prior to the scheduling of an imaging study, the radiologist may select the most targeted exam to maximize clinical value while minimizing cost and radiation risk.	C	[8,24]

REFERENCES

1. Behrens SB, Deren ME, Matson A, Fadale PD, Monchik KO. Stress fractures of the pelvis and legs in athletes: A review. *Sports Health: A Multidisciplinary Approach.* 2013;5(2):165–174.
2. Birrer RB, O'Connor FG. *Sports Medicine for the Primary Care Physician*, 3rd edn. Boca Raton, FL: CRC Press; 2004.
3. Blackmore CC, Emerson SS, Mann FA, Koepsell TD. Cervical spine imaging in patients with trauma: Determination of fracture risk to optimize use. *Radiology.* 1999;211(3):759–765.
4. Bogner EA. Imaging of cervical spine injuries in athletes. *Sports Health.* 2009;1(5):384–391.
5. Byrnes KR, Wilson CM, Brabazon F et al. FDG-PET imaging in mild traumatic brain injury: A critical review. *Frontiers in Neuroenergetics.* 2014;5:13.
6. Chou R, Qaseem A, Snow V et al. Diagnosis and treatment of low back pain: A joint clinical practice guideline from the American College of Physicians and the American Pain Society. *Annals of Internal Medicine.* October 2, 2007;147(7):478–491.
7. Clark AJ, Auguste KI, Sun PP. Cervical spinal stenosis and sports-related cervical cord neurapraxia. *Neurosurgical Focus.* 2011;31(5):E7.
8. Coris EE, Zwygart K, Fletcher M, Pescasio M. Imaging in sports medicine: An overview. *Sports Medicine and Arthroscopy Review.* 2009;17(1):2–12.

9. Fazel R, Krumholz HM, Wang Y et al. Exposure to low-dose ionizing radiation from medical imaging procedures. *The New England Journal of Medicine*. 2009;361(9):849–857.
10. Fredericson M, Jennings F, Beaulieu C, Matheson GO. Stress fractures in athletes. *Topics in Magnetic Resonance Imaging: TMRI*. 2006;17(5):309–325.
11. Haldeman S, Kohlbeck FJ, McGregor M. Risk factors and precipitating neck movements causing vertebrobasilar artery dissection after cervical trauma and spinal manipulation. *Spine*. 1999;24(8):785–794.
12. Hanson JA, Blackmore CC, Mann FA, Wilson AJ. Cervical spine injury: A clinical decision rule to identify high-risk patients for helical CT screening. *American Journal of Roentgenology*. 2000;174(3):713–717.
13. Hoffman JR, Mower WR, Wolfson AB, Todd KH, Zucker MI. Validity of a set of clinical criteria to rule out injury to the cervical spine in patients with blunt trauma. National Emergency X-Radiography Utilization Study Group. *The New England Journal of Medicine*. 2000;343(2):94–99.
14. Hollenberg GM, Beitia AO, Tan RK, Weinberg EP, Adams MJ. Imaging of the spine in sports medicine. *Current Sports Medicine Reports*. 2003;2(1):33–40.
15. Hosey RG, Fernandez MMF, Johnson DL. Evaluation and management of stress fractures of the pelvis and sacrum. *Orthopedics*. 2008;31(4):383–385.
16. Jeyamohan S, Harrop JS, Vaccaro A, Sharan AD. Athletes returning to play after cervical spine or neurobrachial injury. *Current Reviews in Musculoskeletal Medicine*. 2008;1(3–4):175–179.
17. Kim YH, Lee PB, Lee CJ, Lee SC, Kim YC, Huh J. Dermatome variation of lumbosacral nerve roots in patients with transitional lumbosacral vertebrae. *Anesthesia and Analgesia*. 2008;106(4):1279–1283.
18. Laker SR, Concannon LG. Radiologic evaluation of the neck: A review of radiography, ultrasonography, computed tomography, magnetic resonance imaging, and other imaging modalities for neck pain. *Physical Medicine and Rehabilitation Clinics of North America*. 2011;22(3):411–28–vii–viii.
19. Lee KP, Carlini WG, McCormick GF, Albers GW. Neurologic complications following chiropractic manipulation: A survey of California neurologists. *Neurology*. 1995;45(6):1213–1215.
20. Leone A, Cianfoni A, Cerase A, Magarelli N, Bonomo L. Lumbar spondylolysis: A review. *Skeletal Radiology*. 2010; 40(6):683–700.
21. Mettler FA, Huda W, Yoshizumi TT, Mahesh M. Effective doses in radiology and diagnostic nuclear medicine: A catalog. *Radiology*. 2008;248(1):254–263.
22. Moeller JL. Pelvic and hip apophyseal avulsion injuries in young athletes. *Current Sports Medicine Reports*. 2003; 2(2):110–115.
23. Montgomery SP, Erwin WE. Scheuermann's kyphosis—Long-term results of Milwaukee braces treatment. *Spine*. 1981; 6(1):5–8.
24. Orchard JW, Read JW, Anderson IJF. The use of diagnostic imaging in sports medicine. *The Medical Journal of Australia*. 2005;183(9):482–486.
25. Paajanen H, Alanen A, Erkintalo M, Salminen JJ, Katevuo K. Disc degeneration in Scheuermann disease. *Skeletal Radiology*. 1989;18(7):523–526.
26. Rothwell DM, Bondy SJ, Williams JI. Chiropractic manipulation and stroke: A population-based case-control study. *Stroke; A Journal of Cerebral Circulation*. 2001;32(5):1054–1060.
27. Seidenberg PH, Beutler AI. *The Sports Medicine Resource Manual*. Philadelphia, PA: Saunders; 2008.
28. Seyfert S. Dermatome variations in patients with transitional vertebrae. *Journal of Neurology, Neurosurgery, and Psychiatry*. 1997;63(6):801–803.
29. Smith WS, Johnston SC, Skalabrin EJ et al. Spinal manipulative therapy is an independent risk factor for vertebral artery dissection. *Neurology*. 2003;60(9):1424–1428.
30. Smith DH, Johnson VE, Stewart W. Chronic neuropathologies of single and repetitive TBI: Substrates of dementia? *Nature Publishing Group*. 2013;9(4):211–221.
31. Sofka CM. Imaging of stress fractures. *Clinics in Sports Medicine*. 2006;25(1):53–62–viii.
32. Stiell IG, McKnight RD, Greenberg GH et al. Implementation of the Ottawa ankle rules. *Journal of the American Medical Association*. 1994;271(11):827–832.
33. Swischuk LE. *Imaging of the Cervical Spine in Children*. New York: Springer Science & Business Media;2002.
34. Toledo E, Lebel A, Becerra L et al. The young brain and concussion: Imaging as a biomarker for diagnosis and prognosis. *Neuroscience and Biobehavioral Reviews*. 2012;36(6):1510–1531.
35. Torg JS, Naranja RJ, Pavlov H, Galinat BJ, Warren R, Stine RA. The relationship of developmental narrowing of the cervical spinal canal to reversible and irreversible injury of the cervical spinal cord in football players. *The Journal of Bone and Joint Surgery. American Volume*. 1996;78(9):1308–1314.
36. Tribus CB. Scheuermann's kyphosis in adolescents and adults: Diagnosis and management. *The Journal of the American Academy of Orthopaedic Surgeons*. 1998;6(1):36–43.
37. Valerio J, Illes J. Ethical implications of neuroimaging in sports concussion. *The Journal of Head Trauma Rehabilitation*. 2013;27(3):216–221.
38. Weiss HR, Turnbull D, Bohr S. Brace treatment for patients with Scheuermann's disease—A review of the literature and first experiences with a new brace design. *Scoliosis*. 2009;4:1–17.
39. Wenger DR, Frick SL. Scheuermann kyphosis. *Spine*. 1999;24(24):2630–2639.
40. Wheeless CR. *Wheeless' Textbook of Orthopaedics*; 1996. Available at http://www.wheelessonline.com/.
41. Yao K, Haque T. The Ottawa knee rules—A useful clinical decision tool. *Australian Family Physician*. 2012; 41(4):223–224.

19 Musculoskeletal Ultrasound

Sean W. Mulvaney

CONTENTS

TABLE 19.1
Key Clinical Considerations

1. Musculoskeletal ultrasound is a valuable skill for the optimal performance of musculoskeletal medicine and is used to diagnose injuries to ligaments, tendons, muscles, bones, and nerves.
2. Musculoskeletal ultrasound is a safe point-of-care imaging modality.
3. Musculoskeletal ultrasound–guided procedures are more accurate and more efficacious than nonguided (clinically guided) injections.
4. Musculoskeletal ultrasound is a skill that takes time and training to achieve a baseline competency.
5. Musculoskeletal ultrasound has many specific advantages over other imaging modalities, including improved safety, readily available comparison views of the unaffected side, and the ability to look at a structure with multiple views including dynamic and resisted view.

19.1 INTRODUCTION

Musculoskeletal (MSK) ultrasound (US) is used to diagnose injuries to ligaments, tendons, muscles, bones, and nerves.[32] Although the physical exam is the standard approach to any MSK injury, some aspects of the physical exam lack of both sensitivity and specificity,[33] including even being able to accurately palpate a knee joint line or an acromioclavicular joint.[27] There are many advantages to utilizing MSK US including the ability of the provider performing the evaluation of the patient to perform the diagnostic imaging at the point of care,[31] the ability to perform a dynamic exam, the ability to find many MSK injuries with the same or better accuracy as a magnetic resonance imaging (MRI)[11,35] (at a significant reduction in cost), and the ability to accurately guide percutaneous treatments,[32] all with improved safety over other imaging modalities. As the cost of US machines becomes more affordable and the image quality continues to improve, physicians that have MSK US as a portion of their practice will realize clear benefits (Table 19.1).

19.2 ADVANTAGES OF MUSCULOSKELETAL ULTRASOUND

One of the chief benefits of diagnostic US is having it available at the point of care instead of as a separate medical event, as is the case with other imaging modalities.[19] Elements of the history and physical exam help the clinician form a differential diagnosis. This differential diagnosis focuses on the US exam and helps confirm or eliminate potential etiologies of the patients' pain in the same visit, especially when delays impact the quality of care, such as confirming Achilles tendon ruptures (see Figures 19.1 and 19.2).

Comparison views of the unaffected side are readily available, which in the case of anatomic variations or comparing growth plates in children may be critical to making a correct diagnosis. Many US units are portable, allowing one machine to serve more than one exam room or even one location. Diagnostic US has been shown to be a sensitive, specific, and cost-effective means to diagnose many common MSK disorders.[20,25,26]

Clinical Pearl

Using US to compare a painful limb to the unaffected side facilitates rapid initial assessment of growth plates in suspected fractures in skeletally immature patients.

The ability of US to perform a real-time dynamic exam of a soft-tissue structure in motion, or while under tension, is unique in medical imaging. Many movement disorders and soft-tissue disruptions are only apparent while the injured structure is in motion either with or without resistance;[15] compare this to MRI where the structure of interest is usually only available in a single static nonstressed view. US has been found to be as accurate as MRI in the detection of rotator cuff tears[35] (see Figures 19.3 and 19.4).

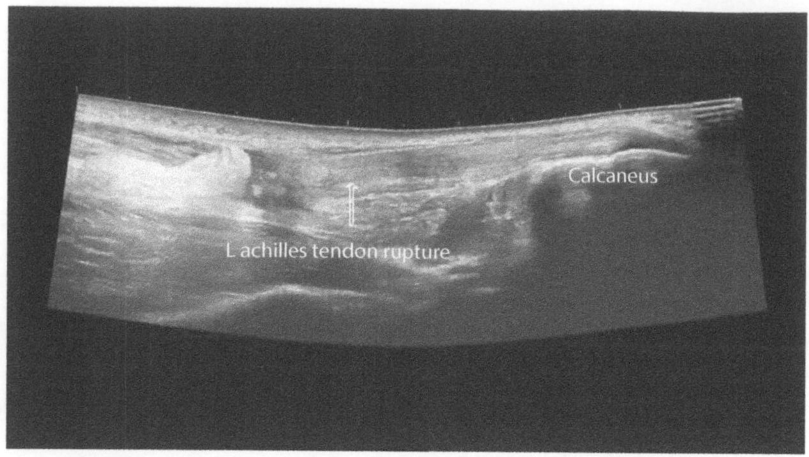

FIGURE 19.1 Achilles tendon rupture in long axis.

US imaging is thought to be safe even in children and neonates.[1] There are no known significant adverse effects of US imaging. Although this is our current understanding of US, it is prudent to use US only when medically indicated and even then adhering to the ALARA (as low as reasonably achievable) principle for US exposure. US is safe especially when compared to other imaging modalities; x-ray and computerized tomography (CT) scan have significant exposure to ionizing radiation with its well-documented risks of iatrogenic neoplasms.[2] The use of iodinated contrast is associated with anaphylactic shock.[7] MRI, although still thought to be safe, is being evaluated for previously unrecognized risks,[3] and this is beyond the risks associated with gadolinium contrast used in MRI and its association with gadolinium-associated nephrogenic systemic fibrosis.[29]

With the possible exception of CT guidance, with its significant ionizing radiation, for certain injections, US is unmatched for precisely guiding needles to soft-tissue pathology.[13,14] It has also been found to be as useful and accurate for many injections previously done under fluoroscopic or CT guidance, including some spine applications.[16,17] Although skills at accurately guiding a needle need to be developed first, needle guidance is relatively straightforward and allows for confirmation of needle placement in the tissue or joint of interest. Using precisely guided low-volume (1–2 mL of 1% lidocaine) diagnostic blocks can help determine the patients' specific pain generator in situations where several etiologies of the patients' pain are possible.

US also enjoys a significant cost savings over other soft-tissue imagining modalities such as CT or MRI.[31] US is not effected by, nor does it effect, metallic implants. US can safely and accurately assess tissue around artificial joints and implanted medical devices. Fluids, such as hematomas or joint/bursa effusions, are readily visible and easily aspirated with US.

US is excellent for imaging nerves and locating nerve injuries[23,34] and does not have the multiweek delay from acute injuries that are required for accurate assessment with

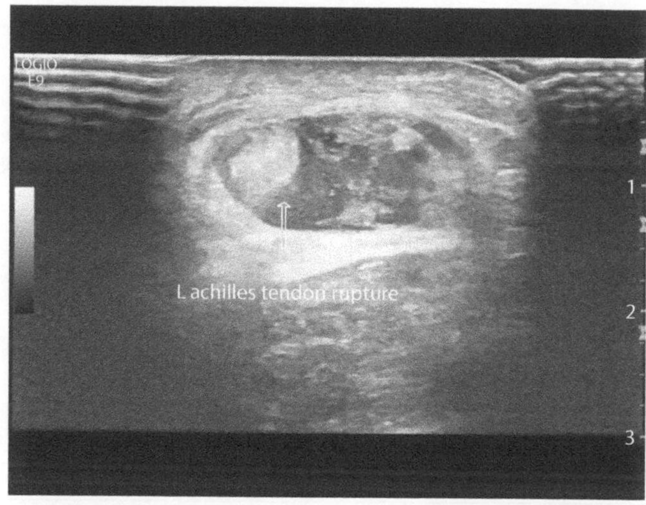

FIGURE 19.2 Achilles tendon rupture in short axis.

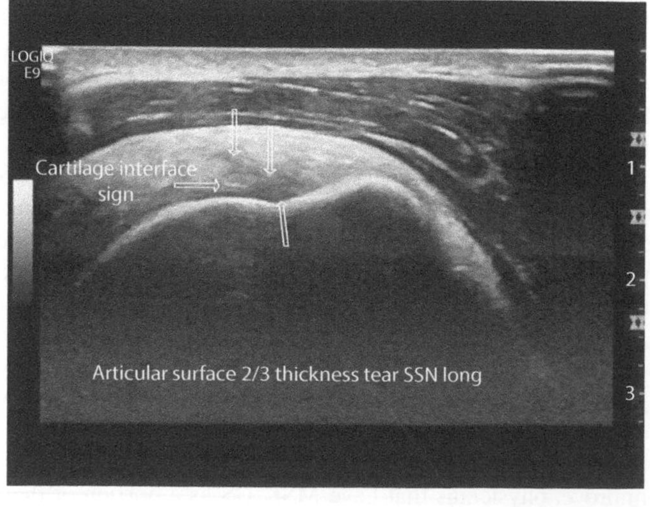

FIGURE 19.3 Supraspinatus tendon partial thickness tear in long axis.

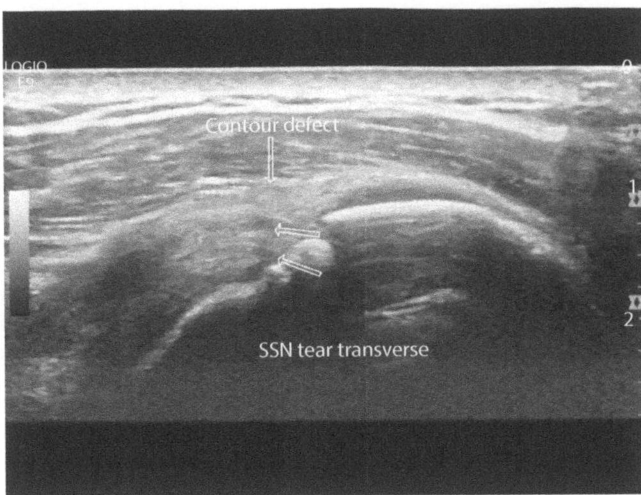

FIGURE 19.4 Supraspinatus tendon partial thickness tear in short axis.

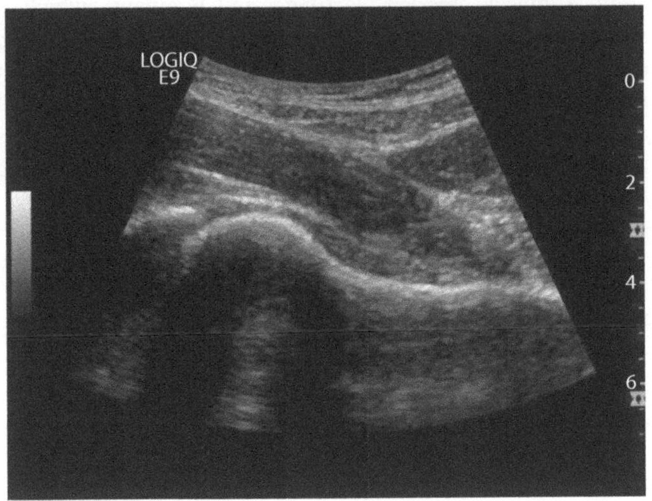

FIGURE 19.5 Normal hip in long axis.

nerve conduction studies.[6] In many cases, nerve cross-sectional area correlates with electromyography data to confirm a peripheral neuropathy.[36] US is especially useful and straightforward for venous or arterial vascular access for blood draws or catheter placement, especially on patients that were previously "hard sticks" (see Figures 19.5 and 19.6).

19.3 LIMITATIONS OF MUSCULOSKELETAL ULTRASOUND

Most US limitations stem from the physics of using sound reflections to construct a real-time image. Chief among US limitations is the signal attenuation that is associated from the increased distance the US pulse has to travel in large or obese patients. This increased sound attenuation results in decreased image resolution and needle visualization in larger patients. US waves do not efficiently transmit through interfaces between areas of significantly different densities, such as between soft-tissue structures and bowel gas, or between soft tissue and bone. US can only outline the surface of osseous structures, and although in some cases this can be used to positively identify fractures, US cannot be used to rule out or further characterize fractures. For some types of fractures, such as rib fractures, US is at least as accurate at identifying a fracture as x-ray. In many cases, intra-articular and labral pathology is difficult to identify with US and the exam is limited; however, this limitation can be mitigated somewhat by specific views and dynamic exams. In the case of the knee meniscus, US was found to be as accurate as MRI for identifying meniscal tears.[11]

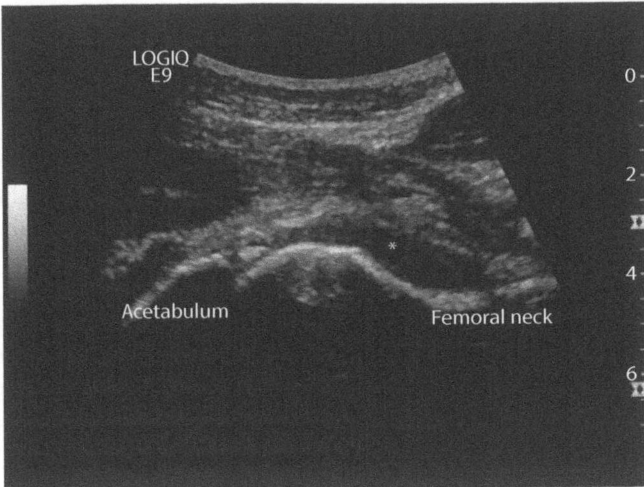

FIGURE 19.6 Hip with effusion in long axis.

Clinical Pearl

Recent studies have found US to be at least as accurate as MRI for identifying rotator cuff tears and knee meniscal tears.

Aside from the limitations of using sound waves for medical imaging, there are other limitations with US. Becoming a proficient MSK sonographer and proficient at US-guided injections requires a significant investment in time, effort, and, in many cases, money. Even if you are already very familiar with MSK anatomy and the anatomy in orthopedic surgical planes, there is still a significant learning curve with understanding the specific cross-sectional anatomy, in multiple planes, in standard US images. There are many MSK courses available, with varying quality and costs. However, it will require many hours of hands-on application of MSK US to develop even basic scanning skills. A good-quality portable US with two transducers can cost up to $40,000 or more. Another limitation is that even if you correctly identify surgical pathology on your exam, and obtain and record excellent images, the orthopedic surgeon may require an MRI in addition to your scan report (unless the surgeon is well known to you and you have a history of accurate exams with their patients).

19.4 KEY ELEMENTS OF ULTRASOUND PHYSICS

A basic understanding of the physics in US is important for understanding both how to properly adjust the US machine and how to properly interpret the US image. MSK US is based on the physics of sound as the transducer-generated sound waves pass through soft tissue and then reflects back to the transducer. Piezoelectric crystals arranged on the transducer vibrate and produce sound waves when electrical current passes through them. These emitted sound waves travel through the soft tissue, and a small fraction of these waves are reflected back to the transducer, which is no longer emitting, but in a listening mode. When the reflected sound waves return to the transducer, they vibrate the piezoelectric crystals, which produce an electric current that is processed by the US machine to construct an image in near real time.

The resolution or quality of the US image depends on both lateral resolution and axial resolution. Lateral resolution is the ability to detect structures that are parallel to the transducer footprint (to determine between two reflectors side by side at the same depth). Axial resolution is the ability to resolve structures in line with the transducer footprint (in the same axis at different depths). The number of piezoelectric crystal elements (also referred to as lines of sight) on a transducer determines the lateral resolution. The number of crystals is fixed at the time of manufacture and largely determines the cost and quality of a transducer and ultimately the quality of the US image. The elements (lines of sight) can all fire at once, creating a sound wave that travels straight down, but they can also be fired in close sequence from right to left and left to right to create sounds wave fronts that advance at a diagonal to the transducer face. These diagonal waves help a linear transducer footprint create multiple wave fronts that create an image with much more detail than is possible with one (straight down) wave front. By having the computing power to process these multiple reflecting lines of sight, the software is able to generate a significantly more detailed 2D image on the display screen. This sequence processing is referred to as "multibeam" or "crossbeam" imaging.

Axial resolution is the ability to resolve between two reflectors in line with the transducer footprint (in the same axis at different depths) and is limited by the physics of sound. Although high-frequency waves produce better axial resolution, they lose energy more quickly as the emitted sound strikes more reflectors (tissues) and the emitted wave is more rapidly attenuated. Attenuation of the emitted sound wave is the result of the loss of energy, due to refraction, reflections, absorption, and friction (heat production). Higher frequency sound waves result in improved resolution but less tissue penetration. By using lower-frequency sound waves, the emitted sound wave will hit fewer reflectors as it goes deeper into tissue and will be subject to less attenuation; however, it will have less axial resolution. Achieving the optimal balance between resolution (high frequency) and penetration (lower frequency) is required to achieve the best image of a structure at a given depth.

Clinical Pearl

Higher frequencies produce US images with better resolution and are suited to shallow targets within 3 cm of the skin. Lower frequencies are less subject to attenuation and have better penetration producing better images of deeper targets.

This limitation in axial resolution is due to the limitations imposed by the formula:

$$\text{Constant} = \text{Frequency} \times \text{Wavelength}.$$

The constant used is the velocity of sound in tissue (dermis, adipose, muscle, tendon, cartilage, and ligament), which is approximately 1540 m/s. Frequency refers to the time between emissions of sound waves. Since the position of any object measured with US can be determined only to an accuracy of about one wavelength, the limitation on image resolution is imposed by wavelength. The resolution required in diagnostic US is 1 mm or less.

$$\text{Therefore, Frequency} = \text{Constant/Wavelength}.$$

In this case, frequency = 1540 m/s per 0.001 m, which equals 1.54×10^6 m/s or 1.54 mHz. Therefore, 1.54 mHz will yield a resolution of about 1 mm before significant attenuation degrades this.

Contemporary transducer technology emits multiple (broadband) frequencies near simultaneously to generate the most useful real-time US image by maximizing potential resolution (using some higher frequencies) and penetration (using some lower frequencies). The particular mix of high and low frequencies may be manually or automatically selected depending on the particular US machine used. The mix of frequencies is based on the depth of the structure of interest, with the frequencies emitted for deeper structures viewed weighted toward lower frequencies and vice versa with superficial structures.

19.4.1 Anisotropy

Anisotropy is an angle-dependent artifact that produces an appearance of false absence in a fibrillar structure that is actually present. Artifacts are any visible structures in an image that do not correlate directly with the actual tissue. US best interprets echosignatures when the transducer is positioned directly perpendicular to a structure. The artificial lack of signal (artifact) caused by the loss of perpendicular positioning is termed *anisotropy* and is a significant challenge in interpreting MSK US.

Clinical Pearl

Understanding how the artifact of anisotropy affects the US image is the critical step in avoiding incorrect interpretation of the US image. Failure to understand artifact leads to incorrect diagnosis of tendon tears, interpreting tendons as being absent when they are present, or even diagnosing the anechoic ellipse on the image as a fluid-filled cyst.

Anisotropy is an artifact producing property of compact bundles of fibers as found in ligaments, tendon, muscle, and nerve tissue. Anisotropy is the most important artifact in MSK US and should always be considered when viewing a potential tear in a structure. An anisotropic artifact can be produced with tilts of the transducer as small as 3°–7° perpendicular to the axis of the fibrillar structure being viewed. Anisotropy can be produced both longitudinal and transverse to the fibrillar tissue and is particularly pronounced on curving fibular structures, such as the curving insertion of a tendon or ligament. One of the techniques for determining if a hypoechoic area in a tendon is a tear is to keep the transducer perpendicular to the tendon (not the skin surface) as it curves into an insertion, in addition to viewing the suspect structure in an orthogonal view. The physics behind anisotropy is not completely understood; however, we do know that the greater the fibrillar or fascicular density of the tissue, the more sensitive that tissue is to the artifact of anisotropy. This property can be useful and can assist in determining tissue type when viewed with US. The order of common MSK tissues from most subject to anisotropy to least subject to anisotropy is as follows: ligament (very compact), tendon (compact), muscle (loosely compact), and nerve (very loosely compact).

19.4.2 Volume Averaging

Volume averaging is another essential concept that is necessary to interpreting a US image. The transducer emits a relatively thin 3D shaft of sound, about 1 mm thick. The input from this 3D "shaft of sound" is processed and "volume averaged" to a 2D image on the US display. During this processing of 3D data to a 2D constructed image, some of the data are lost or "averaged out." Volume averaging explains why partial thickness tears require an astute sonographer to identify them, because if 25% of the tendon under the transducer is absent or torn, the processed image may still appear to be normal. Perhaps that torn section of tendon would appear slightly more hypoechoic (darker) than the surrounding tendon. This relative hypoechoic state is due to reduced attenuation as the sound passes through the area of decreased tissue (the tear). When 50% of the tendon is torn, the image would look fairly normal in gross structure but more hypoechoic and less fibrillar than the surrounding normal tendon. When 75% of the tendon under the transducer is torn, the image appears significantly more hypoechoic but still appears to have a small amount of tendon echotexture. Understanding volume averaging explains how an abnormal tendon can appear relatively normal.

One of the more potentially frustrating consequences of volume averaging is that needle visualization can be challenging. When a needle is guided under the probe in long axis or "in plane," needle visualization is expected. However, due to volume averaging unless the needle in precisely in the center of the thin shaft of sound projected from the transducer, the needle may not be visualized. If the needle is placed on the outer 25% (right or left) of the projected sound slice, the needle is volume averaged out of the display image and not visible.

19.4.3 Through Transmission Enhancement

When a sound wave passes through relatively less echodense material, it will be less subjected to attenuation and will result in a relatively stronger reflection back to the transducer. For example, if a sound wave passes through a fluid-filled cyst lying over a bone, the image of the bone beneath the fluid-filled cyst will appear brighter than the adjacent bone. In the case of a tear in a tendon, the structure immediately deep to this tear will exhibit a relatively hyperechoic (brighter) echosignature. Through transmission enhancement is useful to help identify partial thickness tears, fluid interfaces, and tenosynovitis. In the case of a defect in a tendon overlying cartilage, through transmission enhancement produces an artifact of a more intense hyperechoic signal beneath the defect referred to as "crescent sign" or "cartilage interface sign."

19.4.4 Ultrasound Image

Echosignature of bone, ligaments, tendons, muscles, and other soft tissues is based on the degree of absorption versus reflection of the sound waves. On a US image, tissues are described as anechoic (black on the US display) (e.g., hyaline cartilage or fluid), hypoechoic (nearly black or blacker than the surrounding structures), echoic (tendon), and mixed echogenicity (muscle). Isoechoic refers to tissues of similar densities, while hyperechoic tissue appears as white or nearly white on the US display (e.g., cortical surfaces, dense fascial layers, or metallic hardware).

The US appearances of different MSK tissues have specific standard descriptions. Muscles in transverse (short axis) have a "starry night" appearance, while in longitudinal are described as having a pinnate pattern. Muscles are further described as having a loosely compact (fibrillar) pattern. Tendons in transverse and longitudinal have a compact fibrillar pattern. Ligaments in transverse have a very compact fibrillar pattern, while in longitudinal are classically described as having a "trilaminar" (white–black–white) appearance. Nerves in transverse are described as having a "fascicular" or "bundle of grapes" appearance, while in longitudinal view, nerves are described as having a "striated" (unevenly stripped) fascicular appearance.

19.5 ULTRASOUND EQUIPMENT AND SETTINGS

There are many excellent portable US machines currently available. Some machines will have more simplified controls available to adjust an image, which is an advantage to the new sonographer, while other machines will have the standard controls for diagnostic US machines that allow the skilled sonographer more flexibility to refine the US image. Here are the five key adjustments common to most US machines that will usually get you an acceptable image:

Depth adjustment: The depth should be increased or decreased to cover only the tissue of interest as well as any key boney landmarks used to confirm the anatomy. The idea is to have the tissue of interest in view without extraneous tissue in the image.

Gain: Gain adjusts the intensity of the acoustic pulse emitted by the piezoelectric crystals with the result being a stronger echo return. Increasing gain can enhance the detection of weak reflectors. Gain determines the brightness or darkness of the US image. Think of gain like you would turn up the volume on a stereo. If the room is noisy (brightly lit), you may need more volume (signal intensity) to hear the music. However, if the volume is too loud, you will miss the nuances of the music, just as your image will be too coarse with too much (inappropriate) gain. This is why the typical diagnostic US suite is dimly lit, so the sonographer can achieve the highest quality (nuanced) image. When performing procedures in a well-lit room, increasing the gain is appropriate and generally will not significantly degrade the image. The sonographer should use enough gain to adequately illuminate the target tissue, just do not overdo it. There will also be a "far gain" and "near gain" controls to adjust the brightness of the bottom or top half of the image separately if required to better visualize the target tissue. If you have adjusted the gain and the image looks worse, there is usually an "automatic gain" button, which when pressed will get you back to the machine initial setting for gain.

Frequency: Most current transducers are "broadband" transducers and are able to utilize a limited range of frequencies to optimize image quality. Higher frequencies generally work best on superficial structures, and lower frequencies generally yield the best image on deeper structures. However, you may have to check which frequencies yield the best image in certain situations, for instance, when viewing the plantar fascia, although it is a shallow structure, often lower frequencies will yield a better image. Often the highest frequencies will not produce the best image of the needle, and once the target tissue has been identified, the frequencies can be reduced if a guided injection is going to be performed to optimize needle visualization.

Focal zones: A focal zone is created when the transducer focuses the sound waves more at certain depths within the image. In effect, you are telling the US precisely where, within the depth range you have selected, your target tissue is. Bracketing the target tissue with focal zones just above and below it will yield the best image. More focal zones require additional image processing power, which results in reducing the frame rate at which the generated image is refreshed. This reduced frame rate is more significant in applications where motion is critical such as echocardiograms where the image of the beating heart will appear to move in a choppy fashion at a slower frame rate. However, for MSK US applications, three or even four focal zones will not significantly affect the apparent frame rate of the static tissue being viewed, and as long as the transducer is moved slowly and smoothly, it will result in a more processed image with better resolution. Some US machines may simplify this process of setting focal zones and frequencies by having preselected settings that optimize resolution or penetration within the depth selected.

Transducers: Two types of transducers are needed for performing MSK US. The first transducer is a broadband high-frequency (8–15 mHz) linear transducer with a footprint 30–50 mm long; this will cover most of the scanning done within 4 cm of the skin. It has excellent resolution but limited penetration and limited field of view. This workhorse transducer is useful for shoulders, upper extremities, lower leg and feet, neck, and superficial vessels and nerves. The next transducer needed is a broadband low-frequency (1–5 MHz) curvilinear transducer with about 60 mm of footprint. This transducer has excellent penetration for deeper structures (over 4 cm) and a much wider field of view due to the curved shape of the footprint. The wider field of view helps with orienting to the anatomy. It does not have the resolution of the high-frequency probe. This transducer is required for hips, thighs, shoulders (in large individuals), spine, and abdomen. In heavy individuals, it will have even more utility. One transducer cannot cover the range of requirements for MSK US; both are required. There are times when a small-footprint (20–25 mm), high-frequency linear transducer is useful for hands, wrists, and ankles; however, this falls into the nice-to-have category of equipment, and these requirements can be met with the longer footprint linear transducer described earlier.

A wheeled US cart with adjustable height is required for proper positioning of the US machine. A multitransducer connector facilitates easy transitioning between different transducers but is not required. A foot pedal control is an inexpensive and highly useful option for saving the images you feel best represent the procedure, especially while both hands are engaged while performing a guided injection.

19.6 SCANNING BASICS

The goal is to be able to control the transducer with relaxed precision to achieve the best image possible. The following key steps are needed to achieve this goal:

Adjust the US machine. Before you start to scan the patient, and keeping in mind your anatomic target, set your estimation of depth, frequency, gain, and focal points; these can be adjusted once you start to scan as needed, but select a solid starting point.

Adjust the patient. Position the patient so that you can perform the required scan in a relaxed, ergonomic posture, with either sonographer sitting or standing. The patient should be in a relaxed position that facilitates them staying still. Use bolsters as needed to support the patient. Use a procedure table with adjustable height. If appropriate to the scan, have the patient facing the US machine to facilitate explaining any significant findings. Consider how you will conduct any dynamic scans.

Adjust the position of the US machine. This is important and often overlooked. Generally, the patient should be positioned directly between the sonographer and the US machine so that the sonographer does not have to turn their head to see either the US display or the patients' anatomy being scanned. Adjust the height of the US cart. This is an important step when performing real-time US-guided injections. Attempt to have the US machine in arms reach. If this is not possible, the use of a foot pedal control is recommended (available as a relatively inexpensive option on many machines) to control the "freeze image" and "save image" settings.

Control the transducer. This is the most critical step. To scan well, use the thumb and index finger to control the probe, and use the other three fingers to form a stable base of contact with the patient's skin. By having a good base of contact with the patient and the transducer in relaxed control, the image will stay steady. By being in relaxed control, the transducer will not inadvertently slide with small movements of the patient nor will the hand holding the transducer become fatigued and start to inadvertently slide off target. For even marginally skilled scanning, the transducer hand and arm must be relaxed; this allows the subtle fine control required to yield good consistent images. By having a wide base of contact with the patient, the sonographer will be able to use light pressure on the transducer face yet stay in control. By using light pressure, subtle fluid-filled bursa, hematomas, and veins will be able to be appreciated, which would often otherwise be obscured by being collapsed while using heavier pressure. Move smoothly while scanning, and move in a distinct axis when adjusting the transducer. A long-axis slide is sliding the transducer along its longest axis; a short-axis slide is moving along the shortest axis; a rotation is rotating the transducer on its central axis, while a pivot is rotating the transducer with one side of the probe remaining fixed. Avoid tilting the probe as a general rule; once you start "using the transducer like a flashlight" and tilting the probe to attempt to find a target or a needle, you create nonstandard anatomical cross sections and compound angles, which are much more difficult to reliably orient. Move the transducer standard anatomic planes when possible (transverse or cross-sectional, sagittal or longitudinal, coronal). While scanning, consider sonopalpation. Sonopalpation is placing a palpating finger between the transducer and the skin to specifically palpate the (potentially painful) structure of interest to help confirm the patient's pain generator.

19.7 ULTRASOUND-GUIDED INJECTIONS

Multiple studies have been published validating the fact that even in the hands of experienced specialists, US-guided injections are not only more accurate than clinically guided (blind) injections[4,5,8,10,12,18] but also result in improved clinical outcomes.[4,21,22,24,28,30] This has been documented even in commonly performed injections such as knee joint injections.[12] "Does US needle guidance affect the clinical outcomes" was addressed by Sibbet et al. in a randomized controlled study of 148 painful joints that were randomized to intra-articular corticosteroid injection by conventional palpation-guided or sonographic image–guided injection. Relative to conventional palpation-guided methods, sonographic guidance resulted in 43% reduction in procedural pain ($p > 0.001$), 58% reduction in absolute pain scores at the 2-week outcome ($p > 0.001$), 75% reduction in significant pain ($p > 0.001$), and 62% reduction in nonresponder rate. Sonography also increased the detection of effusion by 200% and volume of aspirated fluid by 337%. They concluded that sonographic guidance significantly improved clinical outcomes.[30]

19.7.1 Injection Procedures

Whatever equipment you use, especially the transducers, it must be cleaned before and after each procedure with a cleaner approved by both the US machine manufacturer and the specific medical facility. Some medical cleaning products will damage the transducer face and significantly degrade the image and reduce the life span of this expensive piece of equipment, so make sure the cleaner is approved for the transducer.

A low-risk preparation would consist of cleaning the transducer (and letting it dry for the approved amount of time for the cleaner used), wide skin preparation with an alcohol or chlorhexidine product, wearing sterile gloves and applying sterile gel, or using only the still moist skin preparation product as the US coupling medium. For higher-risk injections (catheter placements, hip joints, injections requiring multiple skin penetrations) or injections in immunocompromised patients, strongly consider using sterile transducer covers in addition to skin preparation, sterile draping, sterile US gel, and sterile gloves. The use of US gel is not recommended for any guided approach to neuraxial structures.[9]

All of the tenants of the "scanning basics" section especially apply when performing US-guided injections. Proper positioning of the patient and US machine is the first step. A procedure table with adjustable height facilitates the use of healthy ergonomic posture for the injector. The table should have enough space all around it to facilitate proper positioning of the US machine. An assortment of pillows and bolsters will allow you to place the patient in a position of repose; this is important with guided injections because the tendency of the patient will be to move away from the noxious stimulus of the needle. Any movement on the part of the patient will significantly both increase the difficulty of the procedure and reduce safety if needle visualization cannot be continuously maintained.

A stable and relaxed transducer hand with a broad but light base of contact with the patient is a critical element of reliable and reproducible guided injections. This point cannot be overstated. Usually, the needle is controlled with the dominant hand, either with a "hand-on-syringe" or with a "hand-on-needle" technique. The significant advantage of a "hand-on-syringe" technique is that the injector has the feedback from the syringe plunger on the injection pressure and can synthesize the injection pressure with the real-time US image. This "pressure" feedback can be critical, chiefly for the reason that the US image on the screen is only a computer-generated approximation of the needle location due to volume averaging. In other words, although the image is usually accurate, it is not 100% accurate, and just because the needle tip appears to be in a structure, it may not actually be there. For example, if you see your needle tip in a fluid-filled bursa and you expect a very low-resistance injection, but your injection pressure is higher than you think it should be, your needle tip may actually be in another structure, or your needle tip may be occluded. When injecting into what appears to be a relatively intact tendon, there should be some significant resistance to the injectate. If you are injecting a tendon and you have confirmed the location of your needle tip in two planes and the injection pressure is low, this would be an important secondary sign of significant tendinopathy or even of a significant tear. Either way, if the injection pressure is not what you anticipated, stop and reassess the injection and strongly consider repositioning the needle. A disadvantage of "hand on syringe" is that performing a one-handed aspiration can be challenging while keeping the needle in position.

With the "hand-on-needle" technique, the injector holds the needle, usually by the hub, while a connector tube is attached to the syringe held by an assistant. This facilitates improved needle control, especially with deep or otherwise challenging injections. This technique can work well with a knowledgeable and experienced assistant that can provide reliable feedback on aspiration and injection pressures. Assuming the role of the assistant, controlling the syringe affords an element of control and safety when mentoring other providers in guided injections and ensures both reliable aspirations before injecting and injection pressures consistent with expectations.

There are three methods of real-time US guidance. (The modifier "real-time" with US guidance specifically applies to using the US to track the needle into the target tissue and differentiates it from just "ultrasound guidance," which may mean that the US was used only to template the skin and record the depth of the target tissue.) There are long-axis (or in-plane) injections, short-axis (or out-of-plane) injections, or a diagonal combination of short- and long-axis injections. With long-axis (in-plane) injections, the needle is inserted along the longest axis of the transducer footprint. The entire length of the needle (which is in the viewing frame) is in view. Long axis is the best view for confirming depth, allows the entire anatomy that the needle is passing through to be viewed, and is a view readily understood by patients. Short-axis injections are very useful but more difficult to visualize. In short-axis (out-of-plane) injections, the needle enters the skin perpendicular to the long axis of the transducer. In short axis, only the tip of the needle is visible as a dot when the needle is advanced into the thin "plane or shaft of sound" projected by the transducer. Short-axis injections allow for precise left–right alignment over a structure, such as for vascular access, and are useful for when a long-axis approach would be suboptimal, such as entering a small superficial joint. Sometimes, a long-axis view is desirable but not able to be achieved due to anatomy, such as when the calf muscle size constrains injecting into an Achilles tendon insertion in long axis. In this case, a combined short- and long-axis diagonal view can be used to see more of the needle approaching the tendon insertion in long axis than could otherwise be achieved.

For more advanced injections, deeper injections (over 3.5 cm), or injecting to a precise location (such as along a nerve or near an artery), confirm the location of the needle tip by viewing it in both long- and short-axis views before injecting. The goal is to be comfortable switching between short- and long-axis views (the concept of orthogonal views in x-ray radiology) during an injection to confirm the needle position and to take advantage of the strengths of each technique thus (nearly) overcoming the physical limitation of volume averaging. When the injectionist has achieved relaxed control of the transducer hand, they will no longer worry about not being able to "find" the needle. This is not to say that good needle visualization is always easy, or even achievable, even by very skilled injectionists. With steep injections, the amount of sound reflected off of the needle back to the transducer drops off logarithmically as steepness increases. Some patients have very echodense tissue and even otherwise straightforward injections become challenging. Some areas of the body are very challenging to get good needle visualization, such as the paravertebral space.

One of the largest challenges in training a new injectionist is getting them to look down at their hands during an injection and not up at the screen. The injection is achieved by having a precise view of the target tissue with the transducer hand and then precisely placing the needle into that exact view with the needle hand. Unfortunately for beginning injectionists, these two things must happen simultaneously; you cannot have a good image of the target and then scan for a good image of the needle. Guiding a needle is a precise physical skill that takes practice and experience, like throwing a baseball accurately. The US image *only confirms what the hands are doing* and then helps to provide accurate terminal guidance to the target tissue. When you are having a difficult time finding the needle, look down at your hands.

Clinical Pearl

Looking down at your hands is the critical step to injecting well. No matter how expensive the US machine was, the US transducer will never image the needle unless it is perfectly under the transducer. If you find yourself unable to locate the needle, pull the needle out, take a breath, look down at your hands, and start over. The US image only confirms what has happened with your hands.

With long-axis injections, one of the chief impediments to placing the needle precisely into the view of the target tissue is a lack of awareness of eye dominance. We each have a dominant eye. To check for eye dominance, make a small circle with your thumb and index finger and extend your arm out in front of you. Pick a distant target (across the room, across the field) and with both eyes open, view the target through the circle your fingers create. Now close one eye then open it and close the other eye. The target will only remain in the circle formed by your fingers when viewed with your dominant eye. This eye dominance can result in the needle being slightly off center, even though it appears to you to be exactly in the center of the transducer. By being aware of your own tendency to always be to the left or right of the shaft of sound, you can "precorrect" your needle insertion point.

Another common guidance mistake during long-axis injections is the tendency to cross through the "imaging plane" (the shaft of sound projected from the transducer) from right to left at a slight diagonal for a right-hand-dominant person. This will result in partial needle visualization; however, the tip will cross out of the image plane. If you are advancing the needle and the needle tip appears to be visible but you do not see the tip advancing, you have crossed the image plane. One way to spot this is to always have the bevel of the needle facing the transducer during injections; the bevel of the needle has a distinct appearance and positively identifies the tip of the needle. To correct the tendency to cross the imaging plane, first be aware of it then compensate for it by tucking in the elbow of the hand driving the needle and lining the needle up perfectly parallel with the center axis of the transducer. Just because your skin entry point is in the center of the long-axis view does not mean the rest of the needle is properly lined up.

With short-axis injections, being left or right of the intended target is obvious. The chief issue with short-axis injections is that you do not have a view of the tissue the needle is going through. The other issue is that as you are advancing a needle in short axis, once you see the hyperechoic "dot" that represents the needle tip coming into the "imaging plane" being projected by the transducer, *you must stop* and not advance any further. If you continue to advance in a mistaken attempt to "go deeper," the image will remain unchanged, but the needle tip will be advancing into nonvisualized tissue. To perform a short-axis injection, have the bevel of the needle facing the transducer; this will facilitate an enhanced echo return to the transducer. Start with the transducer centered over the target tissue; many transducers have a mark on them indicating the center of the transducer footprint. With short-axis injections, it is very helpful if your machine has a "centerline" function or even using "M-mode," which projects a line down the center of the image. Line up your target tissue on this projected centerline. The needle entry point must be perpendicular to the center of the transducer. Especially for deeper injections, approach the target in planed stages. First, enter the skin at a shallow angle and advance the needle under the transducer to confirm that you have selected an accurate skin entry point and are lined up over the target. Then, estimate the (steeper) angle that will place the needle about half of the depth required to reach the target and advance the needle until you see the hyperechoic dot of the needle tip coming into the plane of the US beam. Each time you adjust the angle, the needle must be withdrawn nearly to the skin. With these first two angles confirmation of being over the target, estimate the steeper angle required to reach the target and advance the needle. If you have advanced the needle at too steep of an angle, you may not see the needle at all; stay aware of your depth, look at your hands, and make sure things still look reasonable. Deep short-axis injections can be challenging. A method of locating your needle tip in short axis is to vibrate or gently peck the needle tip as you perform a short-axis slide along the length of the needle until the tip is identified.

With each procedure, record the best possible image of the needle in the target tissue for the medical record. This will be useful if your medical records are ever audited to prove you actually performed the procedure you billed for.

19.8 MUSCULOSKELETAL ULTRASOUND IN THE CLINIC

In some clinical settings, specific credentialing in MSK US and US-guided injections may be required by some insurance plans for successful reimbursement. There is an individual provider qualification available through the American Registry for Diagnostic Medical Sonography MSK certification as well as a specific facility accreditation available through the American Institute of Ultrasound in Medicine. Although neither individual certification nor facility accreditation may be required, check with the insurance providers to see if one or both of these are mandatory for successful reimbursement for ICDM codes relating to diagnostic US or US-guided injections. When initiating new procedures, it is also reasonable to inform your medical malpractice insurance provider (Table 19.2).

TABLE 19.2
SORT: Key Recommendations for Practice

Clinical Recommendation	Evidence Rating	References
Musculoskeletal ultrasound–guided procedures are more accurate and more efficacious than nonguided (clinically guided) injections.	A	[24,28,30]
Musculoskeletal ultrasound can be used to diagnose injuries to ligaments, tendons, muscles, bones, and nerves.	A	[20,35,36]
Musculoskeletal ultrasound is about as accurate as MRI for diagnosing rotator cuff tears.	B	[35]
Musculoskeletal ultrasound is about as accurate as MRI for diagnosing knee meniscal tears.	C	[11]
Dynamic ultrasound exams can detect pathology not visible with static view imaging.	C	[15]

REFERENCES

1. Aiken CE, Lees CC. Long-term effects of in utero Doppler ultrasound scanning—A developmental programming perspective. *Medical Hypotheses.* April 2012;78(4):539–541.
2. Albert JM. Radiation risk from CT: Implications for cancer screening. *American Journal of Roentgenology.* July 2013;201(1):W81–W87.
3. Arthurs OJ, Bjørkum AA. Safety in pediatric imaging: An update. *Acta Radiology.* 2013;54(9):983–990.
4. Berkoff DJ, Miller LE, Block JE. Clinical utility of ultrasound guidance for intra-articular knee injections: A review. *Clinical Interventions in Aging.* 2012;7:89–95.
5. Bloom JE, Rischin A, Johnston RV et al. Image-guided versus blind glucocorticoid injection for shoulder pain. *Cochrane Database System Review.* 2012;8:CD009147.
6. Boon A. Ultrasonography and electrodiagnosis: Are they complementary techniques? *PMR.* May 2013;5(5 Suppl.): S100–S106.
7. Brockow K, Sánchez-Borges M. Hypersensitivity to contrast media and dyes. *Immunological Allergy Clinical North America.* August 2014;34(3):547–564.
8. Chavez-Chiang NR, Delea SL, Norton HE et al. The outcomes and cost-effectiveness of intraarticular injection of the rheumatoid knee. *Rheumatology International.* 2012;32(2):513–518.
9. Chin KJ, Karmakar M, Peng P. Ultrasound of the adult thoracic and lumbar spine for central neuraxial blockade. *Anesthesiology.* 2011;114:1459–1485.
10. Choudur HN, Ellins ML. Ultrasound-guided gadolinium joint injections for magnetic resonance arthrography. *Journal of Clinical Ultrasound.* 2011;39(1):6–11.
11. Cook JL, Cook CR, Stannard JP, Vaughn G, Wilson N, Roller BL. MRI versus ultrasonography to assess meniscal abnormalities in acute knees. *Journal of Knee Surgery.* August 2014;27(4): 319–324.
12. Curtiss HM, Finnoff JT, Peck E, Hollman J, Muir J, Smith J. Accuracy of ultrasound-guided and palpation-guided knee injections by an experienced and less-experienced injector using a superolateral approach: A cadaveric study. *PMR.* 2011;3(6):507–515.
13. Daley EL, Bajaj S, Bisson LJ, Cole BJ. Improving injection accuracy of the elbow, knee, and shoulder does injection site and imaging make a difference? A systematic review. *American Journal of Sports Medicine.* March 2011;39(3): 656–662.
14. Epis O, Bruschi E. Interventional ultrasound: A critical overview on ultrasound-guided injections and biopsies. *Clinical and Experimental Rheumatology.* January–February 2014; 32(1 Suppl. 80):S78–S84.
15. Feuerstein CA, Weil L Jr, Weil LS Sr, Klein EE, Fleischer A, Argerakis NG. Static versus dynamic musculoskeletal ultrasound for detection of plantar plate pathology. *Foot and Ankle Specialist.* July 15, 2014;7(4):259–265.
16. Galiano K, Obwegeser A. Ultrasound-guided versus computed tomography-controlled facet joint injections in the lumbar spine. *Regional Anesthesia and Pain Medicine.* 2007;32(4):317–322.
17. Galiano K, Obwegeser A. Ultrasound guidance for facet joint injections in the lumbar spine. *Anesthesia and Analgesia.* 2005;101(2):579–593.
18. Gokalp G, Dusak A, Yazici Z. Efficacy of ultrasonography-guided shoulder MR arthrography using a posterior approach. *Skeletal Radiology.* 2010;39(6):575–579.
19. Hedelin H, Goksör LÅ, Karlsson J, Stjernström S. Ultrasound-assisted triage of ankle trauma can decrease the need for radiographic imaging. *American Journal of Emergency Medicine.* December 2013;31(12):1686–1689.
20. Klauser A, Tagliafico A, Allen GM et al. Clinical indications for musculoskeletal ultrasound: A Delphi-based consensus paper of the European society of musculoskeletal radiology. *European Radiology.* 2012;22:1140–1148.
21. Lee HJ, Lim KB, Kim DY et al. Randomized controlled trial for efficacy of intra-articular injection for adhesive capsulitis: Ultrasonography-guided versus blind technique. *Archives of Physical and Medical Rehabilitation.* 2009;90(12):1997–2002.
22. Makhlouf T, Emil NS, Sibbitt WL et al. Outcomes and cost-effectiveness of carpal tunnel injections using sonographic needle guidance. *Clinical Rheumatology.* 2014;33(6):849–858.
23. Mulvaney S. Ultrasound guided percutaneous neuroplasty of the lateral femoral cutaneous nerve for the treatment of meralgia paresthetica: A case report and description of a new ultrasound guided technique. *Current Sports and Medical Reports.* 2011;10(2):99–104.
24. Naredo E et al., A randomized comparative study of short term response to blind injection versus sonographic-guided injection of local corticosteroids in patients with painful shoulder. *Journal of Rheumatology.* 2004;31(2):308–314.
25. Ottenheijm R, Jansen MJ, Staal B, Bruel AVD, Weijers RE, deBie RA, Dinant GJ. Accuracy of diagnostic ultrasound in patients with suspected subacromial disorders: A systematic review and meta-analysis. *Archives of Physical and Medical Rehabilitation.* 2010;90:1616–1625.
26. Parker L, Nazarian LN, Carrino JA, Morrison WB, Grimaldi G, Frangos AJ, Levin DC, Rao VM. Musculoskeletal imaging: Medicare use, costs, and potential for cost substitution. *Journal of American College Radiology.* 2008;5:182–188.
27. Rho ME, Chu SK, Yang A, Hameed F, Lin CY, Hurh PJ. Resident accuracy of joint line palpation using ultrasound verification. *PMR.* 2015; 6(10):920–925
28. Sage W, Pickup L, Smith TO et al. The clinical and functional outcomes of ultrasound-guided vs landmark-guided injections for adults with shoulder pathology—A systematic review and meta-analysis. *Rheumatology.* 2013;52(4):743–751.

29. Schlaudecker J, Bernheisel C. Gadolinium-associated nephrogenic systemic fibrosis. *AFP.* 2009;80(7):711–714.
30. Sibbet WL, Peisajovich A, Michael AA et al. Does sonographic needle guidance affect the clinical outcome of intraarticlular injections. *Journal of Rheumatology.* 2009;36:9.
31. Sivan M, Brown J, Brennan S, Bhakta B. A one-stop approach to the management of soft tissue and degenerative musculoskeletal conditions using clinic-based ultrasonography. *Musculoskeletal Care.* 2011;9(2):63–68.
32. Smith J, Finnoff JT. Diagnostic and interventional musculoskeletal ultrasound: Part 2. Clinical applications. *PMR.* 2009;1:162–177.
33. Swain MS, Henschke N, Kamper SJ, Downie AS, Koes BW, Maher CG. Accuracy of clinical tests in the diagnosis of anterior cruciate ligament injury: A systematic review. *Chiropractic and Man Therapy.* August 1, 2014;22:25. eCollection 2014.
34. Tagliafico AS, Michaud J, Marchetti A, Garello I, Padua L. US imaging of the musculocutaneous nerve. *Skeletal Radiology.* October 2010;8:7701953.
35. Teefey SA, Rubin DA, Middleton WD et al. Detection and quantification of rotator cuff tears. Comparison of ultrasonographic, magnetic resonance imaging, and arthroscopic findings in seventy-one consecutive cases. *Journal of Bone and Joint Surgery American.* 2004;86-A(4):708–716.
36. Ziswiler HR, Reichenbach S, Vögelin E, Bachmann LM, Villiger PM, Jüni P. Diagnostic value of sonography in patients with suspected carpal tunnel syndrome: A prospective study. *Arthritis & Rheumatism.* 2005;52(1):304–311.

20 Common Laboratory Findings in an Athlete

Collin G. Hu and Shawn F. Kane

CONTENTS

TABLE 20.1
Key Clinical Considerations

1. Laboratory studies should be used in conjunction with a good history and physical examination to rule out or confirm a diagnosis.
2. Athletes may have laboratory results that are abnormal compared to a sedentary individual but are normal for athletes due to physiological changes.
3. All abnormal laboratory findings must take into account an athlete's potential physiology and should be repeated to confirm its finding.

20.1 INTRODUCTION

Musculoskeletal presentations can be very challenging for the primary care provider; referred pain, psychological overlay, comorbid illness, and autoimmune disease are just several entities that can confound the correct diagnosis. In conjunction with a good history and physical examination, laboratory findings can help confirm a diagnosis, rule out disease, and provide insight into the overall health of a patient. In the athletic population in particular, lab findings that may be abnormal in a nonathlete may be completely normal in an athlete and vice versa. This chapter will look at commonly ordered labs and their usefulness as they pertain to musculoskeletal and sports medicine. It will also highlight unique lab results normal to an athlete, detail unique clinical problems defined by a laboratory abnormality, and discuss follow-up considerations for potential abnormal labs (Table 20.1).

20.2 BASIC METABOLIC PANEL

20.2.1 Sodium

Sodium is an important electrolyte and mineral that helps regulate the body's fluid balance, in addition to assisting with the function of both nerves and muscles. Sodium is generally the first component of the basic metabolic panel that is reported; normal results for this test are 135–145 mEq/L; however, different laboratories use different values for "normal" (see Table 20.2). There are no described physiologic differences in normal sodium levels between athletes and nonathletes; however, the primary care provider should be aware of the clinical entity of exercise-induced hyponatremia.

Exercise-induced hyponatremia (sodium <135 mmol/L) is an abnormality not uncommonly seen in athletes after prolonged endurance exercise. Presentation can range from an asymptomatic incidental finding to very severe symptomatology that can progress to intracranial swelling and death. Mild symptoms include headache, malaise, nausea, fatigue, and confusion. Severe hyponatremia (<130 mmol/L) can include seizures, respiratory arrest, increased intracranial pressure, coma, and, as previously identified, death.[1]

Symptomatic hyponatremia has been found in 0.1%–4% of athletes involved in prolonged endurance exercise; however, athletes have also been known to be hyponatremic and been completely asymptomatic.[1] Though hyponatremia can be found in elite athletes, it is more prevalent in female and recreational

TABLE 20.2
Basic Metabolic Panel: Normal Values

Sodium	135–145 mmol/L	No physiologic difference in normal sodium levels has been noted between athletes and nonathletes. Exercise-induced hyponatremia is commonly seen in endurance athletes.
Potassium	3.4–5.0 mmol/L	
Chloride	96–112 mmol/L	
Bicarbonate	21–34 mmol/L	
Blood urea nitrogen (BUN)	4–20 mg/dL	No correlation found between BUN levels, muscle injury from eccentric exercise, or long-term creatine supplementation.
Creatinine	–1.2 mg/dL	Athletes tend to have higher serum creatinine compared to sedentary individuals. Endurance athletes are known to have significantly decreased levels. Baseline Cr levels not influenced by training or competition.
Glucose (nonfasting)	70–108 mg/dL	

athletes.[2,3] It has also been found in races longer than 8 hours but is rarely seen in events lasting less than 4 hours.[4]

Clinical Pearl

Symptomatic hyponatremia is directly related to race duration, with ultra-endurance events posing the greatest risk to athletes.

Three principal factors play a role in causing hyponatremia in athletes: inadequate suppression of antidiuretic hormone, salt depletion, and excess fluid intake during exercise.[5] Inadequate suppression of antidiuretic hormone is commonly known as syndrome of inappropriate antidiuretic hormone. This causes decreased urine output, increased fluid retention, and thereby leads to hyponatremia via fluid overload.[6] Up to 1800 mL of sweat can be lost per hour with the relative sodium content of sweat ranging from 25 to 75 mEq/L.[3] However, sweat is hypotonic, and if an athlete does not drink fluids, the end result will actually cause hypernatremia.

Clinical Pearl

Hyponatremia in athletes is caused by inadequate suppression of antidiuretic hormone, excessive hypotonic fluid intake, and hypotonic salt loss.

It is sweat loss in conjunction with excessive hypotonic fluid intake and inadequate suppression of antidiuretic hormone that eventually causes hyponatremia. Most athletes with mild asymptomatic exercise-induced hyponatremia will have variable weight loss.[5,7] On the other hand, symptomatic hyponatremic athletes tend to gain weight secondary to being overhydrated on free water.[5,7] Prompt recognition of an athlete suffering from symptomatic hyponatremia and appropriate treatment with hypertonic saline is critical in avoiding adverse outcomes.

20.2.2 Blood Urea Nitrogen

Blood urea nitrogen (BUN) is a measurement of protein breakdown within the body and can be used to help monitor kidney function. The normal range for BUN is 6–20 mg/dL (see Table 20.2). The usual ratio of BUN to creatinine concentration in serum is 10:1.[8] However, this ratio can increase for multiple prerenal causes including volume depletion (i.e., dehydration), high-protein diets, and even sepsis.

After eccentric exercise, BUN has been found to be significantly decreased from baseline, and there is a small positive correlation between creatinine kinase and BUN 4 days postexercise. Though overall, no correlation has been found between BUN levels, muscle injury from eccentric exercise, and long-term creatine supplementation.[9,10]

20.2.3 Creatinine

Creatinine (Cr) is a breakdown product of creatinine phosphate in muscle and is excreted unchanged by the kidneys. It is routinely used to evaluate renal health. The common reference range for Cr is 0.6–1.2 mg/dL. In general, athletes have been shown to have a statistically significantly higher serum creatinine compared to sedentary individuals, due to increased muscle mass.[11] However, endurance athletes have been shown to have significantly decreased levels of serum creatinine compared to a sedentary population. This is thought to be due to chronic hypervolemia, which is commonly found during pregnancy and with endurance athletes.[12] Current research shows that baseline creatinine levels are not influenced by training or competition.[13] A set reference range for creatinine in athletes is not currently recommended. Instead, consecutive creatinine levels should be drawn. At least one should be drawn prior to training and competition in order to have baseline values.[11] An elevated baseline Cr warrants a urine analysis to determine if there is any protein spilling.

Clinical Pearl

Creatinine levels should be drawn prior to training and competition in order to have baseline values.

20.3 LIVER AND MUSCLE ENZYMES AND PROTEINS

The liver works to process blood, metabolize nutrients, produce proteins, detoxify harmful substances, and many other functions. As the liver is damaged, it releases enzymes into the blood stream that can be measured by several blood tests (see Table 20.3). The most commonly measured liver enzymes include aspartate aminotransferase (AST) and alanine aminotransferase (ALT).

20.3.1 Aminotransferases

ALT and AST are generally considered to be the most useful markers for liver damage. ALT comes almost exclusively from the liver, while AST is also found in muscle in addition to the liver. There is no significant difference in concentration of these enzymes between sedentary healthy individuals and athletes.[14] The American Gastroenterology Association defines mild transaminase elevations as AST and/or ALT of less than 5 times normal and severe elevations as greater than 15 times. Table 20.4 lists common etiologies of AST and ALT elevations.

Strenuous exercise and trauma can break down muscle and therefore can lead to an increase in aminotransferase levels. Studies have shown significant increase in AST levels after exercise and only minimal increases in ALT levels.[15] Increases in AST levels have been seen in association with muscle tissue damage during contact sports, such as American football and generic muscle cramping.[16,17] It can also be associated with alcohol-related liver injury, especially with an AST/ALT ratio greater than two. Nonalcoholic steatohepatitis (NASH) can also present with similar symptoms as alcohol liver injury; however, the AST/ALT ratio may be closer to one. This should be considered when there is little to no alcohol consumption in the athlete's history.[18] Ultrasound may be useful in determining liver pathology secondary to alcohol consumption, and a liver biopsy is necessary to diagnose NASH.

TABLE 20.3
Normal Reference Ranges for Common Liver and Muscle Tests

Alanine aminotransferase (ALT)	6–43 U/L	Elevations of ALT associated with over-the-counter medications, supplementations, and increased body mass index.
Aspartate aminotransferase (AST)	10–40 U/L	Elevations of AST levels associated with muscle tissue damage during contact sports.
Lactate dehydrogenase (LDH)	100–250 U/L	
Myoglobin	3–70 μg/mL	Increased levels noted after extreme competitions such as marathons and in diseases such as rhabdomyolysis.
Creatine kinase (CK)	M: 50–260 U/L F: 30–235 U/L	Postmarathon runners can have a 14-fold increase in CK and remain elevated for 4–5 days. Persistent CK above 1000 U/L, even with rest, warrants a full evaluation.

TABLE 20.4
Common Etiologies of Aspartate Aminotransferase and Alanine Aminotransferase Elevations

Hepatitis
- Autoimmune
- Infectious

Toxins
- Alcohol
- Drugs
- Industrial
- Hemodynamic disorders

Fatty infiltration
- Alcohol related
- Nonalcohol related

Muscle injury
- Exertional rhabdomyolysis
- Heat stroke or injury

Iron or copper overload

Alpha1 antitrypsin deficiency

Source: Adapted from Kane, S. F. and Cohen, ML. *Curr. Sports Med. Rep.*, 8(2), 77, 2009.

Mild elevations in ALT have a wider differential that can include both infectious and autoimmune etiologies. Common causes include taking supplements, over-the-counter medication, viral hepatitis, autoimmune hepatitis, hereditary hemochromatosis, Wilson's disease, alpha$_1$-antitrypsin disease, celiac sprue, and an elevated body mass index (BMI).[18,19] Measuring serum iron and total iron biding capacity may help determine hemochromatosis. Obtaining a 24 hour urine test measuring for copper excretion is used to diagnose Wilson's disease. Serum antigliadin and antiendomysial antibodies are used to diagnose celiac sprue. Finally, alpha$_1$-antitrypsin deficiency, though an uncommon cause for elevated ALT, can be confirmed by the lack of a peak in alpha globulin bands on serum protein electrophoresis.

With elevated ALT levels, an athlete's BMI must also be kept in mind, along with supplement use. Both ALT and AST levels have been found to be elevated in athletes who have abused anabolic androgenic steroids, all of which are metabolized by the liver. In fact, ALT and AST levels have been found to be two times higher in steroid abusing bodybuilders.[19]

Clinical Pearl

Elevated transaminases should illicit further investigation into an athlete's medications, supplement use, alcohol consumption, and potential toxin and blood exposures.

The cause of 85% of cases involving elevated transaminases can be determined by a good history and physical examination; however, the remaining 15% may require further clinical work-up.[18] Over-the-counter and prescription medications, nutritional and sports supplements, and alcohol, as well as toxins and blood exposures, should all be taken into account when evaluating elevated transaminases. With athletes, elevated AST should be considered from muscles and elevated ALT from potential liver pathology.

20.3.2 Myoglobin

Myoglobin is a protein found in the muscle that helps bind oxygen and iron. However, it can be found in the blood stream especially after muscle damage. This is especially true in athletes that have rhabdomyolysis. It can also be elevated after extreme competitions such as marathons, with one study recording an average 19-fold peak increase in myoglobin.[20] Another study demonstrated a sevenfold increase in myoglobin from baseline on day 1 after competition and even twofold, increase on day 2.[21] It has a half-life of 2–3 hours, and therefore, serum levels can return to baseline within 6–8 hours. Myoglobin can be found in urine once the serum levels of myoglobin have reached 1.5 mg/dL.[22] However, a lack of myoglobin in urine does not mean that pathology, such as rhabdomyolysis, is not present.[23]

20.3.3 Creatine Kinase

Creatine kinase (CK) is used for cellular energy and transfer and is a useful marker for muscle damage. CK has three distinct isoenzyme forms, MM, MB, and BB. Normal skeletal muscle has 99% MM isoenzyme and only a trace amount of MB, whereas cardiac tissue has the highest concentration of CK-MB.[24] Serum CK levels are dependent upon different factors including gender and ethnicity. Women tend to have a lower baseline of CK compared to males; however, they have also been found to present with a higher CK peak and relatively greater increase in serum CK after exercise.[25] Ethnicity can also play a role in serum CK levels. In fact, healthy black people can have a serum CK level greater than 70% compared to white people.[26] Research has shown that this may be due to increased CK activity in all tissues in the black population during both high and fluctuating energy demands.[26]

Clinical Pearl

The classic triad of rhabdomyolysis of muscle pain, weakness, and dark urine is seen in less than 50% of patients. Patients will generally have CK levels at least five times the upper limit, and a lack of myoglobin in the urine does not rule out this disease.

Elevation of CK-MB can be found not only in individuals with pathology, such as myocardial infarction, but also in elite athletes and in individuals who just completed an extreme exercise such as a marathon.[27] Studies have shown postmarathon runners to have a 14-fold increase in CK and can remain elevated for 4–5 days.[20] With rhabdomyolysis, CK will be at least five times the upper limit of normal and is usually entirely of MM. CK can be found to increase within 2–12 hours following injury but reaches its peak within 1–3 days.[28] Usually, a decline in CK will be seen in 3–5 days after the muscle injury. CK's half-life is roughly 1.5 days, with it consistently declining 40%–50% of the previous day's value.[29] Regardless, an athlete with a persistent CK above 1000 U/L, even with rest, warrants a full evaluation.

Myoglobin and CK are both useful markers for muscle damage, including rhabdomyolysis. However, care must be taken in diagnosing pathology solely from these markers. With high-intensity exercise and competition, it is not uncommon for these labs to be found elevated even days after the event. Therefore, the athlete's history, their training regimen, and other laboratory findings all need to be evaluated in determining true pathology.

20.4 COMPLETE BLOOD COUNT

A complete blood count measures a patient's hemoglobin (Hb), hematocrit (Hct), white blood cells (WBC), and platelets that are circulating. Through technology, we can also determine the count and size of cells, including a mean corpuscular volume (MCV), and even the variation in cell size, or red cell distribution width (RDW). Further analysis of WBC can determine the percentage of neutrophils, lymphocytes, monocytes, eosinophils, and basophils[30] (see Table 20.5).

20.4.1 Neutrophils

Neutropenia in an athlete can be a benign finding that may be benign in certain populations. Known as benign neutropenia, it is most commonly seen in athletes of African and Middle Eastern descent, is an autosomal dominant trait, and has been hypothesized as being a protector against malaria.[31] If an isolated decrease in WBC count with neutropenia is found, recheck the lab once or twice to ensure it is chronic. If a parent has similar lab findings, then it can be assumed that the athlete has ethnic benign neutropenia. This condition is benign and does not carry with it any increased risk for infection, even though an absolute neutrophil count (ANC) may be as low as 800–1200 cells/uL. This is the reason why currently there is no recommendation to screen an athlete's WBC.

TABLE 20.5
Normal Reference Ranges for Complete Blood Cell Count

White blood cell (WBC) count	3.2–10.8 k/μL	Currently no recommendation to screen athletes WBC.
Hemoglobin (Hb)	13.1–18.6 g/dL	Body adapts to an athlete's increased oxygen demand by increased hemoglobin levels.
Hematocrit (Hct)	38.1–54.1%	Levels tend to be lower in the athletic population at rest but elevated during exercise.
Platelet count (Plt)	125–352 k/μL	
Mean corpuscular Hb concentration	32.9–35.5 g/dL	
Mean corpuscular volume	79.7–97.6 fL	

20.4.2 Hemoglobin (Hb) and Hematocrit (Hct)

Athletes generally have higher oxygen demand secondary to training and competition compared to sedentary individuals. The body adapts to an athlete's increased oxygen demand by increasing hemoglobin levels and total red blood cell (RBC) mass. This is especially true with endurance athletes.[32] Current studies show that erythropoiesis causes an increase in total RBC mass and may be stimulated by several factors. These include renal hypoxia, release of growth factors, and androgen use.[33] It has also been well studied that people living at a high altitude have an increase in Hb, RBCs, MCV, Hct, and reticulocyte count, all of which can explain the benefits of high-altitude endurance training.

Clinical Pearl

Individuals living at a high altitude have elevated Hb, RBC, MCV, Hct, and reticulocyte percentage.

Hematocrit tends to be lower in athletes than sedentary individuals secondary to increased plasma volume.[32] After exercising, plasma and blood volume increases rapidly, causing a decrease in hematocrit.[34] This rise in plasma volume is due to the body's compensatory release of antidiuretic hormone and aldosterone activation due to water loss during training. An elevated plasma volume also causes "sports anemia," which is a misnomer and not a true anemia. This will present with a decreased hematocrit but an elevated hemoglobin and total RBC mass compared to sedentary individuals.[33]

Clinical Pearl

Sports anemia presents as a low hematocrit level due to elevated plasma levels. This is not a true anemia.

However, when exercising, athletes tend to have an elevated hematocrit. This is due to fluid loss from sweating, secretion of lactic acid, and other metabolites causing a shift of fluid into the interstitial space and increased capillary hydrostatic pressure.[35] Of note, male and female African athletes are known to have marginally lower Hb levels, ~5 g/L, compared to Caucasian athletes.[36]

An athlete's normal hemoglobin and hematocrit can be significantly different from the sedentary population. When assessing abnormal values, a body's adaptation to high-intensity training, supplement use, and even the sea level at which an athlete trains all need to be taken into account in determining potential pathology. There is insufficient research into whether there is significant difference in WBC and platelet counts between the athlete and sedentary population.

20.5 FERRITIN

Recommended daily allowance for dietary iron in the adult male is 8 mg/day, and for menstruating, nonpregnant females, the recommendation is 18 mg/day. The higher daily allowance in women is to account for basal iron losses from menstruation.[37] Ferritin reflects the amount of iron stores in the body and can be used as a marker for iron deficiency. One ng/mL of ferritin corresponds to roughly 5–9 g of iron. In postpubertal males, the mean value of plasma ferritin is 90 ng/mL, and in females, it is 25–30 ng/mL during their reproductive years.[38]

Several studies have indicated ferritin concentration of <20–35 ng/mL as a good baseline for iron supplementation and an adequate level for maintenance.[39–41] Iron deficiency has been shown to decrease intracellular metabolic function, cognitive function, hemoglobin formation, immune function, and overall sports performance.[42]

Clinical Pearl

Normocytic athletes with low iron levels, who are treated with iron supplementation, have shown an increased maximal performance capacity and endurance.

It is well known that athletes will benefit from iron supplementation when they are both iron deficient and anemic. However, studies have also shown that normocytic athletes with low iron levels who receive iron supplementation have increased maximal performance capacity and endurance without changing their RBC volume.[43,44] Athletes should be treated with iron supplementation not only to prevent anemia but also to treat potential impaired aerobic performance.

Of note, ferritin is an acute-phase reactant and may be elevated due to several different causes including vigorous exercise and even an inflammatory illness.[42] Therefore, measurements of ferritin must be postponed in patients who may be in an inflammatory state, such as postexercise or those with a febrile illness. It has been recommended that routine screening be completed for male endurance athletes and female athletes in general.[40,45,46]

20.6 GLUCOSE 6-PHOSPHATE DEHYDROGENASE

Glucose 6-phosphate dehydrogenase (G6PD) deficiency occurs where there is a mutation in the x-chromosomal G6PD gene. The protein is critical as an antioxidant defense system that works against the formation of reactive oxidant species. Individuals can suffer from severe acute hemolytic anemia from taking certain drugs that are known oxidative agents, such as nitrofurantoin, primaquine, and even fava beans.[47,48] Theoretically, it is possible that athletes with G6PD deficiency have erythropoietin less able to withstand oxidative stress and therefore are more prone to acute hemolytic anemia. However, research has shown that athletes with G6PD deficiency do not experience a rise in oxidative stress compared to nondeficient athletes during high-intensity exercise.[47] Therefore, G6PD-deficient athletes may participate in high-intensity muscle-damaging activities, without any negative impact on muscle function or hemolysis.[49]

Clinical Pearl

Athletes with G6PD deficiency may participate in high-intensity exercises and activities without any negative impact.

20.7 SICKLE-CELL ANEMIA AND SICKLE-CELL TRAIT

Prevalence of sickle-cell trait is 8%–10% in the African American population.[50] It can also be found in persons from Mediterranean countries, Turkey, the Arabian Peninsula, and the Indian subcontinent.[51] It is currently recommended that all newborns be screened for hemoglobinopathies.[52] There are several variants to sickle-cell disease with the most common being homozygous sickle-cell disease (hemoglobin SS disease), double heterozygous sickle hemoglobin C disease (hemoglobin SC disease), and the sickle β-thalassemias.[51] Patients with sickle-cell trait are carriers of this recessive condition. These individuals will have one normal hemoglobin gene and one hemoglobin S gene.

Sickle-cell trait can be tested through several different methods. The National Collegiate Athletic Association (NCAA) recommends a hemoglobin solubility test at a minimum.[53] This test works by adding a reagent in blood. Compared to other hemoglobins, hemoglobin S is insoluble and therefore will appear cloudy instead of clear. However, this test will not distinguish between sickle-cell disease, sickle-cell trait, and other hemoglobin variants.[53] Instead, hemoglobin electrophoresis is used to differentiate between different hemoglobin types. When an electrical charge is applied to a gel, the hemoglobin will migrate through the gel at different rates. This is considered the most accurate test to determine if an athlete has sickle-cell trait.[53]

Hemolysis is commonly associated with sickle-cell disease; however, there is a spectrum of severity in regard to symptoms and anemia. Patients with β°-thalassemia and homozygous sickle-cell disease can present with the highest severity, whereas β+-thalassemia is the mildest variant followed in severity by sickle hemoglobin C disease.[51] Thalassemia should be suspected in patients with microcytosis or hypochromia without known iron deficiency.

Athletes with sickle-cell trait are for the most part asymptomatic. However, it has been linked to sudden death due to exertion sickling.[54] Risk factors for sudden death in patients with sickle-cell trait include heavy exercise with poor physical conditioning, dehydration, increased ambient temperature, and training at high altitudes.[54] Sickle-cell trait should not bar any athlete from exercising or participating in sports according to the American College of Sports Medicine (ACSM) and the National Athletic Trainers' Association (NATA). However, acclimatization to temperature, humidity and altitude, good hydration, and gradual conditioning can all help combat complications in athletes with sickle-cell trait.[55] There is currently no consensus from the ACSM or the NATA to screen athletes for sickle-cell trait, though the NCAA does require that all new student athletes participating in Division I, II, and III sports be screened for sickle-cell trait.[56] Regardless, it is recommended that all team physicians and athletic trainers be educated on sickle-cell trait, the risk factors for complications, and understanding serious complications associated with sickle-cell trait, though rare.[57,58]

Clinical Pearl

Sickle-cell trait should not limit an athlete from exercising or participating in sports. Athletic trainers and team physicians should be educated on this disease, its risk factors, and possible complications.

20.8 VITAMIN D

Low vitamin D is common in athletes, and levels below 25 ng/mL warrant replacement.[59] The recommendation is to keep vitamin D levels between 40 and 100 ng/mL.[60] Little is known regarding the direct impact of vitamin D deficiency on an athlete's performance, though research has found a correlation between decreased vitamin D levels and stress fractures.[61] If supplementing, athletes should be monitored to ensure that there are no adverse effects.[61] Monitoring should occur biannually specifically during the late summer and winter nadir.[62]

20.9 SEXUALLY TRANSMITTED DISEASE

20.9.1 Chlamydia

The current U.S. Preventive Service Task Force (USPSTF) recommendation is to routinely screen all sexually active women aged 25 years and younger for chlamydial infection.

There is currently no recommendation by the USPTF for or against screening the male population, though studies have found that male athletes are more sexually active compared to nonathletes[63] and are in fact more likely to have unprotected sex compared to female athletes.[64] Therefore, male athletes are at a higher risk for chlamydia and, in addition to sexually active females, should have a urine chlamydia screen.

Clinical Pearl

Male athletes along with females <25 years old should have a urine chlamydia screen.

20.9.2 Human Immunodeficiency Virus

The risk of transmitting human immunodeficiency virus (HIV) during athletic competition is very low. One study concluded that the chance of HIV transmission during professional American football is less than one per 85 million game contacts.[65] HIV is tested through detection of serum or salivary antibody to HIV by enzyme-linked immunosorbent assay (ELISA) and confirmed by Western blot. Currently, there is no medical or public health need to screen athletes for HIV.[66] In fact, the American Academy of Pediatrics recommends that all athletes with HIV be allowed to participate in all sports.[67] Regardless, all coaches, trainers, athletes, and officials should be educated on infection control, first aid, and basic hygiene.[66]

Clinical Pearl

Athletes with HIV should be allowed to participate in all sports.

20.10 URINE ANALYSIS

Urine analysis is one of the most commonly ordered laboratory studies secondary to low cost and easy availability.[68] Though relatively common, most of the time lab abnormalities are not clinically significant.[18] The most common abnormalities are hematuria, proteinuria, and bacteriuria[68] (see Table 20.6).

20.10.1 Hematuria

Microscopic hematuria is defined as three or more RBCs per high-power field during microscopic exam of the urinary sediment. Macroscopic hematuria is defined as blood noted in the urine under cross-examination. Asymptomatic hematuria occurs from 0.19% to 21% in adults and 3% to 4% in children 6–15 years old and therefore is a relatively common finding.[69] Though common, majority of the time hematuria is a benign finding. It is associated with significant renal disease in approximately 20% of adults and rarely in children.[70] There are no studies regarding the prevalence of hematuria in the athlete population compared to the sedentary population. However, it has been suggested that the prevalence may be higher in athletes secondary to foot-strike hemolysis, renal ischemia, and skeletal muscle damage.[70]

If a patient's hematuria is found to be due to a benign cause, such as recent vigorous exercise, menstrual contamination, recent intercourse, or trauma, a repeat urinalysis should be completed 48 hours after stopping the offending cause.[71] If the hematuria resolves, no further work-up is necessary. Urinary sediment should be examined for red cell casts or dysmorphic red cells, which can be associated with glomerular bleeding.[69] Differential diagnosis for glomerular bleeding includes IgA nephropathy and thin basement membrane disease, both of which warrant further work-up by a nephrologist. Isolated hematuria is defined as patients having persistent hematuria, normal history and physical exam, and no evidence of glomerular bleeding. This does not warrant further evaluation, though these patients should be followed for the development of hypertension or proteinuria.[18]

TABLE 20.6
Normal Reference Rages for Urine Analysis

Specific gravity	1.003–1.030	
pH	5.0–9.0	
Leukocyte esterase	Negative	
Nitrite	Negative	
Protein	Negative	Postexertion proteinuria is common in athletes, though routinely benign and self-limiting.
Glucose	Negative	
Ketones	Negative	
Urobilinogen	0.2–1.0 mg/dL	
Bilirubin	Negative	
Blood	Negative	Hematuria may be higher in athletes secondary to foot-strike hemolysis, renal ischemia, and skeletal muscle damage.
White blood cell UA	0–5/High-power field	
Red blood cell UA	2/High-power field	

Clinical Pearl

If hematuria is possibly due to a benign cause, a repeat urine analysis should be obtained 48 hours after stopping the offending cause.

Hematuria can also be associated with infection, especially in the presence of pyuria and bacteriuria. In this setting, a repeat urinalysis should be obtained in 6 weeks to look for complete resolution. A complete urologic evaluation must be initiated if hematuria persists with pyuria and bacteriuria present.[72]

20.10.2 Hemoglobinuria

Hemoglobinuria is present when a urine dipstick is positive for blood, but no RBCs or RBC casts are present on microscopy. It is commonly associated with hemolysis of RBCs causing excessive free circulating hemoglobin. In the athletic population, hemoglobinuria can present as foot-strike hemolysis, also known as march hemoglobinuria. It has been found in endurance athletes, military trainees, and athletes participating in impact sports. It can become worse as the training distance increases; however, research has shown that march hemoglobinuria is transient and benign.[73]

20.10.3 Proteinuria

The normal amount of protein in urine should be less than 150 mg/dL, and a urine dipstick reads positive when there is more than 300–500 mg/dL. Therefore, this test is specific but not very sensitive.[18] Postexertion proteinuria is common in athletes, though routinely benign and self-limiting.[74] Transient proteinuria, secondary to exercise, dehydration, fever, and stress, is the most common diagnosis.[18,27] However, athletes can also have orthostatic proteinuria and persistent proteinuria. A repeat urinalysis is obtained 48 hours after stopping the offending factors; if the urinalysis is normal, the diagnosis is transient proteinuria, and no further work-up is necessary.[74]

Orthostatic proteinuria occurs mostly in the pediatric population and is rare in patients over 30 years old. With orthostatic proteinuria, there is elevated protein excretion in the upright position and normal protein excretion in the recumbent position.[18] Diagnosis is made by obtaining a urinalysis and a protein to creatinine ratio from the first morning void. Patients are instructed to void before going to bed and then lay recumbent until the sample is taken. A normal urinalysis and protein to creatinine ratio is diagnostic for orthostatic proteinuria, and no further work-up is necessary. However, an abnormal urinalysis and protein to creatinine ratio is diagnostic for persistent proteinuria and further urologic evaluation is necessary.[18]

20.11 SYNOVIAL FLUID ANALYSIS

Synovial fluid analysis is used to diagnose bacterial infections or synovitis due to crystals. There are several indications to draw an analysis. The American College of Rheumatology (ACR) clinical guidelines state that any unexplained inflammatory synovial fluid, especially in a febrile patient, should be considered infected until proven otherwise.[75] The ACR further recommends that an analysis be completed to rule out septic arthritis specifically in febrile patients who have an established arthritis.[75] In patients where infection is less likely, unexplained swelling of a joint, bursa, or tendon is grounds for synovial fluid aspiration and analysis. Finally, the last indication for an analysis would be in a patient who may have a crystal disease, i.e., gout, causing inflammation, although no association has been found between moderate distance running and an increase in synovial fluid.[76]

Clinical Pearl

Unexplained inflammatory synovial fluid should be considered infected until proven otherwise.

Clinical Pearl

There is no association between moderate distance running and increased synovial fluid.

20.11.1 Characteristics

There are several components to a synovial fluid analysis. The fluid is first inspected for its gross characteristics. Normal synovial fluid may be highly viscous, clear, acellular, with one-third the protein concentration that is in plasma; however the glucose concentration may be very similar to plasma.[77]

20.11.2 Microscopic Examination

Under microscopic examination, the fluid is analyzed for a white cell count and differential, is examined for crystals, underwent a Gram stain, and cultured. A patient's chance of having septic arthritis increases as the synovial fluid white cell count increases. In adults, as the white cell count increased from 25,000 mm^{-3} to over 50,000 mm^{-3} to over 100,000 mm^{-3}, the positive likelihood ratio of septic arthritis increased from 2.9 to 7.7 and finally to 28, respectively.[78] The positive likelihood ratio of septic arthritis is 0.32 for a synovial white cell count of less than 25,000 mm^{-3}.[78] However, a lower synovial white cell count may be seen in immunocompromised patients along with joints infected by specific bacteria.[75] On differential of the white cell count, patients with a bacterial joint infection will have greater than 75% polymorphonuclear leukocytes.[79] Eosinophils found in the differential may indicate a parasitic infection, neoplasm, allergy, or Lyme disease.[80,81]

When concerned for septic arthritis, a Gram stain and culture may also be obtained. A Gram stain will help determine if the offending organism is Gram positive or Gram negative, as well as identify common organisms. The sensitivity of a Gram stain is between 50% and 70% for nongonococcal bacterial arthritis; however, it is less than 10% in gonococcal arthritis.[82] In addition to obtaining a Gram stain, a culture of the synovial fluid can further be used to differentiate what bacteria may be infecting the joint. However, if there is concern for a possible gonococcal arthritis, organisms may not be cultured in routine culture media.[83] In fact, less than 50% of cultures of synovial fluid tend to be positive in patients with gonococcal arthritis.[84] Therefore, joint aspirate must be specifically cultured for *Neisseria gonorrhoeae* when it is suspected.

Clinical Pearl

Synovial fluid must be specifically cultured for *N. gonorrhoeae* if clinically suspected.

20.11.3 Crystal Examination

Examinations of the synovial fluid for monosodium urate (MSU) and calcium pyrophosphate dihydrate (CPPD) crystals are another part of the synovial fluid analysis. MSU crystals are referred to as negatively birefringent, are needle shaped, and may appear yellow when seen under certain filters applied to a microscope. CPPD crystals, on the other hand, are considered to have a positive birefringence, are rhomboidal in shape, and may appear blue.

20.12 SERUM RHEUMATOLOGIC TESTS

Rheumatologic tests are useful in confirming a potential diagnosis. Understanding the indications, sensitivity, specificity, cost, and clinical utility ensures that these tests are appropriately ordered and therefore decrease potentially unnecessary evaluations.

20.12.1 Rheumatoid Factor

Testing is completed using an IgM antibody against a crystallizable fragment (Fc) portion of IgG. It can be noted in several rheumatologic and nonrheumatologic diseases. This test is useful with patients who may have rheumatoid arthritis. Up to 80% of patients with rheumatoid arthritis will have a positive RF; however, 20% of patients who have rheumatoid arthritis may be seronegative.[85] Specificity of RF for rheumatoid arthritis is from 80% to 95%, with the sensitivity approximately 10% in patients with polymyositis to more than 90% in those with Sjögren's syndrome or cryoglobulinemia.[86] Though in the athletic population, RF has been found to be significantly elevated 72 hours after an ultramarathon, similar to an acute-phase reactant.[87]

Clinical Pearl

Rheumatoid factor has been found to be elevated 72 hours after an ultramarathon.

20.12.2 Antinuclear Antibodies

Indirect immunofluorescence is used to detect antibodies that bind to different nuclear antigens. Results are reported as titers with the greater the titer the more likely the result is true positive. The ratio 1:20 or 1:40 is commonly seen as positive; however, patients with rheumatologic syndromes rarely have low titers.[88] Antinuclear antibodies (ANA) are commonly positive in patients with connective tissue disease; however, the sensitivity varies among different types of disease.[88] Patients with systemic lupus erythematosus and drug-induced lupus have sensitivity near 100%, with the specificity for systemic lupus erythematosus approximately 90%.[88] Of note, the seroprevalence of ANA has been found to be increased in weight lifters.[89]

Clinical Pearl

The seroprevalence of ANA has been found to be increased in weight lifters.

20.12.3 Anti-Double-Stranded DNA

Anti-double-stranded DNA (anti-dsDNA) can be specific for SLE; however, only 60% of patients with the disease have positive anti-dsDNA.[90] This lab finding also correlates with lupus nephritis, whereas the levels of anti-dsDNA correlate with the disease severity of SLE.[91] Testing is, therefore, recommended in patients with a positive ANA test and clinical suspicion for SLE.[91]

20.12.4 Antihistone

This lab finding can be useful in patients with a positive ANA and history of drug exposure that may cause a medication-induced lupus.[91] It is very sensitive but nonspecific for medication-induced lupus.[91] Procainamide and isoniazid are two medications that are commonly implicated in medication-induced lupus.

20.12.5 Anti-Small-Nuclear Ribonucleoproteins

There are several anti-small-nuclear ribonucleoproteins (anti-snRNPs) that have been investigated. Anti-Smith is a commonly ordered antibody and is very specific for SLE; however, it may only be detected in 20%–50% of patients.[92] Anti-U1 snRNP is another study that is ordered and can help diagnose mixed connective tissue disease. Therefore, this antibody should be tested in patients with a positive ANA and who may have concern for SLE or a mixed connective tissue disease.

20.12.6 Anti-Ro and Anti-La

These antibodies are commonly seen in patients with Sjögren's syndrome and can also be found in 40% of patients with SLE.[93] Therefore, this test can also be helpful in patients presenting with symptoms of SLE and can also help confirm the diagnosis of Sjögren's syndrome.

20.12.7 Anticentromere

A positive test for anticentromere antibodies is strongly correlated in patients with Raynaud's phenomenon and CREST syndrome.[88] This antibody can be found in 22%–36% of patients with scleroderma.[92] Therefore, this test may be helpful when attempting to diagnose a patient with scleroderma.

20.12.8 Erythrocyte Sedimentation Rate

Erythrocyte sedimentation rate (ESR) is a diagnostic criterion in patients with polymyalgia rheumatica and temporal arteritis, with a sensitivity of 80% for polymyalgia rheumatica and 95% for temporal arteritis.[94–96] It can also be useful in staging rheumatoid arthritis, with a sensitivity of 50% in patients with symptoms of rheumatoid arthritis.[97] However, the specificity of an elevated ESR is low, thus limiting its use as a diagnostic test[91] (Table 20.7).

TABLE 20.7
SORT: Key Recommendations for Practice

Clinical Recommendations	Evidence Rating	References
No correlation between blood urea nitrogen levels, muscle injury from eccentric exercise, or long-term creatine supplementation.	B	[9,10]
An athlete with persistent CK above 1000 U/L, even with rest, warrants a full evaluation.	C	
Routine screening of ferritin levels should be completed for male endurance athletes and female athletes in general.	A	[40,45,46]
Iron-deficient athletes who are normocytic have shown increased maximal performance capacity and endurance when placed on an iron supplementation.	A	[43,44]
G6PD-deficient athletes may participate in high-intensity muscle-damaging activities without any negative impact.	B	[47,49]
Team physicians and athletic trainers should be educated on sickle-cell trait, risk factors for complications, and understanding serious complications associated with sickle-cell trait.	C	[57,58]
Sickle-cell trait should not bar and athlete from routine sports participation.	C	[55]
Vitamin D levels below 25 ng/mL warrant replacement.	C	[59]
Male athletes along with females less than 25 years old who are sexually active should have a urine chlamydia screen.	A	[63,64]
Athletes with HIV should be allowed to participate in all sports.	A	[64]
Unexplained inflammatory synovial fluid in a febrile patient is considered infective until proven otherwise.	B	[75]

REFERENCES

1. Speedy DB, Noakes TD, Rogers IR et al. Hyponatremia in ultradistance triathletes. *Medicine and Science in Sports and Exercise.* 1999;31(6):809–815.
2. Noakes TD, Norman RJ, Buck RH et al. The incidence of hyponatremia during prolonged ultraendurance exercise. *Medicine and Science in Sports and Exercise.* 1990;22(2):165–170.
3. O'Connor RE. Exercise-induced hyponatremia: Causes, risks, prevention, and management. *Cleveland Clinic Journal of Medicine.* 2006;73(Suppl 3):S13.
4. Hiller W. Dehydration and hyponatremia during triathlons. *Medicine and Science in Sports and Exercise.* 1989; 21(5 Suppl):S219–S221.
5. Noakes TD, Sharwood K, Speedy D et al. Three independent biological mechanisms cause exercise-associated hyponatremia: Evidence from 2,135 weighed competitive athletic performances. *Proceedings of the National Academy of Sciences of the United States of America.* 2005;102(51):18550–18555.
6. Murray B, Stofan J, Eichner ER. Hyponatremia in athletes. *Sports Science.* 2003;88:88.
7. Noakes T. Hyponatremia in distance runners: Fluid and sodium balance during exercise. *Current Sports Medicine Reports.* 2002;1(4):197–207.
8. Andreoli TE, Gregory Fitz J, Benjamin I et al. *Andreoli and Carpenter's Cecil Essentials of Medicine.* Philadelphia, PA: Elsevier Health Sciences; 2010.
9. Kreider RB, Melton C, Rasmussen CJ et al. Long-term creatine supplementation does not significantly affect clinical markers of health in athletes, in Clark JF (ed.) *Guanidino Compounds in Biology and Medicine.* New York: Springer; 2003, p. 95–104.
10. Martin RP, Haskell WL, Wood PD. Blood chemistry and lipid profiles of elite distance runners. *Annals of the New York Academy of Sciences.* 1977;301(1):346–360.
11. Banfi GF, Massimo Del, Serum creatinine values in elite athletes competing in 8 different sports: Comparison with sedentary people. *Clinical chemistry.* 2006;52(2):330–331.
12. Lippi G, Brocco G, Franchini M et al. Comparison of serum creatinine, uric acid, albumin and glucose in male professional endurance athletes compared with healthy controls. *Clinical chemistry and laboratory medicine.* 2004;42(6):644–647.
13. Gerth J, Ott U, Fünfstück R et al. The effects of prolonged physical exercise on renal function, electrolyte balance and muscle cell breakdown. *Clinical Nephrology.* 2002;57(6):425–431.
14. Banfi G, MorelliP. Relation between body mass index and serum aminotransferases concentrations in professional athletes. *The Journal of Sports Medicine and Physical Fitness.* 2008;48(2):197–200.
15. Lippi G, Schena F, Montagnana M et al. Significant variation of traditional markers of liver injury after a half-marathon run. *European Journal of Internal Medicine.* 2011;22(5):e36–e38.
16. Hoffman JR, Maresh CM, Newton RU et al. Performance, biochemical, and endocrine changes during a competitive football game. *Medicine and Science in Sports and Exercise.* 2002;34(11):1845–1853.
17. Maddali S, Rodeo SA, Barnes RP et al. Postexercise increase in nitric oxide in football players with muscle cramps. *The American Journal of Sports Medicine.* 1998;26(6):820–824.
18. Kane SF, Cohen MI. Evaluation of the asymptomatic athlete with hepatic and urinalysis abnormalities. *Current Sports Medicine Reports.* 2009;8(2):77–84.
19. Banfi G, Colombini A, Lombardi G et al. Metabolic markers in sports medicine. *Advances in Clinical Chemistry.* 2012;56:2.

20. Ohman EM, Teo KK, Johnson AH et al. Abnormal cardiac enzyme responses after strenuous exercise: Alternative diagnostic aids. *British Medical Journal* (Clinical Research ed.). 1982;285(6354):1523.
21. Kupchak BR, Volk B, Kunces L et al. Alterations in coagulatory and fibrinolytic systems following an ultra-marathon. *European Journal of Applied Physiology.* 2013; 113(11):2705–2712.
22. Huerta-Alardín AL, Varon J, Marik PE. Bench-to-bedside review: Rhabdomyolysis—An overview for clinicians. *Critical Care.* 2005;9(2):158–169.
23. Melli G, Chaudhry V, Cornblath DR. Rhabdomyolysis: An evaluation of 475 hospitalized patients. *Medicine.* 2005; 84(6):377–385.
24. Neumeier, D. Jockers-Wretou E. Tissue specific and subcellular distribution of creatine kinase isoenzymes, in *Creatine Kinase Isoenzymes.* Springer; 1981, p. 85–131.
25. Miles MP, Clarkson PM, Smith LL et al. 948 serum creatine kinase activity in males and females following two bouts of eccentric exercise. *Medicine & Science in Sports & Exercise.* 1994;26(5):S168.
26. Brewster LM, Coronel CMD, Sluiter W et al. Ethnic differences in tissue creatine kinase activity: An observational study. *PLoS One.* 2012;7(3):e32471.
27. Miller M. Muscle enzymes in the evaluation of neuromuscular disease, in UpToDate 2008: Waltham, MA.
28. Miller M. Clinical manifestations and diagnosis of Rhabdomyolysis, in UpToDate2012: Waltham, MA.
29. Mikkelsen T, Toft P. Prognostic value, kinetics and effect of CVVHDF on serum of the myoglobin and creatine kinase in critically ill patients with rhabdomyolysis. *Acta Anaesthesiologica Scandinavica.* 2005;49(6):859–864.
30. Tefferi A, Hanson CA, Inwards DJ. How to interpret and pursue an abnormal complete blood cell count in adults, in *Mayo Clinic Proceedings.* Rochester, MN: Elsevier, 2005; 80(7):923–936.
31. Eichner ER. Sports medicine pearls and pitfalls: Benign Neutropenia in athletes. *Current Sports Medicine Reports.* 2009;8(4):162–163.
32. Sharpe K, Hopkins W, Emslie KR et al. Development of reference ranges in elite athletes for markers of altered erythropoiesis. *Haematologica.* 2002;87(12):1248–1257.
33. Mairbäurl H. Red blood cells in sports: Effects of exercise and training on oxygen supply by red blood cells. *Frontiers in Physiology.* 2013;4:9–21.
34. Sawka MN, Convertino VA, Eichner R et al. Blood volume: Importance and adaptations to exercise training, environmental stresses, and trauma/sickness. *Medicine and Science in Sports and Exercise.* 2000;32(2):332–348.
35. Convertino V. Fluid shifts and hydration state: Effects of long-term exercise. *Canadian Journal of Sport Sciences* (*Journal canadien des sciences du sport*). 1986;12(Suppl 1):136S–139S.
36. Perry GS, Byers T, Yip R et al. Iron nutrition does not account for the hemoglobin differences between blacks and whites. *The Journal of Nutrition.* 1992;122(7):1417–1424.
37. *Dietary Supplement Fact Sheet: Iron*, Office of Dietary Supplements, National Institutes of Health, February 19, 2015; Available from: http://ods.od.nih.gov/factsheets/iron-health-professional/. Accessed June 24, 2015.
38. Valberg L. Plasma ferritin concentrations: Their clinical significance and relevance to patient care. *Canadian Medical Association Journal.* 1980;122(11):1240.
39. Newhouse I, Clement D. Iron status in athletes. *Sports Medicine.* 1988;5(6):337–352.
40. Rodenberg RE, Gustafson S. Iron as an ergogenic aid: Ironclad evidence? *Current Sports Medicine Reports.* 2007;6(4):258–264.
41. Zoller H, Vogel W. Iron supplementation in athletes—First do no harm. *Nutrition.* 2004;20(7):615–619.
42. Rowland T. Iron deficiency in athletes: An update. *American Journal of Lifestyle Medicine.* 2012;6(4):319–327.
43. Friedmann B, Weller E, Mairbaurl H et al. Effects of iron repletion on blood volume and performance capacity in young athletes. *Medicine and Science in Sports and Exercise.* 2001;33(5):741–746.
44. Hinton P, Sinclair L. Iron supplementation maintains ventilatory threshold and improves energetic efficiency in iron-deficient nonanemic athletes. *European Journal of Clinical Nutrition.* 2006;61(1):30–39.
45. Arne L, Peter JJ, Lars E et al. Consensus statement: The International Olympic Committee (IOC) Consensus Statement on periodic health evaluation of elite athletes March 2009. British Journal of Sports Medicine. 2009;43:631–643.
46. DellaValle DM. Iron supplementation for female athletes: Effects on iron status and performance outcomes. *Current Sports Medicine Reports.* 2013;12(4):234–239.
47. Jamurtas AZ, Fatouros IG, Koukosias N et al. Effect of exercise on oxidative stress in individuals with glucose-6-phosphate dehydrogenase deficiency. *In Vivo.* 2006;20(6B):875–880.
48. *Unsafe to Take.* 1996 [cited May 2014]; Available from: http://www.g6pd.org/en/G6PDDeficiency/SafeUnsafe/DaEvitare_ISS-it
49. Theodorou AA, Nikolaidis MG, Paschalis V et al. Comparison between glucose-6-phosphate dehydrogenase-deficient and normal individuals after eccentric exercise. *Medicine and Science in Sports and Exercise.* 2010;42(6):1113–1121.
50. Motulsky AG. Frequency of sickling disorders in US blacks. *The New England Journal of Medicine.* 1973;288(1):31–33.
51. Wethers DL. Sickle cell disease in childhood: Part I. Laboratory diagnosis, pathophysiology and health maintenance. *American Family Physician.* 2000;62(5):1013–1020, 1027–1028.
52. Lees C, Davies S, Dezateux C. Neonatal screening for sickle cell disease. *Cochrane Database of Systematic Reviews*, 2000;2:CD001913.
53. Harmon KG, Drezner JA, Klossner D et al. Sickle cell trait associated with a RR of death of 37 times in national collegiate athletic association football athletes: A database with 2 million athlete-years as the denominator. *British Journal of Sports Medicine.* 2012;46(5):325–330.
54. Kark JA, Posey DM, Schumacher HR et al. Sickle-cell trait as a risk factor for sudden death in physical training. *New England Journal of Medicine.* 1987;317(13):781–787.
55. ACSM and NCAA Joint Statement on Sickle Cell Trait and Exercise, in *National Collegiate Athletic Association* 2013, National Collegiate Athletic Association.
56. Klossner D. *2013–14 NCAA Sports Medicine Handbook.* Indianapolis: National Collegiate Athletic Association; 2013.
57. *ACSM Current Comment: Sickle Cell Trait*, 2007, American College of Sports Medicine.
58. Anderson SE. *Consensus Statement: Sickle Cell Trait and the Athlete*, 2007, National Athletic Trainer's Association.
59. Trojian TH. To screen or not to screen: Commentary and review on screening laboratory tests in elite athletes. *Current Sports Medicine Reports.* 2014;13(4):209–211.
60. Larson-Meyer DE, Willis KS. Vitamin D and athletes. *Current Sports Medicine Reports.* 2010;9(4):220–226.

61. Moran DS, McClung JP, Kohen T et al. Vitamin D and physical performance. *Sports Medicine.* 2013;43(7):601–611.
62. Larson-Meyer E. Vitamin D supplementation in athletes; 2013.
63. Habel MA, Dittus PJ, De Rosa CJ et al. Daily participation in sports and students' sexual activity. *Perspectives on Sexual and Reproductive Health.* 2010;42(4):244–250.
64. Huang J-H, Jacobs DF, Derevensky JL. Sexual risk-taking behaviors, gambling, and heavy drinking among US college athletes. *Archives of Sexual Behavior.* 2010;39(3):706–713.
65. Brown LS, Drotman DP, Chu A et al. Bleeding injuries in professional football: Estimating the risk for HIV transmission. *Annals of Internal Medicine.* 1995;122(4):271–274.
66. Mast EE, Goodman RA, Bond WW et al. Transmission of blood-borne pathogens during sports: Risk and prevention. *Annals of Internal Medicine.* 1995;122(4):283–285.
67. Nelson M et al. Human immunodeficiency virus acquired immunodeficiency syndrome (aids) virus in the athletic setting. *Pediatrics.* 1991;88(3):640–641.
68. Patel DR, Torres AD, Greydanus DE. Kidneys and sports. *Adolescent Medicine Clinics.* 2005;16(1):111–119, xi.
69. Grossfeld GD, Litwin MS, Wolf JS et al. Evaluation of asymptomatic microscopic hematuria in adults: The American Urological Association best practice policy—Part I: Definition, detection, prevalence, and etiology. *Urology.* 2001; 57(4):599–603.
70. Grossfeld GD, Litwin MS, Wolf JS Jr et al. Evaluation of asymptomatic microscopic hematuria in adults: The American Urological Association best practice policy—Part II: Patient evaluation, cytology, voided markers, imaging, cystoscopy, nephrology evaluation, and follow-up. *Urology.* 2001;57(4):604–610.
71. Cohen RA, Brown RS. Microscopic hematuria. *New England Journal of Medicine.* 2003;348(23): 2330–2338.
72. Jones GR, Newhouse I. Sport-related hematuria: A review. *Clinical Journal of Sport Medicine.* 1997;7(2):119–125.
73. Deitrick R. Intravascular haemolysis in the recreational runner. *British Journal of Sports Medicine.* 1991;25(4):183–187.
74. Lindberg U, Claesson I, Hanson LA et al. Asymptomatic bacteriuria in schoolgirls: VIII. Clinical course during a 3-year follow-up. *The Journal of Pediatrics.* 1978;92(2):194–199.
75. Shmerling R et al. Guidelines for the initial evaluation of the adult patient with acute musculoskeletal symptoms. *Arthritis and Rheumatism.* 1996;39(1):1–8.
76. Kingston A-R, Toms AP, Ghosh-Ray S et al. Does running cause metatarsophalangeal joint effusions? A comparison of synovial fluid volumes on MRI in athletes before and after running. *Skeletal Radiology.* 2009;38(5):499–504.
77. Russell A. *Synovial Fluid Analysis.* Waltham, MA: UpToDate; 2014.
78. Margaretten ME, Kohlwes J, Moore D et al. Does this adult patient have septic arthritis? *Journal of the American Medical Association.* 2007;297(13):1478–1488.
79. Shmerling RH, Delbanco TL, Tosteson AN et al. Synovial fluid tests: What should be ordered? *Journal of the American Medical Association.* 1990;264(8):1009–1014.
80. Dougados M. Synovial fluid cell analysis. *Baillière's Clinical Rheumatology.* 1996;10(3):519–534.
81. Kay J, Eichenfield AH, Athreya BH et al. Synovial fluid eosinophilia in Lyme disease. *Arthritis & Rheumatism.* 1988;31(11):1384–1389.
82. Shmerling RH. Synovial fluid analysis. A critical reappraisal. *Rheumatic Diseases Clinics of North America.* 1994;20(2):503–512.
83. Sharp JT, Lidsky MD, Duffy J et al. Infectious arthritis. *Archives of Internal Medicine.* 1979;139(10):1125–1130.
84. Wise CM, Morris CR, Wasilauskas BL et al. Gonococcal arthritis in an era of increasing penicillin resistance: Presentations and outcomes in 41 recent cases (1985–1991). *Archives of Internal Medicine.* 1994;154(23):2690–2695.
85. Shmerling RH, Delbanco TL. The rheumatoid factor: An analysis of clinical utility. *The American Journal of Medicine.* 1991;91(5):528–534.
86. Shmerling R. Rheumatic disease: Choosing the most useful diagnostic tests. *Geriatrics.* 1996;51(11):22–6, 29–30, 32.
87. Semple S, Smith LL, McKune AJ et al. Alterations in acute-phase reactants (CRP, rheumatoid factor, complement, Factor B, and immune complexes) following an ultramarathon. *South African Journal of Sports Medicine.* 2004;16(2):17–21.
88. Peng S, Hardin J, Craft J. Antinuclear antibodies. *Textbook of Rheumatology.* 1997;1:250–266.
89. Calabrese LH, Kleiner SM, Barna BP et al. The effects of anabolic steroids and strength training on the human immune response. *Medicine and Science in Sports and Exercise.* 1989;21(4):386–392.
90. Reeves W, Satoh M, Wang J et al. Systemic lupus erythematosus. Antibodies to DNA, DNA-binding proteins, and histones. *Rheumatic Diseases Clinics of North America.* 1994;20(1):1–28.
91. Lane SK, Gravel JW, Jr. Clinical utility of common serum rheumatologic tests. *American Family Physician.* 2002; 65(6):1073–1080.
92. Moder KG. Use and interpretation of rheumatologic tests: A guide for clinicians. in *Mayo Clinic Proceedings.* Elsevier; 1996.
93. Harley J, Scofield R, Reichlin M. Anti-Ro in Sjogren's syndrome and systemic lupus erythematosus. *Rheumatic Diseases Clinics of North America.* 1992;18(2):337–358.
94. Fauchald P, Rygvold O, Øystese B. Temporal arteritis and polymyalgia rheumatica: Clinical and biopsy findings. *Annals of Internal Medicine.* 1972;77(6):845–852.
95. Gonzalez-Gay MA, Rodriguez-Valverde V, Blanco R et al. Polymyalgia rheumatica without significantly increased erythrocyte sedimentation rate: A more benign syndrome. *Archives of Internal Medicine.* 1997;157(3):317–320.
96. Sox HC, Liang MH. Diagnostic decision: The erythrocyte sedimentation rate guidelines for rational use. *Annals of Internal Medicine.* 1986;104(4):515–523.
97. Wolfe F, Michaud K. The clinical and research significance of the erythrocyte sedimentation rate. *The Journal of Rheumatology.* 1994;21(7):1227–1237.

21 Nerve Conduction Studies and Electromyography

Jason Friedrich and Venu Akuthota

CONTENTS

TABLE 21.1
Key Clinical Considerations

1. Electrodiagnostic (EDX) testing serves as an extension of the neuromuscular physical exam to better localize and characterize a lesion within the peripheral nervous system, including anterior horn cell, nerve root, plexus, peripheral motor nerves, large fiber sensory nerves, neuromuscular junction, and muscle fibers.
2. A typical EDX consultation will include two complementary parts: nerve conduction studies and needle electromyography (EMG).
3. The quality of an EDX consultation is dependent on the skill level of the consultant, as clinical judgment is required throughout the study.
4. To optimize the value of an EDX study, the referring provider should formulate a clinical differential diagnosis prior to the study such that a more specific question can be answered.
5. Timing matters when considering EDX testing. Most nerve injuries are optimally tested between 1 and 3 months after onset. A severe traumatic nerve injury may be tested immediately then serially to monitor for spontaneous recovery.

21.1 INTRODUCTION

Although the patient history and physical examination remain the most important steps for the identification of a nerve injury, electrodiagnostic (EDX) testing can augment the clinical evaluation to better localize and characterize suspected nerve pathology. Whereas imaging studies assess structural anatomy, EDX studies assess nerve physiology and provide information about the function of the peripheral nervous system (PNS). However, findings from an EDX study should not be viewed in isolation but rather need to be interpreted in the full clinical context. EDX studies are highly dependent on the quality of the examiner as clinical judgment is required throughout the study (Table 21.1).[1–3,5,7,8]

Most EDX evaluations involve two complementary parts: nerve conduction studies (NCS) and needle electromyography (EMG). NCS yield information about electrical conduction along large fiber motor and sensory nerves. Needle EMG samples muscle fibers with a small needle electrode and can provide information regarding the entire motor unit from the anterior horn cell in the spinal cord to the muscle fibers it eventually innervates. The term "electromyography" or "EMG" is often inappropriately used to describe all components of the EDX evaluation but should properly be reserved for describing only the needle examination.[2]

This chapter will provide an overview of peripheral nerve anatomy and pathophysiology of nerve injury, as they relate to EDX testing. At the conclusion of the chapter, the reader will be able to describe the indications for ordering EDX testing, understand the value and limitations of NCS and EMG, and be able to effectively utilize an EDX report.

21.2 APPLIED ANATOMY OF THE PERIPHERAL NERVOUS SYSTEM

EDX studies evaluate the PNS, both afferent sensory nerves and efferent motor nerves, including the lower motor neuron pathway[7,8] (see Figure 21.1).

Standard EDX testing provides little information about the integrity of the central nervous system (CNS) or upper motor neuron pathway.

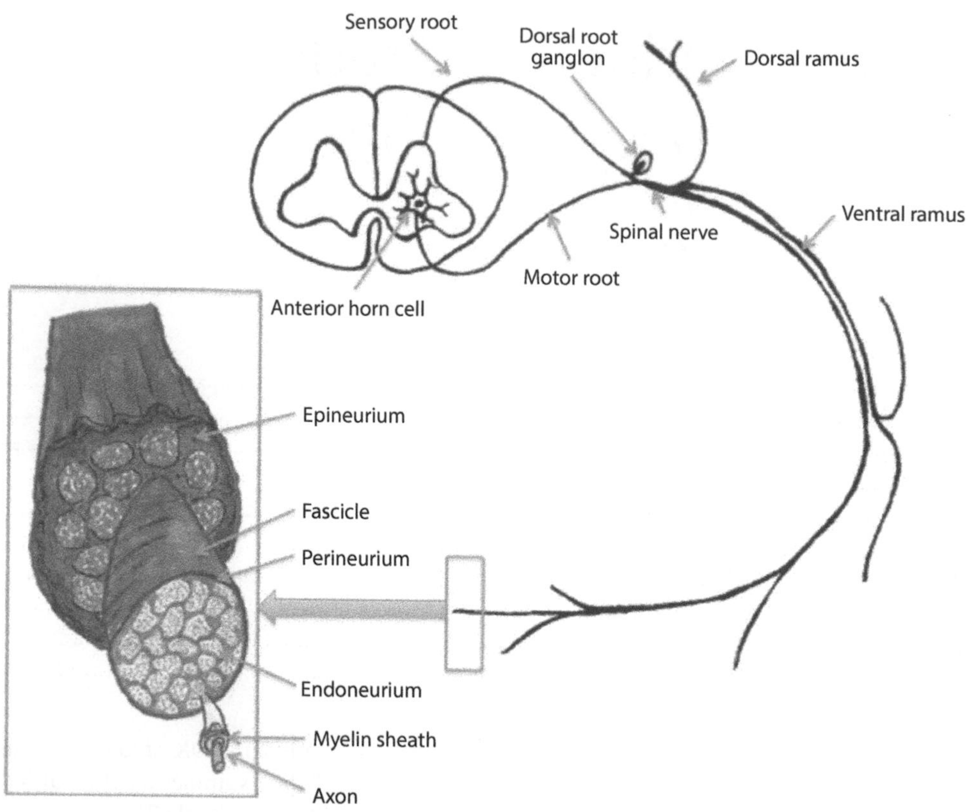

FIGURE 21.1 Anatomy of the peripheral nerve. (From Akuthota, V. and Friedrich, J.M., in O'Connor, F. et al. (eds.), *ACSM's Sports Medicine: A Comprehensive Review*, American College of Sports Medicine, Philadelphia, PA, 2013. Online Supplement.)

Within the PNS, the afferent sensory pathway begins with cutaneous receptors forming sensory axons, which coalesce to form pure sensory nerves or bundle with motor axons to form mixed nerves.[2] From the periphery, the sensory fibers travel through specific portions of nerve plexuses (e.g., brachial plexus, lumbosacral plexus) to their cell bodies in the dorsal root ganglion (DRG), usually located within the intervertebral foramina. Moving proximal from the DRG, the sensory fibers form dorsal roots in preparation for synapse in the dorsolateral spinal cord. This pathway is evaluated during NCS of pure sensory or mixed nerves.

The *efferent motor pathway* (i.e., the lower motor neuron pathway) starts at the anterior horn cells within the gray matter of the ventral spinal cord. Motor fibers form a ventral root and exit the spinal canal via intervertebral foramina as spinal nerves, subsequently dividing into ventral and dorsal rami. The motor fibers in the ventral rami then traverse their respective plexuses and become peripheral motor nerves, which ultimately synapse at specific limb muscles through neuromuscular junctions. The dorsal rami motor fibers innervate the paraspinal musculature in a segmental distribution based on their spinal level; thus, these fibers do not contribute to the brachial or lumbosacral plexuses. At neuromuscular junctions, acetylcholine is transported to the muscle membrane to induce an all-or-none action potential. This lower motor neuron pathway is evaluated during NCS of motor or mixed nerves, from the point of stimulation to the recording site over a muscle. A *motor unit* is defined as an anterior horn cell, its axon, and all the muscle fibers it innervates. Individual motor units can be evaluated during the needle EMG with voluntary muscle activation.[2,3]

Within the motor and sensory pathways of the PNS, there still exists a heterogeneous group of nerve fibers, roughly categorized by fiber size and presence of myelin. NCS only test the largest and fastest fibers (Type 1, A-α fibers). Myelin is made from Schwann cells in the PNS and serves as insulation for the axon, decreasing resistance and capacitance and allowing more rapid conduction down the axon.[8] Thus, injury to the myelin slows down conduction velocity.

Clinical Pearl

EDX studies do *not* test pain directly. In the PNS, pain conduction occurs via small and unmyelinated C-fibers, which are not assessed with NCS. A patient can experience true neuropathic pain and have a normal EDX study. When neuropathic pain is associated with a large fiber nerve injury, then EDX can help localize the source of this pain.

21.3 APPLIED PATHOPHYSIOLOGY OF PERIPHERAL NERVE INJURY

Peripheral nerve injuries are categorized by injury to the myelin sheath alone (i.e., the insulation of the nerve) or to the axon (i.e., the nerve fiber proper). Seddon classification divides traumatic peripheral nerve injuries into neurapraxia, axonotmesis, and neurotmesis.[1–3,8]

Neurapraxia is a comparatively mild injury that affects only the myelin sheath and causes focal conduction slowing or *conduction block (i.e., failure of axonal conduction past a segment of demyelination)* as a result of current leakage.[18] Although the myelin is injured, the axons remain in continuity. This results in motor or sensory loss from impaired conduction across the demyelinated segment. However, impulse conduction is normal distal to the injury, where the myelin remains intact.[2,3]

Clinical Pearl

The presence of conduction block on NCS is often a positive prognostic indicator as myelin damage recovers faster than axonal injury.

Because the axon is intact, the needle EMG will be normal. For example, a runner with true tarsal tunnel syndrome often experiences a neurapraxic injury of the tibial nerve branches due to repeated traction injury with the foot in pronation.[2] More generally, demyelination injuries can occur with focal nerve entrapments (e.g., carpal tunnel syndrome) or with more systemic peripheral polyneuropathies as either a patchy process (e.g., Guillain–Barre syndrome) or a diffuse process (e.g., diabetic peripheral polyneuropathy).[2,3]

Axonotmesis and *neurotmesis* refer to axonal injury with *Wallerian degeneration* ("dying back") of nerve fibers disconnected from their cell bodies. These types of injuries result in loss of nerve conduction at the site of injury and distally. Axonotmetic injuries involve damage to the axon, with some preservation of the surrounding stroma (endoneurium, perineurium, epineurium), whereas neurotmetic injuries imply complete disruption of the enveloping nerve sheath. EDX studies typically cannot distinguish axonotmesis from neurotmesis.[2,18] Athletes can experience a variety of axonal nerve injuries, such as axillary nerve injury following shoulder dislocation. More generally, most toxic and metabolic peripheral polyneuropathies (such as alcohol-induced neuropathy) tend to produce more of an axonal than demyelinating injury.

Recovery is possible from both neurapraxic and axonal injuries, though the timeline differs and degree of recovery depends on the cause, severity, and location of the injury. In general, neurapraxic injuries can recover over weeks to months through regeneration of myelin from Schwann cells. Axonal injuries can improve over months to years through both *terminal sprouting* (i.e., intact axons take over adjacent denervated muscle fibers) and *axonal regrowth*.[8,18] Sensory recovery is thought to be slower than motor recovery in most instances.

Clinical Pearl

Axonal regrowth occurs at a rate of 1 mm/day or 1 in./month from cell body to target muscle.

21.4 WHAT ARE THE ROUTINE EDX STUDIES?

When you refer to an EDX evaluation, you can typically expect your patient to receive both NCS and needle EMG. Each part of the evaluation has its own strengths and shortcomings; therefore, it is imperative that a well-trained consultant performs EDX studies and can recognize sources of error during testing and not overcall diagnoses.[1–3]

Clinical Pearl

EDX conclusions should be based on a pattern of abnormalities rather than an isolated finding.

21.4.1 Nerve Conduction Studies

NCS may be performed on motor, sensory, or mixed nerves to help determine the speed of conduction and number of functioning axons. A stimulator is used to deliver a current through the skin to depolarize the underlying nerve. The nerve transmits this impulse, which is then recorded by a surface electrode and measured. Both motor and sensory NCS test only the fastest, myelinated axons of a nerve.[5,13,14] Motor nerves are stimulated at accessible sites and the *compound motor action potential (CMAP)* is recorded over the motor points of their target muscles. Motor points represent regions of high concentration of neuromuscular junctions, typically in the central muscle belly. Deep motor nerves and deep proximal muscles are more difficult to examine.[10] Sensory nerves can be studied along the physiologic direction of the nerve impulse (*orthodromic*) or opposite the physiologic direction of the afferent input (*antidromic*). A stimulated sensory nerve produces the recorded *sensory nerve action potential (SNAP)*. Frequently, sensory nerves are tested within mixed nerves, such as the plantar nerves, and produce a mixed nerve action potential (MNAP).

CMAP, SNAP, and MNAP waveforms are analyzed and interpreted by the clinician. Waveform parameters include amplitude, latency, and conduction velocity. In general, *amplitude* measurement evaluates the number of functioning axons in a given nerve, and for motor nerves, the number of muscle fibers activated. *Latency* refers to the time (millisecond) from the stimulus to the recorded action potential. With motor NCS, latency accounts for peripheral nerve conduction (distal to the site of stimulation), neuromuscular junction transition time, and muscle fiber activation time.[8] With sensory nerves, latency measures only the conduction time within the segment of nerve stimulated. *Conduction velocity* is calculated by dividing the distance traveled by the impulse conduction time. For motor nerves, the segment between a distal and proximal stimulation site is used for the calculation of true conduction velocity as the neuromuscular junction time and muscle depolarization time can then be subtracted out.[8] In general, a normal motor nerve conduction velocity is >50 m/s in the upper limbs and >40 m/s in the lower limbs, accepting some variability for age and height.

Clinical Pearl

If prolonged latency or slowing of conduction velocity is reported, think myelin injury. If reduced amplitude is reported, think axonal injury (unless conduction block is also present).

21.4.2 Late Responses

Late responses are a type of nerve conduction study. Whereas routine NCS typically evaluate distal nerve segments, late responses, such as the H reflex and F wave, travel the full length of a nerve.[2,3] The most common *H reflex* is the electrophysiological analog to the ankle stretch reflex. It measures sensory and motor conduction along the S1 nerve root pathway.[11] A latency difference of at least 1.5 ms is significant in most laboratories. Amplitude of <50% compared with the uninvolved side is also significant. However, since the amplitude of this reflex is sensitive to contraction of the plantar flexor muscles, amplitude changes without associated latency abnormalities may not be pathological and should be interpreted with caution.[17]

Clinical Pearl

Cool limb temperatures slow conduction velocity, prolong latencies, and increase amplitudes on NCS. Limb temperatures should be reported. Normal limb temperatures are >30°C in lower limbs and >32°C in upper limbs.

The *F wave* is a late muscle potential that represents conduction up and down a motor nerve to the anterior horn cell and back, without any sensory contribution.[11] Like the H reflex, F wave studies examine long nerve pathways, which consequently obscure small focal abnormalities. Abnormalities of F wave values may be due to an injury anywhere along the pathway evaluated; thus, specificity is limited.

21.4.3 Needle Electromyography Examination

The needle EMG examination can characterize disorders of the motor unit (lower motor neuron pathway), but not the sensory pathway. When an injury is present to the motor unit, the EMG can often help localize it to the anterior horn cell, nerve root, plexus, peripheral nerve, neuromuscular junction, or muscle fiber. This component of the EDX evaluation includes needle EMG of muscles at rest (to detect potential axonal injury) and with volitional activity (to evaluate voluntary motor unit morphology and recruitment).[6]

At rest, muscles are studied for *abnormal spontaneous activity*. Of these abnormal waveforms, the most common are *fibrillation potentials* and *positive sharp waves*. They are found when the muscle tested has been denervated or injured.[8] The term "denervation potentials" should be avoided, as muscle membrane instability can also occur with local muscle trauma or inflammatory muscle diseases.

Clinical Pearl

Fibrillations and positive sharp waves are graded on a scale from 0 (absent) to 4+ depending on the amount of abnormal activity present. While a grading of 4+ probably represents more severe injury than 1+, other grades are more subjective and may or may not correlate with clinical severity.

Complex repetitive discharges (CRDs) are also common and represent ephaptic spread of a spontaneous discharge ("crosstalk") from a single muscle fiber to neighboring fibers.[2,3] CRDs may be present in the setting of long-standing cycles of denervation and reinnervation. *Fasciculation potentials* represent spontaneous discharges of an entire motor unit; thus, they are much larger than fibrillations and positive waves and can sometimes be grossly observed as muscle twitches. They can be found in a variety of benign or malignant conditions. Benign fasciculations may be found in athletes following heavy exercise, dehydration, anxiety, fatigue, coffee consumption, or smoking. [1–3]

When muscles are studied during contraction, *motor unit action potentials (MUAPs)* may be analyzed. Motor unit analysis offers a good opportunity to distinguish between neuropathic and myopathic processes, based on MUAP morphology and recruitment pattern differences.[1–3]

EMG may also help differentiate acute from chronic neuropathic conditions. The amplitude of fibrillation potentials can estimate a nerve injury as occurring for less than or more than 1 year (with smaller potentials for the latter).[15] This can be particularly helpful in identifying an acute or chronic nerve injury. Chronic nerve injuries may additionally show large-amplitude, long-duration, polyphasic MUAPs, representative of reinnervation through terminal sprouting or nerve regrowth.[17,18]

21.5 WHY ORDER EDX STUDIES?

The previous sections have provided an overview of nerve anatomy, pathophysiology, and the basis for EDX testing. This and the following sections aim to provide some practical guidelines to effectively utilize EDX studies, including indications and timing for testing, referral advice, and some guidance on interpreting the EDX report.

The *indications for EDX* testing vary depending on the clinical context. Of course, clinical recognition of patterns of pain, sensory, or motor abnormalities is the first step toward the identification of a nerve problem.[1–3]

Clinical Pearl

EDX testing is indicated when a motor or sensory deficit is discovered during clinical assessment and requires localization, characterization, confirmation, or ruling out a competing diagnosis.

However, localizing a nerve injury can be difficult with clinical exam alone. For example, an athlete presenting with plantar surface numbness and tingling may have a sciatic nerve lesion anywhere along the course of the sciatic nerve or its branches. EDX studies can be used to localize the injury within the nerve roots, plexus, or peripheral nerves.

Furthermore, EDX testing can help characterize a known nerve injury, offering information about the type of injury, chronicity, and severity, which can help guide prognosis and treatment.[5,17,18] Because EDX studies examine nerve physiology, they can provide a correlate of nerve function within a region of structural pathology found on imaging studies. EDX testing may also identify an unsuspected concomitant and overlapping pathological process. For instance, in a type of "double-crush syndrome" coexisting ulnar neuropathy may be found in a patient with a clinical C8 radiculopathy causing some overlapping motor and sensory deficits in the hand.

EDX studies can differentiate a neurapraxic injury from axonal degeneration, which has important implications for the timeline of recovery (Table 21.2). NCS can determine if neurapraxic injury is present and can analyze CMAP motor amplitudes to estimate the proportion of surviving axons. In the absence of conduction block, side-to-side amplitude difference of >50% likely represents significant axonal loss. Generally, the greater the percentage of surviving axons, the better the prognosis.[1,2,18]

Needle EMG evaluation of volitional motor units can also offer prognostic information.[1–3,18] Of course, if no motor units are detected during the early stages and NCS do not reveal conduction block, a severe axonal injury is present and full recovery is unlikely. After a couple of months, motor unit analysis can demonstrate the presence of early reinnervation by means of terminal reorganization or sprouting from preserved axons,[18] indicating an incomplete nerve injury and providing some cautious optimism for at least partial recovery.

In conjunction with the clinical history, the acuteness and chronicity of a nerve lesion may also be assessed with EMG using fibrillation amplitude measurement and motor unit analysis.[1–3,15] This information may have a significant impact on the aggressiveness of treatment for the nerve injury and can be helpful for identifying an acute or chronic injury. For instance, an athlete may have some persistent symptoms from an old lumbar radiculopathy and experience some worsening or recurrence of usual symptoms. EDX testing can be helpful to determine if a new injury has occurred.

21.5.1 Contraindications

There are no absolute contraindications to testing because portions of the exam can still be completed even if certain specific tests need to be avoided. Proximal stimulation at erb's point (often used when evaluating for brachial plexopathy)

TABLE 21.2
Classification of Nerve Injury and Electrodiagnostic Correlate

Injury Type	Pathology	EDX Correlate	Prognosis
Neurapraxia	Myelin injury	CV slows across injured segment; reduced amplitude proximal, but normal distal; needle EMG normal (except possible reduced recruitment)	Recovery in weeks to months
Axonotmesis	Axonal injury, with variable stromal disruption	Reduced amplitude proximal and distal; abnormal spontaneous activity; abnormal voluntary motor units	Longer recovery (months to years) and more variable
Neurotmesis	Nerve severed	No waveform proximal or distal; abnormal spontaneous activity; no recruited motor units	Poor recovery, surgery required

Source: Adapted from Akuthota, V. and Friedrich, J.M., Electrodiagnostic testing in the runner, in: Wilder, R. et al., eds., *Running Medicine*, 2nd edn., Healthy Learning, Monterey, CA, 2014.

Note: CV, conduction velocity; EMG, electromyography.

should be avoided in patients with a pacemaker. Needle EMG should be avoided in regions at risk for infection, including limbs with open wounds, anasarca, or lymphedema or near an AV fistula.[1–3]

Clinical Pearl

Anticoagulation is not a contraindication to needle EMG, though clinical judgment is used in higher-risk muscle groups.

21.6 WHEN TO ORDER EDX STUDIES

When considering EDX testing, the duration of symptoms is important. If an EDX study is performed too early or too late, certain findings will not be detectible[1–3] (see Table 21.3).

With acute traumatic nerve injuries, serial EDX testing, including an immediate study, may be helpful to determine the extent of injury. NCS can provide some limited information regarding the presence of a specific nerve injury immediately. Within 9–11 days, NCS can differentiate conduction block from axonotmesis, which provides early prognostic information. Before this time, the distal segment NCS may be normal in both neurapraxic and axonal injuries. A study at 1 month can utilize information from both NCS and EMG. If EMG is performed too early (i.e., less than 2–3 weeks after the initial injury), spontaneous muscle fiber discharges (i.e., positive sharp waves and fibrillations) may not have had time to develop. If the EMG is performed too late (i.e., more than 3–6 months after the initial injury), reinnervation from collateral sprouting may have stabilized the muscle membrane and halted spontaneous muscle fiber discharges.[1–3] The proximal muscles are reinnervated first (as early as 3 months), followed by distal muscles in a length-dependent fashion. For most insidious nerve injuries, testing anywhere between 1 and 3 months post onset will be adequate for diagnosis. For severe traumatic injuries, it is reasonable to test immediately, at 1 month, 3 months, and 6 months, to best define the evolution of injury and recovery. Repeat testing is only necessary if it will change the management of the patient, such as consideration for surgical exploration after a period of watchful waiting for spontaneous recovery.

Clinical Pearl

A poorly performed EDX study can be very misleading and delay proper diagnosis and treatment.

21.7 HOW TO GET THE MOST OUT OF AN EDX REFERRAL

Of course, the first step in ordering an EDX consultation is to formulate a clinical differential diagnosis and a specific question to be addressed by EDX testing. The referral should then be placed to a well-trained electrodiagnostician. The needle EMG in particular should *always* be performed by a physician well trained in EDX medicine, most often a physiatrist or a neurologist with special interest in neuromuscular diseases.

TABLE 21.3
Timing of Wallerian Degeneration, Nerve Recovery, and EDX Findings with Axonal Injury

Time	Nerve Degeneration	Nerve Recovery	NCS correlate	Needle EMG correlate
Day 0	None	None.	Abnormal across lesion; Normal distal to lesion	Decreased recruitment
Day 3	NMJ impaired	Nodal and terminal sprouts begin to form.		
Day 9	Motor axons lost		Distal segment CMAP drops	Increased insertional activity
Day 11	Sensory axons lost		Distal segment SNAP drops	
Day 14				Large fibs/PSWs in proximal followed by distal muscles
Day 21		Terminal sprout reorganization.		
Week 6–8			CMAP/SNAP increasing	Nascent reinnervation potentials followed by polyphasic MUAPs, followed by large-amplitude/long-duration MUAPs
Week 16		Axonal regrowth, 1mm/day, 1 in/month.		
Week 20				
Year 1				Smaller and potentially absent fibrillations
Year 2		Muscle no longer viable.		

Sources: Adapted from Akuthota, V. and Casey, E., Diagnostic tests for nerve and vascular injuries, in: Akuthota, V. and Herring, S.A., eds., *Nerve and Vascular Injuries in Sports Medicine*, Springer, New York, 2009; Akuthota, V. and Friedrich, J.M., Chapter 11: Electrodiagnostic testing in the runner, in: Wilder, R. et al., eds., *Running Medicine*, 2nd edn., Healthy Learning, Monterey, CA, 2014; Akuthota, V. and Friedrich, J.M., Chapter 20: Electrodiagnostic testing, in: O'Connor, F. et al., eds., *ACSM's Sports Medicine: A Comprehensive Review*, American College of Sports Medicine, Philadelphia, PA, 2013.

Note: CMAP, compound muscle action potential; fibs, fibrillation potentials; MUAPs, motor unit action potentials; NMJ, neuromuscular junction; PSWs, positive sharp waves; SNAP, sensory nerve action potential.

The EDX report can provide some insight into the quality of the electrodiagnostician.

21.7.1 Interpreting the EDX Report

While a comprehensive EDX consultation should integrate the history, physical exam, and EDX findings into a meaningful diagnosis, the referring provider may still need to correlate the EDX conclusion with their own working clinical diagnosis. Therefore, the ordering provider should understand not only the indications for ordering EDX testing but also the limitations and common pitfalls of EDX tests including being able to recognize a poor-quality study (see Table 21.4).

When an EDX report comes back, the first step is to determine if the referral question was addressed. This can often be determined by reading the diagnostic conclusions. If not, then look at the data to see what was tested. Were both NCS and needle EMG performed, and if not, is there an explanation? Perhaps most critical is whether or not the EDX findings correlate with the clinical findings. If there is a discrepancy, then some commentary should follow. Inconsistencies may have as much importance in the treatment of the patient as consistent results.[1–3] Ideally, the report should also give the referring provider the degree of confidence in the electrophysiological diagnosis, such as "definitive," "probable," and "possible." A diagnosis of an S1 radiculopathy by an H reflex alone will carry much less weight than abundant abnormal spontaneous activity in the S1 myotome and corresponding paraspinals.[1–3] One abnormal finding should not make the diagnosis if other evidence points to a different diagnosis.

When possible, the report should provide sufficient evidence to rule out alternative diagnoses and to identify superimposed conditions. Chronicity should be discussed, as well as compared to prior studies when available. Of course, the more specific the question to be answered, the higher yield the result from the study. For instance, a study is likely to be of higher quality and value if a patient is sent for evaluation of a suspected acute peroneal nerve injury versus L5 radiculopathy, rather than the same patient sent for "leg pain" or "numbness."

When utilizing EDX information, keep in mind that the most important measure of recovery is the patient's functional improvement on clinical exam.[1–3] Results from EDX studies can lag behind clinical improvement and incidental EDX findings do occur. For example, a patient may have electrophysiological evidence of a median neuropathy at the wrist on NCS, but should not undergo carpal tunnel release surgery unless they have clinical carpal tunnel syndrome.

TABLE 21.4
Checklist for Evaluating the EDX Report

- Was your specific question answered?
- Are the stated clinical findings consistent with your evaluation?
- Is the EDX conclusion consistent with clinical findings? If not, is this explained?
- Are appropriate negative findings described?
- Is there sufficient data to rule out alternative diagnoses?
- Were both NCS and EMG performed? If not, is there explanation?
- Is the presence of partial or complete conduction block described?
- Were limb temperatures monitored and recorded?
- Were cool limbs warmed?
- Are individual measures reported?
- Are normal values provided?

Sources: Akuthota V, Friedrich JM. Chapter 11: Electrodiagnostic testing in the runner. In: Wilder R, O'Connor F, Magrum E, eds. *Running Medicine*, 2nd edn. Monterey, CA: Healthy Learning, 2014; Albers JW. Numbness, tingling, and weakness. *AAEM Annual Assembly*, Vancouver, Johnson Printing Company, 1999.

Note: EDX, electrodiagnostic; EMG, electromyography; NCS, nerve conduction studies.

Clinical Pearl

An athlete should not be kept out of sport purely because of persistent EDX abnormalities if they are performing well on clinical testing in simulated sports activities.[1–3,10]

21.8 LIMITATIONS

EDX testing has many limitations and should not be performed on every patient with neurologic signs or symptoms.[1–3] Some diagnoses are unequivocal and treatment should be initiated without delay. As stated previously, EDX testing does not provide information about CNS disorders (i.e., upper motor neuron lesions), nor does it evaluate small fiber neuropathies, or certain types of muscle diseases that only affect Type II fibers (such as steroid-induced myopathy). EDX tests are timing and severity dependent and cannot rule out all possibility of a nerve injury. As with any diagnostic test, there can be incidental findings and false positives. The probability of one false-positive result increases with the number of tests performed: 12% probability if 5 tests performed and 20% if 9 tests performed. Therefore, EDX conclusions need to be based on a pattern of abnormalities, not on an isolated finding.[2,3,7]

Limitations, sources of error, and other pitfalls of NCS and EMG are summarized in Table 21.5.

Several limitations can be exemplified by the following scenario: you refer someone for testing for a suspected clinical C6 radiculopathy causing pain specifically in the lateral arm and sensory alteration over the index finger and thumb. While specific, EDX testing lacks sensitivity for radiculopathy and needle EMG may be normal. Furthermore, as part of the routine evaluation, the ulnar nerve may be tested and show some slowing of nerve conduction across the elbow (a test often wrought with measurement error). The report might state mild ulnar neuropathy across the elbow as the only EDX abnormality. Clearly, this patient does not have a symptomatic ulnar neuropathy, nor does this diagnosis correlate with your clinical suspicion of a C6 radiculopathy.

TABLE 21.5
Limitations and Sources of Error for EDX Studies

	Nerve Conduction Studies	Electromyography
Intrinsic limitation	• Can only test large/myelinated fibers • Anomalous innervation	• Time-dependent findings • Prior surgery or muscle trauma in region tested • Only can test Type I muscle fibers
Technical or physician error	• Cool limb temperature • Inadequate or excessive stimulation • Improper machine or electrode setup • Measurement error • Volume conduction to nearby nerve • Inadequate number of tests • Diagnosis based on isolated abnormality	• Poor technique • Incorrect interpretation of waveforms/sounds (e.g., classifying normal end plate spikes as fibrillations) • Inadequate number of muscles tested to localize the injury • Inadequate number of fibers tested within a muscle • Diagnosis based on isolated abnormality
Patient factors	• Age, height, obesity, edema, involuntary muscle contractions	• Poor cooperation or effort

Clinical Pearl

EDX testing can augment a clinical evaluation, but cannot and should not replace clinical judgment.

Athletes, especially runners, are often sent for EDX evaluation of suspected nerve injury in the foot or ankle. Relative to other body regions, EDX study of the foot may yield less definitive results due to some special challenges testing this region of the body.[2,3] Nonetheless, NCS and needle EMG of the foot intrinsic muscles by an experienced electromyographer can be useful in the evaluation of suspected nerve entrapment of the foot and ankle.[2,3,9,16]

21.9 SUMMARY

EDX testing serves as an extension of the physical exam to better localize and characterize a suspected nerve injury and are highly dependent on the quality of the consultant. EDX studies evaluate the PNS (anterior horn cell, nerve root, plexus, sensory, and motor peripheral nerve, neuromuscular junction and muscle fibers). EDX testing can help define the pathophysiology of a nerve injury and better characterize the location, duration, severity, and prognosis. The timing of EDX testing is important as some needle EMG findings may take 2–6 weeks to develop. The limitations of NCS and EMG need to be kept in mind when performing and interpreting EDX studies (Table 21.6).

TABLE 21.6
SORT: Key Recommendations for Practice

Clinical Recommendation	Evidence Rating	References
EDX testing should only occur following a clinical exam and establishment of a clinical differential diagnosis.	C	
If EDX findings do not correlate with the clinical problem, question the relevance of the EDX findings, consider technical error, reexamine the patient, and avoid treating an EDX abnormality that does not fit the clinical presentation.	C	
Question any EDX conclusion based on an isolated finding. EDX conclusions should be made based on a pattern of abnormalities.	C	
Be cautious with EDX conclusions based on provocation EDX testing (i.e., testing limbs in provocative positions). These techniques have not been validated with sound research and are prone to measurement error.	C	
Anticoagulants and antiplatelet agents should not be routinely discontinued for needle EMG. Clinical judgment on the part of the electromyographer is required in unique higher-risk situations.	A	[12]

REFERENCES

1. Akuthota V, Casey E. Diagnostic tests for nerve and vascular injuries. In: Akuthota V, Herring SA, eds. *Nerve and Vascular Injuries in Sports Medicine*, New York: Springer; 2009.
2. Akuthota V, Friedrich JM. Chapter 11: Electrodiagnostic testing in the runner. In: Wilder R, O'Connor F, Magrum E, eds. *Running Medicine*, 2nd edn. Monterey, CA: Healthy Learning; 2014.
3. Akuthota V, Friedrich JM. Chapter 20: Electrodiagnostic testing. In: O'Connor F, Casa D, Davis B, et al., eds. *ACSM's Sports Medicine: A Comprehensive Review.* Philadelphia, PA: American College of Sports Medicine; 2013.
4. Albers JW. Numbness, tingling, and weakness. *AAEM Annual Assembly*, Vancouver: Johnson Printing Company; 1999.
5. Chémali KR, Tsao B. Electrodiagnostic testing of nerves and muscles: When, why, and how to order. *Cleveland Clinic Journal of Medicine.* 2005;72(1):37–48.
6. Daube JR, Rubin DI. Needle electromyography. *Muscle Nerve.* 2009;39(2):244–270.
7. Dillingham, TR. Electrodiagnostic medicine II: clinical evaluation and findings. In: Braddom RL, ed. *Physical Medicine & Rehabilitation*, 3rd edn. Philadelphia, PA: Elsevier; 2007.
8. Dumitru D. *Electrodiagnostic Medicine.* Philadelphia, PA: Hanley and Belfus; 2001.
9. Dumitru D, Diaz CA, King JC. Prevalence of denervation in paraspinal and foot intrinsic musculature. *American Journal of Physical Medicine & Rehabilitation.* 2001;80(7):482–490.
10. Feinberg JH. The role of electrodiagnostics in the study of muscle kinesiology, muscle fatigue and peripheral nerve injuries in sports medicine. *Journal of Back and Musculoskeletal Medicine.* 1999;12:73–88.
11. Fisher MA. H reflexes and F waves: Fundamentals, normal and abnormal patterns. *Neurologic Clinics.* 2002;20(2): 339–360, vi.
12. Gertken JT, Patel AT, Boon AJ. Electromyography and Anticoagulation. *PM&R.* 2013;5S(Suppl 1):S3–S7.
13. Gooch CL, Weimer LH. The electrodiagnosis of neuropathy: Basic principles and common pitfalls. *Neurologic Clinics.* 2007;25(1):1–28.
14. Horowitz SH. The diagnostic work-up of patients with neuropathic pain. *Medical Clinics of North America.* 2007; 91(1):21–30.
15. Kraft GH. Fibrillation potential amplitude and muscle atrophy following peripheral nerve injury. *Muscle Nerve.* 1990;13(9):814–821.
16. Park TA, Del Toro DR. Electrodiagnostic evaluation of the foot. *Physical Medicine & Rehabilitation Clinics of North America.* 1998;9(4):871–896, vii–viii.
17. Press JM, Young JL. Electrodiagnostic evaluation of spine problems. In Gonzalez G, Materson RS, eds. *The Nonsurgical Management of Acute Low Back Pain.* New York: Demos Vermande; 1997. p. 191–203.
18. Robinson LR. AAEM minimonograph 28: Traumatic injury to peripheral nerves. *Muscle & Nerve.* 2000;23(6):863–873.

22 Exercise Testing

Russell D. White and George D. Harris

CONTENTS

TABLE 22.1
Key Clinical Considerations

1. The two most important factors in the analysis of patients undergoing exercise testing are the pretest prevalence of disease and the sensitivity and specificity of the selected test.
2. The selection of the protocol should be determined by the patient's cardiac risk factors: the patient's daily activities, cognitive status, age, weight, nutritional status, and mobility.
3. The examiner should stop the exercise test when the patient has reached maximal effort (Borg scale) or exhibits clinical signs to terminate.
4. Maximal test sensitivity is achieved with the patient supine postexercise. The examiner should auscultate the patient immediately for any abnormal heart findings such as a new-onset heart murmur or third heart sound.

22.1 INTRODUCTION

Exercise and activity depend on the physiologic functioning of the skeletal and cardiac muscle in the body. Muscle fatigue is based on (1) genetic characteristics, (2) training of the individual athlete, and (3) presence or absence of disease states that may adversely affect either cellular metabolism or overall functioning of the exercising body tissues. Patients with coronary artery disease (CAD) may have a combination of diseased cardiac muscle, localized vascular disease in the myocardium, or ischemia/infarction to a region of the heart affecting cardiac ejection fraction and cardiac output. This abnormal function can manifest clinically as poor exercise duration, electrocardiograph (ECG) changes of ischemia, and overall poor exercise duration with formal exercise testing. In general, maximal aerobic power decreases with age but can be maintained by active training and absence of disease states (Table 22.1).

22.2 INDICATIONS

There are limitations for recommending exercise testing for everyone choosing to begin an exercise program. However, one often discovers occult heart disease in many "asymptomatic" patients who instinctively exercise slightly below their "clinical" threshold for symptoms. In addition, one is able to appropriately develop an exercise program based on the objective testing in the studied patient. The American College of Sports Medicine (ACSM) has published recommendations for exercise testing prior to the beginning of an exercise regimen.[1] Activity level is divided into moderate or vigorous activity. Moderate activity is 3–6 METs or 40%–60% $VO_{2\ max}$, while vigorous activity is >6 METs or 40%–60% $VO_{2\ max}$. Those persons who want to perform moderate activity *and* are at high risk or want to perform vigorous activity and are at a moderate or high risk *require* an exercise test prior to initiating that level of exercise. Exercise testing in low-risk, asymptomatic males is usually not indicated unless there are specific risk factors. Although there is no chronological age for routine screening of individuals, the ACSM recommends that low-risk men and women (less than 45 and 55 years of age, respectively) be exempted from routine screening. Cautioned is advised since some individuals less than these ages may have coronary heart disease and symptoms. One *must* classify them according to the aforementioned criteria and *not* based solely on the individual's age and sex.

Additional indications for exercise testing are (1) evaluation of the patient with chest pain with activity even when you doubt cardiovascular disease, (2) determining the prognosis and severity of known cardiovascular disease, (3) evaluation and risk stratifying a patient after myocardial infarction (MI), (4) early detection and diagnosis of labile hypertension, (5) evaluating arrhythmias in a "controlled environment," (6) assessing a patient's functional capacity, or (7) determining the degree of heart failure in a given patient.[2]

Clinical Pearl

Many "asymptomatic" patients with heart disease instinctively exercise slightly below their "clinical" threshold for symptoms.

22.3 CONTRAINDICATIONS/COMPLICATIONS

When assessing a patient with chest pain, a thorough medical history can provide significant information toward the development of a differential diagnosis, while the physical exam further delineates the underlying cause. Determining further testing must rely on the inherent accuracy of the test defined by the sensitivity and specificity, the benefits versus risks to the patient, and any absolute versus relative contraindications for the test.[3]

Two important factors in the analysis of patients undergoing exercise testing are the pretest prevalence of disease and the sensitivity and specificity of the test. The pretest evaluation determines when and how to study an asymptomatic patient in whom the risk for coronary heart disease is low and there is an increase in false-positive findings.[4] When deciding how to study an asymptomatic patient for coronary disease, each patient must be properly evaluated by the history and physical examination as well as stratified by age, gender, symptoms (typical angina, atypical angina, nonanginal chest pain, no symptoms), and major risk factors (diabetes mellitus, hypertension, dyslipidemias, smoking).[4,5]

Multiple cohort studies have demonstrated that screening exercise tolerance testing identifies only a small proportion of *asymptomatic* persons (up to 2.7% of those screened) with severe coronary artery obstruction who may benefit from revascularization.

The *absolute contraindications* to performing exercise testing include a recent significant change in the resting ECG, recent MI (within 2 days) or other acute cardiac event, history consistent with unstable angina, uncontrolled cardiac arrhythmias causing symptoms or hemodynamic compromise, documented severe left main artery disease, severe symptomatic aortic stenosis, uncompensated congestive heart failure, an acute pulmonary embolus or pulmonary infarction (within 3 months), suspected or confirmed dissecting aneurysm, an acute infection, hyperthyroidism, severe anemia, acute myocarditis or pericarditis, and an uncooperative patient.[6]

The relative contraindications include those situations in which the risks involved with performing the procedure may outweigh the benefits. These patients require careful evaluation and a cardiology consultation in some cases; other patients may have underlying conditions that require correction or stabilization before testing. Relative contraindications to exercise testing include any known history of left main artery stenosis; moderately stenotic valvular heart disease; electrolyte abnormalities (e.g., hypokalemia, hypomagnesemia); severe arterial hypertension (systolic greater than 200 mmHg or diastolic greater than 110 mmHg); asymmetrical septal hypertrophy; hypertrophic cardiomyopathy or other forms of outflow tract obstruction; compensated heart failure; the presence of a ventricular aneurysm; any uncontrolled metabolic disease (e.g., diabetes mellitus, thyrotoxicosis, or myxedema); patients with high-degree atrioventricular heart block; tachy-brady arrhythmias; chronic infectious disease (e.g., mononucleosis, hepatitis, AIDS); high degree of atrioventricular block (second-degree Mobitz II or third-degree block); neuromuscular, musculoskeletal, or rheumatoid disorders that prohibit exercise; and any mental or physical impairment leading to inability to exercise adequately.[3,6]

Clinical Pearl

Multiple cohort studies have demonstrated that screening exercise tolerance testing identifies only a small proportion of *asymptomatic* persons (up to 2.7% of those screened) with severe coronary artery obstruction who may benefit from revascularization.

22.4 EQUIPMENT AND PERSONNEL

Necessary equipment for exercise testing includes (1) an exam table for patient preparation and recovery after the test, (2) an exercising device (e.g., treadmill, stationary bicycle or arm ergometer), (3) an ECG recording device, and (4) a monitor for evaluating the heart rate and rhythm in real time. In addition, (1) a defibrillator, (2) acute cardiac life support (ACLS) equipment, and (3) ACLS medications (crash cart) are necessary. Testing personnel, including a physician or mid-level provider trained in exercise testing and an assistant, should be ACLS trained and certified. In the United States, most testing is done with the treadmill, while in Europe, studies are commonly done with the stationary bicycle. In patients unable to walk or bike due to lower extremity disease, stroke, or amputation, studies can be done with arm ergometry but blood pressure measurements are cumbersome. One may select alternative testing, for example, pharmacologic chemical testing, in these patients.

22.5 EXERCISE PROTOCOLS/SPECIAL TESTING

There are standard protocols with specific speed and grade intervals available for each type of testing (e.g., treadmill, a bicycle, or a stepping device). Exercise testing performed in the United States tends to use a continuous, instead of an intermittent, format that varies in the amount of work applied and the duration of effort required. The patient is not allowed to rest but instead experiences a progressively increasing workload allowing for the patient's peak aerobic capacity or end point to be attained earlier.[7] The selection of the protocol should be determined by the patient's cardiac risk factors; the patient's daily activities, current fitness level, cognitive status, age, weight, nutritional status, and mobility. A number of patients seen in medical offices are high-risk patients who have several cardiovascular risk factors, are poorly conditioned, have had a previous MI, or have several cardiovascular risk factors.[2] The chosen protocol should include continuous ECG monitoring (during pretest, active testing, and posttest recovery), a type of activity to match the patient's ability, a varied workload, repeated blood pressure measurements in each stage or period, a method to estimate the aerobic requirements of tested individuals, maximum safety and minimum discomfort, and the highest possible specificity and sensitivity.[7,8] Various treadmill protocols have been developed for inducing and detecting ECG changes consistent with myocardial ischemia.[8,9] Regardless of the selected protocol the total exercise time needs to be at least 8–12 minutes.

Selecting the correct protocol is dependent on the patient's ability to perform exercise and the rationale for testing. A maximal exercise test provides the most information since the patient performs true maximum effort (greater than 10 METS) and reaches the personal point of exhaustion rather than a predicted level of exercise defined from age-determined heart rate tables. In post-MI patients, who need to be tested prior to discharge from the hospital, a low-level protocol (a submaximal test) is selected to evaluate for dysrhythmias or ischemia occurring at low levels of activity. The goal is 65% of the maximum predicted heart rate (MPHR) or 5 METs. An individual requires an exercise intensity of at least 5 METs to carry out the activities of daily living.

Worldwide, the *Bruce protocol* is the most common protocol used for exercise testing and comprises 66% of all routine clinical tests performed.[7,10]

Clinical Pearl

Worldwide, the Bruce protocol is the most common protocol used for exercise testing and comprises 66% of all routine clinical tests performed.

This protocol begins with a 3 minute stage of walking at 1.7 mph at 10% grade (Stage 1) and has the energy expenditure estimated to be 4.8 METs. The speed and incline increase with each stage; the incline is incremented 2% every 3 minutes and the speed is incremented 0.8 mph every 3 minutes until the treadmill reaches 18% grade and 5 mph.[11,12] At each stage, the blood pressure and heart rate are recorded along with a Borg scale (perceived exertion) at the end of each stage (Table 22.2).[13]

The procedure is continued until the patient reaches peak exercise or develops complications (e.g., arrhythmias, chest pain, ST-segment changes). If the patient achieves <85% of his MPHR and no abnormalities are found, the results are *inconclusive* (MPHR = 220 − Age ± 12 beats for 95% confidence limits for one (1) SD). If there is a plateau of the heart rate (failure of the heart rate to increase in response to an increasing workload), this portends a poor outcome and a greater incidence of complications and the test should be terminated.[8] This vigorous protocol approach with significant changes in workloads between stages allows for high exertional levels to be reached rapidly. Unfortunately, these changes are not physiologic and Stage 4 of this protocol frequently is awkward, that is, difficult for the patient to choose between running and walking, rendering different oxygen consumption rates. In some studies, it has been found to have a poor correlation with measured gas analysis.[8]

TABLE 22.2
Bruce Protocol[8,10]

Stage*	Speed (mph)	Grade (%)
1	1.7	10
2	2.5	12
3	3.4	14
4	4.2	16
5	5.0	18
6	5.5	20
7	6.0	22

*Each stage is 3 minutes.

The *modified Bruce protocol* was designed to provide a lower initial increment. However, it decreases moderately the capacity of peak exercise due to peripheral fatigue secondary to the first stage of low intensity. When compared to the standard Bruce protocol, the modified Bruce protocol inserts two 3 minute stages before entering the standard Bruce protocol and maintains the same speed as the grade is increased during Stage 0 and Stage 1/2. At Stage 1, the patient is at the same grade and speed as present in the standard Bruce protocol. It is ideal for those patients who are less fit or less active. Since many patients can perform METs of work but not at the speed required for the standard Bruce protocol, this protocol allows them to exercise 8–12 minutes and achieve the METs required for a proper physiologic response.

Clinical Pearl

The Ramp protocol allows for a more physiologic assessment, an unperceivable change experienced by the participant, and correlates well with $VO_{2\,max}$ gas analysis.

The *Ramp protocol* allows for a more physiologic assessment, an unperceivable effort change experienced by the participant, and correlates well with $VO_{2\,max}$ gas analysis. With this protocol, once a target MET workload is selected, total exercise time is set at 8–12 minutes for a physiologic response. The computer then selects the speed and grade to achieve the defined target workload. The grade and speed can be programmed to increase every 6 seconds in alternating fashion. Furthermore, the Ramp modification of the Bruce protocol can be performed and the subject achieves equivalent hemodynamic goals but with greater duration and achieved METs. In studies, patients exercised longer with the Ramp protocol than with the Bruce protocol and achieved an optimal duration for the exercise test of approximately 10 minutes—the goal for an optimal exercise test.[14,15] Patients prefer the Ramp protocol with respect to comfort and ease to perform. Myers et al. determined that the ratio of oxygen uptake to work rate is greater with Ramp protocols than with conventional protocols that involve large increments in work.[15]

22.6 TESTING ATHLETES

Testing athletes is similar to testing other individuals, but one must select the appropriate testing protocol.[16] Several protocols accommodate the much higher fitness level in athletes and include the Bruce protocol, Astrand protocol, Costill protocol, Ramp protocol, and the Astrand–Storer–Davis protocol for competitive cyclists. Athletes gauge their training based on their competitive sport. Triathletes may evaluate their training program by alternating running with cycling protocols in the exercise laboratory.

The patient preparation, management of the exercise test, recovery, and interpretation of the test results are the same as with any other study subject. The only difference is that athletes require protocols that are more demanding to gather essential information in 8–12 minutes of total exercise.

The Bruce protocol has often been used and can be selected for athletes. The subject may easily exercise into Stage 6 or Stage 7 of this protocol. The Astrand protocol is another protocol for the well-trained subject. Here, the subject selects the ideal *personal speed* at which to run and then the grade is gradually increased. This protocol "fits" the personal speed of the runner and is very popular. In contrast, the Costill protocol begins with a 10 minute warm-up and then increases in grade every 2 minutes until exhaustion. The Ramp protocol permits a "variable" speed and/or grade to fit within a 10–15 minutes period of time and still be customized to the individual runner. This protocol may be more physiologic for the individual. Last, one may select a Storer–Davis protocol for the trained competitive cyclists.

22.7 PERFORMING THE EXERCISE TEST

The objective for testing the patient is to learn the maximum about the patient's pathophysiological causes of exercise limitation with the greatest accuracy, the least patient stress, and in the shortest time frame.[8,9,14,17] The physician should perform a pretest evaluation and select the proper protocol prior to scheduling the test. A medical history of the patient's symptoms and past medical problems is the most important aspect of patient evaluation. The chest pain symptoms should be defined and characterized as angina, atypical angina, or atypical chest pain, and any associated history or symptoms of exercise-induced syncope or near syncope, significant left ventricular outflow obstruction, uncontrolled congestive heart failure or unstable angina, viral myocarditis, or pericarditis noted. Any major risk factor for CAD, including a history of smoking, hypertension, hyperlipidemia, diabetes mellitus, obesity, as well as family history of sudden death during exercise should be recorded.[18] Results from any previous exercise test should be reviewed and the patient is queried of any problems with prior testing. It is especially important to discuss any recent interval change in any chest pain pattern or medical history before initiating exercise testing. The examiner should (1) explain the test to the patient and the risks involved, (2) delineate other options for evaluation, and (3) obtain written consent.

Prior to selecting the exercise protocol, one must select a maximal or submaximal exercise test. If one chooses a symptom-limited maximal stress test, the patient is in control and ultimate information is obtained. If the ECG and blood pressure are normal and the patient follows the Borg scale of perceived exertion, very little risk is posed for the patient. The use of rating scales for perceived exertion is often helpful in the assessment of patient fatigue.[6,19] One can instruct the patient in using either the Borg RPE Scale (the classic 15-grade scale) or the nonlinear 10-grade scale (the Borg CR10 Scale; Borg's Perceived Exertion and Pain Scales, Human Kinetics, Champaign, IL).[19–21] Prior to performing the exercise test, a pretest cardiovascular examination should include bilateral blood pressure measurements, notation of pulse pressure, simultaneous radial–femoral pulse evaluation, carotid upstroke evaluation, and careful auscultation of the second heart sound. Any systolic murmurs suggestive of aortic stenosis or hypertrophic cardiomyopathy or any signs of uncompensated congestive heart failure or extra heart sounds should be noted. A review of the patient's medications is necessary and beneficial. The patient should be reminded to take their routine medications except beta-blockers or calcium channel blockers prior to exercise testing. The exception to this recommendation deals with those patients with documented CAD since these individuals do better during exercise with beta-blockers by achieving a higher workload.[7] Patients taking calcium channel blockers also perform at higher workloads even though their systolic blood pressure and heart rate decrease for a given level of exercise.[7,22] The patient is instructed to not smoke and to eat little or no food for at least 2 hours before testing. The patient should wear comfortable clothes and shoes for the test and should avoid applying body oils or lotions that might interfere with attaching the electrodes.

During each stage of exercise and recovery, the ECG, heart rate, and blood pressure are monitored and recorded. The examiner should warn the patient of upcoming stage changes and query the patient's perceived level of effort (Borg scale). The exercise test is stopped when the patient has reached maximal effort (Borg scale) or exhibits clinical signs to terminate. Symptom-limited testing with the Borg CR10 Scale has been recognized as an important aid when the treadmill test is used to assess functional capacity.

The patient is monitored continuously for transient rhythm disturbances, ST-segment changes and other electrocardiographic manifestations of myocardial ischemia.[23] A 12-lead

ECG tracing is obtained during the last minute of each stage of exercise, at the point of maximum exercise testing, at 1 minute in recovery, and then every 2 minutes during the recovery phase (e.g., 1, 3, 5, 7 minutes). The blood pressure is obtained and recorded with each ECG tracing.

The patient is informed that he/she is in charge and may stop the test at any time. Otherwise, test termination requires clinical evaluation and judgment concerning the status of the patient. The absolute indications to terminate exercise testing are (1) the presence of an acute MI or suspicion of MI; (2) the onset of progressive angina or anginal equivalents; (3) exertional hypotension, decrease in systolic blood pressure (20 mmHg) with increasing workload or a decrease below the baseline standing systolic blood pressure prior to test, accompanied by signs or symptoms indicating poor left ventricular function and poor cardiac output; (4) serious dysrhythmias, for example, ventricular tachycardia; (5) signs of poor perfusion (pallor, cyanosis, nausea or cold, clammy skin); (6) central nervous system symptoms (ataxia, vertigo, visual or gait problems, and confusion); (7) failure of increasing heart rate response with increasing workload; (8) technical problems with monitoring the ECG or equipment failure; or (9) the patient requests to stop.[24]

The *relative* indications to terminate exercise testing are pronounced ECG changes from baseline, including more than 2 mV of horizontal or downsloping ST-segment depression or 2 mV of ST-segment elevation; progressive or increasing chest pain; pronounced fatigue, shortness of breath or wheezing; development of leg cramps or intermittent claudication; an hypertensive response (systolic blood pressure greater than 250 mmHg or diastolic blood pressure greater than 115 mmHg, supraventricular tachycardia; or exercise-induced bundle branch block that cannot be distinguished from ventricular tachycardia.[23] During the recovery phase, the patient should be placed immediately in the supine position or allowed a "cooldown walk" and then placed in a chair. Maximal test sensitivity is achieved with the patient placed supine postexercise. Without delay, the examiner should auscultate the patient for a new-onset heart murmur or third heart sound. In addition, one should auscultate the lungs for any evidence of exercise-induced bronchospasm, which might be a cause of chest pain complaints. During the recovery phase, the blood pressure and ECG recordings are obtained at 1 minute and then every 2 minutes. The heart rate recording at 1 minute postexercise and the 3 minutes systolic BP/peak BP ratio has been correlated with overall mortality and prognosis.[25,26] The patient is observed carefully until the vital signs are stable and any observed ST-segment changes have returned to baseline. This may require 8–10 minutes. It is important to watch carefully for any "recovery-only" ST-segment depression in the recovery period.[27] One may consider administration of sublingual nitroglycerin after placing the patient supine, monitoring the blood pressure, and observing other vital signs until the ST-segment changes have resolved.

Once the patient is stable, the ECG monitoring equipment can be removed, all of the information is interpreted, the results are conveyed to the patient, and a formal report is completed. Information is valid and more predictable if the patient achieves his personal maximum heart rate determined by high work load (METs), exertional fatigue (Borg scale), and plateau of his heart rate (failure of heart rate to increase in response to an increasing workload).

22.8 INTERPRETATION OF THE EXERCISE TEST

Interpreting the exercise test involves analysis of several parameters. The heart rate and blood pressure response are indicators of the presence, or absence, of cardiac disease. The heart rate is monitored constantly during the exercise test, while the blood pressure is determined at the end of each protocol stage. Physiologically, the systolic blood pressure should increase with increasing workload and the diastolic blood pressure should remain constant or decrease. At peak exercise, well-trained athletes may demonstrate a systolic blood pressure approaching 200 mmHg or greater with the diastolic blood pressure falling to 0–10 mmHg. In contrast, a falling *systolic blood pressure with increasing workload* indicates that heart disease is associated with complications *during* exercise testing and is an indication to *terminate* the exercise test immediately.[23]

22.8.1 Heart Rate Response

With aerobic exercise, the normal heart rate response should increase in a gradual, linear fashion with workload and oxygen uptake and correspond with prognosis. While a well-conditioned individual may demonstrate a delay or an initially slow increase, ultimately the healthy heart rate will rise with the increased workload, that is, increase in slope (grade) and speed. Failure to increase heart rate to at least 120 beats per minute with maximum exercise is defined as chronotropic incompetence. Cole found that the recovery of the maximum heart rate following cessation of exercise also correlates with mortality.[25] Mathematically, this is maximum heart rate minus the recovery heart rate at 1 minute in recovery. In summary, the diseased heart requires more time to recover from exercise (stress) and has a less favorable prognosis.

22.8.2 Blood Pressure Response

The normal blood pressure response to exercise is an increase in systolic blood pressure while the diastolic blood pressure remains stable or decreases with exercise. Exercise-induced hypotension is defined as a fall in *systolic* blood pressure to or below baseline and is indicative of underlying heart disease. A rise in the *diastolic* blood pressure more than 10 mmHg is a hypertensive response to exercise and is abnormal.

22.8.3 Presence/Absence of Symptoms

The most common symptom for termination of the test is fatigue irrespective of the presence or absence of heart disease. Other symptoms include dyspnea, wheezing (objective bronchospasm), claudication, and chest pain. Chest pain may be tightness, aching, or vaguely described pressure by the patient who will often deny chest "pain" when directly questioned. The examiner should instruct the patient to notify the staff if any exercise-related symptoms occur while testing. Watching for nonverbal signs (e.g., frowning, diaphoresis, or gazing downward) could indicate either maximum exercise tolerance or equivalent anginal symptoms.

22.8.4 Evidence for Myocardial Ischemia

The primary indication for myocardial ischemia is depression of the ST segment, which is due to an imbalance of the blood supply and demand to the myocardial muscle. The gradations of ST-segment depression can be grouped into either (1) upsloping ST-segment changes, (2) horizontal ST-segment changes, or (3) downsloping ST-depression. The severity of the myocardial ischemia correlates with the progression of the described three types. Upsloping ST-segment depression is a gradual gradation from normal to abnormal. Some patients with this change will represent false-positive changes, and some will be abnormal changes of ischemia. Often, further evaluation or clinical following is necessary to define which patients are truly developing progressive CAD. Horizontal (2) and downsloping groups (3) usually indicate significant heart disease and are further evaluated.

22.8.5 Arrhythmias

Arrhythmias are common in exercise testing and are divided into simple and complex groups. Simple arrhythmias include premature atrial contractions, atrial tachycardia, atrial flutter, atrial fibrillation, and isolated premature ventricular contractions (PVCs). If these are present at rest and then disappear with exercise, they are considered benign, are not worrisome, and do not usually correlate with underlying CAD. If PVCs (including bigeminy, couplets and ventricular tachycardia [VT]) occur with exercise they are more worrisome and often do indicate CAD.[28] In the French postal workers study, an increase in PVCs (more than 10% of beats during a 30 s ECG) did correlate with a long-term increase of cardiovascular death in men followed for 23 years.[29] In general, *isolated* PVCs do *not* indicate an increased incidence of CAD. When worrisome arrhythmias occur during exercise testing, the test is usually terminated and alternate studies are considered looking for structural changes (e.g., echocardiogram) or occult CAD (e.g., nuclear studies or angiography). When *progressive* occurrence of PVCs or runs of VT occur, these abnormalities represent markers for coronary heart disease with exposure of underlying coronary ischemia and must be evaluated.[30]

22.8.6 Functional Aerobic Capacity

Functional aerobic capacity is *measured* by formal VO_2 testing with gas analysis or is *estimated* by the amount of work (METs) achieved by exercise testing. Greater duration of exercise with increasing workload demands a higher cardiac aerobic capacity. If ECG ischemic changes occur, CAD is suspected. If no ECG ischemic changes occur, one may record the duration of exercise, the MET level achieved and estimate the aerobic capacity. Exercise, in the presence of ischemic heart disease, reveals ECG changes of ischemia, and the individual is unable to achieve the predicted workload capacity (MET level). For each one (1) MET increase in exercise capacity, there is a 12% improvement in survival.[25]

22.9 EXERCISE TESTING REPORT

The exercise testing report should address the following: (1) any symptoms during or after testing, (2) the heart rate and blood pressure response, (3) presence of dysrhythmias, and (4) any evidence for myocardial ischemia. The summary statement should describe the testing procedure followed by the assessment of the results along with any further recommendations.

The assessment includes (1) the presence or absence of ECG ischemia, (2) normal or abnormal heart rate and blood pressure response to exercise, (3) presence or absence of any dysrhythmias, (4) presence or absence of clinical symptoms, maximum aerobic capacity (METs) achieved, and (5) a summary statement concerning the patient's risk for CAD or mortality based on test results. Finally, any recommendation for lifestyle changes, exercise prescription, medical management, or further evaluation or consultation is discussed with the patient.[7]

22.10 SUMMARY

Implementing a pretest evaluation and proper evaluation of the patient via thorough history, physical examination, and risk stratification allows one to safely study patients. The most important precaution is careful pretest patient evaluation and selection of the proper protocol by noting the absolute and relative contraindications prior to testing the patient and seeking proper referral and assessment.

With proper training, graded exercise testing is a useful primary procedure to detect CAD in the outpatient or inpatient setting. This screening diagnostic test provides both diagnostic and prognostic information concerning the risk of cardiovascular disease. The information provided can be used to determine further clinical evaluation, formulate appropriate treatment plans, and develop therapeutic prescriptions for exercise (Table 22.3).

22.11 CODING

22.11.1 ICD-9 Codes

401.1–429.9	Includes hypertension, coronary artery disease, angina, aneurysm of heart and coronary vessels, cardiomyopathy, atrial fibrillation, and heart failure
780.2	Syncope and collapse
786.05	Shortness of breath
786.06	Tachypnea
786.07	Wheezing

TABLE 22.3
SORT: Key Recommendations for Practice

Clinical Recommendation	Evidence Rating	References
In patients who are able to exercise the exercise test is an appropriate first step in evaluating chest pain suspicious for coronary artery disease.	B	[4,6]
Downsloping ST-segment depression during exercise testing and associated typical angina symptoms correlate highly with the presence of significant coronary artery disease.	A	[24,27,30]
A decreasing systolic blood pressure with increasing workload during an exercise test is associated with *severe complications during the test* and is an indication to terminate the exercise test immediately.	A	[24,26,30]

786.5	Chest pain, unspecified
786.51	Precordial pain
786.59	Chest pain, other
V71.7	Observation for suspected cardiovascular disease

22.11.2 ICD-10 Codes

I10	401.1	Essential hypertension
I25.10	414.00	Coronary atherosclerosis of natural vessel without angina
I25.119	413.90	Coronary atherosclerosis of natural vessel with angina
I25.3	414.19	Other aneurysm of the heart (need to add other codes to further identify)
I48.0	427.31	Paroxysmal atrial fibrillation
I48.91	427.31	Unspecified atrial fibrillation
I48.2	427.31	Chronic atrial fibrillation
I50.20	428.20	Unspecified systolic congestive heart failure
I50.30	428.30	Unspecified diastolic congestive heart failure
R55	780.2	Syncope and collapse
R07.9	786.50	Chest pain, unspecified
R07.2	786.51	Precordial pain
R06.02	786.05	Shortness of breath
R06.82	786.06	Tachypnea
R06.2	786.07	Wheezing
R07.89	786.59	Chest pain, other

REFERENCES

1. Pescatello LS, American College of Sports Medicine. *ACSM's Guidelines for Exercise Testing and Prescription.* Philadelphia, PA: Wolters Kluwer/Lippincott Williams & Wilkins Health; 2014.
2. Blair SN, Kohl HW, Paffenbarger RS, Clark DG, Cooper KH, Gibbons LW. Physical fitness and all-cause mortality. A prospective study of healthy men and women. *Journal of the American Medical Association.* 1989;262(17):2395–2401.
3. Herbert DL, Herbert WG, White RD, Froelicher VF. Legal aspects of graded exercise testing. In: *Exercise Testing for Primary Care and Sports Medicine Physicians*, edited by C.H. Evans, R.D. White, 1st ed. New York: Springer; 2009, pp. 255–271.
4. Fowler-Brown A, Pignone M, Pletcher M, Tice JA, Sutton SF, Lohr KN. U.S. Preventive Services Task Force. Exercise tolerance testing to screen for coronary heart disease: A systematic review for the technical support for the U.S. Preventive Services Task Force. *Annals of Internal Medicine.* 2004;140(7):W9–W24.
5. Heart and Stroke Association Statistics. http://www.heart.org/HEARTORG/General/Heart-and-Stroke-Association-Statistics_UCM_319064_SubHomePage.jsp. Accessed October 31, 2014.
6. Fletcher GF, Ades PA, Kligfield P et al. Exercise standards for testing and training: A scientific statement from the American Heart Association. *Circulation.* 2013;128(8):873–934.
7. Ellestad MH. *Stress Testing: Principles and Practice.* 5th ed. Oxford, New York: Oxford University Press; 2003.
8. Harris GD. Exercise testing special protocols. In *Exercise Testing for Primary Care and Sports Medicine Physicians*, edited by C.H. Evans, R.D. White, 1st ed. New York: Springer; 2009, pp. 45–53.
9. Wasserman, K. ed. *Principles of Exercise Testing and Interpretation: Including Pathophysiology and Clinical Applications.* 4th ed. Philadelphia, PA: Lippincott Williams & Wilkins; 2005.
10. Bruce RA. Exercise testing of patients with coronary heart disease. Principles and normal standards for evaluation. *Annals of Clinical Research.* 1971;3(6):323–332.
11. Mark DB, Hlatky MA, Harrell FE, Lee KL, Califf RM, Pryor DB. Exercise treadmill score for predicting prognosis in coronary artery disease. *Annals of Internal Medicine.* 1987;106(6):793–800.
12. Mark DB, Shaw L, Harrell FE, Hlatky MA, Lee KL, Bengtson JR, McCants CB, Califf RM, Pryor DB. Prognostic value of a treadmill exercise score in outpatients with suspected coronary artery disease. *The New England Journal of Medicine.* 1991;325(12):849–853.
13. White RD, Harris GD. Exercise stress testing. In *The Essential Guide to Primary Care Procedures*, edited by EJ Mayeaux. Philadelphia, PA: Wolters Kluwer Health/Lippincott Williams & Wilkins, 2009, pp. 100–108.
14. Buchfuhrer MJ, Hansen JE, Robinson TE, Sue DY, Wasserman K, Whipp BJ. Optimizing the exercise protocol for cardiopulmonary assessment. *Journal of Applied Physiology: Respiratory, Environmental and Exercise Physiology.* 1983;55(5):1558–1564.
15. Myers J, Buchanan N, Walsh D, Kraemer M, McAuley P, Hamilton-Wessler M, Froelicher VF. Comparison of the ramp versus standard exercise protocols. *Journal of the American College of Cardiology.* 1991;17(6):1334–1342.

16. Price DE, Warren ET, White RD. Testing athletic populations. In *Exercise Testing for Primary Care and Sports Medicine Physicians*, edited by CH Evans, RD White, 1st ed. New York: Springer, 2009, pp. 341–351.
17. Harris GD, White RD. Performance of the exercise test. In *Exercise Testing for Primary Care and Sports Medicine Physicians*, edited by CH Evans, RD White, 1st ed. New York: Springer, 2009, pp. 23–44.
18. White RD, Goldschlager NF. Stratifying symptomatic patients using the exercise test and other tools. In *Exercise Testing for Primary Care and Sports Medicine Physicians*, edited by CH Evans, RD White, 1st ed. New York: Springer, 2009, pp. 167–192.
19. Borg GA. Psychophysical bases of perceived exertion. *Medicine and Science in Sports and Exercise*. 1982;14(5):377–381.
20. Borg G. Perceived exertion as an indicator of somatic stress. *Scandinavian Journal of Rehabilitation Medicine*. 1970;2(2):92–98.
21. Borg G, Holmgren A, Lindblad I. Quantitative evaluation of chest pain. *Acta Medica Scandinavica*. Supplementum. 1981;644:43–45.
22. Rice KR, Gervino E, Jarisch WR, Stone PH. Effects of nifedipine on myocardial perfusion during exercise in chronic stable angina pectoris. *The American Journal of Cardiology*. 1990;65(16):1097–1101.
23. Froelicher VF. *Exercise and the Heart*. 5th ed. Philadelphia, PA: Saunders; 2006.
24. White RD, Harris GD. Exercise testing. In *ACSM's Sports Medicine: A Comprehensive Review*, edited by FG O'Connor. Philadelphia, PA: Wolters Kluwer Health/Lippincott Williams & Wilkins, 2013, pp. 136–143.
25. Cole CR, Blackstone EH, Pashkow FJ, Snader CE, Lauer MS. Heart-rate recovery immediately after exercise as a predictor of mortality. *The New England Journal of Medicine*. 1999;341(18):1351–1357.
26. Taylor AJ, Beller GA. Postexercise systolic blood pressure response: Clinical application to the assessment of ischemic heart disease. *American Family Physician*. 1998;58(5):1126–1130.
27. Lachterman B, Lehmann KG, Abrahamson D, Froelicher VF. 'Recovery only' ST-segment depression and the predictive accuracy of the exercise test. *Annals of Internal Medicine*. 1990;112(1):11–16.
28. Udall JA, Ellestad MH. Predictive implications of ventricular premature contractions associated with treadmill stress testing. *Circulation*. 1977;56(6):985–989.
29. Jouven X, Zureik M, Desnos M, Courbon D, Ducimetière P. Long-term outcome in asymptomatic men with exercise-induced premature ventricular depolarizations. *The New England Journal of Medicine*. 2000;343(12):826–833.
30. Evans CH, Ellstad MH. Interpreting the exercise test. In *Exercise Testing for Primary Care and Sports Medicine Physicians*, edited by CH Evans, RD White, 1st ed. New York: Springer, 2009, pp. 81–107.

23 Compartment Pressure Testing

Kristen L. Slappey and Marvin H. Sineath, Jr.

CONTENTS

TABLE 23.1
Key Clinical Considerations

1. When considering which compartments to test for CECS, keep in mind the specific muscles/nerves affected within each compartment and their corresponding action/innervation pattern.
2. A postexertion physical exam that provokes the patient's symptoms can help guide which compartments should be tested to minimize unnecessary invasive procedures.
3. A common reason for failure to obtain accurate pressure readings is improper technique, such as failure of the needle to penetrate through the fascia into the respective compartment.

23.1 INTRODUCTION

A 21-year-old female with a 4-year history of bilateral anterior and lateral leg pain was evaluated in a case study by Diebal et al. for the diagnosis of chronic exertional compartment syndrome (CECS). The patient reported experiencing leg pain and tightness while running, predictably before 0.8 km, which progressed to numbness, pressure, and pain. The symptoms became significant enough to alter her running pattern and eventually force her to stop running secondary to the pain. Her symptoms invariably would resolve after 5–10 minutes of rest. The physical exam demonstrated firmness and tenderness to palpation in both anterior compartments of the leg and decreased dorsiflexion bilaterally (Table 23.1).[8]

This is an example of CECS, defined as an increase in intramuscular pressures resulting in pain, paresthesias, and neuromuscular dysfunction reproduced by exercise. The symptoms arise during a specific interval of activity and subside with rest. It has been estimated that approximately 14%–27% of previously undiagnosed leg pain may be attributable to CECS, and lack of awareness by clinicians results in an average 22-month delay in diagnosis.[2,5] This chapter is dedicated to understanding the technique of compartment pressure testing, which is the gold standard for diagnosing CECS. A more in-depth discussion of the definition, symptomatology, and management of CECS is discussed in other chapters of this book.

Clinical Pearl

CECS should be considered in patients with exertional leg pain, when shin splints or stress fracture is less likely.

23.2 AFFECTED COMPARTMENTS

The most common compartments affected are the anterior and lateral compartments of the leg, accounting for approximately 95% of CECS cases.[1,4,6,11,15] The anterior compartment of the leg contains several muscles, including the anterior tibialis, extensor hallucis longus, extensor digitorum longus, and peroneus tertius, as well as the deep peroneal nerve and anterior tibial artery and vein.[7,10,13] The lateral compartment has fewer muscles, comprising the peroneus longus and brevis muscles as well as the superficial peroneal nerve.[7,10,12] Case reports of CECS in the thigh, foot, upper extremity, and erector spinae musculature are far less common. Therefore, this chapter focuses on testing of the leg compartments.[2]

The decision regarding which compartment to test can be guided by history and physical exam as well as consideration of the contents of each compartment. The anterior compartment primarily affects the anterior tibialis and extensor hallucis muscles and deep peroneal nerve. Thus, clinically the patient will present with weakness in dorsiflexion of the foot, weakness in dorsiflexion of the great toe, and paresthesias over the dorsal first web space. The lateral compartment primarily affects the peroneus muscles and superficial peroneal nerve. Thus, clinically the patient will present with weakness with foot eversion and paresthesias over the dorsal foot, sparing the first web space.[9] Please refer to Table 23.1. The posterior and deep posterior compartments are affected with much less frequency than the anterior and lateral compartments.[7,10,12] Please refer Table 23.2 for the structures affected within these compartments. It has been postulated that the posterior tibialis muscle constitutes a separate compartment, but we have chosen the conventional approach and included it within the deep posterior compartment.

TABLE 23.2
Lower Limb Compartments

Compartment	Muscles	Nerves	Vasculature
Anterior	Anterior tibialis Extensor hallucis longus Extensor digitorum longus Peroneus tertius	Deep peroneal nerve	Anterior tibial artery and vein
Lateral	Peroneus longus Peroneus brevis	Superficial peroneal nerve	None
Superficial posterior	Gastrocnemius Soleus Plantaris tendon	None	None
Deep posterior	Flexor hallucis longus Flexor digitorum longus Posterior tibialis Popliteus	Tibial nerve	Posterior tibial artery and vein Peroneal artery and vein

Sources: Adapted from Detmer, D. et al., *Am. J. Sports Med.*, 13(3), 162, 1985; George, C. and Hutchinson, M.R. *Clin. Sports Med.*, 31, 307, 2012; Hartsock, L. and Barfield, W., *Lower Extremity Rev.*, 2012.

23.3 INDICATIONS, CONTRAINDICATIONS, AND TYPES OF TESTING

Although history and physical exam may raise suspicion for CECS, they are inadequate for making a definitive diagnosis. For this reason, intracompartmental manometry is considered the gold standard for diagnosis.[14]

Indications for CECS testing include complaints of pain in the lower extremity and numbness or weakness located in the specific anatomical area that is not otherwise specified by another diagnosis. The pain occurs at a given interval, distance, or intensity of exercise and resolves with cessation of activity.[7] There are no contraindications for the use of manometry; however, evidence of an active skin infection at the site of testing and patient refusal would preclude the procedure.

There are various types of manometry that can be used to measure lower extremity compartment pressures. Needle techniques described by Reneman et al., or the wick or slit catheter techniques popularized by Scholander et al., are common; however, the Stryker needle technique has been the most widely used and available method for intracompartmental pressure measurement.[15]

Clinical Pearl

If there is concern for CECS, nonurgent compartment testing should be performed.

23.4 TECHNIQUE FOR STRYKER NEEDLE TESTING

The Stryker needle is a handheld device that includes a transducer, amplifier, and display that connects directly to a needle or slit catheter that provides a simplified approach to compartment pressure testing. The patient should be placed in a standardized fashion, in the supine position with the knee at 10°–30° of flexion and the ankle at 20° of flexion so that the results yield the most accurate readings.[14] For the compartment being tested, the needle should be inserted in the midportion of the muscle belly/compartment; see Figures 23.1 and 23.2. Under sterile technique, mark the area prior to needle insertion, and anesthetize the skin with lidocaine or marcaine, ensuring to avoid injecting anesthesia within the compartment. Prior to insertion, the monitor should be zeroed. The needle is inserted through the skin, at a 90° angle, until the needle penetrates the fascia, typically with a popping sensation. Inject approximately 0.5 mL of saline to equilibrate with the interstitial fluids and then obtain a resting pressure. Next, the needle is removed and bandages applied, and the patient is instructed to exercise until symptoms are reproduced, and then repeat pressure measurements are obtained at 1 and 5 minute intervals after the onset of the symptoms. When checking pressure measurements, it is

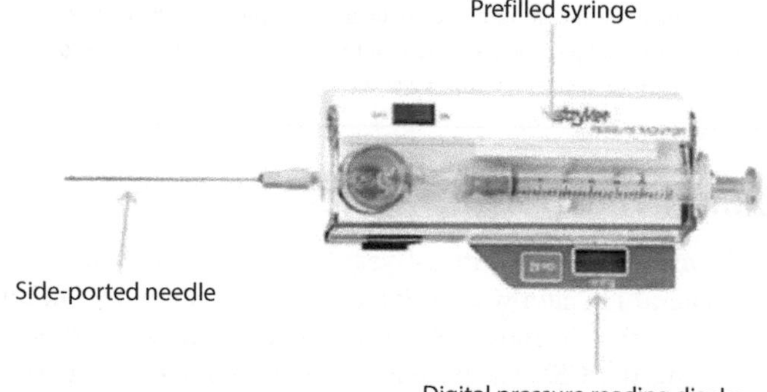

FIGURE 23.1 Stryker needle.

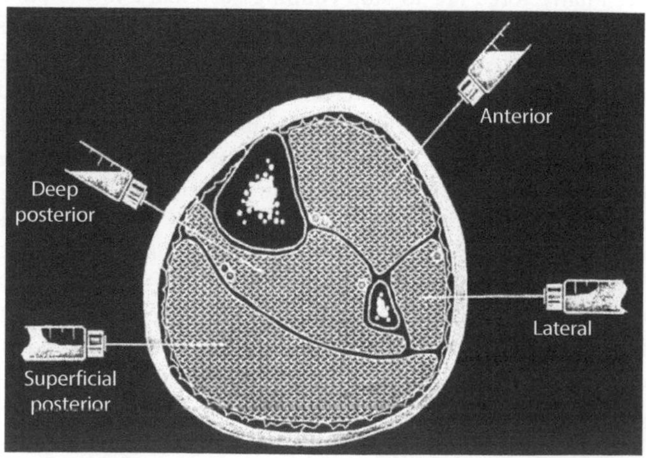

FIGURE 23.2 Compartment testing. (From Hartsock, L. and Barfield, W., *Lower Extremity Rev.*, 2012.)

TABLE 23.3
Compartmental Manometry Measurements for Chronic Exertional Compartment Syndrome

Pedowitz Criteria	
Preexercise	≥15 mmHg
1 minute postexercise	≥30 mmHg
5 minute postexercise	≥20 mmHg

Sources: Frontera, W., *Essentials of Physical Medicine and Rehabilitation*, Hanley & Belfus, Philadelphia, PA, 256, 2002; George, C. and Hutchinson, M.R., *Clin. Sports Med.*, 31, 307, 2012; Pedowitz, R.A. et al., *Am. J. Sports Med.*, 18, 35, 1990.
Note: Diagnosis of CECS is made with one or more of these measurements in the setting of clinical symptoms.

imperative to ensure that the knee and ankle are in a standardized position as this can affect pressure readings.[14] All techniques of intracompartmental pressure testing carry a low risk of infection and can be minimized by using sterile technique. Other complications include pain associated with needle insertion, which can be reduced by the use of local anesthesia.

23.5 INTERPRETATION OF TESTING

Pedowitz criteria (see Table 23.3) are the most widely accepted and utilized tool to diagnose CECS.[13,14] Pedowitz et al. reported one or more of the following as diagnostic for CECS: (1) a resting pressure of 15 mmHg or greater, (2) a 1 minute postexercise pressure of 30 mmHg or greater, or (3) a 5 minute postexercise pressure of 20 mmHg or greater[13,14] (see Table 23.3).

23.6 OTHER DIAGNOSTIC TESTING

Several noninvasive testing modalities are available; however, their clinical utility has not yet been proven and remains under investigation. The most studied noninvasive modalities include magnetic resonance imaging (MRI) and near-infrared spectroscopy (NIRS). Both MRI and NIRS testing should be performed at rest and post-induction of symptoms, similar to the Stryker needle method described earlier.

MRI, specifically T2-weighted imaging, will show increased signal intensity within the affected musculature, indicating edema, and correlates well with increased intracompartmental pressures.[7] MRI has been shown to be more sensitive postexercise.[5] Other findings on MRI suggestive of CECS include fatty infiltration of the muscle (suggesting chronic ischemia), fascial thickening, and muscular swelling.[5]

NIRS measures levels of oxygenated and deoxygenated blood within the muscles. A baseline measurement of oxygenated blood is taken preexercise, and then the ratio of oxygenated to deoxygenated blood postexercise is determined. Measurements that indicate CECS include a delay in returning to oxygenated baseline postexercise as well as a decreased ratio of oxygenated to deoxygenated blood within the muscles postexercise.[5] A cohort study by Brand van den et al. comparing diagnostic value of MRI, NIRS, and intracompartmental pressure testing in 50 patients with CECS found the sensitivity of NIRS to be comparable to intracompartmental pressure testing at 85%. The study also demonstrated MRI to have a lower sensitivity of 77%. Although NIRS testing is equal sensitive for diagnosing CECS compared to the gold standard of intracompartmental pressure testing, its use clinically is precluded by the paucity of spectrometers in most clinical settings (Table 23.4).[3,14]

TABLE 23.4
SORT: Key Recommendations for Practice

Clinical Recommendation	Evidence Rating	References
Pedowitz criteria should be used when evaluating manometry results in the assessment of chronic exertional compartment syndrome.	C	[12]
Intracompartmental manometry with the Stryker needle device is the gold standard to diagnose chronic exertional compartment syndrome in comparison to MRI or NIRS.	C	[3,5,7,13]
Chronic exertional compartment syndrome most commonly affects the anterior and lateral leg compartments versus the posterior or deep posterior compartments of the leg, foot, thigh, upper extremity, or erector spinae.	C	[2,4,6,11,14]

REFERENCES

1. Blackman PG. A review of chronic exertional compartment syndrome. *Journal of the American Academy of Orthopaedic Surgeons*. 2003;11:268–276.
2. Bong MR, Polatsch DB, Jazrawi LM, Rokito AS. Chronic exertional compartment syndrome: Diagnosis and management. *Bulletin (Hospital for Joint Diseases (New York, N. Y.))*. 2005;62(3–4):77–84.
3. Brand van den JGH, Verleisdonk EJMM et al. The diagnostic value of intracompartmental pressure measurement, magnetic resonance imaging, and near-infrared spectroscopy in chronic exertional compartment syndrome: A prospective study in 50 patients. *The American Journal of Sports Medicine*. 2005;33:699–704.
4. Brennan F, Kane S. Diagnosis, treatment options, and rehabilitation of chronic lower leg exertional compartment syndrome. *Current Sports Medicine Reports*. 2003;2:247–250.
5. Brown R, Rosenberg Z. MR imaging of exercise-induced lower leg pain. *Magnetic Resonance Imaging Clinics of North America*. 2001;9(3):544–547.
6. Cook S, Bruce G. Fasciotomy for chronic compartment syndrome in the lower limb. *ANZ Journal of Surgery*. 2002;72(10):720–723.

7. Detmer D, Sharpe K, Sufit RL et al. Chronic compartment syndrome: Diagnosis, management, and outcomes. *The American Journal of Sports Medicine.* 1985;13(3):162–170.
8. Diebal AR, Gregory R, Alitz C et al. Effects of forefoot running on chronic exertional compartment syndrome: A case series. *International Journal of Sports Physical Therapy.* 2011;6:312–321.
9. Frontera W. *Essentials of Physical Medicine and Rehabilitation.* Philadelphia, PA: Hanley & Belfus; 2002, pp. 256–261.
10. George C, Hutchinson MR. Chronic exertional compartment syndrome. *Clinics in Sports Medicine.* 2012;31(2):307–319.
11. Goldfarb S, Kaeding C. Bilateral acute-on-chronic exertional lateral compartment syndrome of the leg: A case report and review of the literature. *Clinics in Sports Medicine.* 1997;7:59–62.
12. Hartsock L, Barfield W. Compartment syndrome following tibial fracture. *Lower Extremity Review.* 2012. Available from http://lermagazine.com/article/compartment-syndrome-following-tibia-fracture. Accessed July 3, 2015.
13. Pedowitz RA, Hargens AR, Mubarak SJ et al. Modified criteria for the objective diagnosis of chronic exertional compartment syndrome of the leg. *The American Journal of Sports Medicine.* 1990;18:35–40.
14. Tucker AK Chronic exertional compartment syndrome of the leg. *Current Reviews in Musculoskeletal Medicine.* 2010;3(1–4):32–37.
15. Verleisdonk E, Schmitz R, Werken C. Long term results of fasciotomy of the anterior compartment in patients with exercise-induced pain in the lower leg. *International Journal of Sports Medicine.* 2004;25:224–229.

24 Neuropsychological Testing in Concussion

Andrea L. Pana

CONTENTS

TABLE 24.1
Key Clinical Considerations

1. There is no one test that is the gold standard for the diagnosis of concussion.
2. The total number of sports concussions may be underestimated as many concussions may be underreported or unrecognized by athletes, parents, or coaches or even underdiagnosed by health-care personnel.
3. Diagnosis and management of concussion is made through an evaluation of signs and symptoms through a comprehensive history and physical exam along with other tests evaluating mental status, cognitive function, gait, and balance.
4. Most concussions will resolve spontaneously, but postconcussive symptoms and clinical recovery patterns vary and not all have a typical course; symptom resolution often precedes cognitive recovery, and there may be risks of returning to activity before complete cognitive recovery.
5. There are many factors that can affect test scores in a concussed athlete as well as recovery from concussion. It is important that the provider interpreting tests and treating the athlete be aware of these factors as they make return-to-play decisions.

24.1 INTRODUCTION

Concussion is defined as a "traumatically induced transient disturbance of brain function and is caused by a complex pathophysiological process."[27] There are an estimated 1.6–3.8 million concussions occurring annually in the United States.[5,19,27] This number may underestimate the total number of sports concussions because many concussions may be underreported or unrecognized by athletes, parents, or coaches or even underdiagnosed by health care personnel.[27,48] There is currently no single test or gold standard in testing for concussion. Diagnosis and management of concussion is made through an evaluation of signs and symptoms through a comprehensive history and physical exam along with other tests evaluating mental status, cognitive function, gait, and balance (Table 24.1).[50]

Neuropsychological (NP) testing in sports concussion began in the 1980s with research by Barth and colleagues using paper-and-pencil testing.[40,49] By the 1990s, the Pittsburgh sports battery evolved and its use spread to professional athletes.[40,49] The sports battery was eventually transformed to computerized use, which allowed more widespread use of NP testing in athletes with concussion.[40] Traditional NP testing evaluates cognitive abilities and psychological functioning as well as limited testing of sensory and motor functioning.[61] The NP protocols used in the assessment of sports concussion consist of neurocognitive measures that evaluate domains of memory and learning, attention and the ability to process information, reaction time, and executive functioning.[19,59,61]

24.2 WHAT IS THE ROLE OF NP TESTING IN SPORTS CONCUSSION?

NP testing in concussion was developed in response to a need to have an objective measure in managing concussion patients. There is no gold standard test for the diagnosis or management of concussion. History, physical exam, balance testing, reaction time testing, sideline NP tests, and more comprehensive tests are tools used in the diagnosis and management of concussion. Genetic markers, fMRI, EEG, and other radiological tests are among some of the tests also being performed in sports concussion patients but are not used routinely.

There are many reasons why NP tests may be useful in the evaluation of concussion. Patients with concussion are often of a wide range of ages, genders, and backgrounds. Although most concussions heal in 7–10 days,[27,43,47,49,50] postconcussive symptoms and clinical recovery patterns vary,[17,25,27] and not all have a typical course with some taking weeks to years to resolve.[25,27] Children and adolescents have been shown to have longer recovery periods.[27,39,50] At this point of time, it is believed that returning an athlete to participation before complete recovery may increase the risk of second concussive injury, a catastrophic event, or chronic, long-term injury.[27,40] While all patients that have a concussive injury may not have long-term consequences, it is unclear from present scientific knowledge which patients are at risk. Therefore, it is prudent to not return any athlete to competition until they have completely recovered symptomatically, cognitively, and physically. Self-reported symptoms are not reliable as a sole indicator of concussion,[6,24,43,80] and symptom recovery may precede cognitive recovery.[6,19,24,36,43,44,46,47,50,58,80] Studies have found that the sensitivity of symptoms in detection of concussion is 64%–68%.[6,80] Athletes may underreport symptoms for several reasons; first, they may blatantly deny symptoms due to internal or external pressures to compete (fear of losing position, losing respect, seeming weak, or letting the team down).[24,48] Second, they may fail to identify or mislabel symptoms when they occur and instead attribute them to other things such as stress, dehydration, a tight-fitting helmet, or something other than a concussion. An athlete may also view it as their baseline functioning, or they may not be aware that symptoms such as fatigue and sleep issues are symptoms of concussion. Finally, an athlete may be truly asymptomatic but still have neurocognitive deficits associated with concussion.[24]

Clinical Pearl

Self-reported symptoms are not reliable as a sole indicator of concussion as athletes may underreport symptoms. Additionally, symptom recovery may precede cognitive recovery.

24.3 TYPES OF NP TESTING USED IN CONCUSSION MANAGEMENT

Neurocognitive or NP testing in athletes can take place on the sidelines or in the office setting. The three main types of NP testing used in concussion are sideline assessment tools/tests, clinician-administered tests, and computerized NP tests.

24.3.1 Sideline Assessment Tools/Tests

Sideline assessment tools are basic NP tests designed for the sideline assessment of athletes with suspected concussions. Sideline NP assessment consists of tests of orientation, memory and concentration, and delayed recall. Serial cognitive assessment along with physical exam changes can be used to follow a patient on the sidelines to assess for improvement or worsening of symptoms and cognitive status (which may indicate a need for further imaging and evaluation to rule out a more extensive injury like an intracranial bleed).

To assess the orientation on the sidelines, Maddocks' questions are traditionally used. These questions were validated in a 1995 study in which Maddocks provided evidence that questions relating to orientation asking about the person, date of birth, age, and month were not sensitive to discriminating between concussed and nonconcussed individuals with P values 0.6–1.0.[42] Instead, questions relating to a recall of recently acquired events (ground, quarter, how far into the quarter, last team to score, team last played, who won last) were sensitive in detecting concussion ($P < 0.001$, except ground <0.004).[42] However, questions of orientation relating to the month, date, day or week, year, and time were found to be somewhat sensitive ($P = 0.06–0.25$) and are used in some sideline assessment tools in addition to Maddocks' questions.[42]

Clinical Pearl

The questions most sensitive in assessing orientation in a concussed athlete are as follows: What ground (field) are we at? What quarter is it? How far are we into the quarter? Which was the last team to score? Who won the last game?

Assessment of memory and concentration is evaluated in tests seen originally in the sideline assessment tool called the Standardized Assessment of Concussion (SAC), which was developed in 1996 in response to the need for a standardized concussion assessment tool.[45] It is a validated assessment tool that is scored and is optimally used when compared to baseline measures.[45] Examples of individual tests in the SAC and other sideline assessment tools that assess memory are three- to five-word memory recall—immediately and at 5 minutes (immediate and delayed memory)—repeating digits backward (up to six digits in some tests), and months of the year backward (concentration). Maddocks' questions and the SAC were later incorporated into the Sport Concussion Assessment Tool (SCAT) developed from the *Second International Consensus Conference on Concussion in Sport*.[49,57] Later, it was modified to become the SCAT2 that consists of eight sections: symptoms, physical signs, Glasgow coma scale, Maddocks' questions, cognitive assessment (SAC)—memory and concentration and delayed recall—balance examination, and coordination examination.[51] The SCAT2 has recently been revised to the SCAT 3 by the 2012 consensus group on concussion (Appendix I). Neither the SCAT2 nor SCAT3 has been validated as a complete tool. Of note, a 2011 study that sought to establish normative baseline values of SCAT2 in high school athletes found that there was a low percentage of high school athletes who were able to recite months of the year backward or repeat five digits backward.[35] In addition, there was a high variability of balance testing with respect to single leg and tandem stance.[35] This is important to consider as one interprets scores of the SCAT2 or SCAT3, particularly if the athlete does not have a baseline score. While these tests do not require a baseline to use them in evaluating a concussed athlete, one must remember that a baseline measurement is needed for their optimal use if one is using them to follow the patient serially. However, these tools are not intended to be used for more than 48 hours after concussion as their sensitivity in detecting concussion sharply declines;[17,45–47] one study showed that the sensitivity of SAC is 80% immediately, 31% at day 1, 23% at day 2, and 9% at day 7.[46]

24.3.2 Clinician-Administered (Paper and Pencil) Tests

Clinician-administered tests are typically administered by a neuropsychologist and consist of batteries that focus on cognitive function (cognitive processing speed [PS], working memory, attention, executive functioning),[19,25,61] but additional tests assessing related psychological functioning can be added in cases where more extensive NP testing may be warranted in a particular patient.[61]

Examples of tests that assess memory would include tests such as the Hopkins Verbal Learning Test, Brief Visuospatial Memory Test, WAIS-III Digit Span Test, WAIS-III Letter–Number Sequencing Test, and Paced Auditory Stimulation Test.[25,61] Examples of tests assessing PS would be Symbol Digit Modalities Test, Wechsler Adult Intelligence Digit Symbol Subtest, Controlled Oral Word Association Test, Paced Auditory Stimulation Test, and Trail Making Test (TMT).[25,61] While executive functioning may be tested with tests such as Stroop Color Word Test, TMT, Wisconsin Card Sorting Test, and Controlled Oral Word Association Test,[25,61] attention is tested in the Trail Making Test-B, Continuous Performance Test, and Stroop Color Word Test.[25,60]

Paper-and-pencil tests have been used for years, and their validity to detect changes in neurocognitive functioning has been well documented.[61] The reliability of the individual tests has been documented in various studies with test–retest reliability measures or intraclass correlation coefficients (ICCs) ranging from 0.39 to 0.93[3,4,19,25,30,79] with most below the ideal reliability of 0.90 and only some above the minimally accepted reliability of 0.60.[5,67] A review of studies involving reliability of paper-and-pencil testing with respect to sensitivity found that there is "some evidence that paper and pencil tests are sensitive to the effects of concussion, at least within the first 5 days."[61] More recent studies on collegiate athletes showed sensitivity to be 43.5%[6] and 23%[49] when tested at 24 and 48 hours, respectively. Another study on Australian Football players reported sensitivities of paper-and-pencil tests to be 17.5% while athletes were still symptomatic and 4.2% when they became asymptomatic.[43] Clinical utility of paper-and-pencil testing has not been demonstrated as most studies have not demonstrated that paper-and-pencil tests can detect concussion once players are asymptomatic.[25,61]

Clinical Pearl

Domains tested in both paper-and-pencil and computer NP batteries include memory (new learning and working memory), cognitive processing, attention, and executive functioning as these are the domains most affected in concussive injury.

24.3.3 Computerized NP Testing

Computerized NP tests used in the evaluation of concussion measure various aspects of memory (new learning), cognitive processing, working memory, or executive functioning. These domains are tested, as they are the functions typically affected by traumatic brain injury.[19]

There are several available computerized NP tests that have been used in the evaluation of sports concussion. The four tests most commonly used in the evaluation of sports concussion are Automated Neuropsychological Assessment Metric (ANAM), Axon Sports Computerized Cognitive Assessment Tool (now called Cogstate CCAT), Headminder, and Immediate Post-Concussion Assessment and Cognitive Test (ImPACT). CNS Vital Signs is a newer test that is available in the sports market, but there are few studies validating this in athletes. The King–Devick test is a computerized oculomotor test that only measures cognitive visual performance[78] and thus is not being included in this discussion of computerized NP tests.

Deciding which test to use in your patient population requires an understanding of what the particular test is intended to do, how it can be used, and what the statistical data are regarding the test in addition to information about administration and interpretation. An overview of these aspects will follow, but detailed explanations are beyond the scope of this chapter.

24.3.3.1 Automated Neuropsychological Assessment Measure

ANAM was developed for serial testing and precision management of cognitive function in the U.S. military.[37,75] It was not specifically developed for sports concussion assessment but a sports medicine battery evolved. The sports medicine battery consists of code substitution, code substitution delayed, continuous performance test, mathematical processing, match to sample, and simple reaction time (SRT).[37,75] These tests measure the domains of verbal and visual memory, attention, concentration, PS, and reaction time.

The statistical support for ANAM testing in sports concussion is variable. Test–retest reliability of individual ANAM subtests in several studies has been shown a range of ICCs for throughput scores to be 0.38–0.96[8,9,37,75] with the majority being below the minimum 0.60. Validity was shown in one study to be good.[8] However, recent studies have brought the sensitivity and specificity of ANAM in sports concussion to be low and questionable.[32,63,66]

24.3.3.2 AXON/CogSport

AXON CCAT (www.axonsports.com) was developed in Australia as a computerized NP test and was first available for use in sports concussion in 2002 (CogSport/Cogstate). AXON CCAT is the online version. This test uses playing cards in a 12–15 minute battery designed to be brief and motivating. It is not intended to be a complete NP battery, but focuses on speed and accuracy to detect change in cognitive measures over time.[1] The four tests making up the AXON CCAT are PS, attention, learning, and working memory.[1,10,77]

Test–retest reliability of AXON has been looked at in intervals of 1 hour to 1 month[9,10,77] with ICCs for speed/reaction time subtests ranging from 0.45 to 0.90[9,10,77] but for accuracy ranging from 0.08 to 0.51.[9,10,77] Validity of Axon/CogSport compared to conventional tests has been evaluated in several studies with Pearson's coefficients ranging from 0.23 to 0.86 for tests measuring speed and 0.02 to 0.38 for those measuring accuracy.[10,72] The sensitivity of the CogSport/Axon battery was shown in one study to be 70.8%[43] while patients were symptomatic, with computerized tests showing deficits 2–3 days longer than symptoms and paper-and-pencil tests.[43]

24.3.3.3 Headminder Concussion Resolution Index (CRI)

Headminder CRI was developed specifically for the assessment of sports-related concussion. The CRI is composed of six subtests, which measure possible cognitive change with tests of attention and reaction time.[21,23,28] These subtests are reaction time, cued reaction time, animal decoding, visual recognition 1, visual recognition 2, and symbol scanning.[21,23,28] Three indices are derived from the subtests: SRT, complex reaction time (CRT), and PS.

There are some data on Headminder's test–retest reliability, but the two studies showed different results. One study showed a 2-week test–retest reliability of 0.65–0.90[23] for the subscores, but the other showed ranges from 0.03 to 0.66,[5] although this test has been criticized for its methodology by some.[70] Validity of Headminder has been looked at in several studies[21,22,72] with a wide range of correlation values on the various tests compared to SRT, CRT, and PS. r values ranged from 0.06 to 0.74 with higher correlations with the PS score (most above 0.60).[21,22,72] Sensitivity of Headminder was found to range from 78.6% to 88% in several studies.[6,21,23]

24.3.3.4 Immediate Post-Concussion Assessment and Cognitive Test (ImPACT)

ImPACT (www.impacttest.com) was developed in the 1990s in Pittsburgh to increase the availability of NP testing in the athletic environment.[71] It is a 20–25 minute test, which assesses symptoms along with cognitive domains of attention span, working memory, sustained and selective attention, response variability, nonverbal problem solving, and reaction time.[24,33,34,70,71] There are six modules that make up the ImPACT test: word discrimination, design memory, Xs and Os, symbol match, color match, and three-letter memory. Each of these tests is individually scored and then used to calculate composite scores of verbal memory, visual memory, PS, reaction time, and impulse control.[24,33,34,54,70,71] A symptom score is also recorded as part of the test.[24,33,34,54,70,71]

The ImPACT test has several studies on reliability with time intervals ranging from 1 day to 2 years.[5,9,18,34,64,65,67,68] The ICCs were 0.29–0.71 at 24–72 hours,[64] 0.67–0.86 at 7 days,[34] 0.50–0.88 at 30 days,[9,68] 0.15–0.88 at 45 and 50 days,[5,65] 0.57–0.85 at 1 year,[18] and 0.46–0.75 at 2 years.[67] Validity shown in studies looked primarily at correlations with reaction time and PS and TMT-A and TMT-B and Digit Symbol tests and found correlation coefficients ranging from 0.44 to 0.70.[34,72] Sensitivity was 79.2% at 1 day,[6] but when combined with symptoms and postural stability, the complete battery had a sensitivity of greater than 90%. In other studies, the sensitivity of ImPACT was found to be 82% and 91% at 72 hours with specificities of 89.4% and 69.1%.[71,73]

24.3.3.5 CNS Vital Signs

CNS Vital Signs is a computerized neurocognitive test battery initially developed as a clinical screening instrument for use in neurological disorders. It comprises seven tests: verbal and visual memory, finger tapping, symbol digit coding, Stroop test, a test of shifting attention, and continuous performance test.[26]

CNS Vital Signs has become available in the last few years for use in the evaluation of sports concussion. There are only a few studies looking at the psychometric properties of the test in the athletic population. Test–retest reliability at 30 days showed ICC measures of 0.29–0.79,[9] while another study (on normal volunteers and neuropsychiatric patients, not athletes) showed correlation coefficients (r) at an average of 62 days to be 0.31–0.87 with most above 0.60.[26] In the same study, the test was found to have moderate concurrent validity.[26] No studies on sensitivity of CNS Vital Signs in sports concussion were noted in our literature review.

24.3.4 Advantages and Disadvantages of Paper-and-Pencil and Computerized NP Tests

Paper-and-pencil tests have the advantage of being a more extensive and thorough validated battery with a low cost of equipment. However, the tests take hours of both athletes and neuropsychologist's time, with a high-cost administration and interpretation.[40,55] They are not ideal for serial use and lack equivalent forms.[49,59] They are subject to interrater biases and practice effects.[49] Paper-and-pencil tests have poor test–retest reliability and cannot measure speed and reaction times as precisely. They must be administered and interpreted by a neuropsychologist, so widespread use in management of all concussions is not feasible.[40,49]

Computerized NP tests have many advantages. They are shorter tests (<30 minutes), they may be administered by athletic trainer staff, and they do not require a physician to be present but allow for instant scoring and instant information to the provider.[49,57] They do not require a neuropsychologist for interpretation. Timing measures of computerized NP tests allow for more precise measures to the 1/100 of a second.[40,49,57,59] There are multiple equivalent forms that decrease practice effects.[49,57] NP tests allow for standardization of stimulus and can be useful for serial testing.[40,49,57] They can be administered on computers in individual or group settings.[40,49,57] Internet-based testing allows for central data storage, analysis, and reporting.[40,49,57] Disadvantages include cost of computers and software and limitations in the domains that are tested in comparison to more extensive paper-and-pencil testing.[55,59]

Clinical Pearl

Key advantages of computerized NP tests are a short administration time (<30 minutes) and ability to precisely measure reaction time to the 1/100 of a second.

24.4 CONSIDERATIONS FOR NP TESTING

24.4.1 Administration of Testing

A qualified health-care professional trained in the administration of that test should administer testing. For computerized NP testing in the collegiate, professional, and high school setting, this role has often been relegated to the athletic trainer. Test atmosphere (temperature and noise), time of day, computer display, practice and learning effects, and administrator expertise may all affect the results of a test.[17,49,57,59]

There are no evidence-based guidelines on the ideal timing of postconcussion NP testing. When to perform the first test, how many tests to perform, and the interval to use between testing sessions are at the discretion of the physician. Some health-care providers will test within 48 hours of concussion to demonstrate the cognitive changes or provide prognostic information (at times to see what functions are affected) or they may also use a test to reaffirm a diagnosis, for example, to prove to the patient, parent, or coach that there is really a concussion as well as guide academic restrictions. Typically, another test is done when the patient is asymptomatic before progression of exertion, although some physicians will progress noncontact exertion as long as the patient remains asymptomatic, and then a retest is done prior to clearance. There is no evidence to support one ideal time for NP testing in a patient who has sustained a concussion.

24.4.2 Baseline Testing

Baseline testing allows for comparison of an athletes' postconcussion test or neurocognitive functioning to their own preconcussion functioning/test. If no baseline testing exists, then age-matched normative data are used. While intuitively it would seem that baseline comparisons are preferable with less error (as an individual is being compared to their own baseline),[16,29] there is one study that shows no significant added benefit.[74] This may be due to the fact that baseline testing can be affected by a variety of internal and external factors.[2,7,11,12,14,15,25,30–32,36,39,41,49,53,54,57,59,62,64,76] Effort has been shown to affect baseline testing[31,76] although it was also shown in studies that it is difficult to "sandbag" a baseline test.[20,69] There is also evidence that administering the test in an individual versus in a group environment affects baseline scores.[54] In addition, studies have shown in-season athletes were less alert and performed lower on baseline testing than out-of-season athletes.[7] Consensus opinion of the Concussion in Sport Group is that baseline testing is not a mandatory aspect of concussion management; however, it may add useful information to the overall interpretation.[50]

24.4.3 Factors Affecting Testing

There are a multitude of factors that can affect both baseline and postconcussive testing; these factors fall into the following categories: psychological, physiological, cultural, premorbid conditions/past history, genetic, methodological, and others (see Table 24.2).[16,25,49,55,57,59] Factors found to have research-based evidence include age,[30,36,39,64] gender,[7,12,14,15] attention deficit disorder,[11,76] SAT scores,[7] fatigue,[7] headache,[53,62,76] dehydration,[56] psychological or emotional distress,[2,32] musculoskeletal injury,[32] effort level,[31,76] or concussive history.[7,11–13,36,54] Also, there is one study that suggests ethnicity to be a factor;[41] however, another author found no difference between ethnic groups when controlling for educational background.[38]

TABLE 24.2
Factors That Affect Neuropsychological Testing

Cultural	Genetic	Methodological
Education Language Previous exposure to use of computers	Age Intelligence Gender Ethnicity Handedness Visual acuity Auditory acuity	Test setting/atmosphere (Temperature, quietness, lack of distractions) Time of day Size of computer display Ease of use of computer mouse Practice/learning effects Random variance/chance History of prior testing Administrator experience/expertise
Physiological	**Pre-existing Medical Issues**	**Psychological**
Fatigue Headache Alertness Sleep Pain Medication Severity of present concussion Nutrition Dehydration Hormonal	History of prior concussions Previous head injuries Preexisting neurological disorder/deficits ADHD or other learning disorder Developmental disorder, neurodevelopmental disorder Personality disorder Drug use Alcohol use	General anxiety Test anxiety Stress Depression Fear Other emotional condition Effort/motivation

24.4.4 Interpretation of Testing

NP testing should be interpreted by a medical provider trained in the use and interpretation of the particular NP testing.[27] Test interpretation requires understanding of patient symptoms, psychometric properties of the test, complex interaction of test data, sources of error, extra test variables, and intra-individual variables.[16,17,27]

24.4.5 Referral to a Specialist

When to refer a patient to a specialist may vary with the experience and training of the initial provider evaluating the patient. The majority of sports concussions are managed by certified athletic trainers and primary care physicians.[52] If a physician does not feel comfortable in the management or has not been trained in the various tests that are utilized in concert to evaluate and manage concussion, they should refer to a sports medicine specialist or neuropsychologist experienced in the treatment of concussion. With respect specifically to NP testing, one may refer to a neuropsychologist for the interpretation of computerized testing if one has no experience in interpreting testing. Second, sports medicine specialists or scores do not make sense with the clinical picture or if they are not improving as expected. Finally, one might refer for further paper-and-pencil testing to evaluate domains not tested in the computerized tests or if patient is experiencing persistent deficits.

24.5 VALUE ADDED BY NP TESTING

A test can have a high reliability or sensitivity but not necessarily add clinical value. For concussion, an NP test would be clinically useful if it is sensitive in detecting neurocognitive impairments after concussion symptoms have resolved. It could also add value if it changes clinical decision making or changes clinical outcomes. Computerized NP testing has been shown in multiple studies to be sensitive to detecting neurocognitive changes beyond the symptomatic phase,[6,19,24,36,43,44,46,47,50,58,80] and the sensitivity increases when one combines computer NP testing with symptoms[80] and balance testing.[6] This is not true of paper-and-pencil testing. Neurocognitive testing also adds information that is useful in clinical decision making—such as with return to play, exercise progression, and school accommodations.[50] It is unknown at this time if utilizing NP testing in concussion management changes short- or long-term outcomes.

24.6 EXPERT OPINION

The *Fourth International Consensus Statement on Concussion in Sport* stated "the science of concussion is evolving and therefore the management and return to play decisions remain in the realm of clinical judgment on an individualized basis."[50] The statement also says that "the application of neuropsychological testing in concussion has been shown to be of clinical value and contributes significant information in concussion evaluation. However, it should not be the sole basis of management decisions."[50] The Team Physician Consensus Statement states that NP testing is "recommended as an aid in clinical decision making but is not a requirement for concussion management."[29] They also state that "NP testing is one component of the evaluation process and should not be used as a stand-alone tool to diagnose, manage or make RTP decisions in concussion."[29] The American Medical Society for Sports Medicine (AMSSM) Position Statement on Concussion in Sport states "neuropsychological tests are an objective measure of brain-behavior relationships and are more sensitive for subtle cognitive impairment than clinical exam."[27] However, they felt that "most concussions can be managed appropriately without the use of neuropsychological assessment."[27] Like the other consensus groups, the AMSSM group also stated "neuropsychological testing should be used only as part of a comprehensive concussion management strategy and should not be used in isolation."[27]

TABLE 24.3
SORT: Key Recommendations for Practice

Clinical Recommendation	Evidence Rating	References
NP testing has been shown to be of clinical value and contributes information to concussion evaluation.	C	[6,19,24,36, 43,44,46,47, 50,58,80]
NP testing should not be used in isolation; it should be used along with the rest of a comprehensive concussion evaluation plan.	C	[27,29,50]
Sideline assessment tools are helpful in the evaluation of a concussed athlete on the sidelines; however, they ideally should be compared to baseline scores and are not meant to be used beyond the initial assessment phase (<48 hours).	C	[17,45–47]
Baseline (NP) testing is not necessary in the evaluation of concussion but may add value, particularly in individuals with risk factors that may make their tests different from normative data.	C	[50]
NP testing should be evaluated by a medical provider trained in the evaluation of the NP test being evaluated.	C	[27]

24.7 CONCLUSION

NP testing has been more widely used in concussion management in recent years. There is no gold standard for the diagnosis of concussion. NP testing has been shown to be of clinical value and adds to decision making in the management of sports concussion. However, NP testing should not be used in isolation and is one tool in the concussion armamentarium. It should be used in concert with physical exam, current and past history, balance testing, and other testing as well as sound clinical judgment (see Table 24.3).

REFERENCES

1. Axon Sports. A medical guide to Axon Sports CCAT. www.axonsports.com. Accessed May 1, 2014.
2. Bailey CM, Samples HL, Broshek DK, Freeman JR, Barth JT. The relationship between psychological distress and baseline sports-related concussion testing. *Clinical Journal of Sport Medicine*. 2010;20(4):272–277.
3. Barr WB. Neuropsychological testing of high school athletes: Preliminary norms and test-retest indices. *Archives of Clinical Neuropsychology*. 2003;18:91–101.
4. Barr WB, McCrea M. Sensitivity and specificity of standardized neurocognitive testing immediately following sports concussion. *Journal of the International Neuropsychological Society*. 2001;7:693–702.
5. Broglio SP, Ferrara MS, Macciocchi SN, Baumgartner TA, Elliott R. Test-retest reliability of computerized concussion assessment programs. *Journal of Athletic Training*. 2007;42(4):509–514.

6. Broglio SP, Macciocchi SN, Ferrara MS. Sensitivity of the concussion assessment battery. *Neurosurgery*. 2007;60(6):1050–1058.
7. Brown CN, Guskiewicz KM, Bieiberg J. Athlete characteristics and outcome scores for computerized neuropsychological assessment: A preliminary analysis. *Journal of Athletic Training*. 2007;42(4):515–523.
8. Cernich A, Reeves D, Sun W, Blieberg J. Automated neuropsychological assessment metrics sports medicine battery. *Archives of Clinical Neuropsychology*. 2007; 22: S101–S114.
9. Cole WR, Arrieux JP, Schwab K et al. Test-retest reliability of four computerized neurocognitive assessment tools in an active duty military population. *Archives of Clinical Neuropsychology*. 2013;28(7):732–742.
10. Collie A, Maruff P, Makdissi M, McCrory P, McStephen M, Darby D. CogSport: Reliability and correlation with conventional cognitive tests used in postconcussion medical evaluations. *Clinical Journal of Sport Medicine*. 2003;13(1):28–32.
11. Collins MW, Grindel SH, Lovell MR et al. Relationship between concussion and neuropsychological performance in college football players. *Journal of the American Medical Association*. 1999;282:964–970.
12. Colvin AC, Mullen J, Lovell MR, West RV, Collins MW, Groh M. The role of concussion history and gender in recovery from soccer-related concussion. *The American Journal of Sports Medicine*. 2009;37:1699–1704.
13. Covassin T, Stearne D, Elbin R. Concussion history and post-concussion neurocognitive performance and symptoms in collegiate athletes. *Journal of Athletic Training*. 2008;43(2):119–124.
14. Covassin T, Swanik C, Sachs M. Sex differences and the incidence of concussions among collegiate athletes. *Journal of Athletic Training*. 2003;38:238–244.
15. Covassin T, Swanik CB, Sachs M, Kendrick Z, Schatz P, Zillmer E, Kaminaris C. Sex differences in baseline neuropsychological function and concussion symptoms of collegiate athletes. *British Journal of Sports Medicine*. 2006;40:923–927.
16. Echemendia RJ, Herring S, Bailes J. Who should conduct and interpret the neuropsychological assessment in sports-related concussion? *British Journal of Sports Medicine*. 2009;43(Suppl I):i32–i35.
17. Echmendia RJ, Iverson GL, McCrea M et al. Advances in neuropsychological assessment of sports-related concussion. *British Journal of Sports Medicine*. 2013;47:294–298.
18. Elbin RJ, Schatz P, Covassin T. One-year test-retest reliability of the online version of ImPACT in high school athletes. *The American Journal of Sports Medicine*. 2011;39:2319–2324.
19. Ellemberg D, Henry LC, Macciocchi SN, Guskiewicz KM, Broglio SP. Advances in sport concussion assessment: From behavioral to brain imaging measures. *Journal of Neurotrauma*. 2009;6(12):2365–2382.
20. Erdal K. Neuropsychological testing for sports-related concussion: How athletes can sandbag their baseline testing without detection. *Archives of Clinical Neuropsychology*. 2012;27:473–479.
21. Erlanger D, Feldman D, Kutner K et al. Development and validation of a web-based neuropsychological test protocol for sports-related return-to-play decision-making. *Archives of Clinical Neuropsychology*. 2003;18(3):293–316.
22. Erlanger DM, Kaushik T, Broshek D, Freeman J, Feldman D, FestaJ. Development and validation of a web-based screening tool for monitoring cognitive status. *The Journal of Head Trauma Rehabilitation*. 2002;17(5):458–476.
23. Erlanger D, Saliba E, Barth J, Almquist J, Webright W, Freeman J. Monitoring resolution of postconcussion symptoms in athletes: Preliminary results of web-based neuropsychological test protocol. *Journal of Athletic Training*. 2001;36(3):280–287.
24. Fazio VC, Lovell MR, Pardini JE, Collins MW. The relation between post concussion symptoms and neurocognitive performance in concussed athletes. *Neurorehabilitation*. 2007;22:207–216.
25. Grindel SH, Lovell MR, Collins MW. The assessment of sport-related concussion: The evidence behind neuropsychological testing and management. *Clinical Journal of Sport Medicine*. 2001;11:134–143.
26. Gualtieri CT, Johnson LG. Reliability and validity of a computerized neurocognitive test battery, CNS Vital Signs. *Archives of Clinical Neuropsychology*. 2006;21:623–643.
27. Harmon KG, Drezner J, Gammons M et al. American Medical Society for Sports Medicine position statement: Concussion in sport. *Clinical Journal of Sport Medicine*. 2013;23(1):1–18.
28. Headminder Website. www.headminder.com. Last accessed May 2, 2014.
29. Herring S, Bergfeld J, Indelicato P et al. Concussion (mild traumatic brain injury) and the team physician: A consensus statement. *Medicine & Science in Sports & Exercise*. 2011;43(12):2412–2422.
30. Hunt TN, Ferrara MS. Age-related differences in neuropsychological testing among high school athletes. *Journal of Athletic Training*. 2009;44(4):405–409.
31. Hunt TN, Ferrara MS, Miller LS, Macciocchi S. The effect on baseline neuropsychological test scores in high school football athletes. *Archives of Clinical Neuropsychology*. 2007;22:615–621.
32. Hutchinson M, Comper P, Mainwaring L, Richards D. The influence of musculoskeletal injury on cognition. *The American Journal of Sports Medicine*. 2011;39(11):2331–2337.
33. ImPACT test website. About impact test: Test features. https://www.impacttest.com. Accessed May 2, 2014.
34. Iverson GL, Lovell MR, Collins MW. Interpreting change on ImPACT following sport concussion. *The Clinical Neuropsychologist*. 2003;17(4):460–467.
35. Jinguji TM, Bompadre V, Harmon KG et al. Sport concussion assessment tool-2: Baseline values for high school athletes. *British Journal of Sports Medicine*. 2012;46:365–370.
36. Johnson EW, Kegel NE, Collins MW. Neurological assessment of sports related concussion. *Clinics in Sports Medicine*. 2011;30:73–88.
37. Kaminski TW, Groff RM, Glutting JJ. Examining the stability of automated neuropsychological assessment metric (ANAM) baseline test scores. *Journal of Clinical and Experimental Neuropsychology*. 2009;31(6):689–697.
38. Kontos AP, Elbin RJ, Covassin T, Larson E. Exploring the differences in computerized neurocognitive concussion testing between African American and White athletes. *Archives of Clinical Neuropsychology*. 2010;25:734–744.
39. Lau B, Lovell MR, Collins MW, Pardini J. Neurocognitive and symptom predictors of recovery in high school athletes. *Clinical Journal of Sport Medicine*. 2009;19(3):216–221.
40. Lovell MR. Management of sports-related concussion: Current status and future trends. *Clinics in Sports Medicine*. 2009;28(1):95–111.
41. Lovell MR, Solomon GS. Psychometric data for the NFL neuropsychological test battery. *Applied Neuropsychology*. 2011;18:197–209.
42. Maddocks DL, Dicker GD, Saling MM. The assessment of orientation following concussion in athletes. *Clinical Journal of Sport Medicine*. 1995;5(1):32–35.
43. Makdissi M, Darby D, Maruff P, Ugoni A, Brukner P, McCrory PR. Natural history of concussion in sport: Markers of severity and implications for management. *The American Journal of Sports Medicine*. 2010;38(3):464–471.

44. McClincy MP, Lovell MR, Pardini J, Collins MW, Spore MK. Recovery from sports concussion in high school and collegiate athletes. *Brain Injury*. 2006;20(1):33–39.
45. McCrea M. Standardized mental status assessment of sports concussion. *Clinical Journal of Sport Medicine*. 2001;11:176–181.
46. McCrea M, Barr WB, Guskiewicz K et al. Standard regression-based methods for measuring recovery after sport-related concussion. *Journal of the International Neuropsychological Society*. 2005;11:58–69.
47. McCrea M, Guskiewicz KM, Marshall SW et al. Acute effects and recovery time following concussion in collegiate football players. *Journal of the American Medical Association*. 2003;290(19):2556–2563.
48. McCrea M, Hammeke T, Olsen G, Leo P, Guskiewitz K. Unreported concussion in high school football players. *Clinical Journal of Sport Medicine*. 2004;14:13–17.
49. McCrory P, Makdissi M, Davis G, Collie A. Value of neuropsychological testing after head injuries in football. *British Journal of Sports Medicine*. 2005;39:i58–i63.
50. McCrory P, Meeuwisse W, Aubry M et al. Consensus statement on concussion in sport: The 4th International Conference on Concussion in Sport, held in Zurich, November 2012. *Clinical Journal of Sport Medicine*. 2013;23(2):29–117.
51. McCrory P, Meeuwisse W, Johnston K et al. Consensus statement on concussion in sport: The 3rd International Conference on Concussion in Sport, held in Zurich. *Clinical Journal of Sport Medicine*. 2009;19(3):185–200.
52. Meehan WP, d'Hemecourt P, Collins CL, Comstock RD. Assessment and management of sports-related concussions in the United States high schools. *The American Journal of Sports Medicine*. 2011;39:2304–2310.
53. Mihalik J, Stump, J, Collins, M, Lovell, M, Field, M, Maroon, J. Posttraumatic migraine characteristics in athletes following sports-related concussion. *Journal of Neurosurgery*. 2005;102:850–855.
54. Moser RS, Schatz P, Neidzwski K, Ott SD. Group versus individual administration affects baseline neurocognitive test performance. *The American Journal of Sports Medicine*. 2011;39:2325–2330.
55. Pana AL. *Neuropsychological Testing in Concussion in ACSM's Sports Medicine: A Comprehensive Review*. Philadelphia, PA: Wolters Kluwer-LWW; 2013. pp. 162–171.
56. Patel AV, Mihalik JP, Notebaert AJ, Guskiewicz KM, Prentice WE. Neuropsychological performance, postural stability, and symptoms after dehydration. *Journal of Athletic Training*. 2007;42(1):66–75.
57. Patel DR, Shivdasani V, Baker RJ. Management of sport-related concussion in young athletes. *Sports Medicine*. 2005;35(8):671–684.
58. Peterson CL, Ferrara MS, Mrazik M, Piland S, Elliott R. Evaluation of neuropsychological domain scores and postural stability following cerebral concussion in sports. *Clinical Journal of Sport Medicine*. 2003;13:230–237.
59. Putukian M. Neuropsychological testing as it relates to recovery from sports-related concussion. *PM R*. 2011;3:S425–S432.
60. Randolph C. Implementation of neuropsychological testing models for the high school, collegiate, and professional sport settings. *Journal of Athletic Training*. 2001;36(3):288–296.
61. Randolph C, McCrea M, Barr WB. Is neuropsychological testing useful in the management of sport-related concussion? *Journal of Athletic Training*. 2005;40(3):139–154.
62. Register-Mihalik JK, Guskiewicz KM, Mann, JD, Shields EW. The effects of headache on clinical measures of neurocognitive function. *Clinical Journal of Sport Medicine*. 2007;17(4):282–288.
63. Register-Mihalik JK, Guskiewicz KM, Mihalik JP et al. Reliable change, sensitivity and specificity in a multidimensional concussion assessment battery: Implications for caution in clinical practice. *The Journal of Head Trauma Rehabilitation*. 2013;28(3):274–283.
64. Register-Mihalik JK, Kontos DL, Guskiewicz KM et al. Age related differences and reliability on computerized and paper-and-pencil neurocognitive assessment batteries. *Journal of Athletic Training*. 2012;47(3):297–305.
65. Resch J, Driscoll A, McCaffrey N et al. ImPACT test-retest reliability: Reliably unreliable? *JAT*. 2013;48(4):506–511.
66. Resch JE, McCrea MA, Cullum CM. Computerized neurocognitive testing in the management of sports related concussion: An update. *Neuropsychology Review*. 2013;23:335–349.
67. Schatz P. Long-term test-retest reliability of baseline cognitive assessments using ImPACT. *The American Journal of Sports Medicine*. 2010;38(1):47–53.
68. Schatz P, Ferris CS. One-month test-retest reliability of the ImPACT test battery. *Archives of Clinical Neuropsychology*. 2013;28:499–504.
69. Schatz P, Glatts C. "Sandbagging" baseline test performance on ImPACT, without detection, is more difficult than it appears. *Archives of Clinical Neuropsychology*. 2013;28:236–244.
70. Schatz P, Kontos A, Elbin RJ. Response to Mayers and Redick: Clinical utility of ImPACT assessment for postconcussion return-to-play counseling: Psychometric issues. *Journal of Clinical and Experimental Neuropsychology*. 2012;34(4):428–434.
71. Schatz P, Pardini JE, Lovell MR, Collins MW, Podell K. Sensitivity and specificity of the ImPACT test battery for concussion in athletes. *Archives of Clinical Neuropsychology*. 2006;21:91–99.
72. Schatz P, Putz BO. Cross-validation of measures used for computer-based assessment of concussion. *Applied Neuropsychology*. 2006;13(3):151–159.
73. Schatz P, Sandel N. Sensitivity and specificity of the online version of ImPACT in high school and collegiate athletes. *AJSM*. 2013;41(2):321–326.
74. Schmidt JD, Register-Mihalik JA, Mihalik JP et al. Identifying impairments after concussion: Normative date versus individualized baselines. *MSSE*. 2012;44(9):1621–1628.
75. Segalowitz SJ, Mahaney P, Santessoa DL, MacGregor L, Dywan J, Willer B. Retest reliability in adolescents of a computerized neuropsychological battery used to assess recovery from concussion. *Neurorehabilitation*. 2007;22:243–251.
76. Solomon GS, Haase RF. Biopsychosocial characteristics and neurocognitive test performance in National Football League players: An initial assessment. *Archives of Clinical Neuropsychology*. 2008;23:563–577.
77. Straume-Naesheim TM, Andersen TE, Bahr R. Reproducibility of computer based neuropsychological testing among Norwegian elite football players. *British Journal of Sports Medicine*. 2005; 39:i64–i69.
78. Tjarks BJ, Dorman JC, Valentine VD et al. Comparison and utility of King-Devick and ImPACT composite score in adolescent concussion patients. *The Journal of Neuroscience*. 2013;334:148–153.
79. Valovich-McLeod TC, Barr WB, McCrea M, Guskiewicz KM. Psychometric and measurement properties of concussion assessment tools in youth sports. *Journal of Athletic Training*. 2006;41(4):391–408.
80. Van Kampen DA, Lovell MA, Pardini JE, Collins MW, Fu FH. The "value added" of neurocognitive testing after sports-related concussion. *The American Journal of Sports Medicine*. 2006;34(10):1630–1635.

25 Footwear Considerations in the Athlete

Jay Dicharry and Patrick J. Depenbrock

CONTENTS

TABLE 25.1
Key Clinical Considerations

1. The goal of any shoe/foot interface is let the foot work: encourage adaptation the ground to achieve shock attenuation and stability during contact, and to provide a stabilize environment to allow intrinsic foot muscles to resupinate the foot for push off.
2. Shoe design can influence an athlete's running mechanics.
3. Incorrect footwear can exacerbate lower extremity dysfunction, while ideal footwear selection can prevent dysfunction.
4. Despite widespread use, running shoe prescriptions that assign stability categories (stability, motion control, cushion) do not prevent pain and injury.
5. The clinician should assess a runner's structural alignment, flexibility, intrinsic muscular stability, and gait before identifying his or her footwear needs.

25.1 INTRODUCTION

Despite the fact that humans are capable of running without shoes and have done so competitively for thousands of years, the vast majority of modern-day athletes choose to wear shoes. Athletes wear shoes to protect feet from surface injury, mitigate the risk of overuse injury, and improve performance. Although athletic footwear is a multibillion dollar business, most footwear recommendations are based on conjecture and unsubstantiated claims.[35] There exists a paucity of independent research to prove or disprove industry claims, especially given the ever-evolving trends in shoe designs. This chapter will review the anatomy and construction of the running shoe, basic types of shoe classification, factors to consider when selecting a running shoe, and an update on recent trend toward barefoot running and minimalist footwear (Table 25.1).

25.2 SHOE CONSTRUCTION AND ANATOMY

The running shoe is divided into three main segments: the upper, outsole, and midsole. The upper, which contains the laces and tongue, secures the shoe to the foot and is made of highly breathable fabric that limits heat buildup around the foot. Plastic molding may be imbedded in the running shoe heel to provide rear-foot support. The rear of the shoe often includes posterior heel tab cutouts, which reduce friction delivered to the Achilles tendon. The contour and shape of the upper should be compliant to adapt around the foot, and the lacing configuration can be varied to minimize pressure spikes on the dorsum of the foot. Proprioceptive contact of the upper plays a role in subjective comfort and ensuring that the shoe can move with the foot.

The midsole is the middle and most functional segment of the shoe. It is composed of a foam layer that provides cushion and support. Midsoles consist primarily of ethyl vinyl acetate, a lightweight material that can be blended to various densities to respond to the needs of the runner. Manufacturers will also infuse this layer with other heavier materials such as polyurethane or thermoplastics to achieve a target balance of weight, support, and cushioning. This material may be uniform, or may change in specific positions in the shoe. For example, motion control and stability shoes typically concentrate high-density material (often of darker color) on the medial aspect of the midsole in attempts to limit foot pronation.[25,35] Some companies develop trademark midsole inserts (e.g., Air, Gel, Torsion, etc.) to provide cushioning, dissipate stress, and minimize weight in their running shoes.

The outermost segment is the outsole. This layer provides traction to the running surface and is typically made of a blend of both blown and carbon rubber material. Carbon rubber composite provides support and durability, while the blown rubber provides cushion. Recently, footwear designs have begun to infuse the midsole with blended rubber to minimize the amount of weight in the outsole itself. The geometry (toe spring, and heel bevels) and the flex grooves in the outsole play an important role in optimizing the compressibility of the midsole during loading.

A lasting connects the upper to the midsole via glue or stitching. The material used in this interface plays a role in rigidity. Board and slip are examples of types of lastings. Board lastings increase torsional rigidity, while slip, or California, lastings favor cushion and flexibility. Features of both board and slip are included in a combination lasting, which is divided into a board-like rear-foot segment and a slip-like forefoot segment.

The insole, or sockliner, of a running shoe is a thin layer of cushion material that envelops the foot surface. The insole lacks functional stability and its cushioning properties are ephemeral, often breaking down after the first week of shoe wear. In the event that an athlete chooses to wear orthotics or shoe inserts, the insole is removed in order to accommodate space taken up by the orthotic.

Shoe last, or shape, is the anatomic foot template around which a manufacturer chooses to construct its footwear. This template varies by brand. As a result, an athlete may find that certain shoe brands are more amenable to his or her foot shape than others. The shape of the last can be straight, curved, or semicurved. A straight last provides greater contact surface for the foot, thus affording more torsional rigidity. A curved last better approximates the shape of a high-arched foot. It adds flexibility and decreases torsional rigidity. A semicurved last combines elements of both templates and is a popular shape for top-selling stability shoes. Typically, a shoe's last is not ostensibly marked by the brand and can even vary within a brand. Likewise, the sum of all the parts of the shoe work together to produce an overall feel. Thus, it is important that an athlete try on multiple shoes between brands and within a brand to confirm ideal fit before making a purchase.

TABLE 25.2
Classification of Running Shoes

Classification	Features
Motion control	• Board lasting • Dense midsole • Straight last • Rear and forefoot postings • Ideal for overpronators/heavy runners
Stability	• Dense midsole • Combination last with semicurve • Rear-foot postings • Forefoot cushion • Ideal for mild pronators/light runners
Cushion	• Slip lasting • Soft midsole • Curved-shape last • Heel and forefoot cushion • Ideal for supinators
Trail	• Stability shoe template • Reinforced with carbon fiber • Ideal for use on uneven surface
Racing flats	• Lightweight • Thin midsole • Minimal posting • Ideal for racing on soft track surface

25.3 SHOE CLASSIFICATION

There are five basic types of running shoe classification: motion control, stability, cushion, trail, and racing flats. Motion control shoes have a board lasting, dense midsole, a straight last, and rear and forefoot postings. They are traditionally prescribed to overpronators and heavy runners (e.g., >180 lb) for the purpose of blunting pronation of hypermobile or unstable feet.[25] This, however, is not without controversy. One small study of 89 randomized female half-marathon runners found that subjects with pronated or highly pronated feet noted significantly increased pain with motion control shoes compared to neutral and stability shoes.[33] Unlike motion control shoes, cushion shoes utilize slip lasting, a curved-shape last, and cushion in the heel and forefoot. Traditionally, cushion shoes are used most often by supinators or underpronators, because it is thought that those with a rigid, inflexible foot lack shock absorption and therefore require shoes that maximize cushioning and flexibility.[19] Stability shoes offer a mix of motion control and cushion features. Like motion control shoes, stability shoes have a dense midsole. However, they also have a combination last with semicurved shape. They may feature slightly postings, thermoplastic inserts, or proprietary materials to achieve a balance of cushioning and foot stability. Stability shoes are aimed at mild pronators. Historically, they are the most popular shoe classification sold by manufacturers, as the bulk of the market falls in the middle of the foot spectrum.[35] Trail shoes, which require increased traction, have unique tread designs in the outsole to improve friction and improve durability. Racing flats are about minimizing weight at all cost. They have a light, thin midsole with very little posting. These features can increase ground reaction forces experienced by runners and therefore necessitate a gradual transition period of wear in order to permit an athlete to acclimate to the increased stress[19] (see Table 25.2).

25.4 SHOE RECOMMENDATION

Overuse injury is influenced by a balance of intrinsic and extrinsic factors. Footwear is an example of a modifiable extrinsic risk factor. Running shoes have the ability to affect running mechanics, exacerbate lower extremity dysfunction, and prevent lower extremity injury.[2,10,11,22–24,29,30,37,41,45] Ideally, an athlete's intrinsic factors such as alignment, stability, flexibility, and muscle imbalance would be assessed prior to selecting a shoe.[25,35] An athlete's foot type, gait, and body habitus should guide a provider's recommendation toward an ideal last configuration. Traditionally, physicians have utilized these factors to recommend an athlete for one of three categories of running shoe: cushioned, stability, or motion control. It should be noted, however, that the prescription of running shoe categories lacks evidence.[28] It should also be noted that current conventions for assigning stability categories have not been shown to prevent pain and injury in runners.[33,34]

Foot structure affects the magnitude of force transmitted to bone and soft tissue structures.[2] The arch of a cavus foot tends to be rigid and stable, transmitting a significant portion of stress up the kinetic chain to shins and knees. Conversely, a flexible, or planus, foot tends to dissipate vertically directed force loads within the foot structure itself. Therefore, the ideal last would increase shock absorption of the cavus hypomobile arch, support the planus arch, and promote mechanics of the neutral foot. As a result, cavus foot types are traditionally shod with a curved-shape last with slip lasting, while flat feet are shod with a straight last, board lasting, firm heel counter, multidensity midsole, and medial heal posting.[9,32]

An athlete's foot type can be determined via floor-level inspection of the barefoot patient from behind. A typical heel in standing position will rest in slight pronation (hindfoot valgus) and rotate into varus position upon plantar flexion. Heels that remain in a valgus position as athlete rises onto his or her toes may reflect hindfoot rigidity and therefore benefit from medial foot support as well as evaluation for cause of instability. Heels that begin, and remain, in varus position are usually high-arched and rigid. These feet likely require footwear that will maximize cushioning. The wet foot test, achieved by having the athlete make an impression with a wet foot upon a paper towel, can help confirm high or low arch alignment of the foot.[25,35] However, the wet foot test has not been shown to provide prescriptive shoe criteria that has minimized injury or improved performance.

A runner's gait is best evaluated on a treadmill with the aid of a video analysis program that permits slow motion playback. Unfortunately, this capability is limited to a paucity of specialty clinics. However, simple inspection of an old pair of running shoes may afford some insight on an athlete's gait. During a typical gait cycle for heel strikers (the majority of runners), the lateral aspect of the heel makes first contact with the running surface.[15] The foot then adapts (pronates) as the body translates forward over the foot, reaching peak pronation just after the heel rises from the ground. Then the foot begins to actively increase its congruency (supinate) as weight is transferred through the first ray for push off.[7] As a result, examination of most neutral-gait runners with a heel strike reveals mild lateral wear over the heel with a uniform pressure distribution over the midfoot. However, significant tread wear and midsole breakdown on the lateral heel and/or medial aspect of the forefoot, suggest that the runner has difficulty intrinsically controlling their foot mechanics. This "overpronation" has been associated with anterior knee pain, plantar fasciitis, metatarsal stress fractures, and tendinopathies of the popliteus, posterior tibialis, and Achilles.[1,3,12,16,27,38,39] Evidence of increased wear over the lateral aspect of forefoot suggests an athlete with under-pronation. Under-pronation has been associated with tibial stress fractures, femoral stress fractures, Achilles' tendinopathy, and plantar fasciitis.[20,31,43]

A runner's weight and weekly running mileage should be considered in choice of shoe and frequency of replacement. Most running shoes are designed for 160 lb males and 125 lb females.[35] Heavier runners, or runners who maintain a higher volume and speed, may benefit from a denser midsole and outsole construction. Midsoles lose 40% of their cushioning ability after 400–500 miles; therefore, most running shoes will require replacement at this point.[27] This replacement interval varies based on the weight of the runner and the durability of the shoe itself. Heavier runners and those with less durable shoes will need to replace their shoes closer to the 250–300 mile mark. Over-worn shoes may alter a runner's gait. Athletes who run in worn shoes with compacted cushioning will modify their form (e.g., increased stance time and joint range of motion) in order to minimize the amount of work done by the joints.[15] These form adaptations may play a role in injury development.

25.5 SHOE-BUYING TIPS

Prospective running shoe buyers should consider several tips before making a purchase. The human foot swells with exercise and prolonged standing. Therefore, a running shoe buyer should shop for footwear in the early evening following a run to accommodate dependent foot swelling.[25,35] This requires selection of a running shoe that is often one half to one full size larger than a standard street shoe. Due to size and fit variability between shoe brands and models, an athlete should try on more than one shoe brand and more than one model when purchasing a shoe.

Once a shoe is securely fastened, one-half inch, or a thumb's width, should fit in the space between the longest toe and the tip of the shoe. The flex point of the toe spring should rest underneath the metatarsal heads. The toe box should be wide enough to allow the forefoot rays to splay without constriction during weight bearing. Given the variability in shoe width between brands, it is important to try on multiple pairs of shoes and jog in each pair in order to determine their level of dynamic comfort. Friction points or areas of discomfort are only likely to worsen with wear and have the potential to precipitate blisters, alter foot shape, and affect normal foot motion. Therefore, the initial in-store fit of the ideal running shoe should be one of complete static and dynamic comfort.

There exists a delicate balance between a competitive runner's desire for lightweight shoes (e.g., racing flats) and appropriately cushioned shoes. While shoe makers have made functional gains in minimizing energy lost through lightweight alterations in materials, the ideal level of cushion remains a subject of debate.[42] A recent study of 12 subjects with preferred midstrike patterns showed a lower metabolic cost of running when using a slight amount of foam cushioning (10 mm). Meanwhile, utilizing either barefoot/minimalist running shoe or a higher thickness of foam cushioning (20 mm) did not have a significant effect. This would suggest that a small amount of cushioning (i.e., 10 mm) can mitigate the increased metabolic power required to inherently cushion the foot on impact. However, there may exist a threshold above which the weight of the cushion itself offsets the cushion it provides. In other words, a little, but not a lot, of cushion may be helpful to competitive runners looking to conserve metabolic power and minimize the weight of their shoe.[13] Runners in search of the ideally cushioned shoe should be made aware that the best shoe may not necessarily be the

TABLE 25.3
Shoe-Buying Tips

1. Replace running shoes every 300–400 miles.
2. Try on prospective new shoes at the end of the day after exercise.
3. Select a shoe that is ½ to 1 full size larger than standard street shoe.
4. Try on more than one shoe brand and more than one shoe model.
5. A thumb's width should fit in between the longest toe and shoe tip.
6. Flex point of the shoe should rest underneath the ball of the foot.
7. Toe box should not constrict forefoot while weight bearing in single-leg stance.
8. Jog in store using prospective shoes to determine the level of dynamic comfort.
9. Do not tolerate friction points (they tend to worsen, not improve, with wear).
10. Subjective comfort is paramount.

most expensive shoe. High-cost running shoes have not been shown to provide superior plantar pressure cushioning compared to low- and medium-cost running shoes; therefore, higher cost is not necessarily indicative of a superior shoe[4] (see Table 25.3).

25.6 MINIMALIST FOOTWEAR

Barefoot running and the use of minimalist footwear continue to attract interest. While studies do not confirm the superiority of one form of running over another, they do demonstrate that shoes allow runners to adopt a gait that is different from that of unshod runners.[6] Barefoot runners tend to strike with their mid- or forefoot. They exhibit a more plantar-flexed ankle on surface contact, shorter stride length, and increased cadence.[14,18,40] This is in contrast to shod runners wearing traditional running shoes, who tend to initiate foot strike with their heel.

Traditional running shoes are built with a 2:1 ratio between the heights of the rear-foot and forefoot, respectively. This ratio affects a runner's contact style and muscle activation. Heel elevation of the traditional running shoe places the ankle joint in a position of poor proprioception during the stance phase.[36] This changes pressure throughout the foot and creates a quad-dominant firing pattern that results in postural changes.[34] Proponents of the traditional running shoe design argue that a reduction in shoe heel height has the potential to precipitate Achilles injury. Several studies, however, show no decrease in Achilles stress with elevated shoe heels, with one study even finding increased injury associated with elevated heels.[8,13,26]

Natural running, or minimalist, shoes feature geometry changes with minimal heel -toe drops (typically 0–4 mm). Minimalist shoes also feature firmer midsoles. Together, these features bias the runner into more of a midfoot/foefoot landing style, as opposed to the heel-first contact style of traditional running shoes with elevated heels.[5,40] Minimal shoes are designed for the purpose of improving proprioceptive feedback and maximizing connective tissue elastic recoil. Barefoot and minimalist shoe proponents point out that high vertical impact peaks and vertical loading rates seen among heel strikers are associated with common running injuries such as patellofemoral pain, plantar fasciitis, and tibial stress fractures. A recent study evaluated the kinematics and kinetics of 14 rear-foot runners with no minimalist shoe experience. These subjects, all of whom were male, ran for 10 minutes on a treadmill at a speed of 3.35 m/s in both a minimalist shoe and a standard shoe. These runners remained as rear-foot strikers in the minimalist shoe, suggesting that runners new to the minimalist shoe do not automatically adopt forefoot or midfoot strike pattern by wearing the minimalist shoe (they did not transition to a non-rear-foot strike pattern). Previous studies suggest that it is possible for rear-foot strikers to adopt and maintain midfoot or mild forefoot strike pattern, but this was done under the auspices of a formal gait retraining intervention. Thus, clinicians should not reinforce the assumption among runners that use of a minimalist shoe alone will precipitate a change in gait.[46] Another study with 75 runners showed that traditional elevated heel, pronation control design shoes significantly increased stress to the hip and the knees.[14] However, it is unknown specifically how much increase in joint stress is causative for injury.

25.7 CONCLUSION

Despite the lack of conclusive data on how best to match runner and shoe type, shoe design does have an effect on runners. Incorrect footwear can exacerbate lower extremity dysfunction and alter running mechanics. Conversely, ideal footwear may prevent injury or assist healing by mitigating tissue stress on impaired structures. Because the prescription of shoe categories to runners is not evidence based, a clinician should not ignore the importance of addressing modifiable intrinsic risk factors. Further, the shoe's effect on the runner is not always mechanical, but can be proprioceptive. Therefore, a dynamic running assessment and evaluation of a runner's structural alignment,

TABLE 25.4
SORT: Key Recommendations For Practice

Clinical Recommendation	Evidence Rating	References
Shoe cost should not supersede sense of dynamic comfort, as high-cost running shoes have not been shown to provide superior cushioning compared to lower-cost running shoes.	C	[4]
Do not rely on stability categorization–based running shoe prescriptions to prevent running pain and injury.	B	[33,34]
In the absence of formal gait retraining, simple use of a minimalist shoe should be relied upon to change a runner's gait.	C	[46]
A small amount of foam cushioning (10 mm) can reduce the metabolic cost of running.	C	[13]

flexibility, and intrinsic muscular stability are encouraged to help identify an athlete's unique footwear needs. Purchasing tips should guide the patient toward trying on multiple shoes to establish a sense of static and dynamic comfort. More research is needed to determine the effects of footwear on injury and performance in the running athlete (Table 25.4).

REFERENCES

1. Andrews JR. Overuse syndromes of the lower extremity. *Clinics in Sports Medicine*. 1983;2:137.
2. Barnes RA, Smith PD. The role of footwear in minimizing lower limb injury. *Journal of Sports Sciences*. 1984;12:341–353.
3. Campbell JW, Inman VT. Treatment of plantar fasciitis and calcaneal spurs with OC-BL shoe insert. *Clinical Orthopaedics*. 1974;103:57.
4. Clinghan R, Arnold GP, Drew TS et al. Do you get value for money when you buy an expensive pair of running shoes? *British Journal of Sports Medicine*. 2008;42:189–193.
5. De Wit B, De Clercq D, Aerts P. Biomechanical analysis of the stance phase during barefoot and shod running. *Journal of Biomechanics*. 2000;33:269–278.
6. Dicharry JM. Barefoot running: Is barefoot better? In: *UVA Running Medicine Conference*. Charlottesville, VA; 2010.
7. Dicharry JM, Franz JR, Croce UD et al. Differences in static and dynamic measures in evaluation of talonavicular mobility in gait. *Journal of Orthopaedic & Sports Physical Therapy*. 2009;39:628–634.
8. Dixon SJ, Kerwin DG. The influence of heal lift manipulation on sagittal plane kinematics in running. *Journal of Applied Biomechanics*. 1999;15:139–151.
9. Foot and ankle update. In *Proceedings of Healthsouth Educational Program*. Charlottesville, VA; 2002.
10. Hardin EC, van den Bogert AJ, Hamill J. Kinematic adaptations during running: Effects of footwear, surface, and duration. *Medicine & Science in Sports & Exercise*. 2004;36:838–844.
11. Hennig EM, Milani TL. Pressure distribution measurements for evaluation of running shoe properties. *Sportverletz Sportschaden*. 2000;14:90–97.
12. Hulkk OA, Orava S. Stress fractures in athletes. *International Journal of Sports Medicine*. 1987;8: 221.
13. Jarvinen TA, Kannus P, Maffulli N et al. Achilles tendon disorders: Etiology and epidemiology. *Foot and Ankle Clinics*. 2005;10:255–266.
14. Kerrigan DC, Franz JR, Keenan GS et al. The effect of running shoes on lower extremity joint torques. *PMR: Journal of Injury, Function, and Rehabilitation*. 2009;1:1058–1063.
15. Kong PW, Candelaria NG, Smith DR. Running in new and worn shoes: A comparison of three types of cushioning footwear. *British Journal of Sports Medicine*. 2009;43:745–749.
16. Kristoff WB, Ferris WB. Runner's injuries. *Physician and Sportsmedicine*. 1979;7: 53.
17. Kryztopher DT, Franz JR, Kram R. A test of the metabolic cost of cushioning hypothesis during unshod and shod running. *Medicine & Science in Sports & Exercise*. 2014;46(2):324–329.
18. Lieberman DE, Venkadesan M, Werbel WA et al. Foot strike patterns and collision forces in habitually barefoot versus shod runners. *Nature*. 2010;463:531–535.
19. Logan S, Hunter I, J Ty Hopkins JT et al. Ground reaction force differences between running shoes, racing flats, and distance spikes in runners. *Journal of Sports Science and Medicine*. 2010;9:147–153.
20. Lutter LD. Shoes and orthoses in the runner. *Techniques in Orthopaedics*. 1990;5:57.
21. Milgrom C, Giladi M, Stein M et al. Stress fractures in military recruits: A prospective study showing unusually high incidence. *Journal of Bone and Joint Surgery (British Volume)*. 1985;65B:732.
22. Milgrom C, Finestone A, Ekenman I et al. The effect of shoe sole composition on in vivo tibial strains during walking. *Foot & Ankle International*. 2001;22:598–602.
23. Nigg BM, Stefanyshyn D, Cole G et al. The effect of material characteristics of shoe soles on muscle activation and energy aspects during running. *Journal of Biomechanics*. 2003;36:569–575.
24. Nigg BM, Stergiou P, Cole G et al. Effect of shoe inserts on kinematics, center of pressure, and leg joint moments during running. *Medicine & Science in Sports & Exercise*. 2003;35:314–319.
25. O'Connor FG, Wilder RP, Nirschl R. *Textbook of Running Medicine*. New York: McGraw-Hill, Medical Publishing Division; 2001.
26. Reinschmidt C, Nigg BM. Influence of heel height on ankle joint moments in running. *Medicine & Science in Sports & Exercise*. 1995;27:410–416.
27. Reinschmidt C, Nigg BM. Current issues in the design of running and court shoes. *Sportverletz Sportschaden*. 2000;14:71–81.
28. Richards CE, Magin PJ, Callister R. Is your prescription of distance running shoes evidence-based? *British Journal of Sports Medicine*. 2009;43:159–162.
29. Roberts ME, Gordon CE. Orthopedic footwear. Custom-made and commercially manufactured footwear. *Foot and Ankle Clinics*. 2001;6:243–247.
30. Roy JP, Stefanyshyn DJ. Shoe midsole longitudinal bending stiffness and running economy, joint energy, and EMG. *Medicine & Science in Sports & Exercise*. 2006;38:562–569.
31. Roy S. How I manage plantar fasciitis. *Physician and Sportsmedicine*. 1983;11:127.
32. Running course. In *Proceedings of Healthsouth Educational Program*. Charlottesville, VA; 2002.
33. Ryan MB, Valiant GA, McDonald K et al. The effect of three different levels of footwear stability on pain outcomes in women runners: A randomised control trial. *British Journal of Sports Medicine*. 2011;45:715–721.
34. Sahrmann S. *Diagnosis and Treatment of Movement Impairment Syndromes*. St. Louis, MO: Mosby; 2002.
35. Seidenberg PH, Beutler AB. *The Sports Medicine Resource Manual*. Philadelphia, PA: Saunders, Elsevier; 2008.
36. Sekizawa K. Effects of shoe sole thickness on joint position sense. *Gait Posture*. 2001;13:221–228.
37. Sharkey NA, Ferris L, Smith TS et al. Strain and loading of the second metatarsal during heel-lift. *Journal of Bone and Joint Surgery*. 1995;77:1050–1057.
38. Simkin A, Leichter I, Giladi M et al. Combined effect of foot arch structure and an orthotic device on stress fractures. *Foot & Ankle*. 1989;10:25.
39. Smart GW, Taunton JE, Clement DB. Achilles tendinosis in runners: A review. *Medicine & Science in Sports & Exercise*. 1980;12:231.
40. Squadrone R, Gallozzi C. Biomechanical and physiological comparison of barefoot and two shod conditions in experienced barefoot runners. *The Journal of Sports Medicine and Physical Fitness*. 2009;49:6–13.
41. Stacoff A, Kalin X, Stussi E. The effects of shoes on the torsion and rearfoot motion in running. *Medicine & Science in Sports & Exercise*. 1991;23:482–490.

42. Stefanyshyn DJ, Nigg BM. Energy aspects associated with sport shoes. *Sportverletz Sportschaden*. 2000;14:82–89.
43. Tory JS et al. Overuse injuries in sport: The foot. *Clinics in Sports Medicine*. 1987;6:291.
44. van Gent RN, Siem D, van Middelkoop M et al. Incidence and determinants of lower extremity running injuries in long distance runners: A systematic review. *British Journal of Sports Medicine*. 2007;41:469–480.
45. Wakeling JM, Pascual SA, Nigg BM. Altering muscle activity in the lower extremities by running with different shoes. *Medicine & Science in Sports & Exercise*. 2002;34: 1529–1532.
46. Willy R, Davis I. Kinematic and kinetic comparison of running in standard and minimalist shoes. *Medicine & Science in Sports & Exercise*. 2014;46:318–323.

26 Gait Analysis

Donald Lee Goss, Robert Alan Whitehurst, and Sean N. Martin

CONTENTS

TABLE 26.1
Key Clinical Considerations

1. When analyzing gait, be sure to observe at least two views in order to observe sagittal and frontal plane mechanics.
2. Gait analysis is an adjunct to a thorough subjective and objective physical exam, and gives a perceptive clinician a good idea of what areas of the body warrant additional testing.
3. Due to individual differences in gait, when attempting to identify gait abnormalities it may be more beneficial to focus on asymmetries between limbs as opposed to perceived irregularities that exist within both limbs.
4. Approximately 80% of runners use a rearfoot strike pattern (RFS), but many runners are often unable to accurately describe their foot strike pattern. Be sure to observe runners in order to accurately obtain their running characteristics.
5. Many runners with anterior chronic exertional compartment syndrome, knee pain, and stress fractures have benefited from transitioning from a rearfoot strike pattern to a non-rearfoot strike pattern (NRFS).
6. No well-designed RCTs have demonstrated that NRFS running reduces injury rates.
7. Using a RFS pattern in minimalist or partial minimalist shoes is not recommended due to potentially injurious ground reaction force rates of loading.

26.1 INTRODUCTION AND HISTORY OF GAIT ANALYSIS

Though man has been observing each other for many years, the science behind observing gait and describing gait began in the seventeenth century with many of the early and famous renaissance scholars and scientists contributing to this body of work including Borelli, Newton, and Descartes as only a very few examples (Table 26.1). Much of the mathematical modeling, geometry, and classical mechanics they employed enabled them to describe and represent gait. At that time, the process was labor-intensive, and little, if any, practical clinical applications developed using their methods. The framework that they laid though has allowed modern scientists, physicians, and clinicians to build upon, improve, and develop new methods for analyzing gait. Of special note, Dr. Vern Inman and his student Dr. Jaqueline Perry have pioneered many of the new techniques and ideas behind analyzing gait[51]:

> Amidst the technical accomplishments is the need to preserve the quality of observational gait analysis. This technique remains the first step in the treatment of patients' gait abnormalities. If the physician fails to identify a problem, the therapeutic need will be missed. Physical therapists use their observational skills for treatment planning and evaluation. Orthotists and prosthetists depend on observation to evaluate the functional success of their devices. The concluding principle is that the purpose of gait analysis is to improve the patient's ability to walk. The analytical technique selected should be in balance with the level of need and objectivity.
>
> **Jacquelin Perry**
> *Gait Analysis: Technology and the Clinician*

With advances in technology like computers, cameras, video, force plates, and EMG along with many others, our ability to acquire and analyze data has increased exponentially.[51–53] Whole labs, businesses, and even institutions are devoted to this area of study. This topic is much too exhaustive to go into any depth in this chapter, but some of the basic concepts and tools for analyzing gait and the techniques for observational gait analysis will be discussed and explored in the subsequent pages. This is by no means an exhaustive work on the subject, and additional reading and material can further enlighten the clinician who is inclined to learn more about this subject.

For our purposes, gait will refer to the movement of a human subject over a solid surface using alternating lower extremity movement patterns. While there are almost as many differences in gait as there are people due to the variability and individuality of each person, there are characteristics of gait that are relatively conserved across the spectrum that we would consider "normal," which we will discuss in this chapter.

For the majority of people, gait is an integral part of daily life. Our method of gait allows us to maintain support and posture of the trunk, upper extremities, and head during movement, allows the control of our foot trajectory for safe ground clearance, and both generate and absorb mechanical energy allowing us to propel ourselves forward in space. It is how we get from point A to point B, which depending on our desires and purpose gives us the ability to participate and access many environments and situations.

Clinical Pearl

With the importance of being able to travel under one's own power and the loss of quality of life when that power is reduced or hampered, knowing how to identify a patients's gait impairment will help you to improve patient satisfaction and overall health.

For many, it is foundational to their exercise and health, their method of travel to and from work and school, and a basic component of their recreational activities. A recent study found that the average American adult takes 5117 steps/day.[4] For most people, it is automatic and unconscious. We decide we want to move and we go. How is this accomplished though? What steps are necessary? And when the ability to have normal gait is impaired, can we identify which steps are affected and by so doing further diagnose the potential cause of the impairment? This chapter will more specifically cover some of the basic steps and tips for analyzing gait, discuss the "gait cycle" and "normal" walking gait, and discuss the phases of running and the differences found between some of the different running styles.

26.2 PRACTICAL TIPS FOR ANALYZING GAIT

A gait assessment should first begin with static observation of the patient. Ideally, the patient should be in athletic clothing with feet and knees exposed. In order to determine if your patient possesses the necessary mobility and stability for normal gait, you may want to screen the patient's lower extremity range of motion (ROM) and strength for adequate hip flexion/extension, knee flexion/extension, and ankle dorsiflexion/plantar flexion. The Thomas test is useful for assessing the flexibility of the hip flexors.[3] The hamstring 90/90 test is a good test for checking hamstring flexibility.[23] Finally, the weight-bearing dorsiflexion test is useful for assessing dorsiflexion ROM.[35]

Next, a quick standing assessment can give you an idea if the patient has excessive genu valgum or varum and/or pes planus or pes cavus.[30] These static postures have been associated with increased incidence of lower extremity injuries.[41]

Another quick standing assessment is to ask the patient to stand on one leg. A positive Trendelenburg sign (when the nonstance hip drops below the stance hip) is indicative of hip abductor weakness on the stance leg. Hip abductor, hip extensor, and hip external rotation weaknesses have been linked to lower extremity injuries.[47–49]

Clinical Pearl

Just as "one view is no view" when looking at radiographs, the same goes for gait analysis.

Whether assessing static posture or active gait, it is imperative to observe from multiple angles.

If a patient is walking overground, have them walk several times and try to observe them from the front, rear, and at least one side. If your patient is walking or running on a treadmill, try to observe them from the front, back, and at least one side (Figure 26.1).

Observing a patient from the side enables you to observe their sagittal plane motion of foot strike, hip ROM, knee ROM, ankle ROM, and the amount of vertical displacement of their center of mass (also known as bouncing or pistoning). A view from the front allows you to see if the patient's feet are toeing in or out excessively. From the front, you can also appreciate the amount of knee valgus or varus, hip abduction/adduction or rotation, and any excessive trunk or upper extremity transverse plane rotation. From the rear view, it is easy to assess the patient's degree of foot and ankle pronation/supination, frontal plane knee motion, and frontal plane hip motion.

As the patient is walking or running, listen for the audible sound of foot strikes. Loud audible foot strikes are associated with greater vertical ground reaction force rates of loading. These greater rates of loading have been linked to stress fractures, plantar fasciitis, and patellofemoral pain syndrome (PFPS).[11,46,58,60]

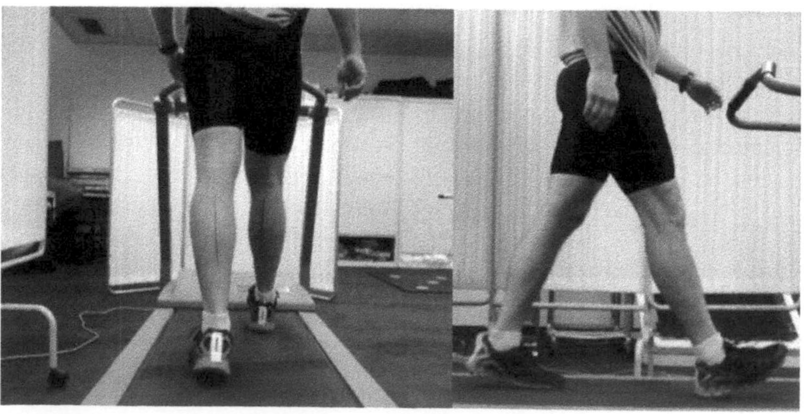

FIGURE 26.1 Anterior and lateral views of treadmill walking.

Adequate runway distance must be a consideration. Having a patient walk inside your examination room is less than ideal. Preferably, take the patient out into the hallway or into a larger open area where you can observe greater than three steps and they can walk at their preferred walking speed. The human eye is fairly good at observing walking gait without assistance. However, the speed of running movement makes it difficult to assess overground or on a treadmill without assistance of some sort of video. Video assessment is also helpful to provide immediate feedback for patients. When considering using video assessment overground, it is helpful to have the camera mounted in a stationary position.

Historically, most cameras, smartphones, and tablets have come with a video camera sampling at 30 frames per second (fps). Recently, more cameras and smartphones have been capable of sampling frequencies of 120–240 fps. These greater sampling frequencies are very helpful when you want to use slow-motion assessment. If you are using your smartphone, you can give the patient immediate feedback after the gait trial. Keep in mind if you are using a camera that there may be a delay to upload video to a computer for viewing. There are many free applications available that the authors have found to be helpful in replaying video in slow motion, measuring angles, and drawing lines on video to aid in patient education. For basic clinical evaluation purposes, it is not necessary to purchase expensive software that is used more in competitive sports and research applications. As the technology of hardware and software continues to improve, video gait analysis should only continue to get easier.

Some final considerations of treadmill use versus overground gait analysis uphill and downhill are as follows:

- Treadmill use will likely increase medial/lateral drift.
- Treadmill use will produce shorter step length, increased step cadence, and likely less knee extension at initial contact.[36]
- Uphill walking and running may produce shorter strides, a more anterior foot strike, and a forward trunk lean.
- Downhill walking and running may produce longer strides, a rearfoot strike, greater ground reaction forces, more knee loading, and a posterior trunk lean into extension.

Clinical Pearl

Gait cycle: Starting with initial contact and stance of one limb through swing and back to right before initial contact and stance of the same limb.

26.3 WALKING

In order to better understand the mechanisms, motions, and forces associated with normal gait, we can break down gait into a series of movements described as "phases of gait" within the "gait cycle." The gait cycle is divided into two periods termed stance and swing. Each limb spends roughly 60% of the cycle in stance and 40% in swing. We will look at one limb at a time, and one cycle of gait will be defined as a full cycle of movement of one limb from the beginning of stance through swing to right before the beginning of stance again. Stance is when the foot is in any contact with the ground, and swing is the portion of gait with no contact with the ground of that limb. In normal walking, the limbs alternate between swing and stance so constant contact with the ground is maintained. There are two periods of double limb support stance within one cycle with alternating swing limb support stances in between. There are eight phases of gait, with five phases in the stance period and three phases in the swing period (Figure 26.2).

The first phase of gait in the stance period is "initial contact" or "heel strike." It is when the foot first contacts the ground. While there are many different types of strides, the majority of people while walking will make first contact with the heel or midfoot. In normal gait, the hip is flexed while the knee is extended and the ankle joint maintains a fairly neutral position. When first contact is made, the anterior compartment muscles of the leg are contracting to maintain neutral or slightly dorsiflexed ankle position, and they will eccentrically lower the foot as the rest of the sole of the foot comes into contact with the ground during the "loading response" phase. Those with weak anterior

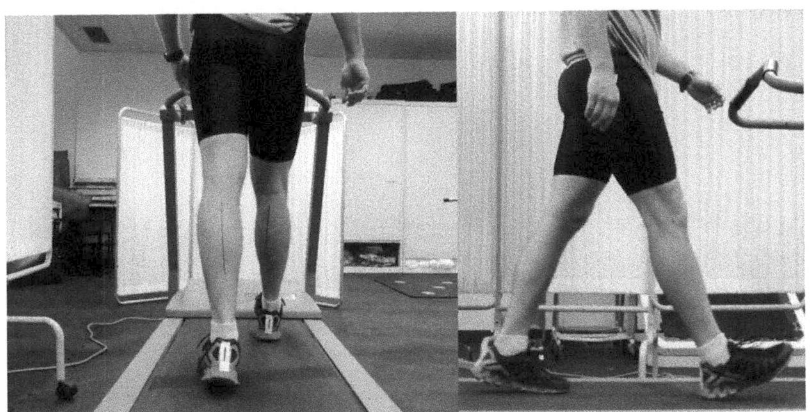

FIGURE 26.2 Walking initial contact.

compartment muscles (tibialis anterior mm, extensor digitorum longus mm, and extensor hallucis longus mm) or nerve damage to the deep fibular nerve will be unable to control the lowering of the foot at the ankle joint, and a characteristic "slap" sound will follow after each initial contact leading to a very quick transition into the next phase of gait. This is frequently termed "foot drop" and is a common finding in many pathological gait patterns. Also, at normal walking speeds, those with an equinus foot will not strike with the heel, and first contact will be made with either the forefoot or midfoot. This is a common gait deviation seen in many neurological conditions like multiple sclerosis, stroke, muscular dystrophy, and Parkinson's disease[1] (Figure 26.3).

Clinical Pearl

Hearing a "slapping" sound after initial contact could be the result of either nerve damage to the anterior fibular nerve or tibialis anterior muscle weakness. Landing on the forefoot instead of the heel during normal walking is usually associated with neurological involvement in adults.

The second phase of gait in stance is termed the "loading response" phase. It is the period of time when the body is in "double stance" and both feet are in contact with the ground until the time that the opposite limb moves into swing phase. The weight of the body is transferred from the opposite leg to the current leg in preparation for that swing. The hip is still flexed, the foot is neutral, but the knee starts to flex as the upper portion of the body continues to move forward in space. The whole foot comes into contact with the ground at this point, the hip extensors are contracting to bring the body forward in space, and the quadriceps are eccentrically contracting while the hamstrings are contracting to maintain the flexed position of the knee joint as the weight of the body is completely transferred to the current limb. During this phase, you want to pay close attention to the foot especially the angle of the hindfoot to the midfoot to the forefoot and observe the arch of the foot. Adult-acquired flatfoot deformity is a pathological condition that presents as pes planus or "flat feet" that may be caused by posterior tibialis tendon insufficiency or ligamentous or capsular weakening.[56] The change in foot positioning can be a source of pain and discomfort and can result in a loss of gait efficiency all through the stance phase of that limb. Pes cavus, which appears as a "high" arch, causes a decrease in the contact surface area of the ground and leads to an increased load on the metatarsal heads when compared to those with more neutral feet.[21] Though neither pes cavus nor pes planus is in and of itself pathological, those who are experiencing new symptoms or whose normal foot structure has changed should be further evaluated to assess whether this finding may be contributing to their symptoms (Figure 26.4).

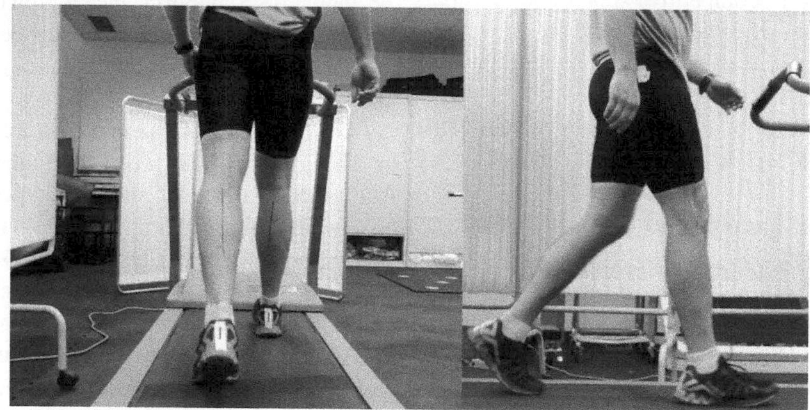

FIGURE 26.3 Walking loading response.

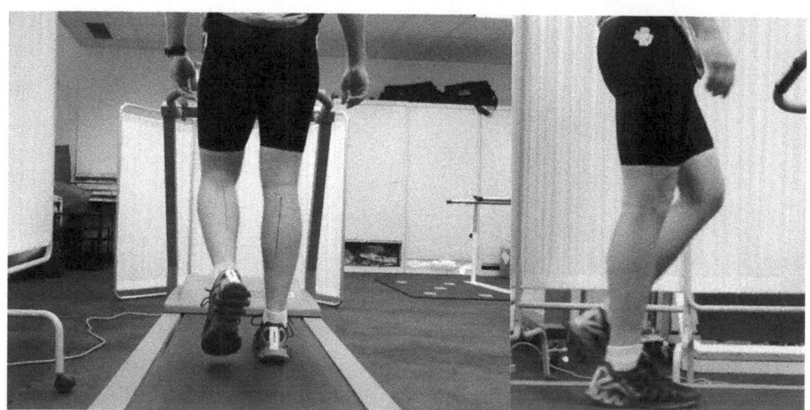

FIGURE 26.4 Walking midstance.

Clinical Pearl

Changes in structure resulting in pes cavus and pes planus can cause abnormal stress to be placed on ligaments, capsules, and muscles and can contribute to changes in gait, loss of metabolic efficiency, and cause pain in various regions.

The third phase of gait is called "midstance" and begins as the opposite foot is lifted, beginning the single limb support interval, and will continue until the center of gravity resides over the forefoot. The hip moves from a state of flexion to slight extension as the knee moves from slight flexion to extension and the foot becomes slightly dorsiflexed. At this point, the weight of the body is maintained solely on the current leg with the majority of the weight and stability being provided by the ligaments and bones with little muscle activity, with the exception of the hip abductors. In order to keep the torso upright, the hip abductors engage and keep the pelvis level in midstance. Those with damage to the gluteus medius or gluteus minimus mm or the superior gluteal nerve can experience a "hip drop" where the opposite pelvis drops down toward the ground during the swing phase of the opposite leg. This is termed a "Trendelenburg's sign" or a "Trendelenburg gait." It can present in two ways, the first being the way that was previously described. There is also a "compensated" Trendelenburg where the person with hip abductor weakness or pain will lean with their trunk to the side of the weak or painful limb during the swing phase of the opposite limb. This enables them to keep their center of mass closer to the stance leg and decrease the moment arm or torque at the hip joint. This test may only be positive, however, with marked weakness of the hip abductors,[34] and a positive test has not yet been fully described or validated.

Clinical Pearl

A common gait deviation is a "Trendelenburg gait" or sign and is characterized by a contralateral drop of the pelvis during the affected limb's stance phase or excessive trunk lean to the side of the affected leg.

The fourth phase of gait is "terminal stance," and it will finish out the single limb (Figure 26.5) support interval. It begins with the heel rising and continues until the initial contact of the opposite foot as it ends the swing portion of the opposite limb. The hip continues to extend, the knee stays predominately extended, and the heel rises while the forefoot maintains contact with the ground. This phase requires the most dorsiflexion of the ankle joint, and those with loss or lack of ROM will compensate by shortening their stride. This is commonly seen after ankle surgery or any time after the ankle/leg has been cast for an extended period of time. It can be caused by ligamentous tightness, scar tissue, or posterior compartment muscle tightness (typically gastrocnemius and/or soleus mm). This can be detected by comparing the step lengths of both limbs, with the involved limb having a decreased length compared to the uninvolved limb. Those who have been hospitalized or wheelchair bound can frequently have bilateral loss of ankle dorsiflexion where a side-to-side comparison is not different, but stride and step length can be compared to the normal table, as well as measuring both active and passive ROMs with a goniometer to detect loss (normal ROM at the ankle is generally 10°–20° depending on extended or flexed knee). Loss of ankle dorsiflexion has also been proposed to increase sheer forces at the knee during landing tasks, increasing the risk of damage to the ACL.[22]

The fifth phase is "preswing" or "toe off." The knee begins to flex, the hip moves from extension to more neutral, and the ankle increases plantar flexion. This phase (Figure 26.6) begins with the opposite limb's initial contact and will continue until toe off. This ends the stance period of gait. It is important to note that the final portion of toe off requires a great deal of toe or hallux extension or dorsiflexion as well as dorsiflexion of the metatarsal phalangeal joint. The plantar fascia on the inferior portion of the foot connects to the big toe and has been described as a "windlass" mechanism that allows for the rigidity of the foot during toe off.[5] The extension of the toe pulls the fascia tight and creates a rigid bar or lever for which the contracting posterior compartment muscles can then use to produce a moment around the ankle joint and metatarsal phalangeal joints aiding in propelling the body forward. Reduction in force at this phase can lead to substantially shorter stride length and walking speed.[25]

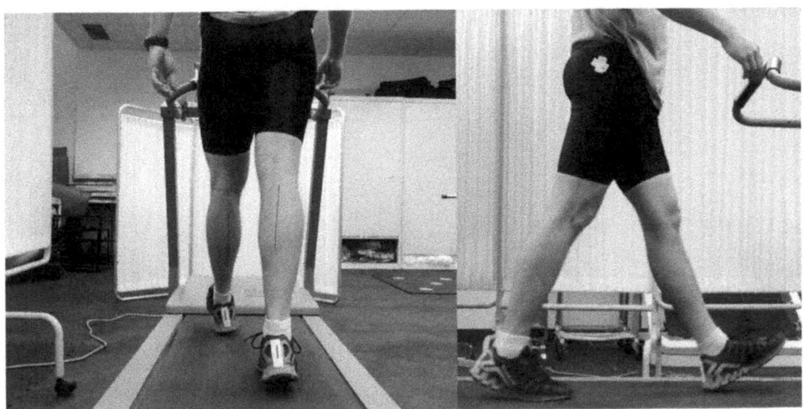

FIGURE 26.5 Walking terminal stance.

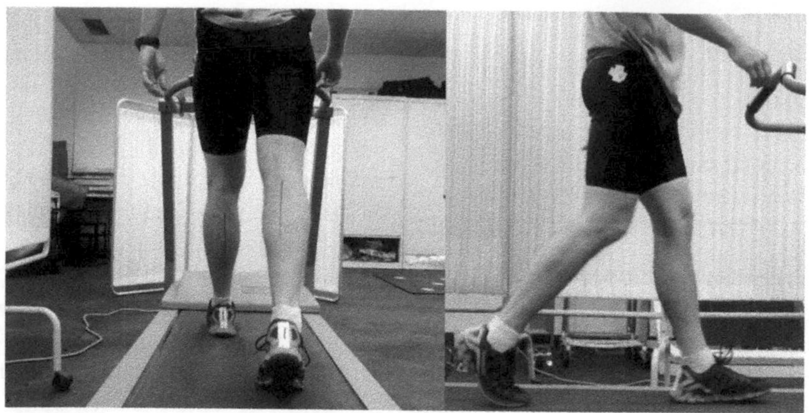

FIGURE 26.6 Walking toe off.

In the sixth phase of gait, the "initial swing" phase, the foot lifts from the floor at the beginning, swings forward through space, and ends when the two feet are close in proximity with each other. The knee maintains flexion, the hip moves from neutral to (Figure 26.7) slightly flexed, and the ankle is transitioning from plantar flexion to neutral. In order to clear the ground, the hip flexes forward causing flexion at the knee so that the neutral foot can clear the ground. In those with foot drop or hip flexor weakness, compensations are commonly seen with either "hip hiking" an exaggerated elevation of the pelvis on the involved side or lateral circumduction at the hip causing the foot to move in an arc away from the body during the swing phase, as strategies for clearing the foot.

Phase seven is "midswing" and continues the forward progress of the foot and ends when the tibia is roughly perpendicular to the floor. The hip is flexing, the knee is flexed from the momentum of the hip, and the ankle maintains a neutral position. This is the phase in which the foot must clear the floor, else the foot will catch and the cycle will be terminated early as the person attempts to "catch" themselves as momentum and balance are unexpectedly changed. Lack of hip strength, knee flexion, or lack of dorsiflexion can all cause a lowered foot. Less tibialis anterior muscle activation is needed to maintain neutral or dorsiflexion of the ankle during midswing than after initial contact, so it is not uncommon to be able to clear the foot yet still hear the characteristic foot slap of someone with a weak or impaired tibialis anterior muscle (Figure 26.8).

The final phase, the eighth, of gait is "terminal swing" (Figure 26.9). The hip ends its flexion and the knee continues the travel of the foot by fully extending. The foot travels forward with the ankle either neutral or slightly dorsiflexed and the phase ends with initial contact. During this phase, the hamstrings are eccentrically contracting to slow down the rapid extension of the knee as it moves from a maximally flexed to fully extended position as it transitions through swing phase and along with hip positioning allows for proper foot placement (see Table 26.1).

Typically, the purpose of human gait is to produce locomotion while maintaining balance. Stride length and cycle time determine the speed of gait and influence front to back balance, while the walking base influences side-to-side balance. Stride is the distance between the back of the foot at the beginning and end of one gait cycle. Cadence is strides per unit of time. The time spent on one limb versus the other is usually equal in the normal population. In those with pain in one limb, a shortened stance phase of that limb will be seen, decreasing the travel distance of the good limb and resulting in what is often described as a "limp" in their gait as they spend as short a time as possible on the bad limb.

Being able to identify and understand "normal" gait is the first step in being able to identify pathological or abnormal gait.

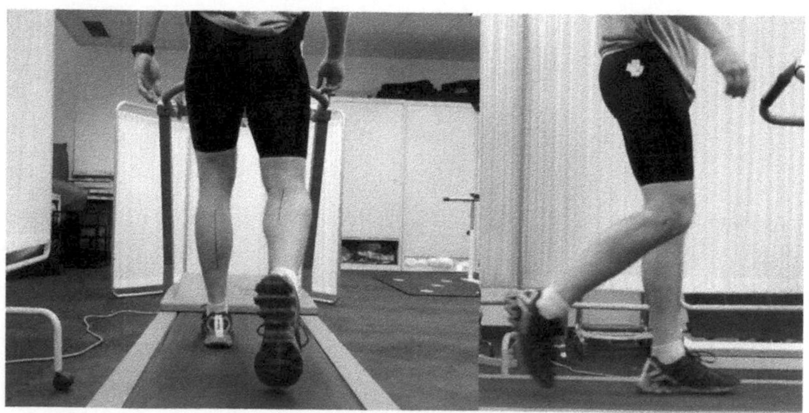

FIGURE 26.7 Walking initial swing.

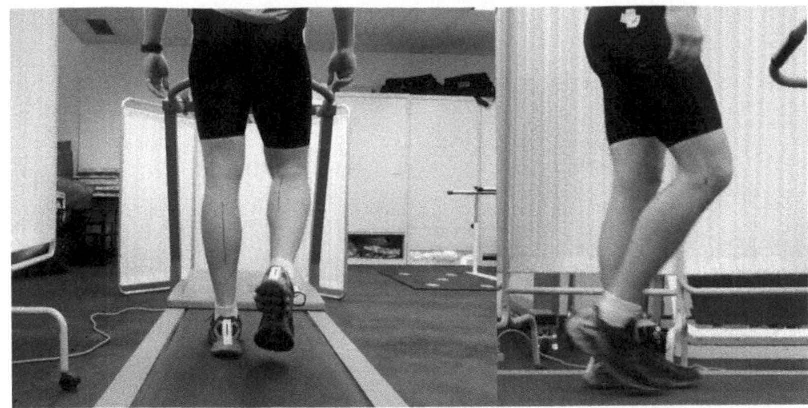

FIGURE 26.8 Walking midswing.

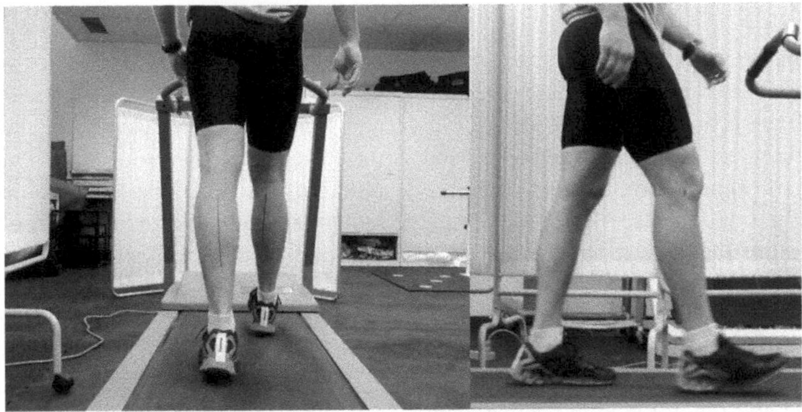

FIGURE 26.9 Walking terminal swing.

Identifying the impairment seen and being able to hypothesize the likely underlying cause is only the first step and allows the clinician to tailor the rest of the exam to better tease out the cause of the abnormality. With both the myriad number of abnormalities and the same presentation from many different causes, an observational gait analysis is almost never enough to positively identify the underlying pathology. Some normal values for many of the parameters discussed in this section have been provided, with the caution that much variability can exist in a completely normal patient and different methods of measuring (measurement tools, landmarks, etc.) can give false positives (see Tables 26.2 through 26.4, Figure 26.10).

TABLE 26.2
Range of Motion in Degrees at Ankle, Knee, and Hip Joint during Different Phases of Gait at Self-Selected Normal Speed (n = 10)

	Ankle	Knee	Hip
Initial contact	0 DF	5 flex	20 flex
Loading response	3 PF	10 flex	15 flex
Midstance	10 DF	10 flex	0 flex
Late stance	17 DF	5 flex	15 ext
Toe off	0 DF	35 flex	12 ext
Preswing	5 PF	55 flex	5 ext
Midswing	5 DF	58 flex	15 flex
Terminal swing	7 DF	10 flex	17 flex

Source: Adapted from Nymark, J.R. et al., *J. Rehabil. Res. Dev.*, 42(4), 523, 2005.

26.4 RUNNING

What makes running different from walking? With walking, one foot is always in contact with the ground and there is a 20% overlap period of double limb stance. With running,

TABLE 26.3
Walking Mean Range of Motion in Degrees at Ankle, Knee, and Hip Overground and on Treadmill at Normal Self-Selected Speed (n = 10)

	Ankle	Knee	Hip	Trunk
Overground	28.3 ± 5.0	64 ± 4.8	38.2 ± 6.4	10.9 ± 2.4
Treadmill	30.9 ± 5.7	61 ± 10	38.3 ± 6.2	10.9 ± 3.1

Source: Adapted from Nymark, J.R. et al., *J. Rehabil. Res. Dev.*, 42(4), 523, 2005.

TABLE 26.4
Normal Gait Speed in Normal Subjects by Male and Female Age Groups from 10 to 79 Years Old

Males				Females			
Age Range (Years)	N	Mean (m/s)	95% C.I. (m/s)	Age Range (Years)	N	Mean(m/s)	95% C.I. (m/s)
10–14	12	1.32	1.20–1.45	10–14	12	1.09	1.02–1.16
15–19	15	1.35	1.28–1.43	15–19	15	1.24	1.14–1.34
20–29	15	1.23	1.17–1.29	20–29	15	1.24	1.15–1.33
30–39	15	1.32	1.24–1.40	30–39	15	1.28	1.18–1.39
40–49	15	1.33	1.28–1.38	40–49	15	1.24	1.17–1.33
50–59	15	1.25	1.16–1.35	50–59	15	1.11	1.02–1.16
60–69	15	1.28	1.21–1.34	60–69	15	1.16	1.07–1.25
70–79	14	1.18	1.10–1.27	70–79	15	1.11	1.05–1.18

Source: Adapted from Oberg, T. et al., *J. Rehabil. Res. Dev.*, 30(2), 210, 1993.

only one foot is ever in contact with the ground, and there is approximately a 20% period of float or flight phase when neither foot is in contact with the ground (Figure 26.11).

Generally, the greater the speed, the longer the float period. Approximately 75%–87% of runners use a rearfoot-strike pattern with the heel making initial contact[31,32,37] (Figure 26.12). Most runners will also demonstrate a more narrow step width than walkers.

Running requires greater ROM and greater eccentric muscle activity than walking to attenuate the larger ground reaction forces. When runners utilize a rearfoot-strike pattern, the knee is relatively extended and the ankle is in relative dorsiflexion upon initial contact. Normal sagittal plane excursion for the ankle, knee, and hip of a rearfoot-striking runner is depicted in Table 26.5.

Typical rearfoot-striking runners contact the ground with the ankle in neutral or slight dorsiflexion. During stance, the ankle is dorsiflexed as the tibia moves over the foot, and then in later stance, the ankle moves into plantar flexion to enable push-off (see Figures 26.13 and 26.14 and Table 26.6).

The knee is near full extension at initial contact and moves into 90°–120° of flexion during stance, depending on the running speed. Typical recreational runners demonstrate approximately 30° of hip flexion at initial contact and 10° of hip extension at toe off. Overall hip excursion increases with greater running velocity.[43]

26.4.1 Barefoot or Minimalist Shoe Running

Barefoot running and other alternative running styles have gained recent popularity, leaving many health-care providers with questions regarding the safety and appropriateness of these techniques for various running populations. In several publications, habitual barefoot runners exhibited a more anterior midfoot- or forefoot-striking pattern, thereby avoiding heel strike.[37] A growing number of barefoot running advocates, teachers, and websites have provided barefoot running instruction since the 2009 publication of the best-selling book *Born to Run* by Christopher McDougall.[40]

Generally, habituated barefoot or minimalist shoe runners use a nonrearfoot-strike pattern with a shortened stride length and greater stride frequency, and the vertical displacement of the center of mass is reduced. [18,19,37] However, one recent study reported habituated barefoot runners using a rearfoot-strike pattern at a self-selected endurance pace.[32] In this section, we will present differences in running form with the two different foot-strike patterns and highlight the literature supporting each running style.

Clinical Pearl

To date, no well-designed prospective studies have demonstrated that running with a more anterior foot-strike pattern is beneficial to prevent running injuries in the general population.

Runners using a nonrearfoot-strike pattern may contact the ground in slight plantar flexion and then move into the same amount of dorsiflexion in midstance followed by maximum plantar flexion at toe off (see Table 26.7).

The knee may be more flexed at initial contact in a runner using a more anterior foot strike (Figure 26.15).

The lower leg is more vertical and the foot contacts the ground under the knee instead of more anterior to the knee as in a rearfoot-striking runner. Hip ROM is similar between runners using either foot-strike patterns (see Figures 26.16 and 26.17).

26.4.2 Patterns of Muscle Activity

Ankle dorsiflexors are more active initially in heel-striking runners.[16] Greater ankle dorsiflexor activity may be problematic in runners with a history of anterior chronic exertional compartment syndrome. When runners use a more anterior foot-strike pattern, ankle plantarflexors are more

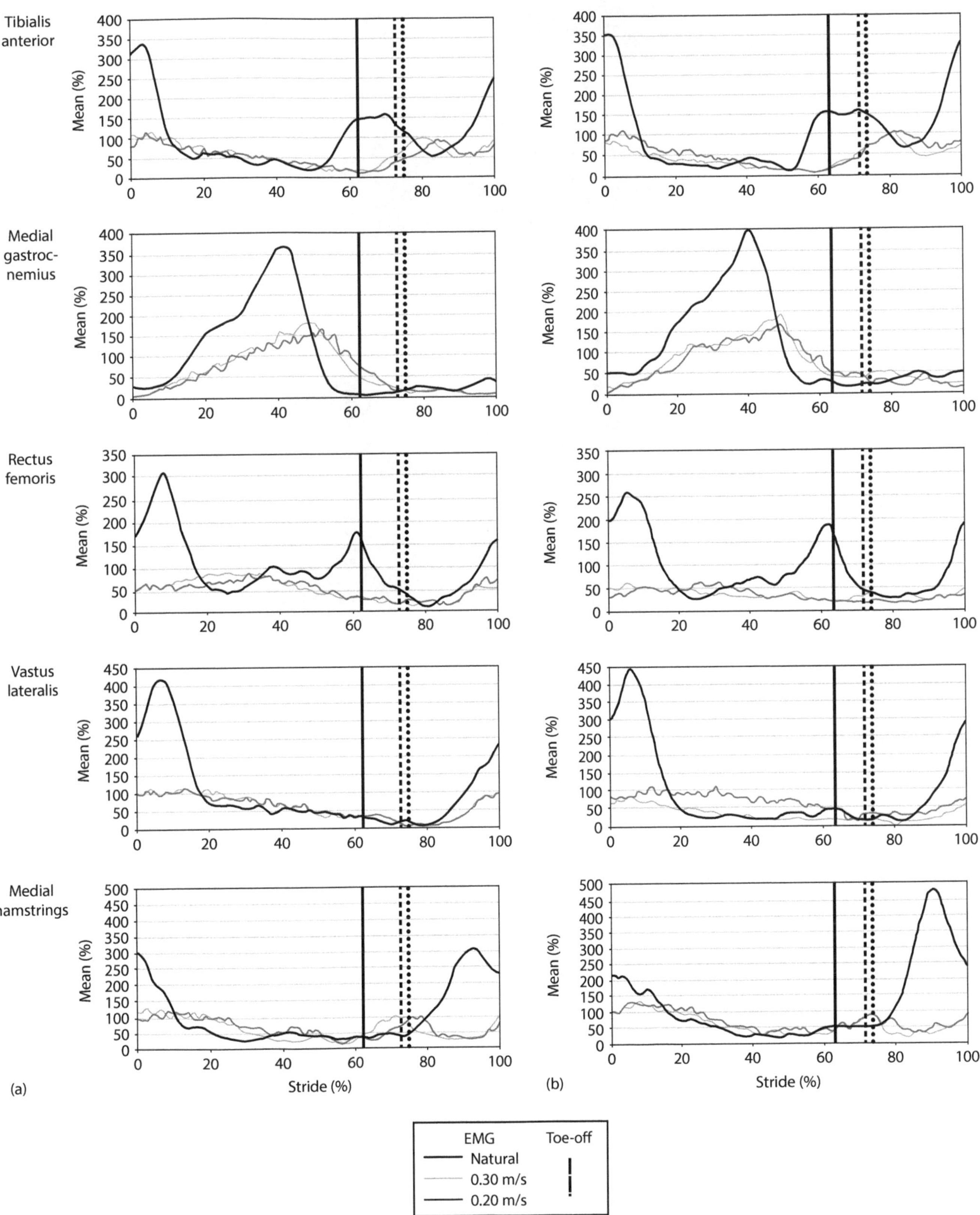

FIGURE 26.10 Ensemble average EMG activity normalized to one gait cycle at three walking speeds (a) overground and (b) treadmill (n = 10). (Reprinted from Nymark, J.R. et al., *J. Rehabil. Res. Dev.*, 42(4), 523, 2005.)

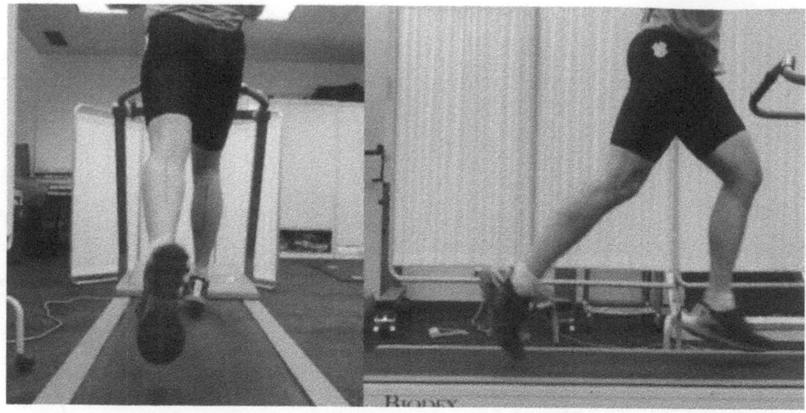

FIGURE 26.11 Running float phase.

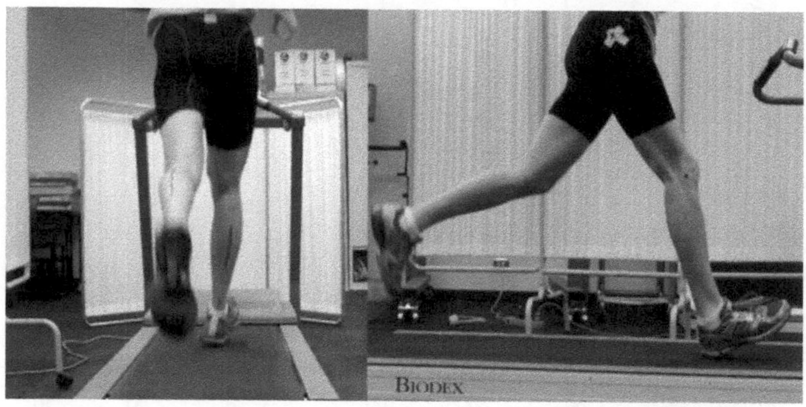

FIGURE 26.12 Rearfoot strike.

TABLE 26.5
Gait Parameter Data from Normal Subjects at Natural Speed (n = 18)

	Overground	Treadmill
Cadence (steps/min)	112.3 ± 9.3	117.8 ± 7.2
Stride length (m)	1.55 ± 0.13	1.47 ± 0.08
Stance (%)	62.1 ± 2.5	63.1 ± 2.4

Source: Adapted from Nymark, J.R. et al., *J. Rehabil. Res. Dev.*, 42(4), 523, 2005.

active at initial contact and perform greater eccentric work to dampen ground reaction forces.[2,26] Consideration should be given to whether this foot-strike pattern is effective for runners with a history of Achilles tendinopathy or gastrocnemius and soleus strains. These runners using an anterior foot strike also spend more time in loading the forefoot, which may be problematic for runners with a history of metatarsal stress fracture or metatarsalgia.[24] Greater eccentric knee extensor work has been observed with runners using a rearfoot-strike pattern due to the greater excursion of the knee from extension into flexion to dampen ground reaction forces.[2,26]

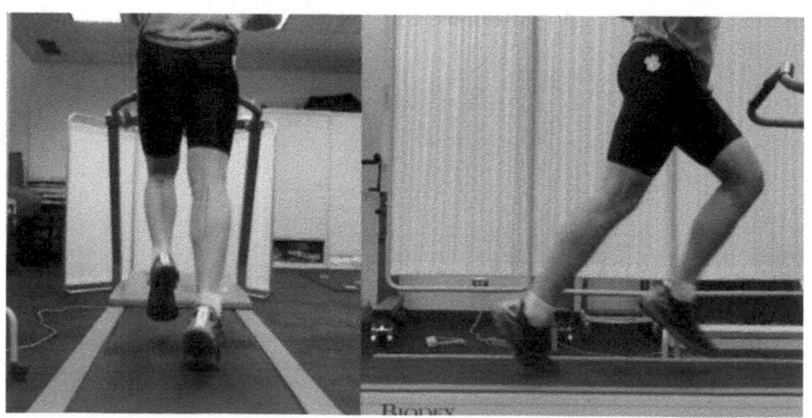

FIGURE 26.13 Running toe off.

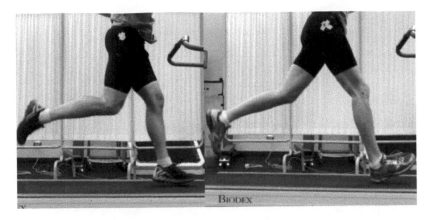

FIGURE 26.14 Running comparison of two foot-strike patterns: midfoot strike on left, rearfoot strike on right.

TABLE 26.6
Running Range of Motion for Rearfoot-Striking Runners

	Ankle	Knee	Hip
Initial contact	0 DF	10 flex	30 flex
Midstance	20 DF	45 flex	0 flex
Toe off	20 PF	10 flex	10 ext

TABLE 26.7
Running Range of Motion for Anterior Foot-Striking Runners

	Ankle	Knee	Hip
Initial contact	5 PF	20 flex	30 flex
Midstance	20 DF	45 flex	0 flex
Toe off	20 PF	10 flex	10 ext

26.4.3 Swing Phase

Muscle activation and ranges of motion are similar in late swing and early to midswing phase between rearfoot strikers and anterior foot strikers. As the ankle moves into plantar flexion at late stance, the plantarflexors are actively pushing off. The ankle dorsiflexors lift the toes, the hamstrings flex the knee, and the hip flexors flex the hip to achieve toe clearance in early swing phase. By midstance, the hip has reached maximum flexion, the quadriceps then prepare to extend the

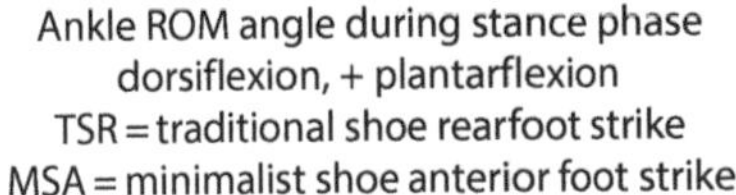

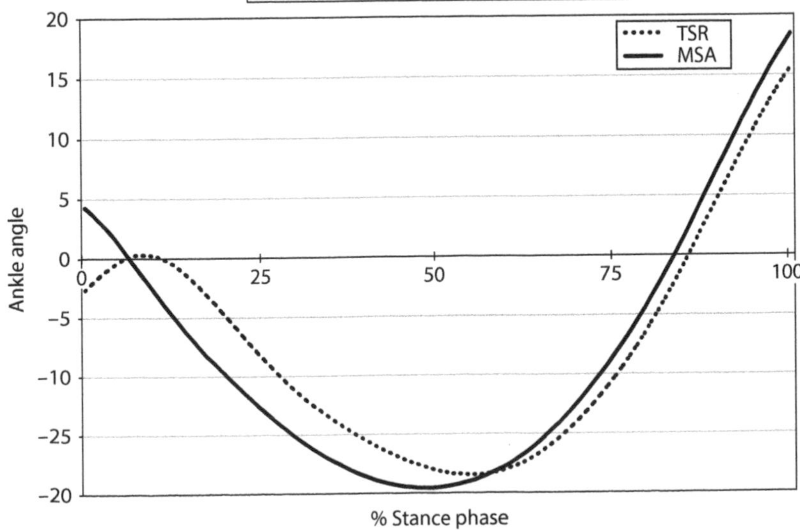

FIGURE 26.15 Ankle range of motion in stance phase for traditionally shod rearfoot strikers and minimalist shoe anterior foot strikers.

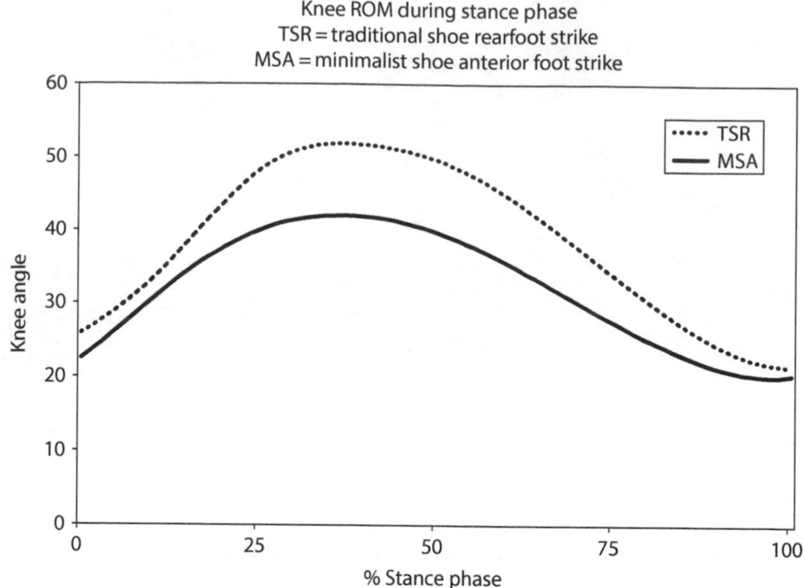

FIGURE 26.16 Knee range of motion in stance phase for traditionally shod rearfoot strikers and minimalist shoe anterior foot strikers.

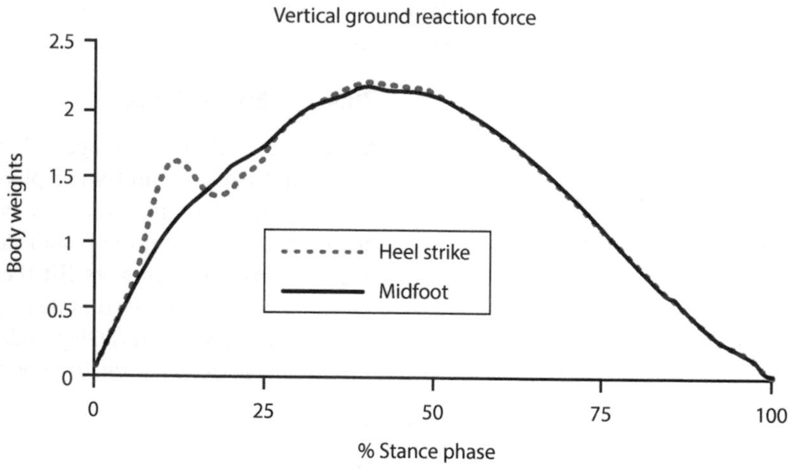

FIGURE 26.17 Vertical ground reaction forces of rearfoot and anterior foot-striking runners.

knee, and the foot prepares for ground contact. In rearfoot-striking runners, the knee is more extended and the ankle is near neutral to slight dorsiflexion (Figure 26.14). Anterior foot striking runners will maintain more knee flexion and activate the plantarflexors in late swing[18] in anticipation to contact the ground with the ankle in slight plantar flexion.

26.4.4 Kinetics

Runners using a rearfoot-strike pattern are likely to produce an impact peak present at approximately 10%–12% of the stance phase on the vertical ground reaction force curve (Figure 26.17).

Clinical Pearl

Typical running peak vertical ground reaction forces are between 1.5 and 3.5 times body weight.

This force is passive in nature and the anterior–posterior component of this impact is generally considered a braking force with the heel strike anterior to the runner's center of mass. The second peak for the vertical ground reaction force occurs between 40% and 50% of the stance phase.[33] This force is more active as the runner pushes off the ground, and the anterior–posterior component is more propulsive in nature with the runner's center of mass superior/anterior to the foot contact. Vertical ground reaction forces increase linearly with increasing running velocity[42] and increasing stride length[13,20,50] and decrease with a faster stride rate or cadence.[9] Runners with a history of injuries may demonstrate greater vertical ground reaction force rates of loading (slope of the vertical ground reaction force curve from approximately 20%–80% of the initial impact peak).[12,46,59,60]

Runners using a rearfoot-strike pattern in bare feet or minimalist footwear have demonstrated greater initial vertical loading rates than shod heel strikers.[14,37] Runners using a rearfoot strike may require greater angular work at the knee[2,26] possibly resulting in greater patellofemoral and tibiofemoral compressive forces and possibly greater risk of knee injury than other running styles with more anterior foot-strike patterns.[2,27,29] Since the knee is the most commonly injured joint in runners,[55] runners with a history of knee injury or osteoarthritis of the knee may benefit from using a running style that avoids a rearfoot-strike pattern.

Most habitual barefoot runners choose to land with a midfoot or forefoot initial foot contact to avoid greater initial loading rates observed with heel striking in bare feet.[15] Using a more anterior foot-strike pattern will likely reduce the vertical ground reaction force rates of loading and eliminate the initial impact peak[26,37] (Figure 26.17). While most runners attempting to run in bare feet or minimalist shoes will convert to a more anterior foot strike, McCarthy et al. reported recently on a sample in which 50% of runners continued to demonstrate a rearfoot-strike pattern 2 weeks after changing to the Vibram FiveFinger shoe.[39] Failing to use a more anterior foot-strike pattern in minimalist running shoes can lead to potentially injurious vertical ground reaction force rates of loading[28,39]). This should be a consideration when you have patients asking you about transitioning to a minimalist shoe. We strongly recommend that they transition to a nonrearfoot-strike pattern in minimalist shoes to avoid these potentially injurious rates of loading. Similar to McCarthy et al. who witnessed that 50% of runners wearing minimalist footwear for 2 weeks were still using a rearfoot-strike pattern,[39] Goss et al. observed that nearly half of all runners wearing minimalist footwear for greater than 6 months still demonstrated a rearfoot-strike pattern.[28]

Clinical Pearl

Not all runners who switch to minimalist footwear will adopt a more anterior foot strike. Do not take your patient's word for it that they have transitioned from a rearfoot to an anterior foot-strike pattern. Watching them run on the treadmill or over ground is strongly recommended to assess their running gait for your own interpretation.

Just as there is no perfect running shoe for everyone, at present, there is little evidence to support recommending a blanket anterior or rearfoot-strike pattern universally for every runner. Prescriptive case studies have demonstrated effectiveness for certain runners with a history of chronic exertional compartment syndrome[17], knee pathology[7], and stress fractures[10] to transition to a more anterior foot-strike pattern. Other authors have reported metatarsal stress fractures in runners switching to minimalist running shoes.[24] The individual patient's past medical history, skeletal alignment, available ROM, and strength should all be evaluated and taken into account when making recommendations on running style selection for patients with a history of lower extremity injury.

Basic locomotion is an important functional capability of human beings. Understanding the components of normal walking and running gait is a helpful tool for any clinician to possess. Being able to assess your patients' gait patterns, to identify asymmetries, and to make recommendations has the potential to genuinely improve their quality of life. A basic understanding of the phases of normal walking and running gait and the evidence supporting different running styles should help a clinician take care of a variety of patient needs. (Table 26.8).

TABLE 26.8
SORT: Key Recommendations for Practice

Clinical Recommendation	Evidence Rating	References
The modified Thomas test has an ICC = 0.92 using a goniometer and an ICC = 0.89 using an inclinometer. Pain with the modified Thomas test with the hip in internal or external rotation (McCarthy sign) has a 92% specificity and 89% sensitivity for labral tears.	C	[6,8]
Tight hamstrings as measured by the hamstring 90/90 test in a population with PFPS had 68% sensitivity and 56% specificity with identifying those likely to benefit from an off-the-shelf foot orthosis.	C	[54]
Weight-bearing dorsiflexion test has a reported ICC = 0.93–0.99, and WBDF measurement immediately after cast removal has low to moderate predictive value on functional measures and outcomes 6 months after cast removal of an ankle fracture.	C	[38]
The Trendelenburg test has a reported 55% sensitivity and 70% specificity in identifying patients with hip osteoarthritis, with an ICC = 0.63–0.69.	C	[57]

REFERENCES

1. Agostini V, Balestra G, Knaflitz M. Segmentation and classification of gait cycles. *IEEE Transactions on Neural Systems and Rehabilitation Engineering: A Publication of the IEEE Engineering in Medicine and Biology Society.* 2013;22(5):946–952.
2. Arendse RE, Noakes TD, Azevedo LB, Romanov N, Schwellnus MP, Fletcher G. Reduced eccentric loading of the knee with the pose running method. *Medicine and Science in Sports and Exercise.* 2004;36(2):272–277.
3. Bartlett MD, Wolf LS, Shurtleff DB, Stahell LT. Hip flexion contractures: A comparison of measurement methods. *Archives of Physical Medicine and Rehabilitation.* 1985;66(9):620–625.
4. Bassett DR, Wyatt HR, Thompson H, Peters JC, Hill JO. Pedometer-measured physical activity and health behaviors in U.S. adults. *Medicine and Science in Sports and Exercise.* 2010;42(10):1819–1825.

5. Bolgla LA, Malone TR. Plantar fasciitis and the windlass mechanism: A biomechanical link to clinical practice. *Journal of Athletic Training*. 2004;39(1):77–82.
6. Burgess RM, Rushton A, Wright C, Daborn C. The validity and accuracy of clinical diagnostic tests used to detect labral pathology of the hip: A Systematic review. *Manual Therapy*. 2011;16(4):318–326.
7. Cheung RT, Davis IS. Landing pattern modification to improve patellofemoral pain in runners: A case series. *The Journal of Orthopaedic and Sports Physical Therapy*. 2011;41(12):914–919.
8. Clapis PA, Davis SM, Davis RO. Reliability of inclinometer and goniometric measurements of hip extension flexibility using the modified Thomas test. *Physiotherapy Theory and Practice*. 2008;24(2):135–141.
9. Clarke TE, Cooper LB, Hamill CL, Clark DE. The effect of varied stride rate upon shank deceleration in running. *Journal of Sports Sciences*. 1985;3(1):41–49.
10. Crowell HP, Davis IS. Gait retraining to reduce lower extremity loading in runners. *Clinical Biomechanics (Bristol, Avon)*. 2011; 26(1):78–83.
11. Davis IM. Do impacts cause running injuries? A prospective investigation; 2010a. Presented at the *American College of Sports Medicine Annual Meeting*, Baltimore, MD, May 2010.
12. Davis IM. Vertical impact loading in runners with a history of patellofemoral pain syndrome; 2010b. Presented at the *American College of Sports Medicine Annual Meeting*, Baltimore, MD, May 2010.
13. Derrick TR, Hamill J, Caldwell GE. Energy absorption of impacts during running at various stride lengths. *Medicine and Science in Sports and Exercise*. 1998;30 (1):128–135.
14. De Wit B, De Clercq D, Aerts P. Biomechanical analysis of the stance phase during barefoot and shod running. *Journal of Biomechanics*. 2000;33(3):269–278.
15. De Witt B, De Clercq D. Timing of lower extremity motions during barefoot and shod running at three velocities. (Cinetique Des Mouvements Des Membres Inferieurs Lors de La Course a Trois Vitesses, Pieds Nus Ou Avec Chaussures.) *Journal of Applied Biomechanics*. 2000;16(2):169–179.
16. Diebal AR, Gregory R, Alitz C, Gerber JP. Effects of forefoot running on chronic exertional compartment syndrome: A case series. *International Journal of Sports Physical Therapy*. 2011;6(4):312–321.
17. Diebal AR, Gregory R, Alitz C, Gerber JP. Forefoot running improves pain and disability associated with chronic exertional compartment syndrome. *The American Journal of Sports Medicine*. 2012;40(5):1060–1067.
18. Divert C, Mornieux G, Baur H, Mayer F, Belli A. Mechanical comparison of barefoot and shod running. *International Journal of Sports Medicine*. 2005;26(7):593–598.
19. Divert C, Mornieux G, Freychat P, Baly L, Mayer F, Belli A. Barefoot-Shod Running Differences: Shoe or Mass Effect? *International Journal of Sports Medicine*. 2008;29(6):512–518.
20. Edwards WB, Taylor D, Rudolphi TJ, Gillette JC, Derrick TR. Effects of stride length and running mileage on a probabilistic stress fracture model. *Medicine and Science in Sports and Exercise*. 2009;41(12):2177–2184.
21. Fernández-Seguín LM, Mancha JAD, Rodríguez RS, Martínez EE, Martín BG, Ortega JR. Comparison of plantar pressures and contact area between normal and cavus foot. *Gait and Posture*. 2014;39(2):789–792.
22. Fong C-M, Blackburn JT, Norcross MF, McGrath M, Padua DA. Ankle-Dorsiflexion Range of Motion and Landing Biomechanics. *J Athl Train*. 2011;46(1):5-10.
23. Gajdosik RL, Rieck MA, Sullivan DK, Wightman SE. Comparison of four clinical tests for assessing hamstring muscle length. *The Journal of Orthopaedic and Sports Physical Therapy*. 1993;18(5):614–618.
24. Giuliani J, Masini B, Alitz C, Owens BD. Barefoot-simulating footwear associated with metatarsal stress injury in 2 runners. *Orthopedics*. 2011;34(7):e320–e23.
25. Goldmann J-P, Brüggemann G-P. The potential of human toe flexor muscles to produce force. *Journal of Anatomy*. 2012;221(2):187–194.
26. Goss DL, Gross MT. A comparison of negative joint work and vertical ground reaction force loading rates between chi runners and rearfoot striking runners. *The Journal of Orthopaedic and Sports Physical Therapy*. 2013;43(10):685–692.
27. Goss DL, Gross MT. Relationships among self-reported shoe type, foot strike patterns, and injury incidence. *US Army Medical Department Journal*. 2012a;25–30.
28. Goss DL, Lewek MD, Yu B, Ware WB, Teyhen DS, Gross MT. 2015. Lower Extremity Biomechanics and Self-Reported Foot-Strike Patterns Among Runners in Traditional and Minimalist Shoes. J Ath Train. 50(6):603–611.
29. Goss DL, Yu B, Lewek MD, Ware WB, Teyhen DS, Gross MT. A comparison of lower extremity joint work and initial loading rates among four different running styles. Dissertation, Chapel Hill, NC: University of North Carolina; 2012b.
30. Gross MT. Lower quarter screening for skeletal malalignment—Suggestions for orthotics and shoewear. *The Journal of Orthopaedic and Sports Physical Therapy*. 1995; 21(6):389–405.
31. Hasegawa H, Yamauchi T, Kraemer WJ. Foot strike patterns of runners at the 15 km point during an elite-level half marathon. *The Journal of Strength and Conditioning Research*. 2007;21(3):888–893.
32. Hatala KG, Dingwall HL, Wunderlich RE, Richmond BG. Variation in foot strike patterns during running among habitually barefoot populations. *PLoS One*. 2013;8(1):e52548.
33. Hreljac A. Impact and overuse injuries in runners. *Medicine and Science in Sports and Exercise*. 2004;36(5):845–849.
34. Kendall KD, Patel C, Wiley JP, Pohl MB, Emery CA, Ferber R. Steps toward the validation of the trendelenburg test: The effect of experimentally reduced hip abductor muscle function on frontal plane mechanics. *Clinical Journal of Sport Medicine*. 2013;23(1):45–51.
35. Konor MM, Morton S, Eckerson JM, Grindstaff TL. Reliability of three measures of ankle dorsiflexion range of motion. *International Journal of Sports Physical Therapy*. 2012;7(3):279–287.
36. Lee SJ, Hidler J. Biomechanics of overground vs. treadmill walking in healthy individuals. *Journal of Applied Physiology (Bethesda, MD, 1985)*. 2008;104(3):747–755.
37. Lieberman DE, Venkadesan M, Werbel WA, Daoud AI, D'Andrea S, Davis IS, Mang'eni RO, Pitsiladis Y. Foot strike patterns and collision forces in habitually barefoot versus shod runners. *Nature*. 2010;463(7280):531–535.
38. Mark H, Herbert R, Stewart M. Prediction of outcome after ankle fracture. *Journal of Orthopaedic and Sports Physical Therapy*. 2005;35(12):786–792.
39. McCarthy C, Porcari JP, Kernozek T et al. Like barefoot, only better. *ACE Certified News*. 2011; 8–12.
40. McDougall C. 2009. *Born to Run*. New York: Alfred A. Knopf.

41. Messier SP, Legault C, Schoenlank CR et al. Risk factors and mechanisms of knee injury in runners. *Medicine and Science in Sports and Exercise*. 2008;40(11):1873–1879.
42. Nigg BM, Bahlsen HA, Luethi SM et al. The influence of running velocity and midsole hardness on external impact forces in heel-toe running. *Journal of Biomechanics*. 1987;20(10): 951–959.
43. Novacheck. The biomechanics of running. *Gait and Posture* 1998;7(1):77–95.
44. Nymark JR, Balmer SJ, Melis EH et al. Electromyographic and kinematic nondisabled gait differences at extremely slow overground and treadmill walking speeds. *Journal of Rehabilitation Research & Development*. 2005;42(4):523–534.
45. Oberg T, Karsznia A, Oberg K. Basic gait parameters: reference data for normal subjects, 10–79 years of age. *Journal of Rehabilitation Research & Development*. 1993;30(2):210–223.
46. Pohl MB, Hamill J, Davis IS. Biomechanical and anatomic factors associated with a history of plantar fasciitis in female runners. *Clinical Journal of Sport Medicine*. 2009;19(5):372–376.
47. Powers CM. The influence of abnormal hip mechanics on knee injury: A biomechanical perspective. *The Journal of Orthopaedic and Sports Physical Therapy*. 2010;40(2):42–51.
48. Souza RB, Powers CM. Differences in hip kinematics, muscle strength, and muscle activation between subjects with and without patellofemoral pain. *The Journal of Orthopaedic and Sports Physical Therapy*. 2009a;39(1):12–19.
49. Souza RB, Powers CM. Predictors of hip internal rotation during running: An evaluation of hip strength and femoral structure in women with and without patellofemoral pain. *The American Journal of Sports Medicine*. 2009b;37(3):579–587.
50. Stergiou N, Bates BT, Kurz MJ. Subtalar and knee joint interaction during running at various stride lengths. *The Journal of Sports Medicine and Physical Fitness*. 2003;43(3): 319–326.
51. Sutherland DH. The evolution of clinical gait analysis part I: Kinesiological EMG. *Gait and Posture*. 2001;14(1):61–70.
52. Sutherland DH. The evolution of clinical gait analysis part II: Kinematics. *Gait and Posture*. 2002;16(2):159–179.
53. Sutherland DH. The evolution of clinical gait analysis part III: Kinetics and energy assessment. *Gait and Posture*. 2005;21(4):447–461.
54. Sutlive TG, Mitchell SD, Maxfield SN et al. Identification of Individuals with Patellofemoral Pain Whose Symptoms Improved after a Combined Program of Foot Orthosis Use and Modified Activity: A Preliminary Investigation. *Physical Therapy*. 2004;84(1):49–61.
55. Van Gent RN, Siem D, van Middelkoop M et al. Incidence and determinants of lower extremity running injuries in long distance runners: A systematic review. *British Journal of Sports Medicine*. 2007;41(8):469–480; discussion 480.
56. Vulcano E, Deland JT, Ellis SJ. Approach and treatment of the adult acquired flatfoot deformity. *Current Reviews in Musculoskeletal Medicine*. 2013;6(4):294–303.
57. Youdas JW, Madson TJ, Hollman JH. Usefulness of the trendelenburg test for identification of patients with hip joint osteoarthritis. *Physiotherapy Theory and Practice*. 2010;26(3):184–194.
58. Zadpoor AA, Nikooyan AA. The relationship between lower-extremity stress fractures and the ground reaction force: A systematic review. *Clinical Biomechanics (Bristol, Avon)*. 2011;26(1):23–28.
59. Zifchock RA, Davis I, Hamill J. Kinetic asymmetry in female runners with and without retrospective tibial stress fractures. *Journal of Biomechanics*. 2006;39(15):2792–2797.
60. Zifchock RA, Davis I, Higginson J et al. Side-to-side differences in overuse running injury susceptibility: A retrospective study. *Human Movement Science*. 2008;27(6):888–902.

27 Maximal Aerobic Capacity

Selasi Attipoe and Patricia A. Deuster

CONTENTS

TABLE 27.1
Key Clinical Considerations

1. Maximal aerobic capacity is an important health measure because it serves as a criterion for assessing cardiorespiratory (or cardiopulmonary) fitness.
2. The gold standard for measuring maximal aerobic capacity is progressive treadmill exercise testing to exhaustion while directly measuring expired gases.
3. The current criteria for documenting attainment of VO_{2max} while directly measuring expired gases are the primary measure of a plateau in VO_2 and/or the secondary measures of blood (or plasma) lactate, RER, heart rate, and perceived exertion.
4. Maximal aerobic capacity can be estimated using maximal or submaximal exercise testing protocols. Submaximal exercise testing protocols reduce risk, testing time, and costs associated with maximal effort exercise tests.
5. Maximal aerobic capacity can also be predicted using nonexercise prediction tests that can be conducted in clinical, commercial, and/or outdoor settings.

27.1 INTRODUCTION

Maximal aerobic capacity (or maximal oxygen uptake [VO_{2max}]) is the greatest amount of oxygen a person can utilize during physical exercise. It is an important health measure because it serves as a criterion for assessing cardiorespiratory (or cardiopulmonary) fitness.[11,30,31,89] Low levels of cardiorespiratory fitness are associated with an increased risk of all-cause mortality, whereas high levels are associated with higher levels of habitual physical activity, which is associated with many health benefits.[73] The measurement of maximal aerobic capacity serves multiple roles: it is a useful measurement for characterizing the functional capacity of the oxygen transport system, serves as an index of maximal cardiovascular and pulmonary function, and significantly reflects endurance performance. The objectives of this chapter are to (1) present important concepts associated with maximal aerobic capacity, (2) provide an overview of measuring and estimating maximal oxygen uptake, and (3) outline expectations of healthcare personnel supervising exercise tests. See Table 27.1 for a summary of key clinical considerations.

27.2 EXPECTED VALUES FOR MAXIMAL AEROBIC CAPACITY

By definition, maximal aerobic power is the highest oxygen intake (VO_{2max}) a person can achieve during exercise and is bounded by the parametric limits of the Fick equation (stroke volume × heart rate × [arterial oxygen − venous oxygen]). Consequently, the absolute value of VO_{2max}, typically expressed in liters per minute ($L{\cdot}min^{-1}$), characterizes cardiovascular function because it highly correlates with cardiac output.[3,58] Absolute values may range from as low as 1.0 $L{\cdot}min^{-1}$ (or lower with cardiovascular disease) to as high as 6 $L{\cdot}min^{-1}$ (or even higher in large, well-trained individuals). Because two individuals of different body weights can have the same absolute values, VO_{2max} is usually normalized for body weights (and expressed as $mL{\cdot}kg^{-1}{\cdot}min^{-1}$) to allow for comparisons between and among different persons. For example, if two men have absolute values of 4.2 $L{\cdot}min^{-1}$, but one weighs 70 kg and the other 95 kg, then their VO_{2max} values normalized for body weight would be 60 $mL{\cdot}kg^{-1}{\cdot}min^{-1}$ for the 70 kg man and 44.2 $mL{\cdot}kg^{-1}{\cdot}min^{-1}$ for the 95 kg man. This relative VO_{2max} provides an indication of an individual's potential for work—particularly tasks that involve running and climbing—and overall endurance. So, the man who weighs only 70 kg is in better shape for physical work because his relative effort at a work level demanding an oxygen intake (VO_2) of 40 $mL{\cdot}min^{-1}$ would only be 66% of his VO_{2max}, whereas the 95 kg man would be operating at 90% of his VO_{2max}. Table 27.2 presents normative data by age and gender from the Cooper Institute; this allows VO_{2max} values to be compared and interpreted in light of the general population.

TABLE 27.2
Normative Maximal Aerobic Capacity (VO_{2max}) Ranges in $mL \cdot kg^{-1} \cdot min^{-1}$ for Men and Women by Age[a]

Age	Poor	Fair	Good	Excellent	Superior
			Men		
20–29	≤41.3	41.4–45.2	45.3–49.8	49.9–54.7	≥54.8
30–39	≤40.1	40.2–44.0	44.1–47.6	47.7–52.9	≥53.0
40–49	≤38.0	38.1–41.7	41.8–45.6	45.7–51.1	≥51.2
50–59	≤35.1	35.2–38.5	38.6–42.5	42.6–47.9	≥48.8
60–69	≤31.9	32.0–35.2	35.3–38.9	39.0–44.2	≥44.3
70–79	≤28.9	29.0–32.0	32.1–35.9	36.0–41.7	≥41.8
			Women		
20–29	≤35.6	36.7–39.0	39.1–43.1	43.2–48.2	≥48.3
30–39	≤34.0	34.1–37.3	37.4–41.7	41.8–46.3	≥46.4
40–49	≤32.5	32.6–35.5	35.6–39.1	39.2–44.2	≥44.3
50–59	≤29.6	29.7–32.4	32.5–35.9	36.0–39.9	≥40.0
60–69	≤26.9	27.0–29.5	29.6–32.5	32.6–36.8	≥36.9
70–79	≤25.6	25.7–28.0	28.1–30.2	30.3–35.0	≥35.1

[a] Modified based on percentile values from *ACSM's Guidelines for Exercise Testing*, 9th edn. Data originally acquired from the Cooper Institute, Dallas, TX.[73]

Clinical Pearl

Maximal aerobic power in absolute values can be used to characterize cardiovascular function because it highly correlates with cardiac output.

27.3 FACTORS AFFECTING MAXIMAL AEROBIC CAPACITY

An individual's VO_{2max} depends on a variety of factors, both intrinsic (e.g., genetics, age, gender, body composition, skeletal muscle characteristics, heart structure and function) and extrinsic (e.g., medications, activity levels, nutritional status, presence of disease, environmental conditions) factors.

Genetics is a dominant intrinsic factor in determining VO_{2max} and can account for 25%–70% of an individual's inherent VO_{2max}.[3,15] However, many other factors—including age, gender, heart structure and function, and properties of skeletal muscle—are also important intrinsic factors.[15] For instance, age is inversely related to VO_{2max}, with VO_{2max} declining at approximately 10% per decade in the absence of regular activity.[41] Also, women tend to have lower VO_{2max} levels than men; values are approximately 15% lower even when matched by activity status. Body composition—in particular, lean muscle mass—is another important factor.[32,40,60,79,86] In fact, the age- and gender-related differences in maximal values can largely be accounted for by differences in body composition. Typical values for men are 25%–50% higher than values for women whether in absolute terms or relative to body weight. However, if the absolute values are normalized for lean body mass instead of total body weight, the differences between men and women are minimal.[79]

The primary extrinsic factor influencing VO_{2max} is physical activity. Training alone can improve[15] and inactivity can markedly compromise VO_{2max}.[20] Whereas exercise training can increase the VO_{2max} of sedentary individuals by 25% over several months,[15] physical inactivity, as characterized by bed rest, can decrease VO_{2max} by as much as 26% after only 21 days.[20] Typically, the magnitudes of increase and decrease are related to the duration of activity/inactivity, initial fitness, and health. Those with higher initial fitness levels appear to decline more than those who are less fit when confined to bed rest over a comparable period.[20] Age-related declines in aerobic fitness can largely be attributed to reduced physical activity.[41] Although other factors affect VO_{2max} (e.g., environmental extremes of altitude, heat, cold, and air pollution, disease processes, nutritional status, and sleep habits),[3,84] participation in physical activity is the best way to improve VO_{2max}.[54] Unfortunately, physical fitness profiles of young men and women today suggest a disturbing worldwide trend of decreased aerobic fitness and increased obesity.[35,41,48,54,55,88]

27.4 MEASURING MAXIMAL AEROBIC CAPACITY WITH MAXIMAL EXERCISE AND ANALYSIS OF EXPIRED GASES

An individual's maximal aerobic capacity can be measured or estimated by a variety of techniques, including treadmill running, cycle ergometry, arm cranking, stair stepping, rowing, and walking.[3,5,9,16,39,51,68,80] Nevertheless, the gold standard is progressive treadmill testing by running the subject to exhaustion while directly measuring expired gases. Pulmonary ventilation is measured by using open-circuit spirometry where the subject breathes through a low-resistance valve with his or her nose occluded.[73] In addition, an electrocardiographic (ECG) recording system is usually used to monitor heart rhythm and ECG changes during exercise and recovery.[74] As such, these tests are usually conducted in clinical or research settings due to high costs associated with sophisticated equipment and the requirement for trained personnel.[73] In these settings, medical supervision is often required. This section will present essential concepts the primary care physician needs to thoroughly assess VO_{2max} when called upon to supervise maximal exercise tests where pulmonary ventilation and expired gases are assessed. This will include a presentation of exercise testing principles to help obtain valid measures of VO_{2max}, a discussion of the two most common exercise modalities (i.e., treadmill tests and cycle ergometer), and an overview of determining the attainment of a valid measure of VO_{2max}.

27.4.1 Principles of Exercise Testing

Certain requirements must be met in order to obtain valid measures of VO_{2max}. First, the exercise must involve large muscle groups.[2] Second, the rate of work must be measurable and reproducible.[2] Third, the mode of exercise should

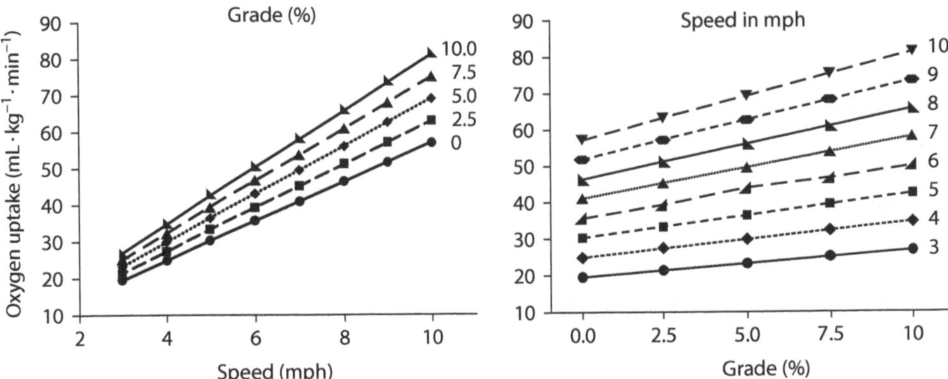

FIGURE 27.1 Oxygen uptake (VO_2) values expected for various treadmill speeds and grades as determined by the American College of Sports Medicine's formulas for metabolic calculations.

be something most people can tolerate.[2] Also, test conditions should be standardized and begin with a warm-up.[2,17] Finally, the test must be independent of the motivation or specific skill sets of the individual.[84] For these reasons, the most common modes for testing in clinical settings include the treadmill and cycle ergometer. Although stair-stepping tests do not require specific skills and have been used for many years, they are not the preferred tests when directly measuring VO_2 because they are uncomfortable and require self-motivation: it is difficult to "drive" a subject to his/her maximum with stair stepping.[2] However, when it involves actual stairs rather than machines, it is useful in field settings and/or under conditions where large numbers of persons need to be tested.

27.4.2 Treadmill Tests for Maximal Aerobic Capacity

A variety of treadmill test protocols have been described and compared[2,7,17,27,33,75,76,84] and, depending on the setting and specific requirements, all are excellent tests. One of the first is a constant grade with increments in speed.[43] However, many nonathletes find this very difficult. Other tests use a constant speed with incremental grade changes (e.g., the Balke[7] and Taylor[84] tests). Kyle et al.[53] described a version of the Taylor test in which the constant speed (6–8 mph) was determined by heart rate after a 10 minute warm-up and the grade (initially 0%) was increased by 2.5% every 2 minutes. Other protocols, such as the Bruce protocol, change both grade and speed.[17] Again, many people find the imposed increases in both speed and grade difficult. Modified versions of all protocols can be used, depending on the population of interest. Clearly, small grade increments and slow speeds are preferred for older and/or deconditioned subjects, whereas larger work increments and higher speeds are suitable for younger and highly active populations. Figure 27.1 provides a range of relative VO_2 (oxygen intake) values expected for various speeds and grades. This information can provide the tester with an estimate of what to expect during a test, despite significant individual variation due to biomechanics, body composition, and other characteristics. Importantly, the protocol selected should be suitable for the individual being tested.

27.4.3 Cycle Ergometer Tests for Maximal Aerobic Capacity

Although treadmill testing principles can be applied to cycle ergometer tests, the cycle ergometer differs from the treadmill in that work rates are independent of body weight, and the two primary variables are cycling rate and resistance. These variables determine the power (work per unit of time), which is expressed in watts. Figure 27.2 shows the linear relation between work rate (in watts) and VO_2 during steady-state cycling (i.e., exercising at a sustainable steady rate) at various work rates. Scientists suggest that VO_2 increases at a rate of 9–11 mL of O_2 per watt.[34,77] Although some variability exists, this relationship can be used to estimate VO_2 when actual measurements are not possible. For cycle ergometer tests, a common cycling rate for these tests is 50–60 revolutions/rotations per minute (rpm), although some subjects find this too slow at low watts. In all cases, the subject should have a warm-up prior to any increase in resistance, with either no or minimal load (25–50 W), depending on the degree of training

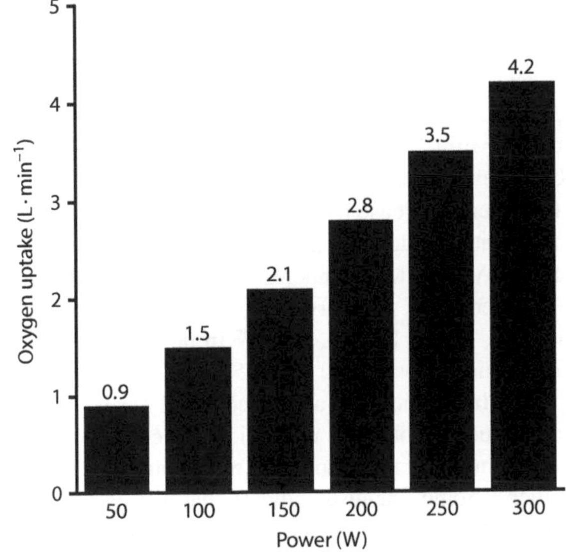

FIGURE 27.2 Expected VO_2 values during cycle ergometry at various power outputs.

and familiarity with cycling. Each progressive stage should be between 1 and 3 minutes, and the step increments can range from 25 to 60 W, depending on the subject population.

Although cycle ergometer tests tend to produce maximal aerobic capacity values that are 5%–20% lower than those from treadmill tests,[1] they offer a few advantages over the latter. First, they are the preferred instrument for use in settings that require repeated examinations over several years because the results are independent of body weight.[3] Second, because subjects/patients sit with the upper body relatively immobile, it is easier to obtain readable ECG tracings and perform studies with indwelling catheters.[3]

27.4.4 Documenting Attainment of Maximal Aerobic Capacity

For accurate maximal aerobic capacity test results, it is important to know whether VO_{2max} has been achieved. The current criteria for determining this include the primary measure of a plateau in VO_2 and/or secondary measures of blood (or plasma) lactate, respiratory exchange ratio (RER), heart rate, and perceived exertion.[22,24,26,45,81]

Clinical Pearl

The current criteria for documenting the attainment of VO_{2max} are the primary measure of a plateau in VO_2 and/or the secondary measures of blood (or plasma) lactate, RER, heart rate, and perceived exertion.

27.4.4.1 Plateau in Oxygen Uptake

The occurrence of a plateau in oxygen intake (VO_2) despite increasing work rates emerged through the work of Hill and Lupton.[71,84] Subsequent research expanded that work and showed that a 2.5% increase in treadmill grade typically resulted in a VO_2 rise of approximately 300 mL·min^{-1}.[84] However, at a certain point, further increases in the exercise (work) rate did not yield the same VO_2 increase. The study concluded that an increase in VO_2 of less than 150 mL·min^{-1}—or 2.1 mL·kg^{-1}·min^{-1} for a higher work rate—marked a plateau in VO_2. They also concluded that a grade increase was preferable to a speed increase for achieving a plateau.

Some critics state that 150 mL·min^{-1} is too large a value and causes VO_{2max} to be underestimated. They have proposed more conservative numbers: increases of <50 mL·min^{-1},[22] 80 mL·min^{-1},[5] and 100 mL·min^{-1}.[47] In lieu of consensus, verification values between 50 and 150 mL·min^{-1} are currently acceptable. In addition, not all subjects will reach a plateau due to factors such as physical restrictions, age, or motivation. In fact, a recent study recommended not using a plateau in VO_2 altogether.[26] Some scientists indicate that it is easy to misinterpret this criterion because of the achievement of several plateaus during a continuous graded exercise protocol.[26,72] The secondary criteria (described in Sections 27.4.4.2 through 27.4.4.5) evolved in response to the issues associated with this primary criterion.

27.4.4.2 Age-Predicted Maximal Heart Rate

The widely recognized linear relationship between heart rate and VO_2 has made the use of a target percentage of the age-predicted maximal heart rate one of the most widely recognized criteria.[24,45] The two most commonly used formulas for estimating maximal heart rate are (220 − age) and (208 − [0.7 × age]).[83] Unfortunately, the predictive accuracy of the equations varies widely; for instance, the interindividual variability of the first equation (i.e., 220 − age) is ±10 to 12 bpm.[73] As such, reliable measures of maximal effort are rarely documented when heart rate is the sole criterion. Thus, heart rate should be used only in conjunction with other secondary criteria (discussed in Sections 27.4.4.3 through 27.4.4.5).[24,26,45]

27.4.4.3 Borg Scale or Rating of Perceived Exertion

The Borg scale is the most widely used method of expressing perceived exertion, although recent data suggest that its validity is lower than previously thought.[19,26] It was designed as a simple linear measure of increase in exercise intensity parallel with the apparent linear increases in VO_2 and heart rate with workload.[13,14] The original scale ranged from 6 to 20, with each number associated with a simple and understandable verbal expression (e.g., 6, no exertion at all; 12 or 13, somewhat hard; 16 and 17, very hard; 20, maximal exertion). The numbers of the scale roughly represent actual heart rate, such that when a person exercises at 130 beats·min^{-1}, the numeric rating of perceived exertion (RPE) is 13. Similarly, a perceived exertion of 19 suggests a heart rate of 190. The scale was not intended to be exact, but rather an aid in the interpretation of perceived exertion. Nevertheless, studies have demonstrated a good correlation between RPE and VO_2.[28,38] In terms of establishing RPE as a criterion, a value of 17 or greater can be considered a positive indicator of maximal effort.

27.4.4.4 Blood Lactate Levels

A rise in blood lactate has also been used to demonstrate a maximal effort, especially in the absence of a true plateau in VO_2.[2,3,5] As the workload continues to rise and the person moves toward a maximal effort, blood lactate levels increase due to an acceleration in glycogen breakdown in muscle, increased recruitment of fast-twitch muscle fibers, reduction in liver blood flow, and elevations in plasma epinephrine concentration.[2,3,5,82] Although identifying a standard cutoff for blood lactate levels has been difficult, scientific data suggest that 8 mM is a reasonable value for use as a criterion.[2,5,22,24,45,81] For example, two well-designed studies found that 78% of their subjects achieved levels greater than 8 mM.[22,81] Thus, although current standards vary, most researchers accept that lactate values of 8 mM or more are indicative of maximal effort. Postexercise blood lactate concentration, compared to some of the other criteria for determining VO_{2max}, is a more objective physiological reflection of high-intensity exercise: it cannot be manipulated, and it has high measurement accuracy.[26] As such, some scientists strongly recommend its use.[26]

27.4.4.5 Respiratory Exchange Ratio

The respiratory exchange ratio (RER) is the ratio of CO_2 volume produced to O_2 volume used, or VCO_2/VO_2. At ratios of 1.0 or below, it is synonymous with respiratory quotient (RQ), an indicator of metabolic fuel or substrate utilization in tissues. RQ typically ranges between 0.7 and 1.0, where a ratio of 0.7 indicates mixed fat utilization, and a ratio of 1.0 indicates exclusive use of carbohydrates.[47] Thus, during low-intensity, steady-state exercise, when fatty acids are the primary fuel, RQ and RER are typically between 0.80 and 0.88. As the intensity of the exercise increases, and carbohydrate becomes the dominant or primary fuel, RQ and RER increase to between 0.9 and 1.0.

Whereas RQ cannot exceed 1.0 (because it reflects tissue substrate utilization), RER commonly exceeds 1.0 during strenuous exercise because it simply reflects respiratory exchange of CO_2 and O_2. During nonsteady-state, strenuous exercise, individuals typically hyperventilate, which results in increased unloading of CO_2 and increases in muscle lactic acid. As additional CO_2 is produced in the buffering of lactic acid, RER is no longer synonymous with RQ (i.e., no longer indicates substrate usage). Instead, RER reflects *both* hyperventilation and blood lactate.[3,24,45,47] Because RER reproducibly increases with exercise intensity, it is used as a criterion for maximal effort. The first study to propose RER as a criterion for VO_{2max} noted that it must be in excess of 1.15 to more accurately assess VO_{2max}.[47] The 1.15 value appears to be reasonable, but not all subjects are able to achieve it. Recent studies have used values from 1.00 to 1.13,[24,45] but at present, there is no clear consensus.

27.4.4.6 Summary: Documenting Attainment of Maximal Aerobic Capacity

To date, no guidelines have been agreed upon, and the criteria used across studies are inconsistent. In fact, many criticize the current VO_{2max} criteria for several reasons. One primary criticism is that the criterion for a plateau in VO_2 was initially established for a discontinuous treadmill test with 2.5% increases in grade. However, the criterion for a plateau has not been redefined for other specific tests; thus, it may not generalize to other maximal exercise testing procedures.[65–67,78]

A group of exercise scientists recently performed a systematic review of criteria used to date and developed new recommendations by age and sex for individuals performing a continuous graded treadmill exercise test[26]. They proposed using only postexercise blood lactate concentrations and RER values based on age and gender, including postexercise blood lactate concentration cutoff values for aged 20–49, 50–64, and ≥65 years, respectively, of 9.0, 6.0, and 4.0 mmol·L^{-1} for men and 7.0, 5.0, and 3.5 mmol·L^{-1} for women. For RER, they proposed 1.10, 1.05, and 1.00 for both men and women in the same age categories.[26]

In summary, if a true plateau can be observed, then it is adequate to establish a true VO_{2max}. However, the attainment of a true plateau is not an absolute prerequisite; some combination of secondary criteria is satisfactory for most purposes. The criteria presented in Table 27.3 can serve as a guide, but at least two, and preferably three, of the secondary criteria should be met.

TABLE 27.3
Criteria for Documenting Attainment of VO_{2max} during a Maximal Effort Test[a]

	Primary criterion
VO_{2max} plateau	Increase in VO_2 < 150 mL·min^{-1} or 2.1 mL·kg^{-1}·min^{-1} with a 2.5% grade increase
	Secondary criteria
Blood lactate	≥8 mM
RER	≥1.15
Heart rate	Increase in heart rate to maximal estimated for age ±10 bpm
Borg scale	≥17

[a] If the primary criterion is not met, then at least two of the remaining four should be met.

27.5 ESTIMATING MAXIMAL AEROBIC CAPACITY WITH SUBMAXIMAL EXERCISE AND ANALYSIS OF EXPIRED GASES

For individuals restricted by pain, fatigue, abnormal gait, and/or impaired balance, direct assessment of VO_{2max} while exercising to volitional exhaustion is not advisable.[26,73] Still, other individuals may simply not be motivated to exercise at maximal levels. In addition, strenuous exercise tests increase the likelihood of adverse cardiac events, especially in elderly and cardiac patients.[26] As a result, submaximal testing protocols have been developed to reduce risk, testing time, and costs associated with maximal effort exercise tests.[26] In this section, we discuss the prediction of maximal aerobic capacity while assessing expired gases during submaximal exercise tests. In a later section, we will discuss prediction methods that do not require measuring expired gases.

A recent review compiled a list of 43 submaximal exercise–based equations that use open-circuit spirometry to predict maximal aerobic capacity.[26] Correlation coefficients for these equations range from 0.57 to as high as 0.92. The majority use heart rate and/or RPE (such as the Borg scale) for the prediction, and little variability has been observed in the predictive accuracy between the two methods.[26] Currently, there is no guidance on the factors to consider when selecting an equation; however, exercise setting, test modality and protocol, and population characteristics should be considered when making a choice. Importantly, all the studies presented in the aforementioned review were graded as weak, so the validity and reliability of the equations may be in question.[26]

Clinical Pearl

Maximal aerobic capacity prediction tests can be conducted in clinical, commercial, and/or outdoor settings. These tests are especially helpful for testing the elderly, children, and people with physical impairments (cardiovascular/pulmonary disease and/or musculoskeletal restrictions) who cannot tolerate maximal exercise tests.

27.6 MONITORING EXERCISE TESTS

As mentioned previously, medical supervision is important when healthy individuals are asked to exercise to exhaustion or when patients/subjects with chronic conditions such as cardiovascular disease are being evaluated.[73] VO_{2max} testing sessions should be monitored by a physician or other properly trained healthcare professional such as a nurse, nurse practitioner, or exercise physiologist/specialist to ensure the safety of the individual and provide care should an adverse event occur. Attending medical personnel must terminate exercise tests with the onset of any of the following indications: drop in systolic blood pressure (SBP) of ≥10 mmHg with an increase in work rate, moderately severe angina, increasing nervous system symptoms such as ataxia and dizziness, signs of poor perfusion, technical difficulties in monitoring the ECG or SBP, the subject's desire to stop, sustained ventricular tachycardia, or ST elevation (+1.0 mm) in leads without diagnostic Q waves.[73]

27.7 PREDICTING MAXIMAL AEROBIC CAPACITY IN THE ABSENCE OF EXPIRED GAS ANALYSIS

Although laboratory measurement is the only way to accurately quantify VO_{2max}, this procedure does pose limitations: the equipment required for direct sampling of oxygen is very expensive to purchase and maintain, the subject must wear a cumbersome/uncomfortable apparatus, the individual performing the test must be well trained, and the nature of a maximal test itself can be limiting to some subjects. In particular, the elderly, children, and people with physical impairments (cardiovascular/pulmonary disease and/or musculoskeletal restrictions) cannot tolerate maximal exercise tests. Finally, large groups cannot be efficiently tested within a reasonable period of time. All of these factors have led to the development of multiple "prediction" tests that can be conducted in clinical, commercial, and/or outdoor settings. Current prediction tests can be divided into three types, depending on the situation: maximal effort prediction tests, submaximal effort prediction tests, and nonexercise prediction tests. Understanding the advantages, disadvantages, and limitations of each type can be important for selecting the most appropriate test for a given environment, a specific population, and/or a particular need.

27.7.1 MAXIMAL PREDICTION TESTS

Maximal prediction tests, although designed to reduce the problems associated with "true" VO_{2max} tests, still require the subject to perform a given protocol to maximal effort. The major difference is that expired gases are not measured; instead, other selected values are collected during the test to predict VO_{2max}. The most common maximal prediction tests involve running a specified distance as quickly or as far as possible within a set time, performing a shuttle/track run, or using time on a treadmill from a standardized maximal treadmill test. However, other modes of exercise such as cycling and stair-stepping can be used.

One of the best known examples of a prediction test is the Cooper 12 minute field performance test.[21] The subject runs on a level surface (usually a measured track) for 12 minutes, the distance (D = meters covered) is recorded, and a predicted VO_{2max} is calculated using a regression equation. Studies have found correlation coefficients (r) between this test and actual VO_{2max} measures of around 0.87–0.89.[21,64] The following regression equation can be used to estimate VO_{2max} from the distance covered in 12 minutes: VO_{2max} (in $mL{\cdot}kg^{-1}{\cdot}min^{-1}$) = D (in m) × 0.02235 − 11.3.

Another commonly used test is the 1.5 mile run. Subjects must complete 1.5 miles in as short a time as possible; the time (T) required to complete the distance is used to predict VO_{2max}.[64,90] Correlations reported between this test and actual VO_{2max} measures range from 0.73 to 0.92.[37,64] The equation for the 1.5 mile run[73] is VO_{2max} in ($mL{\cdot}kg^{-1}{\cdot}min^{-1}$) = 483 ÷ T (in minutes) + 3.5.

Other variations of the 1.5 mile run have been developed, and these tests often include variables other than time.[18,23,37,52,73] For example, the Rockport 1-mile walk test incorporates body weight, age, gender, and heart rate.[37,52,73] Fortunately, all of these tests yield essentially comparable values, so it is incumbent upon the tester to determine which test will be most feasible to conduct.

One other useful test for runners is the shuttle/track run test. Shuttle run tests involve having the individual begin by covering a fixed distance (usually 20–400 m) at a certain speed and time.[6,10,12,56,57,61,69] The individual then must repeat the run multiple times, each time increasing the speed (effectively reducing the allotted time) until the individual can no longer keep pace. The speed achieved can then be used to predict the individual's VO_{2max} from a regression formula. Correlations between values obtained from these tests and actual measurements range from 0.83 to 0.98.[10,56,57,69] One formula used for estimating VO_{2max} from the 20 m shuttle,[57] where S = speed in km/h, is VO_{2max} (in $mL{\cdot}kg^{-1}{\cdot}min^{-1}$) = 5.857 × S − 19.458.

Another way to estimate VO_{2max} is to use the time a person stays on a treadmill for a standardized maximal exercise test. For each of the major maximal effort treadmill protocols, regression equations have been developed to predict VO_{2max} using time.[17,33,75,76] For example, equations (with correlations between 0.86 and 0.92) have been developed for the Bruce protocol with active men, sedentary men, men with coronary heart disease, and healthy adults.[17,33,75,76] One of the more general equations for the Bruce protocol[75] is VO_{2max} (in $mL{\cdot}kg^{-1}{\cdot}min^{-1}$) = 4.326 × T − 4.66, where T = time on treadmill in minutes.

The tests mentioned earlier are all examples of prediction tests involving maximal effort. The first three—the Cooper 12 minute field, 1.5 mile run, and shuttle run—can be performed without the restrictions of the VO_{2max} tests done in the laboratory, whereas the fourth test must be conducted on a treadmill, but without expensive metabolic equipment. Each has a specific utility, depending on the goals and the population of interest, but each also has the inherent problems and/or errors that come with any prediction equation. It must be remembered that prediction equations are typically designed for a specific population and should, therefore, be used with caution. Other variables, including gender, age, and perceived functional ability, can also affect the accuracy of such prediction equations.

27.7.2 Submaximal Prediction Tests

As indicated in a previous section, submaximal effort prediction tests are useful for less-fit individuals who are just starting an exercise program or those recovering from medical conditions who often cannot tolerate a maximal effort. These tests—whether constant load, steady state, or progressive—have at least four advantages over maximal exertion tests. They are physically less demanding, take less time to perform, are safer to conduct, and can often be performed with large groups. However, they do sacrifice a degree of accuracy.

Heart rate provides the theoretical basis behind most submaximal tests,[29] and a majority of submaximal tests use age-predicted maximal heart rate to estimate VO_{2max}. In these predictions, an erroneous estimate of maximal heart rate can markedly affect the outcome. For instance, the age-predicted maximal heart rate tends to underestimate maximal heart rates in older adults,[83] so resulting values from prediction equations can be inaccurate. In addition, underestimating heart rate will recommend that an older adult exercise at higher intensities than they should, which may result in adverse events.[29]

The relation between heart rate and work load is particularly important for progressive, submaximal cycle ergometer protocols. One such protocol utilizes four incremental 2 minute stages, with an initial workload based on the subject's body weight and self-reported activity level.[59] For example, a 95 kg, physically active subject might perform a four-stage protocol at incremental workloads of 50, 100, 150, and 200 W while pedalling at 50 rpm. In contrast, someone less physically active might exercise at 25, 50, 75, and 100 W at 50 rpm. For both, heart rates at each of the work rates would be plotted and the line extrapolated to the estimated maximal heart rate (e.g., 190 or 170 bpm); the point on the line that coincides with age-predicted maximal heart rate would then provide an estimate of VO_{2max} (Figure 27.3). Other progressive tests with known

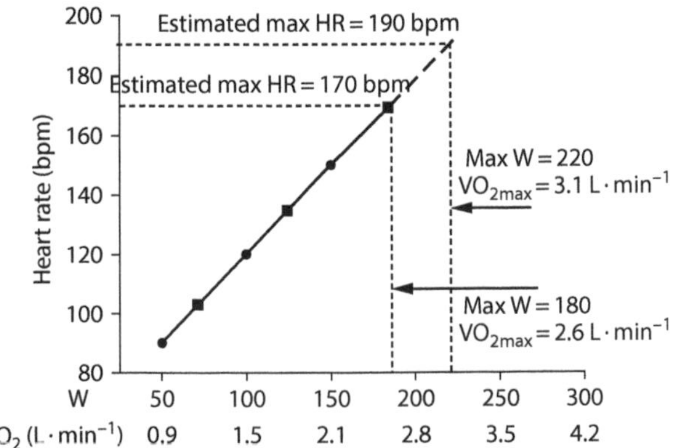

FIGURE 27.3 Extrapolation of VO_{2max} from heart rate and workload on a cycle ergometer test.

workloads have been conducted in a similar manner using stair-steppers,[44] treadmills, and seated rowing machines.[8]

Steady-state submaximal effort tests are also used to predict VO_{2max}. Treadmills, track walking/running, stair steppers, cycle ergometers, bench steps, rowing machines, and squat repetitions have all been used.[4,25,37,44,46,52,85,90] These all maintain a few points in common: all require a steady-state workload and a measure of the subject's heart rate upon test completion. From there, heart rate may be used alone to predict VO_{2max} from a nomogram (i.e., a chart showing numerical relationships)[4,85] or in conjunction with age, weight, gender, and other variables in a regression equation.[25,37,46,52]

In addition to nomograms, regression equations have been developed to predict VO_{2max} based on individuals walking/jogging on a treadmill at submaximal levels,[25] stepping up and down stairs for a set time,[90] and/or jogging one mile on a track.[37] These prediction equations were typically derived from a particular population and set of conditions, so they must be interpreted with caution when being applied to other situations/populations. The equations may not give usable results for a population with different ages, gender, and fitness levels.

Although submaximal prediction tests do not provide the same physiological data as true VO_{2max} tests, they do serve an important role in estimating VO_{2max}. In addition, these tests have high retest precision and are excellent for tracking performance over time.[21] However, all submaximal tests are somewhat variable in their accuracy in estimating VO_{2max} because the predictive value relies on an accurate estimate of maximal heart rate. And yet, as noted previously, both means of estimating maximal heart rate can yield values as much as 20–30 bpm (one standard deviation = ± 10 to 12) higher or lower than the actual maximal heart rate, depending on age and training of the subject.[59,73] Thus, understanding the limitations of the tests and subjects and knowing the goals of the test will allow for the clinician or healthcare provider to select the most appropriate test for estimating aerobic capacity.

27.7.3 Nonexercise Prediction Tests

Equations to predict VO_{2max} without using any exercise at all also exist. These equations to estimate VO_{2max} rely on nonexercise parameters such as age, height, weight, body composition, gender, self-reported level of physical activity, usual intensity of activity, and perceived functional ability to walk, jog, or run given distances.[36,42,49,50,62,63,70,87] One such test uses the ratio between maximum and resting heart rate to predict VO_{2max}.[87] Specifically, divide the subject's maximum heart rate by his/her resting heart rate and multiply the resulting value by 15 to get an estimate of VO_{2max}. These nonexercise prediction tests show promise and have one significant advantage: They can be administered without the requirements of expensive equipment, special supervision, or significant inconvenience to the subject. However, as with all regression equations, they were developed for specific populations and conditions, and using them for other situations is questionable, because certain assumptions were made about the original populations from which they originated.

TABLE 27.4
SORT: Key Recommendations for Practice

Clinical Recommendation	Evidence Rating	References
Terminate exercise tests with the onset of any of the following indications: drop in systolic blood pressure (SBP) of ≥ 10 mm Hg with an increase in work rate, moderately severe angina, increasing nervous system symptoms such as ataxia and dizziness, signs of poor perfusion, technical difficulties monitoring the ECG or SBP, the subject's desire to stop, sustained ventricular tachycardia, or ST elevation (+1.0 mm) in leads without diagnostic Q waves.	C	[73]
When choosing the mode of exercise, ensure that it involves large muscle groups, the rate of work is measurable and reproducible, and most people can tolerate it.	C	[2]
Exercise test conditions should be standardized, begin with a warm-up, and end with a cool-down.	C	[2,17]
Ensure that the exercise test is independent of the motivation or specific skill sets of the individual.	C	[84]
When assessing maximal aerobic capacity with maximal exercise test, ensure that the criteria for attainment of VO_{2max} are met. The primary measure is a plateau in VO_2. Secondary measures of blood lactate, respiratory exchange ratio, heart rate, and perceived exertion should be examined according to the criteria detailed in this chapter.	C	[22,24,26,45,81]
Submaximal exercise prediction tests, rather than maximal exercise tests, are recommended for the elderly, children, people who cannot tolerate maximal efforts, and people with physical impairments or disease conditions.	C	[73]

27.8 SUMMARY

In summary, maximal aerobic capacity—VO_{2max}—is an extremely valuable measure of cardiovascular and pulmonary functions and endurance performance. The strong association between maximal aerobic capacity and multiple health benefits is overwhelming, so knowing VO_{2max} provides an excellent index of health and health risk. It can be directly measured by using standardized maximal treadmill, cycle ergometer, and other protocols, or it can be estimated using either maximal and submaximal exercise prediction protocols or even non-exercise prediction equations. These protocols for predicting VO_{2max} are readily available, and many are extremely easy to administer. Table 27.4 presents a summary of the key recommendations for practice.

REFERENCES

1. American College of Sports Medicine ed. *Guidelines for Exercise Testing and Prescription.* 4th ed. Philadelphia, PA: Lea & Febige; 1991.
2. Astrand PO. Quantification of exercise capability and evaluation of physical capacity in man. *Progress in Cardiovascular Diseases.* 1976;19(1):51–67.
3. Åstrand PO. *Textbook of Work Physiology: Physiological Bases of Exercise.* 4th ed. Champaign, IL: Human Kinetics; 2003.
4. Astrand PO, Ryhming I. A nomogram for calculation of aerobic capacity (physical fitness) from pulse rate during sub-maximal work. *Journal of Applied Physiology.* 1954;7(2):218–221.
5. Astrand PO, Saltin B. Maximal oxygen uptake and heart rate in various types of muscular activity. *Journal of Applied Physiolog.* 1961;16:977–981.
6. Aziz AR, Chia MY, Teh KC. Measured maximal oxygen uptake in a multi-stage shuttle test and treadmill-run test in trained athletes. *The Journal of Sports Medicine and Physical Fitness.* 2005;45(3):306–314.
7. Balke B, Ware RW. An experimental study of physical fitness of Air Force personnel. *US Armed Forces Medical Journal.* 1959;10(6):875–888.
8. Beneke R. Anaerobic threshold, individual anaerobic threshold, and maximal lactate steady state in rowing. *Medicine & Science in Sports & Exercise.* 1995;27(6):863–867.
9. Bergh U, Kanstrup IL, Ekblom B. Maximal oxygen uptake during exercise with various combinations of arm and leg work. *Journal of Applied Physiology.* 1976;41(2):191–196.
10. Berthoin S, Pelayo P, Lensel-Corbeil G, Robin H, Gerbeaux M. Comparison of maximal aerobic speed as assessed with laboratory and field measurements in moderately trained subjects. *International Journal of Sports Medicine.* 1996;17(7):525–529.
11. Blair SN, Kohl HW, 3rd, Paffenbarger RS, Jr, Clark DG, Cooper KH, Gibbons LW. Physical fitness and all-cause mortality. A prospective study of healthy men and women. *Journal of the American Medical Association.* 1989;262(17):2395–2401.
12. Boddington MK, Lambert MI, Waldeck MR. Validity of a 5-meter multiple shuttle run test for assessing fitness of women field hockey players. *The Journal of Strength & Conditioning Research.* 2004;18(1):97–100.
13. Borg GA. Psychophysical bases of perceived exertion. *Medicine & Science in Sports & Exercise.* 1982;14(5):377–381.
14. Borg GA, Noble B. Perceived exertion. In: Wilmore JH, ed. *Exercise and Sport Science Reviews.* New York: Academic Press; 1974, pp. 131–153.
15. Bouchard C, Dionne FT, Simoneau JA, Boulay MR. Genetics of aerobic and anaerobic performances. *Exercise and Sport Sciences Reviews.* 1992;20:27–58.
16. Brahler CJ, Blank SE. VersaClimbing elicits higher VO_{2max} than does treadmill running or rowing ergometry. *Medicine & Science in Sports & Exercise.* 1995;27(2):249–254.
17. Bruce RA, Kusumi F, Hosmer D. Maximal oxygen intake and nomographic assessment of functional aerobic impairment in cardiovascular disease. *American Heart Journal.* 1973;85(4):546–562.
18. Castro-Pinero J, Mora J, Gonzalez-Montesinos JL, Sjostrom M, Ruiz JR. Criterion-related validity of the one-mile run/walk test in children aged 8–17 years. *Journal of Sports Sciences.* 2009;27(4):405–413.

19. Chen MJ, Fan X, Moe ST. Criterion-related validity of the Borg ratings of perceived exertion scale in healthy individuals: A meta-analysis. *Journal of Sports Sciences.* 2002;20(11):873–899.
20. Convertino VA. Cardiovascular consequences of bed rest: Effect on maximal oxygen uptake. *Medicine & Science in Sports & Exercise.* 1997;29(2):191–196.
21. Cooper KH. A means of assessing maximal oxygen intake. Correlation between field and treadmill testing. *Journal of the American Medical Association.* 1968;203(3):201–204.
22. Cumming GR, Borysyk LM. Criteria for maximum oxygen uptake in men over 40 in a population survey. *Medicine and Science in Sports and Exercise.* 972;4(1):18–22.
23. Cureton KJ, Sloniger MA, O'Bannon JP, Black DM, McCormack WP. A generalized equation for prediction of VO_2 peak from 1-mile run/walk performance. *Medicine and Science in Sports and Exercise.* March 1995;27(3):445–451.
24. Duncan GE, Howley ET, Johnson BN. Applicability of VO_{2max} criteria: Discontinuous versus continuous protocols. *Medicine and Science in Sports and Exercise.* 1997;29(2):273–278.
25. Ebbeling CB, Ward A, Puleo EM, Widrick J, Rippe JM. Development of a single-stage submaximal treadmill walking test. *Medicine and Science in Sports and Exercise.* 1991;23(8):966–973.
26. Edvardsen E, Hem E, Anderssen SA. End criteria for reaching maximal oxygen uptake must be strict and adjusted to sex and age: A cross-sectional study. *PLoS One.* 2014;9(1):e85276.
27. Ellestad MH, Allen W, Wan MC, Kemp GL. Maximal treadmill stress testing for cardiovascular evaluation. *Circulation.* 1969;39(4):517–522.
28. Eston RG, Davies BL, Williams JG. Use of perceived effort ratings to control exercise intensity in young healthy adults. *European Journal of Applied Physiology.* 1987;56(2):222–224.
29. Evans HJ, Ferrar KE, Smith AE, Parfitt G, Eston RG. A systematic review of methods to predict maximal oxygen uptake from submaximal, open circuit spirometry in healthy adults. *Journal of Science and Medicine in Sport.* 2015;18(2):183–188.
30. Farrell SW, Fitzgerald SJ, McAuley P, Barlow CE. Cardiorespiratory fitness, adiposity, and all-cause mortality in women. *Medicine & Science in Sports & Exercise.* 2010;42(11):2006–2012.
31. Farrell SW, Kohl HW, Rogers T. The independent effect of ethnicity on cardiovascular fitness. *Human Biology.* 1987;59(4):657–666.
32. Fleg JL, Lakatta EG. Role of muscle loss in the age-associated reduction in VO_{2max}. *Journal of Applied Physiology (1985).* 1988;65(3):1147–1151.
33. Froelicher VF, Jr, Brammell H, Davis G, Noguera I, Stewart A, Lancaster MC. A comparison of three maximal treadmill exercise protocols. *Journal of Applied Physiology.* 1974;36(6):720–725.
34. Gaesser GA, Poole DC. The slow component of oxygen uptake kinetics in humans. *Exercise and Sport Sciences Reviews.* 1996;24:35–71.
35. Gahche J, Fakhouri T, Carroll DD, Burt VL, Wang CY, Fulton JE. Cardiorespiratory fitness levels among U.S. youth aged 12–15 years: United States, 1999–2004 and 2012. *NCHS Data Brief.* 2014(153):1–8.
36. George JD, Stone WJ, Burkett LN. Non-exercise VO2max estimation for physically active college students. *Medicine & Science in Sports & Exercise.* 1997;29(3):415–423.
37. George JD, Vehrs PR, Allsen PE, Fellingham GW, Fisher AG. VO_{2max} estimation from a submaximal 1-mile track jog for fit college-age individuals. *Medicine & Science in Sports & Exercise.* 1993;25(3):401–406.
38. Glass SC, Knowlton RG, Becque MD. Accuracy of RPE from graded exercise to establish exercise training intensity. *Medicine & Science in Sports & Exercise.* 1992; 24(11):1303–1307.
39. Gleser MA, Horstman DH, Mello RP. The effect on VO2 max of adding arm work to maximal leg work. *Medicine and Science in Sports.* 1974;6(2):104–107.
40. Goran M, Fields D, Hunter G, Herd S, Weinsier R. Total body fat does not influence maximal aerobic capacity. *International Journal of Obesity.* 2000;24(7):841–848.
41. Hawkins S, Wiswell R. Rate and mechanism of maximal oxygen consumption decline with aging: Implications for exercise training. *Sports Medicine.* 2003;33(12):877–888.
42. Heil DP, Freedson PS, Ahlquist LE, Price J, Rippe JM. Nonexercise regression models to estimate peak oxygen consumption. *Medicine & Science in Sports & Exercise.* 1995;27(4):599–606.
43. Hill AV, Lupton H. Muscular exercise, lactic acid, and the supply and utilization of oxygen. *QjM.* 1923(62):135.
44. Holland G, Hoffman J, Vincent W. Treadmill vs. steptreadmill ergometry. *Phys Sports Med.* 1990;18:79.
45. Howley ET, Bassett DR, Jr., Welch HG. Criteria for maximal oxygen uptake: Review and commentary. *Med Sci Sports Exerc.* September 1995;27(9):1292–1301.
46. Inoue Y, Nakao M. Prediction of maximal oxygen uptake by squat test in men and women. *Kobe J Med Sci.* April 1996;42(2):119–129.
47. Issekutz BJ, Birkhead NC, Rodahl K. Use of respiratory quotients in assessment of aerobic work capacity. *J Appl Physiol.* January 1, 1962;17(1):47–50.
48. Jackson AS, Sui X, Hebert JR, Church TS, Blair SN. Role of lifestyle and aging on the longitudinal change in cardiorespiratory fitness. *Arch Intern Med.* October 26, 2009;169(19):1781–1787.
49. Jang TW, Park SG, Kim HR, Kim JM, Hong YS, Kim BG. Estimation of maximal oxygen uptake without exercise testing in Korean healthy adult workers. *Tohoku J Exp Med.* 2012;227(4):313–319.
50. Jurca R, Jackson AS, LaMonte MJ et al. Assessing cardiorespiratory fitness without performing exercise testing. *Am J Prev Med.* October 2005;29(3):185–193.
51. Kasch FW, Phillips WH, Ross WD, Carter JE, Boyer JL. A comparison of maximal oxygen uptake by treadmill and steptest procedures. *J Appl Physiol.* July 1966;21(4):1387–1388.
52. Kline GM, Porcari JP, Hintermeister R et al. Estimation of VO_{2max} from a one-mile track walk, gender, age, and body weight. *Med Sci Sports Exerc.* June 1987;19(3):253–259.
53. Kyle SB, Smoak BL, Douglass LW, Deuster PA. Variability of responses across training levels to maximal treadmill exercise. *J Appl Physiol.* July 1989;67(1):160–165.
54. Kyrolainen H, Santtila M, Nindl BC, Vasankari T. Physical fitness profiles of young men: Associations between physical fitness, obesity and health. *Sports Med.* November 1, 2010;40(11):907–920.
55. Lavie CJ, McAuley PA, Church TS, Milani RV, Blair SN. Obesity and cardiovascular diseases: Implications regarding fitness, fatness, and severity in the obesity paradox. *J Am Coll Cardiol.* April 15, 2014;63(14):1345–1354.
56. Leger L, Boucher R. An indirect continuous running multistage field test: The Universite de Montreal track test. *Can J Appl Sport Sci.* June 1980;5(2):77–84.
57. Leger LA, Lambert J. A maximal multistage 20-m shuttle run test to predict VO_{2max}. *Eur J Appl Physiol Occup Physiol.* 1982;49(1):1–12.

58. Levine BD. VO_{2max}: What do we know, and what do we still need to know? *J Physiol.* January 1, 2008;586(1):25–34.
59. Lockwood PA, Yoder JE, Deuster PA. Comparison and cross-validation of cycle ergometry estimates of VO_{2max}. *Med Sci Sports Exerc.* November 1997;29(11):1513–1520.
60. Maciejczyk M, Wiecek M, Szymura J, Szygula Z, Wiecha S, Cempla J. The influence of increased body fat or lean body mass on aerobic performance. *PLoS One.* 2014;9(4):e95797.
61. Mahar MT, Guerieri AM, Hanna MS, Kemble CD. Estimation of aerobic fitness from 20-m multistage shuttle run test performance. *Am J Prev Med.* October 2011; 41(4 Suppl 2):S117–S123.
62. Malek MH, Housh TJ, Berger DE, Coburn JW, Beck TW. A new non-exercise-based VO_{2max} prediction equation for aerobically trained men. *J Strength Cond Res.* August 2005;19(3):559–565.
63. Malek MH, Housh TJ, Berger DE, Coburn JW, Beck TW. A new nonexercise-based VO2(max) equation for aerobically trained females. *Med Sci Sports Exerc.* October 2004;36(10):1804–1810.
64. McNaughton L, Hall P, Cooley D. Validation of several methods of estimating maximal oxygen uptake in young men. *Percept Mot Skills.* October 1998;87(2):575–584.
65. Midgley AW, Carroll S. Emergence of the verification phase procedure for confirming "true" VO(2max). *Scand J Med Sci Sports.* June 2009;19(3):313–322.
66. Midgley AW, Carroll S, Marchant D, McNaughton LR, Siegler J. Evaluation of true maximal oxygen uptake based on a novel set of standardized criteria. *Appl Physiol Nutr Metab.* April 2009;34(2):115–123.
67. Midgley AW, Mc Naughton LR. Time at or near VO_{2max} during continuous and intermittent running. A review with special reference to considerations for the optimisation of training protocols to elicit the longest time at or near VO_{2max}. *J Sports Med Phys Fitness.* March 2006;46(1):1–14.
68. Nagle FJ, Richie JP, Giese MD. VO2max responses in separate and combined arm and leg air-braked ergometer exercise. *Med Sci Sports Exerc.* December 1984;16(6):563–566.
69. Naughton LM, Cooley D, Kearney V, Smith S. A comparison of two different shuttle run tests for the estimation of VO_{2max}. *J Sports Med Phys Fitness.* June 1996;36(2):85–89.
70. Nes BM, Janszky I, Vatten LJ, Nilsen TI, Aspenes ST, Wisloff U. Estimating VO_2 peak from a nonexercise prediction model: The HUNT Study, Norway. *Med Sci Sports Exerc.* November 2011;43(11):2024–2030.
71. Noakes TD. Implications of exercise testing for prediction of athletic performance: A contemporary perspective. *Med Sci Sports Exerc.* August 1988;20(4):319–330.
72. Noakes TD. Maximal oxygen uptake: "Classical" versus "contemporary" viewpoints: A rebuttal. *Med Sci Sports Exerc.* September 1998;30(9):1381–1398.
73. Pescatello LS, Arena R, Riebe D, Thompson PD, eds. *ACSM's Guidelines for Exercise Testing and Prescription.* 9th ed. Philadelphia, PA: Lippincott Williams & Wilkins, 2014.
74. Pina IL, Balady GJ, Hanson P, Labovitz AJ, Madonna DW, Myers J. Guidelines for clinical exercise testing laboratories. A statement for healthcare professionals from the Committee on Exercise and Cardiac Rehabilitation, American Heart Association. *Circulation.* February 1, 1995;91(3):912–921.
75. Pollock ML, Bohannon RL, Cooper KH et al. A comparative analysis of four protocols for maximal treadmill stress testing. *Am Heart J.* July 1976;92(1):39–46.
76. Pollock ML, Foster C, Schmidt D, Hellman C, Linnerud AC, Ward A. Comparative analysis of physiologic responses to three different maximal graded exercise test protocols in healthy women. *Am Heart J.* March 1982;103(3):363–373.
77. Poole DC, Richardson RS. Determinants of oxygen uptake. Implications for exercise testing. *Sports Med.* November 1997;24(5):308–320.
78. Poole DC, Wilkerson DP, Jones AM. Validity of criteria for establishing maximal O_2 uptake during ramp exercise tests. *Eur J Appl Physiol.* March 2008;102(4):403–410.
79. Proctor DN, Joyner MJ. Skeletal muscle mass and the reduction of VO_{2max} in trained older subjects. *J Appl Physiol (1985).* May 1997;82(5):1411–1415.
80. Secher NH, Ruberg-Larsen N, Binkhorst RA, Bonde-Petersen F. Maximal oxygen uptake during arm cranking and combined arm plus leg exercise. *J Appl Physiol.* May 1974;36(5):515–518.
81. Stachenfeld NS, Eskenazi M, Gleim GW, Coplan NL, Nicholas JA. Predictive accuracy of criteria used to assess maximal oxygen consumption. *Am Heart J.* April 1992;123(4 Pt 1):922–925.
82. Stallknecht B, Vissing J, Galbo H. Lactate production and clearance in exercise. Effects of training. A mini-review. *Scand J Med Sci Sports.* June 1998;8(3):127–131.
83. Tanaka H, Monahan KD, Seals DR. Age-predicted maximal heart rate revisited. *J Am Coll Cardiol.* January 2001; 37(1):153–156.
84. Taylor HL, Buskirk E, Henschel A. Maximal oxygen intake as an objective measure of cardio-respiratory performance. *J Appl Physiol.* July 1955;8(1):73–80.
85. Teraslinna P, Ismail AH, MacLeod DF. Nomogram by Astrand and Ryhming as a predictor of maximum oxygen intake. *J Appl Physiol.* March 1966;21(2):513–515.
86. Thakur J, Yadav R, Singh V. Influence of body composition on the dimensions of VO_{2max}. 2010;1(2):72–77.
87. Uth N, Sorensen H, Overgaard K, Pedersen PK. Estimation of VO_{2max} from the ratio between HR_{max} and HR_{rest}—the Heart Rate Ratio Method. *Eur J Appl Physiol.* January 2004;91(1):111–115.
88. Wang CY, Haskell WL, Farrell SW et al. Cardiorespiratory fitness levels among US adults 20–49 years of age: Findings from the 1999–2004 National Health and Nutrition Examination Survey. *Am J Epidemiol.* February 15, 2010; 171(4):426–435.
89. Wei M, Kampert JB, Barlow CE et al. Relationship between low cardiorespiratory fitness and mortality in normal-weight, overweight, and obese men. *Journal of the American Medical Association.* October 27, 1999;282(16):1547–1553.
90. Zwiren LD, Freedson PS, Ward A, Wilke S, Rippe JM. Estimation of VO_{2max}: A comparative analysis of five exercise tests. *Res Q Exerc Sport.* March 1991;62.

Section IV

Injury Management and Rehabilitation

28 General Approach to Musculoskeletal Overuse Injury

Robert P. Wilder, Francis G. O'Connor, and Robert P. Nirschl

CONTENTS

TABLE 28.1
Key Clinical Considerations

1. Overuse injuries commonly occur during a transition in training during which there is an increase in training volume or intensity or a change in the mode of training.
2. Both intrinsic and extrinsic risk factors contribute to overuse injuries. Intrinsic factors include biomechanical, strength, and flexibility imbalances and deficits. Extrinsic factors include equipment, environment, and training patterns. Treatment addresses these factors in addition to injury-specific rehabilitation.
3. Rehabilitation of overuse injuries follows a series of stages including establishment of a correct pathoanatomic diagnosis, controlling pain and inflammation, rehabilitative sport and recreational exercise and general conditioning, and controlling abuse leading ultimately to sports participation.
4. Corticosteroid injections have a limited, anti-inflammatory, role in the treatment of overuse injuries. Anti-inflammatory measures are used to facilitate a comprehensive plan incorporating rehabilitative sport and recreational exercises, general conditioning, and sports-specific training.
5. Return to sports occurs when the athlete has achieved normal flexibility and strength, demonstrates sports-specific function, and is psychologically ready.

28.1 INTRODUCTION

The popularity of sport and recreational exercises has led to the proliferation of associated injuries and illnesses. The literature describing exercise-related disorders is quite robust, as elite and recreational athletes (heretofore grouped as athletes) can be victim to anything from ankle sprains, Achilles tendinitis, and exercise-associated collapse to verbal abuse and dog bites.[15,37,72] The overwhelming majority of injuries that affect athletes, however, are secondary to overuse, with a history of prior injury and inadequate rehabilitation representing important risk factors for future harm.[12,25,47,71] These injuries can be challenging and frustrating for both providers and athletes as the pathophysiology of overuse injuries has yet to be fully elucidated (Table 28.1).[2,3,17]

Athletes by the time they venture to seek medical attention have in all probability sought counsel from exercise colleagues and exhausted multiple interventions and therapies. In addition, while most athletes are willing to adjust and modify training regimens, few are willing to accept prolonged periods of refraining from land sport and recreational exercises. This chapter briefly reviews the epidemiology and etiology of injuries in athletes, with particular attention to overuse injuries, and then details an effective strategy for diagnosing, managing, and rehabilitating injuries in this population. In addition, we discuss the concept of *prehabilitation* and its role in preventing injuries, as well as introduce new orthobiologic interventional therapies.[57,67]

28.2 EPIDEMIOLOGY OF OVERUSE INJURIES

Overuse injuries are thought to be the most commonly encountered sports injuries by primary care providers.[30] Overuse sports injuries have been reported to be twice as frequent as acute injuries with the most common presentation being anterior knee pain.[9] Studies involving sport and recreational exercise clinics have consistently demonstrated that the majority of presenting clinical problems are the result of overuse with patellofemoral disorders being most common.[12,49] Matheson evaluated age as a determinant for presenting injuries in runners and found that patellofemoral dysfunction and stress fractures were more prevalent in young athletes, while metatarsal pain syndromes and plantar fasciitis were more prevalent among older athletes.[53] Additionally, patellofemoral pain and stress fractures are reported more commonly in women than in men; however, this may be more sports specific than gender specific.[7,8] In one study evaluating referrals to a primary care sports medicine clinic, the most common overuse injuries diagnosed included rotator cuff tendonitis (11.7%) and patellofemoral tracking disorders (10.6%), with the latter predominating in running athletes.[14,57]

28.3 WHAT CAUSES OVERUSE INJURIES?

Overuse injuries result from repetitive microtrauma that leads to local tissue damage in the form of cellular and extracellular degeneration; the exact pathophysiology of these disorders remains to be fully elucidated.[2,5,32,57,75] This tissue damage can culminate clinically in tendinitis or tendinosis, stress fracture, joint synovitis, entrapment neuropathies, ligament strains, or myositis.[34,75]

These injuries are most likely to occur when an athlete changes the mode, intensity, or duration of training; a phenomenon that Leadbetter describes as the "principle of transition."[39] Physical training uses prescribed periods of intense activity or *overreaching* to induce the desired goal of *supercompensation* or performance improvement. However, a mismatch between overload and recovery can lead to breakdown on a cellular or systemic level. At the cellular level, repetitive overload on tissues that fail to adapt to new or increased demands can lead to tissue degeneration and overuse injury. It is important to realize that, in theory, this subclinical tissue damage can accumulate for some time before the person experiences pain and becomes symptomatic[39] (shown in Figure 28.1).

Clinical Pearl

Athletes undergoing a transition in training, increasing volume or intensity, or changing the mode of training are particularly at the risk of overuse injury.

On the systemic level, rapid increases in training load without adequate recovery may cause a global "overtraining syndrome."[18] In overtraining syndrome, improper increases in workout loads do not result in *supercompensation*; rather, the individual enters a cycle of performance decrements, fatigue, poor sleep patterns, myalgias, weight loss, and neuroendocrine and immune dysfunctions.[63] Athletes commonly refer to overtraining syndrome as *staleness* or *burn out*. If medical providers fail to recognize the symptoms of this commonly described overtraining syndrome, their athletes risk chronic overuse injuries as well as failed performance, illness, and premature retirement.[18,76]

Both intrinsic and extrinsic risk factors have been described and may contribute to overuse injuries.[56] Intrinsic risk factors are biomechanical abnormalities unique to a particular athlete. High arches, for example, have been demonstrated in military recruits to predispose to a greater risk of musculoskeletal overuse injury than low arches or "flat feet."[20] Genu valgum, excessive Q angle, and genu recurvatum have been reported as risk factors for overuse injuries associated with vigorous training.[19] Intrinsic risk factors, however, have been difficult to reproduce in subsequent studies, as this remains a difficult and challenging area to perform well-controlled studies.[65,73,74] Extrinsic (avoidable) factors that commonly contribute to overload include poor technique, improper equipment, and improper changes in the duration or frequency of activity. These inappropriate changes in activity duration or frequency, or *training errors*, are thought to be among the most common causes of overuse injuries in recreational sport and recreational exercise athletes.[18,25,73] It is also believed that vulnerability to extrinsic overload varies with the intrinsic risk factors of an individual athlete (see Table 28.2).

Sports-acquired deficiencies, categorized as an extrinsic risk factor, actually represent the product of biomechanical abnormalities and training errors. Sports activity can overload an athlete's musculoskeletal system in predictable ways; athletic repetition without proper conditioning can propagate

TABLE 28.2
Risk Factors That Contribute to Overuse Injuries

Intrinsic	Extrinsic
Malalignment	Training errors
Muscle imbalance	Equipment
Inflexibility	Environment
Muscle weakness	Technique
Instability	Sports-imposed deficiencies

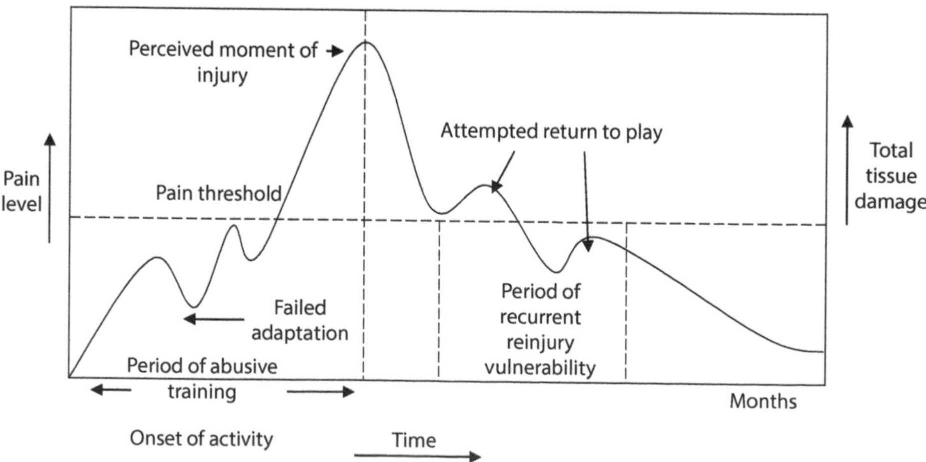

FIGURE 28.1 Profile of chronic microtraumatic soft-tissue injury. (Adapted and reproduced with permission from Leadbetter, W.B., *Clin, Sports Med.* 11(3), 533, 1992.)

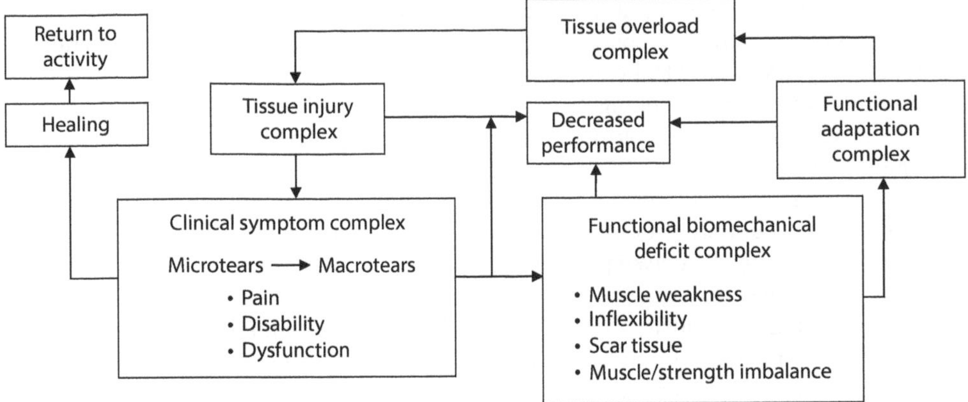

FIGURE 28.2 Vicious overload cycle. This model for the vicious overload cycle is useful for thorough injury evaluation that includes five categories: the tissue injury complex, the clinical symptom complex, functional biomechanical deficits, the functional adaptation complex, and the tissue overload complex. (Adapted and reproduced with permission from Kibler, W.B., et al., *Clin. Sports Med.* 11(3), 661, 1992.)

predictable muscular imbalance and flexibility deficits. For example, biomechanical studies in athletes have identified that hip abductor weakness and inflexibility are clearly associated with iliotibial band syndrome.[24,29] Several authorities have described that gluteus medius weakness not only can be a culprit for the pathology of iliotibial band syndrome but can also result as a consequence of repetitive overload.[13,27] Accordingly, multiple protocols exist that emphasize a restoration of hip abductor strength as core to the rehabilitative effort of the runner with iliotibial band syndrome.[10,28]

Given the complexity of musculoskeletal overload and injury production, the physician must ensure that all aspects of the primary injury and the secondary sites of injury or dysfunction are completely diagnosed.[35] In Kibler's "vicious overload cycle," five interrelated categories require the attention of the clinician: the tissue injury complex, the clinical symptom complex, functional biomechanical deficits, the functional adaptation complex, and the tissue overload complex.[35] Evaluation of the primary and secondary sites of injury (the kinetic chain) in the context of these five categories enables the primary care provider to develop an effective rehabilitation and treatment program (see Figure 28.2).

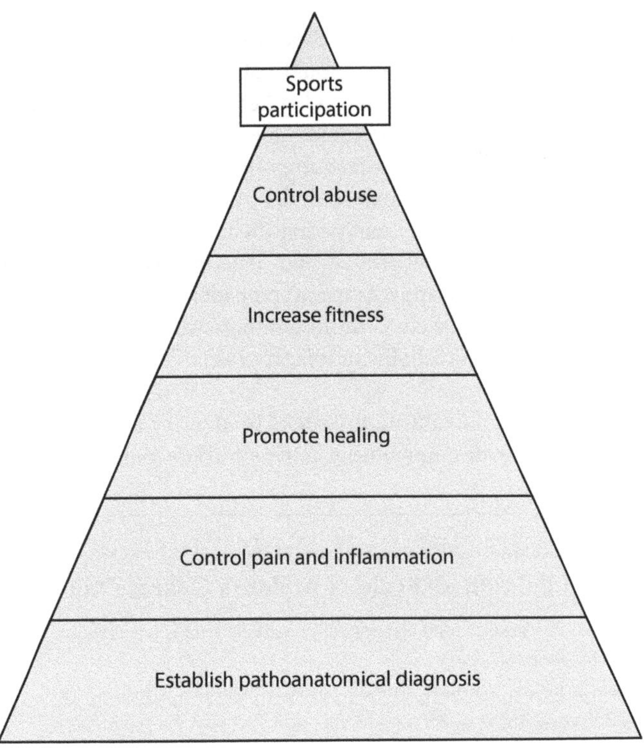

FIGURE 28.3 Nirschl clinic overuse injury pyramid. The five-step pyramid designed to manage overuse injuries and return elite and recreational athletes to sports participation.

28.4 FIVE STEPS TO MANAGEMENT

The diagnosis and management of overuse injuries are best facilitated through a systematic approach. The sports medicine team's responsibilities are to establish a correct pathoanatomic diagnosis and direct rehabilitation, which enlist the expertise of the directing physician, physical therapists, orthotists, athletic trainers, and coaches. We utilize a five-step management pyramid designed to assist providers in systematically diagnosing and managing an athlete to a successful return to sports participation[56] (see Figure 28.3).

28.4.1 Make a Correct Pathoanatomic Diagnosis

Accurate diagnosis and management of most overuse injuries require no more than a good history, physical examination, and selected radiographs. Vague diagnoses, such as "runner's knee" and "shin splints," do not clearly identify the anatomic dysfunction and should be avoided. Diagnoses such as patellar tendinopathy and chronic exertional compartment syndrome more clearly identify the painful, presenting structure. However, even these diagnoses are limited since they may not accurately describe the pathologic process of the injury and offer limited insight into associated dysfunctions that occur along the rest of the kinetic chain.[57]

A thorough history is key to a successful diagnosis as it illuminates the differential and identifies risk factors. The provider should begin the history by asking the athlete questions that identify the *transition* that may have contributed to the overuse. When did the injury first occur? Did you recently purchase new shoes or transition to incorporating barefoot sport and recreational exercises? Have you changed training locations or your training regimen?

Questions should also focus on the quality of the athlete's pain and function. Does the pain occur only with sports activity or also with activities of daily living? Perceived pain phase scales, such as Puffer and Zachazewski's, can often be helpful in classifying injury, determining prognosis, and gauging rehabilitative progress.[62] Type 1 pain occurs after activity only; type 2 occurs during activity, but does not impair or restrict performance; type 3 occurs during activity and is severe enough to interfere with performance; and type 4 is classified as chronic and unremitting. Nirschl's seven-phase pain scale is somewhat more useful because it separates the activities of daily living from sports performance (see Table 28.3).

General health questions should identify recurrent minor illness, sleep patterns, nutritional habits to include the use of supplements, and overall mood states that may provide clues to an overtrained state. Female athletes should be questioned about a history of stress fractures, menstrual abnormalities, and eating habits.[40] These findings are manifestations of the "female athlete triad"; early identification of the triad—eating disorders, amenorrhea, and osteoporosis—allows for interventions that may prevent considerable morbidity.[11,46] Determining an athlete's training intensity and goals helps the physician design a rehabilitation program that fits the patient's athletic objectives.

The physical examination seeks to identify the focal problem and uncover contributing intrinsic abnormalities.[51] Using Macintyre and Lloyd-Smith's concept of *victims and culprits* can be helpful in detailed examination.[48] The victim represents the presenting problem, while the culprit is the dysfunction or anatomic abnormality that created the victim. An example would be gastroc–soleus inflexibility (culprit) contributing to plantar fasciitis (victim). The entire extremity and kinetic chain need to be thoroughly examined for possible "culprits" when evaluating a specific injury. Leg length discrepancies, sacral rotations, hamstring inflexibility, excessive forefoot pronation, and gluteal weakness are only a few of the many potential *culprits* in this case. Assessment of core strength and upper and lower quarter stability should be included. Failure to identify muscle imbalance patterns and structural malalignment often sabotages an otherwise well-planned rehabilitation program.

TABLE 28.3
Nirschl Pain Phase Scale of Athlete's Overuse Injuries

Phase 1. Stiffness or mild soreness after activity. Pain is usually gone within 24 hours.

Phase 2. Stiffness or mild soreness before activity that is relieved by warm-up. Symptoms are not present during activity, but return after, lasting up to 48 hours.

Phase 3. Stiffness or mild soreness before specific sports or occupational activity. Pain is partially relieved by warm-up. It is minimally present during activity, but does not cause the athlete to alter activity.

Phase 4. Pain is similar to, but more intense than, phase 3 pain. Phase 4 pain causes the athlete to alter the performance of the activity. Mild pain occurs with activities of daily living, but does not cause a major change in them.

Phase 5. Significant (moderate or greater) pain before, during, and after activity, causing alteration of activity. Pain occurs with activities of daily living, but does not cause a major change in them.

Phase 6. Phase 5 pain that persists even with complete rest. Phase 6 pain disrupts simple activities of daily living and prohibits doing household chores.

Phase 7. Phase 6 pain that also disrupts sleep consistently. Pain is aching in nature and intensifies with activity.

Clinical Pearl

Examination of overuse injuries should include a thorough screening of flexibility and strength through the kinetic chain including an assessment of core strength and upper and lower quarter stability.

Dynamic testing should include observation of walking, sport and recreational exercises, and sports-specific mechanics. Observational analysis is most commonly employed clinically. Video analysis can be helpful in refractory cases. Finally, the examination should include an evaluation of the sport and recreational exercise shoes, to include past and present shoe wear and orthotics.

Radiographs aid diagnosis and can rule out related injuries such as fractures, tumors, intra-articular abnormalities, or heterotopic calcification. Ultrasound is an evolving diagnostic tool in the outpatient setting and can provide real-time imaging to assist clinicians at the time of patient evaluation (see Chapter 19).[42,52] Only a minority of overuse injuries, including combined pathoanatomic presentations or those with clinical evidence of major soft-tissue disruption, require more advanced imaging techniques, such as MRI or nuclear bone scans. Electromyographic studies and intracompartmental testing can assist when clinically warranted (see Chapters 21 and 23).

28.4.2 Control Pain and Inflammation

Inflammation is required for proper healing of sports injuries; however, an excessive or prolonged inflammatory response can become self-perpetuating and self-destructive. Therefore, controlling or modifying pain and inflammation is traditionally one of the primary goals of initial overuse injury treatment. The literature on overuse injuries, however, has consistently questioned the timing and role of inflammation, with multiple studies confirming the degenerative, noninflammatory nature of tendinopathies.[2,32,33] Numerous authors have subsequently challenged the role of interventions, such as nonsteroidal anti-inflammatory drugs (NSAIDs), in overuse injury management, citing the distinct lack of evidence-based research to guide clinical decision making.[34,38,68] In addition, the choice to use NSAIDs is not without risk as gastrointestinal complications are not uncommon, and NSAIDs have been associated with exertional hyponatremia.[26,43,53,59]

The classic approach to injury initial management, in particular for acute macrotraumatic injuries, is rest, ice, compression, and elevation. Prevention/protection, modalities, and medications are added to the acronym to create PRICEMM (protection, rest, ice, compression, elevation, medication, modalities), which has the potential to be particularly effective in managing overuse injuries. Nearly, all protocols for managing overuse injuries begin with the athlete abstaining from or modifying exposure to abusive activity. Rest, however, does not mean halting all activities. Relative rest protects the injured area, while avoiding the consequences of deconditioning and disuse atrophy. To prevent reinjury and ensure better compliance with rehabilitation programs, we emphasize what recuperating athletes *can do* to enhance healing and maintain fitness rather than what they cannot do. Athletes with lower-extremity injuries, for example, can frequently duplicate land workouts in a swimming pool or an antigravity treadmill.[57]

Clinical Pearl

Relative rest during injury rehabilitation does not necessarily equate to complete rest. Limited conditioning, cross-training, and sports activity may be allowable provided any pain is limited to a mild level and there is no alteration of sports or gait mechanics.

Modalities and medications may assist in controlling pain and inflammation and are frequently incorporated in the treatment of overuse injuries. Their role, however, has yet to be clearly defined.[66,68] Almekinders, in a detailed review of the literature on tendinitis, concluded that current treatment methods may not significantly alter the natural history of disease.[5] We use both approaches to assist in pain control so the patient can make a quick transition from relative rest to rehabilitative sport and recreational exercises. Useful modalities to control inflammation include cryotherapy, iontophoresis, phonophoresis, pulsed ultrasound, and low-level laser (see Chapter 31). When we choose to utilize NSAIDs, we prescribe as the literature currently recommends, for as short as possible with goal being to control pain to facilitate therapeutic sport and recreational exercises.[54]

Though corticosteroids are potent anti-inflammatories commonly prescribed in managing athletic injuries, their employment in treating overuse injuries is controversial, and their role is not clearly supported by objective data.[38,68] They can be used, however, to treat patients who have significant (Nirschl pain phase 5 or greater) or refractory pain. We administer them with caution, however, because corticosteroids in oral and injectable forms are thought to decrease collagen and ground substance production, weaken the tensile strength of tendons, and ultimately result in poorer healing.[38] When injecting steroids near a weight-bearing tendon or intra-articulary, we restrict sports participation for 2–3 weeks. Injecting into weight-bearing tendons is contraindicated. While we do not use corticosteroid injections more than three times a year for an athlete, there is no rigorous research to support or contraindicate more or less frequent use.

Clinical Pearl

Following a steroid injection, the activity of that extremity is restricted for 2–3 weeks. Controlled cross-training is often permissible.

28.4.3 Promote Healing

All too often after successful efforts to control pain and inflammation have been achieved, the runner prematurely returns to participation and is reinjured. In fact, prior studies have demonstrated that failure to properly rehabilitate an athlete after an initial injury is a leading risk factor for recurrent injury.[23,25] Athletes and health-care professionals often fail to appreciate that rest and anti-inflammatory medications do not necessarily result in tissue healing. Clinicians can ensure a successful return to sports only when pain and inflammation control overlaps aggressive efforts to promote healing.[57]

Healing involves the deposition, proliferation, and maturation of collagen-creating, vascular elements and fibroblasts in injured tissue. This healing cascade is best facilitated through a combination of site-specific rehabilitative sport and recreational exercises and general cardiovascular conditioning, the goal of which is to restore injured tissue to normal or near-normal function.[36] Early controlled sport and recreational exercises enhance tissue oxygenation and nutrition, minimize unnecessary atrophy, and align collagen fibers to meet eventual sports-induced stresses. Progress through rehabilitative programs is best accomplished under the direction of a physical therapist or a certified athletic trainer, since each individual regimen is based on the particular injury and the athlete's specific needs.

Successful rehabilitative sport and recreational exercise programs incorporate flexibility and full-motion strengthening of the injured tissue as well as addressing the strength and stability of the entire kinetic chain. For example, the athlete with patellofemoral syndrome typically requires attention to quadriceps and hamstring strength and flexibility. However, complete rehabilitation may require assessment and rehabilitation of the athlete's *core stability*. Weakness in the hip adductors can cause patellar tracking problems by increasing internal rotation of the femur and dynamically increasing the athlete's Q angle. Strength deficits in the abdominal musculature or paraspinous muscles may also predispose the athlete to lower-extremity injury. As closed chain, functional sport and recreational exercises recruit muscles in a more physiologic motor pattern; they are preferred in both core strengthening and in rehabilitation of the primary injured tissue.

Clinical Pearl

A comprehensive rehabilitation prescription should address flexibility (static and dynamic), strength (concentric and eccentric, open and closed chain), core strength, upper and lower quarter stability, general conditioning, and sports-specific training.

Although literature regarding the effectiveness of stretching in injury prevention and enhancing performance remains inconclusive, flexibility in athletes is still commonly employed following soft-tissue injury. Stretching is believed to improve muscle tendon length, to prevent shortening, and to encourage deposition of collagen in a more normal orientation.[6,21]

Good general body conditioning is also important in the promotion of injury healing because it

- Increases regional perfusion through central and peripheral aerobics
- Provides neurologic stimulus to the injured tissue through neurophysiologic synergy and overflow
- Minimizes weakness of adjacent uninjured tissue (decreases or eliminates destructive domino effect)
- Minimizes negative psychological effects
- Minimizes unwanted fat and helps control weight

A good *general body* conditioning program incorporates strength training of uninjured tissues with appropriate forms of aerobic sport and recreational exercises. Sport and recreational exercises commonly used for such conditioning include stationary bicycling, stair climbing, upper body ergometry, and water workouts.

Occasionally, the athlete with an overuse injury will not respond to the typical treatment regimen. These individuals are at high risk of developing a chronic overuse injury, most typically a chronic tendinopathy, which classically responds very poorly to all forms of conservative treatment. However, consistent evidence indicates that a significant percentage of these injuries will respond to eccentric rehabilitation. The most compelling evidence involves patients with chronic Achilles tendinosis.[1,4,50] While the exact healing mechanism of eccentric sport and recreational exercises is not known, preliminary data suggest that it may alter the neovascular proliferation observed in chronic tendinopathy.[3] Most importantly, eccentric sport and recreational exercise training has been demonstrated to facilitate Achilles tendon remodeling.[58]

In addition to eccentric sport and recreational exercises, there are several other interventions currently being utilized that appear to assist in healing by altering tendon structure and facilitating healing. Extracorporeal shock wave therapy has been a controversial intervention in the sports medicine community for treating recalcitrant tendinopathies.[69] Despite early mixed results, there is evidence to support further study in this area, as this modality remains a viable alternative for select cases.[64] Topical nitroglycerin has also been studied for treating tendinopathies, with some evidence to suggest success in treating the runner with chronic Achilles tendinopathy.[31,50,60] The exact roles for these interventions have yet to be determined.

Perhaps the most exciting and promising area in musculoskeletal sports medicine is the emerging field of orthobiologic therapy.[45,67] Agents such as platelet-rich plasma and autologous blood are thought to augment and accelerate the healing response in tendons, as well as ligaments and joints. There have been several studies in elite and recreational athletes evaluating the success of these interventions, with mixed results.[22,41,44] While these interventions offer great promise, the current literature reflects a need for more randomized controlled trials to elucidate treatment algorithms and outcomes.[67]

Rehabilitative sport and recreational exercises generally restore an athlete's previous level of function. However, a few patients may fail to respond to rehabilitation and may require surgery. Patients who fail to improve with conservative therapy, however, should seek a second opinion to be sure that possible *culprits* have been identified and treated before surgery is considered. If surgery is necessary, it should seek to provide a better physiologic environment for renewed rehabilitative effort through resection of pathologic soft tissue and correction of underlying anatomic risk factors. We consider surgery for a patient when his or her

- Rehabilitative program has failed (after 3–6 months)
- Quality of life is unacceptable
- Weakness, atrophy, and dysfunction persist

28.4.4 Increase Fitness

Once healing and rehabilitative sport and recreational exercises have restored damaged tissues to normal strength, a patient's musculoskeletal system requires further strengthening to achieve the supernormal endurance and power required for the demands of sports. These exercises involve sports-specific rehabilitation and general body conditioning (see Chapter 39).[57]

A patient can begin these fitness exercises once he or she achieves pain-free range of motion, and strength and endurance tests indicate a return to the preinjury state. Sports-specific activities work the athlete's target tissues, providing neurophysiologic stimulus and redeveloping proprioceptive skills. Rehabilitation programs should be expanded to incorporate complex movements combining the sagittal, coronal, and transverse planes of motion. Sports-specific agility, speed, and skill drills such as plyometrics, interactive eccentric/concentric muscle loading, dynamic flexibility, anaerobic sprints, and interval training all coordinate interaction of the athlete's antagonistic and supporting muscles. More recently, an emphasis has also been placed on core stability as a component of the overall rehabilitation program of athletes. Proper control of postural stability and lumbopelvic motion is felt to result in less loading of peripheral structures.

28.4.5 Control Abuse

The final step of overuse injury management is to control force loads to the rehabilitated tissue. Controlling tissue overload necessitates modifying both intrinsic and extrinsic risk factors previously identified in the patient's history and physical examination. Effective control of tissue overload includes

- Improving the athlete's sports technique
- Bracing or taping the injured part
- Controlling the intensity and duration of the activity
- Appropriately modifying equipment

Improving the athlete's sports technique is critical since abnormal and improper biomechanics quickly promote reinjury. The information provided from a biomechanical gait analysis may provide subtle insights to correct form and assist a safe return. Bracing and taping can additionally assist in controlling abuse during rehabilitation, in particular when the athlete first resumes sports activity. We have successfully used bracing and taping techniques to treat patients with plantar fasciitis, shin splints, Achilles tendinosis, and patellar tendinopathy.

Training errors, excessive frequency, intensity, and duration, are the principal risk factors for overuse injuries. The clinician must emphasize that more is not always better and explain that overtraining precipitates injury and causes fatigue and decreased performance. Athletes should be encouraged to follow basic training principles of progression and periodization, which imply gradual increases in workload and training cycles that emphasize programmed rest.

Modifying equipment requires paying attention to shoes, sports-specific equipment, and playing or training surfaces. Subtle abnormalities in an athlete's foot biomechanics can contribute to numerous lower-extremity overuse injuries. Physicians should attempt to correct these abnormalities through rehabilitation, proper footwear, and, if necessary, custom orthotics. Lower-extremity injuries, such as plantar fasciitis and stress fractures, often result from poor or hard playing surfaces. An ideal playing surface provides adequate traction, cushion, and evenness so athletes can avoid excessive forces from repetitive pounding, twisting, and turning.[57]

28.4.6 Back in Action

Traditionally, athletes have been allowed to return to activity when they demonstrate full range of motion and when the injured extremity shows 80%–90% of the strength of the uninjured extremity (objectively measured with functional testing). These two criteria, however, are only minimums. Before an athlete returns to activity, the physician, coach, and trainer should consider two other questions:

- Does the athlete demonstrate sports-specific function?
- Is the athlete psychologically ready?

Clinical Pearl

Prior to returning to sports, the athlete should demonstrate normal flexibility and strength and sports-specific function and be psychologically ready.

TABLE 28.4
Relative Activity Modification Guidelines Patient Handout

Certain injuries (such as stress fractures, nerve trauma, or significant soft-tissue injury) necessitate complete avoidance of sport and recreational exercises. During this time, you may be able to participate in certain cross-training activities to maintain your fitness while you are healing. For our runners and sport and recreational exercise athletes, we recommend deep-water running as an ideal form of cross-training during the recovery period. Other lower-impact forms of cross-training such as the elliptical machine, stationary bike, and stair climber may also be utilized to maintain fitness. Discuss cross-training options with your physician so that an optimum level of fitness can be maintained.

While rehabilitating from certain other injuries, however, the athlete is often able to continue sport and recreational exercises at some level in spite of the presence of injury, but it is important not to exceed the appropriate level of sport and recreational exercises so that proper healing is not impeded. We have devised the following relative activity modification guidelines to assist the athlete in gauging how much sport and recreational exercises they can safely do during the recovery period. However, we emphasize that the instructions given by your physician remain the ultimate guidelines to avoid worsening an injury:

1. You may be able to run with some level of discomfort, but the pain should not exceed the mild level. We define mild pain as 0–3 on a 10-point scale. If certain activities cause moderate level pain (4, 5, and 6 on a 10-point scale), you must decrease activity so that sport and recreational exercises produce no more than mild pain. If pain is severe (7–10 on a 10-point scale), you should not run at all.
2. If you find that pain is present only at the beginning of activity and once you warm-up the pain has resolved, most often this represents mild soft-tissue injury. If, however, you find that there is a point at which pain becomes progressively worse, do not attempt to run beyond that point.
3. If you find that the pain causes you to limp or change your gait mechanics in any way, in order to prevent worsening the injury, you must not run at all. Seek the advice of your physician.

Source: Adapted and used with permission from Wilder, R., The Runner's Clinic at UVa, http://www.medicine.virginia.edu/clinical/departments/physical-medicine-rehabilitation/clinical-services/Runners-page, accessed October 17, 2015.

When all involved are satisfied with the answers to these questions, the athlete can safely return to graduated activity. Return to sport and recreational exercises mandates ability to run within the *Relative Activity Modification Guidelines* (see Table 28.4).

28.5 PREHABILITATION AND THE PREPARTICIPATION EXAMINATION

Because overuse injuries can be so perplexing and frustrating to athletes, coaches, trainers, and health-care professionals, many authors have proposed strategies to prevent these injuries through risk factor identification and modification.[25] Kibler, a major proponent of *prehabilitation*, and others believe that physicians can use the preparticipation examination to identify an individual's weaknesses and flexibility deficits, so that preventative sport and recreational exercises may begin before injury occurs. One current strategy being employed in the sports and occupational athlete arena for *prehabilitation* is functional movement screening (FMS).

The FMS was first introduced in 2001 by Cook.[16] The FMS is a unique screening tool that has altered the paradigm of screening for static biomechanical deficiencies, to assessing functional movements. FMS assesses comprehensive movements and core stability to establish an individual's functional platform.

Preliminary studies on the FMS have demonstrated injury predictability in professional and collegiate athletes, firefighters, and military personnel.[47,55,61,70] Functional movement enhancement programs that address deficiencies identified by the FMS have lowered injury rates and reduced lost time due to injury.[55,61] This assessment tool fills the void between traditional pretraining/preplacement health screenings and performance tests by evaluating the individual in a dynamic and functional approach. The reliability of the FMS has been established in a recent study that reported high interrater reliability with weighted kappa values to range from 0.80 to 1.00.[56] At the DSMC, we presently incorporate FMS as a core tool in both the rehabilitative and *prehabilitative* phases of managing the sport and recreational exercise athlete.

28.6 CONCLUSION

The five-step overuse injury pyramid outlines a process of evaluation and management that we have found helpful in treating sport and recreational exercise athletes with overuse injuries. Along with *prehabilitation*, the pyramid provides a functional approach to these injuries, which offers patients the best chance for recovering from injury and maintaining an active life. The field of sports medicine is rapidly exploding with new tools and interventions including imaging modalities, exciting new orthobiologic therapies, and surgical interventions that offer promise to inured elite and recreational athletes. While diagnostic and interventional modalities and tools will alter future treatment algorithms, we believe the basic paradigm outlined in this chapter will remain consistent and helpful in guiding providers who care for injured athletes (Table 28.5).

TABLE 28.5
SORT: Key Recommendations for Practice

Clinical Recommendation	Evidence Rating	References
Corticosteroid injections may be useful for common overuse injuries, however, available evidence suggests their effect is small and short-lived.	Level A	[5, 38, 68]
When injecting corticosteroids near a weight-bearing tendon or introa-articularly, sports participation should be restricted for 2 weeks.	Level C; consensus opinion	[38]
Eccentric exercise has been demonstrated to be a first-line therapy for chronic tendinopathy.	Level B	[1,4,50]

REFERENCES

1. Alfredson H, Lorentzon R. Chronic Achilles tendinosis: Recommendations for treatment and prevention. *Sports Medicine.* 2000;29(2):135–146.
2. Alfredson H, Lorentzon R. Chronic tendon pain: No signs of chemical inflammation but high concentrations of the neurotransmitter glutamate. Implications for treatment? *Current Drug Targets.* 2002;3(1):43–54.
3. Alfredson H, Ohberg L, Forsgren S. Is vasculo-neural ingrowth the cause of pain in chronic Achilles tendinosis? An investigation using ultrasonography and colour Doppler, immunohistochemistry, and diagnostic injections. *Knee Surgery, Sports Traumatology, Arthroscopy.* 2003;11(5):334–338.
4. Alfredson H, Pietilä T, Jonsson P et al. Heavy-load eccentric calf muscle training for the treatment of chronic Achilles tendinosis. *American Journal of Sports Medicine.* 1998;26(3):360–366.
5. Almekinders LC, Temple JD. Etiology, diagnosis, and treatment of tendonitis: An analysis of the literature. *Medicine and Science in Sports & Sport and Recreational Exercise.* 1998;30(8):1183–1190.
6. Amadio PC. Tendon and Ligament, in Cohen IK, Diegelman RF, Lindblad WJ (eds.). *Wound Healing: Biomechanical and Clinical Aspects.* Philadelphia, PA: Saunders; 1992.
7. Arendt EA. Common musculoskeletal injuries in women. *Physician and Sportsmedicine.* 1996;24(7):39–48.
8. Arendt EA. Musculoskeletal injuries of the knee: Are females at greater risk? *Minnesota Medicine.* 2007; 90(6):38–40.
9. Baquie P, Brukner P. Injuries presenting to an Australian sports medicine centre: A 12-month study. *Clinical Journal of Sports Medicine.* 1997;7(1):28–31.
10. Beers A, Ryan M, Kasubuchi K et al. Effects of multi-modal physiotherapy, including hip abductor strengthening, in patients with iliotibial band friction syndrome. *Physiotherapy Canada.* 2008;60(2):180–188.
11. Bonci CM, Bonci LJ, Granger LR et al. National athletic trainers' association position statement: Preventing, detecting, and managing disordered eating in athletes. *Journal of Athletic Trainers.* 2008;43(1):80–108.
12. Brody DM. Sport and recreational exercise injuries. *Clinical Symposia (Summit, NJ: 1957).* 1980;32(4):1–36.
13. Brody DM. Sport and recreational exercise injuries. Prevention and management. *Clinical Symposia (Summit, NJ: 1957).* 1987;39(3):1–36.
14. Butcher JD, Zukowski CW, Brannen SJ et al. Patient profile, referral sources, and consultant utilization in a primary care sports medicine clinic. *Journal of Family Practice.* 1996;43(6):556–560.
15. Childress MA, O'Connor FG, Levine BD. Exertional collapse in the runner: Evaluation and management in fieldside and office-based settings. *Clinics in Sports Medicine.* 2010;29(3):459–476.
16. Cook G. (ed.). *Athletic Body Balance.* New York: Human Kinetics; 2001.
17. Cook J, Khan K. The treatment of resistant, painful tendinopathies results in frustration for athletes and health professionals alike. *American Journal of Sports Medicine.* 2003;31(2): 327–328; author reply 328.
18. Cosca DD, Navazio F. Common problems in endurance athletes. *American Family Physician.* 2007;76(2):237–244.
19. Cowan DN, Jones BH, Frykman PN et al. Rosenstein, and M.T. Rosenstein. Lower limb morphology and risk of overuse injury among male infantry trainees. *Medicine and Science in Sports & Sport and Recreational Exercise.* 1996;28(8):945–952.

20. Cowan DN, Jones BH, Robinson JR. Foot morphologic characteristics and risk of sport and recreational exercise-related injury. *Archives of Family Medicine*. 1993;2(7):773–777.
21. Day C, Khan K. Tendinopathy, in Wilder RP, O'Connor FG, Magrum E (eds.). *Sport and recreational exercise Medicine*. Monterey, CA: Healthy Learning; 2014.
22. de Vos RJ, Weir A, van Schie HT et al. Platelet-rich plasma injection for chronic Achilles tendinopathy: A randomized controlled trial. *Journal of the American Medical Association*. 2010;303(2):144–149.
23. Ekstrand J, Gillquist J. Soccer injuries and their mechanisms: A prospective study. *Medicine and Science in Sports & Sport and Recreational Exercise*. 1983;15(3):267–270.
24. Ferber R, Noehren B, Hamill J et al. Competitive female elite and recreational athletes with a history of iliotibial band syndrome demonstrate atypical hip and knee kinematics. *Journal of Orthopaedic Sports and Physical Therapy*. 2010;40(2):52–58.
25. Fields KB, Sykes JC, Walker KM et al. Prevention of sport and recreational exercise injuries. *Current Sports Medicine Report*. 2010;9(3):176–182.
26. Fournier PE, Leal S, Ziltener JL. Sports injuries and NSAID. *Revue Médicale Suisse*. 2008;4(166):1702–1705.
27. Fredericson M, Cookingham CL, Chaudhari AM et al. Hip abductor weakness in distance elite and recreational athletes with iliotibial band syndrome. *Clinical Journal of Sports Medicine*. 2000;10(3):169–175.
28. Fredericson M, Weir A. Practical management of iliotibial band friction syndrome in elite and recreational athletes. *Clinical Journal of Sports Medicine*. 2006;16(3):261–268.
29. Fredericson M, Wolf C. Iliotibial band syndrome in elite and recreational athletes: Innovations in treatment. *Sports Medicine*. 2005;35(5):451–459.
30. Herring SA, Nilson KL. Introduction to overuse injuries. *Clinics in Sports Medicine*. 1987;6(2):225–239.
31. Hunte G, Lloyd-Smith R. Topical glyceryl trinitrate for chronic Achilles tendinopathy. *Clinical Journal of Sports Medicine*. 2005;15(2):116–117.
32. Kaeding K, Best T. Tendinosis: Pathophysiology and nonoperative treatment. *Sports Health: A Multidisciplinary Approach*. 2009;1(4):284–292.
33. Khan K, Cook J. The painful nonruptured tendon: Clinical aspects. *Clinics in Sports Medicine*. 2003;22(4):711–725.
34. Khan KM, Cook JL, Kannus P et al. Time to abandon the "tendinitis" myth. *British Medical Journal*. 2002;324(7338):626–627.
35. Kibler WB, Chandler TJ, Pace BK. Principles of rehabilitation after chronic tendon injuries. *Clinics in Sports Medicine*. 1992;11(3):661–671.
36. Kibler WB, Chandler TJ, Stracener ES. Musculoskeletal adaptations and injuries due to overtraining. *Sport and Recreational Exercise and Sport Sciences Reviews*. 1992;20:99–126.
37. Koplan JP, Rothenberg RB, Jones EL. The natural history of sport and recreational exercise: A 10-yr follow-up of a cohort of elite and recreational athletes. *Medicine and Science in Sports & Sport and Recreational Exercise*. 1995;27(8):1180–1184.
38. Leadbetter, WB. Anti-inflammatory therapy in sports injury. The role of nonsteroidal drugs and corticosteroid injection. *Clinics in Sports Medicine*. 1995;14(2):353–410.
39. Leadbetter, WB. Cell-matrix response in tendon injury. *Clinics in Sports Medicine*. 1992;11(3):533–578.
40. Lebrun, CM. The female athlete triad: What's a doctor to do? *Current Sports Medicine Report*. 2007;6(6):397–404.
41. Lee TG, Ahmad TS. Intralesional autologous blood injection compared to corticosteroid injection for treatment of chronic plantar fasciitis. A prospective, randomized, controlled trial. *Foot & Ankle International*. 2007;28(9):984–990.
42. Leininger AP, Fields KB. Ultrasonography in early diagnosis of metatarsal bone stress fractures. Sensitivity and specificity. *Journal of Rheumatology*. 2010;37(7):1543; author reply 1543.
43. Lilly KF. Athletes, NSAID, coxibs, and the gastrointestinal tract. *Current Sports Medicine Report*. 2010;9(2):103–105.
44. Logan LR, Klamar K, Leon J et al. Autologous blood injection and botulinum toxin for resistant plantar fasciitis accompanied by spasticity. *American Journal of Physical Medicine & Rehabilitation*. 2006;85(8):699–703.
45. Lopez-Vidriero E, Goulding KA, Simon DA et al. The use of platelet-rich plasma in arthroscopy and sports medicine: Optimizing the healing environment. *Arthroscopy*. 2010;26(2):269–278.
46. Lynch SL, Hoch AZ. The female runner: Gender specifics. *Clinics in Sports Medicine*. 2010;29(3):477–498.
47. Macera, CA. Lower extremity injuries in elite and recreational athletes. Advances in prediction. *Sports Medicine*. 1992;13(1):50–57.
48. Macintyre J, Lloyd-Smith DR. Overuse sport and recreational exercise injuries, in Renström P.A. (ed.). *Sports Injuries—Basic Principles of Prevention and Care*. Boston, MA: Blackwell Scientific Publications; 1993, pp. 139–160.
49. Macintyre JG, Taunton JE, Clement DB. Sport and recreational exercise injuries: A clinical study of 4173 cases. *Clinical Journal of Sports Medicine*. 1991;1:81.
50. Mafi N, Lorentzon R, Alfredson H. Superior short-term results with eccentric calf muscle training compared to concentric training in a randomized prospective multicenter study on patients with chronic Achilles tendinosis. *Knee Surgery, Sports Traumatology, Arthroscopy*. 2001;9(1):42–47.
51. Magrum E, Wilder RP. Evaluation of the injured runner. *Clinics in Sports Medicine*. 2010;29(3):331–345.
52. Malanga GA, Dentico R, Halperin JS. Ultrasonography of the hip and lower extremity. *Physical Medicine & Rehabilitation Clinics of North America*. 2010;21(3):533–547.
53. Matheson GO, Macintyre JG, Taunton JE et al. Musculoskeletal injuries associated with physical activity in older adults. *Medicine and Science in Sports & Sport and Recreational Exercise*. 1989;21(4):379–385.
54. Mehallo CJ, Drezner JA, Bytomski JR. Practical management: Nonsteroidal antiinflammatory drug (NSAID) use in athletic injuries. *Clinical Journal of Sports Medicine*. 2006;16(2):170–174.
55. Minick KI, Kiesel KB, Burton L et al. Interrater reliability of the functional movement screen. *Journal of Strength and Conditioning Research*. 2010;24(2):479–486.
56. O'Connor FG, Nirschl RP, Sobel J. Five-step treatment of overuse injuries. *Physician and Sports Medicine*. 1992; 21(7):128–142.
57. O'Connor FG, Wilder RP, Nirschl RP. Basic management concepts, in Wilder RP, O'Connor FG, Magrum E. (eds.). *Running Medicine, 2nd Edition*. Monterey, CA: Healthy Learning; 2014.
58. Ohberg L, Lorentzon R, Alfredson H. Eccentric training in patients with chronic Achilles tendinosis: Normalised tendon structure and decreased thickness at follow up. *British Journal of Sports Medicine*. 2004;38(1):8–11; discussion 11.
59. Page AJ, Reid SA, Speedy DB et al. Sport and recreational exercise-associated hyponatremia, renal function, and nonsteroidal antiinflammatory drug use in an ultraendurance mountain run. *Clinical Journal of Sports Medicine*. 2007;17(1):43–48.

60. Paoloni JA, Appleyard R, Murrell GAC. Topical glyceryl trinitrate treatment of chronic noninsertional achilles tendinopathy. A randomized, double-blind, placebo-controlled trial. *Journal of Bone and Joint Surgery—American Volume.* 2004;86-A(5):916–922.
61. Peate WF, Bates G, Lunda K et al. Core strength: A new model for injury prediction and prevention. *Journal of Occupational Medicine and Toxicology.* 2007;2:3–11.
62. Puffer JC, Zachazewski JE. Management of overuse injuries. *American Family Physician.* 1988;38(3):225–232.
63. Purvis D, Gonsalves S, Deuster PA. Physiological and psychological fatigue in extreme conditions: Overtraining and elite athletes. *Physical Medicine & Rehabilitation.* 2010;2(5):442–450.
64. Rasmussen S, Christensen M, Mathiesen I et al. Shock-wave therapy for chronic Achilles tendinopathy: A double-blind, randomized clinical trial of efficacy. *Acta Orthopaedica.* 2008;79(2):249–256.
65. Rauh MJ, Macera CA, Trone DW, Reis JP, Shaffer RA. Selected static anatomic measures predict overuse injuries in female recruits. *Military Medicine.* 2010;175(5): 329–335.
66. Rivenburgh DW. Physical modalities in the treatment of tendon injuries. *Clinics in Sports Medicine.* 1992;11(3): 645–659.
67. Sanchez M, Anitua E, Orive G et al. Platelet-rich therapies in the treatment of orthopaedic sport injuries. *Sports Medicine.* 2009;39(5):345–354.
68. Scott A, Khan KM, Roberts CR et al. What do we mean by the term "inflammation"? A contemporary basic science update for sports medicine. *British Journal of Sports Medicine.* 2004;38(3):372–380.
69. Seil R, Wilmes P, Nuhrenborger C. Extracorporeal shock wave therapy for tendinopathies. *Expert Review of Medical Devices.* 2006;3(4):463–470.
70. Strock M, Burton L. Functional testing of military athletes. *Journal of Special Operations Medicine.* 2007;7(2):104–108.
71. van Mechelen, W. Sport and recreational exercise injuries. A review of the epidemiological literature. *Sports Medicine.* 1992;14(5):320–335.
72. Walter SD, Hart LE, McIntosh JM et al. The Ontario cohort study of sport and recreational exercise-related injuries. *Archives of Internal Medicine.* 1989;149(11):2561–2564.
73. Wen DY. Risk factors for overuse injuries in elite and recreational athletes. *Current Sports Medicine Report.* 2007;6(5):307–313.
74. Wen DY, Puffer JC, Schmalzried TP. Lower extremity alignment and risk of overuse injuries in elite and recreational athletes. *Medicine and Science in Sports and Sport and Recreational Exercise.* 1997;29(10):1291–1298.
75. Wilson JJ, Best TM. Common overuse tendon problems: A review and recommendations for treatment. *American Family Physician.* 2005;72(5):811–818.
76. Zaryski C, Smith DJ. Training principles and issues for ultra-endurance athletes. *Current Sports Medicine Report.* 2005;4(3):165–170.

29 Medications and Substances

Scott Flinn

CONTENTS

TABLE 29.1
Key Clinical Considerations

1. Dietary supplements do not require safety and efficacy evaluation and are not held to the same FDA quality control standards.
2. When prescribing medications to elite-level athletes, providers should frequently review the WADA, USADA, and NCAA list of prohibited medications.
3. Some medications on banned lists may be used by obtaining a therapeutic use exemption (TUE) through the sport's governing body.
4. Creatine supplementation has been shown to improve maximal weight lift, performance in very short cycling sprints (less than 10 s), and increase fat-free body mass.[19,68]
5. A recent meta-analysis found that compared with placebo, glucosamine, chondroitin, and the combination did not reduce joint pain or have an impact on joint space.[70]

29.1 INTRODUCTION

Athletes use various pharmacological or nutritional substances in an effort to improve performance and speed recovery from injury. Medications can be over the counter or prescribed. Other substances are sold over the counter as dietary supplements, some of which may be banned by sports governing bodies or be illegal. According to the 1994 Dietary Health and Supplement Health Education Act, substances can be sold without U.S. Food and Drug Administration (FDA) approval as long as the products are labeled and sold as dietary supplements and the label makes no claim as a drug.[25] These substances do not require evaluation for safety or efficacy and are not held to the same quality control standards as FDA-approved drugs.[12] Because the content and purity of these products are not regulated, the product may contain variable amounts of the ingredients listed. For example, a recent study on vitamin D supplements found potency ranging from 9% to 146% of the labeled amount.[41] The authors noted that U.S. Pharmacopeia–verified products are more accurate and less variable (Table 29.1).

29.2 EVALUATING THE EFFICACY OF MEDICATIONS AND SUBSTANCES

Medications and substances can improve performance by affecting one or more of six major components of fitness: aerobic fitness, anaerobic fitness, strength, body composition, psychological factors, and injury recovery. Aerobic fitness is especially important in endurance events and is the ability to produce work using aerobic metabolism that needs oxygen and generally lasts longer than 1 minute and may last for hours. Aerobic fitness comprises two parts, maximal aerobic power and aerobic capacity. Anaerobic fitness activities are fueled primarily through anaerobic metabolism and generally last less than 1 minute. Maximum strength refers to the amount of power that can be generated in a brief burst and is fueled by anaerobic metabolism. It is usually measured by the one repetition maximum. Body composition can affect performance by increasing lean muscle mass so there is more power and less weight that has to be carried in the athletic maneuver. Decreased perceptions of fatigue and pain are psychological factors that can affect performance. Enhanced healing of injuries and quicker recovery from training promote a more rapid return to training and maintenance of fitness.

29.3 COMPETITION CONSIDERATIONS

Athletes are constantly looking for a competitive edge in order to improve their performance and defeat the competition. In an effort to do so, they will try different medications and substances that they think will give them an advantage, even though the product has not been shown to be efficacious, may have serious side effects, and may be banned by that sport's governing body. In an attempt to keep the playing field level, various amateur and professional organizations have instituted drug policies targeted toward substances that may be harmful, illegal, and/or give an unfair competitive advantage. For example, the International Olympic Committee (IOC) regulates substances through the World Anti-Doping Agency (WADA). The U.S. Anti-Doping Agency was formed in 2000 as an independent anti-doping organization for Olympic sports in the United States. The list of banned substances for the IOC can be viewed on the WADA website at http://www.wada-ama.org/en/world-anti-doping-program/sports-and-anti-doping-organizations/international-standards/prohibited-list/.[74] For National Collegiate Athletic Association sports, the policies and lists can be found at http://www.ncaa.org/health-and-safety/policy/drug-testing.[50] Because the lists are continually changing, physicians caring for athletes in these or other organizations should always consult the governing body prior to writing a prescription or suggesting over-the-counter remedies.

Currently, athletes are usually tested through random urine samples, though in the future, hair or blood samples may also be used.

The more commonly used medications and substances are reviewed here. Specific attention is directed to any proven efficacy on performance, safety and side effects, and permission of use by relevant governing bodies (see Table 29.2).

29.4 ANABOLIC STEROIDS, TESTOSTERONE, AND LOW TESTOSTERONE

Anabolic steroids build lean muscle mass and strength when used with a proper training regimen and diet.[1,8,28,30,67] This effect is increased with supraphysiologic doses. Anabolic steroids do not appear to directly improve aerobic power or capacity other than through increases in lean muscle mass. There is evidence that steroids improve healing and allow faster recovery, which enables an increased training volume.[5]

Anabolic steroids increase the risk of myocardial infarction, due in part to their effects on increased blood pressure and adverse effect on lipid profile, particularly by greatly lowering high-density lipoprotein.[26,31] Steroids also induce hirsutism in females[52] and are dose dependent associated with inappropriate increased aggression.[61,53] Testosterone also hastens the closure of epiphyses, which is significant given the studies suggesting up to 4% of high school

TABLE 29.2
Medications and Substances Effects

Medication/Substance	Proven Positive Effects	Proven Negative Effects	Allowable for Competition
Anabolic steroids	Increases lean body mass, improves strength	Increased risk of premature cardiovascular death, hypertension, hirsutism in women, gynecomastia in men	No
Androstenedione and anabolic precursors	None	Similar to the previous entry except no proven early death	No
B-adrenergic receptor agonists, albuterol	Treatment of EIB and other forms of asthma	Tremor, anxiety, palpitations	Yes with TUE
Erythropoietin	Improves oxygen-carrying capacity, aerobic power, aerobic capacity, prolonged time to exhaustion	Myocardial infarction, stroke, renal failure, death	No
Caffeine	Prolonged time to exhaustion	Anxiety, diarrhea	Yes in moderate amounts
NSAIDs	Pain relief	GI bleed Cardiac events	Yes
Creatine	Increases lean body mass, improves burst strength activities	None	Yes
Glucosamine/ chondroitin	None	None	Yes
Human growth hormone	Increases lean body mass, anaerobic capacity	Acromegaly, fluid retention, left ventricular concentric hypertrophy, insulin resistance, abnormal cartilage growth	No
Ephedrine	Improves anaerobic performance and run times in middle distance	Case reports of death and myocardial infarction, anxiety, agitation, palpitations	Yes, check organizing body limits
Pseudoephedrine	None	Similar to ephedrine but no case reports of death/MI	Yes, check organizing body limits

Note: EIB, exercise-induced bronchospasm; GI, gastrointestinal; MI, myocardial infarction; NSAIDs, nonsteroidal anti-inflammatory drugs; TUE, therapeutic use exemption.

students have used anabolic steroids, with half of them starting before the age of 14.[20,63]

Clinical Pearl

Anabolic steroids increase lean muscle mass and are helpful in patients with androgen deficiency, HIV, and other specific conditions but are hazardous and illegal for use for patients without these conditions who are looking to improve athletic performance.

All anabolic steroids and their precursors are banned by WADA, the NCAA, and various other organizations. Additionally, they are a Schedule III controlled substance in the United States, and inappropriate prescribing or usage has resulted in criminal charges. Masking agents are sometimes used to avoid detection during testing, and these masking agents have also been placed on the banned list. Hair testing may provide a more suitable method in the future. Androgen receptor modulators may be developed, which can target specific tissues to get the beneficial effects while limiting adverse effects.

Testosterone decreases as men age though the decline is modest and the clinical consequences have not been well established. It is not known if testosterone treatment reverses decline in function due to aging or if treatment exacerbates testosterone-dependent problem, such as those that occur with the prostate. In two longitudinal studies, testosterone decreased in men in their 60s, 70s, and 80s, and free testosterone decreased even more so.[29,66] Although not causally proven, there are similarities between changes in men as they age and in men with hypogonadism. These similarities include decline in muscle, increase in fat, and decline in muscle strength.[37,49] Interestingly, in hypogonadal men, treating with testosterone enanthate, which is an intramuscular form, improved bench press by 22% and squat by 45%, while treating with transdermal testosterone had no effect on strength.[9,62] Other possible consequences of low testosterone include decline in sexual function, decreased bone mineral density, anemia, and metabolic syndrome.[18,38,56,62]

The Endocrine Society published an evidenced-based clinical practice guideline for testosterone replacement in adult men with testosterone deficiency.[59] They suggest testosterone therapy only for men that have tested low on more than one occasion and have symptoms of deficiency such as decreased libido, depressed mood, anemia, or osteoporosis (SORT C). They recommend that testing should occur first thing in the morning and be repeated twice due to normal variation. If the tests are consistently under 200 ng/dL, pituitary or testicular disease should first be ruled out before diagnosing low testosterone. When considering replacement therapy, they recommend that the target be lower than in younger men in the range of 300–400 ng/dL. The risk/benefit of testosterone therapy must be weighed when determining to initiate and continue therapy. Although prostate cancer is partly testosterone dependent, to date, there have been no definitive studies that show that testosterone replacement therapy has increased the rate of prostate cancer.[22,59] However, the prostate should first be examined and a prostate-specific antigen (PSA) checked and be below 4 ng/mL or below 3 ng/mL if risk factors are present. The exam and PSA should be rechecked 3 months after starting therapy.

There are a number of methods to administer testosterone. Oral supplementation does not work because of the first pass effect as it is metabolized in the liver. Intramuscular shots, gels, buccal tablets, subcutaneous pellets, and a nasal gel are available. Transdermal patches are not currently available in the United States due to skin irritation.

29.5 ANDROSTENEDIONE AND DEHYDROEPIANDROSTERONE

Both androstenedione and dehydroepiandrosterone (DHEA) are precursors to androgens and have been used in an attempt to boost testosterone levels. Androstenedione is one of the few oral substances that are converted into testosterone when ingested. Although it has been shown to increase both testosterone and estradiol after high doses, double-blinded studies have failed to demonstrate any significant change in lean body mass or strength.[69]

DHEA is naturally secreted by the adrenal glands and peaks in puberty. It was banned as a drug by the FDA but still is available as a supplement.[65] When subjects were given DHEA, it did not increase androgen levels in older men but did in older women.[64] DHEA supplementation in younger men increased androstenedione but not testosterone and did not appear to improve protein metabolism.[73] There are few proven side effects from androstenedione and DHEA. Both are currently banned by the NCAA and IOC.

29.6 BETA-ADRENERGIC RECEPTOR AGONISTS

Albuterol and salmeterol are beta2-agonists, which are used widely as bronchodilators for the treatment of many types of asthma, including exercise-induced asthma. Clenbuterol, available by prescription in some countries, is a longer-acting oral β2-agonist. There is some evidence in animal studies that clenbuterol in high doses increases lean body mass and decreases adipose tissue.[55] A study on salbutamol showed increased quadriceps and hamstring strength, while another study on oral albuterol showed strength gains in isokinetic strength training of the knee after 6 weeks of therapy.[15,46] Studies looking to preserve muscle strength in astronauts have shown some benefit from albuterol and exercise.[13,14]

Side effects from albuterol are similar to other sympathomimetics and include tremor, palpitations, tachycardia, and anxiety. Because of their potential ergogenic effects, clenbuterol in all forms and all oral beta-adrenergic medications are banned by the IOC and NCAA. Inhaled forms are allowed with appropriate documentation. Of interest is that the percentage of U.S. Olympic athletes who claimed exercise-induced asthma and were able to use the inhaled products doubled from the 1984 Summer Olympics to over 20% of athletes in the 1996 Summer Games.[72]

29.7 RECOMBINANT ERYTHROPOIETIN AND BLOOD DOPING

By using either recombinant erythropoietin (rEPO) or blood doping, athletes are able to raise their red blood cell mass to improve performance by increasing their oxygen-carrying capacity. This improves both maximal aerobic power and aerobic capacity, allowing longer time to exhaustion.[58] rEPO can last up to six times longer than native human EPO, and the newer continuous erythropoietin receptor activators (CERAs) last up to 20 times longer, providing much greater convenience for patients and allowing for once monthly dosing.[43]

The major immediate risk with blood doping is a transfusion reaction. Both blood doping and rEPO can cause hemoglobin levels to rise abnormally high; hematocrits over 55% can cause hyperviscosity syndrome and sludging of the blood leading to organ failure, stroke, myocardial infarction, and death.[21] Both blood doping and the blood stimulants rEPO and CERA are banned by the IOC and NCAA.

29.8 CAFFEINE

During both aerobic and anaerobic activity, caffeine in usual doses enhances performance, but its effects on strength and power are unclear.[11] It may prolong the time to exhaustion by decreasing perceived exertion.[2]

Clinical Pearl

Caffeine in a usual dosage equal to one or two cups of coffee is legal for use by most governing authorities and does have performance-enhancing capabilities.

However, its effectiveness may not be as great in habitual users or in hot humid environments. There are few side effects to caffeine in normal dosage, though with increased dosage, restlessness, anxiety, diarrhea, and insomnia are common. It does not appear to increase the risk of heat injury.[54] Caffeine is allowed by the NCAA and IOC in usual dosages, which equate to about two cups of coffee.

29.9 NONSTEROIDAL ANTI-INFLAMMATORY DRUGS

Nonsteroidal anti-inflammatory drugs (NSAIDs) are available over the counter and in prescription form and are commonly used to treat acute and chronic injuries. They are thought to meditate the pain and inflammation of injury through their effect on prostaglandins. Their effect on prostaglandins likewise influences their side effect profile, specifically increasing the risk of a serious gastrointestinal (GI) bleed even with short-term use, and with an increased risk of a myocardial infarction.[33,57]

Patients appearing to be at increased risk for a GI bleed include patients with concurrent *Helicobacter pylori* infections and those on medications such as anticoagulants, including aspirin, and corticosteroids.[23,40,48] Many methods that have been attempted to reduce this risk of GI bleed including using COX-2 selective NSAIDs, proton pump inhibitors (PPI), misoprostol, H2 receptor antagonists, and *H. pylori* eradication with variable success.[36]

In addition to GI bleeding risk, some patients have cardiovascular risk and may be on blood thinners. Table 29.2 summarizes the current evidence-based recommendations. Overall, using acetaminophen or limiting the duration of NSAIDs to a few days is the best strategy. If NSAIDs are needed for longer than a few days, the addition of a PPI and/or switching to a COX-2 selective NSAID seems to be the best option. If patients have an increased cardiovascular risk as defined as those with a history of ischemic heart disease, cerebrovascular, or peripheral arterial disease or whose Framingham 10-year risk is greater than 10%, naproxen seems to be the safest choice at this time. However, GI risk must be taken into account as naproxen does increase the risk of a GI bleed. If the patient has risk factors for a GI bleed, such as a history of nonbleeding ulcers or concomitant corticosteroid use, PPIs should be added to the NSAID. If there is no cardiovascular risk, consider a COX-2 for its lower rate of GI bleed; otherwise consider naproxen and a PPI. For the highest-risk GI patients, those with a history of a previous bleeding ulcer, use of a COX-2 plus a PPI may be prudent, even in the face of positive cardiovascular risk factors because the risk of a fatal bleed may be higher than a cardiovascular event. In order to reduce GI bleed risk in patients on chronic NSAID therapy, consideration should be given to *H. pylori* eradication[45] (see Table 29.3).

TABLE 29.3
Limiting NSAID toxicity by NSAID Choice and Adjuvant Treatment

	Negative Cardiovascular Risk	Positive Cardiovascular Risk	Positive Cardiovascular Risk on ASA or Blood Thinners
Negative GI bleed risk	Nonselective NSAID	Naproxen + PPI	Naproxen + PPI
Positive GI bleed risk	COX-2 or nonselective + PPI	Naproxen + PPI	Naproxen + PPI or COX-2 + PPI
History of GI bleed	COX-2 + PPI	COX-2 + PPI	COX-2 + PPI

Notes: In general, NSAIDs should be avoided if possible in patients with a GI bleed risk, cardiovascular risk over 10%, and in patients on blood thinners including aspirin. ASA, aspirin; COX, cyclooxygenase; GI, gastrointestinal; NSAID, nonsteroidal anti-inflammatory drugs; PPI, proton pump inhibitor

29.10 CREATINE

Creatine is a naturally occurring organic acid stored in skeletal muscle. Supplementation with creatine monohydrate results in an increase in available intracellular ATP.[27] Creatine supplementation has been shown to improve maximal weight lift, performance in very short cycling sprints (less than 10 s), and increase fat-free body mass.[19,68] However, creatine does not seem to improve performance in endurance events.[32]

Concerns regarding creatine adverse effects included increased risk for heat injury and kidney damage. Neither of these side effects has been shown in controlled trials.[44] On the contrary, sprinters performing intermittent sprint exercises performed better following 6 days of creatine supplementation.[75] This may be due to additional retention of fluids with creatine supplementation. Creatine use is allowed by the IOC and the NCAA.

29.11 GLUCOSAMINE AND CHONDROITIN SULFATE

Glucosamine and chondroitin sulfate are used by patients to prevent or treat osteoarthritis. Chondroitin sulfate is an important component of cartilage and is produced from extracts of animal cartilage, commonly cow, pig, shark, or fish, and therefore products have a variable composition.[4] Glucosamine is an amino sugar that is made from the shells of crustaceans or by fermenting corn and should not be taken by people with a shellfish allergy. Chondroitin sulfate is commonly mixed with glucosamine in commercial products.

A recent meta-analysis found that compared with placebo, glucosamine, chondroitin, and the combination did not reduce joint pain or have an impact on joint space.[70] Furthermore, industry-sponsored trials showed greater effects than independent trails. Finally, they recommended that the costs of these supplements not be covered and new prescriptions for the medicine be discouraged.

29.12 HUMAN GROWTH HORMONE

Human growth hormone (HGH) is a prescription injectable medication that is used to treat dwarfism, among other conditions, and can increase lean body mass.[10,42]

In a large study using recreational athletes, men were randomly assigned to receive placebo, growth hormone (2 mg/day subcutaneously), testosterone (250 mg/week intramuscularly), or combined treatments, while women were randomly assigned to receive either placebo or growth hormone (2 mg/day).[47] Growth hormone significantly reduced fat mass, increased lean body mass, and improved sprint capacity approximately 6%, in both men and women. The effect was greater in men when both testosterone and growth hormone were administered, resulting in a 9% increase in sprint capacity. However, neither strength, power, nor endurance was enhanced. The effects were reversed 6 weeks after discontinuing growth hormone.

In addition to the potential benefits of increasing lean body mass and sprint capacity, there are limited data that suggest HGH may speed recovery from soft tissue injury. There is an increase in collagen turnover markers in humans.[51] Furthermore, animal studies have shown that tendons heal faster with insulin-like growth factor-1 (IGF-1) administration, which closely parallels what happens with HGH administration.[39]

Clinical Pearl

Growth hormone supplementation in certain medical conditions is helpful. In persons with normal growth hormone levels, supplementation can provide some performance enhancement in sprinting and increase lean body mass. However, this does not come without serious risks.

HGH administration in supraphysiologic doses is not without risk. Excess growth hormone in acromegaly reduces life expectancy approximately 10 years.[3] Growth hormone can cause insulin resistance and hyperglycemia, diabetes, cardiomegaly, hypertension, myopathy, premature epiphyseal closure, sodium retention with swelling of the hands, and carpal tunnel syndrome.[35] Finally, excess HGH induces dysregulated growth of cartilage, which is manifested by the high rate of osteoarthritis present in acromegalics.[71] HGH is banned by WADA and the NCAA.

29.13 EPHEDRINE AND PSEUDOEPHEDRINE

Ephedrine and pseudoephedrine have been commonly used as stimulants by athletes. In a test where subjects with backpacks ran a 10 km run on a treadmill, ephedrine improved run time significantly.[7] When test subjects performed a 30 second bike test, ephedrine improved anaerobic performance.[6] Supplementation with pseudoephedrine 90 minutes before a 1500 m run significantly reduced run times by 2%.[34] However, a single preexercise dose of pseudoephedrine did not improve performance during prolonged exercise over an hour.[24] Furthermore, pseudoephedrine did not improve strength or anaerobic power in a 30 second bike test.[16]

Ephedra commonly causes agitation and anxiety, with case reports of serious side effects including death, myocardial infarction, and cerebrovascular accidents.[60] Pseudoephedrine does not have as high a risk profile but commonly provokes nervousness and palpitations. Stimulants in general are banned by the NCAA and WADA, but ephedrine and pseudoephedrine are legal up to urine concentration of 10 μg/mL and 150 μg/mL, respectively. Because of their potential to be used in the manufacture of methamphetamine, the drugs were regulated in the United States by the Combat Methamphetamine Epidemic Act of 2005 and have limits on daily sales, 30-day purchases, and other restrictions regarding their sale.[17]

In summary, there are many medications and substances that athletes take to try to improve running performance. Some work, some do not. Some are over the counter while

TABLE 29.4
SORT: Key Recommendations for Practice

Clinical Recommendation	Evidence Rating	References
Anabolic steroids increase the risk of myocardial infarction, due in part to their effects on increased blood pressure and adverse effect on lipid profile, particularly by greatly lowering high-density lipoprotein.	B	[26,31]
Treating low testosterone with testosterone supplementation may improve strength, muscle mass, anemia, bone density, and mood.	C	[59]
A single preexercise dose of pseudoephedrine did not improve performance during prolonged exercise over an hour. Pseudoephedrine did not improve strength or anaerobic power in a 30 second bike test.	B	[16,24]
If NSAIDs are needed for longer than a few days, the addition of a proton pump inhibitor and/or switching to a COX-2 selective NSAID seems to be the best option.	C	[345]
During both aerobic and anaerobic activity, caffeine in usual doses enhances performance, but its effects on strength and power are unclear.	B	[11]

others are available through prescription or illegal drug trade. When taken by otherwise healthy individuals, some of these substances can negatively affect life expectancy. Due diligence by the athlete and physician is necessary to avoid complications while maximizing performance (Table 29.4).

REFERENCES

1. American College of Sports Medicine. The use of anabolic-androgenic steroids in sports. *Medicine & Science in Sports & Exercise*. 1987;19(5):453–539.
2. Applegate E. Effective nutritional ergogenic aids. *International Journal of Sport Nutrition*. 1999;9(2):229–239.
3. Ayuk J, Sheppard MC. Does acromegaly enhance mortality? *Reviews in Endocrine and Metabolic Disorders*. 2008;9:33–39.
4. Barnhill JG, Fye CL, Williams DW, Reda DJ, Harris CL, Clegg DO. Chondroitin product selection for the glucosamine/chondroitin arthritis intervention trial. *Journal of the American Pharmacists Association (Washington, DC)*. 2006;46(1):14–24.
5. Beiner JM, Jokl P, Cholewicki J, Panjabi MM. The effect of anabolic steroids and corticosteroids on healing of muscle contusion injury. *The American Journal of Sports Medicine*. 999;27(1):2–9.
6. Bell DG, Jacobs I, Ellerington K. Effect of caffeine and ephedrine ingestion on anaerobic exercise performance. *Medicine & Science in Sports & Exercise*. 2001;33(8):1399–1403.
7. Bell DG, McLellan TM, Sabiston CM. Effect of ingesting caffeine and ephedrine on 10-km run performance. *Medicine & Science in Sports & Exercise*. 2002;34(2):344–349.
8. Bhasin S, Storer TW, Berman N et al. The effects of supraphysiologic doses of testosterone on muscle size and strength in normal men. *The New England Journal of Medicine*. 1996;335:1.
9. Bhasin S, Storer TW, Berman N, Yarasheski K, Clevnger B, Phillips J, Lee W, Bunnell T, Casaburi R. Testosterone replacement increases fat-free mass and muscle size in hypogonadal men. *The Journal of Clinical Endocrinology & Metabolism*. 1997;82:407.
10. Birzniece V, Nelson AE, Ho KK. Growth hormone administration: Is it safe and effective for athletic performance. *Endocrinology Metabolism Clinics of North America*. 2010; 39(1):11–23, vii.
11. Burke LM. Caffeine and sports performance. *Journal of Applied Physics*. 2008;33(6):1319–1334.
12. Butterfield G. Ergogenic aids: Evaluating sport nutrition products. *International Journal of Sport Nutrition*. 1996;6:191–197.
13. Caruso JF, Hamill JL, Yamauchi M, Mercado DR, Cook TD, Keller CP, Montgomery AG, Elias J. Albuterol helps resistance exercise attenuate unloading-induced knee extensor losses. *Aviation, Space, and Environmental Medicine*. 2004; 75(6):505–511.
14. Caruso J, Hamill J, Yamauchi M, Mercado D, Cook T, Higginson B, O'Meara S, Elias J, Siconolfi S. Albuterol aids resistance exercise in reducing unloading-induced ankle extensor strength losses. *Journal of Applied Physiology*. 2005;98(5):1705–1711.
15. Caruso JF, Signorile JF, Perry AC, LeBlanc B, Williams R, Clark M, Bamman MM. The effects of albuterol and isokinetic exercise on the quadriceps muscle group. *Medicine & Science in Sports & Exercise*. 1995;279(11):1471–1476.
16. Chu KS, Doherty TJ, Parise G, Milheiro JS, Tarnopolsky MA. A moderate dose of pseudoephedrine does not alter muscle contraction strength or anaerobic power. *Clinical Journal of Sport Medicine*. 2002;12(6):387–390.
17. Department of Justice Web site [Internet]. CMEA (Combat Methamphetamine Epidemic Act of 2005). Available from https://www.deadiversion.usdoj.gov/meth/. Accessed August 14, 2014.
18. Davidson JM, Chen JJ, Crapo L, Gray G, Greenleaf W, Catania J. Hormonal changes and sexual function in aging men. *The Journal of Clinical Endocrinology & Metabolism*. 1983;57:71.
19. Dempsey RL, Mazzone MF, Meurer LN. Does oral creatine supplementation improve strength? A meta-analysis. *The Journal of Family Practice*. 2002;51(11):945–951.
20. Eaton DK, Kann L, Kinchen S et al. Youth risk behavior surveillance—United States 2005. *MMWR Surveillance Summaries*. 2006;55:1.
21. Eichner ER. Sports anemia, iron supplements, and blood doping. *Medicine & Science in Sports & Exercise*. 1992; 24(9 Suppl):S315–A318.
22. Fernández-Balsells MM, Murad MH, Lane M et al. Clinical review 1: Adverse effects of testosterone therapy in adult men: A systematic review and meta-analysis. *The Journal of Clinical Endocrinology & Metabolism*. 2010;95:2560.
23. Gabriel SE, Jaakkimainen L, Bombardier C. Risk for serious gastrointestinal complications related to the use of nonsteroidal anti-inflammatory drugs. A meta-analysis. *Annals of Internal Medicine*. 1991;115:787–796.

24. Gillies H, Derman WE, Noakes TD, Smith P, Evans A, Gabriels G. Pseudoephedrine is without ergogenic effects during prolonged exercise. *Journal of Applied Physiology.* 1996;81(6):2611–2617.
25. Glade MJ. The dietary supplement health and education act of 1994—Focus on labeling issues. *Nutrition.* 1997;13(11/12):999–1001.
26. Grace F, Sculthorpe N, Baker J, Davies B. Blood pressure and rate pressure product response in males using high-dose anabolic androgenic steroids (AAS). *Journal of Science and Medicine in Sport.* 2003;6(3):307–312.
27. Greenhaff PL, Bodin K, Soderlund K, Hultman E. Effect of oral creatine supplementation on skeletal muscle phosphocreatine resynthesis. *American Journal of Physiology.* 1994;266:E725–E730.
28. Griggs RC, Kingston W, Jozefowicz RF, Herr BE, Forbes G, Halliday D. Effect of testosterone on muscle mass and muscle protein synthesis. *Journal of Applied Physiology.* 1989;66(1):498–503.
29. Harman SM, Metter EJ, Tobin JD, Pearson J, Blackman M. Longitudinal effects of aging on serum total and free testosterone levels in healthy men. Baltimore Longitudinal Study of Aging. *The Journal of Clinical Endocrinology & Metabolism.* 2001;86:724.
30. Hartgens F, Kuipers H. Effects of androgenic-anabolic steroids in athletes. *Sports Medicine.* 2004;34(8):513–554.
31. Hartgens F, Rietjens G, Keizer HA, Kuipers H, Wolffenbuttel BH. Effects of androgenic-anabolic steroids on apolipoproteins and lipoprotein (a). *British Journal of Sports Medicine.* 2004;38(3):253–259.
32. Hickner RC, Dyck DJ, Sklar J, Hatley H, Byrd P. Effect of 28 days of creatine ingestion on muscle metabolism and performance of a simulated cycling road race. *Journal of the International Society of Sports Nutrition.* 2010;7:26.
33. Hippisley-Cox J, Coupland C, Logan R. Risk of adverse gastrointestinal outcomes in patients taking cyclo-oxygenase-2 inhibitors or conventional non-steroidal anti-inflammatory drugs: Population based nested case-control analysis. *BMJ.* 2005;331:1310–1316.
34. Hodges K, Hancock S, Currell K, Hamilton B, Jeukendrup AE. Pseudoephedrine enhances performance in 1500-m runners. *Medicine & Science in Sports & Exercise.* 2006; 38(2):329–333.
35. Holt RI, Sönksen PH. Growth hormone, IGF-I and insulin and their abuse in sport. *British Journal of Pharmacology.* 2008;154:542.
36. Jones R. Gastrointestinal and cardiovascular risks of nonsteroidal anti-inflammatory drugs. *American Journal of Medicine.* 2008;121(6):464–474.
37. Katznelson L, Finkelstein JS, Schoenfeld DA, Rosenthal D, Anderson E, Klibanski A. Increase in bone density and lean body mass during testosterone administration in men with acquired hypogonadism. *The Journal of Clinical Endocrinology & Metabolism.* 1996;81:4358.
38. Kupelian V, Page ST, Araujo AB, Travison T, Bremner W, McKinlay J. Low sex hormone-binding globulin, total testosterone, and symptomatic androgen deficiency are associated with development of the metabolic syndrome in nonobese men. *The Journal of Clinical Endocrinology & Metabolism.* 2006;91:843.
39. Kurtz CA, Loebig TG, Anderson DD, DeMeo PJ, Campbell PG. Insulin-like growth factor I accelerates functional recovery from Achilles tendon injury in a rat model. *American Journal of Sports Medicine.* 1999;27:363–369.
40. Lanza LL, Walker AM, Bortnichak EA, Dreyer NA. Peptic ulcer and gastrointestinal hemorrhage associated with nonsteroidal anti-inflammatory drug use in patients younger than 65 years. A large health maintenance organization cohort study. *Archives of Internal Medicine.* 1995;155:1371–1377.
41. LeBlanc EJ, Perrin N, Johnson JD, Ballatore A, Hillier T. Over-the-counter and compounded vitamin D: Is potency what we expect? *Journal of the American Medical Association.* 2013;173(7):585–586.
42. Liu H, Bravata DM, Olkin I et al. Systematic review: The effects of growth hormone on athletic performance. *Annals of Internal Medicine.* 2008;148:747–758.
43. Locatelli F, Villa G, de Francisco AL, Albertazzi A, Adrogue HJ, Dougherty FC, Beyer U. Effect of a continuous erythropoietin receptor activator (CERA) on stable haemoglobin in patients with CKD on dialysis: Once monthly administration. *Current Medical Research & Opinion.* 2007;23(5):969–979.
44. Lopez RM, Casa D J, McDermott BP, Ganio MS, Armstrong LE, Maresh CM. Does creatine supplementation hinder exercise heat tolerance or hydration status? A systematic review with meta-analyses. *Journal of Athletic Training.* 2009;44(2):215–223.
45. Malfertheiner P, Megraud F, O'Morain C, Hungin AP, Jones R, Axon A, Graham DY, Tygat G. Current concepts in the management of *Helicobacter pylori* infection—The Maastricht 2–2000 Consensus Report. *Alimentary Pharmacology & Therapeutics.* 2002;16:167–180.
46. Martineau L, Horan MA, Rothwell NJ, Little RA. Salbutamol a Beta 2 adrenoceptor agonist increases skeletal muscle strength in young men. *Clinical Science.* 1992;83:615–622.
47. Meinhardt U, Nelson AE, Hansen JL, Birzniece V, Clifford D, Leung KC. The effects of growth hormone on body composition and physical performance in recreational athletes: A randomized trial. *Annals of Internal Medicine.* 2010;152(9):568–577.
48. Micklewright R, Lane S, Linley W, McQuade C. NSAIDs, gastroprotection and cyclo-oxygenase II selective inhibitors. *Alimentary Pharmacology & Therapeutics.* 2003;17:321–332.
49. Murray MP, Gardner GM, Mollinger LA, Sepic SB. Strength of isometric and isokinetic contractions: Knee muscles of men aged 20 to 86. *Physical Therapy.* 1980;60:412.
50. NCAA Web site [Internet]. NCAA Banned Drug List. Available from http://www.ncaa.org/health-and-safety/policy/drug-testing. Accessed August 10, 2014.
51. Nelson AE, Meinhardt U, Hansen JL, Walker IH, Stone G, Howe CJ. Pharmacodynamics of growth hormone abuse biomarkers and the influence of gender and testosterone: A randomized double-blind placebo-controlled study in young recreational athletes. *The Journal of Clinical Endocrinology & Metabolism.* 2008;93:2213–2222.
52. Nevole G. The effect of anabolic steroids on female athletes. *Athletic Training.* 1987;22(4):297–299.
53. Pagonis TA, Angelopoulos NV, Koukoulis GN, Hadjichristodoulou CS. Psychiatric side effects induced by supraphysiological doses of combinations of anabolic steroids correlate to the severity of abuse. *European Psychiatry.* 2006;21(8):551–562.
54. Pasman WJ, van Baak MA, Jeukendrup AE, de Haan A. The effect of different dosages of caffeine on endurance performance time. *International Journal of Sports Medicine.* 1995;16(4):225–230.
55. Prather ID, Brown DE, North P, Wilson JR. Clenbuterol: A substitute for anabolic steroids? *Medicine & Science in Sports & Exercise.* 1995;27(8):1118–1121.

56. Riggs BL, Wahner HW, Seeman E,Offord K, Dunn W, Mazess R, Johnson K, Melton L. Changes in bone mineral density of the proximal femur and spine with aging. Differences between the postmenopausal and senile osteoporosis syndromes. *The Journal of Clinical Investigation.* 1982;70:716.
57. Salpeter SR, Gregor P, Ormiston TM, Whitlock R, Raina P, Thabane L, Topol EJ. Meta-analysis: Cardiovascular events associated with nonsteroidal anti-inflammatory drugs. *American Journal of Medicine.* 2006;119:552–559.
58. Sawka MN, Joyner MJ, Miles DS, Robertson RJ, Spriet LL, Young AJ. American College of Sports Medicine position stand. The use of blood doping as an ergogenic aid. *Medicine & Science in Sports & Exercise.* 1996;28(6):i–viii.
59. Bhasin S, Cunningham GR, Hayes FJ, Matsumoto AM, Snyder PJ, Swerdloff RS, Testosterone MV. Therapy in men with androgen deficiency syndromes: An endocrine society clinical practice guideline. *The Journal of Clinical Endocrinology & Metabolism.* 2010;95(6):2536–2559.
60. Shekelle PG, Hardy ML, Morton SC, Maglione M, Mojica WA, Suttorp MJ, Rhodes SL, Jungvig L, Gagné J. Efficacy and safety of ephedra and ephedrine for weight Loss and athletic performance: a meta-analysis. *Journal of the American Medical Association.* 2003; 289(12): 1537–1545.
61. Silvester LJ. Self-perceptions of the acute and long-range effects of anabolic-androgenic steroids. *The Journal of Strength & Conditioning Research.* 1995;9(2):95–98.
62. Snyder PJ, Peachey H, Berlin J et al. Effects of testosterone replacement in hypogonadal men. *The Journal of Clinical Endocrinology & Metabolism.* 2000;85:2670.
63. Stilger VG, Yesalis CE. Anabolic-androgenic steroid use among high school football players. *Journal of Community Health.* 1999;24(2):131–145.
64. Stricker PR. Sports pharmacology, other ergogenic aids. *Clinics in Sports Medicine.* 1998;17(2):283–297.
65. Sturmi JE, Diorio DJ. Anabolic agents. *Clinics in Sports Medicine.*1998;17(2):375–392.
66. Travison TG, Araujo AB, Kupelian V, O'Donnell A, McKinlay J. The relative contributions of aging, health, and lifestyle factors to serum testosterone decline in men. *The Journal of Clinical Endocrinology & Metabolism.* 2007;92:549.
67. van Marken Lichtenbelt WD, Hartgens F, Vollaard NB, Ebbing S, Kuipers H. Bodybuilders' body composition: Effect of nandrolone decanoate. *Medicine & Science in Sports & Exercise.* 2004;36(3):484–489.
68. Vandebeurie F, Vandeneynde B, Vandenberghe K, Hespel P. Effect of creatine loading on endurance capacity and sprint power in cyclists. *International Journal of Sports Medicine.* 1998;19:490–495.
69. Wallace MB, Lim J, Cutler A, Bucci L. Effects of dehydroepiandrosterone vs. androstenedione supplementation in men. *Medicine & Science in Sports & Exercise.* 1999;31:1788.
70. Wandel S, Jüni P, Tendal B, Nüesch E, Villiger PM, Welton NJ, Reichenbach S, Trelle S. Effects of glucosamine, chondroitin, or placebo in patients with osteoarthritis of hip or knee: Network meta-analysis. *BMJ.* 2010;341:c4675.
71. Wassenaar MJ, Biermasz NR, van Duinen N, van der Klaauw AA, Pereira AM, Roelfsema F, Smit JW, Kroon HM, Kloppenburg M, Romijn JA. High prevalence of arthropathy, according to the definitions of radiological and clinical osteoarthritis, in patients with long-term cure of acromegaly: A case-control study. *European Journal of Endocrinology.* 2009;60:357–361.
72. Weiler JM, Layton T, Hunt M. Asthma in United States Olympic athletes who participated in the 1996 Summer Games. *Journal of Allergy and Clinical Immunology.* 1998;102(5):722–726.
73. Welle S, Jozefowicz R, Statt M. Failure of dehydroepiandrosterone to influence energy and protein metabolism in humans. *The Journal of Clinical Endocrinology & Metabolism.* 1990;71(5):1259–1264.
74. World Anti-Doping Agency [Internet]. World Anti-Doping Agency Prohibited List 2014 [cited March 14, 2014]. Available from https://wada-main-prod.s3.amazonaws.com/resources/files/WADA-Revised-2014-Prohibited-List-EN.PDF.
75. Wright GA. The effects of creatine loading on thermoregulation and intermittent sprint exercise performance in a hot humid environment. *The Journal of Strength & Conditioning Research.* 2007;21(3):655–660.

30 Injections

Christopher J. Lutrzykowski and Robert B. Stevens

CONTENTS

TABLE 30.1
Key Clinical Considerations

1. Injections are safe with appropriate technique and knowledge of the relevant anatomy.
2. Corticosteroid injections provide short-term benefit in the setting of degenerative change and are an effective adjunct to other treatment modalities.
3. Aspiration of a joint is a necessary diagnostic technique in the presence of an unexplained effusion in particular if there is concern for infection.
4. More than one injection into the same location may be necessary to relieve pain but should call into question the diagnosis if there is limited benefit.
5. Injections may be used both diagnostically and therapeutically.

30.1 INTRODUCTION

Injection has been utilized for more than 50 years in the treatment of intra-articular pathology. It is a very commonly used intervention in the diagnosis and treatment of sports-related injury. Injection, in particular corticosteroid injection, is not without controversy, and this has led to alternative treatments involving many other injection materials and techniques (Table 30.1).

The purpose of this chapter is to provide the primary care provider with the indications, risks, benefits, as well as injection techniques for common sports medicine and orthopedic injections that have been described in the literature on an anatomic basis. As corticosteroids have been the mainstay of treatment for many musculoskeletal pathologies, the discussion is predominantly adjusted in that direction.

Injections are easy to learn but should be performed independently only after proper training and technique have been refined. Knowledge of the anatomy of a given injection site is paramount to learning the appropriate techniques. Timing of intervention and judgment on usage is complex and depends on many variables defined by patient presentation.

30.2 INDICATIONS

Specific indications for each injection will be reviewed in detail for each individual location. In general, there are commonly held principles for performing an injection and include both diagnostic and therapeutic purposes.

Diagnostic indications include procedures such as arthrocentesis to evaluate joint fluid for the presence of crystals, infection, blood, bone spicules, and for fluid analysis for inflammatory and infectious causes. Anesthetic injection may be used to differentiate between causes of pain and to provide temporary relief of discomfort. Finally, injection may also be used for imaging studies such as arthrogram.

Therapeutic injection has been the mainstay of treatment for various musculoskeletal complaints for many years. Injection may be used to provide more lasting relief and as an aid to other therapies in the treatment and rehabilitation of sports-related injury. It serves as the vehicle for delivery of corticosteroid and other injection material. Nerve block may be used in a similar fashion to provide long-term relief or to assist in procedures requiring additional procedure time (beyond the scope of this chapter). It may be used to distend joint capsules as in the treatment of adhesive capsulitis and also useful in removing fluid from a distended joint to aid in diagnosis and rehabilitation.

30.3 RISKS AND COMPLICATIONS

When used appropriately and with proper technique, injection is safe with limited side effects demonstrating an overall complication rate of roughly 5% including extra-articular injections.[19] A number of risks and potential complications have been described from injection that should be understood and reviewed with patients at the time of injection (see Table 30.2). Specific requirements regarding informed consent for patients vary to some degree based on location, but it is always reasonable to review and document the indications, expected outcomes, common adverse

TABLE 30.2
Adverse Reaction to Injection

Adverse Reaction	Rate
Infection	Rare: 1/3,000 to 1/50,000
Fat atrophy	Site dependent: closer to skin more common
Cartilage degeneration	Rare
Skin pigment changes (depigmentation more common)	More common with injections closer to skin
Tendon rupture	Rare: avoid injection into tendon, avoid Achilles and patellar tendon injection
Anaphylaxis	Rare: <1%
Facial flushing	Common: 15%
Steroid flare	Common: 10%–25%
Hyperglycemia	Transient: common Clinically significant: rare
Vasovagal reactions	Common

reactions, and potential complications of each injection/procedure performed. Many institutions now require a documented pause (so-called time out) for injections as well. Regardless of format, a well-educated patient assists in the treatment process.

Fortunately, risks and potential complications of injection are rare. These include infection, skin atrophy, depigmentation, cartilage degeneration, tendon rupture, postinjection pain flare, traumatic injection, and systemic reaction. Each of these is reviewed individually.

Infection risk is very low for injections performed with appropriate technique (reviewed subsequently). Infection rates have been listed as high as 1 per 3,000 to as few as every 50,000 injections.[25,109] Staph organisms are reported as the most common in particular *Staphylococcus aureus.* Certainly with the prevalence of methicillin-resistant *S. aureus,* this can be of great concern, but with the limited frequency of infection, this should not be a major barrier to proceeding (see also Section 30.4).[75]

Rates of skin and subcutaneous fat atrophy are difficult to find in the literature, but certainly those injections that are performed closer to the skin are at greater risk. These include but are not limited to interdigital neuroma, common extensor tendon at the elbow, de Quervain's tenosynovitis, and other hand injections. Additionally, skin changes such as depigmentation and rarely hyperpigmentation may occur. While these changes are not inherently dangerous, they can be unsightly and are usually permanent.[18,83]

Concern for cartilage degeneration has led to traditional teaching that injections into joints should be limited to less than three per year. This has unfortunately led to withholding pain-relieving injections, and recent studies have challenged this assertion. Certainly, frequent pain-relieving intra-articular injection should not divert from definitive treatment if available but limiting a patient based solely on number of injections has not been proven.[83,109] There has been an ongoing concern about chondrotoxicity most notably with bupivacaine infusion. Please see section on anesthetics for details on this potential risk.

Tendon rupture rates after injection are lacking in the medical literature. Tendon rupture has been described and is a potential risk with particular emphasis on tendons that have a paratenon rather than tendon sheath (Achilles, patella, etc.). Care should always be exercised to avoid injecting directly into a tendon.[52] Traditionally, patients have been restricted from significant activity of the injected body part, but no specific guidelines exist for duration or period of immobilization.[18,83] It may be prudent to immobilize weight-bearing locations for a lengthier time frame (3–5 days) although data is lacking to support this approach.

Systemic reactions do occur with injection and include anaphylaxis. Providers and staff should be educated on the location of available emergency medication and procedures in the event this happens. Injections may unfortunately be traumatic involving direct injection into the pleural space, intravascular space, local nerves, or other soft-tissue structures including intramuscular injection. These adverse incidents may occur despite appropriate technique but are generally rare.

Facial flushing (independent of intravascular injection) can occur up to 15% of injections with a female patient preponderance.[26,83]

Postinjection flare can occur in up to 25% of patients although this is not well studied. It is thought to be due to crystal deposition around the injection site.[22,78,83] It is typically short duration and self-limited (<24 hours). The flare is typically characterized by pain and occasionally redness at the injection site and can be confused with infection. Oral nonsteroidal anti-inflammatory medications may be helpful in treating this reaction.

Many providers can recount patients with vasovagal reactions associated with injection but no specific rates have been described for this reaction. It is always prudent to prepare for this eventuality.

A risk of hyperglycemia has been reported in diabetics as there is systemic absorption of the corticosteroid. It is difficult to quantify the risk[83] and may be overestimated,[99] but at least transient subclinical elevations in blood glucose can occur.[24] Intra-articular injections typically have a lower risk of this compared to injections that are subcutaneous or adjacent to a tendon/tendon sheath.[39,110] Effects are thought to last for 5–21 days.[100]

30.4 CONTRAINDICATIONS

There are several described contraindications to joint injection and aspiration (see Table 30.3). Obvious skin infection and breakdown at the injection site should preclude injection. Any uncontrolled coagulopathy is a contraindication, however the usual use of common anticoagulants should not prevent injection. Any intra-articular fracture precludes corticosteroid injection, but anesthetic injection may prove beneficial. Injection into a clearly infected joint or bursa is not recommended but aspiration often is necessary. Entry into difficult joints is a relative contraindication and based on provider experience. Corticosteroid injection into an unstable joint is contraindicated as well. Joints that contain prosthetics are a relative contraindication to corticosteroid injection and finally any known hypersensitivity to any component of the injection should require an alternative approach.

TABLE 30.3
Contraindications to Corticosteroid Injection

Skin infection	Fracture
Osteochondral defect	Uncontrolled coagulopathy
Uncontrolled diabetes	Unstable joint
Septic arthritis	

Note: Often, anesthetic injections are utilized to help assist with joint aspiration and reduction. Diabetes is a relative contraindication, and pros/cons of injection must be weighed prior to corticosteroid injection. True incidence of all reactions is unknown. Preparation for worst-case scenario is useful.

TABLE 30.4
Common Injectable Corticosteroid Preparations in the United States

Steroid	Solubility	Dose Equivalent
Methylprednisolone (Depo Medrol)	Soluble	40 mg/mL
Betamethasone sodium phosphate (Celestone Soluspan)	Soluble	3 mg/mL
Triamcinolone acetonide (Kenalog)	Insoluble	40 mg/mL
Triamcinolone hexacetonide (Aristospan)	Insoluble	40 mg/2 mL

Note: No established advantage proven for one steroid versus another. Please note that additional preparations exist that contain higher dosages of corticosteroid (80 mg/mL methylprednisolone).

30.5 EQUIPMENT/INJECTABLE MEDICATIONS

Techniques for skin preparation for injection have varied through the years and as a general rule of thumb have trended away from "sterile" injections. Skin preparation solutions range from alcohol wipes, chlorhexidine/povidone wipe or swabs, to sterile scrub (may still be appropriate in the setting of septic joint). The use of sterile versus nonsterile gloves has also been debated with literature granting support to neither, but specific procedures may favor sterile gloves including joint aspiration. Providers may like the tactile feel of sterile gloves and thus favor their usage.

Typical syringe sizes range from 1 to 50 mL syringes with 3, 5, 10, and 20 mL sizes being the most commonly utilized. Smaller sizes are typically utilized for injection, while larger volume syringes are more commonly used in aspiration. Needle gauges range from larger bore diameters for aspiration and lavage (14–18 g) to smaller sizes for tight joint and tendon sheath spaces (25 g and higher). Length is entirely dependent on the structure and technique utilized. Common lengths range from ½ in. for small joints or tendon sheaths to 5 or 6 in. needles for intra-articular hip and trochanteric bursa injections. Reviewing the available stock of equipment is prudent to preventing delay of definitive care

Drapes, dressings, sponges are all beneficial to have readily available if not right at the bedside. Access to equipment to treat severe reactions is necessary.

Choice of anesthetic invariably is provider dependent but there has been some concern for chondrolysis with longer-acting anesthetics. This has been described predominantly with bupivacaine in continuous infusion post–shoulder surgery and has not been described in detail from injections.[35,86,100,105] However, no minimum dosage causing chondrocyte toxicity has been described and there are alternative injectables limiting the choice of bupivacaine as an anesthetic. Cardiac toxicity also exists with this medication in the event of intravascular injection. The upper limit of dosing for Bupivacaine is 2 mg/kg.

Lidocaine has been the mainstay for anesthetic injection and has a proven track record but is not without risk. Possible side effects/adverse reactions include cardiac toxicity and mental status changes with inadvertent intravascular injection. Time of onset of anesthetic effect is typically 1–5 minutes and duration is 1–2 hours. Upper limit of dosing is 5 mg/kg of lidocaine; dosage above these levels will begin to demonstrate side effects of the medication. In the setting where a multidose vial of anesthetic is used in particular if used for other procedures, it is recommended to draw the anesthetic in advance of the corticosteroid (so-called "clear to cloudy" technique) to limit the possibility of contamination.

Corticosteroid choice has also varied through the years although no reliable preparation exists for each indication (see Table 30.4). Prior recommendations for the use of higher-solubility steroids (betamethasone, dexamethasone, methylprednisolone) for soft-tissue structures and lower solubility agents for joint injections (triamcinolone) have not been proven in all joint injection scenarios, but where good evidence exists, it will be described in the specific joint injection sections. Provider comfort plays a large role in selection of the agent. Purportedly, the corticosteroid treats the inflammatory component of the location being injected. This has been called into question in the setting of certain injections where inflammation has not been demonstrated as a major component of the process. Nonetheless, corticosteroid is still widely held as useful for many injections performed in orthopedics and sports medicine. Injection volumes vary based on the targeted joint or soft-tissue injection and will be reviewed for each location.

30.6 GENERAL TECHNIQUE

General rules for technique can help assist with overall patient and provider satisfaction with the procedure. Keeping both the patient and provider comfortable during the injection procedure goes a long way to performing a successful injection. It is important to have ready access to the location of the injection without placing the patient in an awkward position. Placing the area to be aspirated or injected at eye level of the provider is a useful technique. A provider that is seated or comfortably standing at the level of the area to be injected helps bolster provider confidence. Making sure all available equipment is within ready reach and direct eyesight of the performing provider is important. While not necessary, an assistant can be invaluable especially in the setting of joint aspiration. Repeatedly identifying the landmarks and use of marking pens outlining important structures can be an aid to appropriate injection especially in the learning provider. Use of topical or injectable skin anesthetics is provider dependent; however, spray anesthetics theoretically raise the possible risk of infection, and subcutaneous anesthesia can distort landmarks. As many injections are undertaken with a 22-gauge needle or smaller bore, topical anesthetics may not be necessary. However, topical anesthetic is a comfort to the patient in the setting of joint aspiration with a large bore needle. As was discussed previously, skin prep is variable and often provider experience driven. Data demonstrate no distinct advantage to the use of "sterile prep" technique, but many providers are still using traditional techniques. Drapes are less commonly used but may be necessary for joint aspiration for infection.

As a rule, the needle and syringe should be utilized as an extension of the finger. The needle entry should be confident and quick, perpendicular (unless specified otherwise in the specific joint injection locations listed later in this chapter) to the skin and advanced easily to the site of injection. Aspiration to limit intravascular access is useful. Delivering the anesthetic and corticosteroid combination varies with location. Care should be exercised to avoid direct injection into a tendon; flow of solute must be smooth and unforced. Significant tissue resistance to injection or movement of needle with motion of a tendon necessitates alteration in depth or location of injection. After the injection, the needle should be withdrawn at a comfortable pace to minimize vacuum effect. Application of a bandage is dependent on any blood flow, which typically is minimal.

Any postinjection pain can be treated with nonsteroidal anti-inflammatory drugs (NSAIDs) or acetaminophen. A brief period of immobilization and ice may also prove helpful but usually is unnecessary. Limiting strenuous activity of the location of the injection for at least 72 hours can be beneficial, but rehabilitation may begin quickly.

30.7 SPECIFIC JOINT INJECTIONS

30.7.1 Shoulder Region

30.7.1.1 Acromioclavicular Injection

Injection of the acromioclavicular (AC) joint has been traditionally used to treat degenerative disease of the AC joint in addition to providing relief to a patient with an AC joint separation (anesthetic only).

The important landmarks of the AC joint must be identified and palpated. This includes the distal clavicle and proximal acromion. It may be helpful to delineate the joint space by marking the skin with an indelible ink pen. The acromioclavicular joint is narrow and often angled from lateral to medial. Place the patient in a seated position with the glenohumeral joint adducted and internally rotated, with the forearm resting on the ipsilateral leg. The joint is approached superiorly and laterally and usually at a steep angle (see Figure 30.1). Preinjection radiographs or ultrasound may prove very useful as the AC joint has varying morphology and may be distorted by degenerative arthritis. Typical needle length is from 0.5 to 1.5 in. and needle gauge is usually small; 25-gauge needles are commonly used. Often, the performing provider will meet resistance from the acromion and will have to "walk" the needle medially into the joint. Usually, 0.5 mL of anesthetic and a corresponding amount of corticosteroid are injected into this small joint. The entire 1 mL may prove too much volume for the joint; high resistance is often felt with patient discomfort.

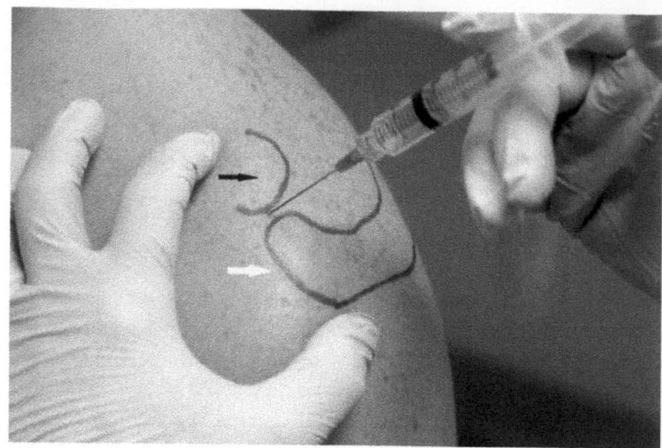

FIGURE 30.1 Acromioclavicular joint injection. The landmarks for the acromioclavicular injection include the distal clavicle (black arrow) and the proximal acromion (white arrow). This injection can be difficult in the setting of advanced arthritis due to distortion of the usual landmarks and a narrowing of the otherwise small joint. Preinjection radiographs may aid in this setting.

While the joint is rather close to the skin and landmarks are often readily palpable, accuracy of this injection in small studies has been reported to be low.[81,111] Presumed reasoning includes small joint space and difficulty navigating joint spurs. Multiple studies show improved accuracy with ultrasound guidance.[17,81,87,93] However, one study comparing efficacy of intra-articular versus periarticular injection found similar outcomes between palpation- and ultrasound-guided injection. However, cross-arm testing was improved with documented intra-articular injection.[94] Overall efficacy remains relatively good although studies remain few with varying results.[46,108] Potential complications mirror those for all joint injection, but it is unusual to enter into other structures given the location of the AC joint. Typically, patients are followed up within 2 weeks to evaluate efficacy. Repeat injections may be necessary.

Clinical Pearl

The AC joint morphology varies from individual to individual and preinjection x-ray is helpful to determining appropriate injection angle and avoidance of joint spurring.

30.7.1.2 Glenohumeral Joint Injection

Glenohumeral joint injection (GHJ) has been used to treat GHJ degenerative changes, inflammatory arthropathy of the GHJ, adhesive capsulitis, and degenerative changes involving the labrum. Accuracy of GHJ injection with tactile guidance has been called into question with rates varying for both anterior and posterior approaches. Multiple studies have compared accuracy rates between palpation guidance and ultrasound guidance, with the majority favoring ultrasound guidance for improved accuracy.[16,28,33,42,80]

The landmarks that must be identified prior to a GHJ joint injection include the coracoid process, humeral head, and acromion process. When using the posterior approach, the examiner identifies the posterolateral corner of the acromion and coracoid process. For the anterior approach, the coracoid, medial aspect of the humeral head, and anteromedial acromion are identified. Internally and externally rotating the humerus aids in identifying this landmark. Marking the skin with pen is recommended for novice providers to help identify landmarks and aid in proprioceptive control.

Usually, a 1.5-in., 22-gauge needle on a 10 mL syringe is used to perform the injection. Skin is prepped (see intra-articular injection discussion in general technique section). Usually, the patient is seated comfortably with the back supported but with shoulder exposed. When using the posterior approach (see Figure 30.2), landmarks are identified as described earlier, and the needle is advanced from just below the posterolateral corner of the acromion process advancing directly toward the coracoid process. In patients with larger body habitus, longer needle lengths are required. Twenty-five-gauge needles may also be used, but at longer lengths, there is increased likelihood of adverse needle deflection caused by soft-tissue obstruction. For the anterior approach, once landmarks have been confidently identified, the needle is introduced approximately 1–1.5 cm below the coracoid process directed perpendicular to the joint. If the needle meets bone resistance, withdraw slightly to remain in the joint. For either approach, aspiration should be performed to assist in avoiding intravascular injection. About 1–2 mL of corticosteroid and 5–10 mL of anesthetic should

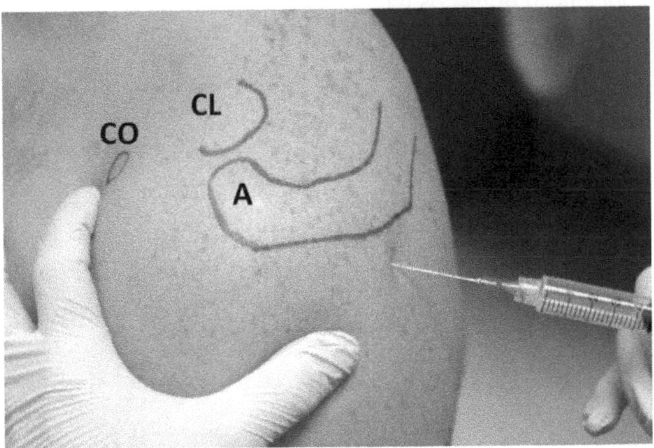

FIGURE 30.2 Subacromial space/bursa injection. The landmarks for this injection include the coracoid process (CO) and acromioclavicular joint bordered proximally by the clavicle (CL) and distally by the acromion (A). The needle enters under the posterolateral corner of the acromion process and is directed toward the coracoid process. Placing the non-dominant thumb on the posterolateral corner of the acromion and index finger on the coracoid process may aid in proprioceptively guiding the needle (hand removed to allow for viewing).

flow smoothly into the joint. If significant resistance is met, repositioning of the needle is required.

Studies have shown benefit of GHJ injection in the treatment of adhesive capsulitis, although one study found a similar response with subacromial injection compared to intra-articular.[77] Less data are available for the treatment of GHJ degenerative changes. Complications are rare and mirror general listing. Concern is raised given the low accuracy rates; brachial plexus and nerves of the upper extremity run fairly close the GHJ joint, and in patients with larger body habitus, landmarks may be harder to find.

Clinical Pearl

Posterior approach: direct your needle from below the posterolateral corner of the acromion toward the coracoid process. For larger patients, longer needles may be required (greater than 1.5 in.).

30.7.1.3 Subacromial Space

Injection into the subacromial space is one of the more common injections performed in musculoskeletal medicine. The indications for the injection include rotator cuff syndrome/impingement syndrome and subacromial bursitis.

Multiple techniques have been described in the literature with two predominant locations noted: the posterolateral and lateral approaches. Some providers prefer an anterior approach, and indeed, at least one study shows improved accuracy compared to the posterolateral approach.[65] However, this is less commonly used and will not be described in detail here.

Using the posterolateral approach, the patient is seated comfortably with the affected shoulder exposed. The shoulder should be adducted and internally rotated; the patient's forearm should be comfortably resting on the ipsilateral thigh. If available, an assistant may apply downward traction on the arm. The posterolateral corner of the acromion process is then identified, and the corresponding recess just below this prominence is palpated. This represents the entry point for the needle. The needle is inserted bevel up utilizing the AC joint as the target. If bony resistance is felt, needle readjustment is necessary, usually in the superior or inferior direction. Needle depth varies based on patient body habitus but ranges typically from 1 to 1.5 cm (see Figure 30.3).

Another common approach is the true lateral approach. The patient is seated similar to the previous description, and the lateral acromion is palpated. Visually bisecting the acromion into halves, the needle is inserted just below the acromion at a 30°–45° angle and advanced 1–1.5 cm but depends on the body habitus of the patient. Occasionally, the examiner may see the adjacent tissue rise as the injection fluid fills the subacromial space.

About 1–2 mL of corticosteroid and 6–9 mL of anesthetic are typically used in the injection. A 1.5-in., 22-gauge needle is typically used, but longer needles may need to be used for larger shoulders. Neither injection location has been favored in the medical literature in a long-standing debate.

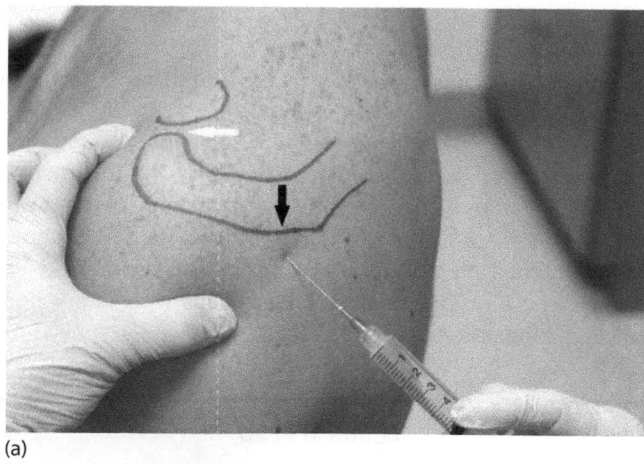
(a)

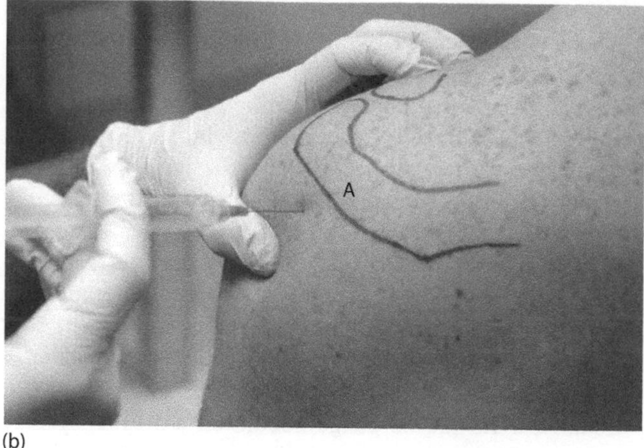

(b)

FIGURE 30.3 Injection into the subacromial space. There are two common injection locations for the subacromial space. (a) The landmarks for this injection include the posterolateral corner of the acromion process (black arrow) and the acromioclavicular joint (white arrow). The needle enters under the posterolateral corner of the acromion and is advanced toward the acromioclavicular joint. Finger position as outlined in glenohumeral joint injection may aid in proprioception with this injection as well. (b) The landmark for the lateral injection is the lateral border of the acromion process. This bony landmark is mentally bisected and the needle enters below the bone in at that location at a roughly 45° angle. The needle is advanced to clear any subcutaneous tissue but is meant to remain superior to the rotator cuff tendons.

Other structures may be inadvertently infiltrated such as the rotator cuff tendons, biceps tendon, and deltoid.

The subacromial injection provides short-term relief of pain to help assist in the treatment process and rotator cuff exercises should be undertaken after 48–72 hours of relative rest. Typical duration of pain relief is from 2 weeks to 2 months. Similar outcomes have been reported with high- or low-dose steroid injections.[45]

Similar to other injections, multiple studies have shown improved accuracy with ultrasound guidance; however, it has yet to be reliably shown that adding radiographic guidance improves outcomes.[30,50] Some studies have compared NSAID to steroid injections with mixed results.[51,71]

Clinical Pearl

Traction on the patient's arm by an assistant may provide better entry into the subacromial space.

30.7.1.4 Biceps Tendon Sheath Injection

The indications for biceps tendon sheath injection include symptomatic biceps tendinopathy. As the biceps tendon is commonly involved in other pathologies of the shoulder (rotator cuff disease, shoulder instability, labral pathology), isolated disease is rare.

The landmarks for the biceps tendon sheath injection are essentially the bicipital groove of the shoulder; this depression is formed between the greater and lesser tuberosities of the humerus and is easily palpated by internally and externally rotating the shoulder while the humerus is adducted to the side. Adding resisted forearm flexion or resisted supination may aid in localizing the tendon.

The injection may be performed seated or supine with the shoulder at 0 degrees of external rotation. The typical approach is in line with the long head of the biceps (longitudinal axis) at a 30° angle with the intent to enter the sheath under the aponeurosis formed by the subscapularis and transverse ligament (see Figure 30.4). If resistance is felt during the injection, repositioning to prevent injection directly into the tendon is warranted.

A 1–1.5 in., 25-gauge needle is typically used for this injection. Insertion depth varies greatly based on body habitus and angle of approach. About 0.5 mL of corticosteroid and 1–2 mL of anesthetic may be used during the injection. Ultrasound guidance can be useful and necessary in some circumstances to assure adequate placement of medication.[41,106] Injection may provide temporary relief of symptoms related to long head of biceps tenosynovitis/tendinopathy.

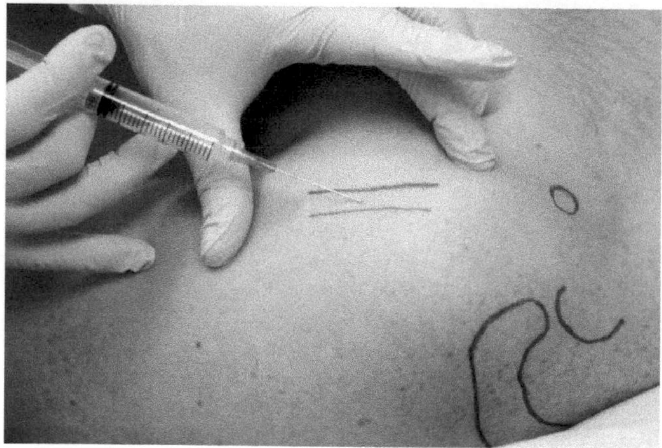

FIGURE 30.4 Injection for biceps tendinopathy. The biceps tendon can be palpated within the bicipital groove formed by the greater and lesser tubercles of the humerus. Internally and externally rotating the shoulder allows the examiner to palpate the tendon as it "rolls" under the fingers. The sheath is represented by the parallel lines above and the injection is meant to enter into the sheath surrounding the tendon but not the tendon itself.

Clinical Pearl

With the arm adducted against the side, the humerus can be internally and externally rotated to aid in identifying the bicipital groove.

30.7.1.5 Trigger Point

Myofascial trigger point injection can be helpful in providing temporary relief of pain associated with trigger points or myofascial pain syndrome. They are commonly located in the shoulder/trapezius muscles but may be found in a number of locations. Detailed description of each location is beyond the scope of this text. The landmarks and clinical anatomy relating to trigger point injection vary by body part to be injected. An excellent working knowledge of local anatomy is paramount to appropriate injection. The technique for trigger point injection varies, but typically, trigger points are palpable as fusiform localized nodules that run in parallel to muscle fibers.

After identifying the nodule, grasping or "trapping" the nodule between thumb and forefinger of the examiner's nondominant hand assists in the injection. The nodule is entered in a perpendicular manner after skin cleansing and depth gauged by proprioception aided by the technique described earlier. Occasionally, a local twitch may be felt when entering the nodule. Needle size and length vary by site but typically range from 1 to 1.5 in. and 25 to 27 gauges. In the past, corticosteroid injection has been used but benefit has been shown with simple anesthetic injection or dry needling.[2,7,103] Needle gauge has not been shown to affect symptom relief or even patient discomfort.[4,118] Efficacy is unclear but short-term relief is the norm at best.[96]

Clinical Pearl

Grasp or pinch the trigger point between the thumb and index finger of your nondominant hand, aiding in your tactile sense of needle positioning.

30.7.2 Elbow Region

30.7.2.1 Lateral Epicondyle

Injection adjacent to the common extensor apparatus is controversial as studies have shown limited long-term benefit. Nevertheless, injection may prove useful in recalcitrant cases and has been used traditionally for the treatment of "lateral epicondylitis." The indication for this injection is common extensor tendinopathy.

The requisite landmarks include the radial head and lateral epicondyle of the distal humerus. The radial head can be easily identified as a bony prominence distal to the lateral epicondyle and should be confirmed with pronation/supination of the forearm (the radial head should roll under the examiners fingers). The extensor carpi radialis brevis (ECRB) tendon is roughly 1 cm distal and medial to the lateral epicondyle and superior to the radial head and is the more common location for tenderness in "tennis elbow."

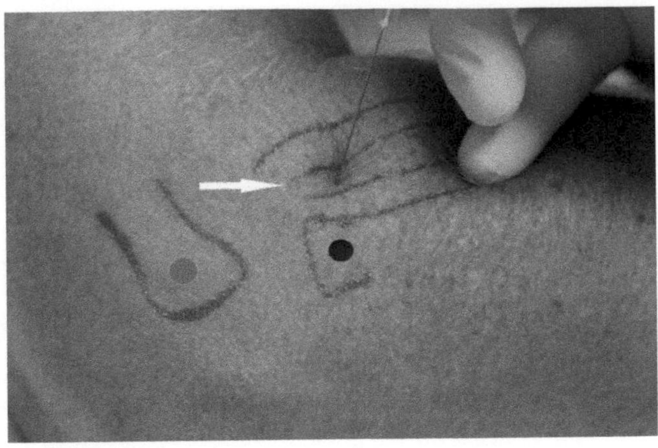

FIGURE 30.5 Injection for common extensor tendinopathy ("tennis elbow"). The landmarks for this injection include the lateral epicondyle (light gray circle), radial head (dark gray circle), and common extensor tendon (white arrow). Direct tendon injection is not recommended.

The injection can be administered in a seated or supine patient with the elbow at 90 degrees of flexion and the forearm supinated (see Figure 30.5). Given the shallow location of the injection, fat atrophy and skin discoloration are a real possibility with this injection; warning the patient prior to injection is useful to limit post injection concerns about cosmetic appearance in the event this adverse outcome occurs. Typically, the area of maximal tenderness is palpated and the needle is inserted in a 30°–45° angle over the extensor tendon aponeurosis. Care must be exercised not to inject directly into the tendon. If resistance is felt during the injection, the needle is repositioned above the tendon. Needle size is usually 1–1.5 in. and 25 gauge. About 0.5 mL of corticosteroid and 1–2 mL of anesthetic may be used. Multiple techniques have been described including needle fenestration, bolus, and peppering the tendon. Use ultrasound guidance to help improve outcome.

The use of various agents has been proposed in place of corticosteroid due to the limited benefit of steroid injection. Overall, steroid injections show some short-term benefit with long-term relief (>3 months) equal to placebo.[10,55,59] Use of autologous blood, protein-rich plasma, or sclerosing agents show varying rates of success, but studies are often methodologically flawed with significant author bias.[55,56,82,88,102,114,121]

Clinical Pearl

Studies have shown good short-term relief from corticosteroid injections, but long-term relief is equivalent to a "wait and see" method. Given the shallow location of the common extensor tendon, fat atrophy and skin discoloration are at relatively higher risk from this injection.

30.7.2.2 Medial Epicondyle

This injection is very similar to the injection for "lateral epicondylitis" and is indicated for the treatment of "medial epicondylitis" ("golfer's elbow"). Very little evidence surrounds the utility of this injection.

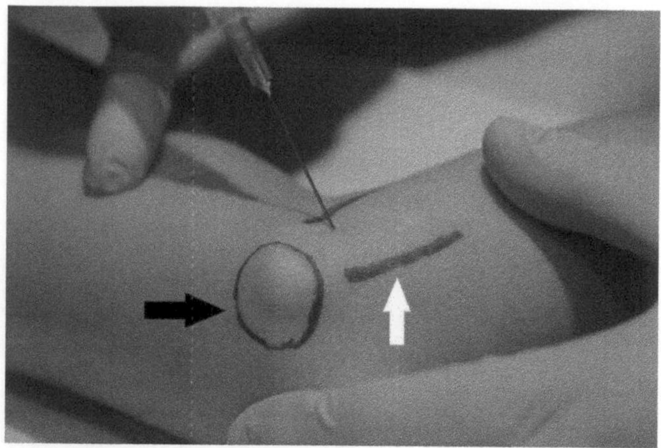

FIGURE 30.6 Injection for "medial epicondylitis." Surgical consultation may be necessary in that setting. The landmarks for this injection include the medial epicondyle (black arrow) and the proximal tendons of the flexor apparatus (white arrow). The needle is directed from superior to inferior.

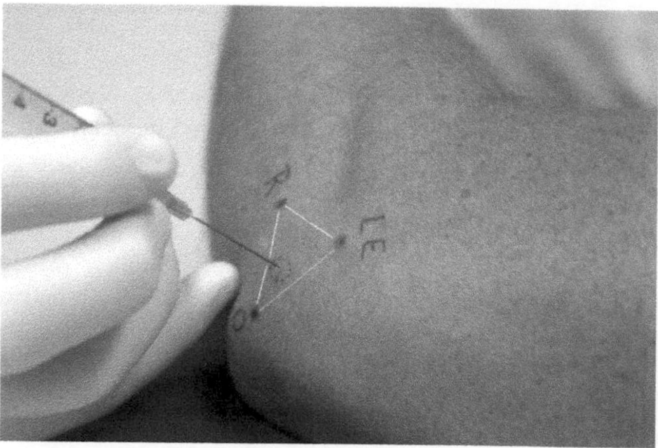

FIGURE 30.7 Intra-articular elbow injection. The radial head (R), lateral epicdondyle (LE), and lateral portion of the olecranon (O) form a triangle that outlines the target for the intra-articular elbow injection.

The medial epicondyle is identified on palpatory exam as is the cubital tunnel beneath the medial epicondyle. Care must be exercised not to enter the cubital tunnel with this injection. The wrist flexor tendons may be palpated just distal, lateral, and anterior to the medial epicondyle and can be identified with wrist flexion (see Figure 30.6). Needle entry, solute composition, and technique are similar to description for lateral epicondylitis injection. Risks are also similar (see risk discussion for lateral epicondylitis).

30.7.2.3 Intra-Articular Elbow

The indications for an intra-articular elbow injection include osteoarthritis or inflammatory arthropathy of the elbow. The landmarks for this injection are bordered proximally by the lateral epicondyle, distally by the radial head and inferiorly by the olecranon process. The center of the triangular area that is formed by these landmarks allows direct access to the intra-articular space of the elbow. If an effusion is present, an area of bogginess will also be palpable.

The patient is either seated or may lie on the contralateral side. The elbow is flexed to 90° and rested comfortably with the shoulder abducted and the elbow on an elevated surface when the patient is seated or resting alternatively, comfortably on the ipsilateral flank if the patient is on their side (see Figure 30.7).

Usually, a 0.5- to 1-in. 25-gauge needle is used with 1 mL of corticosteroid and 2 mL of anesthetic injected. This is a rather shallow location, and care must be made to enter the joint and not into the subcutaneous tissue. Small studies show improved accuracy with ultrasound guidance but equal long-term efficacy.[36,60]

Clinical Pearl

The lateral epicondyle, radial head, and olecranon form a triangle of landmarks, whose center allows direct access to the joint capsule of the elbow.

30.7.2.4 Olecranon Bursitis

The indication for this aspiration and injection include recalcitrant olecranon bursitis swelling that has failed conservative therapy, septic bursitis, and diagnostic aspiration for crystal-induced bursitis.[11] This bursal fluid collection is usually rather obvious over the olecranon process and that is the defining landmark.

The patient may be seated, supine, or prone with elbow flexed. The needle enters into the bursal collection and aspiration is undertaken (see Figure 30.8). Fluid may be sent for crystal evaluation, gram stain, and culture if appropriate. Injection may proceed in the setting of chronic recalcitrant bursal fluid collection as long as no concern for infection is present.

Typically, a 1- to 1.5-in. 18- to 25-gauge needle is utilized for aspiration and injection (typically larger bores for aspiration and injection). Injectable solutions include corticosteroid and anesthetic but need to be used sparingly to limit infection. Repeated injections should be limited due to infection.[14] Surgical consultation may be necessary in that setting.

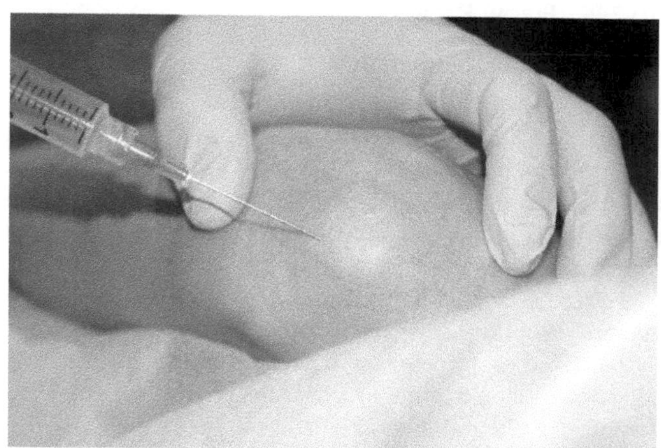

FIGURE 30.8 Injection/aspiration technique for the olecranon bursa. Olecrenon bursal swelling can be easily identified, aspirated, and injected.

Clinical Pearl

The risk of introducing infection into the bursal sack is not inconsequential and added care should be taken to properly cleanse the injection site.

30.7.3 Wrist and Hand Region

30.7.3.1 De Quervain's Tenosynovitis

The indication for this injection is inflammation and pain of the first dorsal compartment containing the tendons of the abductor pollicis longus (APL) and extensor pollicis brevis (EPB). Typically, the area of maximal tenderness is at the radial styloid.

The landmarks to be identified include the anatomic snuffbox (the APL and EPB make up the superolateral border of the snuff box), the radial styloid, and the dorsal tubercle of the radius. Occasionally, the separate tendons may be palpated within the first dorsal compartment just distal to the radial styloid.

Typically, the patient is either supine or seated with the forearm and wrist held in neutral position (thumb pointing to ceiling). Some techniques favor placing a small bolster under the ulnar side of the wrist forcing the wrist into gentle inversion. The location of maximal tenderness is once again identified, and the needle is inserted bevel up at a 45°–60° angle at the radial styloid. If the separate tendons are identified, finding the split can be a good aiming point. The needle is inserted in a cephalad direction (see Figure 30.9). Depth may be difficult to gauge, but typically after at least 5mm of insertion, an attempt to gently administer the fluid should be undertaken. Body habitus must be taken into consideration to avoid shallow injection. Advance or withdraw until fluid flows smoothly; the tendon sheath may fill from distal to proximal. As this injection is quite close to the skin, fat atrophy and skin pallor may occur.

Usually, a 0.5–1 in. 25- or 27-gauge needle is used for the injection. About 0.25–0.5 mL of corticosteroid and similar amount of anesthetic are delivered. Additional amounts are likely to leak into the subcutaneous tissues. Small studies show moderate efficacy with this injection.[49,85] However, a percentage of patients have septated tendon sheaths that prevent a single injection from reaching both tendons, which may lead to incomplete symptom relief or recurrence.[68,72]

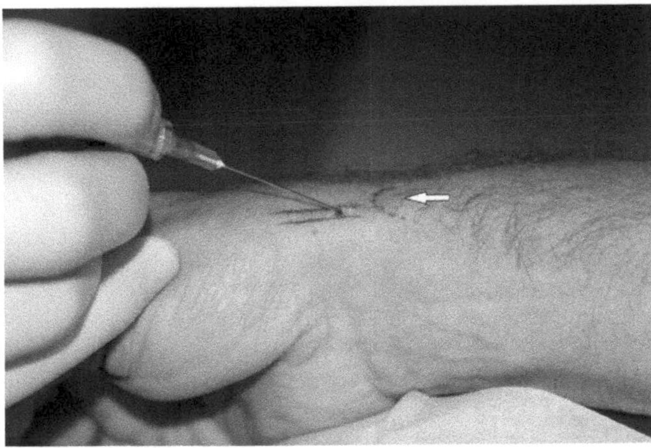

FIGURE 30.9 Injection technique for de Quervain's tenosynovitis. The needle is inserted at a 30°–45° angle into the tendon sheath of the APL and EPB. If a split can be felt between the tendons, this should be the aiming location. The needle is directed toward the radial styloid (see solid arrow) to a depth of 5 mm. Needle may be advanced or withdrawn to allow free flow of fluid.

Clinical Pearl

Inject in a cephalad direction at the radial styloid, where the two tendons split. Monitor for your injectate to flow along the tendon course, filling the sheath.

30.7.3.2 Carpal Tunnel Injection

Carpal tunnel syndrome (median nerve compression) is a common condition and is the indication for this injection. Clinical landmarks that aid in the injection of the carpal tunnel include the palmaris longus (PL) when present, flexor carpi radialis (FCR) tendon, and the proximal wrist crease. The median nerve typically lies between the FCR tendons and the PL or just medial to the midline of the wrist in the case when PL is absent.[101]

As with all injections, the patient and the provider administering the injection must be comfortable. The patient may either be seated or supine on exam table. The supinated forearm should rest on a table or platform and a small bolster should be placed under the dorsal wrist allowing the wrist to relax into slight extension. After landmarks are once again appreciated, the needle is inserted medial to the PL just proximal to the distal wrist crease. In the setting of an absent PL, injecting at the midline of the wrist is a suitable alternative.[101] The angle of insertion is 30° but should be parallel to the angle created by the palm of the hand resting on the bolster (see Figure 30.10). The depth of insertion is usually about 1 cm, and the needle should be directed toward the ring finger. If the patient complains of pain or paresthesia in the median nerve distribution, readjustment prior to injection is necessary. Finger motion may help to avoid injection into the flexor tendons as does readjustment of

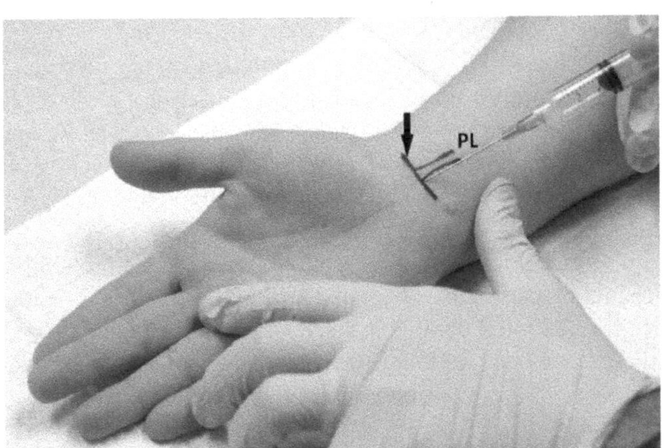

FIGURE 30.10 Injection technique for carpal tunnel syndrome. The landmarks for this injection include the palmaris longus (PL) (when present) and the proximal wrist crease. The needle is directed toward the ring finger and in plane with the angle of the palm of the hand.

the needle should solute not flow freely. Occasionally, a pop may be felt as the transverse carpal ligament is entered.

Typical needle size is 1–1.5 in. and 25–27 gauge. About 1.0 mL of corticosteroid and 1–2 mL of anesthetic may be used for the injection. Carpal tunnel injection has been shown to be effective at least short term.[3,6,47] Patients with less symptoms and smaller cross-sectional area on ultrasound improve more frequently with nonsurgical management.[70] Repeat injection can be beneficial if symptoms recur.[5] Ultrasound guidance may help improve accuracy and efficacy, but studies are mixed in this regard.[62,107]

Clinical Pearl

This is an effective treatment for carpal tunnel syndrome that is often overlooked.

30.7.3.3 First Carpometacarpal and Metacarpophalangeal Joint Injections

Any of the metacarpal phalangeal joints may be injected for the relief of symptomatic osteoarthritis or inflammatory arthritis or to provide anesthesia for reduction of dislocations. The most common location for injection is at the first carpometacarpal (CMC) junction as this is a common site for degenerative change. The anatomy for the first CMC junction injection can be difficult to ascertain due to deformity or body habitus but typically represents the distal margin of the anatomic snuff box over the lateral wrist. Thumb motion and pressure over the proximal first metacarpal accompanied by volar stabilization of the distal first metacarpal aid in locating this joint. Any of the metacarpophalangeal (MCP) joints may be located, usually quite easily at their junction. Moderate distraction may aid in locating the joint line.

The patient is typically resting comfortably with the wrist in neutral (thumb up) for the first CMC injection or on the volar surface for the MCP joint injections. The technique for entering the first CMC space may be aided by outlining the joint with a marker. The skin is entered and the needle advance confidently until entry into the joint or bone is met (see Figure 30.11). Careful manipulation of the first metacarpal bone may aid in locating the joint after needle entry. Needle may need to be "walked" into the joint. MCP joints may be entered either medially or laterally bearing in mind the anatomy of the proximal phalanx and angling the needle accordingly.

The usual amount of steroid is 0.5 mL with a similar amount of anesthetic. This injection uses 0.5-in., 25–27-gauge needles. Limited data exist for accuracy and efficacy. Small studies demonstrated short-term benefit in palpation-guided injection[34,48,90] of the first CMC joint.

Clinical Pearl

This injection is technically challenging. Use of gentle-in-line traction may aid in entering the joint.

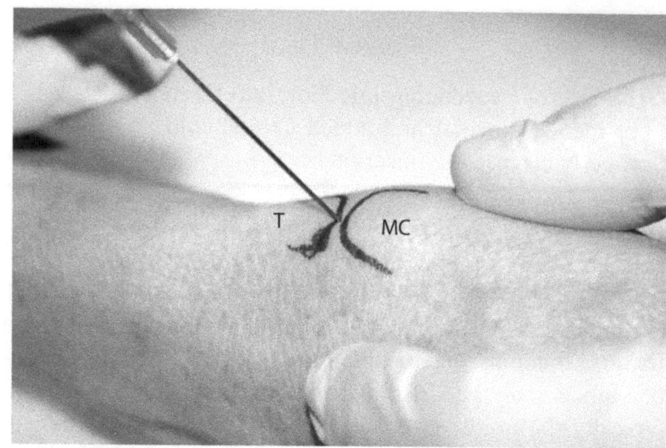

FIGURE 30.11 Injection into first carpometacarpal joint. The landmarks for this injection include the proximal first metacarpal (MC) and the trapezium (T). This can be a challenging injection in the setting of deforming arthritis. The joint space is also narrow.

30.7.3.4 Triangular Fibrocartilage Complex

The indications for this injection include *degenerative tear* of the triangular fibrocartilage complex at the end of the distal ulna, osteoarthritis, or inflammatory arthritis over the same location. The anatomic landmarks include the ulnar styloid process and triquetrum. The superior margin is the FCU tendon.

The patient is typically seated comfortably with the wrist and hand pronated and resting on the table or armrest. Anatomic landmarks are identified and the injection proceeds with the needle entering distal to the ulna styloid process, to the ulnar side of the FCU tendon and angled to aim for the distal radial ulnar joint (see Figure 30.12). Solute should flow freely. Concern about complications from shallow injections also applies to this injection. Typical needle size is 25–27 gauge and length is 0.5 in. About 0.5 mL of corticosteroid accompanied by 0.5–1 mL of anesthetic

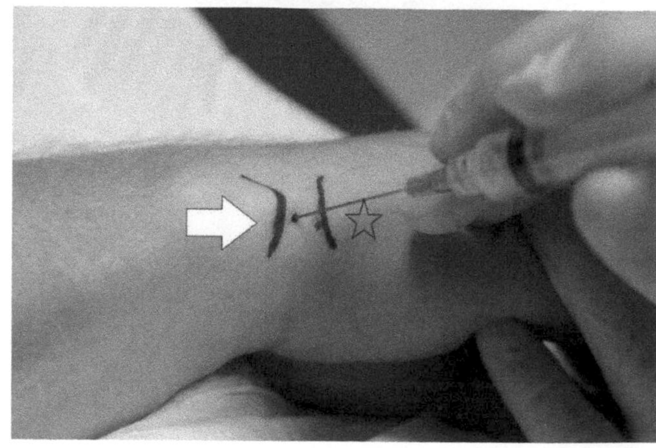

FIGURE 30.12 Injection for degenerative triangular fibrocartilage complex joint pain. Solid arrow is located at the ulnar styloid and hollow star at the triquetrum. The needle enters the hollow formed between these landmarks and is directed to the distal radial ulnar joint to a depth of 0.5–1 cm.

usually suffices. Very limited evidence exists for the accuracy and efficacy of this injection.

Clinical Pearl

This injection can be used in the symptomatic treatment of a *degenerative* triangular fibrocartilage complex tear.

30.7.3.5 Trigger Thumb/Finger

The indications for this injection are stenosing tenosynovitis of the flexor tendons of the fingers and can occur in any flexor tendon.

The landmark that must be appreciated is the A1 pulley. This pulley is often hypertrophied by the ongoing inflammatory response in the flexor digitorum superficialis tendon sheath. The A1 pulley may be appreciated anterior and slightly proximal to the MCP joint(s) and may be tender. A demonstrative pop or triggering of the finger may be noticed.

Typically, the patient is seated but may also be supine with the forearm supinated and the dorsum of the hand resting comfortably on a table or platform. The distal palmar crease is a useful landmark for the injection from a proximal to distal technique. The needle should enter the skin at an oblique angle parallel to the tendon at a depth of about 4–5 mm (see Figure 30.13). Finger motion and attempts to inject may be helpful in assuring the solute is not injected into the tendon directly. A distal to proximal approach may also be used.

Typical needle size ranges from 0.5 to 1.5 in. and 25 to 27 gauge. About 0.5 mL of steroid and a similar amount of anesthetic may be used. The goal is to inject half to all of the solute, but care should be exercised not to "force" the remainder. This injection is considered efficacious by a number of different studies although multiple injections may not be as helpful.[29,74,84,95,97] Diabetics may have a higher failure rate and overall long-term failure rate approaches 30%.[73,95] Rupture of flexor tendons is thought to be rare.[115] Insoluble corticosteroid injection (triamcinolone, methylprednisolone) may be more efficacious than soluble corticosteroid preparations.[73] More than two injections in any year may require surgical intervention.[73,97]

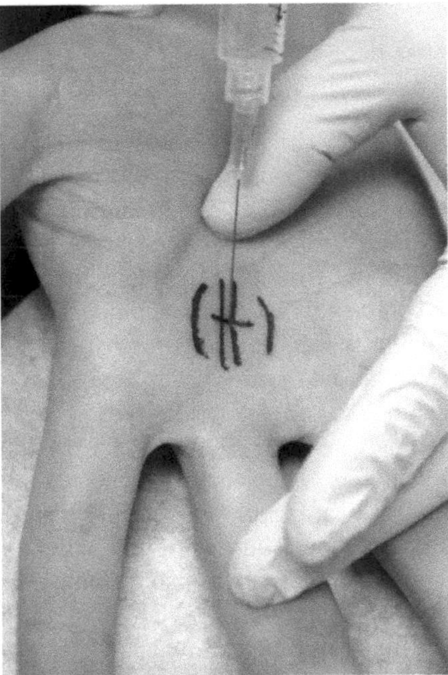

FIGURE 30.13 Injection for trigger finger. The landmarks for this injection include the first metacarpal phalangeal joint (curved lines), the flexor digitorum tendons (vertical lines) and the A1 pulley which can occasionally be palpated when hypertrophied (horizontal line).

Clinical Pearl

Often overlooked, trigger finger injections can provide lasting relief. Care must be exercised to avoid injecting directly into the tendon.

30.7.3.6 Intersection Syndrome

The indications for this injection include inflammation and pain at the junction of the first and second dorsal compartment over the posterolateral wrist. This syndrome is often called intersection syndrome and is much less common compared to de Quervain's tenosynovitis. The anatomic landmarks include the mass of muscle comprising the APL and EPB overlying the tendons of the ECRB and longus and are lateral to Lister's tubercle in anatomic position. If conservative measures fail or if the patient has considerable pain, injection may be undertaken to relieve symptoms.[40,116] The patient is usually seated with the arm resting comfortably in either prone or neutral position. Outlining the distal junction of the compartment may aid in placement of the injection. Extending the wrist and abducting/extending the thumb may aid in locating aiming point for injection. Alternating this technique with forced grip and slight wrist extension may also aid in location of injection. The goal is to inject under the muscle bellies of the APL and EPB but over the ECRB and extensor carpi radialis longus (see Figure 30.14). Usual amount of corticosteroid is 0.5–1 mL with a similar amount of anesthetic.[116] The usual needle length is 1–1.5 cm and bore is usually 25–27 gauge. There is no clear evidence for accuracy or efficacy.

Clinical Pearl

Extending the wrist and abducting/extending the thumb may aid in locating aiming point for injection.

30.7.4 Hip Region

30.7.4.1 Trochanteric Bursitis/Gluteus Medius Tendon

The indications for this injection include recalcitrant trochanteric bursitis or chronic point specific lateral trochanteric pain and tenderness. Prior to the use of musculoskeletal ultrasound, trochanteric bursitis was felt to be common. Gluteus medius and minimus tendinopathy and tears also should be kept in the differential diagnosis as they are common and overlap greatly with the symptoms of trochanteric bursitis.[37]

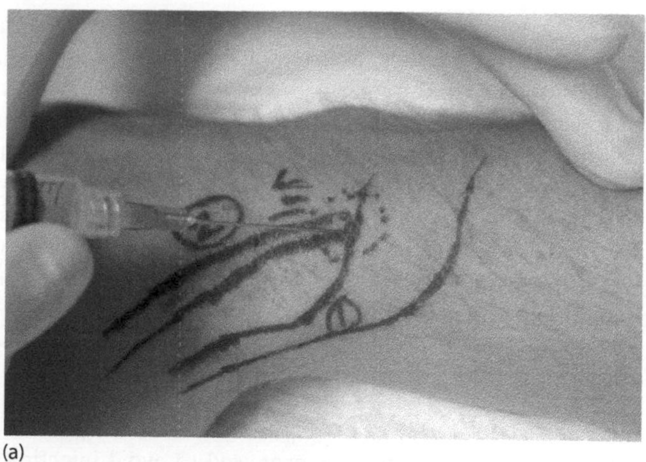

(a)

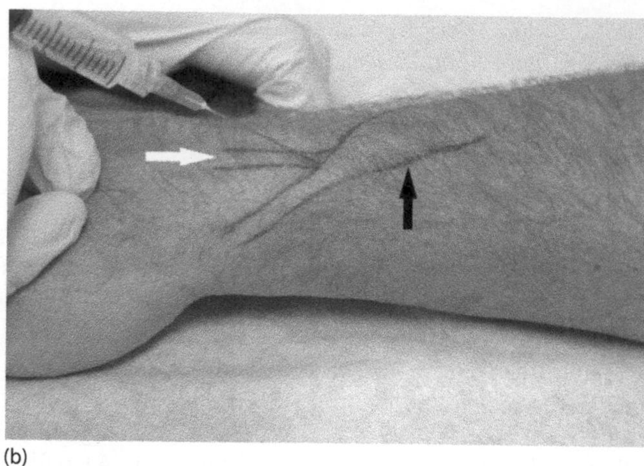

(b)

FIGURE 30.14 Injection for intersection syndrome. This injection occurs between the muscle bellies of the APL and EPB of the rst dorsal compartment (a) and the tendons of the ECRB and ECRL of the second dorsal compartment (b). The aiming location is identied above by the circle and injection is undertaken at the crossing of these compartments.

The landmark to be identified is the greater trochanter of the femur. This is best appreciated by placing the patient in the lateral decubitus position on the contralateral side. The greater trochanter is palpated as the bony prominence over the lateral hip and can be exquisitely tender. The bursa, when enlarged, typically is lateral and slightly posterior to the trochanter.

After the location of maximal tenderness is appreciated, the needle should enter the skin in a perpendicular fashion and advanced confidently to the greater trochanter (see Figure 30.15). The depth of insertion varies by patient body habitus and may range from 0.5 in. to much greater depths (4–5 in.). After contacting the bone, the needle is withdrawn slightly and the injection undertaken. Multiple techniques have been described including bolus injection and peppering.

Needle length is determined by patient body habitus (see previous paragraph regarding depths). Typical needle gauge ranges from 21 to 23 gauge. Needle deflection is a real concern with smaller gauge needles of longer length. Typically, 1 mL of corticosteroid with 2–3 mL of anesthetic is used for the injection. Small studies indicate this injection is modestly effective at least in short term to assist other modalities in treating this diagnosis.[13,20]

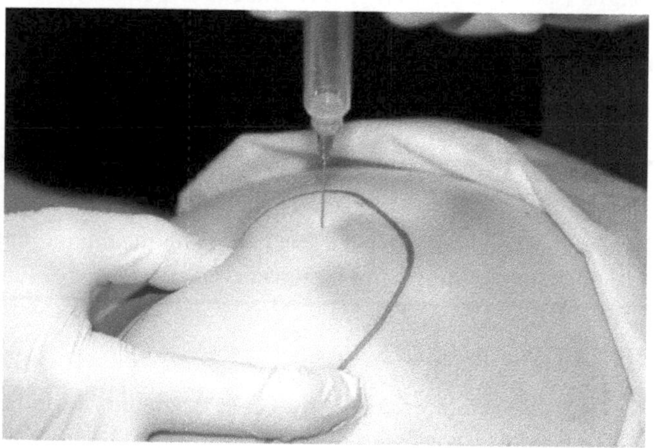

FIGURE 30.15 Injection for trochanteric bursitis. The landmark for this injection is the bony prominence of the greater trochanter (outlined above along with the long axis of the proximal femur). The needle enters the skin in a perpendicular fashion and the needle is advanced to the greater trochanter, withdrawn slightly and the injection is undertaken. Needle lengths may approach 3 in. or longer.

Clinical Pearl

Trochanteric syndrome injection may be best performed under ultrasound guidance if initial injection fails to relieve pain.

30.7.5 Knee Region

30.7.5.1 Intra-articular Knee

Injection of the knee is one of the most common injections in sports medicine and orthopedics. Indications include osteoarthritis, inflammatory arthritis, and joint aspiration.

Multiple different techniques have been described in the literature including both medial and lateral approaches. One of the more commonly utilized injections is through the lateral suprapatellar space. Typically, the patient is supine with the knee slightly flexed (bolster under knee). This area is identified by locating the superolateral aspect of the patella. The space is commonly palpated 1 cm lateral and 1 cm superior to the patellar landmark. The needle is oriented directly medial or toward the trochlea. If bony resistance is met, the needle is withdrawn. Solute should flow smoothly with minimal resistance (see Figure 30.16). This is also a commonly used location for knee joint aspiration.

Another common location for injection is the lateral joint recess slightly lateral to the patellar tendon. The patient is either seated or supine and the recess is identified lateral to the patella and posterior to the patellar tendon just above the joint line. The needle enters this portal and is directed toward the notch of the femur in a posteromedial direction (see Figure 30.17).

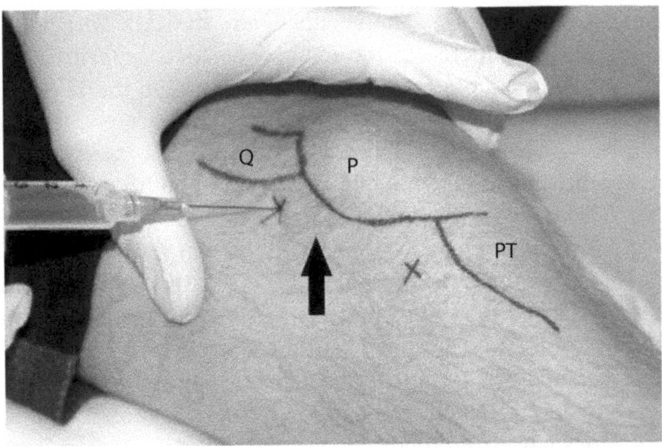

FIGURE 30.16 Superolateral technique for intra-articular knee aspiration/injection. The landmarks for this injection include the lateral aspect of the quadriceps tendon (Q), patella (P), patellar tendon (PT), and the lateral femoral condyle (deep to black arrow). The needle is directed under the patella in the region of the femoral trochlea.

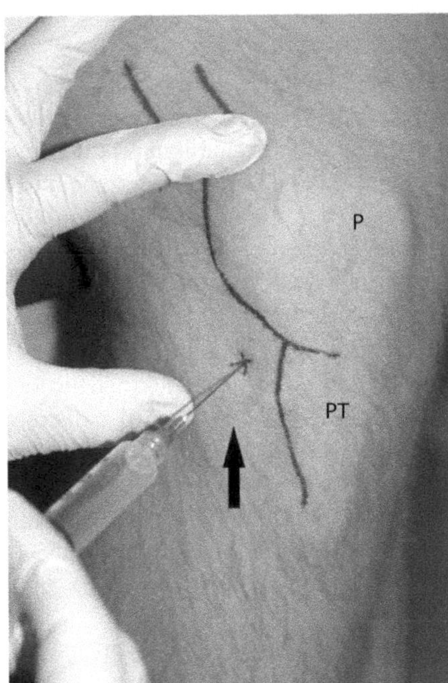

FIGURE 30.17 lateral joint recess technique for intra-articular knee injection/aspiration. The landmarks for this injection include the patella (P), patellar tendon (PTP), and lateral joint line (black arrow). The needle is advanced toward the intracondylar notch and needs to clear Hoffa's fat pad prior to injection.

The depth may be variable based on body habitus but needs to clear Hoffa's fat pad, often slightly more than an inch. The injection of solute must flow easily and smoothly.

Typical needle size for injection is a 1.5 in., 22–25-gauge needle. About 1–2 mL of corticosteroid combined with 2–4 mL of anesthetic is sufficient. Of note, when performing a joint aspiration, larger bore needles (18 or 16 g) and larger syringe volumes (20 mL or greater) are commonly necessary to obtain joint fluid. Typically with larger sized needles, skin anesthesia is necessary for patient comfort.

Multiple studies have been performed on accuracy of injection, and a recent systematic review has helped shed light the most appropriate location for intra-articular knee injection. Of the locations for injection that are palpation guided, the lateral portal(s) appear to be the most accurate location(s) with the superolateral patellar approach reported as the most accurate.[15,60,61,67] Accuracy may improve response to injection but this has not been evaluated in many studies.[67,98] Provider experience may improve accuracy. Medial approaches may be used with less accuracy, but it appears that the medial midpatella approach may prove the most difficult with accuracy rates only approaching a dismal 56% success rate.[32,67] Provider comfort in any approach accompanied by knowledge of more than one location may aid in accurate placement of the needle. Ultrasound or other forms of guidance may aid in needle placement, but accuracy is still very reasonable to perform this injection by visual and palpation confirmed landmarks.[67]

While there does not appear to be an easy way to predict who will respond to corticosteroid injection,[66] short-term benefit has been demonstrated in multiple studies in the setting of osteoarthritis or inflammatory arthritis.[8,12,44] Arthrocentesis for aspiration of joint fluid may be best undertaken in supine position.[120]

Clinical Pearl

The superolateral, lateral midpatella, and superior patellar recess are the most accurate/easiest locations to enter.

30.7.5.2 Pes Anserine Bursa

The pes anserine bursa may become inflamed and often accompanies symptomatic medial joint osteoarthritis. The pes anserinus lies over the medial tibia distal to the joint line and is where the sartorius, gracilis, and semitendinosus insert. The pes anserine bursa is located just proximal to the insertion. There is usually an area of maximal tenderness associated with the syndrome, but the pes anserinus may also be identified by palpation as the patient flexes the knee against resistance.

The pes anserine bursa is the target for the injection (see Figure 30.18). The needle enters the skin just anterior and lateral to the bursa with the needle directed medially and posteriorly. Advance the needle until bone is met and then withdraw slightly. Depth is variable based on body habitus but may be very shallow in those with less subcutaneous tissue (at times 4–5 mm). Aspiration may be helpful with locating the bursa and solute should flow with minimal resistance. Typically, needle size is 1–1.5 in. and 25 g. About 0.5 mL of corticosteroid and 0.5–1 mL of anesthetic is typically used.[1,21,76] Studies on efficacy and accuracy are few but do show at least short-term improvement in pain.[23,58] Ultrasound guidance may be necessary for accurate placement of injection as the pes anserinus is often tender in the setting of medial joint osteoarthritis without a true bursitis present.[11]

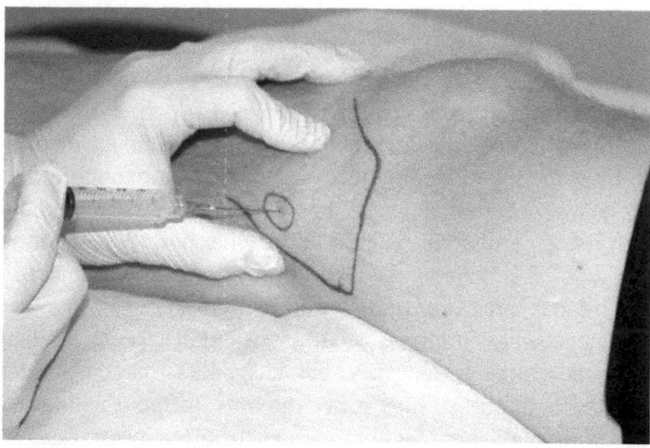

FIGURE 30.18 Injection into the pes anserine bursa. The landmarks for this injection include the medial tibial plateau (solid line) and the pes anserine bursa (circle). The pes anserine complex may be palpable by having the patient flex and adduct the knee gently. The needle is advance until bone is met and withdrawn slightly.

Clinical Pearl

Pes anserine pain is often referred pain from medial joint arthritis. If injection fails to relieve pain, an intra-articular knee injection may prove helpful.

30.7.5.3 Iliotibial Band Friction Syndrome

Iliotibial band (ITB) friction syndrome is a common problem seen in runners and may be injected when recalcitrant. The anatomic landmarks include the lateral femoral epicondyle ridge and the ITB just lateral to that. The superior margin of the ITB may be felt as a ridge lateral to the patella and superior to the joint line over the femoral epicondyle. Flexing and extending the knee may aid in locating the distal ITB.

The patient may be supine or seated for this injection. The knee is typically flexed to 90°, and the point of maximal tenderness is identified. Again, altering knee flexion may help identify this location. The needle enters the skin perpendicularly and is directed to the femoral epicondyle (see Figure 30.19). The intent is to enter the space between the ITB and the lateral epicondyle; this is the location of the bursa. If bone is met, withdraw slightly and attempt aspiration/injection. As with other injections, the fluid must flow smoothly. Care must be exercised not to withdraw too far so as to inject the ITB itself. Typical depths are from 5 mm to 1 cm.

Needle size is usually 1 in. and is typically a 25–27-gauge needle. Corticosteroid volume is 0.5 mL combined with a similar amount of anesthetic. Limited data exist on efficacy and accuracy.[31,38] Short-term benefit may be expected.[38] Complications including distal ITB rupture after repeated injections have been reported.[79]

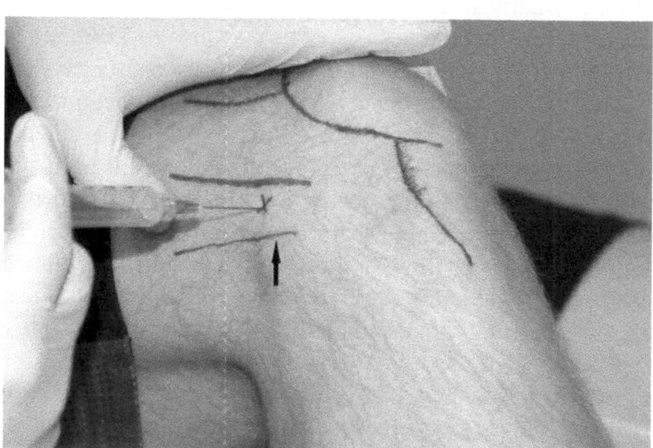

FIGURE 30.19 Injection for iliotibial band friction syndrome. This injection proceeds after identifying the distal ITB (horizontal lines) and the lateral femoral epicondyle (black arrow).

Clinical Pearl

Slight flexion and extension of the knee helps in isolating the superior border of the distal ITB.

30.7.6 Ankle and Foot Region

30.7.6.1 Ankle Joint Injection

Indications for this injection are inflammatory and degenerative conditions of the ankle. It may also be used to provide relief for ankle impingement and arthrocentesis may be used diagnostically.

The ankle joint may be entered anteromedially or anterolaterally.[43,53,112,113] The anteromedial location is the hollow formed by the articulation of the tibial plafond, medial malleolus, and superior talus. The lateral location is formed by the anteromedial border of the fibula, anterolateral border of the tibia, and superior talus.

The patient is usually seated or supine and the foot may either rest on a footrest, table, or rest freely. Ankle distraction may be applied by an assistant if necessary. In either location noted in the preceding text, the needle enters the skin perpendicularly and is directed posteriorly (see Figure 30.20). Continuous aspiration is helpful as the needle advances to know when the joint is entered. The depth of insertion is usually 10–20 mm but may be variable. Solution should flow easily.

A 1.5-in., 25-gauge needle is typically used with larger bore needles reserved for aspiration. About 0.5–1 mL of corticosteroid accompanied by 2–4 mL of anesthetic is common. Accuracy rates are similar with either approach (see references in the previous text). Efficacy is unknown but likely varies based on diagnosis. Typically short term (2–3 months) is expected in the setting of mild degenerative joint disease.

Clinical Pearl

One of the easier and most often overlooked injections/aspirations to perform.

30.7.6.2 First Metatarsal Phalangeal Joint

Pain in the first metatarsal phalangeal joint is very common and often accompanies deformities like hallux valgus, gout,

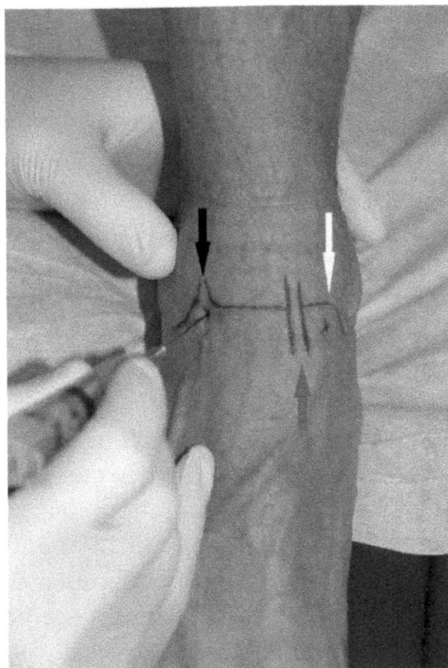

FIGURE 30.20 Intra-articular ankle injection/aspiration. Either the anteromedial (black arrow) or anterolateral (white arrow) portal may be used to enter the ankle joint. The anterolateral approach is bordered by the medial aspect of the fibula, lateral aspect of the tibial and the lateral talar dome. The anteromedial approach is bordered by the arch made by the tibial plafond and medial malleolus superiorly and the talar dome inferiorly. The tibialis anterior represents the lateral margin for this approach (gray arrow).

and degenerative disorders. These diagnoses may limit range of motion compounding the problem. Anatomic landmarks are the head of the first metatarsal, base of the proximal phalanx of the great toe, and extensor tendons of the great toe.

The patient is typically supine, but injection may proceed in a seated fashion. Landmarks are identified and gentle-in-line traction is applied to the great toe. The needle enters at a slight angle (5°) medial or lateral to the extensor tendons and the depth is usually shallow, 5 mm (see Figure 30.21). Aspiration may proceed and needle readjustment may be necessary including "walking" down metatarsal until the joint is entered. Injection is undertaken as a bolus.

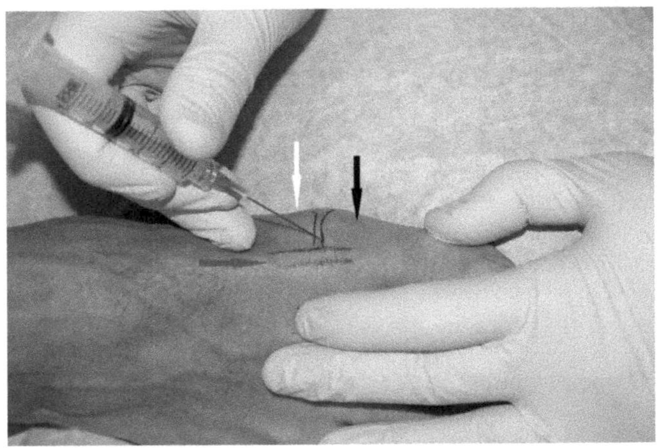

FIGURE 30.21 Injection into the first metatarsophalangeal joint. The landmarks for this injection include the distal first metatarsal head (white arrow), proximal phalanx of the first toe (black arrow), and the extensor hallucis longus tendon (gray arrow). The needle is angled under the flared base of the proximal phalanx and can be difficult in the setting of large joint spurs.

Usual needle length is 1 in. and 25–27-gauge bore. About 0.5–1 mL of corticosteroid accompanied by 0.5–1 mL of anesthetic (total volume should be less than 1.5 mL) may be used. Limited data on accuracy[63] and efficacy exist for this injection.[89]

Clinical Pearl

Gentle-in-line traction may help to open the joint for needle entry.

30.7.6.3 Interdigital "Morton's" Neuroma

The indication is for painful interdigital "Morton's" neuroma. Landmarks are the metatarsal heads and the space between where the interdigital nerves lie. Occasionally, the toes on bordering the neuroma may appear splayed to either side of the neuroma.

The neuroma usually lies in between, just plantar and slightly posterior to the metatarsal heads. Common locations are between the second and third, and third and fourth metatarsal heads, but any space may be involved. The patient may be seated or supine with the foot plantar flexed and resting on the table. The needle enters the skin between the metatarsal heads in a perpendicular fashion on the dorsal surface of the foot and is directed inferiorly (plantar). Occasionally, a pop may be felt as the intermetatarsal ligament is pierced. The location of injection should correspond to the area of maximal tenderness (see Figure 30.22). Depth is approximately 1 cm.

A 25 g, 1 in. needle is utilized for this injection. Typically, 0.5 mL of corticosteroid and 1 mL of anesthetic is used. Fat atrophy and skin hypopigmentation may occur after this injection, especially if repeated given its shallow location. Small studies demonstrate benefit, typically short term.[64,91]

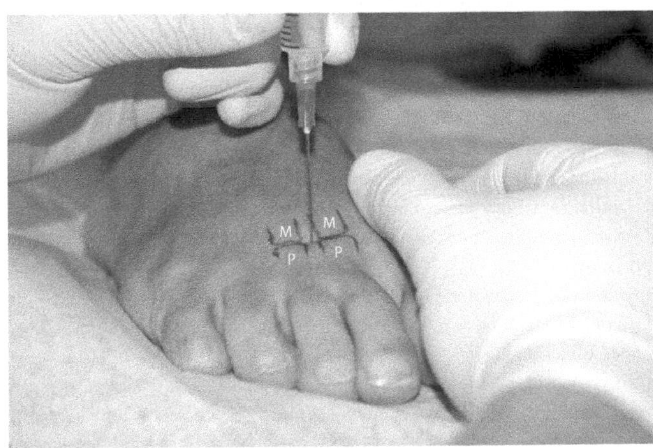

FIGURE 30.22 Injection technique for interdigital neuroma. The landmarks for this injection include the metatarsal heads (M) and proximal phalanxes of the toes (P). The injection is just proximal and directed vertically in a plantar fashion.

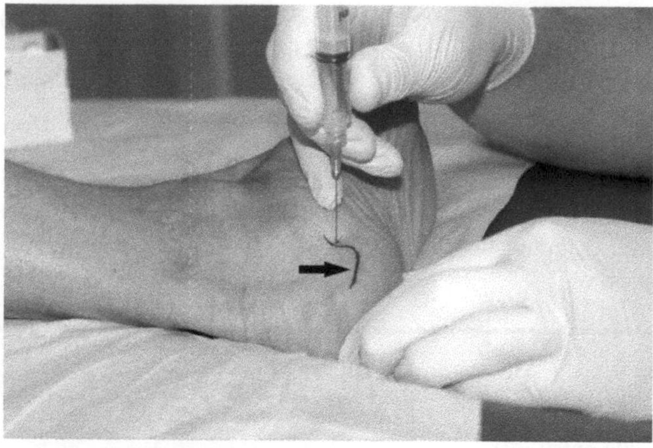

FIGURE 30.23 Injection for plantar "fasciitis." The solid black arrow represents the palpable location of the calcaneal tubercle. The injection is anterior to the tubercle and deep to the plantar fat pad to avoid atrophy.

Clinical Pearl

Risk of atrophy and short-term benefit limit this injection to selected patients that wish to avoid or delay surgery. Frequent injection is not recommended.

30.7.6.4 Plantar Fascia

The indication for this injection is inferior heel pain due to plantar fasciopathy (fasciitis). The calcaneal tubercle is identified both posteriorly and medially. This usually corresponds to the location of maximal tenderness. Occasionally, it is necessary to dorsiflex the ankle and great toe to assist in defining the location.

The patient is typically supine with the foot at the examiners eye level. Two approaches have been traditionally utilized. In the medial approach, the calcaneal tubercle is identified 2–3 cm from the posterior margin of calcaneus. The needle enters the skin from a medial to lateral approach and aiming point is location of maximal tenderness (see Figure 30.23). It is imperative to stay superior/cephalad to the fat pad overlying the calcaneus (avoid a shallow injection) due to worse outcome from fat pad atrophy. Readjustment of the needle may be necessary to find the appropriate location for injection. Significant resistance to injection requires needle repositioning. Flow of solute is not as smooth as typically noted for joint injection but should not require significant force.

An alternate injection technique is to enter the plantar surface of the heel approximately 1 cm distal to point of maximal tenderness. The needle is angled to the point of maximal tenderness and often the needle will contact bone. At this point, the needle should be withdrawn slightly and injection should

TABLE 30.5
SORT: Key Recommendations for Practice

Clinical Recommendations	Evidence Rating	References
Injections are associated with a low rate of infection and overall complication.	A	[19,25,75,109]
Acromioclavicular joint injection can help relieve arthritis pain but may benefit from ultrasound guidance in the setting of joint spurring.	C	[17,46,81,87,93,94,108]
Glenohumeral joint injection may be best suited under ultrasound guidance in particular in those patients with larger body habitus.	B	[16,28,33,42,80]
Palpation-guided subacromial bursa injection compares favorably with image-guided injection.	B	[30,50]
Ultrasound guidance may be necessary to assure accurate needle placement in biceps tendon sheath.	B	[41,106]
Corticosteroid has not been shown to provide benefit in trigger point injection.	B	[2,7,103]
Injection for lateral epicondylitis provides short-term relief only.	B	[10,55,59]
Ultrasound guidance improves intra-articular elbow injection accuracy but with no difference in efficacy.	C	[36,60]
Aspiration and injection of the olecranon bursa is useful after conservative therapy fails.	C	[11]
Corticosteroid injection for de Quervain's tenosynovitis can provide symptom relief.	B	[49,85]
Corticosteroid injection for carpal tunnel syndrome provides at least short-term symptom relief.	A	[3,6,47]
Palpation-guided injection into the first carpometacarpal joint can provide short-term symptom relief.	B	[34,48,90]
Injection for trigger finger/thumb provides relief of symptoms in particular in the nondiabetic patient.	A	[29,74,84,95,97]
Corticosteroid injection for intersection syndrome can provide symptom relief after failure of conservative therapy.	C	[40,116]
Injection for trochanteric syndrome may provide short-term relief.	C	[13,20]
Use of the lateral portals, in particular the superolateral portal, improves accuracy during intra-articular knee injection.	A	[15,60,61,67]
Corticosteroid injection for pes anserine bursitis may provide short-term symptom relief.	C	[23,58]
Injection for distal iliotibial band bursitis may provide short-term symptom relief.	C	[38]
Either the anteromedial or anterolateral portals may be used in intra-articular ankle injection.	A	[43,53,112,113]
Injection of interdigital (Morton's) neuroma may provide short term relief	C	[64,91]
Ultrasound-guided and palpation-guided corticosteroid injection for plantar fasciitis are both efficacious.	B	[9,57,104,119]

proceed. In the author's experience, either approach may be painful and is less tolerated than other injections such as subacromial and intra-articular knee. Topical anesthetic may be necessary. Needle depth for either injection varies by patient but is often more than 1 cm.

Complications include fat pad atrophy and rupture of the plantar fascia. Minimal data on complication rates but are felt to be rare (1%–2%).[54]

A 1.5-in., 25–27-gauge needle is typically utilized for this injection. Corticosteroid volume is usually 0.5 mL and anesthetic is from 1 to 2 mL. Efficacy has been demonstrated in the short term, but long-term benefit is unknown.[27,69] Physical therapy with or without injection may be an effective intervention as well.[92] Previous concern has been raised regarding the use of corticosteroid due to potential harms from this injection, but more recent opinion shows that it is useful. Studies show both palpation- and ultrasound-guided injections are efficacious.[9,57,104,119]

Clinical Pearl

Shallow injections into the plantar fat pad are to be avoided.

CONCLUSION

Injection has been a mainstay procedure for the primary care provider and can be a rewarding experience for both patient and provider when used appropriately. There has been a considerable amount of discussion in the recent literature about solute types, timing of injection, appropriate use of corticosteroid injection when no inflammation is present, utilization of either radiographic or ultrasound guidance, and whether or not any solute should be injected. Additionally, the routine use of corticosteroid injection in the pediatric population has not been recommended (certainly with inflammatory arthritis it may be of benefit). The debate will no doubt be ongoing and lively and help define these questions in the years to come. To date, palpation-guided injection is still very commonly utilized and has shown at least modest success and accuracy (Table 30.5).

REFERENCES

1. Abeles M. Osteoarthritis of the knee: Anserine bursitis as an extra articular cause of pain. *Clin Res* 1983;31:4471–4476.
2. Affaitati G, Fabrizio A, Savini A, Lerza R, Tafuri E, Costantini R, Lapenna D, Giamberardino M. A randomized, controlled study comparing a lidocaine patch, a placebo patch, and anesthetic injection for treatment of trigger points in patients with myofascial pain syndrome: Evaluation of pain and somatic pain thresholds. *Clin Therapeut* 2009;31(4):705–720.
3. Andreu J, Ly-Pen D, Millán I, de Blas G, Sánchez-Olaso A. Local injection versus surgery in carpal tunnel syndrome: Neurophysiologic outcomes of a randomized clinical trial. *Clin Neurophysiol* 2014;125:1479–1484.
4. Ashkenazi A, Blumenfeld A, Napchan U, Narouze S, Grosberg B, Nett R, DePalma T, Rosenthal B, Tepper S, Lipton R. Peripheral nerve blocks and trigger point injections in headache management—A systematic review and suggestions for future research. *Headache* 2010;50(6):943–952.
5. Ashworth N, Bland J. Effectiveness of second corticosteroid injections for carpal tunnel syndrome. *Muscle Nerve* 2013; 48:122–126.
6. Atroshi I, Flondell M, Hofer M, Ranstam J. Methylprednisolone injections for the carpal tunnel syndrome, a randomized, placebo-controlled trial. *Ann Intern Med* 2013;159:309–317.
7. Ay S, Evcik D, Sonel Tur B. Comparison of injection methods in myofascial pain syndrome: a randomized controlled trial. *Clin Rheumatol* 2009;29(1):19–23.
8. Ayhan E, Kesmezacar H, Akgun, I. Intraarticular injections (corticosteroid, hyaluronic acid, platelet rich plasma) for the knee osteoarthritis. *World J Orthop* 2014;5:351–361.
9. Ball E, McKeeman H, Patterson C, Burns J, Yao W, Moore O, Benson C, Foo J, Wright G, Taggart A. Steroid injection for inferior heel pain: A randomised controlled trial. *Ann Rheum Dis* 2013;72:996–1002.
10. Barr S, Cerisola F, Blanchard V. Effectiveness of corticosteroid injections compared with physiotherapeutic interventions for lateral epicondylitis: A systematic review. *Physiotherapy* 2009;95(4):251–265.
11. Baumbach S, Wyen H, Perez C, Kanz K, Uckay I. Evaluation of current treatment regimens for prepatellar and olecranon bursitis in Switzerland. *Eur J Trauma Emerg Surg* 2012; 39(1):65–72.
12. K4. Bellamy N, Campbell J, Robinson V, Gee T, Bourne R, Wells G. Intraarticular corticosteroid for treatment of osteoarthritis of the knee. *Cochrane Datab Syst Rev* 2006; (2):CD005328.
13. Bhagra A, Syed H, Reed D, Poterucha T, Cha SS, Baumgartner T, Takahashi P. Efficacy of musculoskeletal injections by primary care providers in the office: A retrospective cohort study. *Int J Gen Med* April 15, 2013;6:237–243.
14. Blackwell J, Hay B, Bolt A, Hay S. Olecranon bursitis: A systematic overview. *Shoulder Elbow* 2014;6(3):182–190.
15. Bliddal H. Placement of intra-articular injections verified by mini air-arthrography. *Ann Rheum Dis* 1999;58:641–643.
16. Bloom J, Rischin A, Johnston R, Buchbinder R. Image-guided versus blind glucocorticoid injection for shoulder pain. *Cochrane Musculoskeletal* 2012;17(Suppl 1):CD009147.pub2.
17. Borbas P, Kraus T, Clement H, Grechenig S, Weinberg A, Heidari N. The influence of ultrasound guidance in the rate of success of acromioclavicular joint injection: An experimental study on human cadavers. *J Shoulder Elbow Surg* 2012; 21(12):1694–1697.
18. Brand C. Intra-articular and soft tissue injections. *Aust Family Physician* 1990;19:671–682.
19. Brinks A, Koes B, Volkers A, Verhaar J, Bierma-Zeinstra S. Adverse effects of extra-articular corticosteroid injections: A systematic review. *BMC Musculoskelet Disord* 2010;11:206.
20. Brinks A, van Rijn R, Willemsen S, Bohnen A, Verhaar A, Koes B, Bierma-Zeinstra S. Corticosteroid injections for greater trochanteric pain syndrome: A randomized controlled trial in primary care. *Ann Fam Med* May–June 2011; 9(3):226–234. Erratum in: Ann Fam Med. July–August 2011; 9(3):371.
21. Brookler M, Mongan E. Anserine bursitis: a treatable cause of knee pain in patients with degenerative arthritis. *Calif Med* 1973;119:8–10.

22. Caldwell JR. Intra-articular corticosteroids: A guide to selection and indications for use. *Drugs* 1996;52:507–514.
23. Calvo-Alén J, Rua-Figueroa I, Erausquin C. Tratamiento de las bursitis anserina: infiltración local com corticoides frente a AINE: estudo prospectivo. *Rev Esp Reumatol* 1993; 20:13–15.
24. Catalano L, Glickel S, Barron O, Harrison R, Marshall A, Purcelli-Lafer M. Effect of local corticosteroid injection of the hand and wrist on blood glucose in patients with diabetes mellitus. *Orthopedics* 2012;35:e1754–e1758.
25. Charalambous C, Tryfonidis M, Sadiq S et al. Septic arthritis following intra-articular steroid injection of the knee—A survey of current practice regarding antiseptic technique used during intra-articular steroid injection of the knee. *Clin Rheumatol* 2003;22(6):386–390.
26. Cole B, Schumacher H, Jr. Injectable corticosteroids in modern practice. *J Am Acad Orthop Surg* 2005;13:37–46.
27. Crawford F, Atkins D, Young P, Edwards J. Steroid injection for heel pain: Evidence of short-term effectiveness. A randomized controlled trial. *Rheumatology* 1999;38(10):974–977.
28. Cunnington J, Marshall N, Hide G, Bracewell C, Isaacs J, Platt P, Kane D. A randomized, double-blind, controlled study of ultrasound-guided corticosteroid injection into the joint of patients with inflammatory arthritis. *Arthritis Rheumatism* 2010;62(7):1862–1869.
29. Dala-Ali B, Nakhdjevani A, Lloyd M, Schreuder F. The efficacy of steroid injection in the treatment of trigger finger. *Clin Orthop Surg* December 2012;4:263–268.
30. Ekeberg O, Bautz-Holter E, Tveita E, Juel N, Kvalheim S, Brox J. Subacromial ultrasound guided or systemic injection for rotator cuff disease: Randomised double blind study. *BMJ* 2009;338:a3112.
31. Ellis R, Hing W, Reid D. Iliotibial band friction syndrome—A systematic review. *Man Ther* 2007;12:200–228.
32. Esenyel C, Demirhan M, Esenyel M, Sonmez M, Kahraman S, Senel B, Ozdes T. Comparison of four different intra-articular injection sites in the knee: A cadaver study. *Knee Surg Sports Traumatol Arthrosc* 2007;15:573–577.
33. Esenvel C, Ozturk K, Demirhan M, Sonmez M, Kahraman S, Esenvel M, Ozbaydar M, Senel B. Accuracy of anterior glenohumeral injections: A cadaver study. *Arch Orthopaedic Trauma Surg* 2010;130(3):297–300.
34. Fuchs S, Mönikes R, Wohlmeiner, Heyse T. Intra-articular hyaluronic acid compared with corticoid injections for the treatment of rhizarthrosis. *OsteoArthritis Cartilage* 2006;14:82–88.
35. Genovese M. Joint and soft tissue injection: A useful adjuvant to systemic and local treatment. *Postgraduate Med* 1998;103:125–134.
36. Gilliland C, Salazar L, Borchers J. Ultrasound versus anatomic guidance for intra-articular and periarticualr injection: A systematic review. *Physician Sports Med* 2011;39(3):121–131.
37. Grumet R, Frank R, Slabaugh M, Virkus W, Bush-Joseph C, Nho S. Lateral hip pain in an athletic population: Differential diagnosis and treatment options. *Sports Health* May 2010;2:191–196.
38. Gunter P, Schwellnus M. Local corticosteroid injection in iliotibial band friction syndrome in runners: A randomised controlled trial. *Br J Sport Med* 2004;38:269–272.
39. Habib G, Abu-Ahmad R. Lack of effect of corticosteroid injection at the shoulder joint on blood glucose levels in diabetic patients. *Clin Rheumatol* 2007;26:566–568.
40. Hanlon D, Luellen J. Intersection syndrome: A case report and review of the literature. *J Emerg Med* 1999;17:969–971.
41. Hashiuchi T, Sakurai G, Morimoto M, Komei T, Takakura Y, Tanaka Y. Accuracy of the biceps tendon sheath injection: ultrasound-guided or unguided injection? A randomized controlled trial. *J Shoulder Elbow Surg* 2011;20(7):1069–1073.
42. Hegedus E, Zavala J, Kissenberth M, Cook C, Cassas K, Hawkins R, Tobola A. Positive outcomes with intra-articular glenohumeral injections are independent of accuracy. *J Shoulder Elbow Surg* 2010;19(6):795–801.
43. Heidari N, Pichler W, Grechenig S, Grechenig W, Weinberg A. Does the anteromedial or anterolateral approach alter the rate of ankle joint puncture in injection of the ankle? A cadaver study. *J Bone Joint Surg Br* 2010;92-B: 176–178.
44. Hepper C, Halvorson J, Duncan S, Gregory A, Dunn W, Spindler K. The efficacy and duration of intra-articular corticosteroid injection for knee osteoarthritis: A systematic review of level I studies. *J Am Acad Orthop Surg* 2009;10: 638–646.
45. Hong J, Yoon S, Moon D, Kwack K, Joen B, Lee H. Comparison of high- and low-dose corticosteroid in subacromial injection for periarticular shoulder disorder: A randomized, triple-blind, placebo-controlled trial. *Arch Phys Med Rehabil* 2011;92(12):1951–1960.
46. Hossain S, Jacobs L, Hashmi R. The long-term effectiveness of steroid injections in primary acromioclavicular joint arthritis: A five-year prospective study. *J Shoulder Elbow Surg* 2008;17(4): 535–538.
47. Huisstede B, Fridén J, Coert J, Hoogvliet P, European HANDGUIDE group. Carpal Tunnel Syndrome: hand surgeons, hand therapists, and physical medicine and & rehabilitation physicians agree on a multidisciplinary treatment guideline—Results from the European HANDGUIDE study. *Arch Phys Med Rehabil* 2014;95(12): 2253–2263.
48. Jahangiri A, Moghaddam F, Najafi S. Hypertonic dextrose versus corticosteroid local injection for the treatment of osteoarthritis in the first carpometacarpaljoint: A double-blind randomized clinical trial. *J Orthop Sci* 2014;19(5): 737–743.
49. Jeyapalan K, Choudhary S. Ultrasound-guided injection of triamcinolone and bupivicaine in the management of de Quervain's disease. *Skelet Radiol* 2009;38(11):1099–1103.
50. Kang M, Rizio L, Prybicienb M, Middlemasc D, Blacksin M. The accuracy of subacromial corticosteroid injections: A comparison of multiple methods. *J Shoulder Elbow Surg* 2008;17(1):S61–S66.
51. Karthikeyan S, Kwong H, Upadhyay P, Parsons N, Drew S, Griffin D. A double-blind randomised controlled study comparing subacromial injection of tenoxicam or methylprednisolone in patients with subacromial impingement. *J Bone Joint Surg Br* 2010;92-B(1): 77–82.
52. Kennedy JC, Willis RB. The effects of local steroids on tendons: A biomechanical and microscopic correlation study. *Am J Sports Med* 1976;4:11–21.
53. Khosla S, Thiele R, Baumhauer JF. Ultrasound guidance for intra-articular injections of the foot and ankle. *Foot Ankle Int* 2009;30(9): 886–890.
54. Kim C, Cashdollar M, Mendocino R, Catanzariti A, Fuge L. Incidence of plantar fascia ruptures following corticosteroid injection. *Foot Ankle Spec* 2010;3: 335–337.
55. Krogh T, Bartels E, Ellingsen T, Stengaard-Pedersen K, Buchbinder R, Fredberg U, Bliddal H, Christensen R. Comparative effectiveness of injection therapies in lateral epicondylitis: A systematic review and network meta-analysis of randomized controlled trials. *Am J Sports Med* 2013;41(6): 1435–1446.

56. Krogh T, Fredberg U, Stengaard-Pedersen K, Christensen R, Jensen P, Ellingsen T. Treatment of lateral epicondylitis with platelet-rich plasma, glucocorticoid or saline. *Am J Sports Med* 2013;41(3): 625–635.
57. Landorf KB, Menz HB. Plantar heel pain and fasciitis. *Clin Evid* 2008;2: 2–18.
58. Larsson L, Baum J. The syndrome of anserine bursitis: An overlooked diagnosis. *Arthritis Rheum* 1985;28: 1062–1065.
59. Lindenhovius A, Henket M, Gilligan B, Lozano-Calderon S, Jupiter J, Ring D. Injection of dexamethasone versus placebo for lateral elbow pain: A prospective, double-blind, randomized clinical trial. *J Hand Surg* 2008;33(6): 909–919.
60. Lopes R, Furtado R, Parmigiani L, Rosenfeld A, Fernandes A, Natour J. Accuracy of intra-articular injections in peripheral joints performed blindly in patients with rheumatoid arthritis. *Rheumatology* 2008;47: 1792–1794.
61. Luc M, Pham T, Chagnaud C, Lafforgue P, Legre V. Placement of intra-articular injection verified by the backflow technique. *Osteoarthr Cartilage* 2006;14: 714–716.
62. Makhlouf T, Emil S, Sibbitt Jr. W, Fields R, Bankhurst A. Outcomes and cost-effectiveness of carpal tunnel injections using sonographic needle guidance. *Clin Rheumatol* 2014;33: 849–858.
63. Manadan A, Mushtaq S, Block J. Radiocarpal and first metatarsophalangeal intraarticular injection site confirmation with fluoroscopy and review of accuracy of intraarticular injections. *Am J Ther* 2015;22(1): 11–13.
64. Marcovic M, Crichton K, Read JW, Lam P, Slater HK. Effectiveness of ultrasound-guided corticosteroid injection in the treatment of Morton's Neuroma. *Foot Ankle Int* 2008; 29(5): 483–487.
65. Marder R, Kim S, Labson J, Hunter J. Injection of the subacromial bursa in patients with rotator cuff syndrome: A prospective, randomized study comparing the effectiveness of different routes. *J Bone Joint Surg Am* 2012;94(16): 1442–1447.
66. Maricar N, Callaghan M, Felson D, O'Neill T. Predictors of response to intra-articular steroid injections in knee osteoarthritis—A systematic review. *Rheumatology* 2013;52: 1022–1032.
67. Maricar N, Parkes M, Callaghan M, Felson D, O'Neill T. Where and how to inject the knee: A systematic review. *Semin Arthritis Rheum* 2013;43(2): 195–203.
68. McDermott J, Ilyas A, Nazarian L, Leinberry C. Ultrasound-guided injections for de Quervain's tenosynovitis. *Clinical Orthop Rel Res* 2012;470(7): 1925–1931.
69. McMillan A, Landorf K, Gilheany M. Ultrasound guided corticosteroid injection for plantar fasciitis: Randomised controlled trial. *BMJ* 2012;344: e3260.
70. Meys V, Thissen S, Rozeman S, Beekman R. Prognostic factors in carpal tunnel syndrome treated with a corticosteroid injection. *Muscle Nerve* 2011;44: 763–768.
71. Min K, St. Pierre P, Ryan P, Marchant B, Wilson C, Arrington E. A double-blind randomized controlled trial comparing the effects of subacromial injection with corticosteroid versus NSAID in patients with shoulder impingement syndrome. *J Shoulder Elbow Surg* 2013;22(5): 595–601.
72. Mirzanli C, Ozturk K, Esenyel C, Ayanoglu S, Imren Y. Accuracy of intrasheath injection techniques for de Quervain's disease: A cadaveric study. *J Hand Surg* (European Volume) 2012;37(2): 155–160.
73. Mol M, Neuhaus V, Becker S, Jupiter J, Mudgal C, Ring D. Resolution and recurrence rates of idiopathic trigger finger after corticosteroid injection. *Hand* 2013;8:183–190.
74. Murphy D, Failla J, Koniuch M. Steroid versus placebo injection for trigger finger. *J Hand Surg [Am]*. 1995;20: 628–631. Erratum in: J, Hand Surg [Am] November 1995;20: 1075.
75. Murray RJ, Pearson C, Coombs GW, Flexman JP, Golledge CL, Speers DJ, Dyer JR, McLellan DG, Reilly M, Bell JM, Bowen SF, Christiansen KJ. Outbreak of methicillin resistant *Staphylococcus aureus* infection associated with acupuncture and joint injection. *Infect Control Hosp Epidemiol* 2008;39: 859–865.
76. O'Donoghue DH. Injuries of the knee. In: O'Donoghue DH (ed.). *Treatment of Injuries to Athletes*, 4th edn. Philadelphia, PA: W.B. Saunders, 1987;470–471.
77. Oh J, Oh C, Choi J, Kim S, Kim J, Yoon J. Comparison of glenohumeral and subacromial steroid injection in primary frozen shoulder: A prospective, randomized short-term comparison study. *J Shoulder Elbow Surg* 2011;20(7): 1034–1040.
78. Ostergaard M, Halberg P. Intra-articular corticosteroids in arthritic disease: A guide to treatment. *Bio Drugs* 1998;9: 95–103.
79. Pandit S, Solomon D, Gross D, Golijanin P, Provencher M. Isolated iliotibial band rupture after corticosteroid injectionas a cause of subjective instability and knee pain in a military special warfare trainee. *Military Med* 2014;179: e469–e472.
80. Patel D, Nawar S, Hasan S, Khatib O, Sidash S, Jazrawi L. Comparison of ultrasound-guided versus blind glenohumeral injections: A cadaveric study. *J Shoulder Elbow Surg* 2012;21(12): 1664–1668.
81. Peck E, Lai J, Pawlina W, Smith J. Accuracy of ultrasound-guided versus palpation-guided acromioclavicular joint injections: A cadaveric study. *PM&R* 2010;2(9): 817–821.
82. Peerbooms J, Sluimer J, Bruijn D, Gosens T. Positive effect of an autologous platelet concentrate in lateral epicondylitis in a double-blind randomized controlled trial. Platelet-rich plasma versus corticosteroid injection with a 1-year follow-up. *Am J Sports Med* 2010;38(2): 255–262.
83. Pekarek B, Osher L, Buck S, Bowen M. Intra-articular corticosteroid injections: A critical literature review with up-to-date findings. *Foot* 2011;21: 66–70.
84. Peters-Veluthamaningal C, van der Windt D, Winters J, Meyboom-de Jong B. Corticosteroid injection for trigger finger in adults. *Cochrane Database Syst Rev* 2009;21: CD005617.
85. Peters-Veluthamaningal C, Winters J, Groenier K, Meyboom-de Jong B. Randomised controlled trial of local corticosteroid injections for de Quervain's tenosynovitis in general practice. *BMC Musculoskelet Disord* 2009;10: 131.
86. Pfenninger JL. Joint and soft tissue aspiration and injection. In: Pfenninger JL, Fowler GC (eds.), *Procedures for Primary Care Physicians*. St. Louis, MO: Mosby, 1994.
87. Pichler W, Weinberg A, Grechenig S, Tesch N, Heidari N, Grechenig W. Intra-articular injection of the acromioclavicular joint. *J Bone Joint Surg Br* 2009;91(12): 1638–1640.
88. Rabago D, Best T, Zgierska A, Zeisig E, Ryan M, Crane D. A systematic review of four injection therapies for lateral epicondylosis: Prolotherapy, polidocanol, whole blood and platelet-rich plasma. *Br J Sports Med* 2009;43: 471–481.
89. Rakieh C, Conaghan P. Diagnosis and treatment of gout in primary care. *Practitioner* 2011;255: 17–20.
90. Raman J. Intraarticular corticosteroid injection for first carpometacarpal osteoarthritis. *J Rheumatol* 2005;32; 1305–1306.
91. Rasmussen M, Kitaoka H, Patzer G. Nonoperative treatment of interdigital neuroma with a single corticosteroid injection. *Clin Orthop Rel Res* 1996;326: 188–193.

92. Ryan M, Hartwell J, Fraser S, Newsham-West R, Taunton J. Comparison of a physiotherapy program versus dexamethasone injections for plantar fasciopathy in prolonged standing workers: A randomized clinical trial. *Clin J Sport Med* 2014;24: 211–217.
93. Sabeti-Aschraf M, Lemmerhofer B, Lang S, Schmidt M, Funovics P, Ziai P, Frenzel S, Kolb A, Graf A, Schueller-Weidekamm C. Ultrasound guidance improves the accuracy of the acromioclavicular joint infiltration: A prospective randomized study. *Knee Surg Sports Traumatol Arthrosc* 2011;19(2): 292–295.
94. Sabeti-Aschraf M, Stotter C, Thaler C, Kristen K, Schmidt M, Krifter R, Hexel M, Ostermann R, Hofstaedter T, Graf A, Windhager R. Intra-articular versus periarticular acromioclavicular joint injection: A multicenter, prospective, randomized, controlled trial. *Arthroscopy* 2013;29(12): 1903–1910.
95. Schubert C, Hui-Chou H, See A, Deune E. Corticosteroid injection therapy for trigger finger or thumb: A retrospective review of 577 digits. *Hand* December 2013;8: 439–444.
96. Scott N, Guo B, Barton P, Gerwin R. Trigger point injections for chronic non-malignant musculoskeletal pain: A systematic review. *Pain Med* 2008;20(1): 54–69.
97. Sheikh E, Peters J, Sayde W, Maltenfort M, Leinberry C. A prospective randomized trial comparing the effectiveness of one versus two (staged) corticosteroid injections for the treatment of stenosing tenosynovitis. *Hand* 2014;9: 340–345.
98. Sibbitt W, Kettwich L, Band P et al. Does ultrasound guidance improve the outcomes of arthrocentesis and cortico-steroid injection of the knee? *Scand J Rheumatol* 2012;41: 66–72.
99. Slotkoff A, Clauw D, Nashel D. Effect of soft tissue corticosteroid injection on glucose control in diabetics. *Arthritis Rheum* 1994;37(Suppl 9): S347.
100. Stephens M, Beutler A, O'Connor F. Musculoskeletal injections: A review of the evidence. *Am Fam Physician* 2008;78: 971–976.
101. Tallia A, Cardone D. Diagnostic and therapeutic injection of the wrist and hand region. *Am Fam Physician* 2003;67: 745–750.
102. Thanasas C, Papadimitrious G, Charalambidis C, Paraskevopoulos I, Papanikolaou A. Platelet-rich plasma versus autologous whole blood for the treatment of chronic lateral elbow epicondylitis: A randomized controlled clinical trial. *Am J Sports Med* 2011;39(10): 2130–2134.
103. Tsai C, Hsieh L, Kuan T, Kao M, Chou L, Hong C. Remote effects of dry needling on the irritability of the myofascial trigger point in the upper trapezius muscle. *Am J Phys Med Rehabil* 2010;89(2): 133–140.
104. Tsai W, Hsu C, Chen CPC, Chen MJL, Yu T, Chen Y. Plantar fasciitis treated with local steroid injection: Comparison between sonographic and palpation guidance. *J Clin Ultrasound* 2006;34: 12–16.
105. Turner JL, McKeag DB. Complications of joint aspirations and injections. In: Phenninger JL (ed.), *The Clinics Atlas of Office Procedures—Joint Injection Techniques*, vol. 5 (no. 4). December 2002.
106. Ucuncu F, Capkin E, Karkucak M, Ozden G, Cakirbay H, Mehmet T, Guler M. A comparison of the effectiveness of landmark-guided injections and ultrasonography guided injections for shoulder pain. *Clin J Pain* 2009;25(9): 786–789.
107. Üstün N, Tok F, Yagız A, Kizil N, Korkmaz I, Karazincir S, Okuyucu E, Turhanoglu A. Ultrasound-guided vs. blind steroid injections in carpal tunnel syndrome: A single-blind randomized prospective study. *Am J Phys Med Rehabil* 2013;92: 999–1004.
108. Van Riet R, Goehre T, Bell S. The long term effect of an intra-articular injection of corticosteroids in the acromioclavicular joint. *J Shoulder Elbow Surg* 2012;21(3): 376–379.
109. von Essen R, Savolainen HA. Bacterial infection following intra-articular injection. A brief review. *Scand J Rheumatol* 1989;18(1): 7–12.
110. Wang A, Hutchinson D. The effect of corticosteroid injection for trigger finger on blood glucose level in diabetic patients. *J Hand Surg* [Am] 2006;31: 979–981.
111. Wasserman B, Pettrone S, Jazrawi L, Zuckerman J, Rokito A. Accuracy of acromioclavicular joint injections. *Am J Sports Med* 2013;41(1): 149–152.
112. Wisniewski SJ, Smith J, Patterson DG, Carmichael SW, Pawlina W. Ultrasound-guided versus nonguided tibiotalar joint and sinus tarsi injections: A cadaveric study. *PMR* April 2010;2(4): 277–281.
113. Witteveen A, Kok A, Sierevelt I, Kerkhoffs G, van Dijk C. The optimal injection technique for the osteoarthritic ankle: A randomized, cross-over trial. *Foot Ankle Surg* 2013;19: 283–288.
114. Wolf J, Ozer K, Scott F, Gordon M, William A. Comparison of autologous blood, corticosteroid, and saline injection in the treatment of lateral epicondylitis: A prospective, randomized, controlled multicenter study. *J Hand Surg* 2011;36(8): 1269–1272.
115. Yamada K, Masuko T, Iwasaki N. Rupture of the flexor digitorum profundus tendon after injections of insoluble steroid for a trigger finger. *J Hand Surg Eur* 2011 January;36: 77–78.
116. Yonnet G. Intersection syndrome in a handcyclist: Case report and literature review. *Top Spinal Cord Inj Rehabil* 2013;19(3): 236–243.
117. Yoon H, Kim S, Suh Y, Seo Y, Kim H. Correlation between ultrasonographic findings and the response to corticosteroid injection in Pes Anserinus Tendinobursitis Syndrome in Knee Osteoarthritis Patients. *J Korean Med Sci* 2005;20: 109–112.
118. Yoon S, Rah U, Sheen S, Cho K. Comparison of 3 needle sizes for trigger point injection in myofascial pain syndrome of upper- and middle-trapezius muscle: A randomized controlled trial. *Arch Phys Med Rehabil* 2009;90(8): 1332–1339.
119. Yucel I, Yazici B, Degirmenci E, Erdogmus B, Dogan S. Comparison of ultrasound-, palpation-, scintigraphy-guided steroid injections in the treatment of plantar fasciitis. *Arch Orhtop Trauma Surg* 2009;129: 695–701.
120. Zhang Q, Zhang T, Lv H, Xie L, Wu W, Wu J, Wu X. Comparison of two positions of knee arthrocentesis: How to obtain complete drainage. *Am J Phys Med Rehabil* 2012;91: 611–615.
121. Zeisig E, Fahlstrom M, Ohberg L, Alfredson H. Pain relief after intratendinous injections in patients with tennis elbow: Results of a randomised study. *Br J Sports Med* 2008;42: 267–271.

31 Injury Management and Rehabilitation

Principles of Rehabilitation—Physical Therapy in the Treatment of Sports Injuries

Robert M. Barney Poole and Leigh E. Palubinskas

CONTENTS

TABLE 31.1
Key Clinical Considerations

1. Physical therapy is an essential part of recovery and return to participation for injured athletes. The PT is a member of the sports medicine team including the physician, athletic trainer, coach, athlete, and their family.
2. Early referral decreases recovery time and prevents loss of strength and ROM that is detrimental to a speedy return to competition.
3. Physician referral to physical therapy, while not required in all states, is welcomed as a part of the consultation process. When consultation is requested, it should include a diagnosis and general recommendations for treatment and contraindications.
4. PTs are specialized in evaluation and treatment of musculoskeletal issues and may have advanced certifications in sports injury, orthopedics, and neurological conditions.
5. Physical therapy should incorporate the athlete's goals and return to participation in the development of a rehabilitation program. The program may include manual techniques, guided exercise in the clinic to ensure proper strength, balance and coordination, and when appropriate therapeutic modalities. All athletes should have a customized home exercise program in addition to their clinic activities.

31.1 INTRODUCTION

Physical therapy is essential in the treatment of sports injuries and the safe return of an athlete to his or her sport. A sports or orthopedic physical therapist (PT) is specially trained and may be board certified by the American Board of Physical Therapy Specialties of the American Physical Therapy Association. The sports PT has special knowledge of sports' skills, training methods, injury treatment and prevention, exercise physiology, sports psychology, and sports medicine. The orthopedic specialist has specific manual skills including mobilization and manipulation of the spine and peripheral joints. PTs work closely with the athlete and other members of the sports medicine team (see Chapter 2). The PT performs an initial examination of the athlete and determines a diagnosis. A baseline is established from which progress can be measured. Goals are set with the consensus of the athlete, coach, parents, and physician, and a rehabilitation program is specifically designed for that athlete to meet those goals. Ongoing evaluation and modification of the program is necessary to ensure safety and continued progress (Table 31.1).

31.2 REHABILITATION PRINCIPLES

The general goal of any treatment and rehabilitation plan is the return of the athlete to their prior level of competition, as soon as possible. Figure 31.1 depicts an idealized healing curve and rehabilitative program using various therapeutic exercises, modalities, manual skills, and other interventions. Functional progression is used to move the athlete through the recovery process, maximizing function and minimizing reinjury. Phase I (injury period) consists of reduction of the inflammatory process; Phase II (reparative period) promotes optimal healing through therapeutic exercises that are functionally progressive, specific, and balanced. Functional exercises must be constantly monitored and modified during this period to prevent reinjury and/or an increase in inflammation. Phase III (recovery period) is a period of strength and conditioning during which the athlete prepares for entry into regular training and competition. A monitored, functional

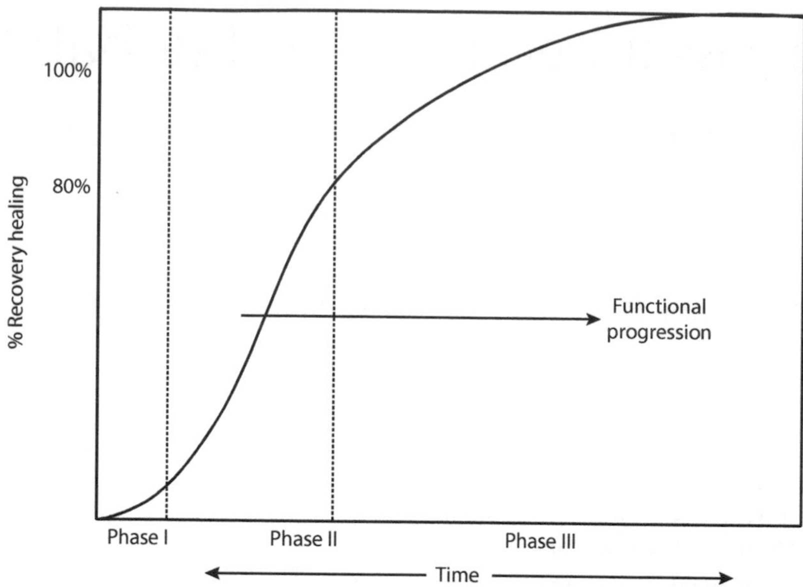

FIGURE 31.1 Under ideal circumstances for healing and rehabilitation, most musculoskeletal injuries progressively improve from the acute phase (I); through the intermediate, reparative phase (II); to the consolidation phase (III). The duration of each phase depends on the severity and type of trauma, rehabilitation program, and risk factors for further injury.

progression of sport-specific and general fitness activities advances the athlete through levels of training. The result is a gradual return to individual or team competition (Figure 31.1).

31.3 REFERRAL TO PHYSICAL THERAPY

Basic first aid of sports injuries occurs on the field or in the training room. A PT or athletic trainer examines the athlete and a diagnosis is determined. The injured athlete may be referred to the team physician for further examination and confirmation of the diagnosis through examination and imaging techniques. When injuries occur, it is important that the team physician be advised as soon as possible. After physician examination, the athlete may be referred to physical therapy for follow-up care. In some states, a written referral to physical therapy is required, but in most states, this is not necessary. A written referral, when required, should be signed by the physician, should include the athlete's name and diagnosis, and may include general recommendations for treatment and safeguards such as weight-bearing status. For examples of how and when to refer to physical therapy, see Table 31.1. A rehabilitation plan of care is developed with input from all members of the sports medicine team. The PT or an athletic trainer may become the coordinator of the athlete's rehabilitation program. Acute injuries may require modality use to decrease swelling and promote healing. An exercise program is important to regain range of motion (ROM) and strength. Table 31.2 provides general guidelines for treatment of some common sports injuries. Constant reevaluation of the athlete and modification of the rehabilitation plan is needed to produce the desired result: the safe return of the athlete to the field (see Table 31.3). Communication among the PT, physician, athlete, athletic trainer, and coach optimizes compliance and the program's success.[5]

31.4 MODALITY USE IN SPORTS INJURY MANAGEMENT

Hippocrates (400 BC) was one of the first proponents of cold as a therapeutic modality to reduce swelling and pain caused by acute trauma.[14] Ice packs, reusable cold gel packs, ice massage, and ice immersion or plunges are techniques frequently used to treat acute sports injuries. Cold application (>15°C) reduces the acute inflammatory response and permits earlier initiation of therapeutic exercise. Temperatures below 15°C should be avoided because the effect can be harmful. The duration of treatment using various forms of therapeutic cold in contact with the skin should not exceed 15–20 minutes and may be repeated every 60–90 minutes until the inflammatory response resolves. An athlete should be cautious if returning to participation after an application of ice because muscle performance may be adversely affected and the protective pain mechanism is blunted, potentially precipitating further injury.[4,21]

Clinical Pearl

Athletes often ask how to apply ice at home. Frozen peas or corn from the grocery store frozen foods section makes a good reusable cold pack for home and can be stored in the freezer when not in use. It should be labeled as a cold pack so it is not mistakenly used for the dinner table. Application of cold should be no longer than 20 minutes.

Therapeutic heat is used to relieve pain, increase circulation, facilitate tissue healing, and prepare stiff joints for manual mobilization/manipulation and tight muscles for exercise. Heat may be applied using moist heat packs or a warm whirlpool.

TABLE 31.2
Treatment Guidelines for Common Sports Injuries

Problem	Acute ((0–72 hours Postinjury)	Chronic (72+ hours Postinjury)
Muscle strains	Ice, gentle ROM	Active exercise, stretching, ultrasound, heat
Ankle sprain	Ice, support,[a] gentle ROM	Active exercise, support,[a] contrast treatments[b]
Knee injuries	Ice, support,[a] gentle ROM	Active exercise, support,[a] contrast treatments[b]
Hip pointer	Ice, support	Stretching, special padding, ultrasound (phonophoresis)
Low back pain	Ice, modalities	Manual techniques,[c] active exercise, heat modalities
Cervical pain	Ice, modalities, gentle ROM	Manual techniques,[c] active exercise, heat modalities
Shoulder injuries	Ice, modalities, gentle ROM, support[a]	Manual techniques,[c] active ROM and exercise, heat modalities
Elbow injuries	Ice, modalities, gentle ROM, support[a]	Manual techniques,[c] active strengthening, iontophoresis
Wrist and finger injuries	Ice, ROM, support[a]	Manual techniques,[c] active strengthening

[a] Support: elastic wrap, athletic taping, splinting, casting.
[b] Contrast treatments: heat followed by cold.
[c] Manual techniques: joint mobilization/manipulation, soft-tissue manipulation, trigger point release.

TABLE 31.3
General Rehabilitative Program Guidelines

- Supervised physical therapy sessions
- Specific rehabilitative active exercise:
  - Early mobilization
  - Active exercise including active range of motion exercises, strength
- Therapeutic modalities as appropriate1. Sport-specific skill and agility training
  - Proprioceptive balance reeducation
  - Cross training to maintain total fitness, flexibility, and strength
  - Correction of biomechanical, equipment, and training errors
  - Return to play

Application time is usually 20 minutes, allowing at least 60–90 minutes between applications. With athletic injuries, heat application can be started after the initial acute phase of injury, or approximately 72 hours after injury.[16] When applying heat, swelling should be monitored. An appropriate form of treatment during the intermediate phase of rehabilitation might begin with moist heat, progress through gentle exercise, and end with an application of cold and compression with a protective wrap to support the injured area. Ultrasound is a form of deep heat that uses high-frequency sound energy to produce changes in tissue temperature as deep as 5 cm. The benefits of therapeutic ultrasound include reduction of muscle spasm and pain relief.[6,12]

Phonophoresis is a technique that uses ultrasound to deliver medication through the skin into the tissues. An anti-inflammatory agent is driven into the inflamed area using high-frequency sound waves. This is commonly used in the treatment of conditions such as bursitis and tendinitis. Most commonly, a 10% hydrocortisone cream is rubbed into the skin, and then a layer of ultrasound coupling gel is applied and ultrasound delivered.[2,7,12]

A variety of pulsed waveforms are available to strengthen and reeducate muscle, reduce pain, and diminish muscle spasm. High-volt pulsed current (HVPC) can be used to recruit muscles that are inhibited by posttraumatic or postsurgical pain and/or edema. The electrical stimulation provides tactile and proprioceptive input while creating active muscle contraction. HVPC promotes motor recruitment and helps diminish muscle atrophy.[17,23]

Transcutaneous electrical nerve stimulation (TENS) is a form of electrical stimulation used to diminish pain. A biphasic waveform is delivered by a small handheld unit powered by a battery. TENS may be helpful in allowing gentle ROM to begin at an earlier stage with less pain.[8,9] Melzack and Wall[15] suggested that TENS stimulates sensory nerves, thereby closing the gate to pain sensation at the level of the spinal cord and preventing that pain from reaching the brain. Other theories suggest that TENS causes a release of endogenous opiates from within the central nervous system.[10,15]

Iontophoresis uses direct current to propel ions of medication into tissue.[3,18] A number of drugs may be used with iontophoresis for specific situations. Dexamethasone sodium phosphate (4 mg/mL) is most often used for treatment of inflamed tissue. With dexamethasone treatment, a negative electrode containing the medication is placed directly over the area to be treated, and the positive electrode is placed approximately 2–4 in. away. The treatment time, with the current adjusted to a comfortable setting (up to 4.0 mA), is 10–20 minutes.[17]

In many states, PTs are using trigger point dry needling to treat myofascial trigger points within injured muscle. Myofascial trigger points are hyperirritable spots within a taut band of contractured skeletal muscle fibers that produce local and/or referred pain when palpated.[22] They also inhibit muscle activation causing weakness in the involved muscle group.[13] Dry needling is performed by inserting a small solid-filament needle through the skin and directly into the trigger point, which breaks up the contraction knots present in the muscle. This technique allows for pain relief and improved flexibility and contractility of the involved muscle. Most patients will have some relief of symptoms after the initial treatment, but it may take several treatments for full relief of pain and return to function.

Therapeutic modalities vary from the simple ice pack to complex and expensive electrical devices. They can be useful in reducing pain, swelling, inflammation, and other effects of sports injuries. They are most effective when applied and monitored by appropriate practitioners and combined with therapeutic exercise into a comprehensive rehabilitation program.

Clinical Pearl

Dry needling or intramuscular manual therapy is an advanced technique used by PTs for the treatment of myofascial trigger points in injured or painful muscles. PTs are required to have additional training in this technique beyond the standard educational curriculum before using it in clinical practice. Not all states allow PTs to perform dry needling, and the minimum requirements for training vary from state to state. It is in the best interest of the athlete and the rehabilitation team to seek out PTs with the highest levels of education and experience with this technique for improved return to function and sport.

Clinical Pearl

Trigger Point Treatment Example

Chronic Lateral Epicondylitis:

A 25-year-old recreational tennis player is referred to physical therapy with chronic lateral epicondylitis. Her pain is located at the lateral epicondyle with referral into her forearm. The patient is treated daily for 10 days with frequent reassessment to determine progress.

Procedure:

1. Localize the area of the lesion by palpation of the lateral epicondyle and wrist extensor muscles.
2. Identify palpable taut bands and trigger points within the wrist extensor muscles.
3. Release trigger points using trigger point dry needling technique.
4. Instruct the athlete in proper technique for eccentric exercise and stretching (refer to Appendix G).
5. Use heat or ice massage for 15 minutes following exercise based on the patient's response to treatment.
6. During subsequent treatments, reevaluate for the presence of trigger points and treat as needed. Once all myofascial restriction is eliminated, continue with strengthening and flexibility with progression to sport-specific activities as tolerated.

31.5 THERAPEUTIC EXERCISE

Restoring flexibility and strength in available ROM is an essential part of any comprehensive rehabilitation program. Without adequate flexibility and joint ROM, normal muscle relationships cannot be reestablished following injury. The first phase of the rehabilitation process is to restore joint ROM without increasing the symptoms of the injury or causing further damage. Gentle active, active-assisted, or passive ROM exercise begins as soon as swelling is under control and comfort allows. During the early stages of the healing process, frequent pain-free ROM minimizes inflammation. Careful attention to the stages of the healing process by continual reexamination is needed in order to appropriately progress the athlete's rehabilitation program.[20] As functionally controlled active ROM increases, gentle stretching exercises begin. The athlete is instructed in proper stretching techniques in order to gain muscle flexibility and maintain functional ROM while building strength.[1,20] Sustained stretching techniques after proper warm-up are the preferred method of stretching. Ballistic stretching, stretching with a bounce at the end of range, may result in micro tears of muscle or fascia and is discouraged.[1]

After functional ROM is restored, the strengthening phase can begin. The three types of strengthening exercises are isometric, isotonic, and isokinetic. Isometric exercises produce muscle force without joint movement. Resistance is adjusted by increasing or decreasing muscle contraction. Isometrics are useful during the acute phase in preventing loss of strength without causing further injury. Also during the acute phase, isometrics can be used to reduce swelling around the joint through the "pumping" action of the muscle. Isometrics promote healing by increasing circulation.

Isotonic exercises strengthen muscles through contraction of muscle fibers against constant resistance. Resistance may be supplied by using strap weights, elastic bands or rubber tubing, free weights, or weight machines. In order to strengthen the muscle isotonically, the load (i.e., resistance) must be increased. When dealing with an injury, increasing the load too soon can cause further injury, thus prolonging the rehabilitation process. A high-repetition, low-weight program is recommended when initiating an isotonic strengthening program. Progressive resistance exercise is one form of isotonic exercise.[19] Progressive resistance exercise is a system of dynamic resistance training in which a constant external load is applied to the contracting muscle and incrementally increased. Many different programs exist but most incorporate 2–3 sets of 6–12. Techniques in which resistance in the early sets is less than in the later sets provide a warm-up for muscles. Techniques in which resistance in later sets is lower than in early sets adapt to muscle fatigue. All techniques call for increasing resistance over time.[11]

In any type of resistance training, especially postinjury training, care is taken to prevent further injury during the healing process. Proper exercise technique through the entire functional ROM is essential to prevent further injury to muscles, the joint capsule, or connective tissue. Exercise that simulates actual athletic activity should be used when possible. Proper warm-up should be emphasized prior to resistive training, and flexibility exercises should be included to maintain functional ROM throughout exercise.

Isokinetic exercise involves muscle contractions through a ROM at a fixed speed. The resistance varies and

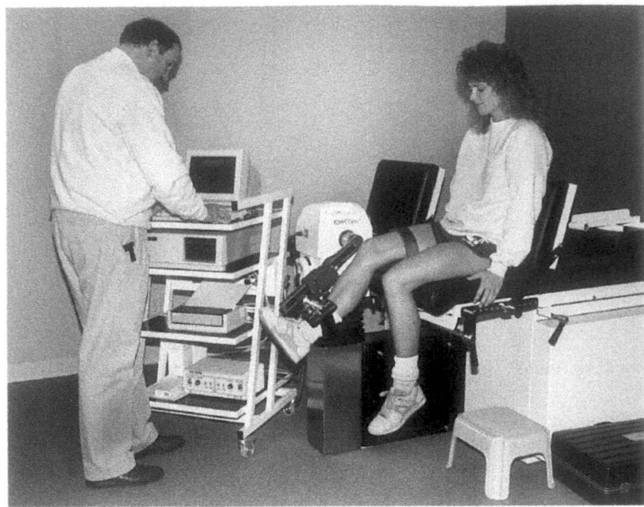

FIGURE 31.2 Isokinetic testing using the KIN-COM®. (Courtesy of Chattanooga Corp., Chattanooga, TN.)

accommodates according to the ability of the muscles to contract. Isokinetic devices load the musculoskeletal unit maximally through the range while taking into account pain, fatigue, and other factors that affect force of muscle contraction. For this reason, it is relatively safe to use isokinetics in postinjury rehabilitation programs. The controlled speed allows muscle training at closer to functional limb speeds (Figure 31.2). The equipment for isokinetic exercise and testing is expensive and requires a good deal of space in the clinic.

In the final phase of rehabilitation, the athlete progresses to sport-specific activities; these are specifically related to activities the athlete will need to perform on the field during practice or competition.[11] Sport-specific activities should include balance or proprioception, coordination, and agility training. Proprioception is the basis for transferring flexibility and strength into agility and skill in competition and is an integral part of preparing the athlete for return to competition. Use of all or parts of actual agility drills used in practice for the athlete's sport may be started at half speed, emphasizing performance skill and confidence, with no increase in symptoms. Also useful in promoting proprioception are activities such as the balance board and one-leg standing for the lower extremity and the use of weighted bats, balls, or other equipment for the upper extremity.

Endurance and conditioning activities for general fitness should be a part of the rehabilitation process and should begin as early as possible. Maintaining the general fitness of the athlete as a whole, while protecting and strengthening the injured area, is essential to a good result and to sustaining motivation. The athlete can continue to work out in the weight room, incorporating aspects of his or her weight routine that do not involve the injured area. Some athletes must also incorporate short bursts of high intensity into their sports. Football players, for instance, should train for short, intense bursts of exercise such as those inherent in their sport; therefore, use of an exercise bike to maintain general fitness should also include short sprint work to help maintain anaerobic capacity.

All activities should begin with proper warm-up and stretching activities. After exercise, a cooldown session should also include stretching, after which ice may be applied as needed to minimize swelling and pain.

31.6 RETURN TO PARTICIPATION

The criteria for the return of an athlete to the playing field include return to normal levels of flexibility, strength, muscle bulk, endurance, agility, skill in sport-specific activities, and psychological factors. Flexibility is determined by assessing muscle length and goniometric joint measurement and is compared with the uninvolved side and with preparticipation physical exam data, if available. Flexibility and strength of agonists and antagonists must be balanced for optimal function. Strength is best evaluated by manual muscle testing. When possible, strength is compared to the uninvolved side. The rehabilitation process is not finished until muscle bulk returns. Although strength may be adequate bilaterally with testing, a difference in muscle bulk may exist. This can be compared bilaterally by a simple circumferential tape measurement above and below the joint line.

Clinical Pearl

An athlete's rehabilitation and return to sport arc not complete until the muscle bulk has returned. Measure muscle circumferentially above and below the joint line, and compare that with the uninvolved side to determine if the muscle bulk is similar.

The athlete is not able to protect adequately against further injury due to decreased endurance and strength until adequate muscle bulk has returned. Coaches and athletic trainers compare the athlete's skill, agility, endurance, and coordination with preinjury levels. The PT provides objective data from both strength and ROM evaluations and evaluation of performance in sports and agility drills. This information is used by the sports medicine team in deciding when to return the athlete to competition. The athlete is a source of some of the most valuable input into the decision to return to participation. Each athlete is different, having his or her own psychological makeup and reaction to injury and rehabilitation; consequently, the return to play is also different for each.[11,19]

31.7 SUMMARY

The sports medicine team consists of the physician, physical therapist, and athletic trainer. Other members might include dieticians, sports psychologists, and exercise physiologists. It is the job of these specialists to evaluate, diagnose, and treat injured athletes. The team goal is to return each athlete swiftly

TABLE 31.4
SORT: Key Recommendations for Practice

Clinical Recommendation	Evidence Rating	References
A careful and comprehensive physical examination designed to identify musculoskeletal conditions in young athletes should be completed prior to treatment.	A	[13]
Referral to physical therapy as part of the athlete's sports medicine team should include a diagnosis, general recommendations for treatment and safeguards such as weight bearing status	C	[5]
Careful attention should be paid to stages of the healing process. Constant re-exam is necessary to make sure the athlete is progressing without further damage	A	[1,20]
Therapeutic exercise is the key to return to functional activity	C	[11,19,20]
Modalities have their place in any rehabilitation program however their use should be limited and used to enhance and progress the athlete's exercise program	A	[2,6,7,12]
Dry needle trigger point release is a new intervention that may be used as part of the progression to treat muscle pain and inhibition and promote improved muscle flexibility.	A	[13,22]

and safely to the playing field. Through the use of therapeutic interventions and constant reevaluation and modification of individualized exercise programs, the athlete is taught how to regain the skills lost to injury and how to prevent further injury (Table 31.4).

ACKNOWLEDGMENTS

The authors thank Judy Koren for her patience and skill in medical writing, Danielle Eidson for her editing skills, and the McCluskey Education and Research Foundation and the Hughston Sports Medicine Foundation and Performance Physical Therapy for their support of this effort. A special thanks to George M. McCluskey, Jr. for his leadership as a pioneer in sports physical therapy and physical therapy private practice and Turner A. Blackburn, Jr. for his mentorship through the years.

REFERENCES

1. Anderson B, Burke ER. Scientific, medical, and practical aspects of stretching. *Clinics in Sports Medicine.* 1991;10(1):63–86.
2. Bare AC, McAnaw MB, Pritchard AE et al. Phonophoretic delivery of 10% hydrocortisone through the epidermis of humans as determined by serum cortisol concentrations. *Physical Therapy.* 1996;76(7):738–749.
3. Bertolucci LE. Introduction of anti-inflammatory drugs by iontophoresis: Double blind study. *Journal of Orthopaedic & Sports Physical Therapy*, 1982;4(2):103.
4. Bleakley CM, Costello JT, Glasgow PD. Should athletes return to sport after applying ice? A systematic review of the effect of local cooling on functional performance. *Sports Med.* 2012;42(1):69–87.
5. Fisher A. Adherence to sports injury rehabilitation programmes. *Sports Med.* 1990;9(3):151–158.
6. Gieck JH, Saliba EN. Application of modalities in overuse syndromes. *Clinics in Sports Medicine.* 1987;6(2):427.
7. Griffin JE, Enternach JL, Price RE, Touchstone JC. Patients treated with ultrasonic driven hydrocortisone and with ultrasound alone. *Physical Therapy.* 1967;47:594.
8. Hillman SK, Delforge G. The use of physical agents in rehabilitation of athletic injuries. *Clinics in Sports Medicine.* 1985;4(3):431.
9. Jensen JE, Etheridge GL, Hazelrigg G. Effectiveness of transcutaneous electrical neural stimulation in the treatment of pain. *Sports Medicine.* 1986;3:79–88.
10. Killian C, Malone I. *High Frequency and High Voltage Protocols.* Minneapolis, MN: Medtronic; 1984, p. 1.
11. Kisner C, Colby LA. *Therapeutic Exercise: Foundations and Techniques.* 4th edn. Philadelphia, PA: F.A. Davis; 2002.
12. Klaiman MD, Shrader JA, Danoff JV, et al. Phonophoresis versus ultrasound in the treatment of common musculoskeletal conditions, *Medicine & Science in Sports & Exercise.* 1998;30(9):1349–1355.
13. Lucas KR, Polus BI, Rich PA. Latent myofascial trigger points: Their effects on muscle activation and movement efficiency. *Journal of Bodywork and Movement Therapies.* 2004;8(3):160–166.
14. Meeusen R, Lievens P. The use of cryotherapy in sports injuries, *Sports Medicine.* 1986;3:398–414.
15. Melzack R, Wall PD. Pain mechanisms: A new theory. *Science.* 1965;150:971.
16. Michlovitz SL. *Thermal Agents in Rehabilitation*, 2 edn. Philadelphia, PA: FA Davis; 1990.
17. Robert D. Transdermal drug delivery using iontophoresis and phonophoresis. *Orthopaedic Nursing.* 1999;19(3):50–54.
18. Ross CR, Segal D. High voltage galvanic stimulation: An aid to postoperative healing. *Current Podiatry.* 1981;34:19.
19. Rutherford OM. Muscular coordination and strength training. *Sports Medicine.* 1988;5:196–202.
20. Sapega AA, Quedenfeld TC, Moyer RA, et al. Biophysical factors in range-of-motion exercise. *Physician and Sportsmedicine.* 1981;9:57.
21. Schmid S, Moffat M, Gutierrez GM. Effect of knee joint cooling on the electromyographic activity of lower extremity muscles during a plyometric exercise. *Journal of Electromyography and Kinesiology.* 2010;20(6):1075–1081.
22. Simons DG, Travell JG, Simons LS. *Travell & Simons' Myofascial Pain and Dysfunction: Upper Half of Body.* Lippincott Williams & Wilkins; 1999.
23. Stamford B. The myth of electrical exercise. *Physician and Sportsmedicine.* 1983;11:144.

32 Fractures and Dislocations

Ronald E. Bowers, Jr.

CONTENTS

TABLE 32.1
Key Clinical Considerations

Dislocations

1. Quick identification of dislocations can be accomplished by noticing the obvious change in the surface anatomy of the joint area.
2. Although rare, neurovascular damage can occur with dislocations. A neurovascular exam *must* be performed at the time of evaluation, right before reduction is attempted, and after reduction is complete.
3. Reduction of dislocations as soon as possible aids in preventing complications.

Fractures

1. Open fractures are an orthopedic emergency and as such emergent consultation is warranted. Closed fractures also can be emergent *if* there is neurovascular compromise. Urgent consultation is warranted in this case.
2. Neurovascular status should be assessed multiple times during examination and treatment and any change noted. If patient goes from neurovascularly intact to deficient, a reason for the change must be addressed. Urgent consultation may be needed if corrective action cannot be rendered appropriately.
3. Angulation and/or displacement may be a reason for neurovascular compromise and should be addressed if the provider is experienced and comfortable with fracture manipulation. Otherwise, consult orthopedics urgently.

32.1 INTRODUCTION

Early proper management of fractures and/or dislocations is important in achieving a good clinical and functional outcome. Evaluation, followed by adequate treatment, is important in reducing patient suffering and preventing possible complications. Achieving anatomic or near anatomic alignment with fractures, as well as reduction of dislocations, is important in assuring good outcomes of healing and functionality. Deciding when it is appropriate to refer the patient to the specialist is based on your personal comfort of handling the injury as well as that of the patient's desires (Table 32.1).

32.2 PRINCIPLES OF DISLOCATION MANAGEMENT

Dislocations are total loss of joint congruity. Subluxation is a slippage of anatomic position such that the joint is not in full congruence.[5,7] Because of the nourishment of the articular cartilage of every synovial joint coming from the synovial fluid and microvasculature of the joint, it is imperative that all dislocations be reduced in a timely manner (less than 6 hours) to prevent potential loss of this function. There may be associated injury to ligaments, articular cartilage, bone, nerves, and blood vessels as well. These must also be examined when a patient presents with a dislocation or subluxation.

32.3 CLINICAL FEATURES OF DISLOCATIONS

Although any dislocation may first appear similar to a fracture, there are several key features that separate the two:

1. *Pain*—Although both fractures and dislocations have pain, the pain associated with dislocation is soft-tissue pain rather than bone pain. This is due to the abnormal positioning of the joint capsule, ligament, and muscles surrounding the joint. Reducing the dislocation back into anatomic position will quickly reduce that pain.

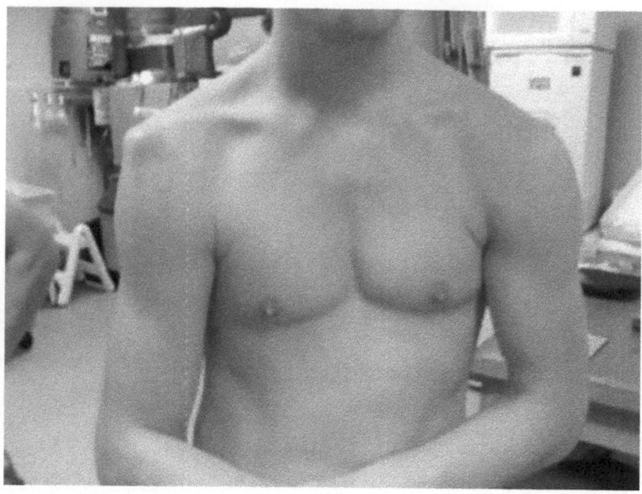

FIGURE 32.1 Dislocated shoulder surface appearance. (From Dr. Rudyard Health Pictures at http://www.rudyard.org/wp-content/uploads/2013/09/dislocated-shoulder-300x225.jpg, accessed January 6, 2015 CC: BY, AC.)

2. *Loss of normal body contour and relationship of bony landmarks*—When a joint is dislocated, the appearance changes as well as the relationship of palpable bony landmarks shifting. For example, when the glenohumeral joint is dislocated, most commonly the dislocation is in an anteroinferior direction. This gives the appearance of a flattened lateral shoulder and loss of normal palpation of the greater tuberosity of the humerus with relation to the acromion (see Figure 32.1).
3. *Loss of motion*—Secondary to joint incongruity and pain, movement of the joint is abnormal at best and limited due to loss of articular cartilage contact as well as correct muscle alignment for proper functional pull.
4. *Positional attitude*—Patients with dislocations will hold that affected joint in a position that is most comfortable for them where the muscle spasms associated with it are least painful. Some joints have diagnostic positions that will aid in the diagnosis of what direction the dislocation has positioned itself—e.g., posterior hip dislocations will appear as the leg is shortened, flexed, adducted, and internally rotated, while an anterior hip dislocation will appear lengthened, abducted, and externally rotated.
5. *Swelling and ecchymosis*—Usually minimal, *unless* there is an associated fracture or vascular compromise. If you note large swelling and ecchymosis, assume there is an associated fracture or vascular damage.
6. *Potential neurovascular compromise*—Although fairly rare, there is a potential for neurovascular compromise due to the malposition of the joint and potential impingement or transection of a nerve or major blood vessel. Each joint has its own neurovascular bundle particular to that joint—e.g., glenohumeral joint and the axillary nerve that runs between the deltoid and coracoid muscles on one side and the rotator cuff on the other. See Chapters 43, 44, 46, and 48 through 51 for specific injury.
7. *Potential ligament and cartilage damage*—With the force required to dislocate any joint, there is potential for damage to the articular cartilage as the bones slide out of position and rub against each other abnormally, as in a Hill–Sachs lesion of the humeral head when it dislocates against the glenoid. Also with this motion, a stretching and potential tearing of the joint capsule and supporting ligaments can also occur.
8. *Fractures can be associated with dislocations*—The worst-case scenario is where not only the joint has dislocated, but there is also an associated fracture to a bone near the joint—e.g., Galeazzi fracture (fracture at the junction of the distal and middle one-third of the radius with a dislocation of the distal ulna at the proximal carpal row) *or* proximal humeral neck fracture with a glenohumeral dislocation. Each of these injuries must be addressed and cared for appropriately (see Figure 32.2).

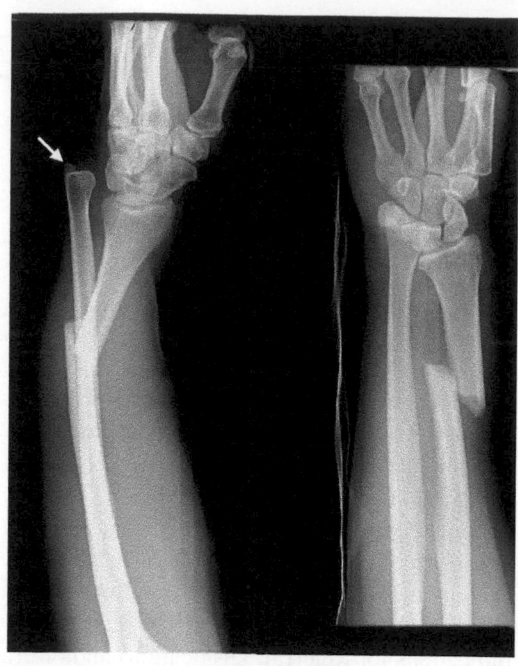

FIGURE 32.2 Galeazzi fracture dislocation. (From "Galeazzi-fraktur 1 THWZ" by Th. Zimmermann (THWZ). Licensed under Creative Commons Attribution-Share Alike 3.0-de via Wikimedia Commons http://commons.wikimedia.org/wiki/File:Galeazzifraktur_1_THWZ.jpg#mediaviewer/File:Galeazzifraktur_1_THWZ.jpg.)

Clinical Pearl

Pain and loss of anatomical contour are the most common presenting findings of dislocations.

32.4 PRINCIPLES FOR REDUCTION OF DISLOCATED JOINTS

1. Generally speaking, the sooner the attempt at reducing the dislocation, the easier it will be. This is because the muscles and soft tissues have not started to adapt to their new positions and are still supple and pliable enough to allow movement of the joint into its appropriate location prior to severe spasm.[2]
2. Always perform a neurovascular evaluation prior to and after all reduction maneuvers.[2]
3. All dislocations require a minimum of two radiographic views oriented at 90° from each other to visualize the joint and bone positions in two planes. The standard views are an anterior to posterior (AP) and lateral. For some joints, special views may be required. Radiographs *must* be taken before and after reduction of the dislocation.[3]
4. Anesthesia (block, conscious sedation, or general) should be used for patient comfort and reduction of muscle contraction. Blocks are good for smaller joints—e.g., digits or carpals. Conscious sedation can be used for most other dislocation reduction attempts. General anesthesia may be required for difficult reductions *or* if an open procedure needs to be done because of nonreducible multiple attempts.[1,2]
5. Reduction of the joint depends on which joint is dislocated. Each joint has special maneuvers to relocate the dislocation into its proper position. The basic principle of reduction is to overcome the muscle contraction with an in-line traction and manipulation by reversing the mechanism of injury.[2] (See individual joints in specific chapters dealing with that joint.)
6. Postreduction care depends, once again, on which joint was dislocated. But a general rule is to splint or sling the affected limb and joint for as short a period as possible so as not to lose range of motion yet not compromise healing. Most soft-tissue healing takes 6 weeks to heal, but gentle motion exercises without muscle contraction are best in assuring the joint does not become stiff and yet allows the soft-tissue capsule and ligaments to heal effectively.[1,2]
7. Most dislocations are put into protective splints/braces following successful reduction of the dislocated joint. Many of these splints/braces have range-of-motion capability that can be locked for protection immediately following the reduction but then unlocked at a specified time when motion can be allowed. Others may be static splints/braces that prevent any motion to allow for complete healing of the soft tissue prior to initiation of motion and rehabilitation[1,2] (see individual chapters for specifics). Braces may be worn following successful rehabilitation for protection against reinjury, especially if returning to a high-level competitive sport.

Clinical Pearl

The basic principle of reduction is to overcome the muscle contraction with an in-line traction and manipulation by reversing the mechanism of injury.

32.5 POTENTIAL COMPLICATIONS FROM DISLOCATED JOINTS

Even though reduction is adequate and timely, there are still potential complications that can occur, some immediately following the reduction and some more long-term sequelae.

Of immediate concern is the condition of the joint capsule and ligamentous and cartilage support. Damage to these can result in an unstable joint construct and recurrence of the dislocation multiple times. Proper assessment of the instability is best done by an experienced provider. Radiographs may demonstrate additional bony pathology—like a boney Bankhardt lesion of the glenoid or a Hill–Sachs lesion in a shoulder dislocation.

Tearing of ligaments of any joint may render that joint unstable and may need repair.[7] If there is any doubt, refer the patient to an orthopedic specialist for evaluation and surgical repair if needed. For example, a tear of the middle patellofemoral ligament of the knee can potentially result in patellar tracking instability that may need repair.

Other potential acute complications are neurovascular structures that may also be damaged during the dislocation or possibly the reduction maneuver.[7] Shoulder anterior dislocation, for example, may cause damage to the axillary nerve; hip dislocation may cause avascular necrosis of the femoral head due to disruption of its blood supply—the extracapsular medial and lateral femoral circumflex arteries, as well as the artery of the round ligament of the femoral head. Careful neurovascular evaluation *must* be done initially, prior to reduction, immediately following the reduction, after return from radiology, and after placement of a splint or brace. Documentation of each neurovascular evaluation should also be done for completeness of the chart and proof of intactness.

Potential long-term sequela from any dislocation is that of damage to the articular cartilage of the joint surfaces and thus progression to osteoarthritis of the joint.[7] Joint stiffness and loss of full range of motion is also possible with many dislocations due to scarring and stiffness of the associated joint capsule, ligaments, or articular cartilage damage. Finger joints, for example, as well as the elbow joint (humeroulnar), are prone to this type of sequela.[7]

Clinical Pearl

An immediate potential complication is that of neural compromise. This can be lessened with a detailed exam.

32.6 REHABILITATION OF DISLOCATED JOINTS

Early motion, once stability is established, is important in preserving range of motion of any joint. All injured tissues go through the healing processes. Depending on the extent of the injury, this may be minimal repair or extensive. The more damage to connective tissue, the more scarring will occur and, hence, contraction of the tissue to a certain degree. Connective tissue proper can be subdivided into dense and loose, each with its own special characteristics. Generally, each is composed of collagen and elastic fibers, water, and cells. Each part of the tissue responds differently to the three phases of healing—inflammatory, proliferative, and remodeling.[7] Without going into great depth here, where to begin rehabilitation is determined by the extent to which motion of the reduced joint has been affected. The more damage, the closer you should follow the recovery and return of function. Age also affects healing. Generally, children will heal faster and more efficiently. An older adult, whose tissue is already changing or has changed, will generally not recover as fully. Referral to a physical therapist is important for lessening this sequela of decreased or lost function. They will utilize joint active and passive range-of-motion exercises, along with other modalities as needed, once the initial injury is deemed stable by the referring physician.[1,2] (See separate chapters for full details.)

Clinical Pearl

Early referral to physical or occupational therapy will help lessen long-term sequelae of joint dislocation.

32.7 DESCRIPTIONS OF FRACTURES

Fractures are classified in several different ways. The purpose is to describe them in such a way as to be able to converse with a specialist accurately so that they know what the fracture looks like and the probable mechanism of injury. Then the specialist will likely know if surgical intervention versus closed care will be warranted.

They should be classified by location on the bone of the fracture—i.e., supracondylar, intertrochanteric, proximal third, or intracondylar. They should be classified by direction of the fracture line—i.e., transverse, oblique, or spiral. They should also be described for bone fragment displacement, angulation, and rotation off from normal. Fractures can be one linear fracture line or they can be comminuted (multiple fracture lines). They can also be *open*, where the skin and soft tissue are disrupted allowing a tract to the fracture or the bone can be totally protruding from its position through the skin.[2] A fracture that does not have communication with the external environment in any way is classified as *closed*. Fractures can also be classified as *pathologic* when the bone fails due to preexisting disease, such as metastatic or primary bone cancers or osteoporosis. Bones can also fracture when too much repetitive stress is placed on them and typically are seen more in military recruits and unconditioned athletes.

Clinical Pearls

Fracture description should include: which bone, where on the bone, simple or comminuted, open or closed, displacement (if any), and angulation (if any).

Children's bones contain more cartilage and therefore are more *flexible* and may only break on one side or even bend without breaking. These are classified as "greenstick" and "plastically deformed," respectively.[1] Because of open growth plates (physis), children's fractures often involve the growth plate (physis) in the fracture patterns. The Salter–Harris (SH) classification system is the most commonly used fracture description system still used today.[1] There have been many added classifications that augment this system, but for primary care providers, the SH is the easiest to use and accepted by all orthopedic specialists (shown in Figure 32.3).

An SH I fracture is a fracture through the growth plate (physis) itself without damage to the structural bone.[1] The physis may sublux or even dislocate if the thick outer periosteum tears. Reduction requires gentle anatomic repositioning to prevent future growth retardation or disruption.

An SH II fracture is the most common physeal fracture. The vector of force in this fracture travels through one side of the physis and exits the other side with a fragment of the metaphysis.[1] Reduction is easier in repositioning because the bone fragment of the metaphysis allows visual confirmation of anatomic realignment on two-view radiographs.

An SH III fracture is a fracture with the vector of force through the epiphysis first followed by the exit through the physis *or* vice versa.[1] This is an interarticular fracture and care to anatomically reduce this fracture is of upmost importance to prevent joint complications later.

An SH IV fracture is a fracture with the vector of force through the metaphysis, physis, and epiphysis.[1] Also called a vertical sheer fracture due to the mechanism of injury, this fracture *must* be anatomically reduced surgically and held in place with hardware (usually pins or K-wires).

An SH V fracture usually is not identifiable at the time of injury. It is a crushing injury to the physis.[1] Evidence of injury may be recognized with a narrowing of the physis when compared to the uninjured side, but this is very subjective. Injury is usually not evident until the injured physis starts to heal and possible bone bridges between the metaphysis and epiphysis develop. Many authors refute this as a separate class because damage to the physis can occur in the other SH classes as well.[2,4]

Clinical Pearl

Damage to a growing physis can result in poor bone growth. Attention to fractures involving the physis is of utmost importance.

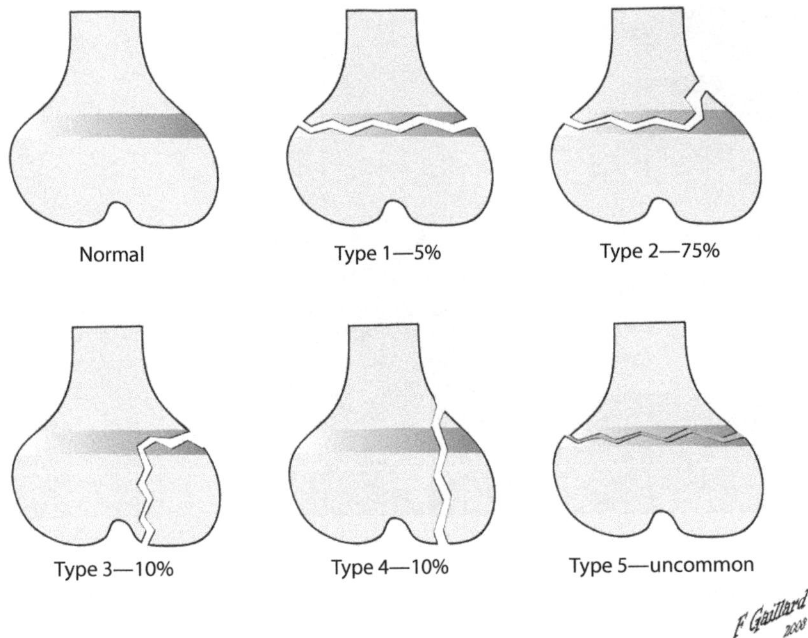

FIGURE 32.3 Salter–Harris classification of children's physeal fractures I–V. (CC: BY, AC courtesy of Dr Frank Gaillard [MBBS, FRANZCR], http://www.frankgaillard.com, accessed January 6, 2015)

32.8 CLINICAL FEATURES OF FRACTURES

Pain is typically the first effect a patient will experience who fractures a bone provided they are neurologically intact.[2] The level of intensity may differ for each individual based on their pain tolerances. Some patients may even ignore the minor pain of some fractures and not seek medical attention. Tenderness may be elicited with gentle palpation of the injured part.

Loss of function is due to either the pain tolerance or deformity of the injured part.[2] Of course, pain goes hand in hand with the deformity and hence lack of use of the injured part due to that pain.

Deformity may or may not be evident in all fractures.[2] The "dinner-fork" deformity of a distal radius fracture, for example, is obvious on observation. However, buckle fractures of a child's distal radius may only have mild edema but will definitely be tender and painful.

Attitude refers to how a patient self-limits and holds the injury so as not to experience pain any more than they are already experiencing.[2] A patient, for example, who fractures a clavicle, will hold the injured side's arm to help take the weight of the extremity from pulling down on the attached clavicle. A patient with a distal radius fracture will cradle the injury with their other arm.

Abnormal mobility may be evident, especially in fractures that have the loss of contact of the fractured ends of the bone(s).[2] Pain is obviously a contributing factor to the lack of motion, but muscles may have lost their ability to contract effectively on the fractured parts to move them.

Crepitus may also be associated with fractures that have multiple fracture components or comminution.[2] Simply moving the fractured part may render an audible or palpable *grinding* of the bones moving over each other abnormally. This should be avoided if possible as it may cause further damage.

Edema of the injured extremity, especially at the fracture site, is common. It can be so bad as to delay surgical intervention or application of a stabilizing cast. A patient may have to wear a rigid splint or external fixator (Ex Fix) until the edema recedes enough to allow for adequate closure or application of a cast without worry of potential compartment syndrome.

Ecchymosis is also common due to disruption of the vascular bed of the surrounding soft tissue. The more ecchymosis that is seen, the more likely there is greater damage to the soft tissue. However, nondisplaced, buckle (torus), or greenstick fractures may show little or no ecchymosis.

Clinical Pearl

The hallmark sins of a fracture are—edema, ecchymosis, deformity, and pain.

32.9 RADIOGRAPHS OF INJURY

Radiographs of all injured bones should be taken *prior* to any manipulation or attempt at reduction. Radiographs should be done such that there are two separate views 90° to each other to identify fully the direction of angulation and/or displacement of the fracture ends[3,4] (see Figure 32.4).

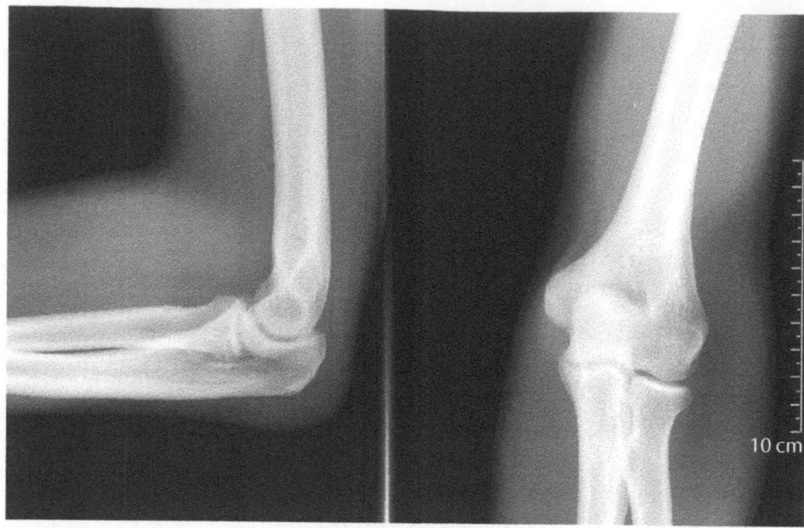

FIGURE 32.4 AP and lateral views of the elbow. (From "Coude fp" by MB–Collection personnelle. Licensed under Creative Commons Attribution-Share Alike 2.5 via Wikimedia Commons http://commons.wikimedia.org/wiki/File:Coude_fp.PNG#mediaviewer/File:Coude_fp.PNG, accessed January 6, 2015.)

This will allow for a better visualization in the care provider's mind as to the extent of angulation and/or displacement and help direct the reduction procedure. There may also be special views required to better visualize a certain aspect of the fracture or joint. Radiographs should also be taken after a reduction is completed and confirm the maneuver was adequate for a proper healing to take place. Radiographs may have to be taken multiple times if there is a failure to adequately reduce the fracture until such attempt the reduction is adequate.

Clinical Pearl

Reduction of a fracture is best done by an experienced practitioner. It is accomplished generally with traction and reversal of the mechanism of injury.

32.10 PRINCIPLES OF ALIGNMENT AND REDUCTION OF FRACTURES

Care of fractures begins with emergent treatment at the location of the injury. This may be accomplished by trained EMS personnel to casual observers who happen to be there at the time of the injury. At this level of care, the guiding principle should be the following: "Above all, do no further harm."[4] This may be accomplished by simply splinting the injury as it is found, without any attempt at manipulation or positional changes. If there is an associated open wound with bone showing, it is best to apply a sterile dressing over the wound and exposed bone, apply the appropriate splint, and evacuate the patient to the nearest emergency care facility.[4] Attempting to "put the bone back under the skin" may potentially do further damage unless you are familiar with the anatomy and potential complications associated with the fracture at hand.

Reduction of closed fractures also has potential damaging consequences.

Reduction of a fracture is best accomplished if done as soon as possible by someone familiar with reduction techniques. To achieve an acceptable reduction, the following three steps can be undertaken (generally speaking): (1) apply traction in the long axis of the limb[2]; (2) reverse the mechanism of injury[2] (if the patient, for example, were to fall on an outstretched hand [FOOSH] falling forward, the resulting fracture could possibly be a Colles or distal radius fracture with dorsal angulation; therefore, to reverse the mechanism of fracture, you would apply the long axis traction while applying a volar-placed fulcrum at the angle of the fracture and applying a volar-directed pressure from the distal end of the radius); and (3) always align the fragment of the fracture that can be controlled with the fragment that cannot.[2] There are so many fracture patterns that could need reductions, which this chapter will not address them, but leave that to the specific chapter that deals with that body part.

Once a fracture has been reduced, some means of holding that reduction must be applied. This can be something as simple as a brace or splint. But many fractures require casting for better protection. Others may be held by an external fixator (Ex-Fix) and some will have to have surgical fixator (pins, screws, and plates) to keep the fracture from displacing while it heals. These cases of course will need to be referred to an orthopedic surgeon for such care (Table 32.1).

32.11 POTENTIAL ACUTE AND CHRONIC COMPLICATIONS OF FRACTURES

32.11.1 Acute Complications of Fractures

There are many more potential acute complications that can occur with any fracture that you might think. With any disruption of the normal bone anatomy of a limb or spine, the surrounding tissues can become involved as well.

Soft tissue can be damaged to a point that it also has to be addressed when treatment is rendered. It can be entrapped in the fracture ends thus preventing good approximation of the bone ends preventing boney healing. It can also have some of its vascular supply disrupted causing a necrosis of the tissue that then must be debrided or revascularized.[2]

Major vascular damage can also occur by the sharp bone ends transecting a vessel, an artery being the worst vessel to damage because it obviously supplies the limb. The provider *must* examine the injured limb checking for distal pulses and capillary refill.[2] If vascular damage is suspected, bedside Doppler ultrasound will help evaluate the vessel further. If a major vessel is involved, it becomes an orthopedic or vascular surgery emergency and must be repaired.

As many neurovascular bundles travel close together, if a vessel is damaged, there may also be a nerve that is damaged as well. Nerve damage can come in many forms:

1. Neuropraxia (first-degree injury), which is much like a bruise to a nerve, is a temporary disruption of nerve function. The axon is intact, but its surrounding myelin sheath may be damaged leading to disrupted transmission. Recovery of function varies from a day to several months.[7]
2. Axonotmesis (second-degree injury) is an injury to the axon of the nerve but with supporting connective tissue intact. Recovery is variable with this injury, depending whether scar tissue interrupts the axon reattachment. Recovery is slow and may take months but usually recovers.[7]
3. Neurotmesis (third-degree injury) is an injury to a nerve with damage to the axon and supportive connective tissue. There is complete loss of both motor and sensory function. There are different grades of *neurotmesis* depending on what part of the supportive tissue is damaged (endoneurium, perineurium, or epineurium) with worsening prognosis with respect to each supportive tissue damaged. Recovery may be complete but is usually a long process. Surgery is almost always indicated for repair. Scarring may prevent full recovery.[7]

Compartment syndrome is also a possible acute complication of fractures.[2] Large bones, like the femur, when broken, can bleed considerably in the closed space of the thigh. When the pressure builds in the compartment from the leaking blood to a point that is greater than the mean arterial pressure of the limb, vascular collapse occurs and potential tissue death if not corrected rapidly. The pressure of compartment syndrome can also put enough pressure on the nerves in the compartment to cause necrosis of the nerve due to the nerve's vascular supply being compromised. Specific signs and symptoms of compartment syndrome will be addressed in another chapter.

Fat embolism syndrome is a potential complication seen with fracture of long bones or crushing fractures. The exact mechanism is not fully understood, but fat emboli or macroglobules enter the bloodstream and can cause damage to the lungs (ARDS), brain (altered mentation—restlessness, disorientation, and possibly marked confusion, stupor, or coma), and kidneys (oliguria).[2] A high index of suspicion is needed to be prepared to treat this potential complication. Onset of symptoms may be immediate or take 2–3 days to appear.

Fracture blisters occur when there is significant soft-tissue trauma associated with the fracture.[2] It typically occurs where the bones are close to the surface of the skin, like an ankle, tibia, and/or elbow. When edema of the tissue becomes too great for the extracellular spaces to hold any more fluid, the fluid leaks out of the skin as blisters. These blisters contain sterile fluid and should be left alone and not ruptured. If they spontaneously rupture, which they many times do, do *not* remove the tissue. Let it heal from the inside and slough the tissue naturally. Just place a sterile dressing over the ruptured blisters until they heal. If there are fracture blisters present, it could delay any surgical fixation until the blisters heal.

Infection is a potential complication of any open fracture.[2] This is why open fractures are orthopedic emergencies. The open fracture is taken to the operating room and meticulously washed out with sterile saline with antibiotics in solution. Typically the fracture is not fixed at that time, but 3 days later at a second washout. Wound cultures are taken before and after each washout.

Converting a closed fracture to an open fracture can occur if the attending provider is not careful in handling the injured limb.[2] If the fracture ends are close to the skin surface when the provider begins manipulation, mishandling can sometimes cause the bone ends to push through the intact skin causing a now open fracture. Care in handling is of utmost importance to prevent this from occurring. Sometimes it is just better to splint a fracture as it lies to prevent unnecessary manipulation. Closed fractures have fewer complications.

Clinical Pearl

Potential acute complications of fractures are: soft-tissue injury, neurovascular injury, compartment syndrome, fat embolism syndrome, fracture blisters, and infection (if an open fracture).

32.11.2 Chronic Complications of Fractures

Despite the provider's best efforts in caring for the patient with a fracture, sometimes chronic complications can occur. These may have to be taken care of when they occur.

Osteomyelitis can be a chronic sequela of open fractures.[2] Despite multiple washouts and intravenous antibiotics, smoldering infections can still occur. This may result in long-term intravenous antibiotics along with debridement of the infected bone. Occasionally infection is difficult to eradicate and placement of antibiotic-impregnated beads will be placed surgically alongside the bone that is infected in an attempt to eliminate the infection more directly.

Malunion of the fracture can occur even though care to align the fracture during the reduction and placement of the cast was taken.[2] The bones can sometimes change their reduced position when the edema subsides and the cast is no longer close-fitting. This is why it is important for the patient to be followed closely until such time as fracture healing is seen on a radiograph taken in the cast. The resulting malunion can be a resulting malalignment, rotational deformity, shortening, or other deformity that is nonanatomic.

Delayed union is classified as a complication because it is less than optimal. There are many causes for a delayed union—tissue interposition, inadequate blood supply to that area of the bone, smoking, diabetes, nonsteroidal anti-inflammatory medications, or overdistracted fracture ends.[2] Delays in healing may mean longer in casts for patients. Casts can have their own complications, mainly of skin issues—ulcers, rashes, and infections. Delays can sometimes be treated with external bone stimulators (which are very costly unfortunately) that may aid in rapidity of healing.

Nonunion is, of course, a complication that every provider wants to avoid. Nonunions come in two different types—hypertrophic and atrophic.[2] Hypertrophic nonunions have radiographic evidence of bone callous showing that the bones were trying to heal but something blocked that healing. This can be soft-tissue interposition or fracture gap from overdistracted bone ends. Atrophic nonunion means there was no attempt by the bone to heal visible on radiographs. This may be due to lack of blood supply to that area of the bone, or necrotic bone ends. Nonunions can have external bone stimulators attempt to restore the osteogenesis of the bone (again, expensive), or surgical debridement of the bone ends, along with bone graft and internal fixation, is the most common way to correct it.

Fractures in or around joints can also end with chronic complications. Avascular necrosis and/or chondrolysis can occur.[2]

Avascular necrosis occurs when there is a disruption of the blood supply to that segment of the bone. In hip fractures, for example, femoral neck fractures that displace more than a few millimeters may disrupt the blood supply to the femoral head and result in osteonecrosis of the femoral head. Another location that can have avascular necrosis occur is the scaphoid bone of the wrist. With only one artery supplying it, if there is displacement of the fracture more than 1 mm, the vascular supply can be disrupted and result in osteonecrosis once again.

Chondrolysis can occur in fractures that involve the joint surface—tibial plateau fractures, acetabular fractures, glenoid fractures, distal humerus fractures, and radial head fractures. Currently there is not much that can be done to restore the cartilage to a healthy state and unfortunately can accelerate the rate of osteoarthritis of that joint.

Loss of range of motion and/or function can be a chronic complication.[2] This can be most troublesome to the patient. Fractures in and around elbows many times have this complication. Early rehabilitation and motion of the joint, as soon as it becomes stable, are important in lessening this complication. Malunions can also lead to loss of function if the resultant angulation of the healed fracture is such that weight-bearing or rotation of the joint is limited due to the healed position. This can sometimes be corrected surgically by an experienced orthopedic surgeon.

Although less common, heterotopic ossification can be seen in fractures that have significant soft-tissue injury.[2] Common sites include acetabular fractures, elbow dislocations, femoral shaft intramedullary nailing, and after total hip arthroplasties. Heterotopic ossification is bone formation in abnormal sites, usually soft tissue. Treatment is done only if there is associated pain from the excess bone being in a place where pressure is applied or if it limits range of motion of the affected joint nearby. Treatment is debridement.

An often missed complication is that of complex regional pain syndrome (CRPS). This complication has many recognized synonyms: reflex sympathetic dystrophy, Südeck's atrophy, causalgia, minor causalgia, mimocausalgia, algodystrophy, algoneurodystrophy, posttraumatic pain syndrome, painful posttraumatic dystrophy, painful posttraumatic osteoporosis, and transient migratory osteoporosis.[2] Its early features are thought to occur as much as 30%–40% of every fracture or surgical trauma but resolves spontaneously with routine treatment and therefore does not represent a separate diagnosis. Common signs and symptoms are as follows: abnormal pain (outside of what is expected following stabilization treatment), swelling (after initial edema resolves), vasomotor and sudomotor dysfunction, contracture, and osteoporosis.[2] Early recognition and treatment of this complication should aid in reducing the duration the patient suffers. Referral to a pain specialist is appropriate.

Clinical Pearl

Potential chronic complications of fractures are: malunion, delayed union, non-union, loss of range of motion or function, CRPS, heterotopic ossification, avascular necrosis (if vascular compromised), and/or chondrolysis and degenerative arthritis (if joint surface involved).

32.12 INDICATIONS FOR REFERRAL: DISLOCATIONS AND/OR FRACTURES

With any dislocation, the primary goal is to reduce the dislocation as soon as possible. Some joints are quick and easy and can be handled by any practitioner, such as proximal interphalangeal (PIP) joints of fingers and generally do not require an anesthetic (digital blocks *can* be used but generally are not). Joints that are larger than fingers usually require at least conscious sedation. This most commonly occurs in an emergency department (ED) where the patient can be

TABLE 32.2
SORT: Key Recommendations for Practice

Clinical Recommendation	Evidence Rating	References
For fractures and/or dislocations, neurovascular evaluation should be performed *before* and *after* any manipulation of the injury or placement of a splint/cast.	C	[1,2,4,6]
A minimum of two radiographic views 90° to each other is imperative in evaluating both dislocations and fractures to assure adequate visualization of the injury.	C	[1–4,6]
Anesthesia appropriate for the injury (block, sedation, or general) should be given for comfort of the patient to aid in preventing patient resistance to the procedure being performed.	C	[1,2,4,6]
Evaluation of injury for any break in the skin communicating with the joint/fracture must be performed to assure there is no open fracture/dislocation that would warrant a surgical emergency.	C	[1,2,4,6]
All patients with fractures and/or dislocations must be followed for potential complications.	C	[1,2,4,6]

monitored properly. That is why it is recommended to send a patient there where definitive care can be provided. If you are the one working in the ED, you may be the one attempting the reduction. So when is the time to refer this patient to the orthopedic specialist? If there is any indication of neurovascular compromise, an open dislocation, or after multiple attempts (usually three) at reduction without success, you should call the specialist to ask them to see the patient. It may be that there is soft-tissue interposition that is keeping the joint from reducing and may mean a trip to the operating room to open the joint to move the tissue out of the way for the reduction to happen. It may just be that you are not comfortable or have never performed a reduction of the joint involved. In that case, referral is appropriate.

For fractures, it is pretty much the same. All open fractures, or fractures with associated neurovascular compromise, should be referred emergently to the specialist. Most other fractures can be splinted safely and referred to the specialist within 3–5 days. If you have experience in handling uncomplicated fractures, such as a buckle fracture, minimally displaced distal radius, fifth metatarsal base fracture, or distal phalanx finger or toe fracture, it is totally acceptable (and appreciated by most orthopedic specialists) to care for the patient yourself.

32.13 CONCLUSION

Careful attention and treatment of dislocations and/or fractures are important in having a good and functional result as well as a happy patient. A solid understanding of the mechanism of injury along with a good thorough physical exam and adequate and appropriate treatment will result in those good outcomes, in most cases. Knowing your limitations and when to refer to the orthopedic specialist also will keep your patient well cared for and happy. Further information about specific fractures and dislocations will be covered in chapters dealing with those topics (Table 32.2).

REFERENCES

1. Beaty JH, Kasser JR. *Rockwood and Wilkins' Fractures in Children*, 7th edn. Philadelphia, PA: Lippincott, Williams, & Wilkins; 2010.
2. Bucholz RW, Court-Brown CM, Heckman JD et al. (Eds.). *Rockwood and Green's Fractures in Adults.* 7th edn. Philadelphia, PA: Lippincott, Williams, & Wilkins; 2010.
3. Greenspan A. *Orthopedic Imaging: A Practical Approach.* 5th edn. Philadelphia, PA: Lippincott, Williams, & Wilkins; 2010.
4. Sarwark JF. (Ed.). *Essentials of Musculoskeletal Care.* 4th edn. Rosemont, IL: American Academy of Orthopaedic Surgeons; 2010.
5. Venes D. (Ed.). *Taber's Cyclopedic Medical Dictionary.* 22nd edn. Philadelphia, PA: F.A. Davis; 2013.
6. Weinstein SL, Buckwalter JA. *Turek's Orthopaedics: Principles and Their Application.* 6th edn. Philadelphia, PA: Lippincott, Williams, & Wilkins; 2005.
7. Whiting WC, Zernicke RF. *Biomechanics of Musculoskeletal Injury.* 2nd edn. Champaign, IL: Human Kinetics; 2008.

33 Splinting and Casting

Jason B. Alisangco, Chad A. Asplund, and Holly J. Benjamin

CONTENTS

TABLE 33.1
Key Clinical Considerations

1. The purpose of splinting and casting is to immobilize, protect, aid in healing, and decrease pain.
2. Immobilization offers three benefits: prevention of loss of position, protection of adjacent structures, and pain relief.
3. Conditions that benefit from immobilization are fractures, sprains, severe soft-tissue injuries, reduced joint dislocations, inflammatory conditions, and deep lacerations across joints and tendon lacerations.
4. The initial approach to casting and splinting involves a thorough assessment of the injury for proper diagnosis to include an exam above and below the injured area.
5. Complications can occur regardless of how long the device is used.

33.1 INTRODUCTION

Musculoskeletal injuries, including bone and soft-tissue injuries, are common in sports medicine and in primary care. Splinting and casting is a valuable skill needed for primary care physicians and those that provide musculoskeletal care. Splints and casts support and immobilize the injured extremity to reduce pain, prevent further injury of tissues in proximity to a fracture, and maintain alignment, which is the first step in healing.[6] Many fractures that are nondisplaced can be stabilized through the use of splinting or casting. Each method has advantages, disadvantages, and specific indications, and it is important to be aware of these characteristics to ensure optimal care to the patient (Table 33.1).

33.2 SPLINTING VERSUS CASTING

Consideration for splinting and castings requires an evaluation of the injury's stage and severity, the potential for instability, risk of complication, and patient's functional requirements. In the primary care setting, splinting is usually more practical and common, and splinting is the preferred method of fracture immobilization in the acute setting.[5] Splints are not circumferential and allow for swelling of the extremity, which will minimize the risk of compartment syndrome. Proper immobilization of a fracture cannot be obtained unless the joints above and below the fracture are immobilized.[7] Casts are circumferential and swelling within the cast increases pressure, potentially increasing risks of compartment syndrome and pressure sores; however, casts immobilize an extremity more completely than splints, which make them the better long-term treatment for fractures (level of evidence C, usual practice).[5,6]

33.2.1 Advantages and Disadvantages of Splinting and Casting

Splinting offers many advantages, including easier application and removal and decreased pressure-related complications due to their noncircumferential property, which allows for the natural swelling that occurs with the initial inflammatory phase. Splints may be static (prevent motion) or dynamic (functional; assist with controlled motion). Several types of splints are available including custom-made and "off-the-shelf" splints.[7] Splints are also more easily removed compared to a cast, which may be an advantage or disadvantage based on the situation. In the initial treatment of fractures, splints are used initially and then replaced by a cast for definitive treatment of unstable fractures.[7]

Clinical Pearl

Splints should be used for the initial treatment of injuries that require air evacuation due to their noncircumferential nature, which will allow for swelling with change in altitude.

Because of their ability to provide more complete immobilization, casting is the mainstay of treatment for most fractures. Casts provide superior immobilization and are reserved for definitive fracture management. However, casting requires more skill and time for application, and if done improperly, complications may occur more commonly than with splinting.

33.3 MATERIALS

Splinting and casting may be performed with a variety of materials to include plaster of Paris, semi-rigid fiberglass (soft cast), and resin-based synthetic materials such as fiberglass. In austere environments or in the wilderness, branches or sticks may be used as splints until definitive care can be provided, but these are only temporizing measures.

Plaster of Paris is traditionally preferred for splints because it is pliable and has longer setting time than fiberglass and produces less heat, which avoids burns and patient discomfort. It is cheaper and has a longer shelf life.[7] Plaster of Paris has been applied using gauze embedded in calcium phosphate powder. Because calcium phosphate is relatively brittle, the mechanical strength of plaster of Paris comes from the integration of layers of gauze embedded with calcium phosphate, which crystallizes and forms an intricate structure upon its making.[9] Plaster of Paris is commonly used postsurgery because of the increased swelling associated with fractures. Plaster of Paris is used as a backslab in the early stages following injury, thus not completely surrounding the limb and allowing the limb to swell. It is considered to be light, relatively soft, and easily removable. Plaster should be used for most routine splinting applications. However, some patients may feel that the plaster is heavy and uncomfortable, which would make ambulation difficult, which would then favor the use of a synthetic material.[3]

Fiberglass is lighter than plaster and is typically used for nondisplaced fractures and severe soft-tissue injuries. Fiberglass is more durable than plaster but has a shorter shelf life and is more expensive than plaster. Despite this, fiberglass is generally preferred for casting by providers who have more experience casting and who treat a larger number of fractures due to its ease of use[7] (see Figure 33.1).

33.4 GENERAL APPLICATION PROCEDURES

When starting the application process, the injured extremity should be assessed, and documentation of skin lesions, neurovascular status, soft-tissue injury, and bony structures should be performed. Neurovascular status should be rechecked following immobilization by cast or splint to ensure that the repositioning has not compromised the neurovascular structures.[7]

During the application process, at least one joint distal to the injury is immobilized to minimize movement of the injured structures. Immobilization of both joints, proximal and distal to the injury, is common and very beneficial, especially for fractures or more severe injuries. Prior to immobilization, fractures should be reduced, and the extremity is placed on its position of function. The extremity should then be padded to prevent skin breakdown and neurovascular compression. Incisions or wounds should be properly treated and covered with a sterile dressing prior to application of the splint or cast.[6]

First, stockinet is placed over the extremity and extended 5–10 cm beyond each end of the intended splint or cast site (shown in Figure 33.2).

The excess is folded back to form a smooth edge once the splint or cast material has been applied. The stockinet should not be too tight and wrinkles must be smoothed. Layers of padding are placed over the stockinet to prevent maceration of the skin and accommodate swelling. Padding is wrapped circumferentially, with each layer overlapping 50% of the previous layer (see Figure 33.3).

Padding should be 2–3 layers thick and extend 2–3 cm beyond the edge of the splint. Extra padding should be placed between digits and over bony prominence. During application, care must be taken to ensure that too much padding is not used as this can compromise the support of immobilization or unduly increase pressure on nerves or other sensitive structures.[7] Padding comes in several widths. In general, padding 2 in. wide is used for the hands, 2–4 in. for upper extremities, 3 in. for feet, and 4–6 in. for lower extremities. Next, the splint or cast material is moistened for appropriate setting time (see manufacturer's

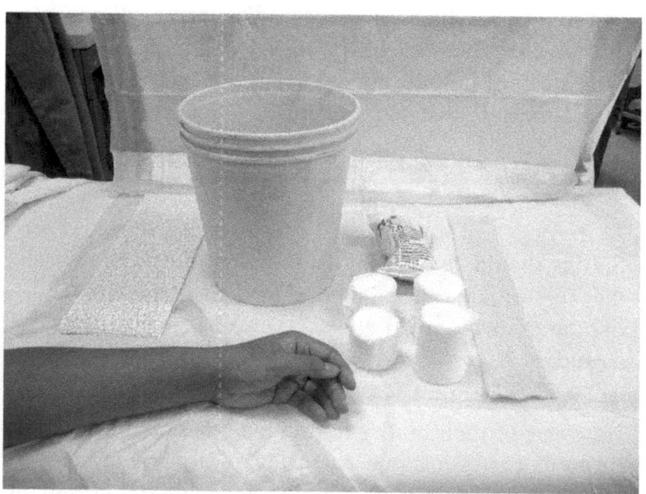

FIGURE 33.1 Fiberglass and materials needed for splinting.

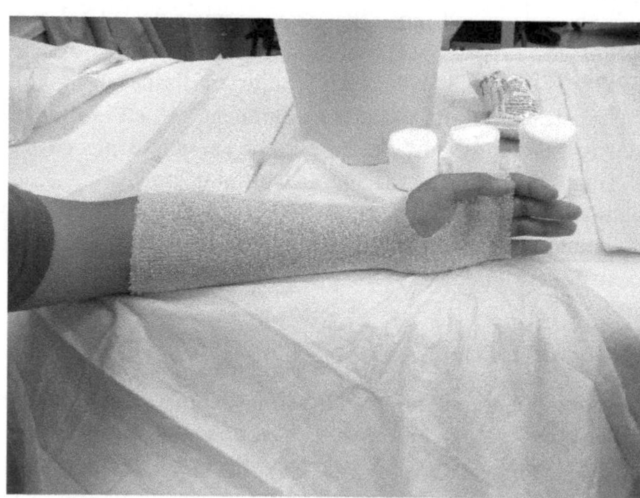

FIGURE 33.2 Stockinet applied, extended 5–10 cm past the edge of the splint.

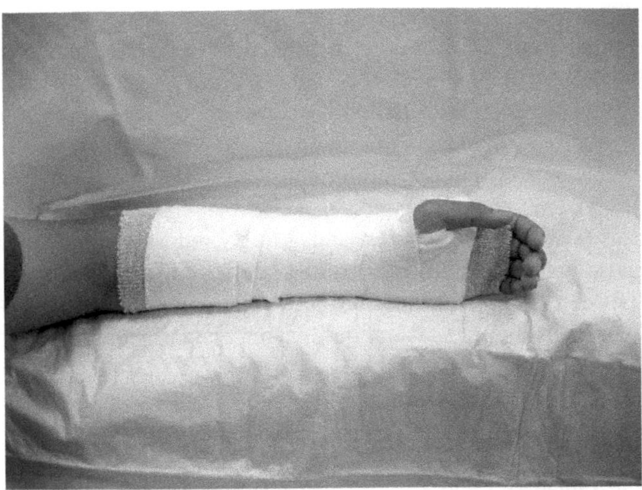

FIGURE 33.3 Padding added, with each layer overlapping 50% of the previous layer.

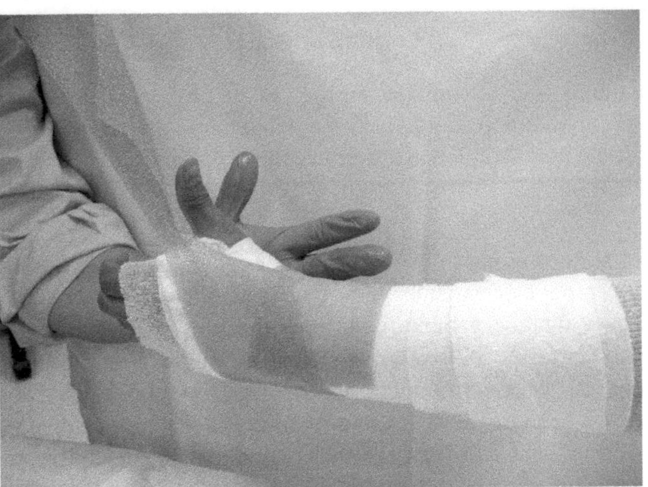

FIGURE 33.4 Fiberglass applied, with each layer overlapping 50% of the previous layer.

recommendations) and to decrease the heat of reaction, to minimize burns on the skin during setting.[6] Casting materials harden faster with the use of warm water compared with cold water. The faster the material sets, the greater the heat produced, and the greater the risk of significant skin burns. Cool water is also recommended when extra time is needed for splint application.

Clinical Pearl

A good rule of thumb is that heat is *inversely* proportional to the setting time and *directly* proportional to the number of layers used.

33.4.1 Splinting

When splinting with plaster of Paris, an additional 1–2 cm of material is required to allow for shrinkage of the plaster material. The splint should be shorter than the padding. The thickness of the splint depends on the patient size, the extremity involved, and the desired strength of the splint. On average, an adult upper extremity should be splinted with 6–10 sheets; lower extremities need approximately 12–15 sheets. In general, the minimum number of layers necessary to achieve adequate strength should be used. The splint material is then submerged in water until the bubbling stops; the excess water is squeezed out to ensure even wetness of all layers of splint material. The material is molded together like a laminate material to achieve improved strength and stability. Next, the splint is placed over the padding and molded to the contours of the extremity. Finally, secure the dry splint to the extremity with an elastic bandage in the distal to proximal direction.[7]

33.4.2 Casting

Fiberglass application for splinting or casting is similar to previously discussed text, with the exception of number of sheets needed—most fiberglass splint material is prepackaged so one thickness is all that is needed. When casting, the fiberglass material is rolled circumferentially around the extremity generally with two layers of material. The width and thickness of the fiberglass casting also depends on the patient size, extremity involved, and desired strength. To prepare the material, it is submerged in water until bubbling stops and is unrolled to the desired casting to immobilize the injury.[7] Fiberglass casting material should go over the stockinet and padding circumferentially with each roll overlapping 50% of the previous layer (described in Figure 33.4).

The stockinet and padding edges should be folded back before the last layer is applied. Excess molding and indentation should be avoided. Open windows should be cut around open wounds for easier monitoring.[7]

33.5 COMPLICATIONS

With the improved practices of internal fixation, splinting and casting have become a lost art with many physicians; in many situations, casts are routinely applied by midlevel providers or cast room technicians. Despite fewer physicians applying splints and casts, it is still important to understand the risks and potential complications that can occur. The risk of morbidity is higher when casts are applied by less experienced practitioners. It is important to properly inform patients of the inherent risks of splinting and casting.[8]

Compartment syndrome is the most serious complication of casting or splinting. It is a condition of increased pressure within a closed space that compromises blood flow and tissue perfusion and causes ischemia and potentially irreversible damage to the soft tissues within that space. If an immobilized patient experiences worsening pain, tingling, numbness, or any sign of vascular compromise such as severe swelling, delayed capillary refill, or dusky appearance of exposed extremities, an immediate visit to the nearest emergency department or urgent care office is indicated for prompt removal of the cast.

Clinical Pearl

Patients who complain of pain out of proportion following cast application should be assumed to have compartment syndrome and should be further evaluated.

Next, thermal or pressure injuries can occur. There are certain groups of patients with higher risk of cast complications. These include patients with an inability to effectively communicate, the obtunded or comatose multitrauma patients, as well as those patients with general or limb block anesthesia because they are unable to feel and respond to pain, such as heat and pressure that may occur during splint and cast application. Additionally, the very young or developmentally delayed are unaware of expressing possible discomfort or fully understand the procedure. Finally, patients with impaired sensation, such as those with spinal cord injuries or medical disorders like diabetes, are at increased risk of excessive heat and pressure injury. Prolonged immobilization may also potentiate osteopenia, which then could lead to poor fracture healing. Patients with spasticity are at risk of developing pressure sores resultant to the increased tone after the cast is applied—as such pressure sores have been noticed in children with cerebral palsy.[8]

To minimize this risk of thermal injury, it is important to understand the thermal dynamics of the casting material. During setup, the conversion of plaster of Paris to the harder gypsum is an exothermic reaction, and the released heat can be transmitted to the patient. The temperature of the moisture system (dip water) and the thickness of the material can affect the amount of heat produced. Thermal injuries increase when the dip water temperature is too hot (>50°C) or the cast is too thick (>24 plies). Fiberglass can cause thermal injury, but the risk is lower.[8]

As earlier, with improper technique, casting can cause compartment syndrome, ischemia, pressure sores, and skin breakdown. Patients should be instructed to return if they experience increased pain following cast application. Upon return they should be evaluated for all neurovascular complaints as soft-tissue swelling can lead to compartment syndrome. Pain may also be due to excessive pressure, which can cause ischemia, skin sores, and skin breakdown. Finally, wet and soiled casts not made with synthetic or waterproof materials can result in skin irritation, skin breakdown, and infection. Foul-smelling casts should be removed to prevent wound skin and wound infection.[8]

33.6 TYPES OF CASTS AND SPLINTS

See Tables 33.2 and 33.3 and Figures 33.5 through 33.8.

33.7 CONCLUSION

Primary care providers can learn to appropriately manage musculoskeletal injuries and fractures if they possess an understanding of the basic principles of immobilization care. Proper management starts with a thorough evaluation of the injured extremity for correct diagnosis and then a thorough neurovascular examination. Depending on the severity and acuity, splinting versus casting or a timely transition with both can aid with immobilization of the fracture for optimal healing and patient comfort. Proper material selection, cast type, and application technique is paramount to minimize possible complications following splint or cast application. If complications occur, it is paramount that providers keep a high level of suspicion for compartment syndrome and thoroughly evaluate patients who experience increased pain following cast application to minimize limb-threatening problems. If casts and splints are used correctly, providers can aid in the healing of their patients and their return back to activity (Table 33.4).

TABLE 33.2
Lower Extremity Splinting and Casting

Region	Type of Splint/Cast	Indications	Pearls/Pitfalls	Follow-Up/Referral
Knee and lower leg	Posterior knee splint	Acute soft-tissue and bony injuries of lower extremity	If ankle immobilization is necessary, splint should be extended to toes.	Days
Ankle	Short leg cast (Figure 33.5)	Isolated nondisplaced malleolar fractures	Compartment syndrome most commonly associated with proximal midtibial fractures.	2–4 weeks
Foot	Short leg cast (Figure 33.5)	Foot fractures: tarsals or metatarsals	Depending on weight-bearing status, it could be walking cast/boot.	2 weeks Refer for displaced/unstable fractures
Ankle	Posterior ankle splint	Severe sprains, isolated nondisplaced malleolar fractures	Splint ends 2 in. distal to fibular head to avoid common peroneal nerve compression.	Less than 1 week Refer for displaced or multiple fractures
Ankle	Stirrup splint	Ankle sprains, isolated nondisplaced malleolar fractures	Mold to site of injury for effective compression.	Less than 1 week

Source: Adapted from Boyd, A.S. et al., *Am. Fam. Physician*, 80(5), 491, 2009.

TABLE 33.3
Upper Extremity Splinting and Casting

Region	Type of Splint/Cast	Indications	Pearls/Pitfalls	Follow-up/Referral
Elbow	Double sugar-tong splint	Acute elbow fracture	Offers greater immobilization against pronation and supination.	Less than 1 week
Proximal forearm and skeletally immature wrist injuries	Long arm posterior splint, long arm cast	Distal humerus, proximal or midshaft forearm fractures	Ensure adequate padding at bony prominences.	1 week Refer for displaced or unstable fractures
Forearm	Single sugar-tong splint (Figure 33.6)	Acute distal radial and ulnar fractures	Used for increased immobilization of forearm.	Less than 1 week Refer for displaced or unstable fractures
Wrist/carpal bones	Volar/dorsal forearm splint	Soft-tissue injuries to hand and wrist Acute carpal bone fractures (except scaphoid) Buckle fracture of radius	Consider splinting as definitive treatment of buckle fractures[10] (level of evidence B, randomized controlled trial (RCT)).	1 week Refer for displaced or unstable fractures Refer for lunate fractures
Wrist/hand	Short arm cast (Figure 33.7)	Nondisplaced fractures of distal radius Carpal bone fractures other than scaphoid		1 week
Finger injuries (excluding thumb)	Buddy tape Aluminum splint Extension block splint Mallet finger splint	Nondisplaced proximal/middle phalynx fractures Distal phalynx fracture Middle phalynx/volar plate fracture Extensor tension avulsion	Encourage active motion. Encourage motion at proximal interphalangeal (PIP)/metacarpophalangeal (MCP) joints. Increase flexion by 15° weekly. Continuous for 6–8 weeks.	2 weeks Refer for angulated, displaced, rotated, or oblique fractures
Thumb, first MCP, carpal bone	Thumb spica splint/cast	Injuries to scaphoid First MCP fractures Stable thumb fractures	Fracture of middle/third of the scaphoid treated with casting Immobilization of thumb with removable splint is preferred by patients and the functional results are comparable to casting[11] (level of evidence B, RCT).	1–2 weeks Refer for angulated, displaced, rotated, or oblique fractures
Ulnar side hand	Ulnar gutter splint/cast (Figure 33.8)	Fourth/fifth phalangeal shaft fractures	Proper positioning of MCP joints at 70–90 degrees of flexion and PIP and distal interphalangeal (DIP) joints at 5–10 degrees of flexion.	1–2 weeks Refer for angulated, displaced, rotated, or oblique fractures
Radial side hand	Radial gutter splint/cast	Second/third proximal shaft fractures	Proper positioning of MCP joints at 70–90 degrees of flexion and PIP and DIP joints at 5–10 degrees of flexion. Recommended for initial immobilization of a displaced distal radial fracture[2] (level of evidence B, RCT).	1–2 weeks Refer for angulated, displaced, rotated, or oblique fractures

Source: Adapted from Boyd, A.S., et al., *Am. Fam. Physician*, 80(5), 491, 2009.

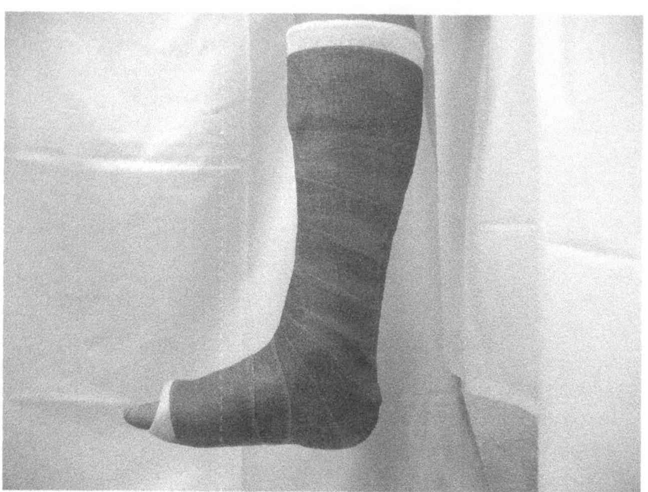

FIGURE 33.5 Short leg cast.

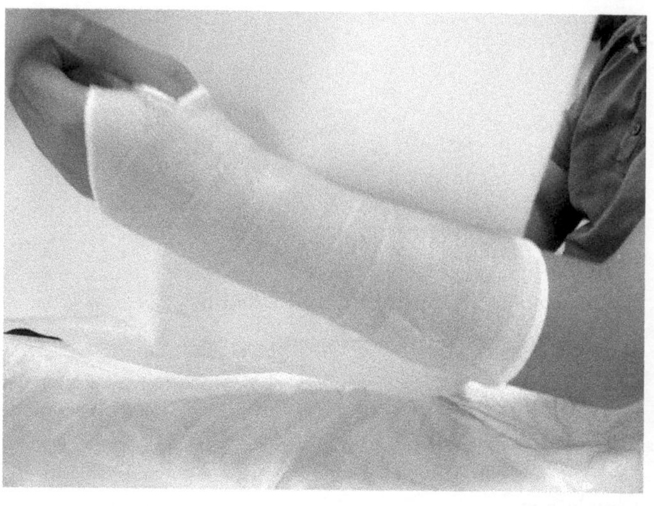

FIGURE 33.7 Short arm cast.

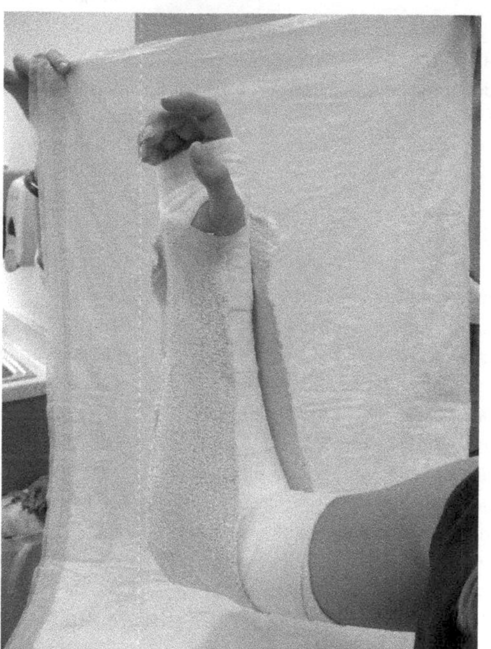

FIGURE 33.6 Simple sugar-tong splint.

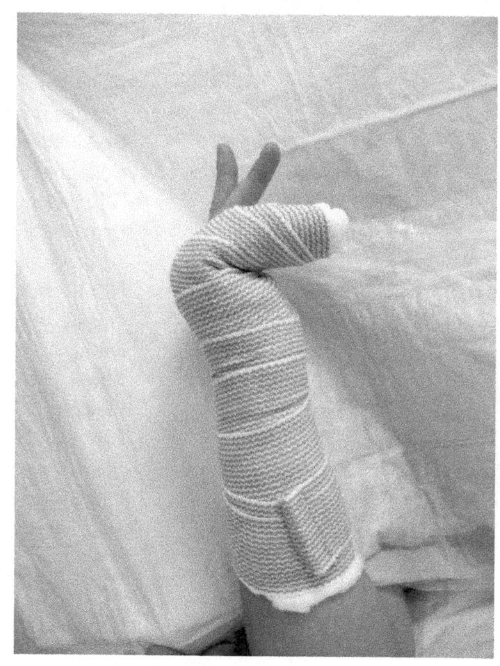

FIGURE 33.8 Ulnar gutter splint.

TABLE 33.4
SORT: Key Recommendations for Practice

Clinical Recommendation	Evidence Rating	References
Splinting is the preferred method of fracture immobilization in the acute care setting.	C	[5]
Casting is the mainstay treatment for most fractures	C	[6]
Plaster of Paris should be used for most routine splinting applications; unless weight, bulk of cast, or time to weight bearing is important, then a synthetic may be the material of choice.	C	[3]
Use of a short arm radial gutter splint is recommended for initial immobilization of a displaced distal radial fracture.	B	[2]
Immobilization of the thumb with a removable splint after a ligamentous injury is strongly preferred by the patient, and the functional outcome is similar to cast immobilization.	B	[11]
Removable splinting is preferable to casting in the treatment of wrist buckle fractures in children	B	[10]

REFERENCES

1. Bakody E. Orthopaedic plaster casting: Nurse and patient education. *Nursing Standard.* 2009;23(51):49–56.
2. Bong MR, Egol KA, Leibman M et al. A comparison of immediate postreduction splinting constructs for controlling initial displacement of fractures of the distal radius: A prospective randomized study of long-arm versus short-arm splinting. *Journal of Hand Surgery.* 2006;31(5):766–770.
3. Bowker P, Powell ES. A clinical evaluation of plaster-of-Paris and eight synthetic fracture splinting materials. *Injury.* 1992;23(1):13–20.
4. Boyd AS, Benjamin HJ, Asplund CA. Splints and casts: Indications and methods. *American Family Physician.* 2009;80(5):491–499.
5. Eiff MP, Hatch R, Calmbach WL (eds.). *Fracture Management for Primary Care*, 2nd edn. Philadelphia, PA: Saunders; 2003, pp. 1–39.
6. Elstrom JA, Virkus W, Pankovich A. *Nonoperative Techniques in Handbook of Fractures.* 3rd edn. Elstrom JA (ed.). New York: McGraw-Hill; 2006, pp. 20–23.
7. Garrison JM, Asplund CA. *Casting and Splinting in ACSM's Sports Medicine: A Comprehensive Review.* O'Conner FG (ed.). Lippincott, Williams & Wilkins; 2012, pp. 549–552.
8. Halanski M, Noonan K. Cast and splint immobilization: Complications. *Journal of the American Academy of Orthopaedic Surgeons.* 2008;16(1):30–40.
9. Oron A, Lindner D, Bergman A et al. Molding significantly affects the mechanical properties of plaster of Paris in orthopaedic use. *Current Orthopaedic Practice.* 2013;24(6): 647–650.
10. Plint AC, Perry JJ, Correll R et al. A randomized, controlled trial of removable splinting versus casting for wrist buckle fractures in children. *Pediatrics.* 2006;117(3):691–697.
11. Sollerman C, Abrahamsson SO, Lundborg G et al. Functional splinting versus plaster cast for ruptures of the ulnar collateral ligament of the thumb. A prospective randomized study of 63 cases. *Acta Orthopaedica Scandinavica.* 1991;62(6):524–526.

34 Mass Participation Event Coverage

Scott W. Pyne

CONTENTS

TABLE 34.1
Key Clinical Considerations

1. Open collaboration, generous support, and mutual respect between the event and medical directors are critical to successful and safe event management.
2. Advanced detailed and diligent medical planning is required to adequately support mass participation events.
3. Scope of care to include treatment algorithms should be discussed, decided, and communicated to all involved early in the planning process.
4. Educating competitors, support, and medical staff regarding medical issues anticipated with the event is highly recommended.
5. Document all patient interactions and complete an after-action report summarizing data to be utilized in subsequent years' planning process.

34.1 INTRODUCTION

A medical infrastructure designed to ensure the safe participation of athletes and staff should be behind every mass participation event. The provision of medical support for these events facilitates an opportunity for community outreach, collaboration with colleagues across the medical continuum of care, service to participants, and often a great deal of personal satisfaction. Mass participation events can be defined as any sporting pursuit involving more participants than a standard two-team competition and frequently involves multiple venues and extensive geographic territory. Common examples are marathons, triathlons, and team sport tournaments and may include long distances and varying terrains and obstacles. Participation has continued to grow and includes not only increased entrants in traditional events but the development of a new series of community sanctioned and unsanctioned combat, obstacle, and adventure challenges. It should be noted that the planning and coverage for these events are separate and unique from that utilized in the planning for mass gathering events such as outdoor concerts, sporting event spectators, and religious pilgrimages.[3,11,27,35,37] Extensive advanced planning is critical to provide safe and effective medical care.[1,2,11,17,25] The medical leader must be adept at communication, planning, collaboration, and sport-specific medical condition diagnosis and management to prevent serious injury or illness to the participants and support staff.[22] The required advanced preparation cannot be underestimated and an intimate understanding of the event rules, goals, peculiarities, and participants will prove invaluable. The requirements for coverage must be considered well in advance of the event to provide optimal number, distribution, and training of medical assets. Having a fully operational emergency action plan is an essential piece for the successful execution of a mass participation event (Table 34.1).[7,42]

34.2 EPIDEMIOLOGY

A key consideration in planning for the coverage of any event is an intimate understanding of the potential medical requirement associated with it. Competitor demographics, course demands, water, speed, terrain, equipment, climate, and temperature are only a few of the variables to be considered. The utilization of the event's past history and that of similar events is often most helpful in planning for the current event. This reinforces the importance of maintaining accurate medical contact statistics from year to year. Focusing on injury type and distribution associated with event duration and location is helpful in staging medical supplies and clinical expertise at sites where their utilization will be optimized.

Clinical Pearl

Discuss the process to stop the event in case of extreme weather or circumstances, develop a written plan, and do not hesitate to act in the best interest of the competitors and support staff.

Increased medical contacts and injury rates have been documented with increasing distance, duration, and temperature.[9,18,20] Injury rates for different events noted in the literature include running (42 km), 1%–20%; running (<21 km), 1%–5%; triathlon (225 km), 15%–30%; Nordic skiing (55 km), 5%; triathlon (51 km), 2%–5%; and cycling (variable), 5%.[23,38,41,47,48] While injury rates are available for individual team sport, multisport, and adventure race events, the variables across these events make generalizations regarding injury rates difficult.[4,6,12–16,26,30,36]

The risk of death for mass participation events is fortunately small, with the likely cause predicted according to the event.[28,29,45] A study evaluating the incidence of cardiac arrest in marathons and half marathons found a rate of 0.54 arrests per 100,000 participants.[24]

34.3 SAFETY CONSIDERATIONS

A shared responsibility of all involved in the conduct of an event is the safety of the participants and support staff. Medical leadership must work closely with event coordinators to assess, mitigate, and provide a safe competition and medical care environment. It should be remembered that these issues are occasionally overlooked by event directors when dealing with competing pressures of finance, sponsorship, and marketing. Contingency plans for all possible safety vulnerabilities must be discussed, agreed upon, and published well prior to the start of the event.[17] A written and signed agreement outlining the roles and responsibilities of all parties is strongly recommended. This responsibility does not end with the competitors but includes the support staff and spectators. The impact of the event on local medical care, medical facilities, and emergency medical services (EMS) must be assessed. Overloading local resources may result in inadequate medical resource availability to the community where the event takes place.

Clinical Pearl

Discuss the process to stop the event in case of extreme weather or circumstances, develop a written plan, and do not hesitate to act in the best interest of the competitors and support staff.

In extreme conditions the event may need to be modified or canceled. Due to the documented increased injury rate with increased environmental temperature, the Twin Cities Marathon has adopted guidance to cancel the event if the temperature reaches a sufficient level.[40] Severe and extreme weather prior to the start or that develops during the event may also necessitate cancelation or modification. The risk and presence of lightening must be anticipated and a plan for the safety of participants and support staff must be developed. The National Oceanic and Atmospheric Administration provides several lightning-specific resources and recommends waiting 30 minutes after the storm has passed to resume athletic events.[33] An appropriate shelter to wait out the storm is important to consider for the participants and support staff, who are many times staged in exposed locations. The shelter from the elements and the provision of food and water should be considered as well.

The safety of the competition field, course, or water must also be closely scrutinized. It is strongly recommended that the medical support staff survey the course and provide input recommending modification of any identified vulnerabilities. Common areas in distance events are the start, transition, and finish.[18,19] All should provide long, wide areas devoid of obstacles, hills, or sharp turns to decrease the risk of falls, excessive crowding, and injury. Water events should optimize the visibility of competitors through the entirety of their participation to lessen the risk of losing a swimmer who may need assistance. Muddy, murky water, strong currents, and obstacles pose increased risk that must be thoroughly addressed. Optimal observation platforms should also be provided. Boats, stand-up paddleboards, or elevated lifeguard chairs may be more effective than kayaks and surfboards in visualizing all competitors. A process of checkpoints for adventure and ultraendurance events is a helpful way to account for all competitors and initiate medical search and aid in a timelier manner.

34.4 CONTINGENCY PLANNING FOR MASS CASUALTY SITUATIONS

Emergency action plans in collaboration with community EMS, fire departments, and law enforcement to deal with the unexpected have gained importance and become the norm especially after the cases of the Marine Corps and New York Marathons following September 11, 2001, and the Boston Marathon after the 2012 terrorist attacks.[5] Prevention of such incidents is a shared responsibility of all involved to include planners, participants, and local community resources. Restriction of access, limitations of bag size, physical screening of personnel and their property, a posture of awareness, and a mechanism to report and investigate areas or items of concern must be considered. Local and federal law enforcement should provide a risk assessment, and cancellation of the event should be considered in circumstances where the safety of the participants cannot be ensured or credible threats to the event have been received. In developing a medical plan and defining a scope of care for mass participation events, contingency planning for mass casualty situations cannot be ignored. Response to an incident and care of injured individuals must be coordinated. Physical, chemical, biological, and nuclear threats and community emergency action plans are often already in place to address these concerns. Inserting the event and its internal resources in this community response, educating support staff, and following the preestablished plan will allow efficient and coordinated response to these unfortunate occurrences.

34.5 MEDICAL CHAIN OF COMMAND

A sole medical director should be identified early in the planning process to serve as a key member of the event team and advisor to the event director. While shared medical responsibility has been utilized at several events, it is preferable to have a single point of contact for the event director, media, and community medical partners to address queries and provide medical direction when required. Several responsibilities of the medical director include advanced planning, event-day medical decision making, and medical troubleshooting.

Since the medical director often cannot be everywhere that medical care is provided, it is helpful to assign a leader to each medical aid station. Ideally, this aid station leader will be well versed in the event specifics, medical support plan, medical assets, and the provision of medical care acting on the behalf of the medical director and serving as the communication point of contact for their area of responsibility.

34.6 MEDICAL PHILOSOPHY

34.6.1 Scope and Level of Care

The scope and level of care for the event must be agreed upon and clearly communicated to all parties prior to the start. This philosophy will set the expectation for all involved; event directors, medical support staff, competitors, EMS, medical facilities, and the local community. It is first important to determine if the medical support will provide care for competitors, support staff, or spectators. The most common arrangement is to provide care to competitors only and utilize a parallel community resource plan for spectators and support staff as needed. A minimal scope of care should include first aid and basic life support with automated external defibrillator availability.[32] Additional services may be provided according to their availability and specific event requirements. It is not unusual for events held in remote locations to establish a higher medical scope of care than is available in the local community. All aid stations need not maintain a similar scope of care, with more advanced services often provided at sites of expected high requirement. The finish aid station for endurance events and those servicing particularly challenging sections of the course universally provide increased services. Familiarization with competition rules will minimize the chance of providing medical interventions and assistance that may inadvertently disqualify the athlete. Likewise medical recommendations about continuation of competition after intervention should be clarified and disseminated.

Early access to advanced cardiac life support (ACLS) is desirable and can be accomplished through partnerships with local EMS and fire and police departments. Mobile units on bicycles, canoes, kayaks, all-terrain vehicle, or golf carts have been successfully utilized at numerous events.

Most community-based EMS are familiar with the Federal Emergency Management Agency's Incident Command System.[13] Elements of this process are often activated to provide support for these events and serve as a real-time drill with direct implications in the event of an emergency situation. Partnerships with these services allow the utilization of their preestablished communication, dispatch, and patient distribution process increasing the efficiency of care.

34.6.2 Medication Plan

The decision to provide medication to competitors must be scrutinized prior to the event and likewise should be published well in advance to address any preconceived expectations of the medical support staff and participants. It is recommended that the choice of medication be kept to a minimum. Many athletes in longer events carry their own medication or have it provided by associates on the course. Without this prior knowledge, overdoses may be inadvertently ingested, leading to untoward events.

Emergency medications, such as aspirin, epinephrine auto-injector, oral glucose, glucagon, inhaled bronchodilators, oxygen, and ACLS medications, should be considered with respect to access through community resources. All medications should be tightly controlled and thoroughly documented when administered.

34.6.3 Laboratory and Intravenous Fluids

Availability of laboratory analysis is often helpful in the appropriate diagnosis and treatment of distressed athletes. Handheld devices, measuring glucose and serum electrolytes, are often utilized to aid in diagnosis and guide treatment.[10] This capability has become the standard in many endurance events and is most helpful in identifying potential life-threatening exercise-associated hyponatremia.

The provision of intravenous fluids (IVs) to competitors should be discussed prior to the event. An IV plan should include indications, fluid composition, site and rate of administration, total volume limits, and follow-up recommendations. Care must be taken to avoid automatic IV administration without an accurate diagnosis because the procedure is not without risks. IV administration with isotonic or hypotonic solution may worsen exercise-associated hyponatremia,[20] and the time taken to prepare and administer an IV may unnecessarily delay the diagnosis of other conditions such as exertional heat stroke or hypothermia.

34.7 STAFFING PLAN

Medical and nonmedical support staffing to match the anticipated requirement is important to ensure optimal medical coverage of the event. Skill sets and numbers of staff will vary depending upon the event and location throughout the course. Previous years' experience and comparison with similar events are the best ways to prepare for staffing number and distribution. A helpful starting point for distance running events has been provided by the American College of Sports Medicine suggesting the following medical personnel per 1000 runners: 1–2 physicians, 4–6 podiatrists, 1–4 emergency medical technicians, 2–4 nurses, 3–6 physical therapists, 3–6 athletic trainers, and 1–3 assistants (see Figure 34.1). Approximately 75% of these medical assets should be staged at the finish area with the others spread throughout the course.[2] Medical staffing makeup should be guided by the event. Orthopedists and emergency medicine physicians and nurses would be a welcome addition to speed and diverse terrain events where head, neck, and limb trauma would be anticipated, while critical care, cardiology, and primary care physicians would be valuable for endurance events. Nonmedical staff is instrumental for their assistance with transporting injured competitors (Figure 34.1), medical care and tracking documentation, crowd control, supply redistribution, and coordination and communication with the event staff. The majority of medical and nonmedical assistants are volunteers although reimbursement for services, travel, and time is occasionally offered. It is recommended to confirm these arrangements and expectations in advance.

Clinical Pearl

Thank medical and staff support personnel for their assistance. Make their experience a positive one and they are more likely to return year after year.

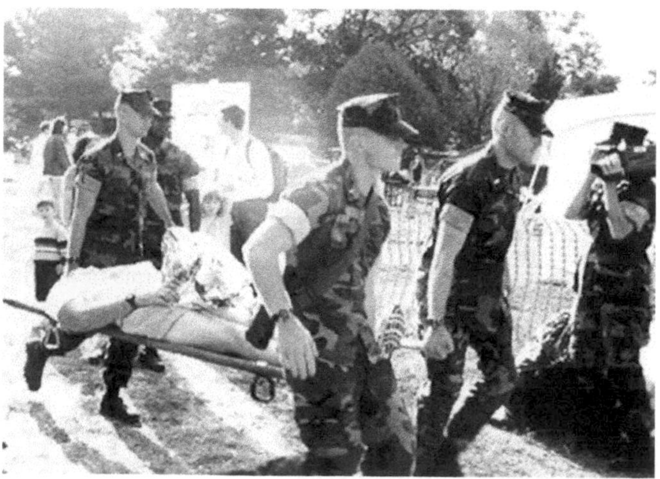

FIGURE 34.1 Nonmedical support staff—U.S. Marine stretcher bearers.

Staff appreciation is important before, during, and after the event. A heartfelt thank you is often more valuable that any T-shirt or memento. Coordinating food and refreshments, securing lavatory facilities, and protecting staff from the elements are positive motivators that will not only enhance the experience but encourage repeat attendance to future events. During and immediately after the event, it is helpful to request feedback from all participants regarding both positive experiences and areas for improvement. The compilation of these data and production of an after-action report is a responsibility of the medical director and should be shared with those who contributed comments, event leadership, and community partners. Colleagues who feel their input is valued are more likely to contribute in the future and encourage others to participate as well.

34.8 EDUCATION

34.8.1 Medical Staff Education

There are several means to educate the medical team regarding the medical philosophy, scope of care, and anticipated requirements based on the particular event. Since the majority of medical care is generally provided in the clinical or hospital setting, it is likely that the medical volunteers will be unfamiliar with the event covered and medical care in the field. Several events offer associated medical conferences with continuing education credits as a means to attract and train interested volunteers. Preevent conferences give the opportunity to educate clinicians on anticipated injuries and illness associated with the event and based upon population-specific information. This provides an opportunity for the medical director to meet many of the volunteers and review the event medical plan in greater detail. If early attendance or conferences are impractical, information can be provided online to include key elements of the plan and medical condition algorithms. On-site orientation and education can also be provided by the medical director and aid station leaders prior to the event. It is best to address questions and concerns in advance, so everyone has a level of understanding of the overall plan prior to a medical emergency.

34.8.2 Competitor Education

Participant education, especially in events with novice competitors, is quite valuable. Scope and availability of care, location of aid stations, medication distribution plan, and common event-associated injuries, illnesses, and warnings can be provided through preevent lectures, question-and-answer sessions, and written or online materials. Preevent provision of medical director contact information is suggested and often helpful for athletes with special needs, physical limitations, or illness. Race-day weather conditions, forecasts, and health warnings have been provided with success at numerous events.[8] Unfortunately, recent events have also necessitated the inclusion of disaster plans and security information.[5]

Public information releases and media interaction are encouraged through collaboration with the event director.

Reassuring the public and participants that their medical needs have been anticipated will add to the community goodwill and generation of mutual support.

34.9 COMMUNICATION PLAN

A critical requirement in the conduct of large athletic events is the ability to communicate with the event director, medical aid stations, competitors, and community resources. Landline telephones, cellular phones, satellite phones, multiple frequency radios, walkie-talkies, short-wave radios, portable advertising signs, bullhorns, messengers, and flags are several means utilized in different situations. Regardless of the primary communication chosen, at least one or more alternate plans should be available. Preevent testing of all plans is important, maintaining awareness that cellular phones and walkie-talkies may be overwhelmed by other users gathered for the event. Amateur ham radio operator clubs are a wonderful resource to provide primary or backup communication.

The communication plan should be coordinated with the event leadership and guidance and prioritization of communication provided to optimize open lines free of clutter. It is helpful to have a separate medical frequency to allow the medical director to communicate with the aid stations individually or as a group. Coordination with community resources must also be established and tested.

Clinical Pearl

Advanced discussions with local community partners, especially medical care assets, enhances mutual understanding of capabilities and limitations and ultimately lays the ground work for improved patient care.

While event and community service leaders often communicate in the coordination of events, communication between the medical director and medical facilities should not be overlooked. The benefit of peer-to-peer medical director discussions with treatment facility clinicians has proven invaluable. Sharing of algorithms, reviewing time-sensitive diagnoses, treatment plans, and field medical capabilities prior to the event will increase the efficiency of treatment provided during and after transport. Direct communication lines for physician-to-physician turnover of patients should be included in the overall plan.

34.10 FINANCES AND LOGISTICS

Mass participation events require sound financial management to successfully meet the intent of the participants, competitors, and support staff. Many events raise a great deal of money for both event organizers and charity organizations. The potential to generate money and corporate marketing should not compromise the safe conduct of the event, and the medical director's attention to this is important throughout the planning process. Many events secure corporate sponsorship from hospitals and health-care systems, which in turn assist with providing medical supplies and often staffing. Care must be taken to ensure that insufficient finances do not result in insufficient medical care. Supply and purchase lists should be prepared very early in planning with the identification of responsible funding entities. Procurement agents should be secured and a plan for supply verification and delivery agreed upon in advance of the event. All contracted services or staff should have signed agreements.

An event or course map should be widely available and distributed. It should clearly identify fluid/food stations, lavatory facilities, medical aid stations, and prominent landmarks. Topographic maps are helpful for adventure and ultradistance events. Maps should be available at the start, throughout the course, and at the medical aid stations. Protected EMS access routes to and from the medical aid stations should be identified. Individuals or entities requiring familiarity with the course or event footprint should perform familiarization prior to the event.

Spacing and location of medical aid stations are determined by many factors. They should be placed in easily visualized and accessible sites off the course or field of play. They should be easily identifiable with signs, placards, or the common Red Cross on a white background. Medical personnel should be easily distinguished from other support staff, commonly using a distinct uniform, shirt, hat, armband, or event credentials. The aid station should not interfere with competitors not requiring aid and should be safe from vehicular traffic and geographic obstacles. Ideally, a separate entrance and exit route would be available for the transportation of those requiring a higher level of care. Often team sport tournaments can be appropriately served through one main medical aid station with roving assets for sideline evaluations, while endurance events may require multiple sites. Out and back courses can utilize similar sites for different directions and some longer and multiday events may have medical assets leapfrog the competitors after they pass to establish a new site further along the course (see Figure 34.2).

The transportation of supplies and personnel before, during, and after the event can be performed by medical or event

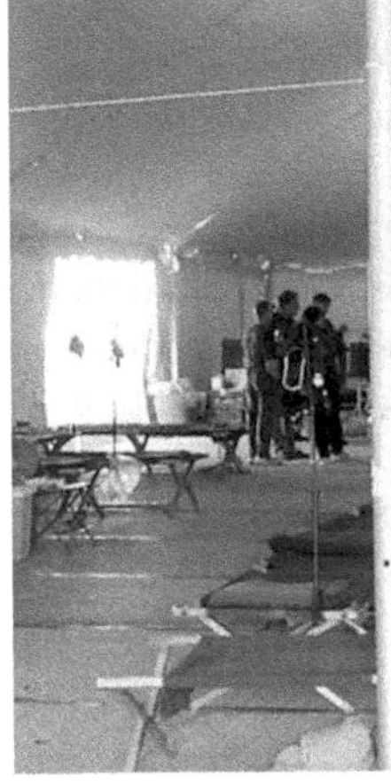
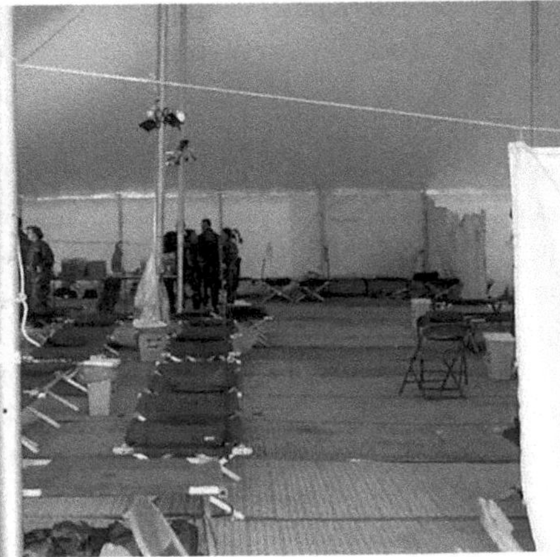 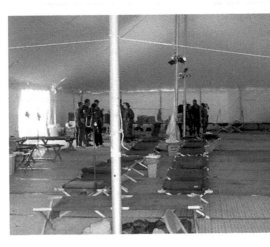

FIGURE 34.2 Finish line medical tent prepared to take casualties.

management. Meeting this requirement must be discussed, agreed upon, and communicated during the planning phase for the event. Assurance that medical supplies, personnel, chairs, cots, tents, and temporary facilities are delivered to the correct place at the correct time is often more daunting that would be initially anticipated. Assigning responsible medical personnel to accompany transportation entities provides greater assurance of the intended delivery. The capability to resupply aid stations during the event must be reviewed. It is often preferable to oversupply rather than face the challenges of movement during the event.

Medical aid stations are important partners with other support entities. They should ensure the security of their surroundings, for example, adequacy of fluids available on the course, and be observant to unexpected injury patterns and communicate any concerns with the event coordinators for assistance and resolution.

34.11 TRANSPORTATION PLAN

The ability to move people, supplies, equipment, and injured competitors requires a great deal of coordination and pre-event planning. Support staff must be promptly transported to their sites in time to set up and be prepared to provide services to competitors. Medical evacuation routes must be secured and protected to ensure efficient and timely transport when required without competing with the event in progress or spectators. Ambulance access to the medical aid station should be clearly identified and the surface sufficient to permit easy entrance and departure. Ground guides to accompany vehicles are strongly advised to prevent accidental injury or damage. Landing zones for helicopter or airplane evacuation should be identified in advance, and local community medical assets will likely be able to assist.

Clinical Pearl

Use the "No one left behind" principle. It is the medical director's responsibility to ensure that all support staff and competitors are returned to their intended destination.

Medical support staff should arrive in enough time to adequately set up and arrange their medical aid station, familiarize themselves with their equipment, and discuss roles and responsibilities. The overall plan should also address how the medical staff departs at the end of the event and accounts for the remaining equipment and unutilized supplies. Depending on the location personal vehicles, public transportation or specified event vehicles can be utilized.

Event competitors who are unable or unwilling to continue often end up at medical aid stations. While they do not require active medical care or transport, they must be provided with a means to return to their vehicle, home, friends, or family. This population is frequently not considered in the transportation plan. Many distance events have a *sweeper* vehicle that follows the last competitor and drives those who abandon the race back to the finish line. Others use public transportation or eventually decide to continue. It is important that the medical aid station not be vacated until all competitors have departed.

34.12 TRIAGE AND TREATMENT GUIDELINES

34.12.1 Treatment Guidelines

Many well-written event-specific guidelines have been published discussing the evaluation and treatment of event-specific diagnoses.[34] The majority of these conditions can be anticipated based on the demands of the event and previous experiences. This preparation is a key element in the planning and education stages of event medical coverage. A common theme regardless of the event is a mechanism to efficiently discern between serious and nonserious casualties. Fortunately, the majority of medical contacts are for nonserious conditions such as sprains, strains, abrasions, and generalized discomfort that can be quickly treated and released.

Severe medical conditions such as cardiac and respiratory arrest, body temperature abnormalities, electrolyte imbalances, near drowning, and head and neck trauma should be quickly separated from nonserious medical conditions. Mental status, accurate body temperature,[39] pulse, respirations, blood pressure, and a rapid neurologic exam are critical in guiding a treatment plan. Serum glucose and sodium levels when available provide additional information. Depending upon the medical scope of care for the event, many severe conditions may be treated in the medical aid station or must be transferred to community medical services. The utilization of treatment algorithms has proven an excellent way to standardize evaluation and care as well as provide education to clinicians who may not be as comfortable with out-of-hospital assessments and treatment.[34] The scope of care for many events includes initial and often definitive treatment for conditions such as heat stroke, heat exhaustion, hypothermia, exercise-associated hyponatremia, and dehydration. The medical director and aid station medical leaders must remain attentive to avoid delays in diagnosing severe medical conditions and transportation to definitive treatment facilities.

The physical layout of the medical aid station to separate severe from nonsevere injuries is a helpful way to organize medical care. Utilizing a common check-in area allows for contact documentation and efficient triage to specific locations of care within the aid station. These areas of care are staffed with clinicians and support staff best suited to address each individual need. Supplies, testing, and treatment areas can also be more readily coordinated and monitored.

Medical holding areas should be considered for competitors who do not require additional treatment but are waiting for transportation and are not quite ready to leave.[34] This allows the injured to gradually acclimatize and recover in a relatively comfortable and safe location. They should be constantly observed for any worsening of their condition and encouraged to make their way back to the postevent areas as soon as possible. Making this area too comfortable may result in overcrowding and common sense principles should be observed.

34.12.2 Exercise-Associated Collapse

Perhaps the most anxiety-provoking condition commonly seen in mass participation events is the collapsed athlete. Fortunately, the majority of cases are the result of predictable physiological events associated with exertion and respond rapidly to positioning with the head down and legs and pelvis elevated position.[18] These athletes generally have normal mental status and suffer more from embarrassment than a lasting medical condition.

Those with altered mental status after positioning should be rapidly evaluated with vital signs to include a rectal temperature for evidence of hyperthermia or hypothermia. A patient with persistent altered mental status and a relatively normal rectal temperature should be treated for exercise-associated hyponatremia until proven otherwise.[18] Access to rapid serum sodium assessment capability can often guide treatment promptly with hypertonic saline.[21,43] Hyperthermic individuals should be cooled as quickly as possible with ice water immersion, and those with hypothermia should be warmed.

34.13 MEDICOLEGAL

Mass participation events hold an ethical responsibility to the competitors and the communities that sponsor them. Event-specific challenges, risks, and goals in addition to support expectations should be clearly communicated before participation. The ability of the competitors and community interest groups to question, seek clarification, and address concerns should be provided. Care must be taken to understand community capabilities and limitations and not inadvertently overload the assets available and reasonably expected. Concerns of increased vehicular traffic, parking, lodging, access to water and food, lavatory facilities, and medical care capabilities with alternate plans must be addressed. Care must be taken that the event does not create a mass casualty situation for the community exceeding their capability and decreasing services to the general population.

The medical director must specifically address medical liability for themselves and event medical personnel. Physicians commonly make four common assumptions when volunteering for sporting or community events: event liability coverage, Good Samaritan legislation, personal medical liability coverage, and prevent injury waivers.[44] General event insurance packages often do not include medical services. Good Samaritan legislation varies from state to state and is designed to protect anyone who renders emergency care without compensation or expectation of compensation. Gross acts of negligence and willful and wanton misconduct and care other than emergent would not be covered by this legislation.[31,44,46] Personal liability policies should be reviewed for inclusion of event coverage. Preevent waivers may not be as protective as physicians would hope as courts generally will not validate a contract that releases a physician from liability in the care on one's patients. A waiver is not a bar against litigation but may be a bar to a successful suit.[43]

The practice of medicine outside the state of licensure requires additional consideration as all states have differing legal licensing provisions applicable when practicing out of state.[44] Laws and regulations governing the EMS systems also differ between states and should be reviewed discussing capabilities and limitations prior to the event.

TABLE 34.2
SORT: Key Recommendations for Practice

Clinical Recommendation	Evidence Rating	References
It is essential to develop an agreement concerning medical care and administrative responsibilities between the medical team and the organizing body.	C	[16]
It is essential to assess potential environmental conditions and site- and event-risk factors.	C	[16]
It is essential to organize the medical team before the event.	C	[16]

34.14 CONCLUSION

Medical care provided for mass participation events can provide a great deal of personal satisfaction utilizing medical training to support athletes, colleagues, and the community. Advanced diligent planning is the core requirement for success. Frequent and effective communication with all parties before, during, and after is critical. Education programs and treatment algorithms are highly recommended to increase medical aid station efficiency and quality of care (Table 34.2).

REFERENCES

1. Anderson JC, Courson RW, Kleiner DM et al. National Athletic Trainer's Association position statement: Emergency planning in athletics. *Journal of Athletic Training*. 2002;37(1):99–104.
2. Armstrong L, Dasa DJ, Millard-Stafford M et al. Exertional heat illness during training and competition. *Medicine & Science in Sports & Exercise*. 2007;39(3):556–572.
3. Baker WM, Simone BM, Niemann JT, Daly A. Special event medical care: The 1984 Los Angeles Summer Olympic experience. *Annals of Emergency Medicine*. 1986;15(2):185–190.
4. Bathgate A, Best J, Craig G et al. A prospective study of injuries to elite Australian rugby union players. *British Journal of Sports Medicine*. 2002;36: 265–269.
5. Biddinger PD, Baggish A, Harrington L et al. Be prepared—The Boston marathon and mass casualty events. *The New England Journal of Medicine*. 2013;368(21):1958–1960.
6. Borland ML, Rogers IR. Injury and illness in a wilderness multisport endurance event. *Wilderness & Environmental Medicine*. 1997;8(2):82–88.
7. Chiampas G, Jaworski CA. Preparing for the surge: Perspectives on marathon medical preparedness. *Current Sports Medicine Reports*. 2009;8(3):131–135.

8. Cianca JC, Roberts WO, Horn D. Distance running: Organization of the medical team. In *Textbook of Running Medicine*. New York: McGraw-Hill; 2001, pp. 489–503.
9. Crouse B, Beattie K. Marathon medical services: Strategies to reduce runner morbidity. *Medicine & Science in Sports & Exercise*. 1995;28(9):1093–1096.
10. Davis DP, Videen JS, Marino A et al. Exercise associated hyponatremia in marathon runners: A two-year experience. *The Journal of Emergency Medicine*. 2001;21(1):47–57.
11. Delaney JS, Drummond R. Mass casualties and triage at a sporting event. *British Journal of Sports Medicine*. 2002; 36:85–88.
12. Elias SR. 10-year trend in USA Cup soccer injuries: 1988–1997. *Medicine & Science in Sports & Exercise*. 2001;33(3):359–367.
13. FEMA Web site. Incident command resources. www.fema.gov/incident-command-system-resources. Accessed July 13, 2015.
14. Grange JT, Bodnar JA, Corbett SW. Motocross medicine. *Current Sports Medicine Reports*. 2009;8(3):125–130.
15. Greenland K. Medical support for adventure racing. *Emergency Medicine Australasia*. 2004;16(5–6):465–468.
16. Hecht SS, Burton MS. Medical coverage of gymnastics competitions. *Current Sports Medicine Reports*. 2009;8(3):113–118.
17. Herring SA, Bergfeld JA, Boyajian-O'Neill LA et al. Mass participation event management for the team physician: A consensus statement. *Medicine & Science in Sports & Exercise*. 2004;36(11):2004–2008.
18. Holtzhausen LM, Noakes TD. Collapsed ultraendurance athlete: Proposed mechanisms and an approach to management. *Clinical Journal of Sport Medicine*. 1997;7(4):292–301.
19. Holtzhausen LM, Noakes TD. The prevalence and significance of post exercise (postural) hypotension in ultramarathon runners. *Medicine & Science in Sports & Exercise*. 1995;27(12):1595–1601.
20. Hiller WD, O'Toole ML, Fortess EE et al. Medical and physiological considerations in triathlons. *The American Journal of Sports Medicine*. 1987;15(2):164–168.
21. Hsieh M. Recommendations for treatment of hyponatremia at endurance events. *Sports Medicine*. 2004;34(4):231–238.
22. Jaworski CA. Medical concerns of marathons. *Current Sports Medicine Reports*. 2005;4(3):137–143.
23. Jones BH, Roberts WO. Medical management of endurance events: Incidence, prevention and care of casualties. In *ACSM's Guidelines for the Team Physician*. Philadelphia, PA: Lea & Febiger; 1991, pp. 225–286.
24. Kim JH, Malhotra R, Chiampas G et al. Cardiac arrest during long-distance running races. *New England Journal of Medicine*. 2012;366:130–140.
25. Kleiner DM, Glickman SE. Considerations for the athletic trainer in planning medical coverage for short distance road races. *Journal of Athletic Training*. 1994;29:145–147.
26. Lorish TR, Rizzo TD Jr, Ilstrup DM, Scott SG. Injuries in adolescent and preadolescent boys at two large wrestling tournaments. *The American Journal of Sports Medicine*. 1992;20(2):199–202.
27. Ma OJ, Millward L, Schwab RA. EMS medical coverage at PGA tour events. *Prehospital Emergency Care*. 2002;6(1): 11–14.
28. Maron BJ, Poliac LC, Roberts WO. Risk for sudden cardiac death associated with marathon running. *Journal of the American College of Cardiology*. 1996;28:428–431.
29. Maron BJ. Sudden death in young athletes. *The New England Journal of Medicine*. 2003;349(11):1064–1075.
30. Martinez JM. Medical coverage of cycling events. *Current Sports Medicine Reports*. 2006;5(3):125–130.
31. Morris E. Liability Under Good Samaritan Laws. American Academy of Orthopaedic Surgeons. http://www.aaos.org/news/aaosnow/jan14/managing3.asp. Accessed May 5, 2014.
32. Nichol G, Stiell IG, Laupacis A et al. A cumulative meta-analysis of the effectiveness of defibrillator-capable emergency medical services for victims of out-of-hospital cardiac arrest. *Annals of Emergency Medicine*. 1999;34(4):517–525.
33. NOAA Lightning Safety website: www.lightningsafety.noaa.gov/sports.htm. Accessed May 5, 2014.
34. O'Connor FG, Pyne SW, Brennan FH. Exercise-associated collapse: An algorithmic approach to race day management part I of II. *The American Journal of Sports Medicine*. 2003;5:221–217, 229.
35. Parrillo SJ. Medical care at mass gatherings: Considerations for physician involvement. *Prehospital and Disaster Medicine*. 1995;10(4):273–275.
36. Pendergraph B, Ko B, Zamora J et al. Medical coverage for track and field events. *Current Sports Medicine Reports*. 2005;4(3):150–153.
37. Perron AD, Brady WJ, Custalow CB et al. Association of heat index and patient volume at a mass gathering event. *Prehospital Emergency Care*. 2005;9(1):49–52.
38. Roberts WO. A 12-yr profile of medical injury and illness for the Twin Cities Marathon. *Medicine & Science in Sports & Exercise*. 2000;32(9):1549–1555.
39. Roberts WO. Assessing core temperature in collapsed athletes: What's the best method? *Physician and Sportsmedicine*. 2000;28(9):71–76.
40. Roberts WO. Determining a "do not start" temperature for a marathon on the basis of adverse outcomes. *Medicine & Science in Sports & Exercise*. 2010;42(2):226–232.
41. Roberts WO. Exercise-associated collapse in endurance events. A classification system. *Physician and Sportsmedicine*. 1989;17:49–57.
42. Ronneberg KR, Roberts WO. Strategies to prevent sudden death in mass participation events. In *Preventing Sudden Death in Sport and Physical Activity*. Burlington, MA: Jones & Barlett; 2011, pp. 253–267.
42. Rosen MH, Kirven J. Exercise associated hyponatremia. *Clinical Journal of the American Society of Nephrology*. 2007;2:151–161.
44. Ross DS, Ferguson A, Herbert DL. Action in the event tent! Medical-legal issues facing the volunteer event physician. *Sports Health*. 2003;5(4):340–345.
45. Schwabe K, Schwellnus M, Derman W et al. Medical complications and deaths in 21 and 56 km road race runners: A 4-year prospective study in 65 865 runners—SAFER study I. *British Journal of Sports Medicine*. 2014;48:912–918.
46. Stewart PH, Agin WS, Douglas SP. What does the law say to good Samaritans? A review of good Samaritan statues in 50 States and on US airlines. *Chest*. 2013;143(6):1774–1783.
47. Tang N, Kraus CK, Brill JD et al. Hospital-based event medical support for the Baltimore marathon, 2002–2005. *Prehospital Emergency Care*. 2008;12(3):320–356.
48. Zijlstra JA. Medical consequences of the 15th eleven-cities skating marathon. *Nederlands Tijdschrift voor Geneeskunde*. 1998;142(7):331–335.

35 On-Field Emergencies

Meghan F. Raleigh

CONTENTS

TABLE 35.1
Key Clinical Considerations

1. Preparation for on-field emergencies includes establishing and rehearsing an emergency response plan, having proper equipment and supplies, and being familiar with the nature of potential emergencies
2. On-field assessment begins with a rapid trauma assessment using ATLS management. The athlete should remain in the position in which he or she is found on the field unless prone or has loss of consciousness (LOC), in which case he or she should be presumed to have a c-spine injury and should be logrolled to a supine position
3. Rarely, traumatic head injury results in epidural hematomas, scull fracture, or intracerebral bleeding. Any head injury warrants immediate evaluation and frequent reassessment. Athletes with LOC, focal neurologic deficits, GCS <15, or clinical deterioration should be immediately transported to a higher level of care for further evaluation
4. The leading cause of death in athletes on the field is SCA and is most commonly from congenital cardiovascular disease. The cornerstone of treatment for SCA is immediate recognition, CPR, and early defibrillation
5. Risk factors for EHI include dehydration, recent illness, poor fitness, and sleep deprivation. Signs and symptoms are nonspecific, and high index of suspicion must be had. The treatment used is active and passive cooling, while EMS for suspected heat exhaustion or heat stroke

35.1 INTRODUCTION

Though the majority of sports-related injuries are musculoskeletal, catastrophic injuries and death, while rare, do occur. The National Center for Catastrophic Sport Injury Research (NCCSIR) reports that in the 30 years from 1982 to 2012, there were 2061 such catastrophic sports-related injuries, the majority (81%) of which were at the high school level and were directly related to the activities of the sport (67%).[17] Of these 2061 recorded events, 41% were fatal, and of the nonfatal 1204 events, 47% resulted in permanent severe dysfunctional disability, while 53% had full recovery (Table 35.1).[17]

Noncatastrophic emergencies such as allergic reactions, asthma exacerbations, and severe musculoskeletal injuries occur more frequently and should be recognized and treated immediately. Prompt recognition of medical emergencies and coordination of the field-side physician (FSP) with athletic trainers and emergency response technicians in conjunction with a well-rehearsed emergency response plan are crucial to minimizing catastrophic outcomes.

35.2 PRE-EVENT PLANNING

The most important step of planning sideline medical coverage is pre-event planning; this includes having an emergency response plan. Responsibilities of the FSP include being aware of or developing the emergency response plan as well as coordinating its rehearsal.[7] Knowing available resources including staff, emergency equipment, means of transportation, hospital services, and phone access is paramount. On-site responders should understand how to communicate with local EMS, and ideally, there should be practice of the response plan before athletic events. All potential responders should be trained in CPR/AED use. The response team should know where to access essential medical equipment such as an AED for early defibrillation, spine board, cervical collar, medications, and telephone.[6]

35.3 MEDICAL BAG

The American College of Sports Medicine recommends that the FSP should have a standardized medical bag with, at a minimum, the following items (see Table 35.2),[6] which may be assembled by the FSP or as a commercially available field-side medical bag (for example, the FIFA Medical Emergency Bag that is required on the sidelines of all FIFA World Cup games).[4] The contents should reflect necessary tools and medication for the FSP to treat anticipated medical emergencies, to include pediatric sizes of equipment and doses of medication if covering this demographic. Essential supplies, medications, and equipments include items that provide life-saving care (anaphylaxis, sudden cardiac arrest [SCA], spinal cord injury, and heat injury).[6] In addition, it is desirable to have supplies to provide sideline care for nonemergent injuries as well (lacerations, dislocations, eye and dental injuries).[6] The contents of the medical bag should be reviewed on a regular basis, expired medications replaced, and emergency supplies should be easily identified and accessible. The contents of the medical bag need to contain sport-specific equipment (i.e., helmet removal tools for football coverage) and should be adjusted accordingly.

TABLE 35.2
Medical Bag

Paperwork
- Medial bag inventory and supply location
- Copy of emergency response plan and relevant phone numbers
- Sideline concussion assessment
- Prescription pad and pen

Personal protective equipment
- Gloves
- Protective goggles
- Pocket mask
- Earplugs

General
- Oral fluid replacement
- Normal saline

CV
- AED (in bag or separate)
- Disposable razor
- Bag-valve mask
- LMA
- BP cuff

Epinephrine 1:1000 in prefilled autoinjector

Head, neck, and neurological
- Cervical collar and spine board
- Protective goggles
- Contact solution
- Dental kit
- Eye kit
- Face mask removal tool
- Penlight
- Nasal packing

Metabolic
- Blood glucose kit and test strips
- Glucose

Extremities
- Tourniquet
- Sterile gauze
- Splints
- Tape
- Elastic bandages
- Bandage scissors

Skin
- Steri-Strips
- Sutures/laceration kit
- Staple kit/removal

Sources: Dvorak, J. et al., *Br. J. Sports Med.*, 47, 1199, 2013; Herring, S.A. et al., *Med. Sci. Sports Exerc.*, 44, 2442, 2012.

35.4 ON-FIELD ASSESSMENT

The FSP should observe practice and games from an appropriate location in order to manage game-day injuries and medical problems. The provider should also be aware of environmental and playing conditions that could affect the athletes.[6] Any on-field assessment of an injured athlete should be rapid and focused and follow the basics of ATLS management.[14] Minor injuries requiring evaluation may be attended to by the athletic trainer who should call the FSP onto the field if needed. The athletic trainer and the FSP should discuss scenarios for which the trainer feels comfortable evaluating solo, with the caveat that the FSP would enter the field for any emergent or serious injury.

If the athlete has loss of consciousness or is prone, the athlete should be presumed to have a cervical spine injury and should be logrolled to a supine position while maintaining cervical spine stabilization (see Section 35.6). Otherwise, the athlete should be left as he or she is found for further assessment.[14]

Once the athlete has had a focused exam, a more thorough secondary survey should take place, either on the field, sideline, or the training room, depending on the injury and the environmental conditions. After assessment and management of injuries or medical problems have taken place, the FSP should determine the athlete's same-game return to play and notify the appropriate parties about the condition.[13]

35.5 RESPIRATORY COMPROMISE

35.5.1 Asthma

As the prevalence of asthma in athletes increases, so do the odds of having a severe asthma exacerbation. Triggers include environmental exposures, exercise, and allergens, though sometimes a specific trigger cannot be identified. Symptoms include cough, wheezing, shortness of breath, chest tightness, and increased work of breathing. The first-line treatment for an acute asthma exacerbation on the sideline is giving two puffs of a short-acting beta-2 agonist (albuterol) using a spacer. If symptoms do not improve or begin to worsen, epinephrine 0.3 mg for adults or 0.15 mg for pediatric patients (defined as weight <25 kg) should be administered intramuscularly or subcutaneously. Autoinjector pens are commercially available in both adult and pediatric doses. Any athlete who is not responding to albuterol should have EMS evaluation.

35.5.2 Pneumothorax

Tension pneumothorax is a true emergency requiring immediate treatment. It occurs when air enters the pleural space but is unable to escape and is usually the result of trauma. Suspicion of tension pneumothorax requires immediate needle decompression in the second intercostal space, midclavicular line, or anterior axillary line, without waiting for radiographic confirmation.

35.5.3 Laryngeal Fracture

Laryngeal fracture is a rare complication of direct trauma to the anterior neck. Signs are nonspecific and include soft tissue swelling, stridor, crepitus, hoarseness, or palpable fracture. Establishing and maintaining an airway with early intubation is critical as soft tissue swelling may cause airway obstruction.

35.6 HEAD INJURY

Head injuries in sports competition are common, and the grand majority of them are concussions. According to the NCCSIR database, there have been fewer than 10 deaths from head and neck injuries per year over the past 25 years.[17] Initial evaluation of a head injury involves eliminating cervical spine injury, serious traumatic brain injury, and removing the athlete from play.[19]

Though rare, skull fracture or intracerebral bleeding may result from direct or indirect head injury. The athlete should be evaluated for skull depression, focal neurologic deficits, pupillary asymmetry, ecchymosis in the periorbital area (raccoon eyes), ecchymosis behind the ear (Battle's sign), CSF rhinorrhea, and hemotympanum. If any of these are present or the athlete has a Glasgow Coma Scale (GCS) <15, they should immediately be transported to a higher level of care.

Epidural hematoma makes up 1%–2% of head trauma cases in the United States and occurs most commonly after a direct blow to the skull. It results from a tear of the middle meningeal artery. Most people with epidural hematoma experience a loss of consciousness. Those who maintain consciousness often complain of severe headache and vomiting and may go on to have seizures. Treatment is emergent surgical decompression, as deterioration often occurs very quickly following the inciting head injury.

Concussion is a disturbance in brain function caused by direct or indirect force to the head that may or may not include loss of consciousness.[19] Clinical symptoms of concussion are nonspecific and may include headache, nausea, dizziness, photophobia, fatigue, balance disturbances, and disorientation (see Chapter 40). Loss of consciousness occurs in less than 10% of athletes.[15] While symptoms generally are present immediately following injury, there may be a several-hour delay, making reassessment of an athlete with any head injury paramount.

The initial evaluation for any head injury is a rapid assessment at the point of injury beginning with compressions, airway, breathing (CABs) and a cervical spine injury assessment. Once any serious cervical spine injury is ruled out, the athlete should be evaluated for mental status changes or balance deficits by doing an initial neurologic examination. A sideline or training room assessment of cognitive function and memory testing in addition to a more thorough physical exam should be performed. Several sideline tools are available for concussion assessment, the most common being the SAC and the Sport Concussion Assessment Tool 3 (SCAT3).

Once a concussion is diagnosed, the athlete should be removed from play and should not return to play on the same day.[16] Though in rare circumstances some professional athletes may be allowed same day return to play, it is not recommended to do so.[16] If there is any doubt as to a diagnosis of concussion, it is best to err on the side of keeping the athlete from playing. Any athlete with concussion should be reevaluated frequently and monitored for new symptoms or deterioration. Additional evaluation in the emergency department with neuroimaging should be done for any athlete with a focal neurologic deficit or if their condition worsens.

A rare but serious complication of a first concussion is a second head injury before the first one is resolved, known as second impact syndrome. This is thought to occur from a catecholamine surge from a second impact to the head causing cerebral edema, increased intracranial pressure, and ultimately coma or death.[19] Treatment of suspected second impact syndrome requires immediate intubation, hyperventilation, administration of an osmotic diuretic such as mannitol, and transport to a higher level of care.[14]

35.7 SPINAL INJURY MANAGEMENT

Spinal cord injury is potentially catastrophic and life changing for the injured athlete. Any athlete with an altered level of consciousness, concerning mechanism of injury, neck pain, boney tenderness on examination, or neck/upper back trauma, should be presumed to have a cervical spine injury.[15]

The focus for managing head and neck injuries on the field is to prevent further injuries.[15] After rapid assessment of CAB, the athlete must be immobilized to accomplish this. If prone or unconscious, the athlete should be logrolled by a four- or five-person team with one person at the athlete's head and the other members at the torso, hips, and legs. The person at the head maintains in-line stabilization of the cervical spine while the spine board is moved into position and directs the rest of the team. If the athlete is wearing a helmet, it should be carefully removed to allow complete assessment. This may require tools depending on the helmet. If the helmet is removed, shoulder pads should be removed as well to avoid any unnecessary extension of the neck. After cervical immobilization, further assessment and transport to a higher level of care for possible imaging as indicated should take place.

Evaluation for cervical spine injury can be ruled out and the patient may be moved if peripheral strength and sensation are normal, there is absence of asymmetric spasm or spinal tenderness, there is normal isometric neck strength and active range of motion of the neck, and the Spurling test is normal.[19] This evaluation should be performed without moving the head or neck. If there are any distracting injuries, concern for intoxication, altered level of consciousness, focal neurologic deficits, or midline tenderness, cervical spine injury cannot be ruled out. The athlete should be secured with a cervical collar and backboard and transported to a higher level of care with neuroimaging capabilities.[19]

35.8 SUDDEN CARDIAC ARREST

SCA is the leading cause of death in athletes during exercise[3] and is estimated to occur in approximately 1.2 in 100,000 college student athletes.[13] The prevalence of SCA is five times more common in African-American athletes than whites (3.8 vs. 0.7 in 100,000 athletes, $p < 0.01$)[13] though the risk remains low and is on par with deaths from suicide and drug abuse. The most common cause of SCA is congenital cardiovascular disease, specifically hypertrophic cardiomyopathy (HCM) or congenital coronary artery anomalies. The preparticipation exam is critical for identifying athletes who may be at risk for HCM or coronary artery anomalies by recognizing a family history of early sudden cardiac death and doing a thorough dynamic cardiac exam.

The cornerstone of SCA management is systematic ACLS treatment that requires immediate recognition, CPR, and early defibrillation. Delays in defibrillation decrease survival of cardiac resuscitation, with survival decreasing 10% per minute that defibrillation is delayed in the absence of CPR but 3%–4% with CPR.[11] The FSP should be alerted to any athlete with symptoms that could be indicative of cardiovascular disease (i.e., presyncope, exertional chest pain, dyspnea, or unusual fatigue).[14] Kramer and colleagues recommend that any football player who collapses without contact from another player should be treated as though he or she has SCA until proven otherwise to prevent delays in care.[8]

SCA resulting from a blunt blow to the chest wall is known as commotio cordis. It is seen most commonly in baseball, lacrosse, hockey, and softball due to a direct blow to the chest from the involved ball or puck, though it may occur in other sports.[10] Though the actual incidence is unknown. there are approximately 10–20 cases of commotio cordis reported annually, with almost all of them affecting adolescents.[10] Sudden death is instantaneous and athletes are most often found in ventricular fibrillation (VF), though the impact is usually not of sufficient force to cause structural injury to the heart.[12] Survival is most likely to occur with prompt recognition, initiation of CPR within 3 minutes of inciting event, and treatment of VF with early defibrillation with an AED.[12]

Athletes with a history of sudden cardiac death who survive are not absolutely excluded from future athletic participation. A stepwise approach has been suggested by Piantanida et al. taking into account the athlete's desire for return to play and the risks of repeat cardiac events, focusing on the athlete's ultimate well-being.[18]

35.9 EXERTIONAL HEAT ILLNESS

Exertional heat illness (EHI) is a spectrum of diseases that include exercise-associated muscle cramping, heat exhaustion, and heat stroke. It is the third most common cause of death in athletes.[2] Risk factors for EHI include dehydration, recent illness not being acclimatized to hot or humid climates, poor fitness, certain medications, obesity, and sleep deprivation,[1] though EHI can affect healthy individuals as well. The signs and symptoms are nonspecific and may include nausea, muscle cramping, headache, confusion, chills, or collapse. The FSP must maintain a high index of suspicion for EHI and obtain a core temperature for any athlete suspected of having heat injury. The gold standard for core temperature measurement for suspected EHI is obtaining a rectal temperature.

Heat stroke presents with nonspecific symptoms but differs from less-severe heat injury in that there is thermoregulatory failure and, however, there is thermoregulatory failure and CNS dysfunction. Core temperature is greater than 104°F, which may be the only notable difference between heat exhaustion and heat stroke on the sideline evaluation. Life-threatening sequelae including brain injury, DIC, rhabdomyolysis, renal failure, and liver failure may result if not treated immediately.[2] EMS should be contacted immediately for suspected heat stroke.

Treatment of heat stroke includes both active and passive cooling by any means possible. This includes removing the athlete from the heat; removing uniform and clothing, utilizing ice packs around the neck, groin, and axilla; and using cool water sprays and fans.[2] Oral hydration with electrolyte-containing sports drinks is preferred over that with water.[2] Intravenous fluids may be necessary if hypovolemia is a concern; however, caution should be used to avoid overhydration.[14] Rapid cooling using cold water immersion may be considered for athletes with core temperatures greater than 104°F.[2]

35.10 ANAPHYLAXIS

Anaphylactic reactions are rapid onset systemic hypersensitivity reactions that can be life threatening if not recognized and treated promptly. Causes of anaphylaxis include exercise, certain foods, insect venom, and idiopathic anaphylaxis. Symptoms can target any organ system but typically include urticaria or angioedema, dyspnea, flushing, headache, nausea, palpitations, hypotension, and syncope.[9] Severe anaphylaxis can lead to pulmonary edema and cardiovascular collapse.

Treatment begins with securing the airway, removing any suspected trigger, and continuing with CABs. EMS should be notified. Oxygen, if available, should be administered, followed by epinephrine 0.3 mg subcutaneously or intramuscularly for adults or 0.01 mg/kg in children (not to exceed 0.3 mg). If bronchospasm is present, B2-agonists should be administered, preferably by nebulizer. Antihistamines and glucocorticoids may also be given while awaiting transport to definitive care.[14]

35.11 MUSCULOSKELETAL INJURY

The majority of sports-related injuries are musculoskeletal injuries and for the most part do not require emergent medical attention. The athletic trainer can attend to minor musculoskeletal injuries on the field and should call the FSP out if additional evaluation is needed.

Injuries requiring immediate FSP evaluation include fractures and dislocations. Simple dislocations (i.e., shoulder, elbow, digits) may be reduced on the sideline if the FSP is confident of the diagnosis, feels comfortable with the reduction, and is able to provide postreduction management. The affected joint should be immobilized and the athlete should not return to play the same day. If unable to reduce the joint, the athlete should be referred for further care.

Fractures can be categorized as open or closed. Open fractures consist of a soft tissue break with communication between the broken bone and the skin, predisposing to infection. Any suspicion of an open fracture should prompt covering the overlying soft tissue with a moist dressing, splinting the affected site, and transport to the nearest emergency department for orthopedic evaluation as they often require washout in the operating room.[14] Closed fractures should be splinted in the position in which they are found. All fractures should prompt a detailed neurovascular assessment. If there is distal vascular compromise, gentle reduction on the field may be attempted to restore perfusion while awaiting transport to definitive care.

Two serious but rare dislocations that require immediate specialty evaluation are knee and hip dislocations. Knee dislocations occur by high-energy mechanism of injury and often reduce by themselves. The concern is that there can often be neurovascular injury to the popliteal artery and the peroneal nerve. Examination is often nonspecific, with immediate swelling and instability.[20] High clinical suspicion must be had to diagnose a knee dislocation and referral for orthopedic and vascular surgery is warranted immediately. Hip dislocations also tend to be caused by high-energy mechanisms of injury as well. If not reduced promptly, there is risk for subsequent avascular necrosis of the femoral head, so again recognition and treatment are key.[20]

35.12 LIGHTNING

Lightning is a hazard during outdoor sporting events especially during summer months. Though the majority of lightning injuries are nonfatal, there is a broad spectrum of injury depending on how lightning strikes the body. When it is fatal, the cause of death is usually cardiac arrest.

Lightning injury by direct strike causes the most injury due to the amount of energy passing through the body, though injuries may also be due to side splash, contact injury, ground current, or blunt trauma from being thrown. Injuries are electrical in nature[13] but may vary greatly depending on the mechanism.[5]

The evaluation of athlete with lightning injury should begin with an assessment of safety of the rescue team. Athletes should be removed to a safe place and quickly be evaluated for apnea, asystole, shock, fractures, and burns. Victims who are pulseless and are apneic should receive attention first; the so-called reverse triage as CPR may restore circulation if performed early.[21]

TABLE 35.3
SORT: Key Recommendations for Practice

Clinical Recommendation	Evidence Rating	References
FSP should be familiar with and coordinate rehearsal of the emergency response plan with athletic trainers, coaches, and emergency responders.	C	[2,5,7,13]
On-field assessment of a down athlete with LOC or in prone position should presume to have a cervical spine injury.	C	[13]
Evaluation of traumatic head injury involves eliminating cervical spin injury and serious traumatic brain injury and removing the athlete from play.	C	[5,13,14,17]
Head injury to include concussion should have frequent reevaluation.	C	[5,13,14,17]
Evaluation of cervical spine injury is not accurate if there are distracting injuries, intoxication, altered level of consciousness, focal neurologic deficits, or midline tenderness.	C	[17]
Management of SCA is a systematic ACLS treatment with immediate recognition, CPR, and early defibrillation	A	[3,5,8,10,13]

35.13 SUMMARY

In summary, though life- and limb-threatening emergencies are rare, proper preparation, recognition, and treatment can improve the outcomes. Practicing the emergency response plan and reviewing how to treat the aforementioned emergencies are critical to ensure that all responders are working together (Table 35.3).

REFERENCES

1. American College of Sports Medicine, Armstrong LE, Casa DJ et al. American College of Sports Medicine position stand. Exertional heat illness during training and competition. *Medicine & Science in Sports & Exercise.* 2007;39(3):556–572.
2. Boden BP. Catastrophic sports injuries. In O'Connor F (ed.), *ACSM's Sports Medicine: A Comprehensive Review.* Philadelphia, PA: Lippincott Williams & Wilkins; 2013, pp. 84–91.
3. Borjesson M, Pelliccia A. Incidence and aetiology of sudden cardiac death in young athletes: An international perspective. *British Journal of Sports Medicine.* 2009;43:644–648.
4. Dvorak J, Kramer EB, Schmied CM et al. The FIFA medical emergency bag and FIFA 11 steps to prevent sudden cardiac death: Setting a global standard and promoting consistent football field emergency care. *British Journal of Sports Medicine.* 2013;47:1199–1202.

5. Fitch RW, Cox CL, Hannah GA et al. Sideline emergencies: An evidence-based approach. *Journal of Surgical Orthopaedic Advances.* 2011;20(2):83–101.
6. Herring SA, Putukian M, Kibler WB. Sideline preparedness for the team physician: A consensus statement—2012 Update. *Medicine & Science in Sports & Exercise.* 2012; 44(12):2442–2445.
7. Herring SA, Putikan M, Kibler WB. Team physician consensus statement: 2013 Update. *Medicine & Science in Sports & Exercise.* 2013;45(8):1618–1622.
8. Kramer FB, Botha M, Drezner J et al. Practical management of sudden cardiac arrest on the football field. *British Journal of Sports Medicine.* 2012;46:1094–1096.
9. Lieberman P, Camargo CA, Bohlke K et al. Epidemiology of anaphylaxis: Findings of the American College of Allergy, Asthma and Immunology Epidemiology of Anaphylaxis Working Group. *Annals of Allergy, Asthma & Immunology.* 2006;97(5):596–602.
10. Link, M. Commotio cordis: Ventricular fibrillation triggered by chest impact-induced abnormalities in repolarization. *Circulation: Arrhythmia and Electrophysiology.* 2012;5:425–432.
11. Link M, Atkind D, Passman R et al. Part 6: Electrical therapies: Automated external defibrillators, defibrillation, cardioversion, and pacing: 2010 American Heart Association Guidelines for Cardiopulmonary Resuscitation and Emergency Cardiovascular Care. *Circulation* 2010;122(Suppl 3):S706–S719.
12. Madias C, Maron BJ, Link MS. Commotio cordis. *Indian Pacing and Electrophysiology Journal.* 2007;7(4):235–245.
13. Maron BJ, Haas TS, Murphy CJ et al. Incidence and causes of sudden cardiac death in U.S. college athletes. *Journal of the American College of Cardiology.* 2014;63(16):1636–1643.
14. May JA, Crown LA, Gaertner MC. Field-side emergencies. In O'Connor F (ed.), *ACSM's Sports Medicine: A Comprehensive Review.* Philadelphia, PA: Lippincott Williams & Wilkins; 2013, pp. 84–91.
15. McAlindon RJ. On field evaluation and management of head and neck injured athletes. *Clinics in Sports Medicine.* 2002;21(1):755–763.
16. McCrory P, Meeuwisse W, Johnston K et al. Consensus statement on concussion in sport: The 3rd International Conference on Concussion in Sport held in Zurich, November 2008. *Journal of Athletic Training.* 2009;44(4):434–448.
17. Mueller FO, Cantu RC. NCCSIR thirtieth annual report. National Center for Catastrophic Sports Injury Research: Fall 1982—Spring 2012. Chapel Hill, NC: National Center for Sports Injury Research; 2012.
18. Piantanida NA, Oriscello RG, Pettrone FA et al. Sudden cardiac death: Ethical considerations in the return to play. *Current Sports Medicine Reports.* 2004;3(2):89–92.
19. Scorza KA, Raleigh MF, O'Connor FG. Current concepts in concussion: Evaluation and management. *American Family Physician.* 2012;8(2):123–132.
20. Skelley NW, McCormick JJ, Smith MV. In-game management of common joint dislocations. *Sports Health.* 2014;6:246–255.
21. Zafren K, Durrer B, Henry JP et al. Lightning injuries: Prevention and on-site treatment in mountains and remote areas. Official guidelines of the International Commission for Mountain Emergency Medicine and the Medical Commission of the International Mountaineering and Climbing Federation (ICAR and UIAA MEDCOM). *Resuscitation.* 2005;65:369–372.

36 Injury Prevention

Sarah De La Motte, Peter Lisman, and Christopher J. Sardon

CONTENTS

TABLE 36.1
Key Clinical Considerations

1. It is important to be familiar with the risk factors associated with musculoskeletal injury as well as the prediction and prevention strategies commonly implemented in athletic settings.
2. Intrinsic and extrinsic risk factors must be identified. Of those risk factors, modifiable factors have the potential to be modified through specific training and/or lifestyle interventions.
3. Poor compliance in injury prevention training programs is a significant problem. Physicians must incorporate potential performance gains in these programs in order to get athletes to "buy in" to the program.
4. Avoid sudden increases in exercise intensity. Do not exceed running 40 miles/week or increases in distance of more than 10%.
5. Neuromuscular training programs must be performed a minimum of twice a week for 6 weeks in order to obtain any benefit.

36.1 INTRODUCTION

Prevention of musculoskeletal injuries (MSKIs) is a primary concern for health care professionals, such as athletic trainers, physical therapists, and physicians, responsible for the care of athletes and other physically active individuals. This initiative is especially challenging given the multifactorial etiology of injury in these populations. Over the years, research has identified numerous risk factors for sports- and training-related injuries. More recent work has suggested that the number and severity of these injuries may be potentially reduced through specific injury prediction and exercise intervention strategies. It is important for the primary care sports physician to be familiar with the risk factors associated with MSKI as well as the prediction and prevention strategies commonly implemented in athletic settings. This chapter will initially review current evidence regarding the multiple risk factors associated with MSKI. The chapter will then discuss several injury prediction and prevention strategies commonly used by sports medicine practitioners (Table 36.1).

36.2 RISK FACTORS FOR MSKI

Research has identified numerous etiologic risk factors associated with incidence of MSKI in physically active individuals. The identification of these factors represents an initial key step in the injury prevention process for the sports medicine clinician. Traditionally, risk factors are classified as being either intrinsic or extrinsic. Intrinsic factors can be described as inherent characteristics of the individual and include age, gender, previous history of injury, and present levels of physical fitness. On the other hand, extrinsic factors are external to the individual and include variables such as training methodologies, playing or occupational surfaces, and the protective equipment or footwear worn during activity. In addition to the aforementioned classification, risk factors can be categorized as either "nonmodifiable" or "modifiable." Nonmodifiable factors cannot be altered through training modifications or other intervention strategies. Common examples include age, prior history of injury, and the specific anatomical characteristics of an individual. Conversely, modifiable factors have the potential to be modified through specific training and/or lifestyle interventions. For example, an appropriately prescribed training program and dietary intervention can positively influence the health-related components of physical fitness of an individual. The current evidence regarding select intrinsic and extrinsic risk factors associated with injury is discussed as follows (see Table 36.2).

36.2.1 Intrinsic Risk Factors

36.2.1.1 Age

Research has provided equivocal evidence on the effects of age on training-related injuries. Knapik et al.[44] reported that male army recruits aged 25.0–29.9 years had an elevated risk of injury compared to those <20 years old; injury incidence was even greater among those aged ≥30 years. Similar findings have been reported among Federal Bureau of Investigation new agent trainees.[45] Conversely, other data have indicated no effect of age on training-related injuries among male and female army basic trainees,[48] and occurrence of stress fractures in U.S. Marine Corps recruits.[79] Nonetheless, it has been

TABLE 36.2
Potential Risk Factors for Injury

Extrinsic Risk Factors	Intrinsic Risk Factors
Nonmodifiable	**Nonmodifiable**
Type of sport played	Age
Level and intensity of competition	Gender
	Previous history of injury
	Previous history of physical activity
	Structural/anatomic factors
Potentially modifiable	**Potentially modifiable**
Training factors	BMI
Playing/occupational surfaces	Percent body fat
Protective equipment and footwear	Tobacco smoking
	Level of cardiorespiratory fitness
	Flexibility/range of motion
	Muscular fitness (strength, endurance, and balance)
	Neuromuscular control and balance

suggested that older recruits may be more susceptible to injury due to age-related declines in fitness and/or a greater likelihood of having a prior history of injury.[44] Similar inconsistent results have been reported in runners[93] and professional soccer players.[27] However, the risk of sports-related injury has been consistently shown to increase in adolescents (>13 years) when compared to younger children, for possible reasons such as increases in level of competition, physicality of play, athlete size, and overall exposure rate.[22]

36.2.1.2 Smoking

The adverse effect of smoking on the incidence of injury has been clearly demonstrated.[33,44,48,73] Male infantry soldiers who were smokers were three times more likely to be injured during training than nonsmokers.[73] Others have reported relative risks (RRs) of 2.0 and 1.8 for training-related injuries in male and female army basic trainees, respectively, who smoked 11–20 cigarettes per day compared with nonsmokers.[48] Furthermore, authors have noted a higher injury risk in male recruits who reported having smoked ≥100 cigarettes in the past or smoking ≥20 cigarettes in the 30 days before training onset.[44]

36.2.1.3 Gender

Females appear to be more prone to training-related injuries than males. For example, injury rates among female army basic trainees have been reported to be 1.5–2.0 times higher than those for males.[5,32,48] In U.S. Military Academy cadets, females had more stress fractures and four times the rate of injuries resulting in hospitalization than males. Civilian studies have also reported an association between gender and several lower extremity MSKI. A recent literature review reported that the rate of noncontact ACL injuries is two to nine times greater in females than males.[92] Importantly, noncontact mechanisms represent the majority of ACL injuries[78] and are especially common in sports such as basketball, soccer, and volleyball.[3] Proposed explanations for the increased risk of ACL injury to female athletes include decreased neuromuscular control of the knee[30] and trunk,[98,99] anatomical considerations such as thickness of the femoral notch ridge and ACL size,[94] generalized joint laxity,[90] and hormonal fluctuations during the menstrual cycle.[100] While female runners also tend to be more prone to medial tibial stress syndrome than their male counterparts,[63] gender has not been shown to influence the incidence of lateral ankle sprains.[7]

36.2.1.4 Previous History of Injury

Previous history of MSKI has been clearly identified as a risk factor for injury. Data from the army have demonstrated that previous history of lower extremity injury is associated with injury during training.[33,44] In soccer players, previous identical injury was found to be a risk factor for lower extremity injuries to the hamstrings,[24] quadriceps,[27] groin,[23] calf,[27] and ankle.[51] Basketball players with a history of an ankle injury had increased ankle injury rates of up to fivefold compared with previously uninjured players.[61] Shelbourne et al.[80] reported that history of ACL reconstruction was especially predictive of subsequent ACL injury of the contralateral knee in women. Literature reviews have also shown that previous history of injury is a strong predictor of future running-related injury in runners.[63,93] Collectively, these findings suggest that individuals suffering lower extremity injuries often experience a cycle of repeated injury. A few proposed reasons for repeat injury include injury-induced functional instability[28] and joint laxity,[60] reduced proprioception,[35] tightness or weakness of injured muscle,[20] and incomplete and/or poor compliance to prescribed rehabilitation.[20]

36.2.1.5 Current Level of Cardiorespiratory Fitness

Cardiorespiratory fitness (CRF), as measured by 1–3 miles maximal effort run times during physical fitness entry tests, has been clearly identified as a strong predictor for training-related injury in military basic trainees.[32,42,48,50] During army basic training, men and women who scored in the slowest quartiles were 1.6–2.2 times more likely to be injured than those in the fastest groups.[32,48] Similar findings have been reported in nonmilitary athletic populations.[86] This relationship is not surprising given the high volume of running and other strenuous physical activities performed during military basic training and sports participation. Individuals with low CRF may perceive physical training as more difficult and may experience an increased level of fatigue in comparison to more fit individuals.

36.2.1.6 Previous History of Physical Activity

Data are less clear on the association between lower levels of previous physical activity and future occurrence of injury. Among military trainees, lower levels of general exercise and sports activity and frequency and length of time running prior to training onset were predictive of injury in some but not all studies.[32,48,49,55] Similar inconsistent results have been found between greater number of years participating in running and occurrence of running-related injuries.[93] Nonetheless, the suggested link between previous history of physical activity and subsequent injury incidence may be due to increases in both muscle[74] and connective tissue strength[40] and bone mineral density[81] that are associated with higher levels of physical activity and exercise of the proper mode, frequency, and duration.

36.2.1.7 BMI and Percent Body Fat

Conflicting evidence exists regarding the role anthropometric characteristics have in relation to training- and sports-related injuries. Data from some military studies indicate a bimodal relationship between BMI and incidence of injury in male but not female army basic trainees.[32,44,48,49] Knapik et al.[44] reported male army recruits with both high (>30 kg/m^2) and low (<18.5 kg/m^2) BMIs were at greater risk for training-related injuries whereas others found no association.[48,49] A large prospective study reported an association between above normal BMI and noncontact ACL injury in female but not male West Point cadets.[90] Findings have also been inconsistent in relation to percent body fat (BF%) and injury incidence in both male and female basic trainees.[32,33,48] In civilian studies, associations have been found between high BMI and both lower extremity injury occurrence in female elite soccer players[64] and medial tibial stress syndrome in runners.[63] In contrast, a large literature review reported that neither BMI nor BF% was associated with the occurrence of training-related stress fractures.[6] Collectively, these findings indicate that additional work is needed to elucidate the potential relationship between body composition and new injury incidence.

36.2.1.8 Select Structural/Anatomic Factors

Research has suggested a link between several anatomical factors and MSKI. Anatomical foot type (pronated, supinated, or neutral) does not appear to be predictive of ankle sprains.[7] In the military, increasing arch height has been found to be predictive of overall injury,[19] whereas both high and low arches,[36] smaller femoral neck diameter,[17] and higher Q angle[18] were associated with stress fractures. In runners, navicular drop was associated with incidence of medial tibial stress syndrome,[63] whereas lower arches were predictive of plantar fasciitis.[70] Foot pronation was not associated with new lower extremity injury in female soccer players.[64] Prospective studies have investigated anatomical risk factors for noncontact ACL injuries in athletic populations. Results suggest an association between new ACL injury and decreased femoral notch width[90,94] and ACL volume[94] and the presence of knee recurvatum or hyperextension.[8] Although evidence has shown females to have smaller ACLs and femoral notch widths than males,[94] which may partially account for their increased incidence of noncontact ACL injury, further work is still needed to determine how these anatomical factors influence injury.

36.2.1.9 Flexibility and Range of Motion

Conflicting evidence has been shown regarding the influence of flexibility/range of motion (ROM) on training- and sports-related injury. Although several military studies have shown a bimodal association between flexibility, as measured by the sit-and-reach test, and training-related injury with both the least and most flexible groups at greater risk for injury than those with average flexibility,[33,48] others have reported that performance on this test did not influence risk of ACL injury.[90] A bimodal relationship has also been reported between hip ROM and injury incidence in female collegiate athletes.[41,46] Recent meta-analyses have suggested that increased hip external rotation ROM was influential in the occurrence of medial tibial stress syndrome in male runners,[63] whereas ROM for inversion, eversion, plantar flexion, and dorsiflexion was not a risk factor for ankle injuries.[96] Clearly, future research investigating the potential link between flexibility/ROM and injury is warranted.

36.2.1.10 Muscular Fitness

Muscular endurance, as measured by performance in sit-up, push-up, and pull-up tests, has been shown to influence training-related injury in military populations.[42,48,50] However, data on the association between muscular strength and injury have been less consistent. Incremental dynamic lift strength was shown to influence injury in some but not all military members.[32,48] Inconsistent results were also found for other strength measurements, such as a 1-RM bench press, handgrip, and isometric upper and lower body strength.[43,48,73] Studies have also investigated the association between strength and injury to specific anatomical sites. Greater concentric plantar flexion strength at high speeds and lower eccentric eversion strength at slower speeds appear to be risk factors for ankle injuries.[96] Low hip muscle strength (external rotation and abduction) has been associated with patellofemoral pain in runners.[15] Muscular strength imbalances, such as bilateral strength differences and atypical agonist-to-antagonist strength ratios, have also been linked to injury. Side-to-side strength differences in knee flexion and hip extension and abduction have been associated with lower extremity injuries in athletes.[41,67] Similar associations have been found between abnormal agonist-to-antagonist strength ratios, such as low knee flexion to extension, hip abduction to adduction, and ankle dorsiflexion to plantar flexion, and lower extremity injuries in this population.[4,57,67]

36.2.1.11 Neuromuscular Control and Balance

Neuromuscular control can be described as the interaction between the nervous and muscular systems to control joint movement and maintain stability in response to a stimulus.[87] Prospective studies have identified ineffective neuromuscular control as a risk factor for ACL injury. Hewett et al.[30] reported that females who injured their ACL demonstrated an increased dynamic knee valgus at landing from a jump-landing task than uninjured athletes. Deficits in neuromuscular control of the trunk have also been noted to be a predictive of knee injuries in male and female athletes, with lateral displacement the greatest risk factor for ACL injury.[98] Poor balance has also been shown to be predictive of lower extremity injury. Poor dynamic balance, as measured by the Star Excursion Balance Test (SEBT), has been shown to be predictive of lower extremity injuries in high school basketball and college football players.[12,69] Similarly, Trojian and McKeag[89] noted an RR of 2.54 for sports-related ankle sprains in high school and collegiate athletes who failed to maintain static balance during a single-leg balance test compared to those who passed the test.

36.2.2 Extrinsic Risk Factors

36.2.2.1 Training Factors

Early studies identified the link between high weekly running mileage and lower extremity injury in male and female distance runners.[52,56] One classic study noted that the incidence of running-related injury was three times higher in men whose running volume was ≥40 miles/week compared to those running <40 miles/week.[56] Another study reported that as duration of running increased from 30 to 45 minutes per workout, the injury rate increased from 24% to 54%.[71] Data from the military have also clearly shown a relationship between running volume and injury incidence. In a study of male army basic trainees, Jones et al.[33] reported that trainees running 11 miles/week experienced 27% more lower extremity injuries than those running 5 miles/week. Importantly, the lower weekly mileage had no significant impact on aerobic fitness gains as measured by run time. In a related study of U.S. Marine Corps recruits, authors reported that injury rates during basic training were greatest during the weeks with the highest hours of vigorous physical training and most hours of running and marching.[1]

36.2.2.2 Protective Equipment and Footwear

Ankle bracing has been shown to be effective in decreasing the prevalence of ankle sprains in basketball and soccer players, especially those with a previous history of ankle injuries. A recent systematic review reported a reduction of ankle injuries by roughly 70% with the use of ankle brace or tape among athletes with a previous history of ankle injury.[21] In a study of military trainees performing parachute landings, authors reported that trainees not wearing ankle braces had a sixfold increased chance of injury in comparison to brace wearers.[2] Prophylactic knee braces are commonly worn by football players to prevent against MCL injury. However, current evidence does not support their use for the prevention of injuries to the MCL, other knee ligaments, menisci, or articular cartilage. Furthermore, the practice of bracing all football players is not endorsed by the American Academy of Orthopaedic Surgeons.[77] Mouthguards have been shown to decrease the risk of sports-related orofacial injury.[10,54,59] A recent meta-analysis noted RRs of 1.6–1.9 for sports-related orofacial injury in athletes not wearing mouthguards in comparison to those who wore the protective device.[47]

Presently, the NCAA only requires mouthguards to be worn by athletes participating in football, ice hockey, men's lacrosse, and women's field hockey. The role of footwear in the incidence of lower extremity injuries has also been examined. With regard to cleats, research has demonstrated that wearing shoes with a fewer number of cleats or shorter cleat height reduced the risk of lower extremity injury in football players.[53] However, shoe type (low or high top) has not been shown to influence the incidence of ankle sprains in physically active populations.[7]

36.2.2.3 Playing/Occupational Surfaces

Research has suggested that the type of playing surface (grass or artificial surfaces) or running surface may impact incidence rates of lower extremity injuries. A recent literature review[95] reported that athletes were more likely to suffer an ankle injury when playing on artificial turf in more than half (8 of 14) of the studies analyzed. However, the evidence was inconclusive for risk of knee injuries and muscle strains. In a separate review, Bennell et al.[6] reported that studies have yet to show an association between training surface and incidence of stress fractures in runners after controlling for the effects of weekly running distance.

36.2.2.4 Sports and Competition Factors

Epidemiological data have clearly shown an association between sports played and risk of injury. In collegiate athletes, the highest frequency of game-related injuries was reported for participants in football, wrestling, men's soccer, women's soccer, men's ice hockey, and women's gymnastics, in that order. When combining all sports, injury rates were higher in games than in practices. Across all seasons, injury rates during practice were higher during preseason than in-season and postseason.[31]

36.3 STRATEGIES FOR MSKI PREVENTION

36.3.1 Role of Education, Leadership, and Compliance

As to be expected, athlete compliance to an injury prevention program directly affects its utility in decreasing injury risk.[84,85] A recent meta-analysis[85] reported that compliance with neuromuscular training programs was an important factor in preventing ACL injury in female athletes. Specifically, authors noted that participants in studies reporting low compliance rates had a fivefold increased chance of ACL injury compared to participants in studies reporting high levels of compliance. Additionally, the evidence suggested that the overall compliance rate to an injury prevention program needs to be >66% in order to decrease ACL injury risk. Alarmingly, two-thirds (four of six) of the reviewed studies reported overall compliance rates less than 50%, which indicates coaches or other leadership personnel (e.g., commanding officers) were not accepting of the intervention. One potential way of improving program compliance is to associate program components with potential sport performance gains. Authors have suggested that this shift in approach may increase "buy-in" from both coaches and players, as players especially tend to be more interested in performing training exercises that focus on performance enhancement than injury prevention.[25] Given these findings, it is important that sports medicine physicians take an active role in educating coaches, as well as those personnel directly responsible for leading the day-to-day injury prevention routine, on the importance of program compliance.

36.3.2 Training Modifications

In order to identify training modifications to prevent MSKIs, a physician must understand the types of injuries that are frequently seen in a particular sport or activity. For these purposes, we will look at endurance training, agility sports, and contact sports separately.

Endurance sports, like running marathons or triathlons, often lead to overuse injuries. The most commonly observed injuries seen in these athletes are patellofemoral pain syndrome, stress fractures, medial tibial stress syndrome (shin splints), plantar fasciitis, iliotibial band syndrome, and Achilles tendinopathy.[34] Limiting the overall mileage per week that a runner runs can easily be modified to prevent overuse injuries. Multiple studies have identified that running ≥40 miles/week has an increased risk of injury.[91] Although excessive mileage per week has an increased risk of injury, it has also been demonstrated that sudden increases in the intensity of exercise leads to an increased risk of injury. This has led to many sports medicine physicians promoting no more than a 10% increase in exercise volume per week. Although sports medicine physicians commonly recommend this, the literature has not supported any statistically significant differences in injury prevention between standard training programs and graded (10% rule) training programs.[9] Although the 10% rule has not been proven in the literature to reduce injuries, it is a good baseline to discuss with patients in order to prevent excessive increases in exercise volume.

Clinical Pearl

Avoid sudden increases in exercise intensity
Do not exceed running 40 miles/week

Agility sports, like soccer and basketball, provide a completely different genre of injuries compared to endurance sports. Although overuse injuries can be seen, more acute injuries are of greater concern. Commonly found injuries in these sports consist of muscle or ligament sprains or tears, meniscal damage, and bone fractures. Although these injuries are often unavoidable, there are a few training modifications that can help reduce the risk.

Neuromuscular training programs are rapidly being developed with the goal of injury prevention. The idea behind these training programs is to improve lower extremity and core muscle fitness and to increase neuromuscular function so that athletes evade positions that increase their susceptibility to injury. Research conducted on these training programs primarily focused on ACL injury prevention; however, these principles can be applied for general lower extremity injury prevention in agility sports. Neuromuscular training programs consist of strength, balance, plyometrics, and flexibility training. When these different aspects of training are performed alone, there is little evidence to suggest a decrease in injuries. However, when these training modalities are combined, they demonstrate a decreased incidence of lower extremity injuries.[58] It is important to keep in mind that an athlete must participate in a neuromuscular training program twice a week for 6 weeks in order to ensure any benefit from the program.[29] While most neuromuscular training programs focus mainly on the ability of the muscles to avoid injury prone situations, it is important for these programs to also incorporate teaching proper techniques for cutting and landing motions. The combination of knowing these proper techniques and training your muscles to avoid injury prone situations will maximize the injury preventing benefit of a neuromuscular training program.

Clinical Pearl

You must perform a neuromuscular training program a minimum of twice a week for 6 weeks in order to obtain any benefit from the program

Contact sports, like football and rugby, have many of the same injuries as agility sports. However, concussions, neck injuries, and dislocated shoulders are of particular concern to the physician since they can result in permanent disabilities. Training modifications can be designed to help prevent these injuries from initially happening and/or recurring. For instance, proper tackling techniques should be taught by coaches in order to prevent the athlete from putting themselves in risky positions. In addition, the proper management after an initial injurious event can prevent future occurrences from happening. A specific example is the return to play guidelines for concussions. This is a topic that is widely discussed in Chapter 40; nevertheless, it confers the gradual reintroduction of an athlete to the athletic field once their postconcussive symptoms resolve.

36.3.3 Equipment Modifications

Although training modifications can significantly reduce the risk of injury, equipment modifications can also play a significant role. Footwear is one of the easiest modifications that can be made; however, there is continued debate as to the role of shoes in injury prevention. Current recommendations are for shoes to be comfortable and appropriate for the athlete's foot shape.[72] If a patient has difficulty finding a shoe that is appropriate for their shoe shape, orthotics may be an appropriate adjunct (see Table 36.3).

While these are the current recommendations, there is little evidence in the literature to support these endorsements. Conversely, there is significant evidence to support that new running shoes lose their shock-absorbing capabilities after running 250–500 miles.[16] Therefore, it is important to advise patients to get new running shoes once they have met these limits.

An increasingly popular trend seen in runners is barefoot running or minimalist shoes. The theory behind the benefits of this running style is that it shortens a runner's gait leading to a midfoot or forefoot strike, rather than the rearfoot strike seen in traditional running shoes. In theory, this would

TABLE 36.3
Appropriate Footwear Recommendations for Foot Shape

Foot Shape	Shoe Recommendation
Pes planus (overpronators)	Minimize foot motion and maintain foot in neutral position.
Neutral foot shape	Maintain neutral foot shape.
Pes cavus (oversupinators)	Extensive cushioning.

Source: Data from Reinschmidt, C. and Nigg, B.M., *Sportverletzung Sportschaden: Organ der Gesellschaft fur Orthopadisch-Traumatologische Sportmedizin*, 14, 71, 2000.

decrease the impact delivered to the foot, knee, and hips. There is very little evidence to promote or negate this trend, which is important for the physician to convey to the patient. Although the evidence is bare, there are a few case reports that propose an increased risk of metatarsal stress fractures, especially in a rapid transition from traditional running shoes to barefoot or minimalist shoes.[13]

Athletes in agility-based sports must weigh multiple factors when selecting cleats. In addition to comfort and foot shape, the athlete must take into consideration the shoe–surface interface. Multiple studies have revealed that a higher incidence of traction between the shoes and the playing surface correlated with an increased occurrence of ACL injuries. This is due to increasing torsional forces on the tibia as the shoe gets caught on the surface during pivoting motions. Therefore, an athlete can reduce their risk of injury by choosing a shoe with fewer cleats.[53,88]

Ankle injuries are a commonly encountered problem among athletes that can potentially be prevented by using ankle braces or taping. As previously discussed, studies have clearly demonstrated that individuals with a history of ankle injury can significantly decrease their chance of recurrence by wearing an ankle brace or taping their ankle.[21] However, the data do not support a clear preventative impact of these interventions on patients without previous ankle injuries.

Clinical Pearl

Ankle bracing and taping helps prevent recurrent ankle injuries; it does not prevent initial injuries

The surface that a runner chooses to run on can also impact the risk of injury, especially overuse injuries like stress fractures. For example, a runner is more likely to develop a stress fracture when running on cement when compared to a treadmill or other soft surface.[62] Harder running surfaces place more stress on the bones and joints, thus making them more prone to injury. Therefore, a physician should recommend the use of treadmills or running on grass for long distance runs if possible.

Concussions are possibly the most controversial topic when it comes to injury prevention. As we are learning more about the negative long-term health effects of repeated brain trauma, the need for equipment modifications to prevent concussions is becoming more important. However, the current literature on the use of helmets and mouthguards for concussion prevention do not suggest there is a significant preventive effect.[26] Although current studies do not show any hard evidence for the protective effects of helmets and mouthguards, the severity of these injuries necessitates that physicians continue to promote their use. This is a hot topic that will continue to evolve over the coming years; therefore, it is imperative that physicians remain up to date on the latest research.

36.3.4 Intrinsic Factors

There are intrinsic factors of each athlete that makes them more or less likely to develop injury. In many cases, these factors are incapable of being changed. For example, an athlete can't change their Q angle or gender. However, there are some intrinsic factors that an athlete can improve with training over time. As previously stated, examples include cardiovascular fitness, bone density, and neuromuscular training.

Improving cardiovascular fitness is an important intrinsic factor that an athlete can improve. With improved cardiovascular fitness, an athlete can delay the onset of fatigue and help prevent MSKIs. Fatigue in an athlete is accompanied by an increase in joint laxity due to decreased proprioception.[76,82] These proprioceptors are responsible for stabilizing the muscles of the joint, and when fatigue sets in, these proprioceptors become less proficient and the joint loses sense of where it is in relation to the rest of the body. This lack of "self-control" leads to the increase in joint laxity and exposes the joint to a higher risk of injury, particularly the ACL. In addition to altered proprioception, the stabilizing muscles of the lower extremity joints have a delayed onset of action while fatigued, thus further making joints like the knee less stable and more susceptible to injurious movements.[65] Therefore, it is important for an athlete to improve their cardiovascular fitness and to recognize when they are fatigued in order to try and avoid putting themselves in situations that would increase their risk of injury.

Clinical Pearl

Fatigue leads to unstable joints thus increasing the risk of injury. Improving cardiovascular fitness decreases the onset of fatigue, thus decreasing the risk of injury.

Bone density is another intrinsic risk factor that can be altered if individual attention is given. This is particularly important in young female athletes as well as postmenopausal women, since osteoporosis is commonly seen in these populations. Increasing bone density in these populations is important because it will help to lower the risk of stress fractures. It is recommended that all women age 65 or older get a DEXA scan to screen for bone mineral density. In addition, women under the age of 65 with specific risk factors (low body weight, previous history of fracture, smoking history, etc.) should also be screened. In young female athletes, particularly gymnasts, osteoporosis is a concern due to low body weight and nutritional deficiencies. It is important for a physician to have a high index of suspicion for the female athlete triad since it has additional significant health concerns in addition to increased fracture risk.

Prevention of osteoporosis and subsequent fractures is aimed at maximizing peak bone mass and minimizing bone loss. Maximizing peak bone mass occurs mostly during adolescents. This can be achieved by maintaining adequate nutrition (particularly vitamin D and calcium), exercising to maximize bone accumulation during the growth phase, maintaining a normal weight, and avoiding smoking and excessive alcohol consumption. As we age, our body slowly loses bone mineral density at a relatively stable rate. It is important for older athletes, particularly postmenopausal women, to make interventions to slow this rate down and decrease their risk of developing fractures. In order for adults to preserve as much of their bone mineral density, they must regularly do weight-bearing exercises, maintain adequate nutrition, stop smoking, use only moderate amounts of alcohol, and prevent falls.[97] For women who have significantly lowered bone mineral densities, pharmacological treatment with bisphosphonates or raloxifene may be necessary.

The final intrinsic factors that can be altered in athlete in order to prevent injury are balance, proprioception, strength, and flexibility. The neuromuscular training programs previously discussed target all of these areas in order to maximize the ability of the athlete to avoid positions that increase their risk of injury.

TABLE 36.4
American College of Sports Medicine (ACSM) Dietary Recommendations

Dietary Component	Recommendation
Calories	Exercising individuals should consume no fewer than 1800–2000 kcal/day. • Insufficient calories can lead to • Reduced muscle mass and bone density • Delayed recovery • Increased fatigue • Increased risk of injury
Carbohydrates	Important for maintaining blood glucose during exercise and replenishing muscle glycogen. • 6–10 g/kg body weight of carbohydrates per day
Protein	Endurance athletes need 1.2–1.7 g/kg body weight of protein per day.
Fat	Healthy fats are a source of energy and provide essential fatty acids and fat-soluble vitamins. • Should comprise 20%–35% of total calorie intake.
Hydration	Drink 16–24 oz of fluid for every pound lost during exercise. For endurance exercise like marathons, it is also important to replace electrolytes.

Source: Data from Rodriguez, N.R. et al., *Med. Sci. Sports Exerc.*, 41(3), 709, 2009.

36.3.5 Nutrition

The role of nutrition and energy balance is an often overlooked aspect of injury prevention. As stated previously in regard to bone mineral density, inadequate intake of calcium and vitamin D predispose athletes to stress fractures. However, a diet consists of many more nutritional factors can have an impact on injury prevention. While there is no specific diet that is best for injury prevention, maximizing nutritional intake can improve performance and recovery from injury. Dietary recommendations as stated by the American College of Sports Medicine are laid out in Table 36.4.

Importantly, recommendations have also been made regarding the timing of nutrient intake following strenuous exercise or sport participation.[10,37] Research suggests consuming 12–15 g of protein and 50–75 g of carbohydrate within 60 minutes of exercise cessation to enhance glycogen resynthesis and help begin the repair of any activity-induced muscle damage.[10] As you can see, nutrition plays a key role in injury prevention since adequate nutrition helps to optimize performance, maintain muscle mass and bone density, and improve recovery from fatigue and/or injury.

36.4 SUMMARY ON INJURY PREVENTION

Injuries are often unavoidable but there are many ways in which an exercising individual can minimize their risk. The four categories that can be modified in order to maximize the potential to avoid injury are training modifications, equipment modifications, intrinsic factor modification, and nutrition optimization. Each of these areas can have a significant impact on injury prevention, and it is the duty of the physician to educate athletes and active individuals on how to maximize their performance and prevent themselves from getting injured (see Figure 36.1).

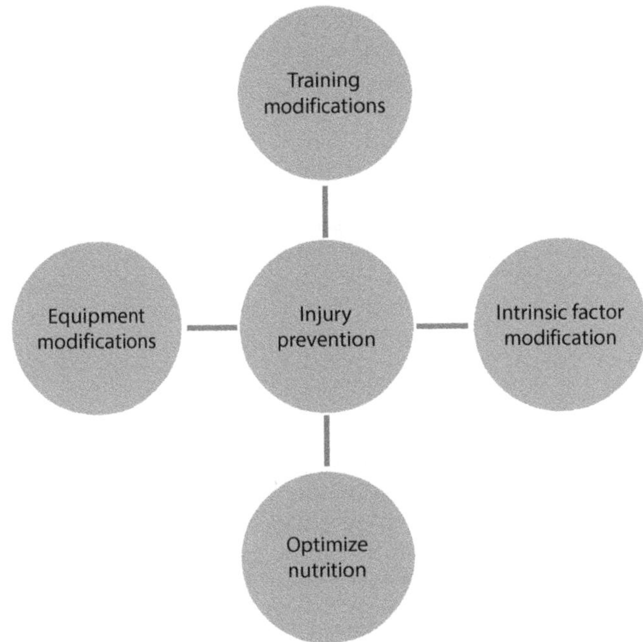

FIGURE 36.1 The four factors of injury prevention.

TABLE 36.5
Association between Functional Movement Assessments and Musculoskeletal Injuries

Study	Subject Characteristics	FMA	Outcome Measure	Injury Definition	Study Results
Kiesel et al.[38]	46 NFL players	FMS	FMS composite score	Membership on the injured reserve and time loss of 3 weeks; surveillance time was one full season.	Significant risk factor for injury: composite FMS score ≤14 (OR 11.67; 95% CI = 2.47–54.52).
Chorba et al.[14]	38 female division II athletes participating in soccer, volleyball, or basketball	FMS	FMS composite score	Injury occurred in practice or game over the course of one season and injury required medical attention or athlete sought advice from ATC, ATS, or physician.	Significant risk factor for injury (All subjects): FMS score ≤14 (OR 3.85; 95% CI = 0.98–15.13) and subjects without prior ACL injury (n = 31): FMS ≤ 14 (OR 4.58; 95% CI = 0.99–21.12)
O'Connor et al.[66]	874 male marine officer candidates	FMS	FMS composite score	Injury occurred during 6-week (n = 447) or 10-week (n = 427) officer candidate school training; injury classifications: any injury, overuse injury, serious injury.	Significant risk factor for any injury: FMS score ≤14 (OR 2.0; 95% CI = 1.3–3.1, p = 0.002) and serious injury (OR 2.0; 95% CI = 1.0–4.1, p = 0.05); no association between FMS score ≤14 and overuse injury
Butler et al.[11]	108 firefighters	FMS	FMS composite score	Injury causing the recruit to miss 3 consecutive days of training due to musculoskeletal pain during 16-week firefighting academy.	Significant risk factor for injury: FMS score ≤14 (OR 8.31; 95% CI = 3.2–21.6)
Kiesel et al.[39]	238 NFL players	FMS	FMS composite score; presence of at least 1 asymmetry in individual FMS test	Injury resulting in any time loss from either practice or preseason game during one full preseason period.	Significant risk factor for injury: FMS score ≤14 (RR 1.87; 95% CI = 1.20–2.96) and presence of ≥1 asymmetry (RR 1.80; 95% CI = 1.11–2.74)
Plisky et al.[69]	235 high school basketball players (130 males, 105 females)	SEBT	Reach distance (average of the right/left limb in cm) and reach distance R/L difference for anterior, posteromedial, and posterolateral directions; composite reach distance (%)	Injury to the lower extremity (including the hip but not the lumbar spine or SI joint) that occurred during practice or game over the course of one season.	Significant risk factor for injury: anterior R/L reach distance difference ≥4cm (OR 2.5; $p < 0.05$) and composite reach distance <94% of limb length (OR 6.5; $p < 0.05$)
Butler et al.[12]	59 NCAA football players	SEBT	Reach distance (average of the right/left limb in cm) and reach distance R/L difference for anterior, posteromedial, and posterolateral directions; composite reach distance (%)	Injury to the lower extremity (noncontact mechanism) that required medical attention and resulted in time loss of >1 day from activity over the course of one season.	Significant risk factor for injury: ROC curve analysis determined a cut-off point of 89.6% limb length in identifying injury (positive likelihood ratio 3.5; 95% CI = 2.4–5.3)
Smith et al.[83]	64 high school and collegiate athletes participating in soccer, football, rugby, gymnastics, lacrosse, or volleyball (20 males, 44 females)	LESS	LESS score	Injury to the ACL (noncontact mechanism) during season.	No association between LESS score and noncontact ACL injury

Note: ATC, certified athletic trainer; ATS, student athletic trainer; CI, confidence interval; OR, odds ratio; ROC, receiver operating characteristic; SI, sacroiliac.

36.5 FUTURE DIRECTIONS: FUNCTIONAL MOVEMENT ASSESSMENTS

MSKIs are a leading cause of morbidity in physically active populations. Recently, clinicians and researchers have been using functional movement assessments (FMAs) in attempt to predict injury risk in athletic and military populations. These assessments are used to identify deficiencies in balance, core stability, flexibility, mobility, and overall neuromuscular control. Initial results have indicated that several commonly used FMAs, such as the Functional Movement Screen (FMS), SEBT, and the Landing Error Scoring System (LESS), have some utility in predicting risk of MSKI in these populations (see Table 36.5).

The FMS consists of seven individual tests (squat, hurdle step, forward lunge, shoulder mobility, active straight leg raise, push-up, and rotary stability) that attempt to capture the quality of fundamental movement patterns and presumably identify an individual's functional limitations or asymmetries. Individual tests are scored on a 0–3 ordinal scale, with 3 being best and 0 being given when pain is present during the movement. Scores are based on the participant's ability to complete each movement in a free and unrestricted manner. Overall FMS scores can range from 0 to 21.[38] To date, research has suggested that athletes and military members with a composite FMS score ≤14 have an increased risk for MSKI in comparison with those with scores >14.[11,14,38,39,66]

The SEBT allows clinicians to assess dynamic balance by challenging participants' lower extremity flexibility, strength and coordination, and overall core stability, during specific movement patterns. In short, participants are required to maintain a single-leg stance while they simultaneously reach their contralateral limb in specific directions (e.g., anterior, posteromedial, posterolateral). Reach distance is measured and normalized as a percentage of limb length.[69] Initial results suggest that anterior reach asymmetries ≥4 cm and composite reach distances <90%–94% of limb length are associated with increased lower extremity injury risk.[12,69]

The LESS attempts to identify high-risk movement patterns during performance of a standardized jump-landing task. In short, participants jump forward from a box 30 cm high to a distance of half their body height. Sagittal and frontal plane images are recorded, and 17 items are subsequently scored to identify the number of "errors," or high-risk movement patterns. Initial results have indicated no association between LESS score and ACL injury risk.[83]

Collectively, research has suggested some utility in using FMAs to predict MSKI risk in athletic populations. However, little evidence exists regarding the utility of FMA-guided interventions in decreasing injury incidence.[68] From the clinicians' viewpoint, it is equally important that results from these assessment tools can be used to direct corrective exercise strategies targeting the identified movement deficiencies, with these interventions ultimately decreasing the overall incidence of injury (see Table 36.5).

TABLE 36.6
SORT: Key Recommendations for Practice

Clinical Recommendation	Evidence Rating	References
Athletes should follow a gradual progression of running distance and intensity, especially when beginning a training program. Particular caution is warranted with excessive running mileage per week (>40 miles).	A	[69,78]
Athletes, particularly those participating in agility-based sports, should include neuromuscular and proprioceptive training as part of the overall conditioning efforts.	A	[15,69,80]
Athletes with a previous history of ankle injury should wear an ankle brace or tape their ankles when participating in sports or high-risk training activities.	A	[64,69]
Athletes should consume 12–15 g of protein and 50–75 g of carbohydrate within 60 minutes of exercise cessation to enhance glycogen resynthesis and help begin the repair of any activity-induced muscle damage.	A	[69,92]

Source: Adapted from Bullock, S.H. et al., *Am. J. Prev. Med.*, 38, S156, 2010.

36.6 SUMMARY

Numerous risk factors are associated with sports- and training-related MSKIs in physically active individuals. It is important for the sports medicine physician to work with other members of the sports medicine team (e.g., athletic trainer, physical therapist, strength and conditioning coach, and coach) in identifying athletes at greater risk for injury. Injury prevention strategies, such as prophylactic bracing/taping, training modifications, and specific neuromuscular training programs, can then be implemented to decrease injury risk. For the previously injured athlete, it is especially important that health care providers take a proactive approach to injury prevention to reduce the potential risk for a cycle of repeat injury (Table 36.6).

REFERENCES

1. Almeida SA, Williams KM, Shaffer RA et al. Epidemiological patterns of musculoskeletal injuries and physical training. *Medicine & Science in Sports & Exercise.* 1999;31(8):1176–1182.
2. Amoroso PJ, Ryan JB, Bickley B et al. Braced for impact: Reducing military paratroopers' ankle sprains using outside-the-boot braces. *Journal of Trauma.* 1998;45(3):575–580.
3. Arendt E, Dick R. Knee injury patterns among men and women in collegiate basketball and soccer. NCAA data and review of literature. *American Journal of Sports Medicine.* 1995;23(6):694–701.

4. Baumhauer JF, Alosa DM, Renstrom AF et al. A prospective study of ankle injury risk factors. *American Journal of Sports Medicine.* 1995;23(5):564–570.
5. Bell NS, Mangione TW, Hemenway D et al. High injury rates among female army trainees: A function of gender? *American Journal of Preventive Medicine.* 2000;18(3 Suppl):141–146.
6. Bennell K, Matheson G, Meeuwisse W, Brukner P. Risk factors for stress fractures. *Sports Medicine.* 1999;28(2):91–122.
7. Beynnon BD, Murphy DF, Alosa DM. Predictive factors for lateral ankle sprains: A literature review. *Journal of Athletic Training.* 2002;37(4):376–380.
8. Boden BP, Sheehan FT, Torg JS et al. Noncontact anterior cruciate ligament injuries: Mechanisms and risk factors. *Journal of the American Academy of Orthopaedic Surgeons.* 2010;18(9):520–527.
9. Buist I, Bredeweg SW, van Mechelen W et al. No effect of a graded training program on the number of running-related injuries in novice runners: A randomized controlled trial. *American Journal of Sports Medicine.* 2008;36(1):33–39.
10. Bullock SH, Jones BH, Gilchrist J et al. Prevention of physical training-related injuries recommendations for the military and other active populations based on expedited systematic reviews. *American Journal of Preventive Medicine.* 2010;38 (1 Suppl):S156–S181.
11. Butler RJ, Contreras M, Burton LC et al. Modifiable risk factors predict injuries in firefighters during training academies. *Work.* 2013;46(1):11–17.
12. Butler RJ, Lehr ME, Fink ML et al. Dynamic balance performance and noncontact lower extremity injury in college football players: An initial study. *Sports Health.* 2013;5(5):417–422.
13. Cauthon DJ, Langer P, Coniglione TC. Minimalist shoe injuries: Three case reports. *Foot (Edinburgh, Scotland).* 2013; 23(2–3):100–103.
14. Chorba RS, Chorba DJ, Bouillon LE et al. Use of a functional movement screening tool to determine injury risk in female collegiate athletes. *North American Journal of Sports Physical Therapy.* 2010;5(2):47–54.
15. Cichanowski HR, Schmitt JS, Johnson RJ et al. Hip strength in collegiate female athletes with patellofemoral pain. *Medicine & Science in Sports & Exercise.* 2007;39(8):1227–1232.
16. Cook SD, Kester MA, Brunet ME. Shock absorption characteristics of running shoes. *American Journal of Sports Medicine.* 1985;13(4):248–253.
17. Cosman F, Ruffing J, Zion M et al. Determinants of stress fracture risk in United States Military Academy cadets. *Bone.* 2013;55(2):359–366.
18. Cowan DN, Jones BH, Frykman PN et al. Lower limb morphology and risk of overuse injury among male infantry trainees. *Medicine & Science in Sports & Exercise.* 1996;28(8):945–952.
19. Cowan DN, Jones BH, Robinson JR. Foot morphologic characteristics and risk of exercise-related injury. *Archives of Family Medicine.* 1993;2(7):773–777.
20. Croisier JL. Factors associated with recurrent hamstring injuries. *Sports Medicine.* 2004;34(10):681–695.
21. Dizon JM, Reyes JJ. A systematic review on the effectiveness of external ankle supports in the prevention of inversion ankle sprains among elite and recreational players. *Journal of Science and Medicine in Sport.* 2010;13(3):309–317.
22. Emery CA. Injury prevention and future research. *Medicine & Science in Sports & Exercise.* 2005;49:170–191.
23. Engebretsen AH, Myklebust G, Holme I et al. Intrinsic risk factors for groin injuries among male soccer players: A prospective cohort study. *American Journal of Sports Medicine.* 2010;38(10):2051–2057.
24. Engebretsen AH, Myklebust G, Holme I et al. Intrinsic risk factors for hamstring injuries among male soccer players: A prospective cohort study. *American Journal of Sports Medicine.* 2010;38(6):1147–1153.
25. Finch CF, White P, Twomey D, Ullah S. Implementing an exercise-training programme to prevent lower-limb injuries: Considerations for the development of a randomised controlled trial intervention delivery plan. *British Journal of Sports Medicine.* 2011;45(10):791–796.
26. Graham R Rivara FP, Ford MA et al. (eds.). Protection and prevention strategies. *Sports-Related Concussions in Youth. Improving the Science, Changing the Culture.* Washington, DC: National Academies Press; 2014, pp. 239–273.
27. Hagglund M, Walden M, Ekstrand J. Risk factors for lower extremity muscle injury in professional soccer: The UEFA Injury Study. *American Journal of Sports Medicine.* 2013;41(2):327–335.
28. Hertel J. Functional instability following lateral ankle sprain. *Sports Medicine.* 2000;29(5):361–371.
29. Hewett TE, Ford KR, Myer GD. Anterior cruciate ligament injuries in female athletes: Part 2, a meta-analysis of neuromuscular interventions aimed at injury prevention. *American Journal of Sports Medicine.* 2006;34(3):490–498.
30. Hewett TE, Myer GD, Ford KR et al. Biomechanical measures of neuromuscular control and valgus loading of the knee predict anterior cruciate ligament injury risk in female athletes: A prospective study. *American Journal of Sports Medicine.* 2005;33(4):492–501.
31. Hootman JM, Dick R, Agel J. Epidemiology of collegiate injuries for 15 sports: Summary and recommendations for injury prevention initiatives. *Journal of Athletic Training.* 2007;42(2):311–319.
32. Jones BH, Bovee MW, Harris JM, 3rd et al. Intrinsic risk factors for exercise-related injuries among male and female army trainees. *American Journal of Sports Medicine.* 1993;21(5):705–710.
33. Jones BH, Cowan DN, Tomlinson JP et al. Epidemiology of injuries associated with physical training among young men in the army. *Medicine & Science in Sports & Exercise.* 1993;25(2):197–203.
34. Junior LC, Carvalho CA, Costa LO et al. The prevalence of musculoskeletal injuries in runners: A systematic review. *British Journal of Sports Medicine.* 2011;45(4):351–352.
35. Katayama M, Higuchi H, Kimura M et al. Proprioception and performance after anterior cruciate ligament rupture. *International Orthopaedics.* 2004;28(5):278–281.
36. Kaufman KR, Brodine SK, Shaffer RA et al. The effect of foot structure and range of motion on musculoskeletal overuse injuries. *American Journal of Sports Medicine.* 1999;27(5):585–593.
37. Kerksick C, Harvey T, Stout J et al. International Society of Sports Nutrition position stand: Nutrient timing. *Journal of the International Society of Sports Nutrition.* 2008;5:17.
38. Kiesel K, Plisky PJ, Voight ML. Can serious injury in professional football be predicted by a preseason functional movement screen? *North American Journal of Sports Physical Therapy.* 2007;2(3):147–158.
39. Kiesel KB, Butler RJ, Plisky PJ. Prediction of injury by limited and asymmetrical fundamental movement patterns in american football players. *Journal of Sport Rehabilitation.* 2014;23(2):88–94.
40. Kjaer M, Langberg H, Miller BF et al. Metabolic activity and collagen turnover in human tendon in response to physical activity. *Journal of Musculoskeletal and Neuronal Interactions.* 2005;5(1):41–52.

41. Knapik JJ, Bauman CL, Jones BH, Harris JM, Vaughan L. Preseason strength and flexibility imbalances associated with athletic injuries in female collegiate athletes. *American Journal of Sports Medicine.* 1991;19(1):76–81.
42. Knapik JJ, Brosch LC, Venuto M et al. Effect on injuries of assigning shoes based on foot shape in air force basic training. *American Journal of Preventive Medicine.* 2010;38 (1 Suppl):S197–S211.
43. Knapik JJ, Jones SB, Sharp MA et al. A prospective study of injuries and injury risk factors among army wheel vehicle mechanics. Defense Technical Information Center, 2006. Availabe at http://www.dtic.mil/dtic/tr/fulltext/u2/a451589.pdf (Accessed August 18, 2014).
44. Knapik JJ, Graham B, Cobbs J et al. A prospective investigation of injury incidence and risk factors among army recruits in combat engineer training. *Journal of Occupational Medicine and Toxicology.* 2013;8(1):5.
45. Knapik JJ, Grier T, Spiess A et al. Injury rates and injury risk factors among Federal Bureau of Investigation new agent trainees. *BMC Public Health.* 2011;11:920.
46. Knapik JJ, Jones BH, Bauman CL et al. Strength, flexibility and athletic injuries. *Sports Medicine.* 1992;14(5): 277–288.
47. Knapik JJ, Marshall SW, Lee RB et al. Mouthguards in sport activities: History, physical properties and injury prevention effectiveness. *Sports Medicine.* 2007;37(2):117–144.
48. Knapik JJ, Sharp MA, Canham-Chervak M et al. Risk factors for training-related injuries among men and women in basic combat training. *Medicine & Science in Sports & Exercise.* 2001;33(6):946–954.
49. Knapik JJ, Swedler DI, Grier TL et al. Injury reduction effectiveness of selecting running shoes based on plantar shape. *The Journal of Strength & Conditioning Research.* 2009;23(3):685–697.
50. Knapik JJ, Trone DW, Swedler DI et al. Injury reduction effectiveness of assigning running shoes based on plantar shape in Marine Corps basic training. *American Journal of Sports Medicine.* 2010;38(9):1759–1767.
51. Kofotolis ND, Kellis E, Vlachopoulos SP. Ankle sprain injuries and risk factors in amateur soccer players during a 2-year period. *American Journal of Sports Medicine.* 2007;35(3):458–466.
52. Koplan JP, Powell KE, Sikes RK et al. An epidemiologic study of the benefits and risks of running. *Journal of the American Medical Association.* 1982;248(23):3118–3121.
53. Lambson RB, Barnhill BS, Higgins RW. Football cleat design and its effect on anterior cruciate ligament injuries. A three-year prospective study. *American Journal of Sports Medicine.* 1996;24(2):155–159.
54. Lieger O, von Arx T. Orofacial/cerebral injuries and the use of mouthguards by professional athletes in Switzerland. *Dental Traumatology.* 2006;22(1):1–6.
55. Lisman P, O'Connor FG, Deuster PA et al. Functional movement screen and aerobic fitness predict injuries in military training. *Medicine & Science in Sports & Exercise.* 2013;45(4):636–643.
56. Macera CA, Pate RR, Powell KE et al. Predicting lower-extremity injuries among habitual runners. *Archives of Internal Medicine.* 1989;149(11):2565–2568.
57. Magalhaes E, Silva AP, Sacramento SN et al. Isometric strength ratios of the hip musculature in females with patellofemoral pain: A comparison to pain-free controls. *The Journal of Strength & Conditioning Research.* 2013; 27(8):2165–2170.
58. Mandelbaum BR, Silvers HJ, Watanabe DS et al. Effectiveness of a neuromuscular and proprioceptive training program in preventing anterior cruciate ligament injuries in female athletes: 2-year follow-up. *American Journal of Sports Medicine.* 2005;33(7):1003–1010.
59. Marshall SW, Loomis DP, Waller AE et al. Evaluation of protective equipment for prevention of injuries in rugby union. *International Journal of Epidemiology.* 2005;34(1): 113–118.
60. Martin DE, Kaplan PA, Kahler DM et al. Retrospective evaluation of graded stress examination of the ankle. *Clinical Orthopaedics and Related Research.* 1996(328):165–170.
61. McKay GD, Goldie PA, Payne WR et al. Ankle injuries in basketball: Injury rate and risk factors. *British Journal of Sports Medicine.* 2001;35(2):103–108.
62. Milgrom C, Finestone A, Segev S et al. Are overground or treadmill runners more likely to sustain tibial stress fracture? *British Journal of Sports Medicine.* 2003;37(2):160–163.
63. Newman P, Witchalls J, Waddington G et al. Risk factors associated with medial tibial stress syndrome in runners: A systematic review and meta-analysis. *Open Access Journal of Sports Medicine.* 2013;4:229–241.
64. Nilstad A, Andersen TE, Bahr R et al. Risk factors for lower extremity injuries in elite female soccer players. *American Journal of Sports Medicine.* 2014;42(4):940–948.
65. Nyland JA, Shapiro R, Caborn DN et al. The effect of quadriceps femoris, hamstring, and placebo eccentric fatigue on knee and ankle dynamics during crossover cutting. *Journal of Orthopaedic & Sports Physical Therapy.* 1997;25(3):171–184.
66. O'Connor FG, Deuster PA, Davis J et al. Functional movement screening: Predicting injuries in officer candidates. *Medicine & Science in Sports & Exercise.* 2011;43(12):2224–2230.
67. Orchard J, Marsden J, Lord S, Garlick D. Preseason hamstring muscle weakness associated with hamstring muscle injury in Australian footballers. *American Journal of Sports Medicine.* 1997;25(1):81–85.
68. Peate WF, Bates G, Lunda K et al. Core strength: A new model for injury prediction and prevention. *Journal of Occupational Medicine and Toxicology.* 2007;2:3.
69. Plisky PJ, Rauh MJ, Kaminski TW et al. Star Excursion Balance Test as a predictor of lower extremity injury in high school basketball players. *Journal of Orthopaedic & Sports Physical Therapy.* 2006;36(12):911–919.
70. Pohl MB, Hamill J, Davis IS. Biomechanical and anatomic factors associated with a history of plantar fasciitis in female runners. *Clinical Journal of Sport Medicine.* 2009;19(5):372–376.
71. Pollock ML, Gettman LR, Milesis CA et al. Effects of frequency and duration of training on attrition and incidence of injury. *Medicine & Science in Sports & Exercise.* 1977;9(1):31–36.
72. Reinschmidt C, Nigg BM. Current issues in the design of running and court shoes. *Sportverletzung Sportschaden: Organ der Gesellschaft fur Orthopadisch-Traumatologische Sportmedizin.* 2000;14(3):71–81.
73. Reynolds KL, Heckel HA, Witt CE et al. Cigarette smoking, physical fitness, and injuries in infantry soldiers. *American Journal of Preventive Medicine.* 1994;10(3):145–150.
74. Rhea MR, Alvar BA, Burkett LN et al. A meta-analysis to determine the dose response for strength development. *Medicine & Science in Sports & Exercise.* 2003;35(3):456–464.
75. Rodriguez NR, Di Marco NM, Langley S. American College of Sports Medicine position stand. Nutrition and athletic performance. *Medicine & Science in Sports & Exercise.* 2009;41(3):709–731.

76. Rozzi SL, Lephart SM, Fu FH. Effects of muscular fatigue on knee joint laxity and neuromuscular characteristics of male and female athletes. *Journal of Athletic Training.* 1999;34(2):106–114.
77. Salata MJ, Gibbs AE, Sekiya JK. The effectiveness of prophylactic knee bracing in american football: A systematic review. *Sports Health.* 2010;2(5):375–379.
78. Serpell BG, Scarvell JM, Ball NB et al. Mechanisms and risk factors for noncontact ACL injury in age mature athletes who engage in field or court sports: A summary of the literature since 1980. *The Journal of Strength & Conditioning Research.* 2012;26(11):3160–3176.
79. Shaffer RA, Brodine SK, Almeida SA et al. Use of simple measures of physical activity to predict stress fractures in young men undergoing a rigorous physical training program. *American Journal of Epidemiology.* 1999;149(3):236–242.
80. Shelbourne KD, Gray T, Haro M. Incidence of subsequent injury to either knee within 5 years after anterior cruciate ligament reconstruction with patellar tendon autograft. *American Journal of Sports Medicine.* 2009;37(2):246–251.
81. Silva CC, Goldberg TB, Teixeira AS et al. The impact of different types of physical activity on total and regional bone mineral density in young Brazilian athletes. *Journal of Sports Sciences.* 2011;29(3):227–234.
82. Skinner HB, Wyatt MP, Hodgdon JA et al. Effect of fatigue on joint position sense of the knee. *Journal of Orthopaedic Research.* 1986;4(1):112–118.
83. Smith HC, Johnson RJ, Shultz SJ et al. A prospective evaluation of the Landing Error Scoring System (LESS) as a screening tool for anterior cruciate ligament injury risk. *American Journal of Sports Medicine.* 2012;40(3):521–526.
84. Steffen K, Emery CA, Romiti M et al. High adherence to a neuromuscular injury prevention programme (FIFA 11+) improves functional balance and reduces injury risk in Canadian youth female football players: A cluster randomised trial. *British Journal of Sports Medicine.* 2013; 47(12):794–802.
85. Sugimoto D, Myer GD, Bush HM et al. Compliance with neuromuscular training and anterior cruciate ligament injury risk reduction in female athletes: A meta-analysis. *Journal of Athletic Training.* 2012;47(6):714–723.
86. Taimela S, Kujala UM, Osterman K. Intrinsic risk factors and athletic injuries. *Sports Medicine.* 1990;9(4):205–215.
87. Teyhen D, Bergeron MF, Deuster P et al. Consortium for health and military performance and American College of Sports Medicine Summit: Utility of functional movement assessment in identifying musculoskeletal injury risk. *Current Sports Medicine Reports.* 2014;13(1):52–63.
88. Torg JS, Quedenfeld TC, Landau S. The shoe-surface interface and its relationship to football knee injuries. *Journal of Sports Medicine.* 1974;2(5):261–269.
89. Trojian TH, McKeag DB. Single leg balance test to identify risk of ankle sprains. *British Journal of Sports Medicine.* 2006;40(7):610–613; discussion 613.
90. Uhorchak JM, Scoville CR, Williams GN et al. Risk factors associated with noncontact injury of the anterior cruciate ligament: A prospective four-year evaluation of 859 West Point cadets. *American Journal of Sports Medicine.* 2003;31(6):831–842.
91. van Gent RN, Siem D, van Middelkoop M, et al. Incidence and determinants of lower extremity running injuries in long distance runners: A systematic review. *British Journal of Sports Medicine.* 2007;41(8):469–480; discussion 480.
92. Voskanian N. ACL Injury prevention in female athletes: Review of the literature and practical considerations in implementing an ACL prevention program. *Current Reviews in Musculoskeletal Medicine.* 2013;6(2):158–163.
93. Wen DY. Risk factors for overuse injuries in runners. *Current Sports Medicine Reports.* 2007;6(5):307–313.
94. Whitney DC, Sturnick DR, Vacek PM et al. Relationship between the risk of suffering a first-time noncontact ACL injury and geometry of the femoral notch and ACL: A prospective cohort study with a nested case-control analysis. *American Journal of Sports Medicine.* 2014;42(8):1796–1805.
95. Williams S, Hume PA, Kara S. A review of football injuries on third and fourth generation artificial turfs compared with natural turf. *Sports Medicine.* 2011;41(11):903–923.
96. Witchalls J, Blanch P, Waddington G et al. Intrinsic functional deficits associated with increased risk of ankle injuries: A systematic review with meta-analysis. *British Journal of Sports Medicine.* 2012;46(7):515–523.
97. Wolff I, van Croonenborg JJ, Kemper HC et al. The effect of exercise training programs on bone mass: A meta-analysis of published controlled trials in pre- and postmenopausal women. *Osteoporosis International.* 1999;9(1):1–12.
98. Zazulak BT, Hewett TE, Reeves NP et al. Deficits in neuromuscular control of the trunk predict knee injury risk: A prospective biomechanical-epidemiologic study. *American Journal of Sports Medicine.* 2007;35(7):1123–1130.
99. Zazulak BT, Hewett TE, Reeves NP et al. The effects of core proprioception on knee injury: A prospective biomechanical-epidemiological study. *American Journal of Sports Medicine.* 2007;35(3):368–373.
100. Zazulak BT, Paterno M, Myer GD et al. The effects of the menstrual cycle on anterior knee laxity: A systematic review. *Sports Medicine.* 2006;36(10):847–862.

37 Protective Equipment

Melissa L. Givens

CONTENTS

TABLE 37.1
Key Clinical Considerations

1. Protective equipment is critical in injury prevention.
2. Protective equipment is useful in both direct contact and indirect contact sports.
3. Sports-specific equipment should be used ensuring proper fit, wear, and proper maintenance.

37.1 INTRODUCTION

Protective equipment is essential for preventing serious injuries or reducing severity of injury. Proper selection, fitting, and maintenance of equipment are critical to ensure protective equipment functions as intended. Protective equipment use is typically associated with contact and collision sports; however, injury can also be mitigated in sports with indirect contact (Table 37.1).

Protective equipment can be off the shelf or customized. Advantages of off-the-shelf equipment include immediate use and possible cost savings. However, proper sizing may be an issue, and this is where customized equipment offers an advantage. Modification of equipment to provide a more comfortable or functional fit may result in loss of protective properties. Additionally, the modifier of the equipment may become liable if injury ensues. Injury liability as a result of equipment inadequacy or defect may fall to the manufacturer.

As a result of concerns for safety standards and potential legal ramifications of injury in relation to equipment use, several organizations are involved in standard development and implementation (see Table 37.2). The National Operating Committee on Standards for Athletic Equipment (NCOSAE) developed voluntary testing standards in an effort to reduce head injuries. Testing standards are available for football and lacrosse helmets and facemasks, ice hockey helmets, and baseball/softball batting helmets. The National Collegiate Athletic Association (NCAA) and National Federation of State High School Association (NFSHSA) adopted the NCOSAE standards for reconditioning and recertification; however, the standard is not a warranty, only a statement that the particular helmet has met the requirements of a performance test when it was manufactured or retested.

Knowledge of sports-specific equipment, to include required/recommended equipment in addition to forbidden equipment, is a key component to ensuring minimal risk of injury for the athlete. Users should adhere to manufacturers' instructions and maintain equipment in accordance with guidelines. Equipment inspection should be routinely performed throughout the season to ensure durability and maintenance of proper fit.

37.2 HEAD AND FACE PROTECTION

The first use of football helmets was reportedly during the Army–Navy game in 1893, but helmet use was not required until 1939 in the NCAA and 1940 in the National Football League (NFL). Head injuries continued to rise despite mandatory helmet use and it was not until 1973 that NOCSAE implemented the first football helmet safety standards.[28] Helmets are specifically designed to protect against the high-energy impacts that result in injuries such as skull fractures and subdural hematomas. It is well documented that the adoption of football helmet standards and use of helmets in high-risk sports results in reduced brain injury-related fatalities and morbidity.[11,16] Helmets also provide protection against soft tissue injury to the head and face as demonstrated by Marshall when comparing injuries to rugby players in comparison with American football players.[25] The ability of helmets to protect against concussion is a much more controversial subject. Concussion injury is often the result of low-energy, linear, and rotational acceleration and deceleration forces. Helmet design is evolving to take account of the forces associated with concussion injury but robust data are not yet available to define the clinical effect of these design evolutions.[12] It is important to understand this limitation of standard head protection in regard to direct collision sports.

Face guards have reduced the number of facial injuries, but there is no evidence to support the theory that face shields reduce concussion risk. Concern is often expressed that face

TABLE 37.2
National Organizations Involved in Protective Equipment Issues

American National Standards Institute	www.ansi.org
American Society for Testing and Materials	www.astm.org
Athletic Equipment Manufacturers Association	www.equipmentmanagers.org
Hockey Equipment Certification Council	www.hecc.net
National Athletic Trainers Association	www.nata.org
National Collegiate Athletic Association	www.ncaa.com
National Association of Intercollegiate Athletics	www.naia.org
National Federation of State High School Athletic Association	www.nfhs.org
National Operating Committee on Standards for Athletic Equipment	www.nocsae.org
Sporting and Fitness Industry Association (formerly Sporting Goods Manufacturers Association)	www.sfia.org
U.S. Consumer Product Safety Commission	www.cpsc.gov

shields may increase concussion risk as the head is more likely to be used as initial point of contact.[12] One study noted that impact to the face shield resulted in higher rotational forces that may translate into greater risk for concussion.[40]

The American Dental Association recommends "mouth protectors for use by participants in sporting and recreational activities with some degree of injury risk and at all levels of competition".[4] Ready-made (stock) mouth guards offer the least protection in contrast to mouth-formed (boil and bite) or custom guards. A well-fitted mouth guard will prevent injury to the teeth and may possibly mitigate concussive forces with impacts to the jaw; however, the data do not support that mouth protectors prevent concussion.[6,9,19,20]

Ear guards are used in wrestling, water polo, and boxing to prevent ear irritation and, ultimately, deformity. A study by Schuller revealed wrestlers are less likely to wear ear guards during practice than competition despite the decreased risk of injury or permanent disfiguration associated with ear guard use.[36]

Athletics are a common etiology for ocular trauma but fortunately the incidence has decreased with use of protective equipment.[26] Glasses may provide some protection if properly fitted but may slip on sweat and fog, detract from peripheral vision, or interfere with headgear. Lenses should be case hardened to crumble instead of splinter on contact. Contact lenses do not fog, degrade peripheral vision, or affect headgear, but there is risk of corneal irritation or lens displacement during play. Eye glasses and guards should be worn in sports with fast-moving projectiles recognizing that the trade-off may be some limitations in vision. Polycarbonate eye shields are available for multiple kinds of headgear. Lenses should be at least 3 mm thick polycarbonate plastic. Nylon sports frames are specifically designed so the lens projects forward when struck instead of posteriorly toward the eye. Athletes with only one functioning eye should wear eye protection for all sports.[2]

37.2.1 Football

Football helmets used at the high school or collegiate level must be certified by NOCSAE. Helmets are marked with exterior labels indicating that the helmet is not designed to strike an opponent. Labeling also indicates that athletes participate at their own risk and that accidental injury may occur, regardless of protective equipment.[27]

There are two basic types of helmets: (1) padded and (2) air and fluid filled. Air-filled helmets are susceptible to change at altitude. Helmet fitting should be performed with wet head to simulate sweat. Follow manufacturer instruction for proper fit, but basic guidelines are as follows: (1) The frontal crown of the helmet should sit one to two fingerbreadths above the eyebrows, (2) the player should be able to extend the neck without impingement by the back of the helmet, (3) grasping the helmet and attempting to rotate it on the head should result in minimal movement, (4) jaw pads should be snug enough to prevent lateral rocking, and (5) the chin strap should have balanced tension on both sides with a snug fit. Proper fit should be routinely checked throughout the season.

Neck rolls may reduce head acceleration and force loads to the cervical spine based on biomechanical analysis; however, robust data on injury prevention are lacking.[34] Mouth guards are also required equipment and regulated use has resulted in a 50% decline in injuries to the mouth.[19,20]

37.2.2 Ice Hockey

The NCAA requires hockey players to wear helmet, facemask, and an internal mouthpiece. The Canadian Standards Association (CSA) must approve ice hockey helmets. Ice hockey helmets are designed to withstand high-velocity impacts (stick or puck) and high-mass low-velocity impacts. Face masks used in high school must meet Hockey Equipment Certifications Council and American Society for Testing Material standards. Face shields in hockey significantly reduce the risk of facial or dental injury without increasing risk of head or neck injury.[5] Throat protection is optional but recommended for goalies due to increased risk.

37.2.3 Baseball

The NCAA requires a double earflap helmet certified by NOCSAE for all batters and base runners. Little league baseball requires helmets for batter, catchers, base runners, first and third base coaches, and on-deck hitters.[24] While the ability of baseball helmets to prevent concussion has not been established, baseball helmets have been shown to reduce injury.[29]

37.2.4 Boxing and Mixed Martial Arts

Controversy exists in regard to boxing headgear and concussion risk. The Amateur International Boxing Association

(AIBA) made the decision to remove headgear for elite fighters, much like their professional counterparts, but still requires headgear for amateur fighters not at the elite level.[18] Argument exists that protective gear may encourage stronger impacts leading to an increased risk of cumulative concussion, or softening the blow may allow the athlete to endure more headshots thus suffering more cumulative injury. Impact dosage studies indicate that padded headgear or gloves decrease cumulative linear dosage and that padded headgear/glove combination has the greatest impact on reducing multiple parameters of injury risk.[7]

37.3 TRUNK AND THORAX PROTECTION

Trunk protection is essential in many sports and is intended to protect regions that are exposed to impact forces including bony protuberances, shoulders, chest cavity, and genitalia. Hip and buttock protection is required in collision and high-velocity sports. Hip and coccyx pads should cover the greater trochanter, iliac crests, and coccyx. Pads may be snap-on, girdle, or wraparound pads.

While proper equipment can protect from injury, there can be increased risks such as use of equipment as an implement in producing trauma or increasing the risk of heat injury, so a balance of necessity versus risk must be found. It is also important to recognize that protective equipment may impede resuscitative efforts because equipment must be removed to provide adequate cardiopulmonary resuscitation (CPR).[13]

37.3.1 Football, Ice Hockey, and Lacrosse Shoulder Pads

There are two types of shoulder pads: cantilevered and noncantilevered. The cantilevered pads are bulkier and designed to provide greater protection as opposed to noncantilevered pads that are less restrictive and provide better range of motion but at the expense of protection. Properly fitted shoulder pads should extend so the inside pad covers the tip of the shoulder, and the neck opening should allow the athlete to raise their arms overhead without pads sliding forward or back. The straps should hold securely in place without causing restriction of friction points. Epaulets and cups should cover the deltoid and allow adequate arm movement. Additional padding may be used for additional protection.

37.3.2 Baseball

Commotio cordis is the second highest cause of death in athletes under 14. Both pitchers and catchers are at risk. Chest protectors for batters and even the bulky chest protectors for catchers do not reliably prevent commotio cordis, so the focus should be on mitigating the risk of balls to the chest and having resuscitation equipment such as an automated external defibrillator (AED) readily available.[13] Chest protectors for catchers do aid in blunting injury from pitches, fouls, and collisions.[3]

37.3.3 Sports Bras

Sports bras are designed to minimize breast movement with the goal of preventing stretching of Cooper's ligament and minimizing breast discomfort associated with running and jumping. Sports bras designed to both elevate and compress breasts have been shown to reduce exercise-induced breast discomfort and bra discomfort in women with larger breasts.[30]

37.3.4 Groin and Genital Protection

Hard cup protection is required for sports involving high-velocity projectiles but should be considered for use in contact sports. Padding to the groin in sports with compressive risk to the perineum such as cycling may decrease compressive nerve symptoms; however, data showing benefit are related to seat padding and not padded shorts.[23]

37.4 SPINE AND LOWER EXTREMITY PROTECTION

Spine protection is most commonly considered in regard to weight lifting. Weight lifting belts can be considered for use during maximal or near maximal lifts above 80% of one repetition maximum.[22] There are also some benefit for submaximal lifts when muscular fatigue limits the supportive capacity of the spinal stabilizers.[21] This is especially important in exercises in which the spinal erectors work against high resistance (squat, dead lift) and in exercises that may result in spinal hyperextension (military press). However, beltless training ensures the spinal stabilizers are engaged and strengthened in order to provide appropriate support in the absence of a lifting belt.[17]

Lower extremity protection may involve selective use of bracing in addition to shin guards and proper footwear. Proper footwear is sports specific but some general principles for proper shoe fit apply universally. The shoe toe box should have adequate space (1/2–3/4 in. from the toe to the front of the shoe). Both feet should be measured when fitting as differences may affect sizing. Fit is best done at the end of the day to allow for swelling and footwear should be tried in approximate conditions of use. The shoe should break at the widest part, which coincides with the ball of the foot.

Shin guards should be worn in soccer and field hockey. The guard should extend the entire length of the tibia. While protection from tibia and fibula fractures is not absolute, shin guards do protect against lower extremity contusions and may reduce anterior compartment syndromes associated with such injuries.[10,35] Different shin guard materials provide varying degrees of protection.[15]

Bracing has been extensively studied in both knee and ankle stability with conflicting results. Bracing may be rehabilitative following injury or functional to provide added support. Knee bracing in football has been shown to increase the risk of anterior cruciate ligament (ACL) injury, but other studies have shown a trend toward reduction of medial collateral ligament (MCL) injuries.[1,33,38] The position statement of the American Academy of Orthopedic

Surgeons, "Prophylactic knee braces may provide limited protection against injuries to the MCL in football players. Scientific studies have not demonstrated similar protection to other knee ligaments, menisci, or articular cartilage," was retired in 2008, and there is currently no consensus statement. Ankle bracing has been shown to have a greater benefit in athletes with prior history of ankle sprain. Cost analysis shows that bracing is less expensive than taping.[32] While bracing may reduce the incidence of ankle injury, it has not been shown to reduce severity of injury.[39]

37.5 SUMMARY

Protective equipment represents a multibillion-dollar industry with projected growth as risk mitigation becomes increasingly important.[7] While some evidence-based recommendations are available for judicious use of protective equipment, there are large gaps in knowledge in regard to the risk–benefit analysis of required or recommended equipment. Ongoing research is necessary to further define the most appropriate use of equipment to protect the athlete from injury. Education in proper selection and fit is important to ensure equipment functions as intended. Future collaboration among industry, athletic organizations, regulatory agencies, and medical professionals is essential to advance the science of protection in sports (Table 37.3).

TABLE 37.3
SORT: Key Recommendations for Practice

Clinical Recommendation	Evidence Rating	References
Knowledge of sports-specific equipment, to include required/recommended equipment in addition to forbidden equipment, is a key component to ensuring minimal risk of injury for the athlete.	C	
Helmets should be worn in high-risk sports to protect against high-velocity injuries understanding that protection from concussion may be limited.	A	[10,15,20]
Mouth guards should be worn in both sports and recreational activities with some degree of risk in order to protect against dental injury.	A	[16,17]
Athletes in sports with risk for ocular trauma should wear eye protection. Athletes with only one functioning eye should wear eye protection in all sports.	A	[2,23]
Shin guards should be worn in sports with risk of lower extremity trauma to reduce shin contusions and possibly reduce risk of fracture and compartment syndrome.	B	[9,28]
Ankle braces should be considered in patients who have suffered previous ankle injury to reduce the risk of recurrent injury.	B	[26]

REFERENCES

1. Albright JP, Powell JW, Smith W et al. Medial collateral ligament knee sprains in college football: Effectiveness of preventive braces. *The American Journal of Sports Medicine.* 1994;22(1):12–18.
2. American Academy of Ophthalmology. Protective eyewear for young athletes. Joint Policy Statement American Academy of Pediatrics and American Academy of Ophthalmology. 2003. http://www.aao.org/about/policy/upload/Protective-Eyewear-for-Young-Athletes.pdf. Accessed April 15, 2014.
3. American Academy of Pediatrics. Policy Statement: Baseball and Softball. *Pediatrics.* 2012;129(3):842–856.
4. American Dental Association. Statement on athletic mouthguards. http://www.ada.org/1875.aspx. Accessed April 11, 2014.
5. Aspplund C, Bettcher S, Borchers J. Facial protection and head injuries in ice hockey: A systematic review. *British Journal of Sports Medicine.* 2009;43(13):993–999.
6. Barbic D, Pater J, Brison RJ. Comparison of mouth guard designs and concussion prevention in contact sports: A multicenter randomized controlled trial. *Clinical Journal of Sport Medicine* 2005;15(5):294–298.
7. Bartsch AJ, Benzel EC, Miele VJ et al. Boxing and mixed martial arts: Preliminary traumatic neuromechanical injury risk analyses from laboratory impact dosage. *Journal of Neurosurgery.* 2012;116:1070–1080.
8. BCC Research. Protective Sports Equipment: The North American Market. July 2013.
9. Benson BW, Hamilton GW, Meeuwisse WH et al. Is protective equipment useful in preventing concussion? A systematic review of the literature. *British Journal of Sports Medicine.* 2009;43(Suppl 1):i56–57.
10. Boden BP, Lohnes JH, Nunley JA et al. Tibia and fibula fractures in soccer players. *Knee Surgery, Sports Traumatology, Arthroscopy.* 1999;7(4):262–266.
11. Cantu RC, Mueller FO. Brain injury related fatalities in American football. *Neurosurgery* 2003;52(4):846–852.
12. Daneshvar DH, Baugh CM, Nowinski CJ et al. Helmets and Mouthguards: The role of personal protective equipment in preventing sports related concussions. *Clinics in Sports Medicine.* 2011;30(1):145–163.
13. Del Rossi G, Bodkin D, Dhanani A et al. Protective athletic equipment slows initiation of CPR in simulated cardiac arrest. *Resuscitation* 2011;82(7):908–912.
14. Doererr JJ, Haas TS, Estes NA 3rd et al. Evaluation of chest barriers for pretection against sudden death due to commotio cordis. *American Journal of Cardiology.* 2007; 99(6):857–859.
15. Francisco AC, Nightingale RW, Guilak F et al. Comparison of Soccer Shin guards in preventing tibia fracture. *American Journal of Sports Medicine.* 2000;28(2):227–233.
16. Haider AH, Saleem T, Bilaniuk JW et al. An evidence based review: Efficacy of safety helmets in the reduction of head injuries in recreational skiers and snowboarders. *Journal of Trauma and Acute Care Surgery.* 2012;73(5):1340–1347.
17. Harman E, Rosenstein R, Frykman P et al. Effects of a belt on intra-abdominal pressure during weight lifting. *Medicine & Science in Sports & Exercise.* 1989;21:186–190.
18. International Boxing Association. AIBA Open Boxing Competition Rules. August 23, 2013. http://www.aiba.org/documents/site1/docs/Rules/AOB%20Competition%20Rules%20-%20August%2023%202013.pdf. Accessed April 11, 2014.
19. Knapik JJ, Marshall SW, Lee RB et al. Mouthguards in sports activities: History, physical properties, and injury prevention effectiveness. *Sports Medicine.* 2007;37(2):117–144.

20. Kvittem B, HArdie NA, Roettger M et al. Incidence of orofacial injuries in high school sports. *Journal of Public Health Dentistry*. 1998;58(4):288–293.
21. Lander JJ, Hundley J, Simonton RL. The effectiveness of weight belts during multiple repetitions of the squat exercise. *Medicine & Science in Sports & Exercise*. 1992;24:603–608.
22. Lander JJ, Simonton RL, Giacobbe J. The effectiveness of weight belts during the squat exercise. *Medicine & Science in Sports & Exercise*. 1990;22:117–124.
23. Leibovitch I, Mor Y. The vicious cycling: Bicycling related urogenital disorders. *European Urology*. 2005;47:277–287.
24. Little League Baseball. Equipment Checklist. http://www.littleleague.org/Assets/forms_pubs/asap/Equipment Checklist.pdf. Accessed April 11, 2014.
25. Marshall SW, Waller AE, Dick RW. An ecologic study of protective equipment and injury in two contact sports. *International Journal of Epidemiology*. 2002;31:587–592.
26. May DR, Kuhn FP, Morris RE et al. The epidemiology of serious eye injuries from the United States Eye Registry. *Graefe's Archive for Clinical and Experimental Ophthalmology*. 2000;238(2):153–157.
27. National Collegiate Atheltic Association. Compiled by Klossner D. The NCAA Sports Medicine Handbook. NCAA. 2012.
28. National Operating Committee on Standards for Athletic Equipment. http://nocsae.org/about-nocsae/history-and-purpose/. Accessed April 15, 2014.
29. Nicholls RL, Elliott BC, Miller K. Impact injuries in baseball: Prevalence, aetiology and the role of equipment performance. *Sports Medicine*. 2004;34(1):17–25.
30. McGhee DE, Steele JR. Breast elevation and compression decrease exercise induced breast discomfort. *Medicine and Science in Sports and Medicine*. 2010;42(7):1333–1338.
31. Martin TJ. Technical Report: Knee brace use in the young athlete. *Pediatrics*. 2001;108(2):503–507.
32. Olmstead LC, Vela LI, Denegar CR et al. Prophylactic ankle taping and bracing: A numbers needed to treat and cost benefit analysis. *Journal of Athletic Training*. 2004;39(1):95–100.
33. Rovere GD, Haupt HA, Yates CS. Prophylactic knee bracing in college sports. *American Journal of Sports Medicine*. 1987;15(2):111–116.
34. Rowson S, McNeely DE, Brolinson P et al. Biomechanical analysis of football neck collars. *Clinical Journal of Sport Medicine*. 2008;18(4):316–321.
35. Saartok Tonu. Muscle injuries associated with soccer. *Clinics in Sports Medicine*. 1998;17(4):811–817.
36. Schuller, DE, Dankle SK, Martin M et al. Auricular injury and the use of headgear in wrestlers. *Archives of Otolaryngology – Head and Neck Surgery*. 1989;115(6):714–717.
37. Sigurdsson A. Evidence based review of prevention of dental injuries. *Pediatric Dentistry*. 2013;35(2):184–190.
38. Sitler M, Ryan J, Hopkinson W et al. The efficacy of prophylactic knee brace to reduce knee injuries in football. A prospective randomized study at West Point. *American Journal of Sports Medicine*. 1990;18(3):310–315.
39. Sitler M, Ryan J, Wheeler B et al. The efficacy of semirigid ankle stabilizer to reduce acute ankle injuries in basketball. A randomized clinical study at West Point. *American Journal of Sports Medicine*. 1994;22(4):454–461.
40. Viano DC, Casson IR, Pellman EJ. Concussion in professional football: Biomechanics of the struck player—Part 14. *Neurosurgery*. 2007;61(2):313–327; discussion 327–318.

38 Complementary and Alternative Medicine for the Sports Medicine Physician

Wayne B. Jonas, Erika S. Reese, and Anthony I. Beutler

CONTENTS

TABLE 38.1
Key Clinical Considerations

1. CAM is increasing in use in the United States; it would help both patients and physicians to partner in these practices.
2. Glucosamine and chondroitin in combination have been shown to have benefit in moderate to severe OA, but have not shown benefit alone.
3. Ephedra is banned by NCAA and is harmful to athletes.
4. Arnica has shown some benefits to short-term pain relief with minimal side effects and could be considered as a treatment for DOMS.
5. Acupuncture may be helpful in the treatment of lateral elbow pain, low back pain, knee and shoulder pain, and Achilles tendinopathy.
6. Massage has shown some benefit in chronic low back pain, DOMS, and OA.

38.1 INTRODUCTION

Western biomedicine (i.e., the medicine practiced in American hospitals) represents just one of the many medical practices and philosophies in the world today. In fact, 80% of the world's population receives their medical care from a system outside of traditional Western biomedicine.[89] These other medical systems and practices are collectively referred to as *complementary and alternative medicine* (CAM), sometimes called complementary and integrative medicine (CIM). CAM practices continue to increase in popularity and prevalence in traditionally Western populations; however, the safety and efficacy of many CAM practices remain undetermined, and the question of how to integrate the evaluation and discussion of CAM therapies in everyday patient care continues to challenge physicians from many specialties. This chapter (1) briefly defines CAM, (2) identifies which segments of the population are likely to use CAM, (3) outlines an ethical and evidence-supported approach for sports medicine physicians to use in evaluating and using CAM therapies or in caring for or counseling with athletes, and (4) summarizes the best efficacy and safety evidence for a few of the myriad CAM therapies used by athletes today (Tables 38.1 and 38.2).

38.2 BRIEF DEFINITION OF CAM

Ayurveda, traditional oriental medicine, and Native American practices predate Western medicine, with spiritualism and traditional oriental medicine both boasting longer histories and larger enrollments than Western medicine.[131] The term CAM is a recent and decidedly Western term that seeks to describe the "broad domain of healing resources ... [including] health systems, modalities, practices, and their accompanying theories and beliefs"[101] that fall outside the theories and treatments typically taught in Western medical schools and practiced in Western hospitals. Table 38.3 provides a CAM classification system based on the terminology used by the National Center for Complementary and Alternative Medicine (now known as the National Center for Complementary and Integrative Health) at the National Institutes of Health.

CAM is exclusionary by definition in that it is Western biomedicine's name for everything that lies outside its bounds. As such, the boundaries of CAM remain imprecise. For example, are glucosamine prescriptions for osteoarthritis and dry needling of chronic tendinosis considered CAM treatments or accepted Western treatments? Indeed, as our understanding of CAM techniques and treatment continues to evolve, so do the boundaries and definitions of what is considered CAM. Still, however, unwieldy and imprecise terms, the words *complementary* and *alternative* do accurately describe the

TABLE 38.2
Summary of Evidence and Recommendations for Common CAM Therapies

CAM Therapy	Purported Benefit	Evidence	Cost[a]	Toxicity (Side Effects)	Cautions (Interactions)[b]	Regulated Substance	Recommended Action
Glucosamine	Relief of osteoarthritis (OA) pain and stiffness, temporomandibular joint (TMJ) dysfunction	Previous trials and meta-analysis showed benefit from glucosamine when compared to placebo in treating OA.[28,31,103,83] Data suggested that pain relief is similar to or better than NSAIDs,[105] especially long term.[80] However recent trials including the GAIT (Glucosamine/chondroitin Arthritis Intervention Trial) have shown no significant benefit except when combined with chondroitin in the treatment of moderate to severe OA, when compared to placebo.[24] A 2010 Meta-analysis in the *Annals of Pharmacotherapy* showed no significant improvement in pain or joint space narrowing when evaluating glucosamine, chondroitin or combination.[140] Limited evidence suggests that glucosamine may slow progression of OA.[97] Most studies involve knee OA, but more limited data suggest that glucosamine may be effective in TMJ syndromes[124] and OA of the spine.[41]	Moderate($1–$2 per day)	Mild gastrointestinal distress, comparable to placebo	Use with caution in diabetics or impaired glucose tolerance (IGT); may increase insulin resistance. Concern for shellfish allergy, but no reactions reported.	No	Consider in treatment of moderate to severe OA and monitor for improvement.
Ephedra(ma huang, herbal ecstasy, teamster's tea, zhong ma huang)	Weight loss, enhanced athletic performance, respiratory conditions, asthma	Small, short-term weight loss (2.7–5.3 kg) over 6 wk–6 mo in patients with BMI < 30 when used with other stimulants (caffeine, guaraná, etc.)[17] Not thought to improve athletic performance[25,30,49,115] unless used in combination with caffeine[15,16] or in very high doses.[25,26]	Low ($0.30–$0.75 per day)	Dizziness, restlessness, anxiety, heart palpitations, tachycardia, hypertension, myocardial infarction, stroke	Adverse effects occur even in healthy patients; capsules often contain impurities, including banned substances.	Banned by the military and International Olympic Committee (IOC) and restricted by FDA.	*Protect* — As negative publicity builds, the number of ephedra-free products increases; however, these may not be any safer than original ephedra products.

(*Continued*)

TABLE 38.2 (*Continued*)
Summary of Evidence and Recommendations for Common CAM Therapies

CAM Therapy	Purported Benefit	Evidence	Cost[a]	Toxicity (Side Effects)	Cautions (Interactions)[b]	Regulated Substance	Recommended Action
Chondroitin	Relief of osteoarthritis, topical use for relief of dry eyes	A recent meta analysis in 2010 found no significant benefit to chondroitin.[140] Several previous trials suggest that chondroitin + NSAIDs is more effective than NSAIDs alone in OA.[75,89] Combination tablets contain glucosamine, manganese, and chondroitin, but it is unclear if combination therapy is better than treatment with any individual component.[126] As stated above, a recent study has shown some benefit with combination glucosamine/ chondroitin in the treatment of moderate to severe OA.[24] Many trials are limited by study quality. Topical uses include FDA-approved product for cornea/cataract treatment (Viscoat®) and investigational treatment for dry eyes.[77]	Moderate ($1–$2 per day); often sold in "joint health" combos	Mild gastrointestinal distress comparable to placebo; combo tablets may exceed safe daily dosage of manganese and cause central nervous system irritability	Potential exists for contamination with diseased animal parts. Use with caution in patients taking anticoagulants (chondroitin has heparinoid structure and may have anticoagulant effects)	No	*Permit* — No adverse effects in 5-year studies; if no clinical effect is noted after 6 to 8 weeks of therapy, discontinue chondroitin (due to moderate cost). Consider risk to benefit in a patient/physician conversation, as benefit is not proven, but adverse effects are not common.
Homeopathy (arnica)	Relief of delayed onset muscle soreness (DOMS)	A recent small study showed decreased pain at 72 hours post exercise but no improvement in performance with the use of arnica in DOMS. Homeopathy is a medical system involving multiple pharmacologic treatments. No single homeopathic treatment has conclusively demonstrated efficacy in DOMS.[39,137,78] A few, small trials have reported positive results in marathon runners;[132,131] similar trials exist that report no such benefit.[138] A recent small study showed decreased pain at 72 hours post exercise but no improvement in performance with the use of arnica in DOMS.[104] Trials are limited by their small treatment groups, the bewildering array of homeopathic remedies, and the differing methods of inducing and defining DOMS.	Low ($0.10–$0.20 per day)	Headaches, fatigue, rash, dizziness, gastrointestinal upset, and increased symptoms reported but not above placebo levels.[27]	Reports of severe allergic reactions appear anecdotal.	Yes. FDA regulates homeopathic remedies in a separate category from dietary supplements but many manufacturers, patients and practitioners do not follow these regulations.	*Permit* — The homeopathic system is too complex to be adequately evaluated with the current evidence; however, costs are low and toxicities minimal in the hands of trained practitioners.

(*Continued*)

TABLE 38.2 (*Continued*)
Summary of Evidence and Recommendations for Common CAM Therapies

CAM Therapy	Purported Benefit	Evidence	Cost[a]	Toxicity (Side Effects)	Cautions (Interactions)[b]	Regulated Substance	Recommended Action
Magnetic field therapy (pulsed electromagnetic field therapy, PEMF)	Decreased pain and stiffness in osteoarthritis	PEMF therapy is already considered a proven remedy for delayed union fractures.[13] Similar fields have been found to stimulate proteoglycan synthesis in chondrocytes,[1,61] which has fueled interest in treatment. Anecdotal accounts abound on Internet sites; however, a recent *Cochrane Review* found only three published articles that met inclusion criteria for their meta-analysis.[61] The meta-analysis concludes that, while PEMF therapy produces statistically significant reductions in knee OA pain and disability, pain and disability from cervical OA is not significantly reduced. Moreover, though statistically significant, the reduction in knee OA symptoms is not likely to be clinically significant. Many questions remain regarding optimum dosage, frequency, and technical specifications of PEMF therapy.	High ($20–$200 per day)	Unknown; effects of PEMF treatment on body tissues are unknown	Caution is advised in this unregulated arena; high-cost interventions with no proven benefit may create potential for fraud and abuse.	No	*Protect* — High-cost treatment has unknown side effects and uncertain efficacy. Until completion of further study on optimum treatment regimens and long-term effects or toxicities, protect patients from "high-tech" regimens that provide none of the promised relief.
Acupuncture	Decreases in: 1. Lateral elbow pain 2. Low back pain 3. Shoulder pain 4. Knee pain 5. Achilles tendinopathy	Acupuncture can be considered an alternative health care system. The variety of approaches and limited available evidence on each approach makes it difficult completely endorse or refute this system as a whole. However, a recent large individual data meta-analysis showed that MS pain relief from acupuncture is safe and effective beyond placebo.[136] For acupuncture in lateral elbow pain, a 2002 *Cochrane Review*[51] found four small RCTs, all unique enough to preclude combination into a single meta-analysis. The review concludes that no pain decrease has been demonstrated beyond 24 hours and that insufficient evidence exists to support or refute the use of acupuncture in lateral elbow pain. A 2004 systematic review supported the notion that short term relief may be a benefit of acupuncture, but due to heterogeneity of the studies and other limitations, this cannot be firmly concluded.[129]	Variable ($20–$100 per session)	Commonly reported side effects: pain, fatigue, bleeding, fainting, nausea, and dizziness	Pneumothorax, broken needles, and increased risks of infectious disease have been reported but are uncommon in the hands of licensed practitioners.	No	*Permit and Promote* — A preponderance of evidence suggests that acupuncture is effective for postoperative nausea and dental pain. It may have some benefit in short term relief of chronic low back pain.[65] Unfortunately, acupuncture has no proven

(*Continued*)

TABLE 38.2 (*Continued*)
Summary of Evidence and Recommendations for Common CAM Therapies

CAM Therapy	Purported Benefit	Evidence	Cost[a]	Toxicity (Side Effects)	Cautions (Interactions)[b]	Regulated Substance	Recommended Action
		Acupuncture for low back pain is discussed in a 2005 *Cochrane review*, in which 35 RCT's were included, 3 for acute low back pain. There was no proven benefit to acupuncture in acute back pain, but some short term decrease in pain and improvement in function was found in chronic low back pain when compared to control groups. It was also suggested that acupuncture and dry needling may be effective when used in combination with other therapies. This is a change from the previous It was also suggested that acupuncture and dry needling may be effective when used in combination with other therapies.[45] *This is a change from the previous Cochrane Review*,[130] in which 11 RCTs are summarized, most of poor quality. The highest quality RCTs compare acupuncture with placebo or sham acupuncture; of these, one reported positive results[32] and one negative results.[46] Shoulder pain is another area where acupuncture has shown some benefit. A 2008 multicentre randomized controlled trial showed that single-point acupuncture in adjunctive treatment with physiotherapy shows improvement in pain and function when compared to physiotherapy alone. This study compared single-point acupuncture and physiotherapy to mock tens and physiotherapy.[135] Yet another RCT found no difference between corticosteroid injections and acupuncture combined with home exercises in treating subacromial impingment.[62] A recent RCT evaluating acupuncture compared to eccentric exercises using a VISA-A questionnaire and VAS for evaluation of acupuncture in the treatment of chronic Achilles tendinopathy found potential benefit in pain and activity with acupuncture.[62] Recently, a large individual data meta-analysis demonstrated that acupuncture was safe and effective for musculoskeletal pain beyond placebo (sham) acupuncture.[136] A recent RCT evaluating acupuncture compared to eccentric exercises using a VISA-A questionnaire and VAS for evaluation of acupuncture in the treatment of chronic Achilles tendinopathy found potential benefit in pain and activity with acupuncture.[155]					efficacy in lateral elbow pain. It may have some benefit in short term relief of chronic low back pain.[58] It may have effect in osteo-arthritis; however, compare to lower cost treatments. Patients should be permitted to use acupuncture for OA with a warning regarding potential for high costs. Recent data suggests some benefit for chronic Achilles tendinopathy, and shoulder pain and may be considered as a treatment option.

(*Continued*)

TABLE 38.2 (*Continued*)
Summary of Evidence and Recommendations for Common CAM Therapies

CAM Therapy	Purported Benefit	Evidence	Cost[a]	Toxicity (Side Effects)	Cautions (Interactions)[b]	Regulated Substance	Recommended Action
St. John's wort	*Oral:* antidepressant, anxiolytic, insomnia, adjunct to weight loss *Topical:* wound healing, anti-inflammatory cream	Considerable, but not unanimous evidence for efficacy in mild–moderate depression.[60,143,47,79] Antidepressant efficacy is better than placebo, similar to low-dose tricyclic antidepressants (TCAs)[100,151] and slightly less effective than selective serotonin reuptake inhibitors (SSRIs).[18,112] St. John's wort should not be used in severe depression, as higher dosages increase the risk for potentially severe skin reactions. Preliminary evidence suggests that St. John's wort may be effective in obsessive–compulsive disorder (OCD).[123] St. John's wort has *in vitro* antibacterial, antiviral, and anti-inflammatory properties that would support its topical use;[110,111] however, no clinical data exist.	Low ($0.10–$0.50 per day)	Insomnia, restlessness, agitation, anxiety, mild GI distress, headache; daily dose over 2 g (5 mg hypericin) increases risk for potentially severe photodermatitis; fewer side effects than TCAs and SSRIs	Multiple, potentially severe herb–herb and herb–drug interactions (TCAs, triptans, oral contraceptives, anti-HIV drugs, warfarin, digoxin) are possible. Combined use with other antidepressants may increase risk for serotonin syndrome.	Not banned by athletic regulatory agencies; banned by government in France. United Kingdom, Japan, and other European governments are investigating.	*Permit* — Acceptable in monitored patients with mild–moderate depression with simple medical regimens if patient prefers it over conventional treatments and is not on other medications with which it interacts.
Ginkgo leaf (*Ginkgo* seed is also used as a supplement, but has different purported efficacies and toxicities than *Ginkgo* leaf)	*Oral:* slows onset of dementia and memory loss, relieves claudication and premenstrual syndrome (PMS) *Topical:* used to treat chilblains (mild cold injury) and improve blood flow in wound healing	Majority of evidence indicates some effect in stabilizing or slowing dementia progression.[74,72,133] In other countries, *Ginkgo* is the treatment of choice for dementia,[72] with effects similar to cholinesterase inhibitors used in the United States.[94] *Ginkgo* appears effective in increasing cognitive function in middle-aged individuals without complaints of memory loss.[106,121] *Ginkgo* + *P. ginseng* may be even more effective for this indication (see below). *Ginkgo* also appears to increase walking distance in patients with vascular claudication[99,101] Insufficient clinical evidence exists to evaluate the other purported benefits of *Ginkgo* therapy.	Moderate ($1–$2 per day)	Mild gastrointestinal upset, palpitations, constipation, headache, skin reactions; diarrhea, vomiting, and weakness in larger doses; serious spontaneous bleeding and seizures reported with *Ginkgo* use	Does not "reverse" dementia and is not a cure for Alzheimer's. Use with extreme caution in patients on anticoagulants or antiplatelet therapy. Avoid in patients with seizure disorder or with other drugs that lower seizure threshold.	No	*Permit* — Acceptable in monitored patients without medical contraindications if patient prefers it over conventional drug treatments; contraindicated in patients on anticoagulants.

(*Continued*)

TABLE 38.2 (*Continued*)
Summary of Evidence and Recommendations for Common CAM Therapies

CAM Therapy	Purported Benefit	Evidence	Cost[a]	Toxicity (Side Effects)	Cautions (Interactions)[b]	Regulated Substance	Recommended Action
Creatine	Increases lean body mass, improves strength, improves athletic performance	Considerable, but not unanimous, support exists for an ergogenic effect in repetitive strength tasks lasting <30 sec;[146,21,134] this effect may be most pronounced in individuals with low to normal levels of endogenous muscle creatine.[53] Increased body mass may impair performance in endurance events. Caffeine consumption may negate ergogenic effects of creatine supplementation.	Low ($0.25–$0.75 per day)	Common side effects: gastrointestinal upset, diarrhea, cramping; reported side effects: cardiomyopathy, renal failure, arrhythmias, rhabdomyolysis	Use with caution with other nephrotoxic drugs (i.e., NSAIDs, cyclosporine, aminoglycosides)	No; the National Collegiate Athletic Association (NCAA) prohibits universities from providing creatine for their athletes.	*Permit* — Can be used after discussion of risks and benefits in healthy patients in appropriate events. Not appropriate for use in athletes with kidney disease, pediatric athletes, or athletes prone to dehydration or heat injury.
Massage therapy	1. Relief of delayed onset muscle soreness, minimize strength loss after exercise 2. Osteoarthritis treatment 3. Low back pain	A few, small trials show mixed results for preventing DOMS with post-exceptional massage therapy. Most studies suffer from small sample sizes. Three trials report a significant positive effect of massage on DOMS;[53,125,10,116] three others show no significant effect or have such severe methodological flaws that their results cannot be interpreted.[107,36,141] A recent review concluded that, while massage is a promising therapy for DOMS, larger, more rigorous trials are required.[38] A 2006 RCT of 68 adults receiving massage vs delayed treatment showed improvement in WOMAC (Western Ontario and McMaster Universities Osteoarthritis index) pain and function scores as well as VAS (visual analogue scale) improvements. However cost effectiveness has not been analyzed adequately.[98] Massage has also proved promising for low back pain. A 2008 Cochrane review of 13RCT's showed benefit in pain and function with massage when compared to other therapies such as sham, joint mobilization, relaxation therapy, physical therapy, acupuncture and self-care. This was applicable to patients with subacute and chronic non-specific low back pain. A barrier to care, however, may be the potential cost for massage therapy. High costs could make it less accessible for patients. This was applicable to patients with subacute and chronic non-specific low back pain. A barrier to care, however, may be the potential cost for massage therapy. High costs could make it less accessible for patients.[44]	High; greatest effects found in repeated massage sessions for 48 to 92 hours post-exercise	No known toxicities	None	No	*Permit* — Despite high cost and questionable efficacy, no major harmful effects have been reported from massage.

(*Continued*)

TABLE 38.2 (*Continued*)
Summary of Evidence and Recommendations for Common CAM Therapies

CAM Therapy	Purported Benefit	Evidence	Cost[a]	Toxicity (Side Effects)	Cautions (Interactions)[b]	Regulated Substance	Recommended Action
Spinal manipulation	Relief of low back pain and low back stiffness; allows more rapid return to play following low back injury	A 2011 RCT of 60 patients with chronic non specific low back pain showed improvement in pain and disability scores through SMT when compared to sham (control). The study also suggests greater benefit in maintained SMT over a 9 month period. Bulk of evidence suggests that spinal manipulation is at least as effective as conventional treatment for low back pain.[6,7,86,73] A 2011 RCT of 60 patients with chronic non specific low back pain showed improvement in pain and disability scores through SMT when compared to sham (control). The study also suggests greater benefit in maintained SMT over a 9 month period.[113] A Cochrane review of 26 RCT's however states that when compared to other interventions, SMT is not clinically different. There has been some evidence to suggest improved short term benefits in pain and function, but this is difficult to conclude based on quality of evidence.[108] Whereas a previous review noted that 9 of 10 RCTs with the highest quality scores concluded that spinal manipulation was better than the control treatments.[7] However, justifiable concern still exists for differences in manipulation techniques and case reports of severe complications.[73] Some authors distinguish between sciatica and low back pain (LBP). Most of these discourage manipulation for sciatica; however, insufficient evidence exists to support or refute this view.[114]	High; *New England Journal of Medicine* reviewed 8 visits in 12 wks (may be covered by insurance)	None	Rare reports of stroke, paralysis, or spinal cord damage in the literature, but almost exclusively from C-spine manipulation. No severe complications reported in over 15,000 patients enrolled in RCTs.[7]	No	*Permit* — In the hands of a competent practitioner, L-spine manipulation is safe and likely effective, although it is higher cost than conventional treatment.
Cromium picolinate	Increases muscle mass, decreases body fat, improves glycemic control in diabetes, lowers cholesterol, treats mild depression	Increased muscle and decreased fat were suggested by early, poorly designed studies.[128,81] Better, newer studies suggest no ergogenic or fat-burning effect.[58,71] Improved glycemic control and lipid profiles are produced in diabetic patients;[5,42] time to effect and size of effect depend on daily dose. Promising initial studies have been done on chromium in depression, but more data are needed.[85]	Low ($0.10–$0.30 per day)	Cognitive and motor dysfunction Sleep changes, mood changes, headaches	Not a cure for diabetes; some concern for DNA mutagenic effects with high-dose, long-term use[119]	No	*Protect* — Minimal toxicity and low cost with short-term use are outweighed by risk of DNA mutations and no proven limited benefits of long-term chromium use.

(*Continued*)

TABLE 38.2 (*Continued*)
Summary of Evidence and Recommendations for Common CAM Therapies

CAM Therapy	Purported Benefit	Evidence	Cost[a]	Toxicity (Side Effects)	Cautions (Interactions)[b]	Regulated Substance	Recommended Action
Panax ginseng (different species of *ginseng* are not equivalent and in many cases are not even biologically related; the data reported here are for *Panax ginseng*, the most commonly used *ginseng*)	Improve athletic performance, increase cognitive function, and treatment of many other ailments	Multiple studies suggest no enhanced athletic performance with oral *ginseng* use.[9,90,3,37] *P. ginseng* use has not been shown to improve memory,[117] but *P. ginseng* + *Ginkgo* may be effective in improving memory in healthy, middle-aged people.[142] Minimal clinical evidence suggests that *ginseng* might be effective in diabetes mellitus treatment,[118] in decreasing cancer risk,[154] in improving mood,[35] and in preventing influenza and the common cold.[109]	Low ($0.25–$0.75 per day)	Insomnia, tachycardia, palpitations, mastalgia, vaginal bleeding, amenorrhea	Intensifies effects of other stimulants (caffeine, guaraná, tea); *ginseng* has hormonal (estrogenic) effects; continuous, long-term (>3 mo) use is not well studied.	No	*Permit* — Studies suggest minimal toxicity in short-term use. Long-term use is questionable due to risk of estrogen-like effects and minimal reported benefits of *ginseng*

[a] Cost data from www.epocrates.com and www.drugstore.com, unless otherwise referenced.

[b] The authors are grateful to the owners of the Natural Medicines Comprehensive Database who made their database available. Herbal toxicities and interactions are from this database, unless otherwise referenced.

utilization of these practices by individuals in Western society. Survey data suggest that less than 5% of those who use CAM do so exclusively or as an alternative to conventional biomedicine.[9] The remaining 95% utilize CAM to complement, or in addition to, conventional medical treatment.

38.3 WHO USES CAM?

Two decades ago, Americans spent more than $27 billion out of pocket annually on CAM, and this rose to $36 billion in 2007.[13,38,55] Visits to CAM practitioners rose from 400 million per year in 1990 to 600 million per year in 1996. In the year 2000, visits to CAM providers rose to 65 visits per 1000 population per month. Primary care clinicians saw 113 visits per 1000 population per month in that same time period.[55] CAM use rates hover around 40%–50% of the population in the United States, United Kingdom, and Australia and reach 75% in France. Recent National Health Interview Survey (NHIS) data from 2007 showed that one in every nine children used CAM therapy.[13] With 100 million Americans supplementing their diets with vitamins, herbs, minerals, and amino acids, perhaps the more appropriate question is "Who doesn't use CAM?"

Many large, well-designed surveys reveal that CAM users tend to be better educated, wealthier, and more likely to have a chronic disease or chronic pain than CAM nonusers.[2,9,22,91,165] Minorities, especially African-Americans, are less likely to use CAM, while women are more likely to use CAM. CAM users are more likely to hold a holistic philosophy toward their health. Interestingly, dissatisfaction with conventional care does not predict those who use CAM as a complement to conventional medicine; however, mistrust of and disaffection with conventional medicine are more common in those who use CAM exclusively (alternatively), as is a desire to retain control over one's health care.[22,38,55,91]

The population of many developing countries relies on CAM practices for most or all of their health care needs.[106] And, even in countries dominated by Western biomedicine, the public employs CAM practices in the treatment of a wide array of major and minor medical problems. Popular and multiple CAM remedies exist for minor ailments such as colds, acne, muscle pain, and arthritis. On the other side of the disease spectrum, 50%–70% of patients with cancer and 50% of those with human immunodeficiency virus will utilize CAM therapies over the course of their illness.[24] According to the NHIS of 2002 and 2007, CAM use increased from 35% to 37% in those not affected by cancer and from 39% to 44% in those affected by cancer.[13,14] Data in 2007 also showed an increase in use of acupuncture, deep breathing, massage, meditation, naturopathy, and yoga.[13] Yeh et al.,[165] however, note an important distinction in their recent study of CAM use in patients with diabetes mellitus. While 57% of those with diabetes used CAM therapies in a year, only 20% used these therapies to treat their diabetes. Yeh notes that CAM use is likely to be less in maladies where the population believes that traditional medicine has a good understanding of the disease process and effective treatments for the disease itself.

38.4 USE OF CAM AMONG ATHLETES

Athletes use CAM therapies to enhance performance and to speed return to play following an injury. Caffeine, creatine, guaraná, and *Ginkgo biloba* are just a few examples of substances with purported performance-enhancing effects. Microcurrents, electrical stimulation, iontophoresis, spinal manipulation, magnets, and acupuncture represent a smattering of the myriad of treatments used to control pain and speed the athlete's return to the playing field. The high pressure and high stakes of athletic competition demand heightened vigilance on the part of the sports medicine physicians to ensure the safety of those entrusted to their care.[157]

38.5 ROLE OF THE SPORTS MEDICINE PHYSICIAN IN CAM

Sports medicine physicians should help patients make informed choices about CAM treatments and therapies, just as they would assist their patients in decisions involving conventional medical treatments. While many effective strategies may be employed in advising CAM patients, the strategy proposed by Jonas[73] suggests that the physician's counsel should vary depending on the patient and treatment being discussed. Specifically, the sports medicine physician should *protect*, *permit*, *promote*, and *partner* with their patients regarding CAM practices.[71]

38.5.1 Protecting Patients from Risk

Not surprisingly, conventional physicians are frequently faced with questions about the safety of CAM. Many CAM practices present minimal risk to the patient when performed by competent providers; however, two of the most popular CAM practices in the United States, herbal and high-dose vitamin supplementation, have potential for serious, even fatal toxicities.[33] Many patients harbor the false assumption that "natural" equals "safe." A very public example of the risk of some CAM supplements and the naiveté of many athletes occurred with the death of Steve Bechler. A professional pitcher for the Baltimore Orioles, Bechler's collapse and death during spring training of 2003 was at least partially due to the diet herb ephedra.[113] Hence, the sports medicine physician should remind his patients that many known pharmacologically active herbs have real effects, real side effects, and relatively narrow therapeutic indices. Examples of these herbs include foxglove (digoxin), belladonna, ergot (ergotamine), and colchicum (colchicine). Even in the absence of direct toxicity, polyconventional and poly-CAM pharmacy creates the potential for herb–herb, drug–drug, and drug–herb interactions that can be serious.[48] Also problematic is the lack of quality control in herbal and nutritional supplements. Contamination, varying potencies, differing absorption rates, and other quality issues with adequately regulated supplements have been well documented.[33]

Many CAM treatments involve minimal risk for direct toxicity, including biofeedback, meditation, prayer, and

TABLE 38.3
Classification of CAM Systems, Therapies, and Modalities

CAM Domains	Examples
Alternative health care systems	Traditional oriental medicine
	Acupuncture
	Ayurveda
	Homeopathy
	Naturopathy
	Chiropractic medicine
	Native American practices
	Tibetan medicine
Biological and diet therapies	Herbal therapies
	Orthomolecular medicine (megavitamin therapy)
	Special diets (macrobiotics, low-fat diets, high-carbohydrate diets)
	Nutritional biologic supplements (shark cartilage, bee pollen, glucosamine)
	Herbal medicine
	Antineoplastons
	Cell treatment
	Chelation therapy
	Neural therapy
Manual healing	Massage therapy
	Alexander method
	Acupressure
	Biofield therapy
	Chiropractic medicine
	Osteopathy
	Reflexology
	Feldenkrais
	Rolfing
Mind–body control	Meditation
	Yoga
	Hypnosis
	Biofeedback
	Guided imagery
	Prayer and mental healing
	Activity therapies (art therapy, dance therapy, music therapy, humor therapy)
Energy therapies	Therapeutic touch
	Qigong and Tai Chi
	Reiki
Bioelectromagnetic applications	Magnetic field therapy

Sources: Jonas, W.B. and Chez, R.A., Complementary & alternative medicine, in: *Current Diagnosis & Treatment in Family Medicine*, South-Paul, J., Matheny, S., and Lewis, E. (eds.), Lange, New York, 2004, pp. 698–706; Najm W. Traditional Chinese medicine, in *Textbook of Primary Care Medicine*, Noble, J. et al. (eds.), St. Louis, MO, Mosby, 2001, pp. 133–134.

acupuncture (see Table 38.3). But even these innocuous practices may indirectly cause harm if used in place of more effective treatments or outside qualified medical judgment. While the patient must be allowed to make the final decision regarding which therapies to pursue, the physician should detail the direct and indirect risks (as well as benefits) associated with all therapeutic options (see Table 38.2).

Ephedra (ma huang) acts as a stimulant to raise heart rate, blood pressure, and central nervous system awareness.[28,65,126] Studies of ephedra and other drugs in its class show no performance-enhancing benefit at therapeutic dosages used in colds or asthma or at even twice therapeutic dosage.[21,28,34,54,126,133] Performance enhancement may occur at dosages greater than three times therapeutic[53] or when ephedra is combined with caffeine[16–18]; however, at these higher dosages, ephedra has effects similar to those seen in methamphetamine use, with side effects of stroke, mania, cardiac arrhythmias, and death.[62] Caffeine is known to potentiate the effects and side effects of ephedra,[166] and caffeine and ephedra combinations have been banned by the U.S. Food and Drug Administration since 1983[44]; however, many dietary supplements circumvent this ban by combining "natural" ephedra sources with guaraná, an herbal form of caffeine. Natural ephedra product purity is predictably poor. A recent review of 20 ephedra-containing herbal supplements showed that the majority contained many different types and quantities of various ephedra alkaloids.[61] Five supplements contained norpseudoephedrine, a schedule IV controlled substance. The total ephedra content of each capsule ranged from 0% to 154% of the stated label content.[30] The systemic use of ephedra-containing products, including cold remedies, is banned by the National Collegiate Athletic Association and International Olympic Committee. Clearly, then, because performance enhancement occurs only in dosages or combinations with serious side effects and given the possibility of violating antidoping regulations, sports medicine physicians should protect their patients against ephedra supplementation (Level of Evidence A, randomized controlled trials [RCTs]).

38.5.2 Permitting the Use of Unproven Therapies

Many physicians feel uncomfortable allowing their patients to engage in unproven therapies; however, if the therapy has little potential toxicity and is not used as an alternative to a proven more efficacious treatment, the wise physician should consider the effects of spontaneous healing and placebo-like (meaning and context) effects.[96] Even if this relief comes through nonquantifiable spiritual means or a placebo effect, it will still be welcomed by the patient and should be accepted by the physician as well. Ideally, the physician should blend and utilize the specific and nonspecific factors in all remedies to maximize patient benefit and comfort.[96] Homeopathic arnica (a CAM treatment frequently used for muscle bruising and soreness[43]) represents a therapy that can often be safely permitted by the sports medicine physician (Level of Evidence B, nonrandomized clinical trial). Assuming that homeopathy is not used as an alternative to a proven therapy, its potential for toxicity is low and the risk of side effects virtually zero. Though toxicity from the compounds used in homeopathy may be theoretically possible, the dilute solutions and tiny doses employed make this unlikely.[95] The risk from biologic contamination is also quite low as many homeopathic remedies are diluted with high concentrations of alcohol. Homeopathy involves a system of individual prescription that emphasizes holism and seeks to treat patients based on their temperament, personality, and emotional responses, as well as their medical diagnoses.[77] The sports physician should permit the integration of CAM therapies that "are neither harmful nor expensive, but that may enhance [these] non-specific healing factors."[76]

38.5.3 Promoting Proven CAM Therapies

Sports medicine physicians should promote safe, effective, and proven therapies to their patients, regardless of the medical system from which these treatments originate. As medical knowledge continues to expand, patients and physicians find themselves with more treatment options and more information about the efficacy of different treatment strategies. Sports medicine physicians should guide their patients to safe, effective, and proven treatments. Glucosamine treatment for knee osteoarthritis is an example of a CAM therapy that should be permitted and possibly promoted. In animal and *in vitro* models of osteoarthritis, glucosamine improves cartilage metabolism, rebuilds damaged cartilage, and demonstrates some anti-inflammatory properties.[138] A previous meta-analysis of glucosamine treatment concluded that glucosamine supplementation demonstrated a moderate to large effect on osteoarthritis symptoms.[90] The Glucosamine/chondroitin Arthritis Intervention Trial (GAIT) analysis recently performed however showed benefit with combination glucosamine/chondroitin in the treatment of moderate to severe OA, but not in mild, and neither individually used showed improvement.[27] The cost of glucosamine supplementation is relatively high (approximately $1/day) when compared with generic ibuprofen ($.05/day) but is substantially lower than commonly prescribed, once daily NSAIDS and the new COX-2 inhibitors, which typically cost in excess of $2/day of therapy (drug prices from *The Medical Letter*[94] and epocrates.com[10]). Other than mild gastrointestinal upset, glucosamine has no known side effects or toxicities. Clearly, then, sports medicine physicians should present glucosamine supplementation as a possible alternative for their patients with osteoarthritis (Level of Evidence A, meta-analysis of RCTs).

Another CAM therapy that has now been proven safe and effective for musculoskeletal pain is acupuncture. A large meta-analysis has demonstrated that its effects are greater than placebo[149] and several large comparative studies show that its effect size is often greater than standard, conventional approaches.[160–163] Acupuncture should be routinely considered as a primary therapy for musculoskeletal pain provided it is desired and affordable by the patient and available from a qualified practitioner.

38.5.4 Partnering with Patients Who Use CAM

Over 60% of patients who use CAM do not inform their physicians that they are using CAM treatments.[38] This CAM communication gap between physicians and their patients results in a wasteful, as well as potentially dangerous, environment. Effective partnering requires that physicians understand why patients choose alternative practices, that physicians have access to reliable data detailing the safety and efficacy of CAM practices, and that physicians actively question, listen to, and communicate with patients about their CAM use.[70] Patients use CAM therapies for a variety of reasons. They may be enticed by marketing schemes or by anecdotal success stories from friends. Partnering with these patients may require an explanation of the role of science in medicine and encouragement that they incorporate good evidence into their health-care decisions.[73] However, studies suggest that these patients represent the minority of CAM users. Most patients choose CAM because conventional therapies have significant side effects or risks, have not been effective in relieving their condition, or are out of harmony with their emotional or spiritual values.[9,37,38] These same studies also show that CAM users are more likely to be educated than ignorant, more likely affluent than poor, and more likely holistic and spiritual than merely neurotic. In short, many patients that use CAM practices exhibit character traits that incline them to actively participate in their medical care. The physician who chooses to repudiate all knowledge and to discourage discussion of CAM practices will likely alienate their patients and not be delivering good patient-centered care.

Effective partnering also requires that the physician have access to reliable information on the safety and efficacy of CAM practices. While a comprehensive database of all reviews of CAM treatments is not yet a reality, several commercial sources are available. The Cochrane Collection conducts and publishes systematic reviews of RCTs for all health-care practices, CAM or traditional. The abstracts of the *Cochrane Reviews* are available free of charge at www.cochrane.org.[45] Full text reviews can be ordered online or viewed online on a fee basis. An additional source of information is the Natural Medicines Comprehensive Database. This source deals mostly with herbal and vitamin supplementation and has separate editions for medical professionals and consumers. Both versions may be viewed online as a subscription service at www.naturaldatabase.com.[100] Additional resources for CAM information are listed in Table 38.4. Equally important to information access, however, is the physician's system for evaluating the evidence, applying the evidence responsibly to their patient population, and finally assisting each patient to make health-care decisions based on the best available information for that individual.

38.6 EVALUATING THE EVIDENCE

So how do we evaluate the overwhelming mountain and sometimes embarrassingly small molehill of relevant medical evidence? The first important step is to realize that evidence

TABLE 38.4
Sources of CAM Information for Health-Care Practitioners

Source of CAM Information	Description	Where to Go
The Cochrane Library	*Database of Systematic Reviews:* Systematic reviews of RCT of CAM and conventional therapies *Controlled Trials Register:* Extensive bibliographic listing of controlled trials and conference proceedings	www.cochrane.org[45] gateway.ovid.com[107]
Natural Medicines Comprehensive Database	Comprehensive listing and cross-listing of natural and herbal therapies; separate "all known uses" and "effectiveness" sections, safety ratings, mechanisms of action, side effects, herb–drug interactions, and review of available evidence	www.naturaldatabase.com[100]
National Library of Medicine	Powerful search engine that allows searches of PubMed and all government guidelines combined; includes "synonym and related terms" option	*Search engine:* hstat.nlm.nih.gov[64] *Individual guidelines:* www.guideline.gov[3]; www.cdc.gov/[25]publications
Focus on Alternative and Complementary Therapies (FACT)	*Quarterly Review Journal* of CAM therapies. Contains evidence-based reviews, focus articles, short reports, news of recent developments, and book reviews on complementary medicine.	www.exeter.ac.uk/[45]FACT
PubMed Clinical Queries Search Engine	Includes clinical queries filter to limit search results (click Clinical Queries on the left blue banner to access the filter); for the most comprehensive search, use the key words "complementary medicine"	www.pubmed.org[145]
National Center for Complementary and Integrative Health	*Clinical trials section:* Listing of clinical trials indexed by treatment or by condition; cross-linked to www.clinicaltrials.gov[144] and PubMed[145]	www.nccam.nih.gov[99]

comes in many different types and forms. For the sake of discussion, we will say that evidence is like food. We all want good food to eat, and we all want good evidence on which to base medical decisions. So what makes food and medical evidence good? We can easily agree on basic standards for purity and hygienic preparation for food. Contaminated food causes sickness instead of sustaining health. Similarly, tainted evidence may overstate findings, make false claims, or be misleading in other ways. Instead of enlightenment, impure evidence can lead to epidemics of error. (An overview of the important process of distinguishing evidence from propaganda and advertisement is provided in Box 38.1.) However, outside of these basic standards of hygiene, what constitutes good food or good evidence depends largely upon our own objectives and personal biases. For example, many people believe that the ideal diet of good food can be described by the food pyramid. The food pyramid provides a hierarchy of what types of foods should be emphasized in an individual diet (e.g., grains and vegetables being preferred over meats; eating more fruit and less sugar and fat), but this hierarchy does not hold for all individual situations. Good food for individuals with diabetes mellitus, celiac sprue, or lactose intolerance may require substantial modifications to the food pyramid. Planning party refreshments for a 7-year-old's birthday may require abandoning the hierarchy all together!

Evidence-based medicine (EBM) attempts to establish a hierarchy for medical evidence (Figure 38.1). In the hierarchy of EBM, case series represent a lower grade of evidence. Higher grades, in order of ascendance, are observational studies, nonrandomized trials, and then RCTs, with systematic reviews or meta-analysis representing the pinnacle or highest form of evidence. The hierarchy of EBM is based on the scientific method, which uses experimentation and observation to establish causal links between intervention and outcome. In many circles, EBM has become nearly synonymous with good medicine; meta-analyses and RCTs now connote good evidence. However, the evidence hierarchy of EBM only provides good answers for certain clinical questions. EBM is unquestionably useful for establishing a specific treatment (CAM or conventional) as the cause for clinical improvement and for determining the relative efficacies of different therapies. RCTs can provide clear quantification of the risks and benefits of CAM treatments compared to another CAM treatment, compared to conventional treatment, or compared to placebo treatment. However, because RCTs depend on the controlling or freezing of many variables that does not occur in practice and because they are difficult to sustain over long periods of time they less valuable for the study of chronic disease.[83]

Clinical outcomes research is a less-recognized source of good evidence on which to base patient counseling and clinical decisions. Outcomes research is more like clinical practice, as it involves a wide range of patient quality of life data and longer periods of time.[152] Rather than looking for a specific, therapeutic cause and measurable effect, outcomes research provides the probability of a therapeutic effect and how large or small that effect is in routine clinical care.

The best type of evidence to use in evaluating a specific CAM treatment depends on the nature of the therapy, the type of information desired, and the individual patient (see Figure 38.2). RCTs provide essential safety and risk–benefit data for therapies that are potentially costly, toxic, or high risk. For low-risk therapies or treatments used in chronic conditions, clinical outcome data can provide information on the probability and magnitude of long-term benefit or harm.[72]

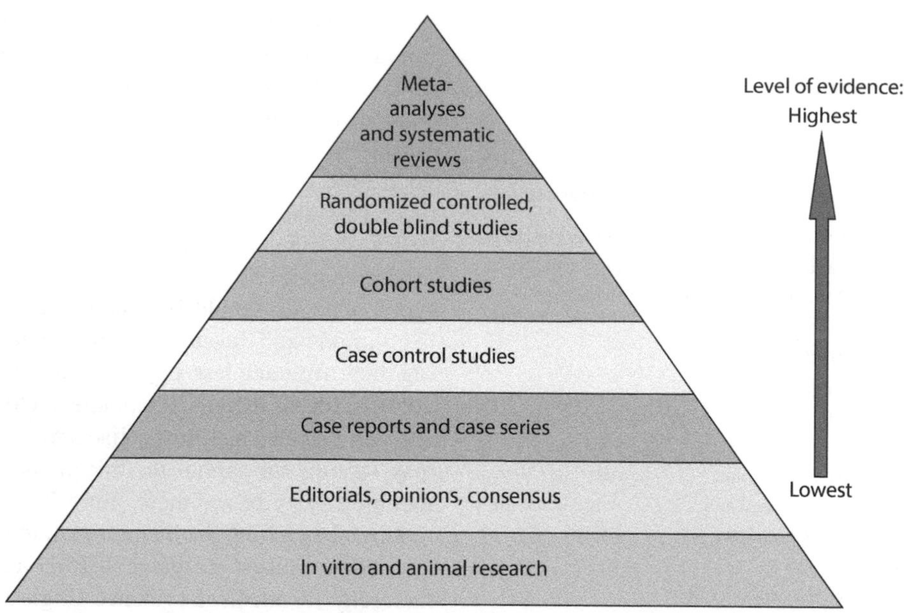

FIGURE 38.1 The evidence hierarchy established by EBM may be conceptualized as a pyramid.

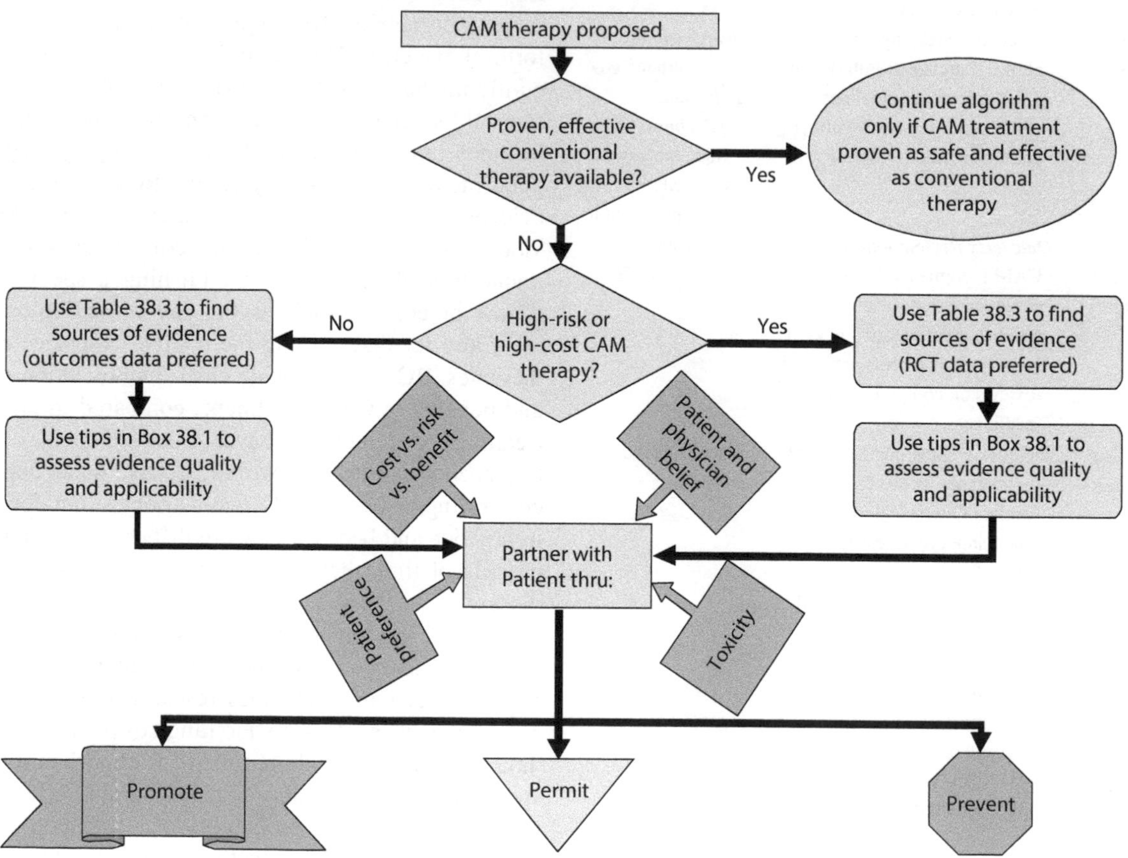

FIGURE 38.2 Flowchart of CAM decision-making process.

The patient's individual beliefs (e.g., prior plausibility) can also influence the evaluation of a CAM treatment.

Jonas and Chez[75] suggest building an evidence *house* instead of an evidence *hierarchy*. The evidence house would have a room for mechanism of action studies, a room for pharmacokinetics, and a room for RCTs and systematic reviews. The house would also have a room for outcome studies of long-term data and a room for clinical relevance. Regulatory authorities and basic scientists may be most interested in the RCT and pharmacokinetic rooms, while health-care providers and patients may be more interested in the outcomes room. Each room, like each type of evidence, serves a different purpose, but every room should be constructed from materials of the highest quality. The house of evidence concept emphasizes that if we select one type of evidence at the exclusion of others we will make important clinical decisions based on incomplete information.[74]

38.7 CONCLUSIONS

Effective patient–physician partnering requires that the sports medicine physician carefully evaluate good evidence from many sources to protect, permit, or promote specific CAM therapies. Understanding who chooses CAM treatments and why they choose CAM can allow physicians from all disciplines to close the CAM communication gap. Providing evidence-supported answers to CAM questions will allow sports medicine physicians to continue to deliver a high standard of quality and compassionate care to their uniquely motivated patients (Table 38.5).

Box 38.1

EVALUATING MEDICAL EVIDENCE

Evaluating the medical evidence is an important skill for sports medicine physicians and physicians in all disciplines. A complete discussion of how to read a research paper is beyond the scope of this chapter, but several such comprehensive guides have been published and are available.[26,57,59,103,105,158] The following steps provide a brief overview of a literature assessment strategy designed to assist the sports medicine physician in evaluating the quality of published evidence. The specifics of evaluating an RCT differ from the evaluation of qualitative or outcomes research; however, the basic questions are the same for both processes and will be treated jointly in an effort to provide a concise and practical guide to evaluating the medical evidence. The method outlined here is adapted from Greenhalgh and Taylor's series *How To Read a Paper.*[59] By using these five questions to evaluate published evidence, the sports medicine physician can estimate the quality of an individual article or assess the body of evidence that exists for a specific CAM or conventional treatment.

38.8 EVALUATING A RANDOMIZED CONTROLLED TRIAL

38.8.1 Did the Study Ask a Valid Question?

The first step in evaluating a research publication is to ask whether the research question is an important one. Or, more specifically, does the study address an issue that matters to you and your patient? For example, if a 25-year-old female patient wants to know about using homeopathy to decrease muscle soreness after running a marathon, an RCT comparing homeopathy to conventional antiemetics for the treatment of hyperemesis gravidarum is not likely to be helpful in answering her question. The study should also measure valid clinical endpoints rather than presumed biochemical markers, for example, a trial demonstrating a decrease in muscle calmodulin levels in rats receiving a homeopathic solution is intellectually interesting but clinically unconvincing. A more useful trial would be an RCT that measured perceived muscle soreness in marathon runners receiving either homeopathy or saline drops.

38.8.2 Who Is the Study About?

No matter how appropriate the research question and how well designed a study may be, the results will only be applicable if the study population is similar to the patient. Ask yourself the following questions[59]:

Who was included in the study? Does the study group's age, education, and gender match that found in your clinical practice?

Who was excluded from the study? Were patients with comorbid disease excluded from the study? Was the level of comorbid disease higher in the study than in your sports medicine practice?

Did the subjects receive a realistic level of care? Were the study patients given extensive patient education? Did they have increased access to health-care providers and health-care support as a result of their being in the study? Did the sponsoring company provide equipment that would not be available to your patients?

While none of these issues may be sufficient to completely invalidate the results or reproducibility of a study, they may raise issues about the applicability of the study data to patients in your practice.

38.8.3 Does the Study Design Match the Study Question?

Another valid question is if the research method is appropriate to the study question. RCTs are structured experiments that compare one or more interventions with each other or placebo. They seek to address attribution. RCTs are useful for asking quantitative research questions of "how many" or "how much" of this compared to that. An appropriate RCT question would be "Does 100 mg of saw palmetto or 2 mg of terazosin yield greater improvement in urinary stream in 50-year-old men?" If the studied outcome is more qualitative—"Why do 50-year-old men complain of more nocturia than 60-year-old men?"—then an RCT is less likely to be appropriate.

The length of follow-up in the study is another important variable. A study comparing the analgesic properties of capsaicin cream with codeine in postoperative patients may only require a 48–72 hours follow-up period; however, a study that examines the effect of *Ginkgo* supplementation on memory loss should involve years of follow-up. A classic example that illustrates this need for long-term follow-up in studies examining chronic therapies is Vaz's report on the efficacy of glucosamine compared to ibuprofen in osteoarthritis.[87] Vaz showed that after 2 weeks of therapy, patients with knee osteoarthritis who were treated with ibuprofen had less knee pain than a similar group treated with glucosamine. However, at 4 weeks of therapy, the pain scores of the two groups were relatively similar, and by 6 weeks of therapy, the glucosamine group reported less pain than the ibuprofen group. Thus, studies with inappropriately short lengths, designs, or follow-ups should be viewed with caution.

It is also important to ensure that the study accurately measures what it claims to examine. For example, a study may clam to measure how often sports physicians discuss hormone replacement therapy with oligomenorrheic athletes. But, how did the study measure this frequency? If the investigators reviewed patient records, then the study assumes that medical records are 100% accurate. If the investigators sat in on patient visits, the presence of an outsider may have influenced this potentially confidential discussion. The issue of how investigators choose to measure human experience leads into the topic of identifying and minimizing bias.

38.8.4 Was Bias Addressed and Minimized?

Bias is almost unavoidable in developing research methods and the interpretation of the results. A comprehensive discussion of bias is too lengthy for inclusion here, but a few of the more obvious questions of bias include the following:

Who is funding the research?

Did the subject recruitment process preferentially select or discriminate against any particular group of patients?

Are the study and placebo groups randomly assigned and statistically similar?

Are outcomes assessed by blinded professionals?

Good research will include a discussion of potential biases or perspectives and what efforts were undertaken to minimize these.[60] Beware of the study that purports to be completely free of bias.

38.8.5 Does the Study Have a Statistical Chance?

A discussion of sample size, effect size, and statistical power is also a mark of a more likely well-done trial. The number of patients needed in a trial depends on how large an effect the investigators expect their intervention to cause. Interventions that cause small effects may require unrealistic numbers of patients to prove their theoretical utility. Worse yet, these small effects may not be clinically significant. For example, a study may claim and prove that meditation and prayer lowered systolic blood pressure by three points; however, this small biologic effect may be clinically negligible. Further, if a measure of clinical importance were to be attempted, the number of subjects needed in such a trial might be nearly impossible to fathom. The statistician's advice is still sage that a trial should be "big enough to have a chance of detecting … a worthwhile effect if it exists, and … be reasonably sure that no benefit exists if it is not found in the trial."[5] While the sports physician may (or may not) entirely understand the statistical theory behind the interplay of sample size, effect size, and statistical power, research that does not contain a discussion of these vital issues must be interpreted with caution.

TABLE 38.5
SORT: Key Recommendations for Practice

Key Clinical Recommendation	Strength of Recommendation	References	Comments
Glucosamine in combination with Chondroitin may have benefit in severe OA. Neither is effective individually.	B	[31,32]	RCT and Meta-analysis
Acupuncture may help in short-term relief of chronic low back pain.	A	[63]	Cochrane Review
Massage may help with subacute and chronic nonspecific low back pain.	A	[108]	Cochrane Review

REFERENCES

1. Aaron RK, Ciombor DM, Jolly G. Stimulation of experimental endochondral ossification by low-energy pulsing electromagnetic fields. *Journal of Bone and Mineral Research.* 1989;4(2):227–233.
2. Adams KE, Cohen MH, Eisenberg D et al. Ethical considerations of complementary and alternative medical therapies in conventional medical settings. *Annals of Internal Medicine.* 2002;137(8):660–664.
3. Agency for Healthcare Research and Quality. http://www.guideline.gov/, accessed September 3, 2015.
4. Allen JD, McLung J, Nelson AG et al. Ginseng supplementation does not enhance healthy young adults' peak aerobic exercise performance. *The Journal of the American College of Nutrition.* 1998;17(5):462–466.
5. Altman D. *Practical Statistics for Medical Research.* London, U.K.: Chapman & Hall; 1991.
6. Anderson RA, Cheng N, Bryden NA et al. Elevated intakes of supplemental chromium improve glucose and insulin variables in individuals with type 2 diabetes. *Diabetes.* 1997;46(11):1786–1791.
7. Andersson GB, Lucente T, Davis AM et al. A comparison of osteopathic spinal manipulation with standard care for patients with low back pain. *The New England Journal of Medicine.* 1999;341(19):1426–1431.
8. Assendelft WJ, Koes BW, Knipschild PG et al. The relationship between methodological quality and conclusions in reviews of spinal manipulation. *Journal of the American Medical Association.* 1995;274(24):1942–1948.
9. Astin JA. Why patients use alternative medicine: Results of a national study. *Journal of the American Medical Association.* 1998;279(19):1548–1553.
10. athenahealthservice. http://www.epocrates.com/, accessed September 3, 2015.
11. Bahrke MS, Morgan WP. Evaluation of the ergogenic properties of ginseng. *Sports Medicine.* 1994;18(4):229–248.

12. Bale P, James H. Massage, warmdown and rest as recuperative measures after short term intense exercise. *Physiotherapy in Sport.* 1991;13:4–7.
13. Barnes PM, Bloom B, Nahin RL. Complementary and alternative medicine use among adults and children: United States, 2007. *National Health Statistics Reports.* 2008;(12):1–23.
14. Barnes PM, Powell-Griner E, McFann K et al. Complementary and alternative medicine use among adults: United States, 2002. *Advance Data.* 2004;(343):1–19.
15. Bassett CA, Pawluk RJ, Pilla AA. Augmentation of bone repair by inductively coupled electromagnetic fields. *Science.* 1974;184(4136):575–577.
16. Bell DG, Jacobs I. Combined caffeine and ephedrine ingestion improves run times of Canadian Forces Warrior Test. *Aviation, Space, and Environmental Medicine.* 1999;70(4):325–329.
17. Bell DG, Jacobs I, Zamecnik J. Effects of caffeine, ephedrine and their combination on time to exhaustion during high-intensity exercise. *European Journal of Applied Physiology.* 1998;77(5):427–433.
18. Bell DG, Jacobs I, McLellan TM et al. Reducing the dose of combined caffeine and ephedrine preserves the ergogenic effect. *Aviation, Space, and Environmental Medicine.* 2000;71(4):415–419.
19. Boozer CN, Nasser JA, Heymsfield SB et al. An herbal supplement containing Ma Huang-Guarana for weight loss: A randomized, double-blind trial. *International Journal of Obesity and Related Metabolic Disorders* 2001;25(3):316–324.
20. Brenner R, Azbel V, Madhusoodanan S et al. Comparison of an extract of hypericum (LI 160) and sertraline in the treatment of depression: A double-blind, randomized pilot study. *Clinical Therapeutics.* 2000;22(4):411–419.
21. Bright TP, Sandage Jr, BW, Fletcher HP. Selected cardiac and metabolic responses to pseudoephedrine with exercise. *The Journal of Clinical Pharmacology.* 1981;21(11–12 Pt. 1):488–492.
22. Burge SK, Albright TL. Use of complementary and alternative medicine among family practice patients in south Texas. *American Journal of Public Health.* 2002;92(10):1614–1616.
23. Casey A, Constantin-Teodosiu D, Howell S et al. Creatine ingestion favorably affects performance and muscle metabolism during maximal exercise in humans. *American Journal of Physiology.* 1996;271(1 Pt. 1):E31–E37.
24. Cassileth BR, Lusk EJ, Guerry D et al. Survival and quality of life among patients receiving unproven as compared with conventional cancer therapy. *The New England Journal of Medicine.* 1991;324(17):1180–1185.
25. Centers for Disease Control and Prevention. http://www.cdc.gov/publications/, accessed September 3, 2015.
26. Christakis DA, Davis R, Rivara FP. Pediatric evidence-based medicine: Past, present, and future. *Journal of Pediatrics.* 2000;136(3):383–389.
27. Clegg DO, Reda DJ, Harris CL et al. Glucosamine, chondroitin sulfate, and the two in combination for painful knee osteoarthritis. *The New England Journal of Medicine* 2006;354(8):795–808.
28. Clemons JM, Crosby SL. Cardiopulmonary and subjective effects of a 60 mg dose of pseudoephedrine on graded treadmill exercise. *Journal of Sports Medicine and Physical Fitness.* 1993;33(4):405–412.
29. The Cochrane Group. http://www.cochrane.org/, accessed September 3, 2015.
30. Congeni J, Miller S. Supplements and drugs used to enhance athletic performance. *Pediatric Clinics of North America.* 2002;49(2):435–461.
31. D'Huyvetter K, Cohrssen A. Homeopathy. *Primary Care.* 2002;29(2):407–418, viii.
32. da Camara CC, Dowless GV. Glucosamine sulfate for osteoarthritis. *Annals of Pharmacotherapy.* 1998;32(5):580–587.
33. De Smet PA. Herbal remedies. *The New England Journal of Medicine.* 2002;347(25):2046–2056.
34. DeMeersman R, Getty D, Schaefer DC. Sympathomimetics and exercise enhancement: All in the mind? *Pharmacology Biochemistry and Behavior.* 1987;28(3):361–365.
35. Drovanti A, Bignamini AA, Rovati AL. Therapeutic activity of oral glucosamine sulfate in osteoarthrosis: A placebo-controlled double-blind investigation. *Clinical Therapeutics.* 1980;3(4):260–272.
36. Duplan B, Cabanel G, Piton JL et al. Acupuncture and sciatica in the acute phase. Double-blind study of 30 cases. *Semaine des Hopitaux.* 1983;59(45):3109–3114.
37. Eisenberg DM. Advising patients who seek alternative medical therapies. *Annals of Internal Medicine.* 1997;127(1):61–69.
38. Eisenberg DM, Davis RB, Ettner SL et al. Trends in alternative medicine use in the United States, 1990–1997: Results of a follow-up national survey. *Journal of the American Medical Association.* 1998;280(18):1569–1575.
39. Ellis JM, Reddy P. Effects of Panax ginseng on quality of life. *Annals of Pharmacotherapy.* 2002;36(3):375–379.
40. Ellison M, Goerhrs C, Hall L. Effect of retrograde massage on muscle soreness and performance [abstract]. *Physical Therapy.* 1992;72:100.
41. Engels HJ, Wirth JC. No ergogenic effects of ginseng (Panax ginseng C.A. Meyer) during graded maximal aerobic exercise. *Journal of the American Dietetic Association.* 1997;97(10):1110–1115.
42. Ernst, E. Does post-exercise massage treatment reduce delayed onset muscle soreness? A systematic review. *British Journal of Sports Medicine.* 1998;32(3):212–214.
43. Ernst E, Barnes J. Are homeopathic remedies effective for delayed-onset muscle soreness: A systematic review of placebo-controlled trials. *Perfusion.* 1998;11:4–8.
44. FDA. New drug status of OTC combination drug products containing caffeine: Phenylpropanolamine, and ephedrine. *Federal Register.* 1982;47(35):344–345.
45. Focus on Alternative and Complementary Therapies (FACT), Wiley Online Library. http://onlinelibrary.wiley.com/journal/10.1111/(ISSN)2042-7166, accessed September 3, 2015.
46. Foerster KK, Schmid K, Rovati LC. Efficacy of glucosamine sulfate in osteoarthritis of the lumbar spine: A placebo-controlled, randomized, double-blind study. *American College of Rheumatology 64th Annual Science Meeting*, Philadelphia, PA, American College of Rheumatology, Atlanta, GA; 2000.
47. Fox GN, Sabovic Z. Chromium picolinate supplementation for diabetes mellitus. *The Journal of Family Practice.* 1998;46(1):83–86.
48. Fugh-Berman, A. Herb-drug interactions. *Lancet.* 2000; 355(9198):134–138.
49. Furlan AD, Imamura M, Dryden T et al. Massage for low-back pain (ABSTRACT/SUMMARY only). *Cochrane Database of Systematic Reviews.* 2008;(4):Cd001929.
50. Furlan AD, van Tulder MW, Cherkin DC et al. Acupuncture and dry-needling for low back pain (ABSTRACT/SUMMARY only). *Cochrane Database of Systematic Reviews.* 2005;(1):CD001351.
51. Garvey TA, Marks MR, Wiesel SW. A prospective, randomized, double-blind evaluation of trigger-point injection therapy for low-back pain. *Spine (Phila Pa 1976)* 1989;14(9):962–964.
52. Gaster B, Holroyd J. St John's wort for depression: A systematic review. *Archives of Internal Medicine.* 2000;160(2):152–156.

53. Gill ND, Shield A, Blazevich AJ et al. Muscular and cardiorespiratory effects of pseudoephedrine in human athletes. *British Journal of Clinical Pharmacology.* 2000;50(3): 205–213.
54. Gillies H, Derman WE, Noakes TD et al. Pseudoephedrine is without ergogenic effects during prolonged exercise. *Journal of Applied Physiology. (1985)* 1996;81(6):2611–2617.
55. Green LA, Fryer Jr, GE, Yawn BP et al. The ecology of medical care revisited. *The New England Journal of Medicine.* 2001;344(26):2021–2025.
56. Green S, Buchbinder R, Barnsley L et al. Acupuncture for lateral elbow pain. *Cochrane Database of Systematic Reviews.* 2000;(1):Cd003527.
57. Greene, L. Using evidence based medicine in clinical practice. *Primary Care* 1998;25(2):391–400.
58. Greenhaff PL. Creatine and its application as an ergogenic aid. *International Journal of Sport Nutrition.* 1995; 5(Suppl):S100–S110.
59. Greenhalgh T, Taylor R. How to read a paper: Papers that go beyond numbers (qualitative research). *BMJ.* 1997;315:740.
60. Greenhalgh T, Taylor R. Papers that go beyond numbers (qualitative research). *BMJ* 1997;315(7110):740–743.
61. Gurley BJ, Gardner SF, Hubbard MA. Content versus label claims in ephedra-containing dietary supplements. *American Journal of Health-System Pharmacy.* 2000;57(10):963–969.
62. Haller CA, Benowitz NL. Adverse cardiovascular and central nervous system events associated with dietary supplements containing ephedra alkaloids. *The New England Journal of Medicine.* 2000;343(25):1833–1838.
63. Hallmark MA, Reynolds TH, DeSouza CA et al. Effects of chromium and resistive training on muscle strength and body composition. *Medicine & Science in Sports & Exercise.* 1996;28(1):139–144.
64. Health Services Technology Assessment Texts (HSTAT), National Library of Medicine. http://www.ncbi.nlm.nih.gov/books/NBK16710/, accessed September 3, 2015.
65. Hoffman BB, Lefkowitz RJ. Catecholamines, sympathomimetic drugs and adrenergic receptor antagonists. *Goodman and Gilman's The Pharmacological Basis of Therapeutics.* J. G. Hardman and L. E. Limbird (eds.). New York: McGraw-Hill; 1996, pp. 221–224.
66. Drugstore. http://www.drugstore.com/, accessed September 3, 2015.
67. Hubner WD, Lande S, Podzuweit H. Hypericum treatment of mild depressions with somatic symptoms. *Journal of Geriatric Psychiatry and Neurology.* 1994;7(Suppl. 1):S12–S14.
68. Hulme J, Robinson V, DeBie R et al. Electromagnetic fields for the treatment of osteoarthritis. *Cochrane Database of Systematic Reviews.* 2002;(1):Cd003523.
69. Johansson K, Bergstrom A, Schroder K et al. Subacromial corticosteroid injection or acupuncture with home exercises when treating patients with subacromial impingement in primary care—A randomized clinical trial. *Family Practice.* 20011;28(4):355–365.
70. Jonas W, Levin J. *Essentials of Complementary and Alternative Medicine.* Philadelphia, PA: Lippincott Williams & Wilkins; 1999.
71. Jonas W, Linde K. Conducting and evaluating clinical research on complementary and alternative medicine. *Principles and Practice of Clinical Research.* J. Gallin (ed.). San Diego, CA: Academic Press; 2002, pp. 401–426.
72. Jonas WB, Linde, K, Walach, H. How to practice evidence-based complementary and alternative medicine. *Essentials of Complementary and Alternative Medicine.* W. Jonas and J. Levin (eds.). Philadelphia, PA: Lippincott Williams & Wilkins; 1999, pp. 72–87.
73. Jonas WB. Alternative medicine—Learning from the past, examining the present, advancing to the future. *Journal of the American Medical Association.* 1998;280(18):1616–1618.
74. Jonas WB. The evidence house: How to build an inclusive base for complementary medicine. *The Western Journal of Medicine.* 2001;175(2):79–80.
75. Jonas WB, Chez RA. Is the complementary and alternative medicine intervention evidence-based? a users' guide to the medical literature. *Primary Care Update OB/GYNS.* 2001;8(5):178–185.
76. Jonas WB, Chez RA. Complementary & alternative medicine. *Current Diagnosis & Treatment in Family Medicine.* J. South-Paul, S. Matheny, and E. Lewis (eds.). New York: Lange; 2004, pp. 698–706.
77. Jonas WB, Kaptchuk TJ, Linde K. A critical overview of homeopathy. *Annals of Internal Medicine.* 2003;138(5):393–399.
78. Kaats GR, Blum K, Fisher JA et al. Effects of chromium picolinate supplementation on body composition: A randomized, double-masked, placebo-controlled study. *Current Therapeutic Research.* 1996;57:747–756.
79. Kleijnen J, Knipschild P. Ginkgo biloba for cerebral insufficiency. *British Journal of Clinical Pharmacology.* 1992; 34(4):352–358.
80. Koes BW, Assendelft WJ, van der Heijden GJ et al. Spinal manipulation for low back pain. An updated systematic review of randomized clinical trials. *Spine (Phila Pa 1976)* 1996;21(24):2860–2871; discussion 2872–2873.
81. Le Bars PL, Katz MM, Berman N et al. A placebo-controlled, double-blind, randomized trial of an extract of Ginkgo biloba for dementia. North American EGb Study Group. *Journal of the American Medical Association.* 1997;278(16):1327–1332.
82. Leeb BF, Schweitzer H, Montag K et al. A metaanalysis of chondroitin sulfate in the treatment of osteoarthritis. *The Journal of Rheumatology.* 2000;27(1):205–211.
83. Lewith G, Walach H, Jonas W. Balanced research strategies for complementary and alternative medicine. *Clinical Research in Complementary Therapies.* G. Lewith, W. Jonas, and H. Walach (eds.). London, U.K.: Churchill Livingston; 2002, pp. 3–27.
84. Limberg MB, McCaa C, Kissling GE et al. Topical application of hyaluronic acid and chondroitin sulfate in the treatment of dry eyes. *American Journal of Ophthalmology.* 1987;103(2):194–197.
85. Linde K, Melchart D. Randomized controlled trials of individualized homeopathy: A state-of-the-art review. *Journal of Alternative and Complementary Medicine.* 1998;4(4):371–388.
86. Linde K, Ramirez G, Mulrow CD et al. St John's wort for depression—An overview and meta-analysis of randomised clinical trials. *BMJ* 1996;313(7052):253–258.
87. Lopes Vaz A. Double-blind clinical evaluation of the relative efficacy of ibuprofen and glucosamine sulphate in the management of osteoarthrosis of the knee in out-patients. *Current Medical Research and Opinion.* 1982;8(3):145–149.
88. Lukaski HC, Bolonchuk WW, Siders WA et al. Chromium supplementation and resistance training: Effects on body composition, strength, and trace element status of men. *The American Journal of Clinical Nutrition.* 1996;63(6):954–965.
89. Marty A. Fundamentals of complementary and alternative medicine. *Chest.* 1997;112(6):16-A.
90. McAlindon TE, LaValley MP, Gulin JP et al. Glucosamine and chondroitin for treatment of osteoarthritis: A systematic quality assessment and meta-analysis. *Journal of the American Medical Association.* 2000;283(11):1469–1475.
91. McFarland B, Bigelow D, Zani B et al. Complementary and alternative medicine use in Canada and the United States. *American Journal of Public Health.* 2002;92(10):1616–1618.

92. McLeod MN, Gaynes BN, Golden RN. Chromium potentiation of antidepressant pharmacotherapy for dysthymic disorder in 5 patients. *Journal of Clinical Psychiatry.* 1999;60(4):237–240.
93. Meade TW, Dyer S, Browne W et al. Low back pain of mechanical origin: Randomized comparison of chiropractic and hospital outpatient treatment. *Journal of Orthopaedic & Sports Physical Therapy.* 1991;13(6):278–287.
94. The Medical Letter. The Medical Letter, Inc. http://secure.medicalletter.org/, accessed September 3, 2015.
95. Merrell WC, Shalts E. Homeopathy. *Medical Clinics of North America.* 2002;86(1):47–62.
96. Moerman DE, Jonas WB. Deconstructing the placebo effect and finding the meaning response. *Annals of Internal Medicine.* 2002;136(6):471–476.
97. Morreale P, Manopulo R, Galati M et al. Comparison of the antiinflammatory efficacy of chondroitin sulfate and diclofenac sodium in patients with knee osteoarthritis. *The Journal of Rheumatology.* 1996;23(8):1385–1391.
98. Morris AC, Jacobs I, McLellan TM et al. No ergogenic effect of ginseng ingestion. *International Journal of Sport Nutrition.* 1996;6(3):263–271.
99. National Center for Complementary and Integrative Health. https://nccih.nih.gov/, accessed September 3, 2015.
100. Natural Medicines Comprehensive Database. http://naturaldatabase.therapeuticresearch.com/home.aspx?cs=&s=ND, accessed September 3, 2015.
101. NIH. NIH panel on defining and describing complementary and alternative medicine, CAM Research Methodology Conference, April 1995. *Alternative Therapies in Health and Medicine.* 1997;3(2):49–57.
102. NIH. Acupuncture, NIH Consensus Statement Online 1997 Nov 3–5. Washington, DC: National Institutes of Health; 1997;15:1–34.
103. O'Brien BJ, Heyland D, Richardson WS et al. Users' guides to the medical literature. XIII. How to use an article on economic analysis of clinical practice. B. What are the results and will they help me in caring for my patients? Evidence-Based Medicine Working Group. *Journal of the American Medical Association.* 1997;277(22):1802–1806.
104. Oken BS, Storzbach DM, Kaye JA. The efficacy of Ginkgo biloba on cognitive function in Alzheimer disease. *Archives of Neurology.* 1998;55(11):1409–1415.
105. Onady G, Raslich MA. Evidence-based medicine for the pediatrician. *Pediatrics in Review.* 2002;23(9):318–322.
106. Organization (WHO). WHO traditional medicine strategy: 2014–2023; 2014. Retrieved September 4, 2014, from http://www.who.int/medicines/publications/traditional/trm_strategy14_23/en/.
107. Ovid Technologies, Inc. http://gateway.ovid.com/, accessed September 3, 2015.
108. Pavelka K, Gatterova J, Olejarova M et al. Glucosamine sulfate use and delay of progression of knee osteoarthritis: A 3-year, randomized, placebo-controlled, double-blind study. *Archives of Internal Medicine.* 2002;**162**(18):2113–2123.
109. Perlman AI, Sabina A, Williams AL et al. Massage therapy for osteoarthritis of the knee: A randomized controlled trial. *Archives of Internal Medicine.* 2006;166(22):2533–2538.
110. Peters H, Kieser M, Holscher U. Demonstration of the efficacy of ginkgo biloba special extract EGb 761 on intermittent claudication—A placebo-controlled, double-blind multicenter trial. *VASA* 1998;27(2):106–110.
111. Philipp M, Kohnen R, Hiller KO. Hypericum extract versus imipramine or placebo in patients with moderate depression: Randomised multicentre study of treatment for eight weeks. *BMJ.* 1999;319(7224):1534–1538.
112. Pittler MH, Ernst E. Ginkgo biloba extract for the treatment of intermittent claudication: A meta-analysis of randomized trials. *American Journal of Medicine.* 2000;108(4):276–281.
113. Pugmire L. Tests: Bechler's Death Was Ephedra Related. Los Angeles, CA: Los Angeles Times; 2003. http://articles.latimes.com/2003/mar/14/sports/sp-bechler14, accessed September 3, 2015.
114. Pujalte JM, Llavore EP, Ylescupidez FR. Double-blind clinical evaluation of oral glucosamine sulphate in the basic treatment of osteoarthrosis. *Current Medical Research and Opinion.* 1980;7(2):110–114.
115. Pumpa KL, Fallon KE, Bensoussan A et al. The effects of topical Arnica on performance, pain and muscle damage after intense eccentric exercise (ABSTRACT ONLY). *European Journal of Sport Science.* 2014;14(3):294–300.
116. Qiu GX, Gao SN, Giacovelli G et al. Efficacy and safety of glucosamine sulfate versus ibuprofen in patients with knee osteoarthritis. *Arzneimittelforschung* 1998;48(5):469–474.
117. Rigney U, Kimber S, Hindmarch I. The effects of acute doses of standardized Ginkgo biloba extract on memory and psychomotor performance in volunteers. *Phytotherapy Research.* 1999;13(5):408–415.
118. Rodenburg JB, Steenbeek D, Schiereck P et al. Warm-up, stretching and massage diminish harmful effects of eccentric exercise. *International Journal of Sports Medicine.* 1994;15(7):414–419.
119. Rubinstein SM, van Middelkoop M, Assendelft WJ et al. Spinal manipulative therapy for chronic low-back pain (ABSTRACT/SUMMARY only). *Cochrane Database of Systematic Reviews.* 2011;(2):CD008112.
120. Scaglione F, Cattaneo G, Alessandria M et al. Efficacy and safety of the standardised Ginseng extract G115 for potentiating vaccination against the influenza syndrome and protection against the common cold [corrected]. *Drugs Under Experimental and Clinical Research.* 1996;22(2):65–72.
121. Schempp CM, Pelz K, Wittmer A et al. Antibacterial activity of hyperforin from St John's wort, against multiresistant *Staphylococcus aureus* and gram-positive bacteria. *Lancet* 1999;353(9170):2129.
122. Schempp CM, Winghofer B, Ludtke R et al. Topical application of St John's wort (*Hypericum perforatum* L.) and of its metabolite hyperforin inhibits the allostimulatory capacity of epidermal cells. *British Journal of Dermatology.* 2000;142(5):979–984.
123. Schrader E. Equivalence of St John's wort extract (Ze 117) and fluoxetine: A randomized, controlled study in mild-moderate depression. *International Clinical Psychopharmacology.* 2000;15(2):61–68.
124. Senna MK, Machaly SA. Does maintained spinal manipulation therapy for chronic nonspecific low back pain result in better long-term outcome? *Spine (Phila Pa 1976).* 2011;36(18):1427–1437.
125. Shekelle PG, Adams AH, Chassin MR et al. Spinal manipulation for low-back pain. *Annals of Internal Medicine.* 1992;117(7):590–598.
126. Sidney KH, Lefcoe NM. The effects of ephedrine on the physiological and psychological responses to submaximal and maximal exercise in man. *Medicine and Science in Sports.* 1977;9(2):95–99.
127. Smith LL, Keating MN, Holbert D et al. The effects of athletic massage on delayed onset muscle soreness, creatine kinase, and neutrophil count: A preliminary report. *Journal of Orthopaedic & Sports Physical Therapy.* 1994;19(2):93–99.
128. Sørensen H, Sonne J. A double-masked study of the effects of ginseng on cognitive functions. *Current Therapeutic Research.* 1996;57(12):959–968.

129. Sotaniemi EA, Haapakoski E, Rautio A. Ginseng therapy in non-insulin-dependent diabetic patients. *Diabetes Care.* 1995;18(10):1373–1375.
130. Speetjens JK, Collins RA, Vincent JB et al. The nutritional supplement chromium(III) tris(picolinate) cleaves DNA. *Chemical Research in Toxicology.* 1999;12(6):483–487.
131. Steyer T. Complementary and alternative medicine: A primer. *Family Practice Management.* 2001;8(3):37–42.
132. Subhan Z, Hindmarch I. The psychopharmacological effects of *Ginkgo biloba* extract in normal healthy volunteers. *International Journal of Clinical Pharmacology Research.* 1984;4(2):89–93.
133. Swain RA, Harsha DM, Baenziger J et al. Do pseudoephedrine or phenylpropanolamine improve maximum oxygen uptake and time to exhaustion? *Clinical Journal of Sport Medicine.* 1997;7(3):168–173.
134. Taylor LH, Kobak KA. An open-label trial of St. John's Wort (*Hypericum perforatum*) in obsessive-compulsive disorder. *Journal of Clinical Psychiatry.* 2000;61(8):575–578.
135. Thie NM, Prasad NG, Major PW. Evaluation of glucosamine sulfate compared to ibuprofen for the treatment of temporomandibular joint osteoarthritis: A randomized double blind controlled 3 month clinical trial. *The Journal of Rheumatology.* 2001;28(6):1347–1355.
136. Tiidus PM, Shoemaker JK. Effleurage massage, muscle blood flow and long-term post-exercise strength recovery. *International Journal of Sports Medicine.* 1995;16(7):478–483.
137. Towheed TE, Anastassiades TP. Glucosamine and chondroitin for treating symptoms of osteoarthritis: Evidence is widely touted but incomplete. *Journal of the American Medical Association.* 2000;283(11):1483–1484.
138. Towheed TE, Maxwell L, Anastassiades TP et al. Glucosamine therapy for treating osteoarthritis. *Cochrane Database of Systematic Reviews.* 2005;(2):Cd002946.
139. Trent LK, Thieding-Cancel D. Effects of chromium picolinate on body composition. *The Journal of Sports Medicine and Physical Fitness.* 1995;35(4):273–280.
140. Trinh K, Phillips S, Ho E et al. Acupuncture for the alleviation of lateral epicondyle pain: A systematic review. *Rheumatology (Oxford).* 2004;43(9):1085–1090.
141. Tulder MV, Cherkin DC, Berman B et al. Acupuncture for low back pain. *Cochrane Database of Systematic Reviews.* 2000;(2):Cd001351.
142. Tveiten D, Bruseth S, Borchgrevink CF et al. Effect of Arnica D 30 during hard physical exertion. A double-blind randomized trial during the Oslo Marathon 1990. *Tidsskr Nor Laegeforen.* 1991;111(30):3630–3631.
143. Tveiten D, Bruset S, Borchgrevnink CF et al. Effects of the homeopathic remedy Arnica D30 on marathon runners: A randomized, double-blind study during the 1995 Oslo Marathon. *Complementary Therapies in Medicine.* 1998;6:71–74.
144. U.S. National Institutes of Health, https://www.clinicaltrials.gov/, accessed September 3, 2015.
145. U.S. National Library of Medicine, National Institutes of Health. http://www.ncbi.nlm.nih.gov/pubmed/, accessed September 3, 2015.
146. van Dongen MC, van Rossum E, Kessels AG et al. The efficacy of ginkgo for elderly people with dementia and age-associated memory impairment: New results of a randomized clinical trial. *Journal of the American Geriatrics Society.* 2000;48(10):1183–1194.
147. Vandenberghe K, Goris M, Van Hecke P et al. Long-term creatine intake is beneficial to muscle performance during resistance training. *Journal of Applied Physiology (1985).* 1997;83(6):2055–2063.
148. Vas J, Ortega C, Olmo V et al. Single-point acupuncture and physiotherapy for the treatment of painful shoulder: A multicentre randomized controlled trial. *Rheumatology (Oxford).* 2008;47(6):887–893.
149. Vickers AJ, Linde K. Acupuncture for chronic pain. *Journal of the American Medical Association.* 2014;311(9):955–956.
150. Vickers AJ, Fisher P, Smith C. Homoeopathy for delayed onset muscle soreness: A randomised double blind placebo controlled trial. *British Journal of Sports Medicine.* 1997;31(4):304–307.
151. Vickers AJ, Fisher P, Smith C et al. Homeopathic Arnica 30x is ineffective for muscle soreness after long-distance running: A randomized, double-blind, placebo-controlled trial. *The Clinical Journal of Pain.* 1998;14(3):227–231.
152. Walach H, Jonas W, Lewith G. The role of outcomes research in evaluating complementary and alternative medicine. *Clinical Research in Complementary Therapies.* G. Lewith, W. Jonas, and H. Walach (eds.). London, U.K.: Churchill Livingston; 2002, pp. 29–45.
153. Wandel S, Juni P, Tendal B et al. Effects of glucosamine, chondroitin, or placebo in patients with osteoarthritis of hip or knee: Network meta-analysis. *BMJ.* 2010;341:c4675.
154. Wenos JZ, Brilla LR, Morrison MJ. Effect of massage on delayed onset muscle soreness. *Medicine & Science in Sports & Exercise.* 1990;22:534.
155. Wesnes KA, Ward T, McGinty A et al. The memory enhancing effects of a Ginkgo biloba/Panax ginseng combination in healthy middle-aged volunteers. *Psychopharmacology (Berl).* 2000;152(4):353–361.
156. Wheatley D. LI 160, an extract of St. John's wort, versus amitriptyline in mildly to moderately depressed outpatients—A controlled 6-week clinical trial. *Pharmacopsychiatry.* 1997;30(Suppl. 2):77–80.
157. White J. Alternative sports medicine. *Physician and Sportsmedicine.* 1998;26(6):92–105.
158. Williams JK. Understanding evidence-based medicine: A primer. *American Journal of Obstetrics & Gynecology.* 2001;185(2):275–278.
159. Williams MH, Kreider RB, Branch JD. *Creatine: The Power Supplement.* Champaign, IL: Human Kinetics, 1999.
160. Witt CM, Brinkhaus B, Willich SN. Acupuncture. Clinical studies on efficacy and effectiveness in patients with chronic pain. *Bundesgesundheitsblatt Gesundheitsforschung Gesundheitsschutz* 2006;49(8):736–742.
161. Witt CM, Ludtke R, Baur R et al. Homeopathic treatment of patients with chronic low back pain: A prospective observational study with 2 years' follow-up. *The Clinical Journal of Pain.* 2009;25(4):334–339.
162. Witt CM, Pach D, Reinhold T et al. Treatment of the adverse effects from acupuncture and their economic impact: A prospective study in 73,406 patients with low back or neck pain. *European Journal of Pain.* 2011;15(2):193–197.
163. Witt CM, Manheimer E, Hammerschlag R et al. How well do randomized trials inform decision making: Systematic review using comparative effectiveness research measures on acupuncture for back pain. *PLoS One* 2012;7(2):e32399.
164. Woelk H. Comparison of St John's wort and imipramine for treating depression: Randomised controlled trial. *BMJ.* 2000;321(7260):536–539.
165. Yeh GY, Eisenberg DM, Davis RB et al. Use of complementary and alternative medicine among persons with diabetes mellitus: Results of a national survey. *American Journal of Public Health.* 2002;92(10):1648–1652.

166. Young R, Gabryszuk M, Glennon RA. (–)Ephedrine and caffeine mutually potentiate one another's amphetamine-like stimulus effects. *Pharmacology Biochemistry and Behavior.* 1998;61(2):169–173.
167. Yun TK, Choi SY. Non-organ specific cancer prevention of ginseng: A prospective study in Korea. *International Journal of Epidemiology.* 1998;27(3):359–364.
168. Zhang BM, Zhong LW, Xu SW et al. Acupuncture for chronic Achilles tendnopathy: A randomized controlled study. *Chinese Journal of Integrative Medicine.* 2013;19(12):900–904.
169. Najm W. (2001). Chapter 12: Traditional Chinese medicine. *Textbook of Primary Care Medicine.* Noble J et al. (eds.). St. Louis, MO: Mosby, pp. 133–134.

39 Strength and Conditioning

Scott E. Young

CONTENTS

TABLE 39.1
Key Clinical Considerations

1. Strength and conditioning is not a specific workout but a method of enhancing physiologic development and performance at all levels and ages.
2. Multiple principles, including progressive overload, periodization, and interval training, should be utilized to achieve the greatest results in the safest manner.
3. Older adults should be risk stratified prior to beginning a moderate or vigorous physical fitness program. Those categorized as low risk do not require medical examination or clearance.
4. Exercise is safe and effective in most cardiovascular conditions. Individuals with severe aortic stenosis and left main coronary artery disease should not exercise until treated by an appropriate specialist.
5. Children can safely participate in resistance training programs, provided they begin with a supervised regimen of lower weight and higher repetitions focusing on form over intensity.

39.1 INTRODUCTION

It is important for providers at all levels to understand the basic concepts of strength and conditioning. Whether in the training room or the primary care clinic, patients present with a variety of musculoskeletal complaints. From sporting injuries to degenerative joint disease, many conditions may benefit from the appropriate application of strength and conditioning concepts. These injuries may also be the result of preventable training errors related to strength and conditioning. Having a general knowledge of strength and conditioning concepts will help primary care providers at all levels identify basic training errors, make adjustments to recreational fitness programs, and understand when referral to a strength and conditioning professional is indicated. Furthermore, knowing what modifications need to be made for common special populations can be key to ensuring their success and preventing injury (Table 39.1).

39.2 CONCEPT OF STRENGTH AND CONDITIONING

Strength and conditioning is not a workout. It is not barbells, kettlebells, or a machine found at the local gym. It is a method of physiologic development intended to improve the performance of individuals at all levels. Strength and conditioning involves any activity that is designed to enhance fitness, including but not limited to lifting weights, aerobic activities, plyometrics, and core strength development. This concept can be applied to all individuals, from the geriatric patient unable to perform specific activities of daily living to the elite competitive athlete. All physical activities require both strength and technical skill, whether it's performing an Olympic clean and jerk or rising up off of the toilet. Application of the appropriate strength and conditioning program will enhance performance and prevent injury by developing strength, balance, endurance, and flexibility. A quality-training program will also incorporate appropriate biomechanics to ensure the safety of each activity. Strength and conditioning programs utilize several principles in order to yield the greatest results in the safest manner.

39.3 STRENGTH AND CONDITIONING PERFORMANCE PRINCIPLES

39.3.1 Progressive Overload

Subjecting the body to the same physical stressors over a period of time will lead to the development of exercise tolerance.[26] Progressive overload involves the gradual increase of physiologic stress on the body, preventing the plateauing effect that occurs with adaptation to exercise.[25] Many techniques can be implemented in a training regimen to safely induce progressive overload.

For resistance training, progressive overload can be accomplished by adding to the load (weight), increasing volume, altering rest periods between sets, and changing the speed of each repetition. Volume refers to the number of repetitions and sets performed. Load can be increased by 2%–10% when the individual can perform one or two more repetitions than desired at the current workload for two consecutive training sessions.[4]

For endurance-related fitness activities, increasing the volume, intensity, or frequency of training will result in progressive overload. Volume indicates the time, number of repetitions, or distance, depending on the exercise being performed. Increasing volume in some athletic activities without inducing injury can be challenging. For instance, runners are often told to add no more mileage than 10% per week to prevent running-related injury.[24] This so-called 10% rule has been shown to be ineffective in preventing injuries for a group of novice athletes preparing to run a recreational 4 mile event.[9] It is likely that an individual's ability to tolerate progressive overload to endurance exercise is dependent on many factors and should be tailored to their response to conservative changes in volume.

39.3.2 Periodization

The development of strength, neuromotor skills, and endurance eventually plateaus or even declines if the same stimulus is applied repetitively. The concept of periodization helps to prevent this phenomenon by altering training types, volume, intensity, and rest over varying periods of time.[15] There are three generally recognized periodization cycles: a macrocycle, which lasts an entire training year; a mesocycle, which lasts 3–6 months; and a microcycle, which lasts one to four weeks.[2] This concept can be applied with the purpose of avoiding training plateaus as well as ensuring peak performance at a specific point in time, such as competition. By focusing on various elements of an athlete's fitness demands while maintaining a baseline level of sports-specific skills, overtraining injuries, and plateauing can be avoided. For example, a runner may spend a period of weeks building their base mileage while working on core and muscular strength. This could then be followed by a speed phase where the focus is on decreasing run times, followed by a taper that allows them to be rested and in peak condition on race day. If this same runner attempted to just focus on speed throughout their entire training cycle, it is likely they would arrive at race day overtrained and not able to perform at their best.

Clinical Pearl

Ensure that athletes presenting with overuse injuries or plateaus in performance are applying periodization to their training programs.

Periodization also applies to noncompetitive athletes as well. Cycling the focus of an individual's training on a weekly, monthly, or annual basis helps prevent overtraining, burnout, and plateauing.[22] Periodization should be utilized in all fitness programs regardless of whether or not competition is a factor.

39.3.3 Split Routine

The split routine concept is designed to prevent the same muscles from being used on successive days, or for the same type of training to be performed day after day.[25] For example, a split routine in resistance training may have an athlete perform upper body exercises on Mondays and Thursday and lower body exercises on Wednesdays and Sundays. This allows for maximal training loads and proper muscle recovery.

39.3.4 Interval Training

Interval training is defined by the application of a period of work followed by a prescribed period of lower-intensity recovery. In high-intensity interval training (HIT), the effort during the work phase is much more intense, followed by a recovery interval of varying length. HIT has been demonstrated to be one of the most effective means of improving cardiorespiratory function.[8,21] When performed at 85%–95% maximal heart rate, HIT may nearly double cardiorespiratory fitness compared to moderate-intensity continuous training, even in those with chronic disease.[49] HIT programs can be beneficial for athletes, active nonathletic individuals, as well as sedentary subjects.[27,50] The safety and effectiveness of HIT have been demonstrated in a number of chronic medical conditions including cardiovascular disease (CVD), diabetes, and the metabolic syndrome.[28,48,51]

Several variables can be altered to produce a different exercise stimulus with interval training, including the duration and intensity of work, the length of rest time, and the number of work–rest cycles. HIT intervals have been discussed at all ranges of the intensity spectrum. At near maximal effort, intervals may be as short as 10–20 seconds.[45] Longer, less intense intervals may last from 30 seconds up to a few minutes, depending on the training stimulus desired.[7] Regardless of the duration of work, each interval will be followed by a period of lower-intensity recovery. For each HIT session, exercise selection will determine how strength and cardiorespiratory fitness are affected, while the duration of the interval and recovery period will control the metabolic energy system that is primarily utilized.[23] For instance, intense intervals followed by very short recovery times will utilize the anaerobic glycolytic pathway and allow for the build up of lactic acid. Similarly intense intervals followed by longer recovery periods will afford time for the clearance of lactic acid, allowing the athlete to provide a stronger effort with each interval but still training the anaerobic system. Longer, less intense periods of work (minutes) followed by appropriate rest periods provide an effective stressor for the aerobic energy system without significant anaerobic impact. When designing a strength and conditioning program, the variables in HIT should be manipulated to provide the most activity or energy system-specific stimulus based on the needs of the individual.

Clinical Pearl

HIT can be a safe and effective means of improving cardiorespiratory fitness in athletes, sedentary individuals, and those with chronic medical conditions.

39.4 SPECIAL POPULATION CONSIDERATIONS

Several groups of special populations have unique attributes that require consideration when applying the general concepts of strength and conditioning.

39.4.1 Older Adults

The point at which "old age" begins and when it should be considered for exercise recommendations is not well defined in the literature.[39] In most cases, adults aged 65 years and older as well as those between 50 and 65 years with significant comorbidities or functional limitations should utilize guidelines recommended for older adults.[10] The American College of Sports Medicine (ACSM) classifies participants in one of three categories when determining who should receive exercise testing prior to initiating a fitness program[5]:

- Low-risk individuals have not been diagnosed with cardiovascular, metabolic, or pulmonary disease and are asymptomatic. They have no more than one CVD risk factor. These participants do not require medical examination or clearance prior to beginning a fitness program.[1,41]
- Moderate-risk individuals have not been diagnosed with cardiovascular, metabolic, or pulmonary disease and are asymptomatic. They have two or more risk factors for CVD. These participants may safely begin low- to moderate-intensity physical activity without medical examination or clearance. They should, however, be evaluated prior to beginning intense exercise.[35]
- High-risk individuals have symptoms of or diagnosed cardiovascular, metabolic, or pulmonary disease. These participants should undergo a thorough medical evaluation prior to beginning any organized fitness program.

Clinical Pearl

Individuals aged ≥65 years as well as those between 50 and 65 years with significant comorbidities or functional limitations should utilize exercise guidelines recommended for older adults.

The value of a strength and conditioning program in older adults has been clearly demonstrated in the literature. The proper exercise program can increase strength, functional status, and spontaneous activity.[52] Exercise can also help prevent falls and fall-related injuries.[16] Fitness activities have a positive impact on many chronic diseases, and optimizing physical activity should be considered a key part of treatment for nearly all medical conditions faced by older adults.

The ACSM recommends the following principles when implementing a strength and conditioning program in older adults[5]:

- Large muscle groups used in activities of daily living should primarily be targeted.
- Prescription recommendations generally follow those for adults, with careful consideration of the type of exercise selected based on structural and medical limitations.
- Volume and intensity of exercise should be low at the beginning and progress in a manner tailored to the individual.
- Resistance training may need to precede aerobic training for frail and significantly deconditioned individuals.
- Supervision by personnel trained in the special needs of this population may be indicated, especially when initiating a weight-training program.
- After a period of appropriate progression, older adults should pursue moderate to vigorous activities as tolerated, which may include HIT.

39.4.2 Cardiovascular Disease

Studies comparing moderate-intensity continuous training and HIT in subjects with coronary heart disease (CHD) have found significantly larger increases in VO_{2peak} in the HIT group.[44] VO_{2peak} is the point at which maximum oxygen consumption occurs during exercise and is dependent on effort. VO_{2max} represents the highest attainable rate of oxygen consumption by an individual. An individual's VO_{2peak} may not reach their true VO_{2max} due to submaximal effort. Direct measurement of maximum oxygen consumption is considered the gold standard for aerobic fitness, and increasing levels of aerobic fitness have been associated with reduced mortality.[13,38]

The safety and effectiveness of exercise and interval training in congestive heart failure patients have been demonstrated in several studies.[37,42,51] Exercise intensity has been shown to be an important factor in reversing left ventricular remodeling and improving aerobic capacity in postinfarction heart failure.[51] The careful application of interval training, including HIT, with appropriate supervision can result in many measurable improvements for heart failure patients.

Primary care providers should be aware of cardiovascular conditions where exercise should be avoided. Aortic stenosis (AS) can be the result of congenital malformations or may develop with calcific AS, rheumatic heart disease, or other rare systemic illnesses. Severe AS, defined by a specific pressure gradient and valve area, increases the risk of sudden cardiac death with exercise.[36,47] Patients with severe left main coronary artery disease should also refrain from fitness activities. The 36th Bethesda conference on athletes with cardiovascular abnormalities provides detailed recommendations on several cardiovascular conditions.[32] If there is any concern or uncertainty, patients with CVD should be referred to a cardiologist for further evaluation prior to beginning an organized exercise program.

The ACSM recommends the following principles when implementing a strength and conditioning program for adults with CVD[5]:

- Those at low risk for cardiac events during exercise training should generally use the exercise prescription guidelines for adults, including vigorous fitness activities.
- For those with very limited exercise capacity, multiple short (1–10 minutes) daily sessions should be considered.
- Exercise intensity should be performed below the ischemic threshold (if previously determined), or at a rate of perceived exertion (RPE) of 11–16 on a scale of 6–20.
- Patients with significant CVD, especially those with recent cardiac events, should begin with a carefully supervised exercise program.
- If an implantable cardioverter defibrillator (ICD) is present, intensity should be maintained at least 10 beats/min below the threshold for defibrillation.

39.4.3 Pregnancy and the Postpartum Period

Healthy pregnant women without contraindications to exercise should be encouraged to participate in an appropriate strength and conditioning program. The benefits of exercise to the mother and fetus have been well recognized, as has the reduction in risk of certain pregnancy-related conditions.[11,18,43] There is good evidence to support the reduced risk of preeclampsia with increased physical activity, thought to be a result of a reduction in blood pressure, decreased circulating inflammatory cytokines, and reduced oxidative stress.[3,31,46] Exercise is beneficial in the prevention and management of gestational diabetes mellitus as well.[3,12] The American College of Gynecology (ACOG) published guidelines in 2002 that recommends healthy pregnant women follow the ACSM adult recommendations for exercise.[19] Since that publication new evidence has demonstrated the importance of moderate to vigorous activity, reflected by the evolution of the ACSM guidelines. More intense exercise, such as HIT, requires less time and produces greater cardiovascular and weight loss benefits in pregnant women.[53]

Resistance training is an important part of any strength and conditioning program. As pregnancy progresses into the second and third trimester, there are several modifying factors that women should keep in mind. First, as the amount of circulating relaxin increases, loosened joints may not support heavier weights as well. This could put additional stress on joints and their supporting structures, leading to a higher risk of injury. In addition, heavier free weights may pose a traumatic injury risk to the growing abdomen and uterus. Due to these factors, lighter weights with more repetitions should be utilized.[53] Consideration should also be given to using resistance bands, callisthenic exercises, or other means of avoiding heavier free weights. Utilizing a light resistance training program during the second and third trimester does not have an impact on infant body size or overall health.[6]

Clinical Pearl

Recreational and competitive athletes with uncomplicated pregnancies can continue their normal exercise routines excluding activities at risk of contact or falling, as well as those that require the supine position after the first trimester or involve significant performance of the Valsalva maneuver.

For breastfeeding women, exercising during lactation does not significantly change the volume, protein, lactose, and lipid composition of breast milk when compared to a sedentary control group.[30] Regarding the immunological components of breast milk, moderate exercise does not seem to have a significant effect, while exhaustive exercise may decrease IgA concentrations. However, this change appears to return to baseline within 60 minutes of exercise cessation.[17] The impact of this temporary change is unclear, and breastfeeding women should still follow the ACSM guidelines when developing an exercise program, including the incorporation of vigorous training activities.

The ACSM, along with the ACOG, recommends the following principles for strength and conditioning programs in pregnant women[5]:

- Recreational and competitive athletes with uncomplicated pregnancies can continue their exercise routines with modifications as medically indicated.
- Strength and conditioning programs for healthy women with uncomplicated pregnancies should follow the recommendations published by the ACSM for adults.
- Fitness activities at high risk for contact or falling, such as soccer, hockey, and basketball, should be avoided due to the potential for trauma to the mother and fetus.
- Exercising in the supine position after the first trimester should be avoided due to impeded venous return by the growing uterus.
- Performance of the Valsalva maneuver may decrease oxygen flow to the fetus by increasing intra-abdominal pressure and should be avoided.[29]
- Any vaginal bleeding, chest pain, dizziness, calf pain or swelling, decreased fetal movement or concerns for amniotic fluid leakage should prompt immediate cessation of fitness activities.[18]

39.4.4 Children and Adolescents

Children are defined as being less than 13 years of age, while 13–18-year olds are considered adolescents. This population deserves special consideration due to their skeletal and physiologic immaturity.[20] Due to the lower levels of circulating testosterone, children will often respond to strength and conditioning programs differently than adults. Strength gains are typically the result of neuromuscular recruitment and not muscular hypertrophy, especially in the prepubescent child.[40] The health and fitness benefits of strength and conditioning programs in children and adolescents are well established and can be obtained safely through a supervised training regimen.[14]

Clinical Pearl

The initial focus in a child's training program should be on form, utilizing lower weights and higher repetitions that induce no more than moderate fatigue.

The American Academy of Pediatrics (AAP) and the ACSM recommend the following principles for strength and conditioning programs in children and adolescents[5,34]:

- Due to the relative thermoregulatory immaturity of younger children, fitness programs should be conducted in a thermoneutral environment with proper hydration.
- Children aged 10–12 years may begin a supervised weight-training program. Lower weight should be utilized with higher repetitions, typically between 15 and 20. Heavier weights and maximum lifts should be avoided.[33] The initial focus should be on form in the execution of exercises, inducing no more than moderate fatigue.
- Adolescents, especially those reaching physical maturity (Tanner stage 5), may participate in strength and conditioning programs using adult guidelines under proper supervision. Once proper form and technique is demonstrated, heavier weights and more intense exercise regimens can be pursued.

39.5 CONCLUSION

An appropriately designed strength and conditioning program can provide considerable benefit to all populations, including older adults, pregnant women, and children. By varying the intensity, volume, load, and type of exercise stimulus, maximum neuromuscular and cardiovascular results can be obtained in the safest and most efficient manner. Whether the objective is to run a marathon, reach a new maximum bench press, or ambulate across a room safely, a properly implemented strength and conditioning program can assist athletes of all ages attain their fitness and lifestyle goals (Table 39.2).

TABLE 39.2
SORT: Key Recommendations for Practice

Clinical Recommendation	Evidence Rating	References
For progression of load, the resistance level should be increased by 2%–10% when an individual can perform one to two repetitions over the desired number on two consecutive training sessions.	B	[4]
Single and multijoint movements utilizing both free weights and machines should be included in resistance training programs in older adults.	A	[4]
A low-volume, high-intensity training program can provide moderate improvement in aerobic power in many populations.	C	[50]
Exercise is contraindicated in symptomatic aortic stenosis as the risk of sudden death is high and valve replacement is almost always required.	C	[36]
Asymptomatic individuals without cardiovascular, pulmonary, or metabolic disease and one or less cardiovascular disease risk factor do not require medical evaluation prior to beginning a strength and conditioning program.	B	[5]
Strength and conditioning programs for healthy women with uncomplicated pregnancies should follow the recommendations published by the American College of Sports Medicine for adults.	C	[5,19]

REFERENCES

1. AHA/ACSM Joint Position Statement: Recommendations for cardiovascular screening, staffing, and emergency policies at health/fitness facilities. *Medicine & Science in Sports & Exercise.* 1998;30(6):1009–1018.
2. The team physician and conditioning of athletes for sports: A consensus statement. *Medicine & Science in Sports & Exercise.* 2001;33(10):1789–1793.
3. Impact of physical activity during pregnancy and postpartum on chronic disease risk. *Medicine & Science in Sports & Exercise.* 2006;38(5):989–1006.
4. Progression models in resistance training for healthy adults. *Medicine & Science in Sports & Exercise.* 2009;41(3):687–708.
5. *ACSM's Guidelines for Exercise Testing and Prescription.* Philadelphia, PA: Lippincott Williams & Wilkins; 2010.
6. Barakat R, Lucia A, Ruiz JR. Resistance exercise training during pregnancy and newborn's birth size: A randomised controlled trial. *International Journal of Obesity (London).* 2009;33(9):1048–1057.

7. Buchheit M, Laursen P. High-intensity interval training, solutions to the programming puzzle. *Sports Medicine.* 2013:43;927–954.
8. Buchheit M, Laursen P. High-intensity interval training, solutions to the programming puzzle. *Sports Medicine.* 2013:43;313–338.
9. Buist I, Bredeweg S, van Mechelen W et al. No effect of a graded training program on the number of running-related injuries in novice runners: A randomized controlled trial. *The American Journal of Sports Medicine.* 2008:36(1);33–39.
10. Chodzko-Zajko WJ, Proctor DN, Sing F et al. Exercise and physical activity for older adults. *Medicine & Science in Sports & Exercise.* 2009;41(7):1510–1530.
11. Dempsey FC, Butler CL, Williams FA. No need for a pregnant pause: Physical activity may reduce the occurrence of gestational diabetes mellitus and preeclampsia. *Exercise and Sport Sciences Reviews.* 2005;33:141–149.
12. Dempsey JC, Sorensen TK, Williams MA et al. Prospective study of gestational diabetes mellitus risk in relation to maternal recreational physical activity before and during pregnancy. *American Journal of Epidemiology.* 2004;159(7):663–670.
13. Erikssen G, Liestol K, Bjørnholt J et al. Changes in physical fitness and changes in mortality. *Lancet.* 1998; 352(9130):759–762.
14. Faigenbaum AD, Kraemer WJ, Cameron JR et al. Youth resistance training: Updated postition statement paper from the National Strength and Conditioning Association. *Journal of Strength and Conditioning Research.* 2009; 23(S5):S60–S79.
15. Fleck S. Non-linear periodization for general fitness & athletes. *Journal of Human Kinetics.* 2011;29A:41–45.
16. Gardner M, Robertson M, Campbell A. Exercise in preventing falls and fall related injuries in older people: A review of randomised controlled trials. *British Journal of Sports Medicine.* 2000;34:7–17.
17. Gregory RL, Wallace JP, Gfell LE et al. Effect of exercise on milk immunoglobulin A. *Medicine & Science in Sports & Exercise.* 1997;29:1596–1601.
18. Gynecologists ACOG. Exercise during pregnancy and the postpartum period. ACOG committee opinion no. 267. *Obstetrics & Gynecology.* 2002;99:171–173.
19. Gynecologists TACOG. Committee on obstetric practice. Exercise during pregnancy and the postpartum period. *American College of Obstetricians and Gynecologists.* 2002;99:171–173.
20. Hebestreit HU, Oded B-O. Differences between children and adults for exercise testing and prescription. *Exercise Testing and Exercise Prescription for Special Cases.* S. JS. Philadelphia, PA: Lippincott Williams & Williams; 2005.
21. Helgerud J, Høydal K, Wang E et al. Aerobic high-intensity intervals improve VO2max more than moderate training. *Medicine & Science in Sports & Exercise.* 2007;39(4):665–671.
22. Herrick AB, Stone WJ. The effects of periodization versus progressive resistance exercise on upper and lower body strength in women. *The Journal of Strength & Conditioning Research.* 1996;10(2):72–76.
23. Shaw JM, Ford C, Davidson LE. Improving aerobic performance. *Conditioning for Strength and Human Performance.* Chandler TJ, Brown LE. Philadelphia, PA: Lippincott Williams & Wilkins; 2008.
24. Johston CAM, Tauton JE, Lloyd-Smith DR et al. Preventing running injuries: Practical approach for family doctors. *Canadian Family Physician.* 2003;49:1101–1109.
25. Kraemer WJ, Adasms K, Cafarelli E et al. American College of Sports Medicine position stand. Progression models in resistance training for health adults. *Medicine & Science in Sports & Exercise.* 2002:34;364–380.
26. Kraemer WJ, Ratamess N, French DN. Resistance training for health and performance. *Current Sports Medicine Reports.* 2002;1(3):165–171.
27. Laursen PB, Shing CM et al. Influence of high-intensity interval training on adaptations in well-trained cyclists. *Journal of Strength and Conditioning Research.* 2005;19(3):527–533.
28. Little JP, Gillen JB, Percival ME et al. Low-volume high-intensity interval training reduces hyperglycemia and increases muscle mitochondrial capacity in patients with type 2 diabetes. *Journal of Applied Physiology (1985).* 2011;111(6):1554–1560.
29. Lotgering FK, Struijk P, van Doorn MB et al. Errors in predicting maximal oxygen consumption in pregnant women. *Journal of Applied Physiology.* 1992;72(2):562–567.
30. Lovelady CA, Lonnerdal B, Dewey KG. Lactation performance of exercising women. *American Journal of Clinical Nutrition.* 1990;52:103–109.
31. Marcoux S, Brisson J, Fabia J. The effect of leisure time physical activity on the risk of preeclampsia and gestational hypertension. *Journal of Epidemiology & Community Health.* 1989;43:147–152.
32. Maron BJ, Zipes DP. Introduction: Eligibility recommendations for competitive athletes with cardiovascular abnormalities—General considerations. *Journal of the American College of Cardiology.* 2005;45(8):1318–1321.
33. Council on Sports Medicine and Fitness. Strength training by children and adolescents. *Pediatrics.* 2001;107(6):1470–1472.
34. Council on Sports Medicine and Fitness, Council on School Health. Active healthy living: Prevention of childhood obesity through increased physical activity. *Pediatrics.* 2006;117(5): 1834–1842.
35. Gibbons RJ, Balady GJ, Timothy Bricker J et al. Guideline update for exercise testing: Summary article: A report of the American College of Cardiology/American Heart Association Task Force on Practice Guidelines (Committee to Update the 1997 Exercise Testing Guidelines). *Circulation.* 2002;106(14):1883–1892.
36. Bonow RO, Carabello BA, Chatterjee K et al. 2008 focused update incorporated into the ACC/AHA 2006 guidelines for the management of patients with valvular heart disease: A report of the American College of Cardiology/American Heart Association Task Force on Practice Guidelines (Writing Committee to Revise the 1998 Guidelines for the Management of Patients with Valvular Heart Disease): Endorsed by the Society of Cardiovascular Anesthesiologists, Society for Cardiovascular Angiography and Interventions, and Society of Thoracic Surgeons. *Circulation.* 2008;118(15):e523–e661.
37. Meyer K, Samek L, Schwaibold M et al. Interval training in patients with severe chronic heart failure: Analysis and recommendations for exercise procedures. *Medicine & Science in Sports & Exercise.* 1997;29(3):306–312.
38. Moholdt T, Madssen E, Rognmo Ø et al. The higher the better? Interval training intensity in coronary heart disease. *Journal of Science and Medicine in Sport.* 2014;17(5):506–510.
39. Nelson ME, Rejeski W, Blair SN et al. Physical activity and public health in older adults: Recommendation from the American College of Sports Medicine and the American Heart Association. *Circulation.* 2007;116(9):1094–1105.
40. Ozmun J, Mikesky A, Surburg P. Neuromuscular adaptations following prepubescent strength training. *Medicine & Science in Sports & Exercise.* 1994;26:510–514.

41. Pate RR, Paratt M, Blair SN et al. Physical activity and public health: A recommendation from the centers for disease control and prevention and the american college of sports medicine. *Journal of the American Medical Association.* 1995;273(5):402–407.
42. Piepoli MF, Davos C, Francis DP et al. Exercise training meta-analysis of trials in patients with chronic heart failure (ExTraMATCH). *BMJ (Clinical research ed.)* 2004; 328(7433):189.
43. Pivarnik JM, Chambliss HO, Clapp JF et al. Impact of physical activity during pregnancy and postpartum on chronic disease risk. *Medicine & Science in Sports & Exercise.* 2006;38:989–1006.
44. Rogmno O, Hetland E, Helgerud J et al. High intensity aerobic interval exercise is superior to moderate intensity exercise for increasing aerobic capacity in patients with coronary artery disease. *European Journal of Cardiovascular Prevention & Rehabilitation.* 2004;11(3):216–222.
45. Sloth M, Sloth D, Overgaard K et al. Effects of sprint interval training on VO2max and aerobic exercise performance: A systematic review and meta-analysis. *Scandinavian Journal of Medicine & Science in Sports.* 2013;23(6):341–352.
46. Sorensen TK, Williams MA, Lee IM et al. Recreational physical activity during pregnancy and risk of preeclampsia. *Hypertension.* 2003;41:1273–1280.
47. Sorgato A, Faggiano P, Aurigemma GP et al. Ventricular arrhythmias in adult aortic stenosis: Prevalence, mechanisms, and clinical relevance. *Chest.* 1998;113(2):482–491.
48. Tjonna AE, Lee SJ, Rognmo O et al. Aerobic interval training versus continuous moderate exercise as a treatment for the metabolic syndrome. *Circulation.* 2008;118:346–354.
49. Weston KS, Wisløff U, Coombes JS. High-intensity interval training in patients with lifestyle-induced cardiometabolic disease: A systematic review and meta-analysis. *British Journal of Sports Medicine.* 2013.
50. Weston M, Taylor KL, Batterham AM et al. Effects of low-volume high-intensity interval training (HIT) on fitness in adults: A meta-analysis of conrolled and non-controlled trials. *Sports Medicine.* 2014;44(7):1005–1017.
51. Wisløff U, Støylen A et al. Superior cardiovascular effect of aerobic interval training versus moderate continuous training in heart failure patients: A randomized study. *Circulation.* 2007;115(24):3086–3094.
52. Evans WJ. Exercise training guidelines for the elderly. *Medicine & Science in Sports & Exercise.* 1999;31:12–17.
53. Zavorsky GS, Longo LD. Exercise guidelines in pregnancy: New perspectives. *Sports Medicine.* 2011;41(5):345–361.

Section V

Regional Clinical Problems

40 Head Injuries

Robert Hayes and Joel L. Shaw

CONTENTS

TABLE 40.1
Key Clinical Considerations

1. In head injuries, MRI or CT imaging should be reserved for patients where there is prolonged disruption of the athlete's level of consciousness (in some studies, this is more than 30 minutes), focal neurological deficits, or worsening symptoms.
2. Computerized NP assessment has been shown to be helpful as one tool in the assessment of athletes prior to return to play after concussion. It is most beneficial in combination with other clinical evaluation tools and after all clinical symptoms have resolved.
3. A strict 5-day return-to-play protocol should be followed in an athlete only after all concussion symptoms have resolved.
4. There is recent evidence that amantadine can improve cognitive function in pediatric patients with postconcussion syndrome, and that melatonin can be beneficial for sleep disturbances and recovery from traumatic brain injury.
5. The best treatment for traumatic head injuries is prevention of head injuries. In certain sports, this may include helmets (alpine and driving sports) and mouth guards to decrease risk of skull fractures or mouth injuries. The best evidence for prevention of concussion is to enforce rule changes that decrease violence and improve fair play in sports.

40.1 INTRODUCTION

According to the data from the National Electronic Injury Surveillance System, 446,788 sports-related head injuries were treated in U.S. emergency departments (EDs) in 2009. It can be safely assumed that considerably more were managed in an outpatient setting and even more were not reported to medical personnel.[35] In that same study, cycling, football, baseball/softball, and water sports were found to be the sports most likely to lead to head injuries. Sports-related fatal head injuries are rare; concussions, however, are becoming more frequently diagnosed (Table 40.1).[31]

40.2 FUNCTIONAL ANATOMY

Superficially, the anatomy of the head begins with the skin. Beneath the skin are several layers of connective tissue. A simple way to remember the layers of the scalp is the mnemonic SCALP. In this mnemonic, S is skin, C is connective tissue, A is (galea) aponeurosis, L is loose connective tissue, and P is periosteum. The skull comprises the frontal, temporal, ethmoid, zygomatic, and maxilla bones, which are joined by sutures (fibrous joints that only occur in the skull). Within the skull, three protective layers known as the meninges encase the brain. The dura mater is the outermost layer and is the thickest and offers the most protections. Next is the arachnoid mater, followed by the pia mater, the deepest and thinnest layer that acts as the initial barrier to cerebrospinal fluid (CSF) leakage. The CSF has several functions crucial to brain physiology, but the main consideration with respect to head injury is as a cushion or shock absorber for the brain when the skull is in motion.

40.3 CLINICAL EVALUATION

As with most other traumatic injuries, in head injuries, a thorough understanding of the mechanism of injury is critical to correctly predicting what type of pathology may be present. Cervical spine injury must be suspected in every traumatic head injury. Symptoms of neck pain should increase suspicion for a cervical spine injury. Symptoms including rapidly increasing headache severity, emesis, and rapid vision changes should increase suspicion for an intracranial hemorrhage.[17]

Clinical Pearl

With every head injury, the first consideration should be to make sure there is no associated cervical spine injury. No other evaluation of the head injury should occur until the spine status is determined.

40.3.1 Mechanisms of Injury

One of the major considerations in head injuries is direct trauma, but the structure of the head creates some unique stresses to consider. Initially, direct trauma causes a compressive force on the skull. Next, as the brain and meninges shift within the cranial vault relative to the skull, shearing forces are experienced and the brain can also come in contact with the inside of the skull. The force imparted onto the brain is somewhat attenuated by the fact that it is floating in the CSF. Even with the CSF, the brain still may collide with the same side of the skull from which the force originated; this is known as a coup injury. If the force is significant enough as the brain and CSF recoil from the coup injury, they can impact with the opposite side of the skull resulting in what is known as a countercoup injury.[1]

40.3.2 Physical Examination

Acute head trauma should be evaluated in the same way as any other trauma with initial focus being on the airway, breathing, and circulation. As stated earlier, all cases of traumatic head injury require an evaluation of the cervical spine for any injury that may potentially compromise the spinal cord. If there is any altered consciousness noticed on the field, a quick Glasgow coma scale (GCS) may be helpful to differentiate the need to transport to a higher level of care immediately or, if normal, to allow for further evaluation on the sideline. If the athlete is conscious and coherent, there are no significant distracting injuries, no motor or sensory deficits, and no cervical spine tenderness, then the athlete should be moved for further evaluation.[17] If there is any concern for or physical evidence of a possible cervical spine injury, the injured athlete must have their neck immobilized and be placed on a spine board for further evaluation and treatment. If the cervical spine is stable, the athlete should be carefully and slowly moved with assistance as they may have balance problems.[15] Often, the next part of the examination occurs on the sidelines; ideally, the examination should take place in the locker room or other quiet location. At this point, a thorough neurologic examination should be undertaken. This should include evaluation of mental status. If the patient has a significantly diminished level of consciousness, either immediately or delayed, the airway must be maintained and imaging should be considered. This is especially true when the level of consciousness is initially normal and then declines as an intracranial hemorrhage must be suspected. A more thorough evaluation of mental status assesses ability to process information. More information about this can be found in the concussion section. In addition, a thorough inspection and palpation of the head is necessary to evaluate for potential bony defects, lacerations, or palpable/visible hematomas[25] (see Table 40.2).

TABLE 40.2
Glasgow Coma Scale

	Eye	Verbal	Motor
1	Does not open eyes	Makes no sounds	Makes no movements
2	Opens eyes in response to painful stimuli	Incomprehensible sounds	Extension to painful stimuli (decerebrate response)
3	Opens eyes in response to voice	Utters inappropriate words	Abnormal flexion to painful stimuli (decorticate response)
4	Opens eyes spontaneously	Confused, disoriented	Flexion/withdrawal to painful stimuli
5		Oriented, converses normally	Localizes painful stimuli
6			Obeys commands

Notes: GCS score is based on the sum of these three categories. Brain injury is classified as follows: Severe, GCS <9; Moderate, GCS 9–12.; Minor, GCS ≥13.

40.3.3 Imaging

Plain radiography offers little in the diagnosis of head injuries, although x-rays can be helpful when there is concern about associated neck and facial injuries. Imaging is of little value to the diagnosis of concussion alone and, according to the Zurich Consensus Guidelines, a CT scan of the brain is best employed when there is suspicion of an intracerebral or structural lesion such as a skull fracture. In the emergent situation, noncontrasted head CT is the preferred imaging modality at this time. It can quickly identify most emergent intracranial pathology and offer the ability to evaluate for skull fractures. Conveniently, CT scans are also readily available at most moderately sized EDs. Symptoms that would suggest CT imaging would be prolonged disruption of the athlete's level of consciousness (in some studies, this is more than 30 minutes), focal neurological deficits, or worsening symptoms.[25] Another guideline that could be followed is the Canadian Head CT Rule. These guidelines are intended for patients with an isolated head injury. The guidelines suggest a head CT if the patient has any of the following: GCS <15 2 hours after injury, suspected open or depressed skull fracture, any sign of basal skull fracture (hemotympanum, raccoon eyes, CSF otorrhea or rhinorrhea, Battle's sign), more than one episode of vomiting, aged >64 years old, preimpact amnesia of ≥30 minutes, or dangerous mechanism of injury (e.g., fall >1 m).[42,45]

Clinical Pearl

CT or MRI should be used selectively in cases with prolonged disruption of the athlete's level of consciousness (in some studies, this is more than 30 minutes), focal neurological deficits, or atypically worsening symptoms.

40.4 SCALP INJURIES

The chief considerations with scalp injuries are lacerations, abrasions, and contusions. Usually apparent upon inspection, these injuries may signify underlying pathology and associated injuries and warrant a thorough investigation. Superficial contusions rarely require significant intervention unless they encroach on critical structures such as the eyes and ears. Lacerations have the potential to be significant injuries due to the complex vasculature to the head and face. Rapid evaluation and treatment of scalp lacerations will be essential to allow further evaluation and treatment of the injured athlete.

The treatment of scalp lacerations is the same as any other laceration; the increased vascularity of the scalp makes obtaining hemostasis an important first step. Lacerations should be thoroughly irrigated with water and thoroughly investigated to ensure that all foreign bodies are removed. If the laceration occurred on an area that is covered by hair, shaving the area should be considered if it could not be adequately evaluated. The laceration will likely need to be closed to maintain hemostasis; however, bites or obviously infected wounds probably should not be closed. Skin closure can then be performed with any of the common methods: staples, sutures, or skin adhesive. Finally, one must consider the cause of the wound and the complications that could occur from it; bites may warrant antibiotics and tetanus immunization status should be updated.

40.5 CONCUSSION

The fourth Consensus Statement on Concussion defines concussion as, "a complex pathophysiological process affecting the brain, induced by biomechanical forces".[31] It can be caused by either a direct blow to the head or indirect "impulsive" force transmitted to the head from elsewhere. It does *not* require a loss of consciousness. Concussion is diagnosed when a trauma (direct or indirect) involving the head is sustained and characteristic symptoms follow. These symptoms are usually brief, typically resolved in 7–10 days. Typical symptoms taken from the sport concussion assessment tool third edition (SCAT3) are listed in Table 40.3. The pathophysiology of concussion is becoming better and better understood. The force applied is believed to result in a pathophysiologic metabolic cascade. The result of this cascade is a change in ion flow and, eventually, mitochondrial dysfunction within the cells in the brain (see Table 40.3).

TABLE 40.3
Symptoms of Concussion (from SCAT3)

Headache	"Don't Feel Right"
"Pressure in the head"	Difficulty concentrating
Neck pain	Difficulty remembering
Nausea/vomiting	Fatigue/low energy
Dizziness	Confusion
Blurred vision	Drowsiness
Balance problems	Trouble falling asleep
Sensitivity to light	More emotional
Sensitivity to noise	Irritability
Feeling slowed down	Sadness
Feeling like "in a fog"	Nervous/anxious

Physical examination in concussion is primarily utilized to rule out emergent pathology. As such, an examination of the cervical spine and a thorough neurologic exam are essential. If the athlete has lost consciousness, then C-spine precautions should be performed. If the athlete is conscious and concussion is suspected, the athlete should be removed from play for an absolute minimum of the remainder of the day of the injury. This time is used to observe the athlete to look for progressing or developing symptoms and to avoid further devastating injury, such as second impact syndrome, to an already concussed athlete. As such, serial examinations may be necessary. When performing the neurologic exam, the goal is to assess for any signs that could signal a more significant intracranial pathology such as an intracranial hemorrhage. These symptoms or signs would include prolonged disturbance in consciousness, focal neurologic deficits, or worsening symptoms.[17]

Imaging is of little value to the diagnosis of concussion alone, and according to the Zurich Consensus Guidelines, a CT scan of the brain is best employed when there is suspicion of an intracerebral or structural lesion such as a skull fracture. Symptoms that would suggest CT imaging would be prolonged disruption of the athlete's level of consciousness (in some studies, this is more than 30 minutes), focal neurological deficits, or worsening symptoms. Another guideline that could be followed is the Canadian Head CT Rule. These guidelines are intended for patients with an isolated head injury. The guidelines suggest a head CT if the patient has any of the following: GCS <15 2 hours after injury, suspected open or depressed skull fracture, any sign of basal skull fracture (hemotympanum, raccoon eyes, CSF otorrhea or rhinorrhea, Battle's sign), more than one episode of vomiting, aged >64 years old, pre-impact amnesia of ≥30 minutes, or dangerous mechanism of injury (e.g., fall >1 m).[42,45] fMRI shows activation patterns that correlate with symptom severity and recovery in concussion. Although this testing can provide information about mechanisms of injury and cause of concussion symptoms, there is currently not enough information to assist in the assessment and treatment of concussion or related head injuries.[12,39] Studies of other imaging modalities such as PET scan, diffusion tensor imaging, and magnetic resonance spectroscopy show some process but as yet are only helpful in research settings.

Other examinations have been evaluated with inconsistent results. Balance tests such as force plate testing and the balance error scoring system (BESS) have shown some consistent postural deficits in the acute phase (first 72 hours) after a sports-related concussion. The BESS test is a simple test that should be performed initially prior to the season to obtain a baseline score. The test involves three stances, each performed on two separate surfaces. For each position, the athlete should have hands positioned on the iliac crests, eyes closed, and a consistent foot position. The three stance positions are double-leg stance, single-leg stance, and tandem stance. In double leg, both feet are flat on the testing surface about pelvic width apart. Single stance involves standing on the nondominant leg with the contralateral leg held in about 20° of hip flexion, 45° of knee flexion, and neutral frontal plane position. In tandem stance, one foot is placed in front of the other with the heel of the anterior foot touching the toe of the posterior foot. Each stance is performed initially on a firm, flat surface followed by standing on a foam surface. Each position should be held for 20 seconds with 1 point deducted for any moving of the hands off the hips, opening of the eyes, any stumble or fall, movement of the hip past 30° of flexion or abduction, lifting the forefoot or heel off the testing surface, or remaining out of the proper testing position for more than 5 seconds. The maximum number of errors per surface is 10. The maximum total score is 60. After a concussion, these tests should be performed and compared to preseason scores. Return to activity should be delayed until postinjury scores have returned to baseline scores. In patients with atypically prolonged symptoms, persistent postural stability abnormalities may be helpful to show persistent neurologic changes related to motor control. As a result, balance tests may be useful in evaluating whether concussion changes persist.[10,11,16,19,21,22]

At this point, multiple genetic markers (apolipoprotein), genetic factors, cytokine factors (IGF, nerve growth factor), serum biomarkers, and CSF biomarkers (myelin basic protein, tau) have been tested, but currently there is insufficient evidence for use of any of these biomarkers in a clinical setting. Electrophysiological recording techniques (EEGs, evoked response potential, and cortical magnetic stimulation) have demonstrated some reproducible abnormalities, but testing has not been able to consistently differentiate between concussed athletes and normal controls.

40.5.1 Neuropsychological Assessment

The use of neuropsychological (NP) testing has been shown to be helpful in clinical concussion evaluation.[13,14,28] There is evidence that in some cases cognitive recovery may follow clinical symptom resolution.[8] In these cases, NP testing may be helpful to identify athletes whose cognitive deficits are still present as a sign that concussion has not resolved despite complete resolution of physical symptoms or to help in return to play protocol.[7] Several recommendations were made in the Zurich guidelines regarding the use of NP testing. The experts emphasized that NP assessment should not be used as the sole basis of management decisions but instead can be used as additional information in combination with assessments of other clinical findings to be used in a coordinated clinical decision-making process. It was recommended that all athletes should undergo clinical neurological cognitive assessment prior to return to play and that computerized NP screening tools would be a useful addition to the cognitive function evaluation. In most cases, the recommendation is to use NP assessment as further screening once the athlete is asymptomatic. The consensus on baseline NP testing at this point is that it is not mandatory but can be helpful and can provide additional information in the evaluation of a concussed recovering athlete.

Clinical Pearl

Computerized NP testing is most beneficial when used after resolution of symptoms and in combination with a thorough cognitive evaluation by a trained physician.

40.5.2 Treatment

The mainstay of treatment in concussion is physical and cognitive rest. In the school-aged athlete, academic concerns must be addressed as well. Fortunately, most concussions in school-aged athletes do not require the athlete to be held from school, but they may have to delay some work to assure that their grades are not adversely affected by their diminished concentration and other cognitive functions. If school-aged athletes are held from school, the recommendation is to return to full participation in scholastic activities before considering return to sport. This is described as "return to learn before return to sport" in the Zurich Concussion Consensus Statement.[31,40] For this, symptoms are monitored until the athlete becomes asymptomatic. Once the athlete has become asymptomatic at rest, a graded return to play can be initiated. A pattern for this graded return is suggested in the fourth Consensus Statement on Concussion.[31] Stages in this suggested protocol are typically one day in length as long as the athlete remains asymptomatic. Stage 1 is no activity and is maintained until the athlete is completely asymptomatic. Stage 2 has the athlete undergo light, nonimpact aerobic exercise such as swimming or stationary biking. Advancing to stage 3 begins to have the athlete participate in sport-specific exercise without any head impact activities. Examples of this listed in the protocol are skating drills in hockey and running drills in soccer. The next stage has the athlete participate in noncontact training drills requiring more concentration, such as a receiver running routes or an athlete completing drills requiring the athlete to follow patterns or change in direction. The fifth stage has the athlete participate in a full-contact practice. If the athlete is able to advance asymptomatically through all of those stages and continues to do well, they may be cleared to return to full participation (see Table 40.4).

40.5.3 Postconcussion Syndrome

Postconcussion syndrome is a poorly defined condition. One general definition is persistence of cognitive, physical, or emotional symptoms of concussion lasting longer that what is normally expected. Unfortunately, the time frame is not well defined, although the Zurich guidelines described the typical window for resolution of 10 days.[31] There is no definitive consensus on the time frame needed to progress to postconcussion syndrome, although opinions range from 2 weeks to a month.[9,41] The cause appears to be related to a combination of psychogenic and physiologic changes. The diagnosis is made clinically by extensive history with no expected physical exam or imaging changes. Symptoms that appear to correlate with prolonged symptoms include amnesia, migraine symptoms, and noise sensitivity.[15,18,27] Multiple studies also show that athletes

TABLE 40.4
Return-to-Play Protocol

Rehabilitation Stage	Exercise Plan	Goal of Stage
1	Complete physical and cognitive rest	Recovery.
2	Light aerobic exercise (walking, swimming, or stationary bike)	Increase heart rate.
3	Sport-specific exercise (skating drills in hockey, running drills in soccer); no head impact activities	Add movement.
4	Noncontact training drills (e.g., passing drills in football or hockey)	Combine exercise with coordination or cognitive work.
5	Full-contact practice	Restore confidence and allow coaching and athletic training staff to asses function.
6	Return to normal game play	

with several previous concussions (usually three or more) are more likely to develop postconcussion syndrome.[14,37] One study confirmed a significant increase in cognitive deficits in professional football players with previous history of at least three concussions.[23] The most common symptoms include headache, distractibility, and poor concentration with other potential symptoms that include depression, anxiety, personality changes, irritability, and apathy.

Treatment of postconcussion syndrome symptoms is difficult and somewhat controversial due to early and limited clinical studies. Options for treating cognitive deficits include dopaminergic agents such as amantadine, levodopa, and bromocriptine.[34] Some recent studies show clinical benefit for cognitive function with the use of amantadine, especially in pediatric athletes.[4,20]

Mood disorder symptoms are best treated with psychiatric counseling, although there is some support for the use of selective serotonin reuptake inhibitors and buspirone.[41] The first-line treatment for associated sleep disturbances should be sleep hygiene education. Melatonin is a good first choice for treatment of sleep disturbances because it is nontoxic and safe, and it has been shown to help with recovery from traumatic brain injury.[29,43] Trazodone is another option for sleep disturbances in postconcussion athletes.[2] Benzodiazepines and antipsychotics should be avoided due to the potential to exacerbate cognitive changes.[2]

40.5.4 Second Impact Syndrome

Second impact syndrome (SIS) is a controversial but very concerning entity. The proposed pathophysiology is catastrophic cerebral swelling as a consequence of sustaining a second concussive blow while still suffering the sequelae of a first concussion. This usually fatal swelling is due to the loss of autoregulation of brain blood flow. The metabolic cascade of the first injury creates an environment in which an otherwise minor blow results in death from brain herniation due to cerebral swelling.[6]

The possibility of this condition is a major reason for not allowing athletes with concussions to return to play until they are asymptomatic. Some states now require that athletes who have been diagnosed with concussion must have clearance from a qualified medical professional prior to return to play. As such, it is unlikely that an athlete who has reported the initial insult would be allowed back to play during the potential timeframe of risk for SIS. Therefore, it is important to ask an athlete, the athletic trainer, and friends/family of the athlete who has sustained a head trauma whether or not they have sustained previous head trauma, especially in the recent past.[6]

Unfortunately, due to the rapidity of decline, treatment is unlikely to be able to be instituted. However, if SIS is suspected, airway management becomes paramount. Neurosurgery should also be consulted, if possible[6] (see Table 40.5).

TABLE 40.5
Indications for Specialty Referral for Common Head Injuries

Diagnosis	Primary Care Referral Considerations
Scalp lacerations	Any lacerations that extend to the eyes or ears may benefit from evaluation by an appropriate specialist (ENT, ophthalmology, plastic surgeon) for repair.
Concussion	When a primary care physician is uncomfortable with return to sport considerations, progression of activity, or possible escalating symptoms, a referral to a sports medicine physician would be recommended.
Postconcussion syndrome	When symptoms persist past 14–28 days (depending on comfort level), an evaluation by a specialist more comfortable with NP testing would be beneficial. If symptoms are causing significant limitations in school, work, or daily function, such as driving, a referral should be considered. Persistent mood disorder symptoms should lead to a consult with a psychologist. Persistent headaches postconcussion should lead to a consult with a concussion specialist.
Concussive convulsions	In all cases of concussive convulsions, neurology referral should be obtained to rule out epilepsy or complications from the head injury.
Skull fractures	A neurosurgeon should evaluate all skull fractures.
Epidural hematoma	This diagnosis should lead to an immediate neurosurgical consult.
Subdural hematoma	A neurosurgeon should evaluate this condition.
Subarachnoid hemorrhage	A neurosurgeon should evaluate this diagnosis.
Cerebral contusion	A neurosurgeon should evaluate this diagnosis.
Chronic traumatic encephalopathy	A neurologist should evaluate this diagnosis.

40.5.5 Concussive Convulsions

Rarely, when an individual sustains a concussion, convulsions may occur. They appear virtually identical to the typical tonic–clonic seizures associated with epilepsy, although the mechanism is not believed to be similar.[38] They are actually believed to be a result of loss of cortical inhibition. The onset is usually immediate, and they typically last less than 2–3 minutes.[32] One distinguishing characteristic is that they rarely have an associated postictal period. Currently, the long-term prognosis of concussive convulsions is believed to be quite good. There is presently no evidence that concussive convulsions have any significant impact on long-term cognition and no increase in incidence in posttraumatic seizure risk beyond the acute episode.[32]

As with concussion, it does not appear that concussive convulsions are associated with a structural abnormality; therefore, conventional imaging modalities are not helpful. Antiepileptic medications are not indicated and offer no benefit. With the exception of maintaining the airway and protecting the cervical spine, no intervention is typically necessary.[25,38]

40.6 SKULL FRACTURE

Skull fractures, while rare in sports, have the potential to be exceedingly harmful. First, if the fracture is displaced or has fragments, there is a risk of damage to the brain from penetration of the fragments. Second, when the skull is fractured, there is the possibility that the cranial vault can be violated, which can result in a secondary infection. When a skull fracture is found, it should raise considerable suspicion for other underlying intracranial pathology, such as intracranial hemorrhage or contusion.[25]

Potential physical exam findings of skull fracture include mastoid/postauricular ecchymosis (also known as Battle's sign), periorbital ecchymosis (also known as raccoon eyes), hemotympanum, conjunctival hemorrhage, anosmia, otorrhea, and clear rhinorrhea. If skull fracture is suspected, a thorough neurologic and cervical spine examination is necessary.

As with other intracranial pathology, CT scan is the preferred method of evaluation, due to its relative rapidity and prevalence. In addition, given the concern for cervical spine fracture, cervical spine radiographs should also be obtained. When a skull fracture is identified, the athlete should be evaluated by a neurosurgeon to determine what, if any, intervention is needed.

40.7 INTRACRANIAL HEMORRHAGE

40.7.1 Epidural Hematoma

Epidural hematoma is bleeding between the outermost layer of the dura mater and the inner portion of the skull, most commonly due to an injury to the middle meningeal arteries. This high-pressure arterial bleed outside the dura pushes the dura away from the skull giving the characteristic biconvex appearance when imaged.

Due to the nature of epidural hematomas, the physical examination may be completely normal until quite late. Patients with an epidural hematoma may present with normal or altered level of consciousness. Classically, this injury results in an immediate loss of consciousness followed by a return of consciousness, often described as the lucid interval. This is followed by a progressive decline in the level of consciousness and a fairly rapid decline into a comatose state. Suspicion for epidural hematoma during the lucid interval must be based on the severity of force of the injury. Eventually, if left untreated, they can lead to coma and even death. Neurological examination may reveal lateralizing signs, but these can vary depending upon where the bleed occurs (e.g., temporal vs. frontal vs. occipital). If an epidural hematoma is suspected, noncontrast head CT should be pursued.

Clinical Pearl

It is important to have a high clinical suspicion for an epidural hematoma due to the rapid progression and the difficulty to distinguish lucid period. If the severity of force is high, then the physician should have a low threshold to evaluate with further imaging.

When an epidural hematoma is found, emergent neurosurgical consultation should be sought. The definitive treatment for epidural hematoma is surgical decompression.

40.7.2 Subdural Hematoma

Subdural hematoma is bleeding within the outermost layer of the dura mater due to an injury of the bridging veins within the dura. Due to the fact that the vessel injured in this instance is a vein, the bleeding is usually much slower. Because of this slower bleeding and the fact that the bleeding occurs within the dura, subdural hematomas appear as a crescent shape on imaging.[33]

Due to the slower nature of the bleeding, symptoms may take a considerable amount of time to appear. Many of the symptoms are nonspecific, such as dizziness, changes in mental status, nausea/vomiting, ataxia, blurred vision, speech abnormalities, and hearing changes. As with epidural hematoma, examination may vary depending upon where the bleed occurs and how severe the pressure exerted. Lateralizing signs on neurologic examination should prompt a CT scan to evaluate for a space-occupying lesion such as a subdural hematoma.

Treatment of subdural hematomas depends largely upon their severity. As with epidural hematomas, management of subdural hematomas should be done with neurosurgical consultation. Smaller hematomas without significant mass effect and no significant neurologic deficits can be monitored with serial examinations and CT scans. Larger hematomas require surgical decompression.[33]

40.7.3 Intracerebral Hemorrhage

Intracerebral hemorrhage occurs when there is bleeding within the parenchyma of the brain itself. The severity and location of bleeding within the brain parenchyma will determine the extent and type of physical examination findings. One potential clue to this diagnosis would be a severe headache with vomiting.[17] If severe enough, coma and eventually even death can occur. Symptoms may also be associated with increased intracranial pressure. As with all types of intracranial hemorrhage, neurosurgical consultation is mandatory.

40.7.4 Subarachnoid Hemorrhage

Subarachnoid hemorrhage (SAH) occurs when bleeding begins in the subarachnoid space. This is the area between the arachnoid and the pia mater. Symptoms are variable depending upon the severity and specific location of bleeding. The classic symptom of subarachnoid hemorrhage is that of the so-called "worst headache of [their] life." The onset of this headache is rapid, typically described as a "thunderclap headache." In addition, vomiting, seizures, cranial nerve dysfunction, confusion, and decreased level of consciousness may be present. Blood is quite irritating and can cause meningismus as it interacts with the meninges.[24]

The first consideration in SAH is stabilizing the patient and obtaining rapid neurosurgical consultation.

40.7.5 Cerebral Contusion

A cerebral contusion is quite literally a bruise to the brain itself. Unlike concussion, imaging studies will reveal abnormalities consistent with edema and/or cell death in cerebral contusion.

Management of cerebral contusion is largely supportive in most instances, depending upon the location and severity of the specific contusion. However, if the contusion is severe, significant swelling can occur and as such neurosurgical consultation should be obtained.

40.8 CHRONIC TRAUMATIC ENCEPHALOPATHY (DEMENTIA PUGILISTICA)

Chronic traumatic encephalopathy (CTE) is an entity that is believed to be secondary to the cumulative effects of multiple concussions and/or subconcussive blows. It can only be definitively diagnosed at autopsy. The pathophysiology of CTE has been found to be similar to Alzheimer dementia in that it involves neurofibrillary tangle formation. It used to be known as dementia pugilistica due to its association with professional boxers, but it has been found in other athletes who have been subjected to multiple head injuries.[30,36]

Clinically, symptoms of CTE are similar to other dementia symptoms. The most common and consistent symptom is a worsening memory loss with poor concentration and focus. Patients may develop dysarthria, disequilibrium, and eventually cognitive impairment. Deterioration occurs in approximately one-third of cases.[30]

At this time, no evidence-based treatment is available for CTE. The best recommendation would be to prevent it. There is no certainty as to what number of concussions or what level of chronic force can occur before the risk of CTE rises. Clinicians should discuss the risks individually with each patient and consider the risks and benefits of continuing to expose athletes to their sport and the inherent trauma risk that goes with it.

40.9 PREVENTION

Due to the nature of many sports, completely eliminating head injuries is impossible, but it is important to make every effort to decrease the risk of injury. There is no clinical evidence that currently available protective equipment is capable of preventing concussion.[5] Mouth guards have not been shown to decrease the risk of concussion, but they do play a significant role in limiting dental and orofacial injury.[3,26] Helmets have been shown to decrease impact forces to the brain, but this has not been correlated with a reduction in the incidence of concussion. Helmets have been shown to prevent the risk of skull fracture and scalp laceration in activities such as alpine, cycling, motor, and equestrian sports.

Rule changes and modification of athletic aggressiveness and fair play have been proven in specific situation to show a reduction in serious head injuries. One such example where enforcement of rules would be beneficial is in football or soccer athletes. Studies have shown that more than 50% of concussions in soccer are caused by upper limb to head contact.[1] Enforcing the rules in heading situations could decrease the incidence of this specific mechanism of injury. Another example of beneficial enforcement of rules to decrease risk of concussions and head injuries is spearing in American football. Decreasing the prevalence of unnecessary violence and improving fair play in sports should help decrease concussion risk.[44]

40.10 SUMMARY

As noted at the beginning of the chapter, well over 400,000 head injuries were treated in U.S. EDs in 2009. Many head injuries do not present to the ED. In fact, it is estimated that there are up to 3.8 million concussions in the United States each year.[31] In addition, it is estimated that as much as 50% of concussions go unreported.[35] As awareness of the severity of concussion increases, it is hoped that athletes will be more likely to report symptoms, but clinicians must be observant as many athletes may still avoid reporting to stay in the game (Table 40.6).

TABLE 40.6
SORT: Key Recommendations for Practice

Clinical Recommendation	Evidence Rating	References
All cases of traumatic head injury should first be evaluated for cervical spine injury prior to moving to the sidelines and continuing the rest of the clinical evaluation.	C	[17,25,31]
Advanced imaging such as CT scan or MRI should be considered with prolonged disruption of level consciousness, focal or lateralizing neurologic deficits, more than one episode of vomiting, extensive preimpact amnesia, or increasing symptoms.	C	[25,45]
Postural testing such as the BESS has proven beneficial in determining the persistence of symptoms, and return to baseline is associated with ability to return to play.	B	[10,11,16,19,21,22]
Computerized NP testing can be beneficial in a multifactorial approach to return to play and prolonged concussions although, according to the Consensus Statement on Concussion from the Fourth International Conference in Zurich, "at present, there is insufficient evidence to recommend widespread routine use of baseline neuropsychological testing."	C	[31]
Amantadine has proven beneficial in the treatment of cognitive deficits for postconcussion syndrome in pediatric patients.	B	[4,20]
Melatonin has proven beneficial in the treatment for recovery from traumatic brain injury and for treatment of sleep disturbances related to traumatic brain injury.	C	[29,43]

REFERENCES

1. Andersen TE, Arnason A, Engebretsen L et al. Mechanisms of head injuries in elite football. *British Journal of Sports Medicine*. 2004;38(6):690–696.
2. Arciniegas DB, Anderson CA, Topkoff J et al. Mild traumatic brain injury: A neuropsychiatric approach to diagnosis, evaluation, and treatment. *Neuropsychiatric Disease and Treatment*. 2005;1:311–327.
3. Barbic D, Pater J, Brison RJ. Comparison of mouth guard designs and concussion prevention in contact sports: A multicenter randomized controlled trial. *Clinical Journal of Sport Medicine*. 2005;15(5):294–298.
4. Beers SR, Skold A, Dixon CE et al. Neurobehavioral effects of amantadine after pediatric traumatic brain injury: A preliminary report. *The Journal of Head Trauma Rehabilitation*. 2005;20:450–463.
5. Benson BW, Hamilton GM, Meeuwisse WH et al. Is protective equipment useful in preventing concussion? A systematic review of the literature. *British Journal of Sports Medicine*. 2009;43(Suppl I):i56–i67.
6. Bey T, Ostick B. Second impact syndrome. *The Western Journal of Emergency Medicine*. 2009;10:6–10.
7. Bleiberg J, Cernich AN, Cameron K et al. Duration of cognitive impairment after sports concussion. *Neurosurgery*. 2004;54:1073–1078; discussion, 8–80.
8. Broglio SP, Macciocchi SN, Ferrara MS. Sensitivity of the concussion assessment battery. *Neurosurgery*. 2007;60(6): 1050–1057.
9. Brown SJ, Fann JR, Grant I. Postconcussional disorder: Time to acknowledge a common source of neurobehavioral morbidity. *The Journal of Neuropsychiatry & Clinical Neurosciences*. 1994;6(1):15–22.
10. Cavanaugh JT, Guskiewicz KM, Guiliani C et al. Detecting altered postural control after cerebral concussion in athletes with normal postural stability. *British Journal of Sports Medicine*. 2005;39:805–811.
11. Cavanaugh JT, Guskiewicz KM, Stergiou N. A nonlinear dynamic approach for evaluating postural control: New directions for the management of sport-related cerebral concussion. *Sports Medicine*. 2005;35:935–950.
12. Chen JK, Johnston KM, Collie A et al. Association between symptom severity, cogsport tests results and functional MRI activation in symptomatic concussed athletes. *Clinical Journal of Sport Medicine*. 2004;14:379.
13. Collie A, Darby D, Maruff P. Computerised cognitive assessment of athletes with sports related head injury. *British Journal of Sports Medicine*. 2001;35:297–302.
14. Collins M, Grindel S, Lovell MR et al. Relationship between concussion and neuropsychological performance in college football players. The NCAA Concussino Study. *Journal of the American Medical Association*. 1999;282(10):964–970.
15. Collins M, Iverson GL, Lovell MR et al. On-field predictors of neuropsychological and symptom deficit following sports-related concussion. *Clinical Journal of Sport Medicine*. 2003;13(4):222–229.
16. Davis GA, Iverson GL, Guskiewicz KM et al. Contributions of neuroimaging, balance testing, electrophysiology, and blood markers to the assessment of sport related concussion. *British Journal of Sports Medicine*. 2009;43(Suppl 1):136–145.

17. Delaney, JS. Strategies for management of acute mild head injury. *Clinical Journal of Sport Medicine.* 2007;17:332–333.
18. Dischinger PC, Ryb GE, Kufera JA. Early predictors of post-concussive syndrome in a population of trauma patients with mild traumatic brain injury. *The Journal of Trauma.* 2009;66(2):289–296.
19. Fox ZG, Mihalik JP, Blackkburn JT et al. Return of postural control to baseline after anaerobic and aerobic exercise protocols. *Journal of Athletic Training.* 2008;43:456–463.
20. Green LB, Hornyak JE, Hurvitz EA. Amandtadine in pediatric patients with traumatic brain injury: A retrospective, case-controlled study. *American Journal of Physical Medicine & Rehabilitation.* 2004;83:893–897.
21. Guskiewicz KM. Assessment of postural stability following sport-related concussion. *Current Sports Medicine Reports.* 2003;2:24–30.
22. Guskiewicz KM. Balance assessment in the management of sport-related concussion. *Clinics in Sports Medicine.* 2011;30(I):89–102.
23. Guskiewicz KM, Marshall SW, Bailes J et al. Recurrent concussion and risk of depression in retired professional football players. *Medicine & Science in Sports & Exercise.* 2007;39(6):903–909.
24. Hop JW, Rinkel GJ, Algra A et al. Case-fatality rates and functional outcome after subarachnoid hemorrhage: A systematic review. *Stroke.* 1997;28(3):660–664.
25. Kelly KD, Lissel HL, Rowe BH et al. Sport and recreation-related head injuries treated in the emergency department. *Clinical Journal of Sport Medicine.* 2001;11:77–81.
26. Labella CR, Smith BW, Sigurdsson A. Effect of mouth guards on dental injuries and concussions in college basketball. *Medicine & Science in Sports & Exercise.* 2002;34(I):41–44.
27. Lau B, Lovell MR, Collins MW. Neurocognitive and symptom predictors of recovery in high school athletes. *Clinical Journal of Sport Medicine.* 2009;19(3):216–221.
28. Lovell MR. The relevance of neuropsychological testing for sports-related head injuries. *Current Sports Medicine Reports.* 2002;1:7–11.
29. Maldonado MD, Murillo-Cabezas F, Terron M et al. The potential of melatonin in reducing morbidity-mortality after craniocerebral trauma. *Journal of Pineal Research.* 2007;42:1–11.
30. McCrory, P. Sports concussion and the risk of chronic neurological impairment. *Clinical Journal of Sport Medicine.* 2011;21:6–12.
31. McCrory P, Meeuwisse WH, Aubry M, Cantu B, Dvořák J, Echemendia RJ et al. Consensus statement on concussion in sport: *The Fourth International Conference on Concussion in Sport* held in Zurich, November 2012. *British Journal of Sports Medicine.* 2013;47(5):250–258.
32. McCrory, PR and Berkovic, SF Concussive convulsions: Incidence in sport and treatment recommendations. *Sports Medicine.* 1998;25(2):131–136.
33. Meagher RJ, Young WF, Lutsep HL et al. Subdural hematoma. Medscape. March 1, 2013; http://emedicine.medscape.com/article/1137207-treatment#aw2aab6b6b2.
34. Meehan W. Medical therapies for concussion. *Clinics in Sports Medicine.* 2011;30(1):115–119.
35. Meehan W, Mannix R et al. The prevalence of undiagnosed concussions in athletes. *Clinical Journal of Sport Medicine.* 2013;23:339–342.
36. Meheroz R, Jordan B. The cumulative effect of repetitive concussion in sports. *Clinical Journal of Sport Medicine.* 2001;11:194–198.
37. Moser RS, Schatz P, Jordan BD. Prolonged effects of concussion in high school athletes. *Neurosurgery.* 2005; 57(2):300–306.
38. Perron, AD, Brady, WJ and Huff, JS. Concussive convulsions: Emergency department assessment and management of a frequently misunderstood entity. *Academic Emergency Medicine.* 2008;8:296–298.
39. Ptito A, Chen JK, Johnston KM. Contributions of functional magnetic resonance imaging (fMRI) to sport concussion evaluation. *NeuroRehabilitation.* 2007;22:217–227.
40. Purcell L. What are the most appropriate return to play guidelines for concussed child athletes? *British Journal of Sports Medicine.* 2009;43(Suppl I):51–55.
41. Putukian M, Echemendia RJ. Psychological aspects of serious head injury in the competitive athlete. *Clinics in Sports Medicine.* 2003;22(3):617–630, xi.
42. Ropper AH, Gorson KC. Concussion. *The New England Journal of Medicine.* 2007;356(2):166–172.
43. Samantaray S, Das A, Thakore NP et al. Therapeutic potential of melatonin in traumatic central nervous system injury. *Journal of Pineal Research.* 2009;47:134–142.
44. Shaw NH. Body checking in hockey. *CMAJ.* 2004;170(I):15–16.
45. Stiell IG, Wells GA, Vandemheen K et al. The canadian CT head rule for patients with minor head injury. *Lancet.* 2001;357(9266):1391–1396.

41 Oral–Maxillofacial Injuries

Charles W. Webb and Sean C. Robinson

CONTENTS

TABLE 41.1
Key Clinical Considerations

1. Airway, breathing, and circulation are essential when assessing maxillofacial injury.
2. High incidence of cervical spine injuries are associated with maxillofacial injury; thus, consideration of cervical spine precautions during initial assessment is essential.
3. Decreased visual acuity necessitates ophthalmological consultation.
4. Prevention is paramount to decrease maxillofacial injuries.
5. One should have a low threshold to consult surgical colleagues for maxillofacial fracture management.

41.1 INTRODUCTION

Maxillofacial injuries are among the more common injuries in athletics. These injuries involve the facial bones, nasal bones, eyes, ears, and dentition. They can have both profound cosmetic and psychological impact on the athlete. This chapter will review the signs and symptoms, treatment, and return-to-play protocols for the most common injuries involving the eyes, ears, nose, facial bones, and teeth (Table 41.1).

Sporting activities have inherent risk of facial injury due to impacts from other competitors, projectiles, and collisions with the playing surface. Facial injuries comprise about 19% of all sports-related injuries seen in a primary care practitioner's office.[23] Rates of injury vary depending on age and gender, with the majority of sports-related facial injuries occurring in males aged 10–29 years.[23] Ball sports also have a higher incidence of facial injuries.[8] With the addition of the mandatory use of face masks and mouth guards in football and hockey along with protective eyewear in women's lacrosse, the number of severe facial injuries has declined dramatically.[8,20,23,24]

Clinical Pearl

Evaluation of oral–maxillofacial injuries always starts with airway, breathing, and circulation. Spine precautions should always be considered.

The management of an athlete with facial injuries begins with the essential airway, breathing, and circulation assessment. Athletes may have false teeth, mouth guards, or other objects that are airway hazards and must be removed to ensure a patent airway. Cervical spine precautions must be observed in all head injuries, especially if the player has been rendered unconscious. The history should cover the mechanism of injury to assess for related injuries and the presence of any other past injuries to the patient's facial area. Most facial injuries are the result of direct trauma. The physical exam should include observation, palpation, visual acuity, extraocular range of motion, pupillary response, and fundoscopic evaluation. Most important is a specific evaluation of the injured structures. Observation includes evaluation of facial symmetry, bruising, lacerations, or swelling. Bruising around the mastoid process is called a battle sign and suggests basilar skull fracture; one may also see raccoon eyes or periorbital ecchymosis. Observation of the nares includes the septum, which can be seen with an otoscope or a nasal speculum, mainly looking for any bluish tinted bulge, which can represent a hematoma. Inspection for any type of fluid drainage mainly assessing for possible spinal fluid is essential. Palpation should include the orbital rim, nasal bones, maxillary bones, mandible, temporomandibular joint (TMJ), mastoid process, and the upper and lower jaws.

Imaging is usually of limited value. X-rays may be helpful in determining the presence of a facial fracture; however, computed tomography (CT) is the gold standard. Return-to-play guidance is based upon the history physical examination and will be addressed with each individual injury through this chapter.

41.2 OCULAR INJURIES

41.2.1 Eyelid Lacerations

These lacerations are common because the skin in this area is thin and typically the first to absorb impact.[6] There are two types of lacerations commonly encountered in sports medicine: full-thickness and eyelid margin.[6] First, eyelid margin repairs require an ophthalmologist because proper function of the lid depends on the repair. Malposition of the eyelid can cause chronic corneal irritation and interfere with the tear drainage system.[6] Repairs of these lacerations should be done in operation room with microsurgical equipment. Second, full-thickness lacerations of the eyelid require special attention not only to rule out penetrating globe injuries but also to ensure proper future function of the levator muscle.[6] In order to identify full-thickness laceration, the eyelid should be everted to look for fat protruding within the wound.[25] If one suspects a full-thickness laceration, consultation with an ophthalmologist is required.[6]

41.2.2 Orbital Fractures

Orbital fractures rarely require emergent surgical repair, but additional injuries that require emergent evaluation are often present. Fractures of the orbit can result in the damage of all the structures of the eye to include nerves, blood vessels, periocular muscles, and lacrimal glands. It is estimated that 22%–29% of orbital fractures are associated with ocular injury.[2] Visual acuity should always be evaluated and if there is loss of acuity, immediate ophthalmology referral is indicated.

Clinical Pearl

Evaluation of visual acuity is essential and any loss of acuity requires immediate ophthalmology referral.

There are two types of orbital fractures: blowout (pure) fractures and orbital (impure). Blowout fractures only involve the orbital walls and are most common.[2] These fractures may cause entrapment of the orbital soft tissues and result in enophthalmos (posterior displacement of the eye) and limited vertical or horizontal eye movement. Orbital blowout fractures occur when larger objects strike the orbit in such a way to case the orbital floor to give way. This can cause enophthalmos, diplopia (typically with upward gaze), and paresthesias over the face, secondary to infraorbital nerve injury. The classic triad of symptoms is diplopia (restrictive strabismus), infraorbital numbness (damage to the infraorbital nerve), and periocular ecchymosis. Enophthalmos is the result from loss of the support structures for the globe and the intraorbital tissues. This may be immediately obvious, with the orbital contents sinking into the maxillary sinus, or may not be apparent for weeks to months after the initial trauma, secondary to orbital edema or hematoma. Diplopia may result from periocular tissues being trapped in the maxillary sinus due to negative pressure or from restriction of the extraocular muscles from direct trauma or secondary to swelling. When an orbital fracture is diagnosed, the patient should be started on systemic antibiotics for prophylaxis against sinus flora. Surgical consult should be made if there is concern for long-term sequel. CT scan can aid in this decision process. Counseling the athlete to avoid nasal blowing is important to decrease further trauma and spread of infection.

TABLE 41.2
Stepwise Return-to-Play Protocol in Maxillofacial Fractures

Step	Activity	Days
1	No activity	<20
2	Light aerobic exercise	21–30
3	Noncontact training drills	31–40
4	Full-contact training drills	>41

Note: The athlete should progress to the next step only if completely asymptomatic at the current step. If symptoms develop, the athlete should drop back to the previous asymptomatic step and try to progress after 7 days.[19]

Impure or orbital fractures can involve any combination of orbital walls along with the involvement of one of three orbital rims.[2] Orbital fractures often involve other fracture patterns such as zygomatic complex, Le Fort fractures, and/or nasoorbital ethmoid fractures.[2] When multiple fractures are seen, one should consider further surrounding structure damage as the degree of force in these injuries is high and a low threshold for surgical referral is recommended. Orbital roof fractures are uncommon because of the thick superior aspect of the orbit. These fractures require immediate surgery as communication with brain contents can occur through the frontal sinus. The lateral wall is usually associated with zygomatic arch fractures. These fractures are known as tripod or trimalleolar fractures and will result in depression of the cheekbone and difficulty opening the job secondary disruptions of the TMJ. Medial wall fractures usually results from damage of the orbital floor and rarely from direct trauma. Periorbital crepitus or subcutaneous emphysema may be present with medial wall fractures.

Return-to-play decisions needed to be discussed with the consulting team, surgical or ophthalmology colleagues, and is typically determined via a case-by-case basis depending on the extent of the injury, surgical repair needed, etc.[19] A potential return-to-play protocol for facial fractures will be discussed in the facial fracture section (see Table 41.2).

41.2.3 Retrobulbar Hematoma

Retrobulbar hematoma can occur after blunt or penetrating facial trauma. Retrobulbar hematoma is also known as retrobulbar hemorrhage and is a rare vision-threatening emergency.[21] Bleeding into the retrobulbar space within the confines of the orbit increases the intraocular pressure and can damage the optic nerve and the globe resulting compression of the retinal vessels and retinal ischemia.[21] This is essentially a compartment syndrome of the eye. The resultant loss of vision is irreversible within 60–100 minutes after the onset of the ischemia.[20] The clinical signs and symptoms of retrobulbar hematoma include the following: pain, nausea, vomiting, decreased vision, proptosis with resistance to retropulsion, chemosis, limited extraocular motility, diplopia, diffuse subconjuntival hemorrhage, increased intraocular pressure, and afferent pupillary defect.[21] Treatment can range from conservative management to emergent surgical decompression pending the severity of the damage. Conservative treatment includes head elevation, ice, and avoidance of aspirin-containing products.[21] Increased intraocular pressures or an afferent pupillary defect requires emergent decompression by an ophthalmologist. Return to play depends upon the severity of the injury.

41.2.4 Subconjunctival Hemorrhage

Subconjunctival hemorrhage is extremely common after blunt ocular trauma and requires no specific treatment as it gradually resolves in 2–3 weeks. Blood will not cover the cornea in the conjunctiva and stops at the lenses. A traumatic subconjunctival hemorrhage may be a sign of less obvious injury, and a thorough ocular and facial evaluation is mandated. An example and picture can found at http://www.aao.org/theeyeshaveit/red-eye/subconjunctival-hemorrhage.cfm.[27]

41.2.5 Hyphema

A hyphema is a collection of blood in the anterior chamber after blunt or penetrating trauma to the orbit causing vessel disruption of the ciliary body and iris.[21] Symptoms include blurred vision, photophobia, and pain. A complete eye exam is mandatory and must include intraocular pressure measurements and a slit lamp evaluation to document fluid levels. This measurement is useful to assess for subsequent active bleeding or secondary hemorrhage. Hyphemas are classified by grades 1–4 based on the volume of blood identified.[21] A grade 1 hyphema refers to the presence of circulating red blood cells that do not layer in the interior chambers, whereas grade 4 refers to a total *8-ball* appearance, with blood completely filling the anterior chamber. Treatment includes placement of an eye shield to help decrease the risk of rebleed, that is, strict bed rest with elevation of the head of the bed to at least 30°. A picture of a hyphema can be seen at http://www.aao.org/theeyeshaveit/trauma/hyphema.cfm.[28] Athlete should not be placed on anti-inflammatory medications. An ophthalmologist should treat with atropine 1% drops two to three times a day. Daily reevaluation is needed to assess for rebleeding and increased intraocular pressures. Activity is restricted for at least 4 days to decrease the risk of rebleeding in the athlete may return to play when resolved.

41.2.6 Uveitis

Traumatic uveitis follows almost any ocular trauma. Despite advancements in therapeutics, the prevalence of blindness secondary to uveitis has not been reduced in the past three decades.[22] The patient will complain of blurred vision, ocular pain, brow ache, redness, photophobia, and headaches. An aqueous flare and cells are often seen in slit lamp evaluation. The intraocular pressure can be decreased secondary to inflammation of the ciliary body or elevated because of obstruction of the trabecular meshwork. It is treated with homatropine two drops four times a day for 1–2 weeks. Steroids may also be used, after consultation with an ophthalmologist.[22]

41.2.7 Corneal Abrasion

A corneal abrasion is a defect to the corneal epithelium caused by trauma, foreign body injury, or contact lens use.[5] These injuries are extremely common in sport. Patients often complain of severe pain in the sensation of a foreign body. On examination, visual acuity maybe normal and the pupil will typically be constricted secondary to a reactive meiosis. Fluorescein staining will demonstrate the area of epithelial defect. An example of a corneal abrasion can seen at http://www.aao.org/theeyeshaveit/trauma/corneal-abrasion.cfm.[29] Special attention should be directed toward looking for the Seidel sign, which is leaking of aqueous humor appreciated with staining.[20] The sign indicates disruption of the globe and an ophthalmological emergency. The eyelids should be everted to look for and remove any foreign body if found. Treatment consists of antibiotic ointment for prophylaxis, lubrication, and narcotic analgesia. Topical NSAIDs may also provide some symptomatic relief. Eye patching is not recommended, as it provides no additional pain relief or acceleration of feelings. Tetanus prophylaxis is only recommended in cases of global perforation and infection.[5]

Clinical Pearl

The Seidel sign is an ophthalmological emergency, as it suggests globe rupture.

41.2.8 Globe Rupture

Globe rupture occurs after blunt injury to the eyes such as from a ball, motor vehicle crash, or an assault.[9] Globe lacerations, essentially global rupture, may occur after trauma from sharp penetrating objects such as a knife for a small high-velocity projectile. Patients with globe injury often complain of pain, redness, tearing, and decreased vision. A subconjunctival hemorrhage, irregular pupil, and iris prolapse through a corneal or scleral wound are possible signs of globe rupture.[21] If a foreign body is visible and protruding out of the globe, it should not be removed. Dilution of the fluorescein by aqueous flow, if seen, a positive Seidel test, confirms globe rupture.[26]

CT of the orbits may be necessary to evaluate for intraocular foreign bodies or orbital wall fractures. For laceration smaller than 1 cm with no other ocular findings, treatment can be initiated in primary care settings with topical antibiotics. Patients should be instructed not to put any more pressure on the eye and limit coughing or straining to prevent stop extrusion of the intraocular contents. A metal shield should be placed over the eye, an antibiotic therapy is initiated (typically oral levofloxacin or moxifloxacin), and the patient should be referred immediately to an ophthalmologist. A tetanus booster should also be administered if indicated.[9]

41.2.9 Foreign Bodies

Intraocular foreign bodies are the most common sports-related eye injuries. It is more common with outdoor sports secondary to dust and debris in the air. Athletes usually will complain of eye irritation, tearing, pain, and a feeling of a sandy/gritty sensation in the eye.[21] A thorough eye exam needs to be done to include eversion of the eyelid and fluorescein staining looking for corneal abrasion. A topical anesthetic may be used to relieve the initial eye pain but should not be administered on a regular basis. Most foreign bodies can be removed using a saline-moistened cotton applicator. If the foreign body is not able to be removed or is embedded, it should be removed using a slip lamp by an ophthalmologist. Metallic foreign bodies often leave a rust ring; these are not to be removed and may necessitate seeing ophthalmology. Most athletes can return to play immediately once the foreign body has been removed and visual acuity has been restored. Eye patching is not recommended and pain medication may be needed. Protective eyewear may be required.[21]

41.2.10 Retinal Detachment

Retinal detachment can occur after any direct trauma to the orbit leading to detachment of the narrow sensory layer of the retina from the underlying retinal pigment epithelium. Retinal detachments are relatively uncommon. Retinal detachments can occur and often from weeks to months after trauma. Up to one-third of cases are being diagnosed 6 weeks after injury.[21] Risk factors include age, ocular trauma, history of cataract surgery, family history of retinal attachment, and a previous retinal attachment in the contralateral eye.[9] Myopia (nearsightedness) is a significant risk factor, especially with patients who have more than three diopters of refractive error, having a 10-fold increase risk.[9,21] Athletes will present complaining of floaters, flashing lights (photopsia), and potentially a blind spot on the edge of the visual field. There is usually a visual field defect in the peripheral vision that may expand over the next few days postinjury. If there is a suspicion of retinal attachment, urgent referral to an ophthalmologist is necessary for a dilated exam. Repair of a retinal attachment requires surgery and is successful 95% of the time.[21] Return to play is dependent upon severity of the injury and visual acuity and may be determined after consultation with an ophthalmologist in more severe cases.

41.2.11 Prevention of Eye Injuries

It is approximated that about 90% of sports-related ocular injuries can be prevented with the proper use of protective eyewear.[20] Polycarbonate lenses provide the most protection that should be mandated in racket sports and for the functionally one-eyed athletes.[11,18] An athlete is considered monocular when the best corrected visual acuity in the weaker eye is less than 20/40.[20] Ice hockey, racket sports, and women's lacrosse have seen dramatic decreases in the number of eye injuries due to the increasing number of athletes required to wear eye protection.[23]

41.3 EAR INJURIES

41.3.1 Auricular Hematoma (Wrestler's Ear, Cauliflower Ear)

Auricular hematoma is the accumulation of blood in the subperichondrial space.[3] This is often seen after blunt trauma and repetitive contusions to the auricle. This trauma allows a blood or serum layer to form between the perichondrium in the cartilage. If left untreated, it leads to cartilage infection resulting in new cartilage and fibrous tissue to form, causing the cosmetic deformity known as cauliflower ear.[3] The athlete will complain of acute throbbing pain, tenderness, and edema over their ear. Physical examination will reveal a swelling or fluctuant area in the cartilaginous area of the outer ear. Treatment includes either needle aspiration or incision and drainage.[3] Prevention of reaccumulation of fluid or blood is necessary to prevent long-term complications.[3] This is done most commonly using bolsters of thermal plastics plant or dental rolls affixed to the pinna via sutures. A bolsterless technique using absorbable mattress sutures to close the dead space following incision and drainage is also acceptable. This technique has the potential advantage of allowing immediate return to activity, whereas the use of bolsters requires removal of the bolsters 7–10 days after administration.[3] Proper headgear and ear protection should always be utilized.

41.3.2 Otitis Externa

Otitis externa, also known as a swimmer's ear or tropical ear, refers to the inflammation or infection of the external auditory canal. There are a number of risk factors: moisture, high environmental temperatures, insertion of foreign objects into the ear (music earbuds, earplugs), and chronic dermatologic conditions.[3,4] Typically, the infectious process begins with disruption of the cerumen in the external auditory canal. Cerumen is the first line of defense against bacteria and infection for the ear. Bacteria, primarily *Pseudomonas aeruginosa* or *Staphylococcus aureus*, most commonly cause otitis externa.[4] Fungal infections account for less than 10% of otitis externa.[4] It is usually unilateral in presentation and peaks between the ages of 7 and 12 years. It is most common in water sport athletes.[4]

Otitis external is classified into three stages. The preinflammatory stage is when dampness in the external ear canal leads to swelling of the skin inside the canal. This weakens the skin obstructed glands from excreting cerumen. Using an otoscope, this stage presents with an ear canal that is white from the effects of moisture and the cerumen is soft and pale.[4] The next stage is the acute inflammatory stage of otitis externa that presents with redness and mild swelling of the external ear canal with mild serous discharge. There will be worsening pain on examination and tenderness on pressing on the tragus or pulling on the pinna; this is the hallmark sign of otitis externa.[3,4] Typically, the tympanic membrane is not involved; if tympanic membrane redness is seen, acute otitis media should be ruled out with mobility testing. The last stage is the chronic stage. Chronic otitis externa is defined as lasting more than a month or recurring four or more times in a calendar year.[4]

Treatment for mild cases including most fungal causes can be done with stringent agents such as 2% acetic acid, 2.75% boric acid, or rubbing alcohol; these may be painful to an already irritated ear canal and considered ototoxic.[4] Moderate-to-severe cases should be treated with topical antibiotics and steroids such as aminoglycosides or fluoroquinolones with hydrocortisone. Fluoroquinolones are the only topical antibiotic approved for use with ruptured tympanic membranes, thus considered safer if one cannot see the tympanic membrane.[4] Treatment duration is variable that usually is only 5–7 days total continuing 2–3 days after symptoms resolve.[3,4] Most athletes will return the water after approximately 1 week. Some studies suggest that we can return to the water 2–3 days after treatment initiation if there is full resolution of pain.[3] Keeping the external ear canal dry can prevent otitis external. This can be done by using swim caps and earplugs or by removing the external water by shaking the head or using a hair dryer.

41.3.3 Exostosis (Surfer's Ear)

Auditory exostosis and osteoid osteomas are benign progressive osseous lesions that present after repetitive cold-water exposure. They are usually multiple and bilaterally symmetrical.[3] Anatomically, they are bony masses covered with cartilage that produce pain with palpation and with cold water exposure. They may present with conductive hearing loss secondary to progressive obliteration of the auditory canal.[3] Surgical borough is needed for excision and advised for large lesions and progressive hearing loss. Protective equipment such as earplugs and swim caps is used for prevention and for treatment in cold-water athletes.[3,14]

41.3.4 Tympanic Membrane Rupture

Tympanic membrane rupture usually occurs secondary to a diving, water skiing, surfing, or slap injury from martial arts or boxing. The signs and symptoms include acute pain, sudden unilateral hearing loss, nausea, vomiting, tinnitus, and vertigo.[4] Small perforations will heal in a month with no specific treatment. Large perforations greater than 80% of the tympanic membrane will not heal spontaneously and should be referred to an otolaryngologist.[4] There is a general recommendation to allow a month for healing of each 10% of the tympanic membrane lost. Antibiotics are only recommended if infection develops; avoidance of ototoxic medications is necessary, i.e., aminoglycosides and acetic acid.[4] Restriction from water sport is recommended until the perforation is completely healed.[4] Typically, otolaryngologists generally wait 3–6 months for healing to occur before considering any type of surgical repair.[14]

41.4 NASAL INJURIES

41.4.1 Nasal Fractures

Nasal fractures are the most commonly fractured bone in the adult face and account for almost 40% of acute bony injuries.[17] Nasal fractures are commonly seen in baseball, softball, rugby, boxing/other martial arts, soccer, and wrestling. These fractures result in varying degrees of deformity based on the mechanism of injury and the direction of the blow. When a nasal fracture is suspected, a thorough assessment of the head and neck is important to rule out other injury. With any facial trauma, importance is placed on airway, breathing, and circulation. The type of blow to the nasal area is helpful to determine the possible fractures. Direct end-on blows or inferior blows usually result in comminuted fractures of the bone and nasal cartilage. Lateral blows (side blows) usually result in displacement of the nasal bones and simple fractures with deviation to the contralateral side.[13] The signs and symptoms of nasal fractures are epistaxis, tearing, severe pain, facial swelling, and ecchymosis. The first visual clues to a potential nasal fracture are asymmetry, swelling, and epistaxis.[13,17] Examination of the potential nasal fracture must include visualization (looking for asymmetry) and palpation (feeling for crepitance), as well as intranasal inspection. Palpation of crepitance or mobility of skeletal parts on palpation is usually diagnostic for fracture. Visualization is best done at the time of injury before swelling has occurred. The intranasal examination evaluates for compound fracture, appearance of septal hematoma, and presence of cerebral spinal fluid (CSF). The double-ring test is a quick way for the primary care physician to detect CSF leakage (see Figure 41.1). The CSF double-ring sign is based on the principle that blood and CSF will disseminate at different rates, due to different fluid densities, creating a *double ring*, one of blood, surrounded by a second ring of CSF.[15]

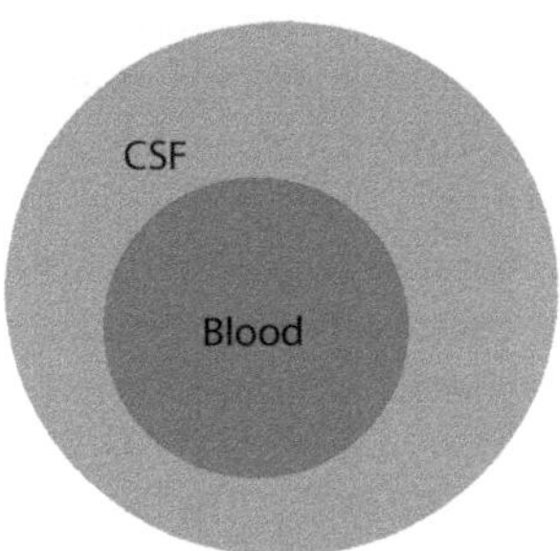

FIGURE 41.1 The double-ring sign is based on the difference of diffusion rates of the blood and CSF. (From Marco, C., *Acad. Emerg. Med.*, 11(1), 75, 2004.)

41.4.2 Double-Ring Sign

Imaging of the nasal bones is rarely helpful in determining the presence of fracture and is not usually required; however, it may prove useful as a medicolegal record of injury.[17]

Clinical Pearl

The double-ring sign can detect for a CSF leak on site or at bedside.

Nondisplaced nasal fractures typically require no treatment. Angulated or displaced nasal fractures may require treatment. The primary care physician may be able to reduce the minimally displaced nasal fracture if done early; however, once swelling has started, the ability to assess the amount of deformity declines and relocation should not be attempted. If relocation is not possible, the athlete will require referral to an otolaryngologist within the next 5–7 days. Relocation is increasingly difficult and usually requires osteotomies for adequate repair after 7–10 days.[13,17] Return to play is not recommended for at least 1 week after nasal fractures, and then external protective devices are recommend for a minimum of 4 weeks after the injury during play.

41.4.3 Septal Hematoma

A septal hematoma is an accumulation of blood between the septal cartilage and the nasal mucosa (perichondrium). In children, these structures are loosely adhered, facilitating hematoma and potential abscess formation.[13] Hematomas are mainly caused by minor trauma of the nasal mucosa and are prone to abscess formation that can lead to a *saddle nose* deformity, as well as other sequela if not treated appropriately.[13,17] The classification of major sequela includes nasal deformation causing important esthetic impairment, deviation of the septum with nasal obstruction, and swelling of the cartilage.[13,17] Minor sequela includes minor esthetic deformities and minimal septal and vault alterations without airway compromise.[13,17] Septal hematomas usually present with a bluish nasal obstruction in one nare, but they can be bilateral.[13] Pain and facial swelling are usually present with theses injuries, and like nasal fractures, they are caused by a traumatic blow to the nose. On physical examination, a bluish bulge is found on the nasal septum on the affected side.[13] Prompt aspiration is the key to successful treatment of septal hematoma. This can be done with an 18–20 gauge needle. Once the hematoma has been drained, the nare is packed for 4–5 days to prevent reoccurrence. It is controversial whether a nasal drain should be utilized.[13] Prophylactic antibiotics are used for 10–14 days to aid in the prevention of abscess. The oral antibiotic should include coverage of *S. aureus*, the most common pathogen isolated. Other pathogens include *Haemophilus influenzae*, *Streptococcus pneumoniae*, and group A β-hemolytic *streptococcus*. Because these are the primary pathogens involved, an antistaphylococcal penicillin or clindamycin is the agent of choice.[13] Otolaryngology referral is required if the bleeding recurs or an abscess forms. Return to play is not recommended until the nasal packing is removed and the chance of rebleeding has diminished.

41.4.4 Epistaxis

The most common nosebleeds originate from the nasal septum and are caused by a disruption of the nasal mucosa overlying the septal vessels (Kiesselbach's plexus).[12] Anterior epistaxis accounts for 90%–95% of nosebleeds.[12] The primary care physician must always consider bony or septal fracture with any traumatic epistaxis, as any force sufficient enough to cause mucosal disruption and bleeding may be sufficient to cause a fracture or dislocation of the nasal skeleton.[10] The signs and symptoms of traumatic anterior epistaxis are pain in the nose and dripping of blood from the nostrils. The treatment is mainly ice and compression at the anterior nose. Another approach is the use of vasoconstrictors, such as topical oxymetazoline hydrochloride or phenylephrine.[10,12] This may decrease the bleeding enough to allow cautery or compression to be utilized, avoiding the potential complications of packing. If this fails, visualization of the bleeding is required so that cautery at the bleeding site can be applied (silver nitrate or electrocautery pen). If cautery is not available or the bleeding site cannot be seen, anterior packing can be applied using gauze with petroleum jelly, expandable cellulose, intranasal tampons, or various pledgets that are commercially available.[12] Complications of nasal packing procedures include septal hematomas and abscesses from traumatic packing, sinusitis, neurogenic syncope during packing, and pressure necrosis secondary to excessively tight packing.[12] Though rarely seen, there may be possibility of toxic shock syndrome with prolonged nasal packing; thus, the use of a topical antistaphylococcal antibiotic ointment on the packing materials is recommended.[10,12] In patients that require packing, referral to an otolaryngologist should be made within 24 hours and antibiotics should be initiated.[10] Return to play with a traumatic anterior nosebleed is a judgment call, as any force sufficient enough to cause bleeding is also capable of inducing a fracture. Care must be taken to rule out nasal fracture and dislocation. If the bleeding is easily controlled and no evidence of fracture is seen, return to play can be granted with a warning about the risk of nasal function being impaired if reinjury occurs.

41.4.5 Posterior Epistaxis

Posterior epistaxis accounts for 5%–10% of all nosebleeds and requires more aggressive intervention.[10] As with anterior epistaxis, the cause of posterior epistaxis can either be traumatic or nontraumatic. Posterior bleeding most likely occurs from the sphenopalatine arterial system in the lateral nasal wall.[10] The signs and symptoms are similar to anterior epistaxis, except that the bleeding drains to the posterior pharynx and care must be taken to protect the airway. On examination, the bleeding site cannot be visualized and the athlete must be evaluated for other facial trauma, such as fractures of the nose and orbit.[10] Bleeding that does not stop with ice and compressions is an indication of posterior origin. This type of bleeding is best treated on the field with topical decongestants. Hemostasis is usually achieved if the clot is removed, and then a topical decongestant (vasoconstrictor) can be sniffed until the athlete can expectorate it from the posterior pharynx; this should be repeated until the bleeding stops.[10] If the bleeding is not controllable in this manner, a small Foley (16–18 Fr.) can be inserted though the nare into the nasopharynx and inflated (10–15 cc saline). Anterior traction is put in place to seat the balloon and tamponade the bleeding. All athletes with posterior epistaxis require evaluation by an otolaryngologist within 24 hours and may require hospitalization.[10] As posterior epistaxis can be massive and has been associated with significant morbidity, the athlete is not allowed to return to play until clearance is obtained from otolaryngology.

41.4.6 Prevention

Most nasal injuries can be prevented using appropriate face masks (football) and other protective gears.[8,23] Care should be taken to ensure proper bracing and masking in athletes that are returning from previous nasal injuries.

41.5 FACIAL BONE INJURIES

41.5.1 Frontal Bone Fractures

The frontal bone creates the outward appearance of the forehead and is considered part of the skull; thus, fracture in this area is considered a skull fracture.[2] The frontal bone is involved in 5%–15% of facial fractures.[2] The frontal sinus is considered the strongest bone in the face, and a considerable amount of forces is required for fracture. Therefore, other craniofacial injuries are present in 56%–87% of frontal bone fractures, stressing the importance of a thorough physical exam.[2] Any rhinorrhea in patients with this fracture is considered a CSF leak until proven otherwise.[2]

Clinical Pearl

Any rhinorrhea in a frontal bone fracture is considered CSF leak until proven otherwise.

These fractures are most commonly diagnosed with CT. These fractures are rarely seen in isolation; thus, prompt surgical consultation is recommended.[2] Approximately, 25% of patients with frontal bone fractures also have ocular injury; therefore, a thorough ocular exam is mandated.[2] Damage to the supraorbital nerve will cause numbness over its distribution. The recommended CT scan is with 2 mm cuts to fully evaluate the frontal bone and sinus.[2] Fractures may be evident on PA/lateral and water's x-rays. Commonly associated injuries with frontal bone fracture include other injury/fracture, CSF leak, nasofrontal duct involvement/damage, ocular injury, and neurological injury. Due to the complexities of these fractures, surgical evaluation and consultation is recommended.

41.5.2 Mandibular Fracture

The mandible is the third most commonly fractured facial bone, behind the nose and the zygoma, respectively.[16] Fracture of the mandible is caused by either direct or indirect blunt trauma or penetrating trauma to the mandible during contact/collision sports. The most common sites of fracture are the condyle and the mandibular angle.[16] Athletes will present with pain, swelling, and inability to chew or completely close their mouth. There may be signs of swelling and ecchymosis, step-off, malocclusion, and deviation of the jaw to the fractured side. Paresthesias of the lower lip may also be present. Bleeding may indicate an open fracture and potentially dental alveolar involvement. Posterior, anterior, and lateral obliques with panoramic and Towne's views are the x-ray images of choice.[16] A CT may be necessary to identify hairline and condylar fractures. Treatment involved temporary immobilization with an elastic bandage and further fixation with intermaxillary wiring may be required. Rehabilitation with jaw fixation includes repetitive activities such as lightweight training, cycling, and swimming. Resumption of full activity, to include contact and collision sports, requires wearing special protection, such as customized mouth guard for an addition of 1–2 months.

41.5.3 Mandibular Dislocation

The mandibular condyles articulate with temporal bone, at the mandibular fossa, forming a sliding hinge joint, the TMJ. Both indirect and direct traumas to the mandible can result in mandibular dislocation.[16] Symptoms include pain, inability to move the jaw well, inability to chew, or the presence of open bite and bite misalignment. The differential diagnosis includes hemarthrosis of the TMJ, fracture of the mandible or zygoma, capsulitis, or injury to the meniscus. Physical examination reveals tenderness over the TMJ, malocclusion, swelling, restriction of jaw motion, and deviation of the jaw to the normal side upon opening. Radiographic evaluation should include panoramic and Towne's views.[16] Arthrogram CT or magnetic resonance imaging of the TMJ may be included to evaluate meniscus integrity.[16] Initial treatment of mandibular dislocation involves rest, ice, compression and elevation, temporary immobilization, and reduction. Reduction is achieved by utilizing posteroinferior directed force with both thumbs of the operator firmly hooked inside the mouth on the third molars.[16] Local or general anesthetics or muscle relaxants are helpful. Often surgical fixation or stabilization is also required if fractures are present. Long-term management entails a soft diet, NSAIDs or other analgesics for 1–2 weeks, and progressive rehabilitation. Graduated return to play including heavy weight training is permitted after the acute phase (7–10 days).[16] Malocclusion, recurrent dislocation, and TMJ arthritis are possible long-term complications.

41.5.4 Zygomatic Fractures

The zygomaticomaxillary (ZMC) complex comprises the lateral and inferior orbital rims, the zygomatic arch, and the ZMC buttress. The ZMC buttress, the zygomaticotemporal buttress, and the zygomaticofrontal buttress are all points of articulation between the facial bones and are common sites of fracture.[2] Fractures in this area are classified into types A, B, and C. Type A fractures are incomplete fractures that are isolated either to the lateral orbital rim or the inferior orbital rim. Type B fractures are the classic tetrapod fractures or simple malar fractures (noncomminuted). Type C fractures are comminuted fractures. The athlete will present with significant swelling, ecchymosis, and pain over the fracture site. Enophthalmos, or malpositioned globe, and subconjunctival hemorrhage are common signs. Deformity might present as palpable emphysema or step-offs over any aspect of the zygomatic complex; however, swelling often obscures it.[2] Diplopia is commonly seen because of extraocular muscle entrapment.[2] The exam may also find sensory defects in the ipsilateral cheek, inferior eyelid, nose, and upper lip (impinged or damaged inferior orbital nerve). It is estimated that 70%–90% of inferior orbital paresthesias are permanent.[2]

CT is the imaging modality of choice or ZMC fractures.[2] Fractures that are minimally or nondisplaced and are not comminuted are usually managed without surgical intervention.[2] However, all fractures of the ZMC complex should be surgically evaluated by a facial surgeon for potential surgery, as even slightly misaligned fractures can lead to asymmetry in the face and poor cosmetic outcomes.[2]

41.5.5 Maxillofacial Injury and Return to Play

Each individual maxillofacial fracture injury requires unique consideration before an athlete is considered to return to sport. It is estimated that after anatomic reduction and stabilization of the fracture, the bone healing begins with an inflammatory hematoma reaction, up to 5 days postfracture, and callus formation can last 4–40 days postfracture.[19] This is then transitioned to a remodeling phase that occurs between 25 and 50 days.[19] Thus, most would advise abstinence from sport for at least 3 weeks after surgical treatment.[19] A return-to-play protocol has been suggested and can be seen in Table 41.2.

Athletes in combat sports are suggested to resume activity after at least 3 months. Continued discussion regarding strict regulations, appropriate training, and the use of protective head equipment is important for basic prevention strategies.

41.6 DENTAL INJURIES

41.6.1 Tooth Avulsion

Tooth avulsion, also referred to as complete luxation, is where a tooth has come completely out of socket and is a dental emergency. Initial management depends first on determining whether the involved tooth is part of the primary or permanent dentition. Primary teeth should not be reimplanted because of risk of damage to the underlying permanent tooth.[16] If the avulsed tooth is a permanent tooth and can be located after traumatic avulsion, the outcome is optimized by immediate reimplantation at the scene.[16] Handling of the tooth is important. The tooth should be handled only by the crown; contact of the root portion of the tooth will cause further damage.[16] Visible contamination should be rinsed with normal saline if available or tap water. Care should be taken to ensure the root is not rubbed or scraped to remove possible debris, as this decreases the chance for successful reimplantation.[16] The tooth can then be placed back in its normal position. It is important to ensure the root if the tooth is in contact with the socket. The athlete should be instructed to bite down on a piece of gauze to hold the tooth in place during transport to the ED or a dentist. If reimplantation cannot be performed, the patient and the tooth should be transported to the nearest dental professional. Hanks' balanced salt solution (HBSS) is the best medium for transport and storage of the tooth and is currently recommended by the American Association of Endodontists.[16] HBSS is available via commercial products and has been shown to maintain periodontal ligament cell viability (essential component for success of reimplantation) for more than 24 hours. It is thought to improve the likelihood of retention of the reimplanted tooth. If HBSS is not available, milk is the second best option and is more readily available. Milk has been shown to provide suitable conditions for periodontal ligament cell self-preservation for up to 3 hours.[16] This has to do with milk's pH and osmolarity compatibility with the tooth and the root. If HBSS or milk is not available, another option would be to transport the tooth in the patient's own saliva.[16] The tooth should not be place back in the athlete's mouth; rather, saliva should be collected in a sterile container with normal saline solution.[16] The tooth can last up to 2 hours in this environment. Water is to be used only as a last resort, and because of its low osmolarity it is not the ideal environment.[16] Return to play is best discussed with a dental professional and a mouth guard is recommended when the athlete returns.

Clinical Pearl

HBSS is recommended for tooth fragment transport.

41.6.2 Tooth Fractures

A tooth fracture is defined as breakage of the tooth structure. It is important to clean the tooth to ensure visibility of the tooth and fracture line. The tooth should be gently rocked back and forth to assess for any accompanied subluxation (loosening) injury. Tooth fractures can be classified as a root fracture, crown fracture involving the dentin, or a chipped tooth.[16] A chipped tooth involves cracking of the enamel surface with no loss of material and is generally not associated with any pain or sensitivity. No emergent intervention is typically required. Fractures that involve only the enamel of the tooth are characterized by the loss of some portion of the normal contour of the tooth. The dentin is typically sensitive

TABLE 41.3
Indications for Specialty Referral for Common Oral–Maxillofacial Injures

Diagnosis	Primary Care Referral Considerations
Ocular	
Eyelid lacerations	Eyelid margin repairs require a referral to an ophthalmologist because proper function of the lid depends on the repair.
Orbital fractures	Loss of visual acuity requires immediate referral to ophthalmology. Any concern for long-term sequel with these fractures should have surgical follow-up.
Retrobulbar hematoma	Immediate referral for decompression is a necessity to save vision.
Corneal abrasion	Ophthalmology referral is indicated if there is a positive Seidel sign, as it suggests a rupture to the globe.
Global rupture	After stabilization with a metal shield to protect the eye, urgent ophthalmology is needed.
Foreign body	If the foreign body cannot be removed or embedded in the eye, then ophthalmology referral is warranted.
Retinal detachment	If retinal detachment is suspected, urgent referral to an ophthalmologist for dilated eye exam is required.
Ear	
Exostosis	If conductive hearing loss is progressing, surgical consult is recommended.
Tympanic membrane rupture	Perforations greater than 80% will not heal spontaneous and referral to otolaryngology is recommended.
Nasal	
Nasal fractures	Any concern for CSF leak should prompt a higher level of care and advanced imaging. Another consideration for nasal fractures is if relocation is not possible, referral to otolaryngology is recommended within 5–7 days.
Septal hematoma	Otolaryngology referral is required if the bleeding recurs or an abscess forms.
Anterior epistaxis	In patients that require packing, referral to an otolaryngologist should be made within 24 hours and antibiotics should be initiated.
Posterior epistaxis	All athletes with posterior epistaxis require evaluation by an otolaryngologist within 24 hours.
Facial	
Frontal fracture	These fractures are rarely seen in isolation and thus prompt surgical consultation is recommended.
Mandibular fracture	Prompt referral to surgical consultation is required, as treatment usually involves immobilization.
Mandibular dislocation	If one suspects concurrent fracture, surgical referral is recommended.
Zygomatic fracture	A facial surgeon should surgically evaluate all zygomatic fractures as slight misalignments can cause poor cosmetic outcomes.
Dental	
Avulsion	Considered a dental emergency. Urgent referral for reimplantation can save the tooth.
Fracture	Fractures involving the dentin require a timely transfer to the emergency department with immediate dental follow-up. Emergent evaluation by a dental provider is required for fractures extending into the pulp.

to cool water or forced air over the tooth and has the appearance of a more yellow tinged or porous. Fractures that only involve enamel, no dentin exposed, are typically not sensitive to temperature or forced air over the tooth. Normal restoration of the contours can be accomplished using the various composite resins or anesthetic purposes. Rough edges from the enamel fracture may be smoothed with an emery board to avoid tongue or mucosal damage until a dentist can see the athlete. Fractures that extend into the dentin are at risk for subsequent inflammation or infection of the pulp cavity potentially leading to tooth loss.[16] These fractures are recognized by the appearance of two different layers of material with the center being more yellow (dentin) and in the outer a more pearly white enamel. The tooth will be sensitive to temperature and forced air exposure. Initial treatment includes providing appropriate covering over the exposed dentin to limit the risk of ongoing contamination and to provide pain relief. A timely transfer to the ED for immediate dental follow-up is recommended. Fractures that extend into the pulp of the tooth are characterized by visualization of pink pulp material at the base of the defect. These are typically very painful and sensitive to temperature and forced air. However, concussion of the nerve from the initial injury may result in an insensate tooth at initial presentation; thus, relying on sensitivity is not recommended.[16] These fractures result in a high risk of pulp necrosis and potential tooth loss. Emergent evaluation by a dental provider is recommended.[16] However, if this is not immediately available, coverage of the tooth with calcium hydroxide, zinc oxide, or glass ionomer composites should be used to prevent further bacterial contamination and mitigate pain.[7,16] These composites are typically stocked in the emergency room. Systemic antibiotics use is not currently recommended[7,16] (Table 41.3).

41.6.3 Prevention

Properly fitted mouth guard should be protective, comfortable, resilient, and causing middle interference to speaking and breathing. Sports that have introduced mandatory use of mouth guards have shown a 60% reduction in dental injuries.[8,23,24] The literature does not currently support mouth guards in the prevention of concussion.[23] Currently the

TABLE 41.4
SORT: Key Recommendations for Practice

Clinical Recommendation	Evidence Rating	References
Ninety percent of sports-related ocular injuries can be prevented with the proper use of protective eyewear.	A	[20]
The use of mouth guards has shown a 60% reduction in dental injuries.	A	[8, 23, 24]
Mouth guards do not prevent concussion.	B	[23]

American Dental Association recommends the use of mouth guard or acrobatics basketball, bicycling, boxing, equestrian sports, extreme sports, field hockey, football, gymnastics, handball, ice hockey, skating, lacrosse, martial arts, racquetball, rugby, skateboarding, skiing, skydiving, soccer, softball, squash, surfing, volleyball, water polo, weightlifting, and wrestling.[8,23,24]

In conclusion, see Table 41.4.

REFERENCES

1. American Dental Association. For the dental patient. The importance of using mouthguards. Tips for keeping your smile safe. *The Journal of the American Dental Association*. 2004;135(7):1061.
2. Boswell KA. Management of facial fractures. *Emergency Medicine Clinics of North America*. 2013;31:539–551.
3. Cassaday K, Vazquez G, Wright J. Ear problems and injuries in athletes. *Current Sports Medicine Reports*. 2014;13(1):22–26.
4. Conover K. Earache. *Emergency Medicine Clinics of North America*. 2013;31:413–442.
5. Deibel J, Cowling K. Ocular inflammation and infection. *Emergency Medicine Clinics of North America*. 2013;13: 387–397.
6. Ducharme J, Tsiaras W. Sports-related ocular trauma. *Medicine & Health Rhode Island*. 2000;83(2):45–51.
7. Elias H, Baur DA. Management of trauma to supporting dental structures, *Dental Clinics of North America*. 2009;53:675–689.
8. Farrington T, Onambele-Person G, Taylor R et al. A review of facial protective equipment use in sport and the impact on injury incidence. *British Journal of Oral and Maxillofacial Surgery*. 2012;50:233–238.
9. Gelston, C. Common eye emergencies. *American Family Physician*. 2013;88(8):515–519.
10. Kasperek Z, Pollock G. Epistaxis: An overview. *Emergency Medicine Clinics of North America*. 2013;31:443–454.
11. Kent J, Eidsness R, Colleaux K et al. Indoor soccer-related eye injuries: Should eye protection by mandatory? *Canadian Journal of Ophthalmology*. 2007;42:605–608.
12. Kuckik C, Clenney T. Management of epistaxis. *American Family Physician*. 2005;71(2):305–311.
13. Kuckik C, Clenney T. Management of acute nasal fractures. *American Family Physician*. 2004;70(7):1315–1320.
14. Lynch J, Deaton T. Barotrauma with extreme pressure in sport: From scuba to skydiving. *Current Sports Medicine Reports*. 2014;13(2):107–112.
15. Marco C. Clinical pearls: Cerebrospinal fluid double ring sign. *Academic Emergency Medicine*. 2004;11(1):75.
16. Murray JM. Mandible fractures and dental trauma. *Emergency Medicine Clinics of North America*. 2013;31:553–573.
17. Navarro R, Romero L, Williams K. Nasal injuries in athletes. *Current Sports Medicine Reports*. 2013;12(1):22–27.
18. Ong H, Barsam A, Morris O et al. A survey of ocular sports trauma and the role of eye protection. *Contact Lens & Anterior Eye*. 2012;35:285–287.
19. Roccia F, Diaspro A, Nasi A et al. Management of sports related maxillofacial injuries. *Journal of Craniofacial Surgery*. 2008;19(2):377–382.
20. Rodriguez J, Lavina A, Agarwal A. Prevention and treatment of common eye injuries in sports. *American Family Physician*. 2003;67(7):1481–1488.
21. Romaniuk V. Ocular trauma and other catastrophes. *Emergency Medicine Clinics of North America*. 2013;31:399–411.
22. Siddique S, Suelves A, Ujwala B et al. Glaucoma and uveitis. *Survey of Ophthalmology*. 2013;58(1):1–10.
23. Trojian H, Mohamed N. Demystifying preventive equipment in the competitive athlete. *Current Sports Medicine Reports*. 2012;11(6):304–308.
24. Zadik Y, Levin L. Does free-of-charge distribution of boil-and-bite mouthguards to young adult amateur sportsmen affect oral and facial trauma? *Dental Traumatology*. 2009;25:69–72.
25. How to evert and eyelid (video clip). Accessed September 3, 2014. http://www.youtube.com/watch?v=5OrsAuyHdK8.
26. Seidel test (video clip). Accessed September 3, 2014. http://www.youtube.com/watch?v=RQhOlVTGbmk.
27. Subconjunctival Hemorrhage. The American Academy of Ophthalmology. Accessed September 14, 2014. http://www.aao.org/theeyeshaveit/red-eye/subconjunctival-hemorrhage.cfm.
28. Hyphema. The American Academy of Ophthalmology. Accessed September 14, 2014. http://www.aao.org/theeyeshaveit/trauma/hyphema.cfm.
29. Corneal Abrasion. The American Academy of Ophthalmology. Accessed September 14, 2014. http://www.aao.org/theeyeshaveit/trauma/corneal-abrasion.cfm.

42 Cervical Spine

Barry P. Boden and David A. Levin

CONTENTS

TABLE 42.1
Key Clinical Considerations

1. Sports with the highest risk of catastrophic spinal injuries are football, ice hockey, wrestling, diving, skiing, snowboarding, and rugby.
2. Acute brachial plexus injuries, burners, are common in American football and involve only one extremity. Any individual with neurologic symptoms in more than one extremity has an SCI until proven otherwise.
3. Axial compression forces to the top of the head can lead to cervical fracture and quadriplegia in any sport.
4. Any medical personnel covering team sports should have a plan for stabilization and transfer of an athlete with a cervical spine injury.
5. The role of methylprednisolone in the treatment of acute SCI requires further evidence-based clinical studies.

42.1 INTRODUCTION

Most cervical spine injuries in sports are stable injuries requiring careful nonoperative treatment. These injuries include cervical strains and transient brachial plexopathy (TBP). Catastrophic spine injuries in sports are rare but tragic events that may lead to permanent disability. The sports with the highest risk of catastrophic spinal injuries are football, ice hockey, wrestling, diving, skiing, snowboarding, rugby, cheerleading, and baseball. A common mechanism of injury for all at-risk sports is an axial compression force to the top of the head with the neck slightly flexed. The authors review the spectrum of cervical spine injuries in the athletic population, common mechanisms of injury, on-field management of the athlete with a cervical spine injury, and sports-specific injuries in the at-risk sports (Table 42.1).

Clinical Pearl

Sports with the highest risk of catastrophic spinal injuries are football, ice hockey, wrestling, diving, skiing, snowboarding, and rugby.

42.2 BRACHIAL PLEXUS INJURIES

Brachial plexus injuries are rare in most sports except football, ice hockey, and wrestling. Most sports-related brachial plexus injuries are compression or traction neurapraxias, which have a favorable prognosis. The differential diagnosis of a brachial plexus injury should include TBP, acute brachial neuropathy (ABN), root avulsion or neurotmesis, disk herniation, cervical cord neurapraxia (CCN), and cervical spine fracture.

42.2.1 Transient Brachial Plexopathy

Most brachial plexus injuries occur in American football players and are referred to as a "burner" or "stinger." The single-season incidence of TBP in American college football players has been reported to be between 6.9% and 50%.[21,40,53,54] One study revealed that 65% of 201 NCAA division III football players had a history of TBP.[54]

Athletes with TBP typically present with acute unilateral upper extremity radicular symptoms from the supraclavicular region to the finger tips. TBP must be differentiated from CCN, which is defined as injury to the spinal cord with neurologic symptoms in at least two extremities. This important clinical point cannot be overemphasized: burners occur in a single arm. Athletes with neurologic symptoms bilaterally or in more than one extremity have a spinal cord injury (SCI) until proven otherwise. On the sidelines, the player with TBP initially presents shaking his arm or holding it at his side as a response to paresthesias and dysesthesias. Weakness is often associated with the injury and may occur on a delayed basis hours to days after the injury.[4,53] Neurologic deficits, if present, usually occur at the C5 or C6 levels as manifested by shoulder abduction (deltoid) and elbow flexion (biceps) weakness. In most instances, the neurologic symptoms only last for several minutes, but may persist for days to months in 5%–10% of athletes.[59] Prolonged symptoms are more common in athletes with multiple episodes. Physical examination usually reveals a normal, painless cervical range of motion.

Three causes of TBP have been proposed: traction, extension–compression, and direct compression (Figure 42.1). Traction is the most frequently hypothesized mechanism to explain the burner phenomenon and usually occurs in younger athletes. The injury mechanism involves a tackling maneuver when the shoulder is depressed with lateral neck flexion to the contralateral side. The extension–compression mechanism typically involves older players with degenerative changes of the cervical spine. The cervical spine is in extension, compression, and rotation toward the affected arm similar to the Spurling's maneuver position. Foraminal narrowing and/or degenerative disk disease have been implicated as causing impingement on the exiting nerve roots.[34,35] Last, the injury may occur as a result of direct compression at the Erb's point where the brachial plexus is most superficial.

Clinical Pearl

Acute brachial plexus injuries, burners, are common in American football and involve only one extremity. Any individual with neurologic symptoms in more than one extremity has a SCI until proven otherwise.

Diagnosis of TBP is usually made by performing a thorough history and physical examination. Electrodiagnostic studies are not indicated for routine cases of TBP as the study often reveals persistent abnormalities even after complete clinical resolution. Rather, electrodiagnostic evaluation is warranted in athletes with symptoms lasting longer than 3 weeks or for those with multiple episodes. The treatment of TBP involves symptomatic measures. Physical therapy may be helpful to strengthen the affected muscles. Athletes should not be allowed to return to contact sports until full painless neck range of motion and complete neurologic recovery are achieved. Prevention of TBP should include a review of tackling techniques instructing the athlete not to tackle with the shoulder dropped and the head laterally rotated toward the contralateral side. Using a neck roll or other equipment to limit neck extension may reduce the incidence of TBP, but is controversial since the cervical spine is placed in a more vulnerable position for axial forces.

42.2.2 Acute Brachial Neuropathy

ABN, also referred to as Parsonage–Turner syndrome, brachial neuritis, and acute brachial radiculitis, is a condition associated with acute shoulder and neck pain that may spread to the forearm region. The painful phase typically lasts between several hours and 3 weeks and is followed by varying degrees of weakness. Weakness may be mild or severe and usually involves the C5 and C6 distributions, especially the deltoid, supraspinatus, and infraspinatus muscles. Signs that should alert the clinician to ABN are onset of symptoms with no trauma, pain that continues despite rest, and dominant arm predominance.[26] Advanced imaging of the cervical spine is warranted to rule out compressive lesions, particularly when neurologic deficits are present. The etiology of ABN is unknown, but may involve an inflammatory process, such as a viral or autoimmune etiology. Treatment in the early painful phase involves rest, a sling, and analgesics. Once the pain has subsided, a course of physical therapy concentrating on passive range of motion and strengthening[79] should be instituted. Most cases are self-limiting and resolve over the course of several months or years.[75] Upper plexus lesions have a more favorable prognosis.[72]

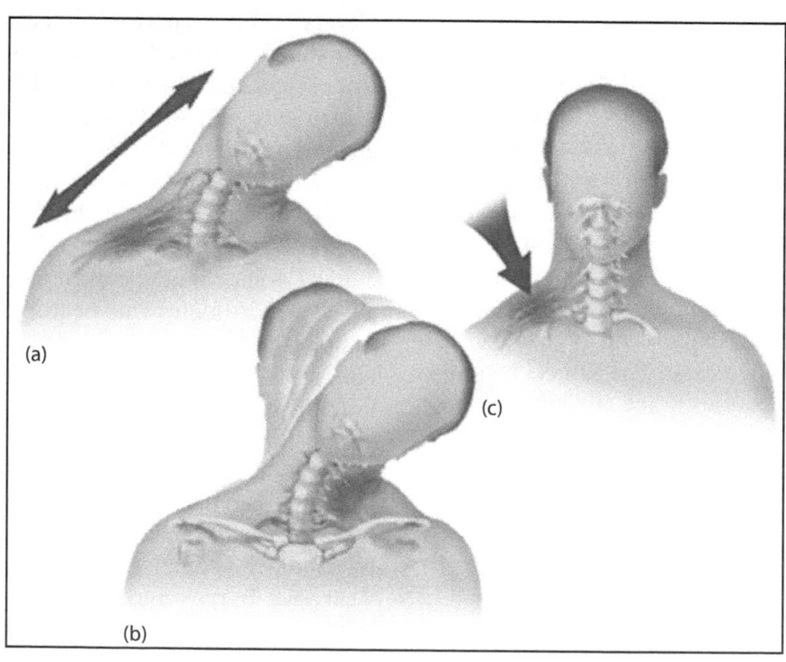

FIGURE 42.1 Illustration of three potential causes of transient brachial plexopathy: (a) traction, (b) extension-compression, (c) direct compression. (Illustration by Renee L, Cannon, 1999.)

42.2.3 Nerve Root Injuries and Neurotmesis

Nerve root avulsions and neurotmesis injuries are rare in athletes but may occur in high-velocity sporting events.[64] Most injuries occur due to severe downward pressure on the shoulder with head flexion to the contralateral side. If the arm is at the side or adducted, injury typically occurs to the upper trunk region; hyperabduction often leads to injury to the lower trunk. Diagnosis is confirmed by MRI. Cervical or shoulder fractures and vascular injuries may be sustained in conjunction with the nerve disruption due to the violent forces necessary to produce this injury. Immediate sensory and motor loss is evident in the affected distribution. Immediate surgical intervention is recommended for patients with a vascular injury or penetrating trauma. In most other cases, surgery is postponed for 3–6 months to allow maximum healing. If significant functional deficits persist, muscle transfer procedures and nerve exploration with direct repair, nerve grafting, and/or neurolysis may be helpful.[37] The prognosis for athletes with root avulsions is poor, and the likelihood of returning to competitive sports is low.

42.3 COMMON CERVICAL SPINE INJURIES

The most common athletic injury to the cervical spine is a strain. Although whiplash injuries with a sudden extension–flexion mechanism are common, any low-grade force to the cervical spine may cause a sprain. Athletes present with paravertebral muscle spasm, occasional limited neck range of motion, and normal neurologic examination. Plain radiographs may reveal loss of normal lordosis. The vast majority of cervical spine strains resolve uneventfully with conservative modalities, including relative rest, anti-inflammatories, muscle relaxants, and physical therapy.

Compression fractures of the cervical spine usually occur at the lower levels. In addition to plain radiographs, flexion–extension radiographs, computed tomography (CT), and/or MRI may be helpful in excluding a more serious injury. Isolated fractures with less than 25% anterior compression can be managed conservatively with a cervical orthosis. Compression fractures with greater than 50% anterior compression may be associated with posterior ligamentous disruption resulting in instability that may require surgical stabilization. An MRI is recommended to rule out posterior soft tissue injury or fracture of the posterior elements of the vertebra, since these injuries may compromise spinal stability.

Avulsion injuries to the spinous process are also known as clay-shoveler's fractures (Figure 42.2). The injuries usually occur in football players and powerlifters, and most commonly occur at the C7 level. The proposed mechanism of injury for clay-shoveler's fractures is forceful flexion of the cervical spine or abrupt contraction of the trapezius and rhomboid muscles. These fractures are stable and can be treated with a cervical orthosis and symptomatic measures. Patients with stable, healed compression or spinous process avulsion fractures who have full, painless cervical range of motion and no neurologic deficits have no contraindications to participate in contact sports.

Cervical disk herniations (Figure 42.3) may occur in athletes in any sport. Symptoms typically include neck pain, restricted cervical motion, radicular symptoms, and sensory and motor deficits. Although neurologic examination can localize the site of the lesion, MRI is appropriate to confirm the diagnosis. Many athletes with a cervical herniated disk respond to nonoperative modalities such as rest, anti-inflammatory agents, a short course of oral corticosteroids, physical therapy, and occasionally epidural steroid injections. When these measures fail or the athlete has a progressive neurologic deficit, surgical decompression is indicated. For far-lateral disk herniations, a minimally invasive posterior foraminotomy can adequately decompress the nerve root. Otherwise, an anterior cervical diskectomy with instrumented fusion is the standard of care. In rare cases, athletes may develop transient quadriplegia or long-tract findings from a large central disk herniation. Anterior diskectomy and interbody fusion is recommended for this condition on an urgent basis.

Although absolute standards for return to play are lacking, guidelines indicate that individuals may return to contact sports after nonoperative treatment of intervertebral disk injuries in patients who are asymptomatic, have no signs of neurologic injury, have full pain-free range of cervical motion, and have no MRI evidence of cervical cord compression.[41,42]

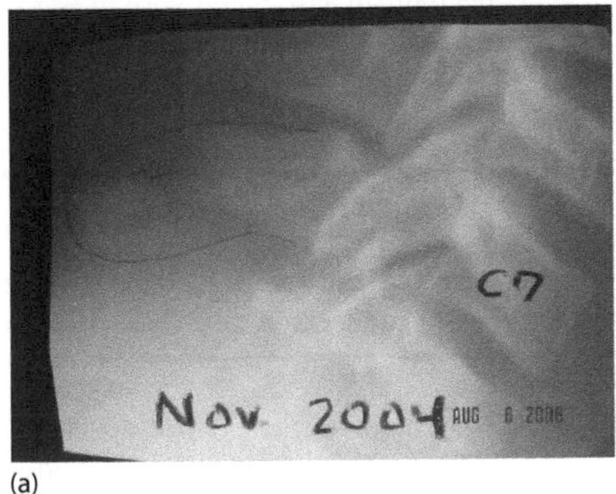

(a)

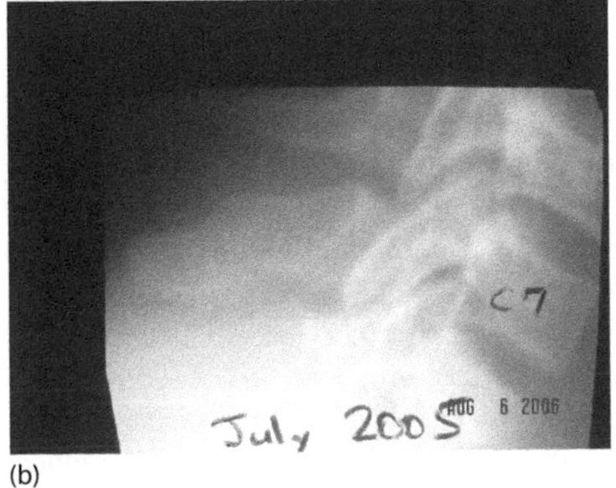

(b)

FIGURE 42.2 (a) C7 spinous process fracture and (b) healed spinous process fracture. (Reprinted from *The Sports Medicine Resource Manual*, Seidenberg, P.H. and Beutler, A.I., Chapter 23: Cervical spine injuries, Boden, B.P., W.B. Saunders, 2008.)

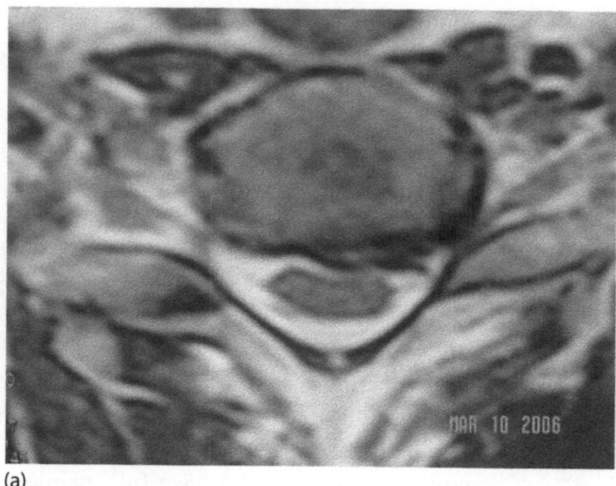

(a)

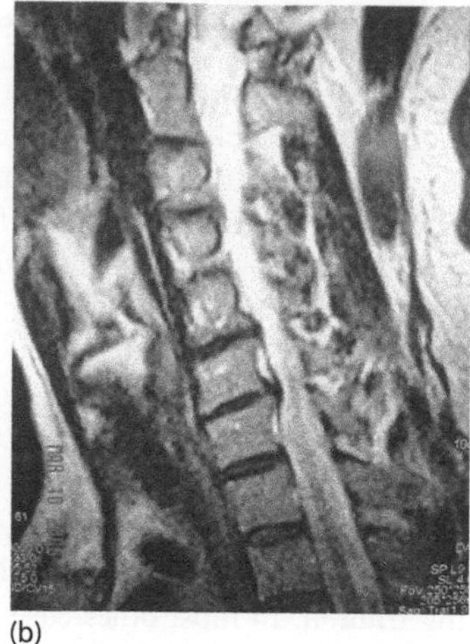

(b)

FIGURE 42.3 (a) Axial and (b) sagittal MRIs of patient with C6–C7 left-sided disk herniation. (Reprinted from *The Sports Medicine Resource Manual*, Seidenberg, P.H. and Beutler, A.I., Chapter 23: Cervical spine injuries, Boden, B.P., W.B. Saunders, 2008.)

The same return-to-play criteria exist for patients following a stable single-level discectomy and fusion. Stable two- or three-level fusion in asymptomatic patients with no neurologic symptoms and full cervical range of motion is a relative contraindication to return to contact sports.[65] Patients with an anterior or posterior fusion of four or more levels and patients with any fusion at C1 should not return to contact sports.[17] While the return-to-play criteria are provided to assist physicians in deciding when to permit or prohibit return to athletic activity, the final decision must be based on the individual, the sport played, and the understanding that further injury is always possible.

42.4 CATASTROPHIC CERVICAL SPINE INJURIES

In the United States, approximately 7% of all new cases of SCI are related to athletic activities.[45] Sports injuries are the second most common cause of SCI in the first 30 years of life.[47] Permanent SCI is much more likely to result from cervical spinal injury than thoracic or lumbar trauma. In a 3-year nationwide survey of all sports in Japan, the incidence of spinal injury was 1.95 per million per year, with a mean age at injury of 28.5 years and 88% occurring in males.[33] Sports identified as placing the participant at high risk for SCI include football, ice hockey, wrestling, diving, skiing, snowboarding, rugby, cheerleading, and baseball.[9] Information on catastrophic injuries in athletes is provided by the National Center for Catastrophic Sports Injury Research (NCCSIR), the National Spinal Cord Injury Statistical Center, the United States Consumer Product Safety Commission (CPSC), and other organizations (see Table 42.2).

The spectrum of catastrophic cervical spine injuries in sports includes unstable fractures and dislocations, CCN (transient quadriplegia), and intervertebral disk herniation.[2] Unstable fractures and dislocations are the most frequent causes of catastrophic cervical spine injury resulting in permanent neurologic sequelae and typically occur in the lower cervical spine, especially at the C5–C6 level. The spinal cord occupies less than half of the canal's cross-sectional area at the level of the atlas, but close to 75% at the lower cervical levels.[51]

TABLE 42.2
Sources of Information on Sport Safety

AACCA	American Association of Cheerleading Coaches and Advisors (www.aacca.org)
CPSC	Consumer Product Safety Commission (www.cpsc.gov)
NCAA	The National Collegiate Athletic Association (www.ncaa.org)
NCCSIR	National Catastrophic Center Sports Injury Research (www.unc.edu/dept/nccsi/)
NCDDR	National Spinal Cord Injury Statistical Center (www.ncddr.org)
NCIPC	National Center of Injury Prevention and Control; Centers for Disease Control and Prevention (www.cdc.gov/ncipc)
NFHS	National Federation of State High School Associations (www.nfhs.org)
NOCSAE	National Operating Committee on Standards for Athletic Equipment (www.nocsae.org)
USA Baseball	USA Baseball (www.usabaseball.com)

The mechanism associated with most catastrophic cervical injuries that result in quadriplegia is an axial force to the top of the head with the neck slightly flexed.[68]

Clinical Pearls

Axial compression forces to the top of the head can lead to cervical fracture and quadriplegia in any sport.

When the neck is in a neutral position, the cervical spine is in a lordotic or extended position, and most energy is dissipated by the paravertebral muscles and the intervertebral disks. However, when the neck is flexed 30°, the cervical spine becomes straight, and the forces are transmitted to the segmented cervical column. Once the maximum compressive deformation is reached, the spine fails in either a flexion (flexion teardrop) or pure compression (burst fracture) mode with a resultant fracture, dislocation, or subluxation. Spinal fragments or the intervertebral disk may retropulse into the spinal canal causing spinal cord damage.

42.5 MANAGEMENT OF THE CERVICAL SPINE–INJURED ATHLETE

Cervical spine trauma can lead to devastating neurologic consequences. Improper care of the athlete's cervical spine on the playing field or during transportation can worsen any SCI. Therefore, the on-site medical team must be prepared to act in an efficient, organized manner. This is best accomplished by a well-trained, rehearsed group of medical personnel. Proper, early care of the athlete with cervical trauma can lead to improved outcomes.[3,67]

Clinical Pearls

Any medical personnel covering team sports should have a plan for stabilization and transfer of an athlete with a cervical spine injury.

42.5.1 Planning and Preparation

There are several principles that should be adhered to by the medical staff responsible for immobilizing and transporting a cervical spine–injured athlete to the hospital:[20]

1. Each school should have an emergency action plan (EAP), including specific details for each athletic facility where practice and competition occur to ensure that appropriate strategies and site-specific procedures are invoked during a time of crisis.
2. An efficient communication system to activate EMS at each athletic venue should be established with a posting of the EAP at each venue, including a list of emergency numbers, facility map with street address, and posting of the specific location of all emergency equipment.
3. All coaches and athletic staff who have contact with student-athletes should be encouraged to train in basic emergency care.
4. An individual, such as the team physician or trainer, should be designated as the leader responsible for supervising on-field management of the injured athlete.
5. The leader must insure that all emergency equipment is available at the site of the potential injury. Necessary equipment includes a spine board, straps to secure the athlete to the spine board, a face mask removal kit, communication devices, and a cardiopulmonary resuscitation (CPR) kit.
6. An ambulance and hospital that are properly equipped and staffed to handle catastrophic cervical spine injuries should be selected in advance of the sporting event.
7. The medical team should practice proper techniques in a mock situation to be fully prepared for an on-field emergency.
8. A decision should be made prior to the event as to which member of the sports medicine team will accompany the athlete during transport.

42.5.2 Removal of Protective Equipment

The National Athletic Trainers' Association formed the Inter-Association Task Force for Appropriate Care of the Spine-Injured Athlete to develop guidelines for proper management of the athlete with a severe spine injury.[36] The task force recommended that in the majority of cases of cervical SCI, the helmet and shoulder pads should not be removed prior to arrival at an emergency room. This rule also applies to youth football athletes since it has been reported that removal of only the helmet leads to increased cervical lordosis compared to removal of the helmet and shoulder pads.[73] Studies of both football and ice hockey players have demonstrated that removal of the helmet or shoulder pads can result in a significant change from the neutral cervical position.[38,50] In rare circumstances, it may be necessary to remove the helmet or shoulder pads prior to transporting the athlete to a hospital. Situations that warrant helmet or shoulder pad removal in the injured athlete are summarized in Table 42.3. It is always best to remove both the helmet and shoulder pads together if either requires removal.[50] In cases where only the helmet can be

TABLE 42.3
Equipment Removal Guidelines

The following situations warrant on-site helmet removal in the injured athlete:

1. If after a reasonable period of time the face mask cannot be removed to gain airway access
2. If the design of the helmet and chin strap is such that even after removal of the face mask the airway cannot be controlled or ventilation provided
3. If the helmet and chin straps do not hold the head securely such that immobilization of the helmet does not also immobilize the head
4. If the helmet prevents immobilization for transport in an appropriate position
5. If the shoulder pads require removal

The following situations warrant on-site shoulder pad removal in the injured athlete:

1. Multiple injuries requiring full access to the shoulder area
2. Ill-fitting shoulder pads resulting in the inability to maintain spinal immobilization
3. CPR requiring access to the thorax that is inhibited by shoulder pads
4. If the helmet requires removal

Source: Adapted from Kleiner, D.M. et al., *Prehospital Care of the Spine-Injured Athlete*, Dallas, TX, National Athletic Trainers' Association, 2001.

removed, occipital padding is recommended to maintain neutral sagittal cervical alignment.[23] For shoulder pad removal, the elevated torso technique has been shown to minimize cervical spine motion compared to the flat torso technique.[29] In the elevated torso technique, an additional assistant lifts the patient's shoulders 30–40° off the ground while the head hold maintains spinal alignment.[29]

Despite the traditional guidelines, there is a new trend to remove the helmet and shoulder pads prior to transport to an emergency facility by at least three rescuers trained and experienced with equipment removal. In these cases, a rigid cervical collar should be applied and manual in-line stabilization maintained until the athlete is stabilized on a full body immobilization device and the athlete's head is properly immobilized to the spine board.

42.5.3 On-Field Assessment and Treatment

The athlete should be treated as though there is a cervical spine injury until proper radiographs can be obtained. The first step in managing the athlete with a cervical spine injury is to immobilize the head and neck in a stable position. The initial evaluation of the injured athlete should assess for any life-threatening conditions using the airway, breathing, circulation, disability or neurologic status, and exposure of the athlete (ABCDE) sequence of trauma care.[3] If a life-threatening problem is identified or suspected, the emergency medical system should be activated. Any unconscious athlete should be assumed to have a cervical spine injury.

42.5.4 Normal Mental Status without Cardiorespiratory Compromise

The most common scenario is an athlete with a cervical injury who is breathing and has a normal mental status. In this situation, the mouth guard should be removed and the airway maintained. The face mask need not be removed initially unless the airway is threatened. If the athlete is breathing and has a normal pulse, the neurologic status and level of consciousness should be assessed. The prone athlete should be carefully logrolled to a supine position, moving the head and trunk as a single unit (Figure 42.4). The leader maintains immobilization of the head by applying slight traction and using the crossed-arm technique. This technique allows for constant immobilization of the head and neck without the leader's arms becoming entangled during the logroll maneuver. In addition to the leader, at least three medical personnel should be available to maintain body alignment during the logroll maneuver. The designated leader controls the head and gives the command for turning (Figure 42.4).

After the athlete is logrolled onto the spine board, the torso of the athlete is secured to the backboard using Velcro straps. The straps are firmly secured allowing enough room for chest movement during breathing. With the leader maintaining cervical stabilization, the face mask is then removed. Removal of the face mask depends on the type of helmet. A cordless screwdriver should be available since it allows for quick removal with minimal helmet motion.[61] A variety of cutting tools should be available in addition to the cordless screw driver to improve the success of face mask removal[25] (Figure 42.5).

The medical team should also be prepared with bolt cutters for the older single- and double-bar masks as well as a sharp knife or scalpel to detach any plastic loops. Although there is currently no standard for loop straps, the ShockBlocker loop strap allows for more efficient face mask removal than other currently available devices.[34] Once the facemask is fully removed, the head is firmly stabilized to the back board. On the leader's count, the spine board is then lifted with a minimum of four assistants, and the patient is placed in the ambulance for evacuation to an emergency room.

42.5.5 Cardiovascular Compromise

If the athlete is not breathing at initial evaluation or stops breathing, an airway must immediately be established. Respiratory distress can be caused by upper cervical SCI with paralysis of the diaphragm. Access to the airway must be accomplished without causing further injury to the spine. The prone athlete is carefully logrolled into a supine position. After the face mask has been removed, rescue breathing according to the standards of the American Heart Association

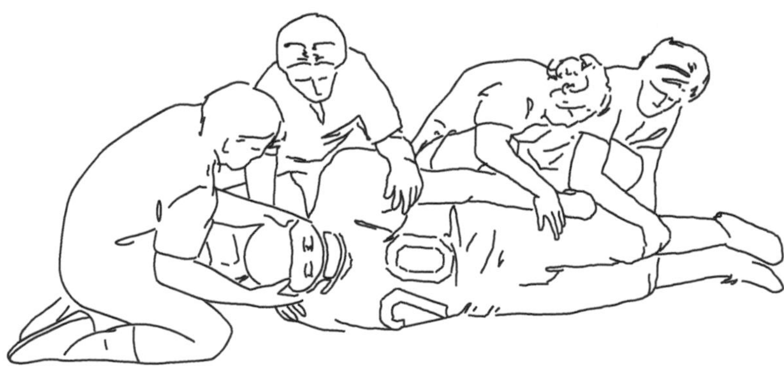

FIGURE 42.4 Proper logrolling technique. A minimum of four individuals is required. The leader uses the cross-arm technique to immobilize the head as the athlete is turned from a prone to supine position onto the spine board. (Reproduced with permission from Torg, J.S. and Gennarelli, T.A., in: DeLee, J.C. and Drez, D. Jr., eds., *Orthopaedic Sports Medicine: Principles and Practice*, Vol. 1. WB Saunders, 1994.)

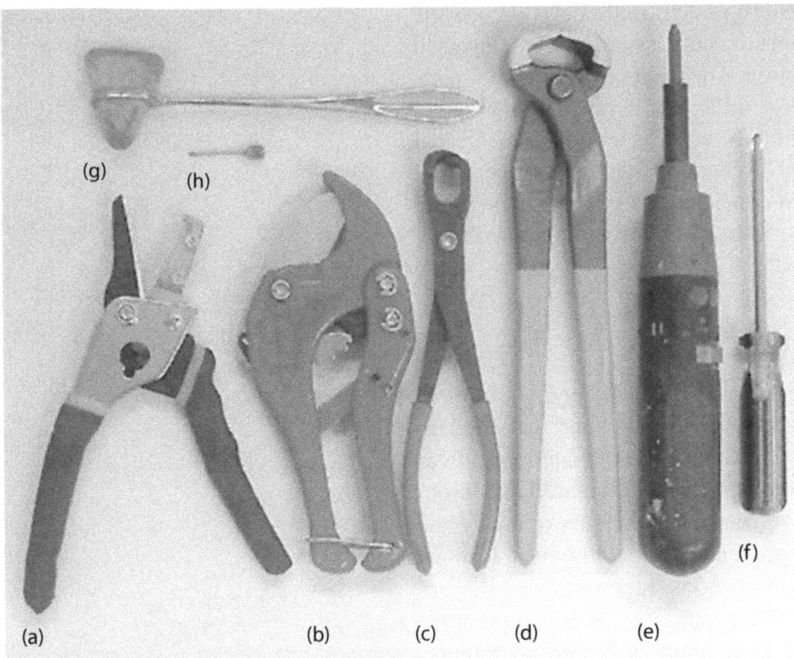

FIGURE 42.5 Essential equipment that should be available to remove the face mask: (a) facemask extractor, (b) PVC pipe cutter, (c) trainer's Angel, (d) wire cutter, (e) electric screwdriver, (f) manual screwdriver, (g) reflex hammer (used to pry away cheek pads), and (h) air pump needle (used to deflate the helmet air bladder). (Reprinted with permission from Waninger, K.N., *Am. J. Sports Med.*, 32, 1331, 2004.)

should be initiated. If the athlete's airway is not open, then a jaw-thrust maneuver is performed. This is accomplished by grasping the angles of the victim's lower jaw and lifting in order to move the tongue away from obstructing the airway. The head-tilt maneuver should be avoided due to the potential for altering cervical alignment. In the athlete who is unresponsive, an oral airway may be necessary to prevent occlusion of the oropharynx.

42.5.6 Emergency Department Management

Once the athlete has been transported to a stable setting in the hospital, care is transferred to the emergency medical staff. The team physician or athletic trainer should assist in the removal of equipment since emergency medical personnel often are not familiar with the protocol. After reevaluating the ABCDEs, radiographs should be performed. Although the traditional protocol was to perform plain radiographs before removal of equipment, this practice has recently been called into question. Football helmets and shoulder pads interfere with radiographic visualization of the cervical spine often leading to undetected pathology.[25] Although controversial, the current trend is that head and shoulder protective gear should be cautiously removed before cervical spine radiographic imaging or at a minimum be removed if radiographs are obscured by protective equipment.[22] In addition, several studies have documented that cervical spine radiographs miss up to 45% of injuries, especially at the upper cervical levels, when compared with CT in trauma victims.[1,48] Therefore, helical CT scans are recommended for complete evaluation of the cervical spine in any athlete with suspected cervical injury.

42.5.7 NEXUS Criteria

The National Emergency X-Radiography Utilization Study (NEXUS) was a large, federally supported, multicenter, prospective observational study designed to examine the sensitivity of various clinical criteria for ruling out significant cervical spine injury. Following a significant mechanism of injury, the study concluded that the cervical spine could be clinically cleared if the following five criteria are met:

1. There is no posterior midline cervical tenderness.
2. There is no evidence of intoxication.
3. The patient is alert and oriented.
4. There is no referable neurologic deficit.
5. There are no painful distracting injuries.

If the injured individual does not meet all five of the aforementioned criteria, further radiographic evaluation is recommended prior to clearing the cervical spine of injury.[28]

42.5.8 Equipment Removal

Prior to removal of the helmet, the chin strap should be unfastened and discarded, the cheek pads should be removed, and/or the air bladder should be deflated. Equipment removal is best accomplished with a minimum of three medical personnel to minimize motion of the cervical spine.[52] The athlete's head is then supported at the occiput by one member of the medical staff while the leader removes the helmet in a straight line with the spine.

The shoulder pads should be removed at the same time as the helmet to avoid excessive flexion or extension of the spine. As the athlete's head and neck are secured, medical personnel gently flex the trunk at the hips approximately 30° so the shoulder pads can be removed. Next, a hard collar is applied to the neck for immobilization. The front of the shoulder pads should be removed to allow CPR and defibrillation, if necessary. Further imaging studies, such as a complete cervical spine series, an MRI, or CT scan, are then performed based on the clinical findings. In conclusion, a clearly defined and coordinated treatment algorithm can improve the outcome of a catastrophic cervical injury.

42.5.9 Role of High-Dose Steroids

Since the early 1990s, the use of high-dose methylprednisolone for the treatment of acute SCI has become the standard of care. In a clinical study by Bracken and coauthors, it was found that patients with acute SCI who were treated with high-dose methylprednisolone within the first 8 hours of injury had significant neurologic improvement at 6-month follow-up compared with a placebo group.[14] The recommended dose of methylprednisolone is an intravenous bolus of 30 mg per kilogram of body weight over 15 minutes, followed 45 minutes later by infusion at 5.4 mg per kilogram per hour for 24 hours. Further improvement in motor function recovery has been demonstrated when maintenance therapy is extended for 48 hours, especially if the initial bolus dose was administered 3–8 hours after injury.[13] Although high-dose methylprednisolone for acute SCI has traditionally been the standard of care, this practice has been questioned. One evidence-based analysis of the published literature on methylprednisolone revealed flaws in data analysis and conclusions with no clear support for the use of methylprednisolone in patients with acute SCI.[16,30] Furthermore, several studies indicated a higher incidence of infectious and respiratory complications with methylprednisolone. Additional randomized trials of pharmacologic therapy for spinal cord resuscitation are necessary. Therefore, methylprednisolone is currently considered an optional treatment, and each patient or patient's family should be consulted on the risks and benefits of the medication prior to use.[16]

42.6 SPORTS-SPECIFIC CONSIDERATIONS FOR CERVICAL SPINE INJURIES

42.6.1 Football

42.6.1.1 Quadriplegia

Football is associated with the highest number of severe cervical injuries per year among all high school and college sports in the United States.[7,19,46,74] While the incidence of head-related fatalities declined in the early 1970s, the number of cases of permanent cervical quadriplegia started to rise. This is likely due to the improved helmets allowing tacklers to strike an opponent using the crown of the head with less fear of self-induced injury. Torg was instrumental in reducing the rate of quadriplegic events by demonstrating that spearing or tackling a player with the top of the head is the major cause of permanent cervical quadriplegia[71] (Figure 42.6). The vast majority of spear tackling injuries occur to defensive players, especially defensive backs.[10,70] A disproportionate number of injuries also occur to players on special teams where the speed of collision is extremely high.[10] In 1976, spearing was banned and the rate of catastrophic cervical injuries dramatically dropped.[68] From 1976 to 1987, the rate of traumatic quadriplegia in football decreased approximately 80%.[68] Other than a spike of 13 quadriplegic injuries in the 1989–1990 academic year, the incidence of injuries has continued to decline through the 1990s.[10] The rate of quadriplegic injuries at the high school and college levels has remained fairly steady in the 1990s and early 2000s at 5.19 per 1 million participants or 1 injury per 192,000 participants.[10]

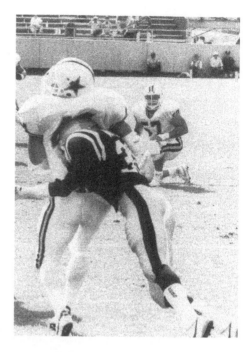

FIGURE 42.6 Photograph of athlete spear tackling with the top of his head. (Reprinted with permission from Torg, J.S. et al., *J. Bone Joint Surg. Am.*, 84, 112, 2002.)

Clinical Pearl

The role of methylprednisolone in the treatment of acute SCI requires further evidence-based clinical studies.

In an effort to reduce the number of quadriplegic injuries, the NCAA strengthened its rule banning spear tackling, effective in the 2005–2006 academic year. The revision removes the word "intentional" from the rule, which makes it easier for referees to call spearing penalties. Under the previous rule, intent was difficult for referees to assess on the field, and the penalty was rarely called. Among the NCAA's efforts to publicize its spearing rule change, the association has produced a poster for locker rooms, a PowerPoint presentation, and a video on the risks, the mechanism of injury, the concept of axial loading, and the prevention of injury by adopting safe tackling techniques.[78] Future epidemiologic data will reveal if this campaign will further reduce the incidence of quadriplegia in football.

Identification of spear tackling as the primary culprit leading to quadriplegic injuries has had a profound effect on reducing this catastrophic injury. Coaches need to continually reinforce proper tackling techniques with the head up. Players should never be allowed to tackle with the head down.

42.6.1.2 Cervical Cord Neurapraxia

CCN is an acute, usually transient, neurologic episode associated with sensory changes with or without motor weakness or complete paralysis in at least two extremities.[68–70] The cervical area is usually pain-free at the time of injury with full painless range of motion. The prevalence has been estimated to be 7 per 10,000 football participants.[68] Complete recovery usually occurs within 10–15 minutes but may take longer. Cervical stenosis is believed to be the primary causative factor predisposing to CCN.[69] The hypothesized mechanism is either hyperflexion or hyperextension of the neck causing a pincer-type compression injury to the spinal cord.[68] New data reveal that there is no one position that is particularly predisposing to a CCN episode and that a variety of mechanisms including axial forces can lead to CCN.[10]

Classification of CCN is based on the neurologic deficit, duration of neurologic symptoms, and pattern of injury.[66] The neurologic deficit may involve motor and/or sensory abnormalities. The grade of injury is based on the duration of neurologic symptoms: Grade I, less than 15 minutes; Grade II, 15 minutes to 24 hours; and Grade III, longer than 24 hours. The pattern of injury is classified as quad, upper only, lower only, or hemi.

An episode of CCN is not an absolute contraindication to return to football. It is unlikely that athletes who experience CCN are at risk for permanent quadriplegia with return to play. Rather, playing technique in which the athlete employs the top of the head for tackling is the primary factor resulting in cervical quadriplegia. There are no known reports of an athlete with a CCN injury returning to football and sustaining a quadriplegic event. However, the number of athletes returning to play after a CCN episode is too low to make a definitive conclusion. Permanent neurologic deficits after a CCN episode are uncommon, but can occur.[15,18] Athletes need to be counseled on an individual basis on the known and potential risks of injury with return to football after a CCN injury.

The overall risk of a recurrent CCN episode with return to football is just over 50% and is correlated with the canal diameter size; the smaller the canal diameter, the greater the risk of recurrence.[69] Athletes with ligamentous instability, neurologic symptoms lasting more than 36 hours, multiple episodes, or MRI evidence of cord defect, cord edema, or minimal functional reserve should not be allowed to return to contact sports.[68]

42.6.1.3 Screening

The Pavlov–Torg ratio was developed as a method of assessing cervical spinal stenosis.[68] The ratio is measured as the diameter of the spinal canal divided by the anteroposterior width of the vertebral body at the midpoint on the lateral radiograph. A ratio of less than 0.8 was proposed as indicating significant spinal stenosis. The ratio has been found to have a high sensitivity for detecting significant spinal stenosis but low specificity, and is a poor predictor of which players will suffer a CCN episode, making it a poor screening tool for athletic participation.[27,49] *Functional* spinal stenosis, defined as loss of CSF around the spinal cord as documented by MRI or CT myelography, is a more accurate method to determine spinal stenosis and risk for CCN.[17] There is currently no cost-effective tool to screen for athletes at risk for CCN; however, all athletes who experience an episode of CCN should undergo appropriate imaging studies to evaluate their risk of recurrence. Preparticipation physicals should specifically query whether an athlete has had a previous neck injury so that appropriate counseling and return-to-play decisions can be made.

42.6.2 Ice Hockey

Although the number of catastrophic injuries in high school and college ice hockey players is low compared with other sports, the incidence per 100,000 participants is high.[46] The majority of spinal injuries in ice hockey are reported to occur to the cervical spine, especially between levels C5 and C7.[43] The most common mechanism of injury is checking from behind and being hurled horizontally into the boards[43,63] (Figure 42.7). Contact with the boards typically occurs to the crown of the player's head subjecting the neck to an axial load.[63] Biomechanical studies have shown that impact velocities as low as 1.8 m/s provided compressive forces from C3 through C5 to 75% of their failure loads in axial compression.[6] It has been demonstrated that skating speeds often reach 12 m/s, and the speed of a sliding skater on ice is approximately 6.7 m/s.[58] Both situations are well above the speeds necessary to cause failure in axial compression.

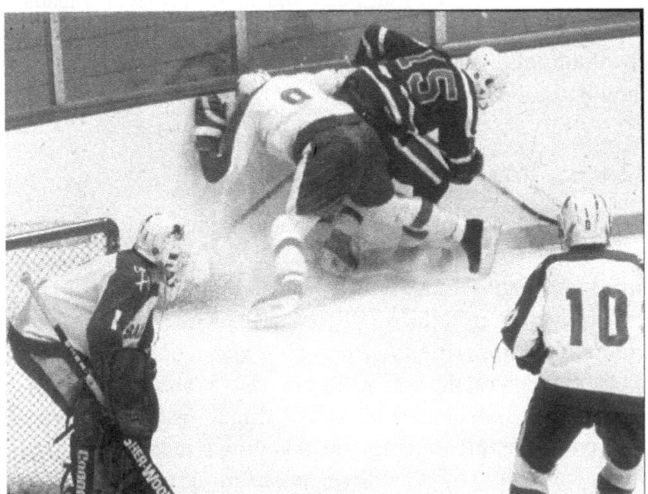

FIGURE 42.7 Illustration of an ice hockey player checked from behind and thrown into boards headfirst. (Courtesy of J.S. Torg, M.D., Philadelphia, PA.)

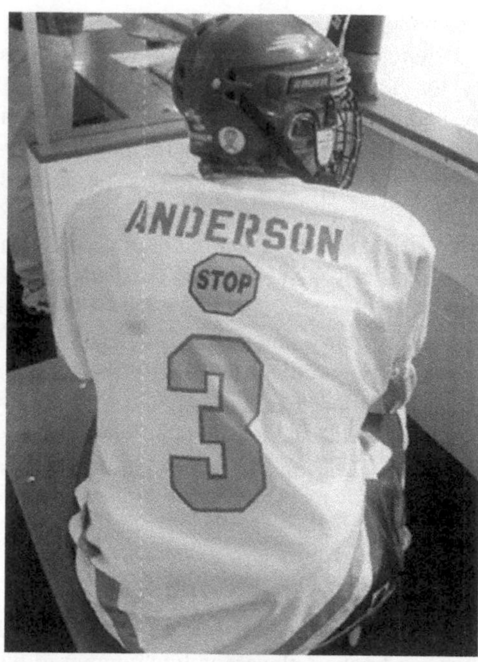

FIGURE 42.8 Safety toward other players (STOP) patch worn on the back of an amateur hockey player as a visual reminder for players not to hit an opponent from behind. (Reprinted with permission from Waninger, K.N., *Am. J. Sports Med.*, 32, 1331, 2004.)

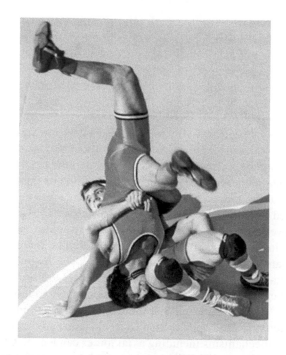

FIGURE 42.9 Wrestler landing on top of head during takedown maneuver. (Courtesy of *Sports Illustrated*.)

A Canadian survey from 1966 to 1993 reported a total of 241 spinal fractures and dislocations in ice hockey.[63] The incidence of major spinal injuries worldwide in ice hockey started to increase significantly in the early 1980s.[5] Data from the SportSmart registry revealed an average of 17 cases a year, with a peak of 26 injuries in 1995.[5] In 1994, the rule against pushing or checking from behind was adopted into the International Ice Hockey Federation rules book[31] (Figure 42.8). As a result of this rule change, the incidence of severe spinal injuries has dramatically decreased since the late 1990s.[5] Padding the boards is an alternative preventive strategy that may be effective. Although it has been suggested that head and facial protection leads to an increased risk of catastrophic spinal injuries, this has never been substantiated.[60] Aggressive play and fighting in hockey should also be discouraged.

42.6.3 Wrestling

Cervical fractures or major cervical ligament injuries constitute the majority of traumatic catastrophic wrestling injuries.[8] There is a trend toward more spine injuries in the low- and middle-weight classes. Most injuries occur in match competitions, where intense, competitive situations place wrestlers at a higher risk.[8] The position most frequently associated with spinal injury in wrestling is the defensive posture during the takedown maneuver (Figure 42.9), followed by the down position (kneeling) and the lying position.[8] There is no clear predominance of any one type of takedown hold that contributes to cervical injuries in wrestling. The athlete is typically injured by one of three scenarios: (1) the wrestler's arms are in a hold such that he or she is unable to prevent himself or herself from landing on his or her head when thrown to the mat; (2) the wrestler attempts a roll but is landed on by the full weight of his or her opponent; and (3) the wrestler lands on the top of his or her head, sustaining an axial compression force to the cervical spine.

General prevention strategies for catastrophic spine injuries in wrestling rely on the referees and coaches. Referees should strictly enforce penalties for slams and gain more awareness of dangerous holds. There is particular vulnerability for the defensive wrestler who may be off balance, have one or both arms held, and then have his opponent land on top of him. Stringent penalties for intentional slams or throws are encouraged. The referee should have a low threshold of tolerance to stop the match during potentially dangerous situations. Coaches can prevent serious injuries by emphasizing safe, legal wrestling techniques such as teaching wrestlers to keep their head up during any takedown maneuver to prevent axial compression injuries to the cervical spine. Proper rolling techniques, with avoidance of landing on the head, need to be emphasized in practice sessions.

42.6.4 Diving

Most catastrophic spinal swimming injuries are related to the racing dive into the shallow end of pools.[46] The injury occurs when a swimmer dives headfirst into the shallow end of a pool and sustains an axial compression injury to the cervical spine (Figure 42.10). The national high school and collegiate associations have implemented rules to prevent injuries during the

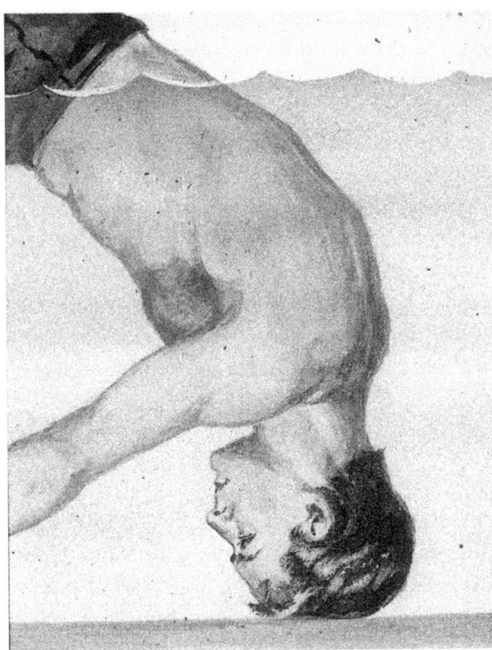

FIGURE 42.10 Diagram of diver landing on top of head while diving into shallow end of pool. (Courtesy of J.S. Torg, M.D., Philadelphia, PA.)

racing dive. At the high school level, swimmers must start the race in the water if the water depth at the starting end is less than 3.5 ft. If the water depth is from 3.5 ft. to less than 4 ft. at the starting end, the swimmer may start in the water or from the deck. If the water depth at the starting end is 4 ft. or more, the swimmer may start from a platform up to 30 in. above the water surface. College rules require a minimum water depth of 4 ft. at the starting end of the pool. During practice sessions where platforms may not be available, swimmers are advised to only dive into the deep end of the pool or to jump into the water feet first.

Many recreational diving injuries go unreported, hampering attempts at improved awareness and water safety. In a retrospective review of traumatic spinal cord injuries presenting to a trauma center in Germany, 7.7% were caused by diving accidents.[57] Ninety-seven percent of the injured patients were male. Inadequate supervision, alcohol use, shallow water, and inexperienced divers are all risk factors for injury.[67] Diving headfirst into shallow or unknown waters was the reported cause in most cases. Many recreational aquatic centers have removed the high board in favor of a water slide to reduce the incidence of spinal cord injuries.

42.6.5 Downhill Skiing/Snowboarding

While the injury rate in skiing is 1.5–4 per 1000 skier-days, the incidence of serious SCI is 0.01 injuries per 1000 skier-days.[44] The location of spinal injuries is fairly evenly distributed between the cervical, thoracic, and lumbar levels.[39] Spinal injuries appear to be increasing among skiers over the last 20 years and tend to occur predominantly in young males. The primary causes of injury are falls caused by poorly groomed slopes, equipment failure, unfavorable weather conditions, overcrowding with skier–skier or skier–snowboarder collisions, skier error, or high speeds with loss of control. The injury rates increase at the end of the day suggesting a link with skier fatigue. Fatality rates for downhill skiers have been estimated to be one per 1.5 million skier-days.[44] Most fatalities result from reckless skiers colliding with a stationary object, most commonly a tree.[44] Although most fatalities are caused by severe head injuries, spinal injuries have also been documented.[44] Enforcement of responsible, safe skiing by the ski patrol is an important factor in preventing injuries.

The incidence of spinal injury in snowboarding has been reported to be fourfold higher than skiing.[62] Jumping is the contributing factor in up to 80% of snowboarding injuries, mostly occurring in the thoracolumbar region.[39,62] Prevention strategies include regulating the downhill runs so snowboarders do not overcrowd the slopes or separating snowboarders from skiers on the slopes. Snowboarders should also be made aware of the potentially deleterious effects of high-risk jumping practices.

42.6.6 Rugby

The lack of protective gear and aggressive style of play in rugby have resulted in a high rate of cervical injury. Scher reported that 10% of serious injuries in rugby involve the cervical spine with spinal cord contusions constituting one-fourth of spinal injuries.[55,56] Cervical spine injuries most frequently occur during the scrum when the opposing packs of tightly bound players come together (engagement).[76] The hooker or central player on the front row suffers the most injuries (Figure 42.11). During engagement, the eight-person scrum may generate forces up to 1.5 tons: the hooker may encounter almost 50% of this force. If engagement does not occur properly or the hooker employs his or her head as a weapon with the neck flexed during contact, a severe

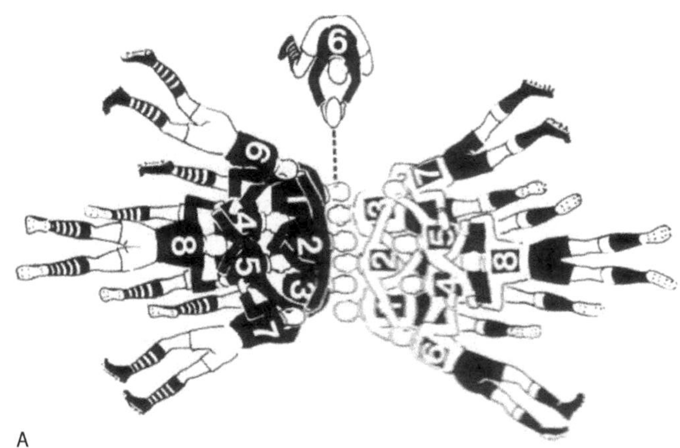

FIGURE 42.11 Diagram of scrum positions: hooker (H), prop (P), flanker (F), second row (SR), and eight-man (8). (Reprinted with permission from Wetzler, M.J. et al., *Am. J. Sports Med.*, 26, 177, 1998.)

cervical injury may result. Preventive methods include avoiding a mismatch in physical size of the hookers, not allowing unskilled players to participate on the front row, and changing the rules of engagement. Sequential engagement or having the front rows engage separately from the pack prevents the second and third rows from thrusting unprepared front-row players into their opponents. An uncontested scrum in which the offensive team is allowed to win the scrum has also been shown to be an effective preventive strategy.[76] There are insufficient data to determine if protective headgear changes the rates of cervical spine injury.

42.6.7 Cheerleading

Over the past 20 years, cheerleading has evolved into an activity demanding high levels of skill, athleticism, and complex gymnastic maneuvers. Compared with other sports, cheerleading has a low overall incidence of injuries, but a high risk of catastrophic injuries. At the college and high school levels, cheerleaders account for more than half of the catastrophic injuries that occur in female athletes.[46] College athletes are more likely to sustain a catastrophic injury than their high school counterparts, which is likely due to the increased complexity of stunts at the college level.[11] In 2000, the Consumer Product Safety Commission estimated a total of 1814 neck injuries in cheerleaders of all ages; 76 of these were cervical fractures.[77]

The most common stunts resulting in catastrophic injury are the basket toss and the pyramid, with the cheerleader at the top of the pyramid most frequently injured.[11] A basket toss is a stunt where a cheerleader is thrown into the air, often between 6 and 20 ft., by either three or four tossers. Less common mechanisms include advanced floor tumbling routines, participating on a wet surface, or performing a mount. The majority of injuries occur when an athlete lands on an indoor hard gym surface.[11]

The high school and college associations have attempted to reduce pyramid injuries by limiting the height and complexity of a pyramid and specifying positions for spotters. Height restrictions on pyramids are limited to two levels in high school and 2.5 body lengths in college. The top cheerleaders are required to be supported by one or more individuals (base) who are in direct weight-bearing contact with the performing surface. Spotters must be present for each person extended above shoulder level. The suspended person is not allowed to be inverted (head below horizontal) or to rotate on the dismount.

Safety measures have also been instituted for the basket toss such as limiting the basket toss to four throwers, starting the toss from the ground level (no flips), and having one of the throwers behind the top person during the toss. The top person (flyer) is trained to be directed vertically and not allow the head to drop backward out of alignment with the torso or below a horizontal plane with the body. Since several injuries have been reported during rainy weather, all stunts should be restricted when wet conditions are present. Floor tumbling injuries can be prevented by proper supervision, progression to complex tumbling only when simple maneuvers are mastered, and spotters as necessary. Mini trampolines, springboards, or any apparatus used to propel a participant have been prohibited since the late 1980s.

Cheerleading coaches need to place equal time and attention on the technique and attentiveness of spotters in practice as they do with athletes' performing the stunts. Pyramids and basket tosses should be limited to experienced cheerleaders who have mastered all other skills and should not be performed without qualified spotters or landing mats.[11]

42.6.8 Baseball

Similar to cheerleading, baseball has a low rate of non-catastrophic injuries, but a relatively high incidence of catastrophic injuries compared with other sports. Severe head injuries are more frequent than spine injuries. The most common mechanism of catastrophic spine injury in baseball is a collision between a base runner and a fielder.[12] Collisions between base runners and fielders often involve the catcher. A typical scenario is a base runner who dives headfirst into a catcher and sustains an axial compression cervical injury.[12] Baseball rules state that the runner should avoid the fielder who has the right to the base path. Unfortunately, this rule is not always enforced when a base runner is racing toward home plate. Since the risk of injury from collisions of a base runner and catcher is significant, and the speed of headfirst sliding has been shown not to be statistically different from feetfirst sliding, the author believes that the headfirst slide needs to be reassessed at the high school and college levels.[32] In Little League Baseball, headfirst sliding is not allowed at any base.

42.7 CONCLUSION

It has been clearly documented that physical activity has numerous health-related benefits. Participation in sports is an excellent way of encouraging physical activity and promote teamwork and camaraderie. While there is an extremely low risk of catastrophic spine injuries in certain organized sports, the cost of catastrophic injury to the injured athlete and to society can be tremendous. In addition to the decreased quality of life for the patient, the lifetime cost for a complete quadriplegic individual can easily surpass $2 million dollars.[39] It has been estimated that the annual aggregate cost of treatment of spinal cord injuries due to sports in the United States in 1995 was close to $700 million.[24] Prevention is the most effective means of reducing the incidence and costs associated with catastrophic spine injuries in sports. Continued research on the epidemiology and mechanisms of catastrophic spine injuries is critical to prevent these injuries (Table 42.4).

TABLE 42.4
SORT: Key Recommendations for Practice

Clinical Recommendation	Evidence Rating	References
Sports with the highest risk of catastrophic spinal injuries are football, ice hockey, wrestling, diving, skiing, snowboarding, and rugby.	A	[21,44,46,71,73]
In the majority of cases of cervical spinal cord injury, the helmet and shoulder pads should not be removed prior to arrival at an emergency room.	A	[51–53]
The overall risk of a recurrent CCN episode with return to football is just over 50% and is correlated with the canal diameter size; the smaller the canal diameter the greater the risk of recurrence.[52]	A	[51–53]
Axial compression forces to the top of the head can lead to cervical fracture and quadriplegia in any sport.	A	[24,41]
Any medical personnel covering team sports should have a plan for stabilization and transfer of an athlete with a cervical spine injury.	C	[27]
High dose steroids is an acute treatment for spinal cord injury to reduce neurologic injury.	B	[40–43]

REFERENCES

1. Babra CA, Taggert J, Morgan AS et al. A new cervical spine clearance protocol using computed tomography. *The Journal of Trauma*. 2001;51:652–657.
2. Banerjee R, Palumbo MA, Fadale PD. Catastrophic cervical spine injuries in the collision sport athlete, part 1: Epidemiology, functional anatomy, and diagnosis. *The American Journal of Sports Medicine*. 2004;32:1077–1087.
3. Banerjee R, Palumbo MA, Fadale PD. Catastrophic cervical spine injuries in the collision sport athlete, part 2: Principles of emergency. *The American Journal of Sports Medicine*. 2004;32:1760–1764.
4. Bateman JE. Nerve injuries about the shoulder in sports. *Journal of Bone and Joint Surgery*. 1967;49A:785–792.
5. Biasca N, WirBiasca N, Wirth S et al. The avoidability of head and neck injuries in ice hockey: An historical review. *British Journal of Sports Medicine*. 2002;36:410–427.
6. Bishop PJ, Wells RP. Cervical spine fractures: Mechanism, neck load, and methods of prevention, in: Castaldi CR and Hoerner, EF (eds). *Safety in Ice Hockey*, volume 2, ASTM STP 1050. Philadelphia, PA: American Society for Testing and Materials; 1989, pp. 71–83.
7. Boden BP. Direct catastrophic injury in sports. *Journal of the American Academy of Orthopaedic Surgeons*. 2005;13:445–453.
8. Boden BP, Lin W, Young M et al. Catastrophic injuries in wrestlers. *The American Journal of Sports Medicine*. 2002;30:791–795.
9. Boden BP, Prior C. Catastrophic spine injuries in sports. *Current Sports Medicine Reports*. 2005;4:45–49.
10. Boden BP, Tacchetti RL, Cantu RC et al. Catastrophic cervical injuries in high school and college football players. *The American Journal of Sports Medicine*. 2006;34:1223–1232.
11. Boden BP, Tacchetti R, Mueller FO. Catastrophic cheerleading injuries. *The American Journal of Sports Medicine*. 2003;31:881–888.
12. Boden BP, Tacchetti R, Mueller FO. Catastrophic injuries in high school and college baseball players. *The American Journal of Sports Medicine*. 2004;12:1189–1196.
13. Bracken MB. Steroids for acute spinal cord injury. *The Cochrane Database of Systematic Reviews*. 2012;1: CD001046.
14. Bracken MB, Shepard MJ, Collins WF et al. A randomized, controlled trial of methylprednisolone or naloxone in the treatment of acute spinal-cord injury: Results of the second national acute spinal cord injury study. *The New England Journal of Medicine*. 1990;322:1404–1411.
15. Brigham CD, Adamson TE. Permanent partial cervical spinal cord injury in a professional football player who had only congenital stenosis. *Journal of Bone and Joint Surgery*. 2003A;85:1553–1556.
16. Bydon M, Lin J, Macki M et al. The current role of steroids in acute spinal cord injury. *World Neurosurgery*. 2013;82:848–854.
17. Cantu RC. Functional cervical spinal stenosis: A contraindication to participation in contact sports. *Medicine & Science in Sports & Exercise*. 1993;25:1082–1083.
18. Cantu RV, Cantu RC. Guidelines for return to contact sports after transient quadriplegia. *Journal of Neurosurgery*. 1994;80:592–594.
19. Cantu RC, Mueller FO. Catastrophic football injuries: 1977–1998. *Neurosurgery*. 2000, 47:673–677.
20. Casa DJ, Almquist J, Anderson SA et al. The inter-association task force for preventing sudden death in secondary school athletics programs: Best-practices recommendations. *Journal of Athletic Training*. 2013 48(4):546–553.
21. Clancy WG Jr, Brand RI, Bergfeld JA. Upper trunk brachial plexus injuries in contact sports. *The American Journal of Sports Medicine*. 1977;5:209–216.
22. Davidson RM, Burton JH, Snowise M et al. Football protective gear and cervical spine imaging. *Annals of Emergency Medicine*. 2001;38:26–30.
23. Decoster LC, Burns MF, Swartz E et al. Maintaining neutral sagittal cervical alignment after football helmet removal during emergency spine injury management. *Spine*. 2012;37(8):654–659.
24. DeVivo MJ. Causes and costs of spinal cord injury in the United States. *Spinal Cord* 1997;35:809–813.
25. Gale SD, Decoster LC, Swartz EE. The combined tool approach for face mask removal during on-field conditions. *Journal of Athletic Training*. 2008;43(1):14–20.
26. Hershman EB, Wilbourn AJ, Bergfeld JA. Acute brachial neuropathy in athletes. *The American Journal of Sports Medicine*. 1989;17:655–659.
27. Herzog RJ, Wiens JJ, Dillingham MF et al. Normal cervical spine morphometry and cervical spinal stenosis in asymptomatic professional football players: Plain film radiography, multiplanar computed tomography, and magnetic resonance imaging. *Spine*. 1991;16:S178–S186.
28. Hoffman JR, Mower WR, Wolfson AB et al. Validity of a set of clinical criteria to rule out injury to the cervical spine in patients with blunt trauma. *New England Journal of Medicine*. 2000;343:94–99.

29. Horodyski M, DiPaola CP, DiPaola MJ et al. Comparison of the flat torso versus the elevated torso shoulder pad removal techniques in a cadaveric cervical spine instability model. *Spine.* 2009;34(7):687–691.
30. Hulbert RJ. The role of steroids in acute spinal cord injury: An evidence-based analysis. *Spine.* 2001;26:539–546.
31. International Ice Hockey Federation (IIHF). *Official Rule Book 1994.* Zurich: IIHF, 1994.
32. Kane SM, House HO, Overgaard KA. Head-first versus feet-first sliding: A comparison of speed from base to base. *The American Journal of Sports Medicine.* 2002;30:834–836.
33. Katoh S, Shingu H, Ikata T et al. Sports-related spinal cord injury in Japan (From the nationwide spinal cord injury registry between 1990 and 1992). *Spinal Cord.* 1996;34:416–421.
34. Kelly JD, Aliquo D, Sitler MR et al. Association of burners with cervical canal and foraminal stenosis. *The American Journal of Sports Medicine.* 2000;28:214–217.
35. Kelly JD, Clancy M, Marchetti PA et al. The relationship of transient upper extremity paresthesias and cervical stenosis. *Orthopaedic Transactions.* 1992;16:732.
36. Kleiner DM, Almquist JL, Bailes J et al. *Prehospital Care of the Spine-Injured Athlete.* Dallas, TX: National Athletic Trainers' Association, 2001.
37. Kline DG. Prospectives concerning brachial plexus injury and repair. *Neurosurgery Clinics of North America.* 1991;2:151–169.
38. LaPrade RF, Schnetzler KA, Broxterman RF et al. Cervical spine alignment in the immobilized ice hockey player: A computed tomographic analysis of the effects of helmet removal. *The American Journal of Sports Medicine.* 2000; 28:800–803.
39. Levy AS, Smith RH. Neurologic injuries in skiers and snowboarders. *Seminars in Neurology.* 2000;20:233–245.
40. Markey KI, Di Benedetto M, Curt WW. Upper trunk brachial plexopathy: The stinger syndrome. *The American Journal of Sports Medicine.* 1993;21:650–655.
41. Maroon JC, Bost JW, Petraglia AL et al. Outcomes after anterior cervical discectomy and fusion in professional athletes. *Neurosurgery* 2013;73(1):103–112.
42. Meredith DS, Jones KJ, Barnes R et al. Operative and nonoperative treatment of cervical disc herniation in national football league athletes. *The American Journal of Sports Medicine.* 2013:41(9):2054–2058.
43. Molsa JJ, Tegner Y, Alaranta H et al. Spinal cord injuries in ice hockey in Finland and Sweden from 1980 to 1996. *International Journal of Sports Medicine.* 1999;20:64–67.
44. Morrow PL, McQuillen EN, Eaton Jr. LA et al. Downhill ski fatalities: The vermont experience. *The Journal of Trauma.* 1998;28(1):95–100.
45. Mueller FO. Introduction, in Mueller FO, Cantu RC, VanCamp SP (eds). *Catastrophic Injuries in High School and College Sports.* Champaign, IL: HK. Sport Science Monograph Series; 1996, pp. 1–4.
46. Mueller FO, Cantu RC. *National Center for Catastrophic Sports Injury Research: Twentieth Annual Report, Fall 1982–Spring 2002.* Chapel Hill, NC: National Center for Catastrophic Sports Injury Research, 2002, pp. 1–25.
47. Nobunga AI, Go BK, Karunas RB. Recent demographic and injury trends in people served by the model spine cord injury care systems. *Archives of Physical Medicine and Rehabilitation.* 1999;80:1372–1382.
48. Nunez DB, Zuluaga A, Fuentes-Bernando DA et al. Cervical spine trauma: How much more do we learn by routinely using helical CT. *RadioGraphics* 1996;16:1307–1318.
49. Odor JM, Watkins RG, Dillin WH et al. Incidence of cervical spinal stenosis in professional and rookie football players. *The American Journal of Sports Medicine.* 1990;18:507–509.
50. Palumbo MA, Hulstyn MJ, Fadale PD et al. The effect of protective football equipment on alignment of the injured cervical spine: Radiographic analysis in a cadaveric model. *The American Journal of Sports Medicine.*;24:446–453.
51. Parke WW. Correlative anatomy of cervical spondylotic myelopathy. *Spine.* 1988;13:831–837.
52. Peris MD, Donaldson WF III, Towers J. Helmet and shoulder pad removal in suspected cervical spine injury: Human control model. *Spine.* 27:995–998; discussion 998–999.
53. Robertson WC, Eichman PL, Clancy WG. Upper trunk brachial plexopathy in football players. *Journal of the American Medical Association.* 1979;241:1480–1482.
54. Sallis RE, Jones K, Knopp W. Burners: Offensive strategy for an underreported injury. *Physician and Sportsmedicine.* 1992;20:47–55.
55. Scher AT. Rugby injuries to the cervical spine and spinal cord: A 10 year review. *Clinics in Sports Medicine.* 1998;17(1):195–206.
56. Scher AT. Rugby spinal cord concussion in rugby players. *The American Journal of Sports Medicine.* 1991;19(5):485–488.
57. Schmitt H, Gerner HJ. Paralysis from sport and diving accidents. *Clinics in Sports Medicine.* 2001;11:17–22.
58. Sim FH, Chao EY. Injury potential in modern ice hockey. *The American Journal of Sports Medicine.* 1978;15:30–34.
59. Speer KP, Bassett FH. The prolonged burner syndrome. *The American Journal of Sports Medicine.* 1990;18:591–594.
60. Stuart MJ, Smith AM, Malo-Ortiguera SA et al. A comparison of facial protection and the incidence of head, neck, and facial injuries in junior A hockey players: A function of individual playing time. *The American Journal of Sports Medicine.* 2002;30:39–44.
61. Swartz EE, Norkus SA, Cappaert T et al. Football equipment design affects face mask removal efficiency. *The American Journal of Sports Medicine.* 2005;33:1210–1218.
62. Tarazi F, Dvorak MF, Wing PC. Spinal injuries in skiers and snowboarders. *The American Journal of Sports Medicine.* 1999;27(2):177–180.
63. Tator CH, Carson JD, Edmonds VE. Spinal injuries in ice hockey. *Clinics in Sports Medicine.* 1998;17:183–194.
64. Taylor PE. Traumatic intradural avulsion of the nerve roots of the brachial plexus. *Brain.* 1962;85:579–601.
65. Torg, JS. Cervical spine injuries. *Orthopedic Knowledge Update: Sports Medicine 3*, Chapter 1, 2004, pp. 1–18.
66. Torg JS, Corcoran TA, Thibault LE et al. Cervical cord neurapraxia: Classification, pathomechanics, morbidity, and management guidelines. *Journal of Neurosurgery.* 1997;87:843–850.
67. Torg JS, Gennarelli TA. Head and cervical spine injuries, in DeLee JC, Drez Jr D (eds). *Orthopaedic Sports Medicine: Principles and Practice.* Philadelphia, PA: WB Saunders Co., 1994, pp. 417–462.
68. Torg JS, Guille JT, Jaffe S. Current concepts review: Injuries to the cervical spine in American football players. *Journal of Bone and Joint Surgery.* 2002;84:112–122.
69. Torg JS, Naranja Jr. RJ, Pavlov H et al. The relationship of developmental narrowing of the cervical spinal canal to reversible and irreversible injury of the cervical spinal cord in football players. An epidemiological study. *Journal of Bone and Joint Surgery.* 1996;78:1308–1321.
70. Torg JS, Pavlov H, Genuario SE et al. Neuropraxia of the cervical spinal cord with transient quadriplegia. *Journal of Bone and Joint Surgery.* 1986;68:1354–1370.

71. Torg JS, Vegso JJ, O'Neill MJ. The epidemiologic, pathologic, biomechanical, and cinematographic analysis of football-induced cervical spine trauma. *The American Journal of Sports Medicine.* 1990;18:50–57.
72. Tracy JF, Brannon EW. Management of brachial plexus injuries (traction type). *Journal of Bone and Joint Surgery.* 1958;40-A:1031–1042.
73. Treme G, Diduch DR, Hart J et al. Cervical spine alignment in the youth football athlete: Recommendations for emergency transportation. *AJSM.* 2008;36(8):1582–1586.
74. Truitt-Cooper M, McGee KM, Anderson DG. Epidemiology of athletic head and neck injuries. *Clinics in Sports Medicine.* 2003;22(3):427–443.
75. Tsairis P, Dyck PJ, Mulder DW. Natural history of brachial plexus neuropathy: Report on 99 patients. *Archives of Neurology.* 1972;27:109–117.
76. Wetzler MJ, Akpata T, Laughlin W et al. Occurrence of cervical spine injuries during the rugby scrum. *The American Journal of Sports Medicine.* 1998;26:177–180.
77. Consumer Product Safety Commission (CPSC) web site. Available at www.cpsc.gov.
78. National Collegiate Athletic Association (NCAA) web site. Available at www.ncaa.org/health-safety.
79. Yang SS, Hershman EB. Idiopathic brachial plexus neuropathy: A review. *Critical Reviews in Physical and Rehabilitation Medicine.* 1993;5:193–201.

43 Sports Injuries: The Shoulder

Kenton H. Fibel, Osric S. King, and Brian C. Halpern

CONTENTS

TABLE 43.1
Key Clinical Considerations

1. The rotator cuff comprises four muscles: supraspinatus, infraspinatus, teres minor, and subscapularis. They can be assessed with specific physical examination tests.
2. External impingement of the shoulder is classically known as "shoulder impingement syndrome" and is the most common soft-tissue injury of the shoulder.
3. Rotator cuff tears are uncommonly seen in a younger person and usually present as tears due to chronic overuse in middle-aged adults.
4. Grade I and II AC joint sprains can be managed conservatively. Grade III sprains can be treated conservatively as well although may need surgical intervention. All Grade IV–VI sprains should be referred for surgical management.
5. Conservative management of clavicle fractures involves pain control and limiting motion at the fracture site with a simple sling, which is preferable to a figure-eight immobilizer. Evaluations made every couple of weeks are appropriate to determine clinical signs of union.
6. The onset of severe shoulder pain with no evidence of infection should raise suspicion for calcific tendinitis in which calcium deposits can be visualized on plain radiographs.
7. There are three recognized forms of thoracic outlet syndrome (TOS): arterial, venous, and neurogenic. Neurogenic TOS is the cause of more than 95% cases of TOS.

43.1 INTRODUCTION

The diagnosis and management of shoulder injuries is often challenging to the examiner. Complaints are typically vague and nonspecific. In addition to isolated musculoskeletal pathology, the etiologies of shoulder symptoms can come from a variety of neurological, inflammatory, and cardiovascular conditions. Determining the cause and treatment relies equally on the history, mechanism of injury, and physical examination. Imaging studies that depend strongly on technique and quality can confirm the diagnosis and help guide management (Table 43.1).

43.2 GENERAL EPIDEMIOLOGY

Most shoulder pain involves the soft tissues (e.g., cartilage and muscle–tendon unit) and occurs in the sedentary and active individual. Many shoulder injuries result directly from repetition as in throwing and racquet sports. Similar damage can result from non-sports-related overhead activities such as painting or ladder climbing. In throwing and racquet sports, shoulder problems can account for more than 50% of injuries.[26] Anterior shoulder problems in these athletes are usually biomechanical and fatigue related. Unless the injury occurred during a traumatic event, most athletic shoulder problems involve the dominant extremity. In sedentary individuals, however, symptoms in the nondominant or inactive shoulder are not uncommon. In an older population, nonmusculoskeletal sources of symptoms can include cardiac, neurologic, primary neoplastic, and metastatic disease, as well as degenerative changes in the glenohumeral joint, rotator cuff, and cervical spine. Age-related changes, poor conditioning, overtraining, and trauma have common injury features. Studies have shown that rotator cuff and deltoid muscle weakness can cause superior migration of the humerus. This impingement of the humeral head against the subacromial arch is the hallmark event that contributes to bursitis and deterioration of the rotator cuff and biceps tendons. Investigations have repeatedly demonstrated subacromial impingement, whether seen in sports or related to poor conditioning, as one of the most common mechanisms of pain.[27]

43.3 ANATOMY

The shoulder girdle comprises the sternoclavicular joint, acromioclavicular (AC) joint, glenohumeral joint, subacromial space, and scapulothoracic space. Movement about all of these articulations allows for the complexity of the throwing motion. Motion exceeds 180° in three planes, with approximately two-thirds of the full elevation occurring at the glenohumeral joint with the remaining third from scapulothoracic motion.[33] The sternoclavicular joint supports the anteromedial clavicle, and the articulation is between the proximal clavicle and superolateral portion of the manubrium. The posterior capsule of the joint is much stronger than the anterior capsule, thus allowing more anterior dislocations. The acromion is the anterior extension of the scapula and has been described as having three shapes based on the degree of its curvature. Type 3 acromion is hooked and has been found to cause or aggravate rotator cuff impingement.[24] The AC joint is between the lateral end of the clavicle and medial surface of the acromion and is associated with an intra-articular meniscus that may be incomplete. The AC ligament provides superior support, but the major stabilizing structures are the coracoclavicular ligaments (the conoid and trapezoid) (Figure 43.1).

Clinical Pearl

The rotator cuff comprises four muscles: supraspinatus, infraspinatus, teres minor, and subscapularis.

The glenohumeral joint is a synovial ball-and-socket joint in which one-third of a spherical humeral head sits in the shallow glenoid process. To improve the containment of the humeral head, the glenoid labrum attaches peripherally around the margin of the glenoid. Thickening of the capsule forms the glenohumeral ligaments: superior, middle, and inferior. They are folds in capsule unlike the distinct ligaments found elsewhere in the musculoskeletal system. The inferior glenohumeral ligament has the most important role in stabilizing the shoulder joint in abduction and external rotation. The four major muscles of the shoulder girdle constitute the rotator cuff: the subscapularis anteriorly, the supraspinatus that begins posteriorly and transverses to the superior aspect of the humeral head, and the infraspinatus and the teres minor posteriorly (Figure 43.2). The subscapularis is responsible for internal rotation of the humerus, the supraspinatus for abduction, and the infraspinatus and teres minor for external rotation.

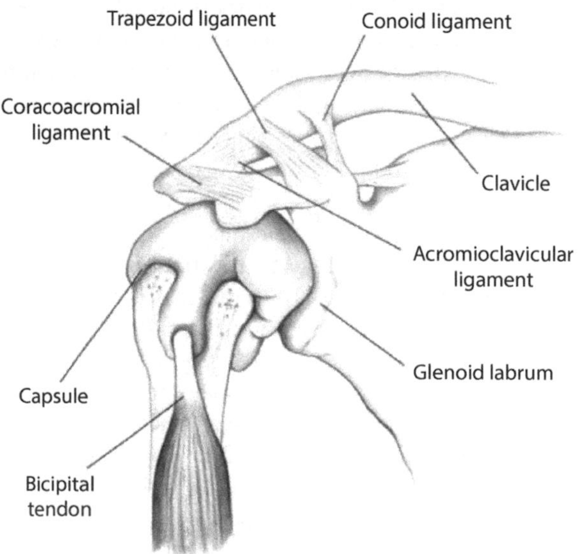

FIGURE 43.1 Ligamentous anatomy of the shoulder.

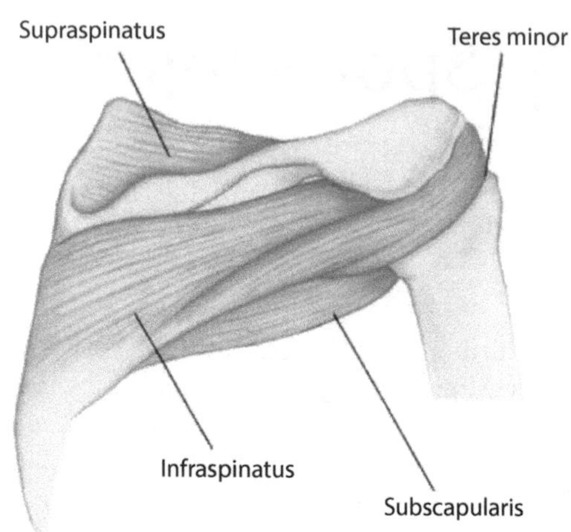

FIGURE 43.2 Rotator cuff muscles.

The subacromial space lies between the acromion and the superior aspect of the humeral head. The supraspinatus and biceps tendon lie adjacent to each other in this space along with the overlying subacromial bursa. The critical area of clearance is under the coracoacromial arch formed by the coracoacromial ligament and the acromion as it distally inserts into the greater tuberosity.[27] Vascular studies have demonstrated a hypovascular zone of the supraspinatus tendon near its distal attachment to the humerus, which may contribute to degenerative tears of the rotator cuff. Likewise, the intracapsular portion of the biceps tendon has a similar hypovascular zone as it passes over the head of the humerus (Figure 43.3). The rotator cuff interval is a triangular space made up of the coracoid process at its base, the anterior margin of supraspinatus tendon as its superior border, and the superior margin of the subscapularis tendon as its inferior border. Within the rotator cuff interval are the long head of the biceps tendon, coracohumeral ligament, superior glenohumeral ligament, and the rotator interval capsule.[51]

43.4 HISTORY AND PHYSICAL EXAMINATION

A description of symptoms should include the quality of the pain, the location, where it radiates, and whether or not it is associated with any swelling or tenderness. Are the symptoms present or worsened with a particular motion, and is the motion restricted? Is there any associated numbness and tingling, which could indicate a brachial plexus injury or an associated

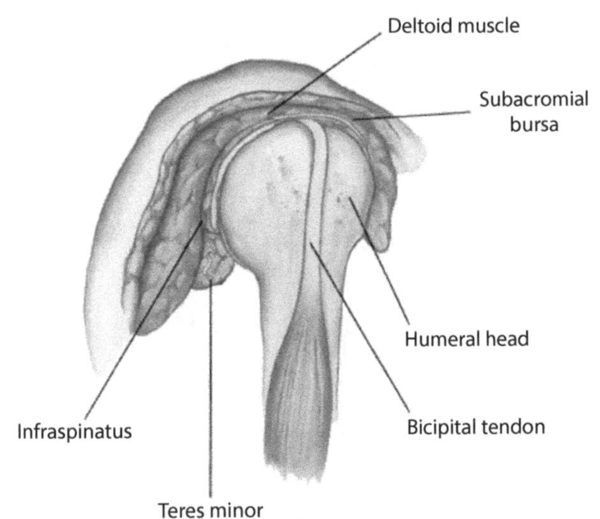

FIGURE 43.3 Lateral view of the shoulder; the bicipital (biceps) tendon runs through the bicipital groove in the head of the humerus.

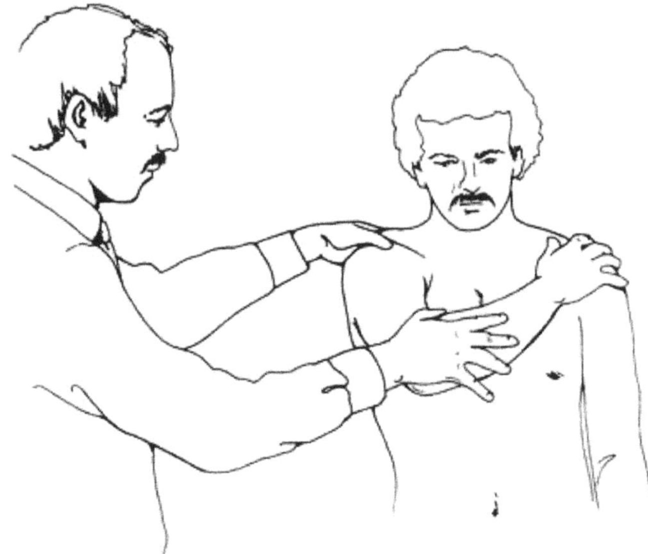

FIGURE 43.4 Crossover test: testing for a sprain of the AC joint.

cervical spine problem? Can the patient recall a traumatic event that preceded the pain? A dull aching discomfort, often felt at night, corresponds with rotator cuff tears, whereas a stabbing, burning pain is more typical of a bursitis or a tendinosis. The location of the pain can be diagnostic. Pain over the AC joint might suggest degenerative disease and, if associated with trauma, might indicate an AC joint sprain. Pain deep in the shoulder may come from rotator cuff involvement, capsular inflammation, arthritic changes, a glenoid labrum tear, or even a humeral head fracture in the setting of trauma.[33]

A popping or catching noise inside the joint can indicate a glenoid labrum tear or biceps subluxation. A history of shoulder instability (described as giving way, slipping, or popping out) suggests subluxation or dislocation of the glenohumeral joint. Anterior dislocations, which make up >90% of shoulder dislocations, occur when a posterior force is exerted onto an abducted, external rotated arm. Congenital ligamentous laxity, anteriorly or posteriorly, can predispose an individual to subluxation events. Both of these occurrences can lead to injury to the cartilaginous glenoid labrum as well as the glenohumeral ligaments that serve to stabilize the shoulder joint. The labrum can also be torn by traction from the biceps tendon (superior labral tear) or impingement between the humeral head and the glenoid cavity. These types of injuries occur in baseball and tennis and often result from a combination of acceleration–deceleration forces and internal–external rotational velocities of the humerus; therefore, it is essential to question the patient regarding what phase of the motion the symptoms occur. A complete review includes obtaining past medical history inquiring about gout, chondrocalcinosis (pseudogout), arthritis, diabetes, neurovascular and metabolic disorders, and neoplastic disease.

The diagnosis is usually confirmed by the physical exam. A few key points for the physical exam include examining the uninjured shoulder, which can serve as a "normal" comparison, and examining the suspected area of injury last as to prevent aggravation of the injury that could lead to false positives of other provocative testing of other structures of the shoulder. Begin the exam with an anterior inspection of both clavicles, AC joints, and overall shoulder contour. Look for asymmetry, ecchymosis, swelling, and atrophy. Palpate the sternoclavicular joint with continued palpation along the clavicle distally feeling for any signs of bony injury such as a step-off or crepitus. Palpate the AC joint for pain, crepitus, and hypermobility in the superior–inferior as well as the anterior–posterior direction, which could represent an unstable joint. Perform the crossover test by placing the hand of the injured shoulder on the uninjured shoulder (Figure 43.4). If there is pain with this maneuver, an AC joint injury probably exists as this motion compresses this joint. Palpate the subacromial space to assess for tenderness. Next, inspect and palpate the posterior rotator cuff muscles. Also check the trapezius and latissimus dorsi muscles, which accentuate rotator cuff movement. A prominent scapular spine suggests posterior rotator cuff atrophy from a complete tear or suprascapular nerve injury. Have the patient push against a wall and note any winging of the scapula, signifying injury to the long thoracic nerve or serratus anterior muscle.

Assess the patient's range of motion (ROM), beginning with abduction, which occurs with glenohumeral and scapulothoracic movement in a 2:1 ratio. For every 3° of shoulder abduction, 2° occurs at the glenohumeral joint and 1 at the scapulothoracic joint.[33] Forward flexion of the shoulder should then be evaluated next. Check internal and external rotation with the arm adducted and again at 90° of abduction while stabilizing the scapula to prevent inaccurate measurements. Internal rotation can also effectively be evaluated by having the patient reach behind their back and seeing how high up their spine they can touch with their thumb recording the level of the spine. Rotator cuff tears, loose bodies, cervical radiculopathy, adhesive capsulitis, and osteoarthritis tend to decrease the glenohumeral motion segment and enhance the scapulothoracic segment during active shoulder elevation. The patient appears to shrug the injured shoulder into abduction denoted as scapular substitution. Testing active and

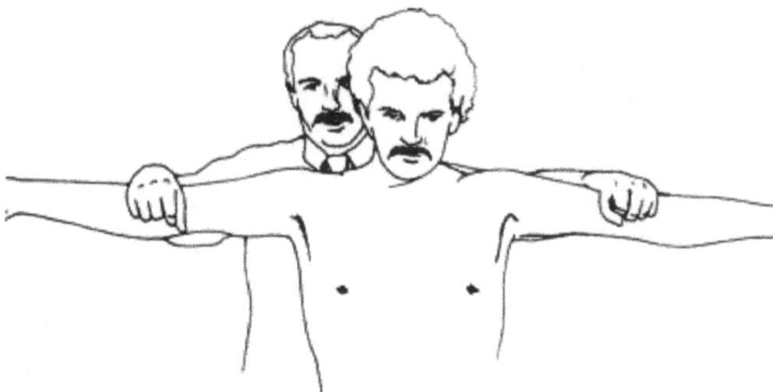

FIGURE 43.5 Supraspinatus test: testing for strength of the supraspinatus and deltoid muscles.

passive ROM is important because it helps to distinguish a rotator cuff tear from adhesive capsulitis or significant glenohumeral osteoarthritis. Remember that conditioned overhand throwers consistently demonstrate increased external rotation of the dominant extremity. Limited internal rotation only can signify a posterior capsular contraction leading to biomechanical dysfunction and internal impingement.

The rotator cuff should be thoroughly evaluated by both strength testing and provocative maneuvers. Injuries to the supraspinatus muscle can be assessed by instructing the patient to abduct their arm and then slowly lower the arm to their side. If they have only pain with this maneuver, it would suggest a tendinitis or partial tear of the supraspinatus; however, if their arm quickly drops to their side during this test, it could represent a complete tear of the supraspinatus. Strength testing of the supraspinatus can be done by applying downward force to the forearm with the shoulder in 90° of abduction, 30° anteriorly toward midline, and full internal rotation with thumb pointing toward the ground (drop arm test, supraspinatus stress test, empty can test) (Figure 43.5). Weakness, pain, or a limited ROM can indicate injury to the supraspinatus muscle or suprascapular nerve.[33] To test for strength of the subscapularis muscle, have the patient internally rotate against resistance with maximum adduction of the arm and elbow flexion to 90° (Figure 43.6). A second test of subscapular strength requires the ability to internally rotate where the patients reach behind their back with the dorsal aspect of their hand against their lower back and attempts to lift their hand away from their back against resistance (Gerber's lift off test). External rotation against resistance with maximum adduction of the arm and the elbow flexed 90° tests the infraspinatus and teres minor muscles (Figure 43.7).[33] Impingement testing is intended to drive the greater tuberosity under the coracoacromial arch and includes the Hawkins test and Neer test. The Hawkins test (Figure 43.8) is performed by internally rotating the humerus with the arm in a forward flexed position at 90° with a positive sign denoted by shoulder pain with this maneuver. The Neer impingement test is performed by internally rotating the arm with the thumb pointing toward the ground, and while stabilizing the scapula, the arm is passively forward flexed up to 180° with a positive sign denoted by shoulder pain recreated with this maneuver. As impingement progresses, refractory tendinosis, wearing of the supraspinatus and biceps

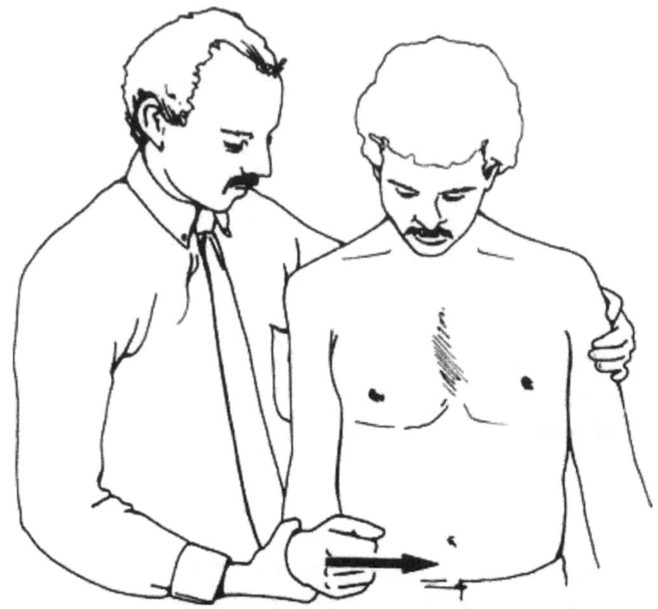

FIGURE 43.6 Testing for strength of the subscapularis muscle.

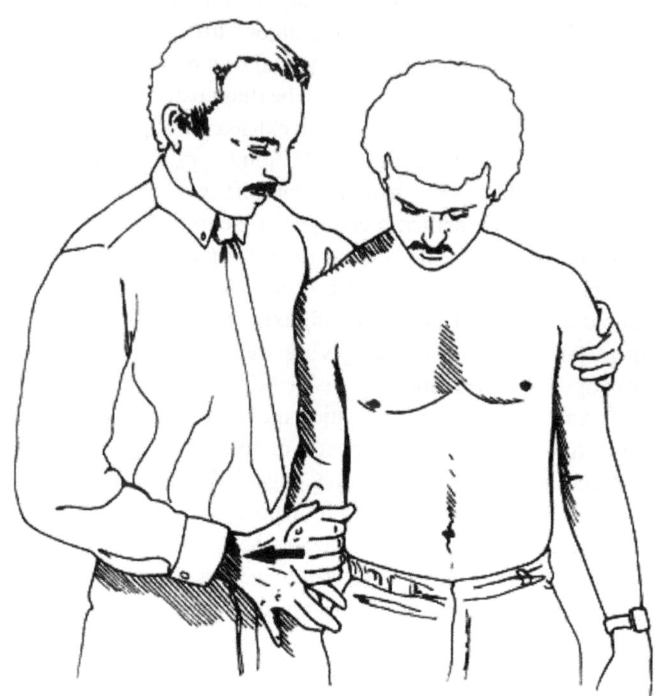

FIGURE 43.7 Testing for strength of the infraspinatus and teres minor muscles.

tendon, and partial or complete thickness rotator cuff tears can occur.[27] A 10 cc injection of 1% lidocaine into the subacromial space can sometimes be used to help differentiate rotator cuff pathology from cervical radiculopathy as the impingement maneuvers can be repeated after the injection with change in findings noted.

The long head of the biceps can be palpated in the bicipital groove when the patient is in the sitting position. With the examiner's finger still in the bicipital groove, the subscapularis tendon can be palpated for tenderness by externally

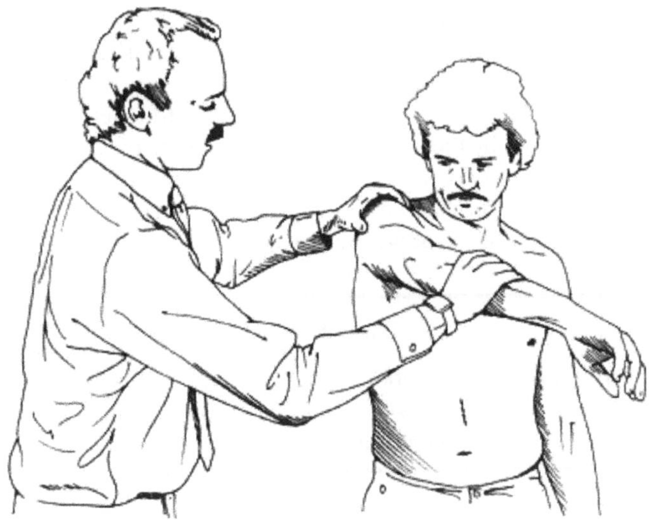

FIGURE 43.8 Impingement test: testing for impingement against the coracoacromial arch.

rotating the humerus. Inspection of the biceps can be useful to identify a complete rupture of the long head by visualizing a "popeye" sign, which is caused by the retracted muscle. If the rupture is in the acute phase, a significant amount of ecchymosis is usually visualized as well. Speed's (straight-arm flexion test, bowling test) and Yergason's test (supination test) are tests that can be used to assess for biceps pathology and the integrity of the tendon. Speed's test is performed by resisting forward flexion of the humerus with the forearm supinated (palm facing upward) with the elbow extended, and a positive sign is when this produces pain in the bicipital groove pain or if decreased strength is appreciated. Yergason's test is performed by having the patient attempt supination and external rotation of the forearm against resistance with the elbow flexed at 90°, and a positive sign is when this produces pain in the bicipital groove or if decreased strength is appreciated.

There are several tests that can be used to evaluate for shoulder instability. Slowly abduct the patient's shoulder with the elbow flexed to 90°. Place your hand on the glenohumeral joint with the fingers palpating the humeral head posteriorly and the thumb anteriorly. With your other hand, support the patient's arm. Using the hand on the patient's shoulder, apply anterior-directed stress to the humeral head, levering it anteriorly (Figure 43.9). Repeat this maneuver at varying degrees of abduction, feeling for anterior subluxation. Place your thumb on the patient's humeral head, flex the arm forward, and direct a posterior stress (Figure 43.10). Feel for any posterior subluxation with your posteriorly placed fingers. Posterior laxity (up to 50%) is often a normal finding in a throwing athlete's shoulder. Multidirectional instability (MDI) presents an often overlooked source of shoulder pain, so the examiner should test for inferior instability as well by applying downward traction on the arm while at the patient's side with elbow in extension. The appearance of a sulcus between the humeral head and lateral acromion is noted as a positive "sulcus sign" and is significant for inferior instability.[33]

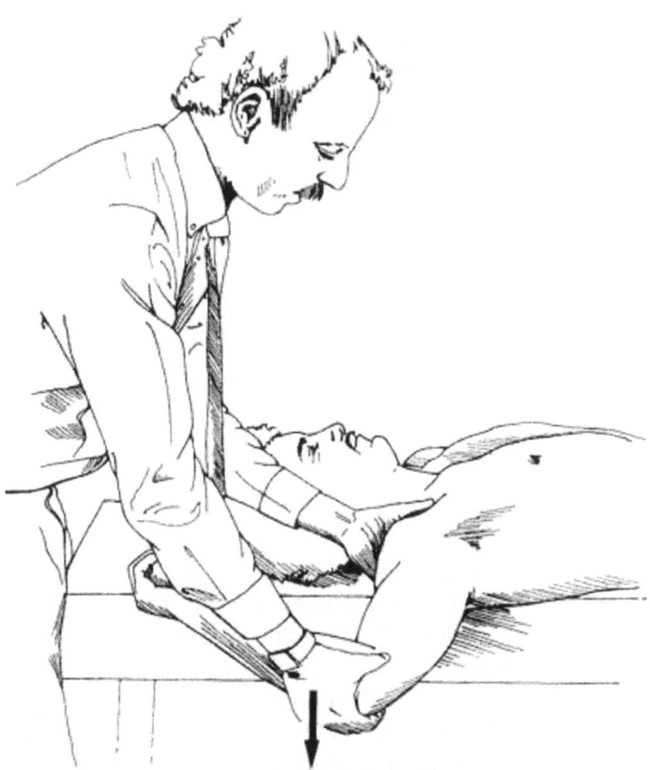

FIGURE 43.9 Testing for anterior subluxation

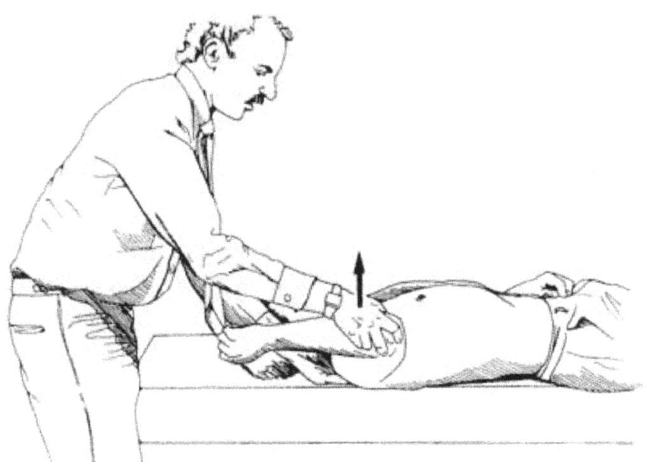

FIGURE 43.10 Testing for posterior subluxation.

A tear of the glenoid labrum can be diagnosed by the clunk test or labral grind test. The clunk test is performed by placing one hand posterior to the humeral head while the other hand rotates the humerus. Bring the arm into full overhead abduction while providing an anterior force to the humeral head. The clunk test is positive when a clunk, pop, or grind is felt in the shoulder as the humerus comes into contact with the labral tear (Figure 43.11). The labral grind test is performed by placing one hand posterior to the humeral head while the other hand brings the shoulder into 90° of abduction with elbow flexed and applies an axial, or compressive, load. The humeral head is then rotated 360° around the glenoid fossa. The labral grind test is positive

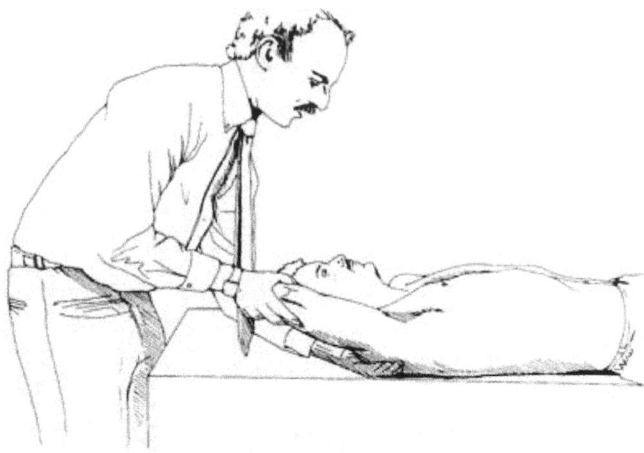

FIGURE 43.11 Clunk test: testing for an anterior labral tear.

when a clunk, pop, or grind is felt in the shoulder at the location of the labral tear. The presence of a superior labral anterior to posterior (SLAP) tear can also be tested with the active compression test (O'Brien's sign). The maneuver consists of having the patient's arm forward flexed to 90°, adducted to 15°, and maximally internally rotated with the thumb pointing toward the ground. The patient is instructed to resist as the examiner applies a uniform downward force. The patient then externally rotates the arm so that the thumb points upward and the maneuver is repeated. The test is positive if pain was felt within the shoulder while the thumb points toward the ground and improved when the thumb pointed upward[46] (Figure 43.12). Another approach to evaluating biceps–labral complex lesions can be done using the "three-pack" examination, which combines bicipital groove palpation, the throwing test, and active compression test (O'Brien's sign).[45] The apprehension–relocation test is also useful in the evaluation of anterior instability and is performed by having the patient lie supine, which helps to stabilize the scapula. The patient's arm is then brought into a position of 90° of abduction with elbow flexed to 90°, while the examiner begins to externally rotate the arm. A positive apprehension sign is denoted by guarding, patient's fear of dislocation as the arm is rotated further into external rotation, or pain in the anterior shoulder. Next, the examiner uses the other hand to apply anterior pressure to the glenohumeral joint in which a positive relocation sign is denoted by resolution of the apprehension sign.

Clinical Pearl

All shoulder examinations should include a neurovascular assessment and a cervical spine evaluation to exclude cervical radiculopathy as the source of shoulder pain.

All examinations must include a neurovascular assessment of the upper extremities and cervical spine evaluation. Brachial, radial, and ulnar pulses should be checked. The neurologic exam should include motor and sensory exams specifically in the axillary, radial, ulnar, and median nerve distributions. Deep tendon reflexes (biceps, C5; brachioradialis, C6; and triceps, C7) should be assessed. A cervical spine examination should include assessing for bony tenderness to palpation, ROM (flexion, extension, lateral flexion, rotation), and Spurling's test. The latter is performed by rotating the head, placing the cervical spine into extension, and then applying axial compression. This should be performed bilaterally, and a positive sign is denoted by radiation of pain into the shoulder or upper extremity with this maneuver.

43.5 DIAGNOSTIC PROCEDURES

There are several modalities to assess shoulder pathology, and each of these have their own benefits and limitations. Plain radiographs (x-rays) are a less expensive, fast modality

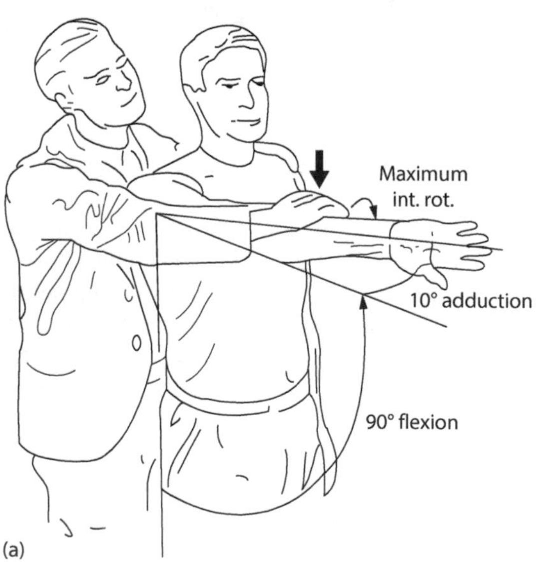

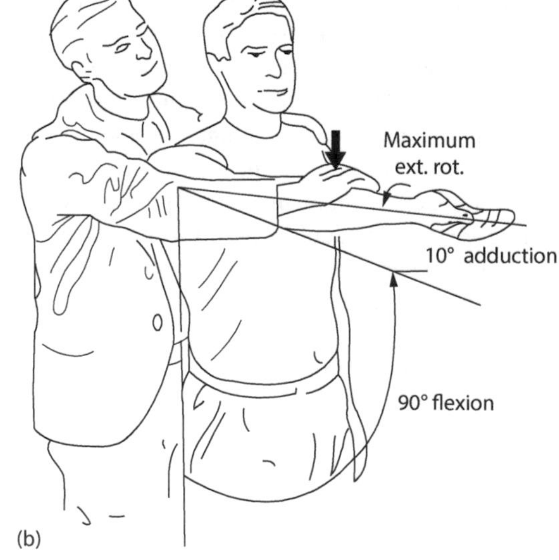

FIGURE 43.12 (a and b) Active compression test.

for initial screening of shoulder pathology, especially in the acute setting in which fractures and dislocations should be ruled out. At least, three views of the shoulder should be obtained with several other views available to assess specific structures and pathology. Frontal views of the shoulder should include an anteroposterior (AP) view with the humerus in neutral position or with it in internal and/or external rotation (often referred to as a "true" AP view). An axillary view or scapular Y view should be included especially in the setting of trauma to better assess the glenohumeral joint and presence of humeral dislocation. A west point axillary view is a modified view that can aid in the detection of a bony Bankart lesion, whereas a Stryker notch view is used for the evaluation of a Hill–Sachs deformity. A suprascapular outlet view is helpful to evaluate shoulder impingement and better assess the anatomy of the acromion.[71] Magnetic resonance imaging (MRI) has improved greatly over the last decade and is now the procedure of choice for evaluating soft-tissue pathology of the shoulder as well as assessing for occult fractures not visualized on plain radiographs. MR arthrography may be utilized to more accurately assess for instability and labral pathology.[71]

Clinical Pearl

Plain radiographs (x-rays) are a useful initial screening of shoulder pathology. At least three views of the shoulder should be obtained. Magnetic resonance imaging is useful in evaluating the soft tissues or identifying occult fractures.

Ultrasound requires expertise, but it can serve as an inexpensive and accessible modality to evaluate the rotator cuff, bursitis, long head of the biceps, and labrum. It can also be used to guide injections and aspirations.[71]

Computed tomography (CT) without contrast can be useful to further evaluate fractures or other bony abnormalities and is most commonly used preoperatively. CT shoulder arthrography is an alternative modality in patients who have a contraindication to MRI, such as having a pacemaker, but ultrasound has become a better option in these instances.[71]

43.6 OVERUSE INJURIES

43.6.1 External Impingement of the Shoulder (Subacromial Bursitis, Shoulder Impingement Syndrome)

Clinical Pearl

External impingement of the shoulder is classically known as "shoulder impingement syndrome" and is the most common soft-tissue injury of the shoulder.

Clinical Pearl

Physical therapy for external impingement of the shoulder should specifically focus on strengthening of the rotator cuff and scapular stabilizers.

When using the term "shoulder impingement," it is important to differentiate between the two different types of shoulder impingement: external versus internal impingement. External impingement of the shoulder is classically known as "shoulder impingement syndrome" and is the most common soft-tissue injury of the shoulder due to repetitive use of the arms above the horizontal plane, such as in throwing and racquet sports, swimming (40%–60% of swimmer's shoulder), weightlifting, and javelin throw.[18,27,44,48] Inflexibility, fatigue, and mechanical and technique errors are risk factors. It typically occurs from repetitive microtrauma during throwing, stroking, and serving, where a dynamic imbalance occurs between the external (rotator cuff muscles) and internal (pectoralis and latissimus dorsi muscles) rotators. This allows the humeral head and its rotator cuff attachments to migrate proximally, which leads to impingement by the undersurface of the acromion and the coracoacromial ligament. Symptoms can also be caused by direct trauma to the acromion and or chronic irritation under the coracoacromial arch due to a hooked (type 3) acromion or subacromial osteophyte. The rotator muscle group consists of the supraspinatus, infraspinatus, subscapularis, and teres minor muscles. Recurrent inflammation of the rotator cuff, especially the avascular area of the supraspinatus tendon, the long head of the biceps tendon, and the subacromial bursa, leads to impingement.[60] Initially, discomfort may be minimal and present deep within the shoulder during activity with no obvious loss of strength. Symptoms progress to significant pain that is frequently worse at night and with overhead movements. Pain-free ROM is restricted, with a painful arc of abduction 70°–120° and positive Neer and Hawkins tests. Also observed are point tenderness over the greater tuberosity and anterior acromion (coracoacromial ligament), tenderness over the biceps tendon proximally in the bicipital groove, positive straight-arm raising test, resisted forward flexion of the humerus with the forearm supinated and the elbow extended (i.e., Speed's test), positive resisted supination forearm test (i.e., Yergason's sign), and weakness of rotator cuff and biceps. Atrophy may be present over the supraspinatus. X-rays tend to be supportive but not diagnostic as they may reveal sclerosis and osteophyte formation on the anterior–inferior acromion, an enlarged or hooked (type 3) acromion, and diminished distance (≤5 mm) between the acromion and proximal humeral head.[3,27] MRI demonstrates excellent visualization of partial and full cuff tears, inflammation of the subacromial bursa and supraspinatus tendon, and tears of the capsule and subscapularis.[56] Ultrasound may also provide visualization of cuff tears and abnormal cuff mechanics. Local anesthetic injection of the subacromial space can be a useful diagnostic tool if it improves shoulder pain and ROM. The differential diagnosis may also include internal impingement of the shoulder, acute traumatic bursitis, subluxating shoulder, arthritis of the AC or glenohumeral joint, cervical disc herniation, adhesive capsulitis, suprascapular nerve injury, glenoid labrum tear, thoracic outlet syndrome, and atraumatic osteolysis of the distal clavicle. Initial treatment consists of relative rest, NSAIDs, and analgesics as needed to control pain. Total rest may be necessary if the patient experiences pain that is sufficiently disabling to affect performance during and after activities. It may be necessary to implement injection therapy with steroid and local anesthesia into subacromial bursa (not recommended for young athletes).[53,68]

Physical therapy improves ROM as well as rotator cuff and scapular stabilizer muscle strength. Modalities such as electric stimulation and ultrasound may help with symptoms but do not necessarily improve healing.[67] Surgical decompression of the subacromial space, acromioplasty, and coracoacromial ligament resection can be considered for patients who fail conservative management.[2,12] Preventive measures include maintaining ROM and strength training of the rotator group[25] as well as improving biomechanics for swimming (avoidance of hand paddles and sprints, increased body roll, and alternation of breathing sides), weightlifting (avoidance of overhead training such as bench and military presses), and pitching (slower "opening up"—turning body toward home plate well ahead of the throwing shoulder).

43.6.2 Internal Impingement of the Shoulder (Posterior Glenoid Impingement)

Internal impingement of the shoulder is due to the entrapment of the rotator cuff between the glenolabral complex and humeral head.[28] It has been mainly described in throwing athletes such as baseball pitches, but other sports requiring repetitive, overhead activities including tennis, volleyball, javelin throw, and swimming are at risk.[35] However, it has also been found to occur in nonathletes as well.[31,69] Young to middle-aged adults are typically affected. Internal impingement is caused by repetitive contact of the greater tuberosity of the humeral head with the posterosuperior glenoid when the arm is abducted and externally rotated. This impinges the rotator cuff and/or labrum.[28] There is not a clear consensus on the exact mechanism, but it has been theorized that a rotational instability in which the shoulder is able to hyperexternally rotate during the late cocking phase places more stress on the anterior capsule. This results in posterior capsular hypertrophy causing increased external rotation and decreased internal rotation or glenohumeral internal rotation deficit (GIRD) termed by Burkhart et al.[15,35] This leads to the central contact point of the glenohumeral articulation to be shifted in a posterosuperior direction causing the supraspinatus tendon, and sometimes the anterior fibers of the infraspinatus tendon, to become entrapped between the humeral head and posterosuperior labrum.[35] The rotator cuff and posterosuperior labrum are interposed between the glenoid rim and greater tuberosity of the humerus. The contact of the rotator cuff on the posterosuperior labrum has been shown to be a normal, physiologic occurrence. However, altered shoulder mechanics can lead to pathologic impingement and inflammation, fraying, or tears of the articular side of the rotator cuff and posterosuperior labrum.[28] Injury to several other structures have been associated with pathologic internal impingement, which include the greater tuberosity, inferior glenohumeral ligament complex, and posterior superior glenoid.[31] The presenting complaint is commonly diffuse posterior shoulder pain that is chronic in nature, although it may be more localized to the joint line.[28] Three stages have been described by Jobe regarding the clinical presentation of internal impingement. In stage I, complaints of stiffness accompany pain specifically in the abducted, maximal externally rotated position. Stage II is denoted by progression to significant posterior shoulder pain with activity. Stage III is when conservative measures fail to result in improvement.[32] The nonathlete, however, is more likely to experience acute posterior shoulder pain following an injury. The most common physical examination findings in a throwing athlete include posterior glenohumeral joint line tenderness, increased external rotation, and decreased internal rotation. Evidence of GIRD, marked by a 30°–40° loss of internal rotation relative to gained external rotation and compared to the contralateral side, should be carefully evaluated. Since there is a high association with other shoulder conditions, a thorough shoulder examination should be performed and include bilateral active and passive ROM, provocative testing for SLAP lesions including the O'Brien's test, and instability testing.[28] A posterior impingement sign was termed by Meister et al., which tests for deep posterior shoulder pain when the arm is brought into abduction 90°–110°, extension to 10°–15°, and maximal external rotation. The sensitivity was 95% and specificity 100% when testing the overhead athletes who had symptoms without sustaining a contact injury.[42] The relocation test can also be used and will create posterior shoulder pain (as opposed to anterior pain with anterior instability) that is relieved with a posteriorly directed force on the humerus.[28] X-rays should be obtained with evaluation using the standard AP, axillary, scapular Y, west point, and Stryker notch view of the shoulder. There have been four associated findings on radiographic imaging with internal impingement, which include exostosis of the posteroinferior glenoid rim (Bennett lesion), sclerotic changes of the greater tuberosity, posterior humeral head osteochondral lesions or cystic "geodes," and rounding of the posterior glenoid rim. Despite awareness of these radiographic findings, MRI remains the gold standard for evaluation with imaging. Findings typical of internal impingement are articular-sided rotator cuff tears of the supraspinatus and/or infraspinatus tendons and posterior superior labral lesions.[35] The differential diagnosis may also include external impingement of the shoulder, full thickness rotator cuff tear, SLAP tear, and anterior instability. Initial treatment consists of relative rest, ice, NSAIDs, and physical therapy including periscapular and rotator cuff strengthening exercises, which should be attempted before surgical intervention. If GIRD is appreciated on exam, a posterior shoulder capsular stretching routine (sleeper stretches) should be implemented.[28] For long-term treatment, a rehabilitation program should be aimed at correcting pathological findings suggested by the physical exam and imaging. If it fails to improve symptoms or if it does not allow the athlete to return to competitive play, then surgical intervention should be considered. Surgical intervention should attempt to address specific pathologic lesions corresponding to the patient's symptoms or that play a role in the complex pathophysiology of internal impingement. A comprehensive diagnostic arthroscopy should be performed for internal impingement because of the high association of other pathologic shoulder conditions.[28] Complications of internal impingement of the shoulder include posterior SLAP tears, microtrauma to greater tuberosity, or posterosuperior rim of the glenoid with some case reports of fractures.[28]

43.6.3 Rotator Cuff Strain (Supraspinatus Tendinitis)

Clinical Pearl

Rotator cuff tears are uncommon to see in a younger person and usually present as tears due to chronic overuse in middle-aged adults.

Acute tears are rare in the young and typically chronic overuse and tears (e.g., skiing fall, body surfing, throwing, and equestrian activities) occur in the "over-45 weekend warrior." Indirect force to the abducted arm and repetitive microtrauma are the usual mechanisms of injury. Acute or chronic tearing of the rotator cuff muscle–tendon unit (see external impingement of the shoulder) is the most common injury. The most common site (critical zone) is the relatively avascular supraspinatus tendon just proximal to the greater tuberosity of the humerus. Acute injury typically presents with significant shoulder pain and the inability to abduct arm against resistance. Presentation of chronic injury includes gradual onset of pain (initially nocturnal, later persistent) and weakness especially with 70°–120° of arm abduction and external rotation, palpable crepitus during supraspinatus abduction, positive impingement sign, full abduction not restored by local anesthetic injection into subacromial space, and variable loss of strength and atrophy of cuff muscles. X-rays are usually normal but may show proximal migration of humeral head, subacromial spurring, and calcific deposits in chronic tears. MRI is the gold standard for evaluating the rotator cuff and is sensitive and specific for partial and complete tears. It is also useful to evaluate the muscle and potential presence of fatty atrophy consistent with a chronic rotator cuff tear. Ultrasound by an experienced user may be helpful in evaluating muscle–tendon integrity and may demonstrate increased hyperemia in the absence of tears. The differential diagnosis may include subacromial bursitis, biceps tendonitis, and cervical radiculopathy. Initial treatment consists of relative rest, ice, NSAIDs, and analgesics. Prolonged physical therapy including ROM and progressive resistance exercises (PREs) should emphasize abduction and external rotation and strengthening scapular stabilizer muscles. Platelet-rich plasma (PRP) may have positive effects in chronic cases. Arthroscopic or open surgery should be followed by physical therapy when conservative (nonoperative) management fails.[67] Complications may include progressing to complete tears. Preventive measure is similar to those described in the External Impingement of the Shoulder section.

43.6.4 Biceps Tendon Problems (Tendinitis, Subluxation/Dislocation, Rupture)

Biceps tendinosis is common in a wide range of throwing, swimming, and racquet sports. In particular, male gymnasts are at risk for biceps tendon injury. Subluxation, dislocation, and rupture often occur on a background of tendinosis, repeated corticosteroid injections, or traumatic injury. Distal ruptures occur predominantly in athletes over 30 years of age. All three pathologies may be associated with an external impingement of the shoulder, rotator cuff disease, or glenohumeral instability. The mechanism of injury is usually repetitive microtrauma (tendinosis); however, acute injury commonly (rupture, subluxation/dislocation) occurs following sudden forceful contraction against resistance or direct blow (e.g., checked baseball swing, fast-pitched softball, arm tackle on a quarterback's passing hand). The biceps tendon originates at the superior border of the labrum (long head) and coracoid process (short head), travels intracapsularly under the transverse humeral ligament covering the intertubercular groove, and inserts into the bicipital tuberosity of the radius. It has a relatively avascular area intracapsularly. A tight, narrow groove, rough supratubercular area, or steep medial wall due to a prominent lesser tuberosity can irritate and inflame the tendon. Chronic inflammation can lead to degenerative rupture. Tears of the transverse humeral ligament in association with a shallow groove or low medial wall can produce subluxation or dislocation. Most subluxations and dislocations are medial, but lateral cases have been reported. Ruptures occur in the muscle–tendon junction in the very young and at the top of the groove in the middle-aged or older athlete; 97% are proximal and 3% are distal.[33] Presentation of this condition commonly occurs in a patient that usually has a significant history of rotator cuff disease or external impingement of the shoulder. Tenderness and crepitus over the bicipital groove can be appreciated, as are vague pain and snapping in the region of the proximal humerus and tendon. The "three-pack" examination can be used to further evaluate for evidence of a biceps–labral complex lesion.[45] A snapping or popping sensation with external rotation indicates subluxation/dislocation; the findings move laterally with external arm rotation or medially with internal rotation. Speed, Yergason, Ludington, and Gilcrest (subluxation/dislocation) tests may be positive. Complete rupture may show ecchymosis and a palpable visible gap in muscle belly (complete rupture) with supination and flexion weakness (40%–50% decrease in distal ruptures, 10%–20% in proximal ruptures). A "popeye" deformity is seen in proximal long-head ruptures (distal movement of muscle mass). There will be antecubital fossa tenderness with a distal rupture. Tunnel views on plain radiographs may show a narrow, shallow groove with osteophytes, tendon calcification, or a prominent lesser tuberosity with tendinosis and subluxation/dislocation. Avulsion fracture may be present in a rupture and x-rays can be helpful to evaluate for a fracture of the lesser tuberosity. Ultrasound is diagnostic for ruptures, associated effusions, and hyperechoic foci (calcifications and loose bodies) seen chronically in tendinosis. MRI is diagnostic for tendon pathology and rupture.[23,65] The differential diagnosis may include external impingement of the shoulder and osteochondral fracture. For conservative management, initially use rest, ice, compression, and elevation (RICE), NSAIDs, and analgesics as needed. For tendinitis, one corticosteroid injection into the biceps sheath may be warranted, and sometimes a PRP injection can be effective. Tenodesis is recommended if patient does not respond to conservative management. For subluxation/dislocation, surgical repair of the transverse humeral ligament is recommended. For rupture, surgical repairs for all distal and proximal ruptures in younger, more athletic patients are recommended; otherwise aside from visual appearance, the majority of older patients will have minimal change in function due to proximal biceps tendon ruptures.[21,50] For preventive measures, the athlete should warm up properly, avoid shoulder-motion extremes, initiate a flexibility and strengthening program (especially of the internal shoulder rotators), and modify technique.

43.6.5 Glenoid Labrum Tears

Glenoid labrum tears may occur from repetitive shoulder motion or acute trauma. In the throwing athlete with repeated anterior shoulder subluxation, tears of the middle and inferior portion of the labrum may occur, leading to instability. Glenoid labrum tears may also result from anterior instability during the release phase of throwing, secondary to the long head of the biceps tendon pulling on the anterior labrum. Weightlifters may also develop glenoid labrum tears from repetitive bench pressing and overhead pressing. Most patients present with nonspecific shoulder pain associated with activity. Complicating the presentation is that the majority of lesions reported in the literature are associated with other shoulder disorders such as rotator cuff tears, AC joint disorders, and instability.[48] The majority of glenoid labral tears occur from traction and compression injuries.[10] Sudden contraction of the biceps can occur with overhead athletes during the release phase of throwing. Compression injuries occur with forceful subluxation or dislocation of the humeral head over the fibrocartilaginous labrum. Tears of the glenoid labrum may also occur from acute trauma such as falling on an outstretched arm. Also, horizontal adduction and internal rotation during the acceleration phase of throwing can damage the labrum by applying a sheering stress across the labrum.[4]

With regard to shoulder instability, MDI occurs on a background of generalized shoulder-capsule laxity, which may be genetic (35%) (e.g., Ehlers–Danlos syndrome) versus environmental (previous trauma, 30%; overuse, 35%).[59] The instability may be voluntary (patient consciously subluxes/dislocates joint) or involuntary. The labrum is a triangular structure located around the periphery of the glenoid. It comprises dense fibrous tissue rather than cartilage[19] and functions as a static stabilizer of the glenohumeral joint.[30,58] The average depth of the articular surface of the glenoid in the transverse plane is 2.5 mm. The labrum serves to deepen the glenoid by an additional 2.5 mm both anteriorly and posteriorly, adding to the static stability of the joint.[9] The glenoid labrum and biceps tendon are closely associated. The long head of the biceps tendon is attached to the superior portion of the labrum and often included in the classification of superior labrum tears. SLAP lesions describe anatomic lesions of the superior glenoid labrum and biceps anchor. Glenoid labrum tears that occur in close proximity to the biceps, in the superior third of the labrum, can demonstrate symptoms similar to those of biceps tendon subluxation. Presentation of a labral tear may include an audible or palpable clunk that can occur as the tear flips in and out of the joint. In throwing athletes, more pain is sensed with release because of the deceleration effect of the biceps pulling on the torn labrum. With other tears, a sense of popping, clicking, or snapping in the joint is experienced during abduction and external rotation (e.g., cocking phase). Anterior humeral joint tenderness and pain with abduction and external rotation are observed. The labral clunk test may be positive along with the active compression test (O'Brien's sign) and the biceps load. Standard x-rays may demonstrate bony abnormalities such as Hill–Sachs and bony Bankart lesions, while other injuries involving the labrum may only have normal-appearing images. In order to further assess for soft-tissue pathology, an MRI of the shoulder should be obtained as it provides excellent evaluation of labral injuries.[60] Especially with a dedicated extremity coil, a good correlation with surgical findings has been found. With the advancements in MRI over the past decade, it has become the gold standard for evaluation of labral pathology with imaging. However, ultrasonography has also been shown to be a useful tool in the evaluation of the glenoid labrum, particularly in excluding tears when the labrum appears normal on sonography.[63] The differential diagnosis may include a rotator cuff tear or impingement. Of patients with MDI secondary to ligamentous laxity, 50%–70% respond to prolonged conservative rehabilitation (6–12 months). MDI secondary to trauma often requires surgical correction. Voluntary MDI secondary to psychological problems is often resistant to all forms of intervention. Initial treatment should consist of RICE and NSAIDs. Conservative management should also include a program to maintain adequate ROM with muscle strengthening exercises, specifically for the posterior rotator cuff muscles (as demonstrated in Figure 43.13). If symptoms do not resolve, these injuries require definitive treatment through surgical intervention.

Chronic instability can lead to disability secondary to arthritis. Preventive measures include teaching proper throwing mechanics with progressive training and conditioning.

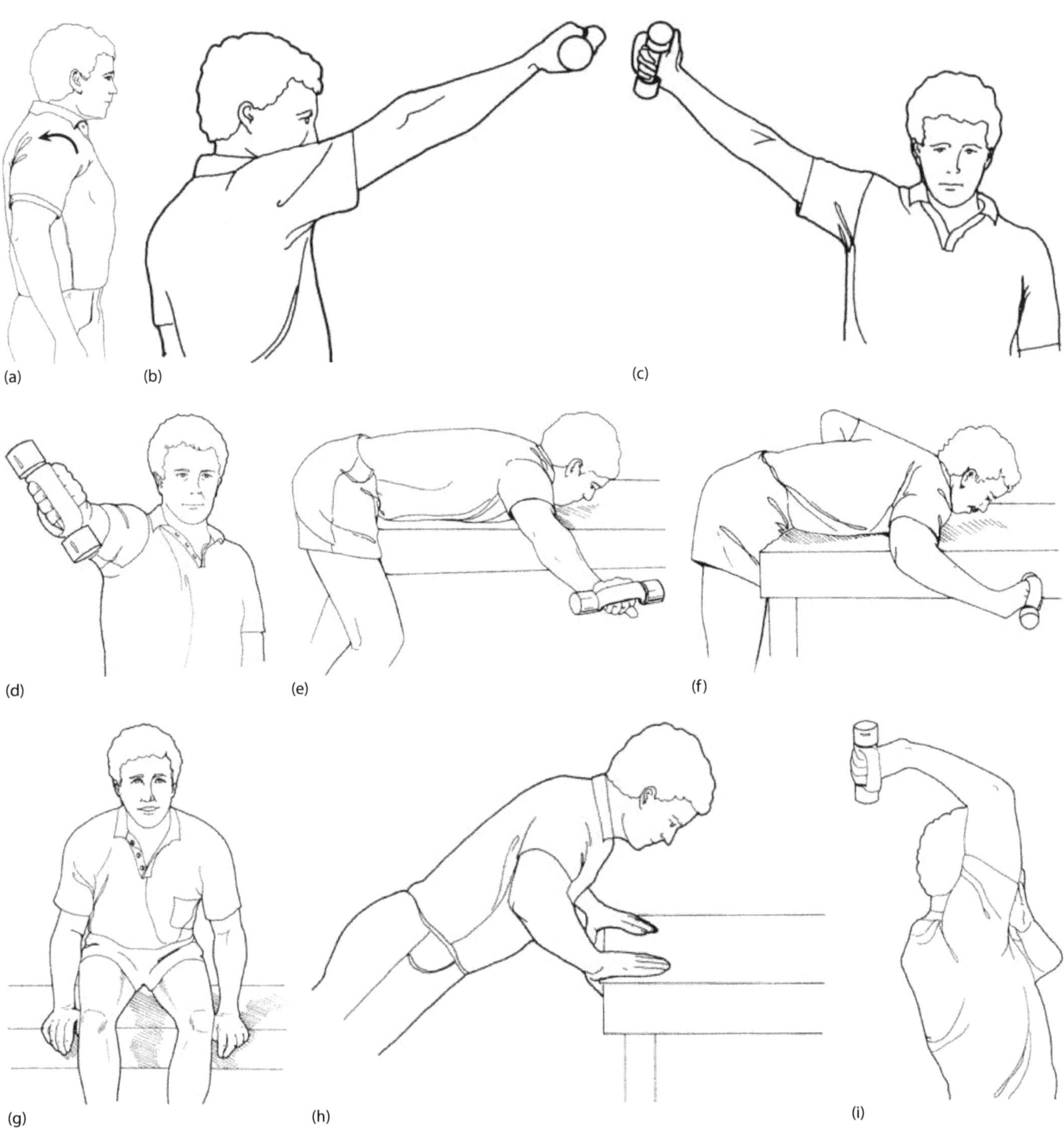

FIGURE 43.13 (a) Shoulder shrug with scapular retraction. (b) Strengthening the anterior portion of the deltoid muscle by forward-flexion exercises. (c) Strengthening the middle portion of the deltoid muscle by abduction exercises. (d) Strengthening the supraspinatus muscle by internally rotating and abducting the humerus. (e) Shoulder position for strengthening the external rotators. (f) Strengthening exercise for the posterior portion of the deltoid muscle and the rotator cuff. (g) Strengthening the shoulder depressor, horizontal adductor, and internal rotator muscles. (h) Modified push-up. (i) French curl exercise for strengthening the triceps muscle. *(Continued)*

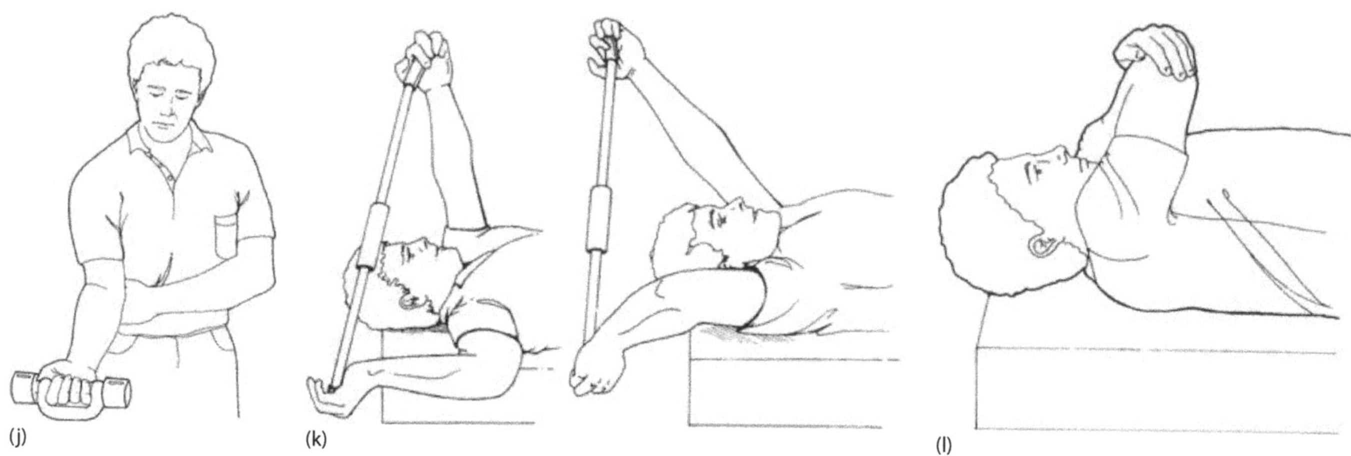

FIGURE 43.13 (*Continued*) (j) Biceps or elbow curl for strengthening the biceps muscle. (k) External rotation flexibility exercises performed with the shoulder abducted from 90° to full abduction. (l) Stretching exercise for the posterior shoulder structures.

43.6.6 Scapulothoracic Problems (Bursitis, Winging)

Scapulothoracic bursitis is common in sports requiring repetitive shoulder motion (e.g., swimming, throwing, and racquet sports). Winging is spontaneous following strenuous activity, such as cycling, swimming, golf, backpacking, or weightlifting, or in collision/contact sports and may be due to long thoracic nerve injury. It is usually caused by high-velocity repetitive microtrauma (shot-putting, back-scratch position during tennis serve) on a background of excessive shoulder motion. Bursitis and winging can also follow direct (e.g., a forceful blow) or indirect (e.g., excessive traction) trauma. Architectural malalignment along the inferior–medial scapular border leads to bursal inflammation. Paralysis of the serratus anterior can follow direct trauma of the long thoracic nerve. Presenting signs and symptoms can include pain, grating, and snapping at the inferior angle of the scapula, which are noted with shoulder elevation. Dull ache or pain can be noted in the shoulder girdle but usually is asymptomatic. Crepitus may be observed with arm elevation when the scapula rolls over the posterior chest wall and a palpable mass at the inferior–medial angle may be best felt with 60° abduction and 30° flexion of the shoulder. Winging occurs when the arm is brought into the elevated position and is emphasized when the patient pushes against a wall with arms extended. Increased pain with contralateral head tilting or ipsilateral arm elevation is noted. AP and lateral views of the proximal humerus in the scapular plane are usually negative. MRI may provide information.

EMG and nerve conduction studies demonstrate conduction delays and denervation if winging is secondary to nerve injury, but findings may be minimal in the first 3 weeks. The differential diagnosis may include a rhomboid strain or cervical radiculopathy. Initial treatment of bursitis consists of NSAIDs, with those not responding can potentially receive injection therapy with both treatments being accompanied by physical therapy (ROM + PREs), specifically focusing on the interscapular musculature. For treatment of winging due to nerve injury, rest and gentle physical therapy (ROM + PREs) should be advised. While recovery may require 2 years, resolution is rarely complete. Winging *per se* should not be a criterion for return to play. Preventive measures include improving sport biomechanics (e.g., reduced shoulder movement during cocking position of tennis serve) and increasing strength of scapular stabilizers.

43.7 TRAUMATIC INJURIES

43.7.1 Sternoclavicular Sprain/Subluxation/Dislocation

The sternoclavicular joint is the only articulation between the upper extremity and axial skeleton yet has the least amount of bony stability of any joint in the body. Sternoclavicular injuries are rare and associated with trauma to the chest or shoulder. They are classified as anterior or posterior, determined by the anatomic position of the medial head of the clavicle in relation to the sternum.[55] Anterior dislocation is more common than posterior, and many dislocations are actually fractures through the physeal plate because the epiphysis at the medial end of the clavicle closes at approximately 23–25 years of age. The mechanism of injury is an indirect force applied from the anterolateral or posterolateral aspect of the opposite or uninjured shoulder. This usually occurs when the athlete falls on the injured shoulder with additional forces applied through the opposite shoulder. Injury can also occur with a direct force to the anteromedial aspect of the clavicle, pushing the clavicle posteriorly behind the sternum into the mediastinum. Disruption of the pulmonary and vascular systems can occur. Injury may consist of tearing of the capsule, intra-articular disc, or costoclavicular ligaments. The injuries can be graded based on severity with Grade I denoting all ligaments are intact and joint is stable, Grade II denoting partial disruption of the sternoclavicular and costoclavicular ligaments leading to subluxation of the sternoclavicular joint, and Grade III denoting complete disruption of the sternoclavicular joint leading to anterior or posterior dislocation. Grade I injuries present with slight swelling and tenderness at the joint, no instability, and mild to moderate pain especially with arm movement. Grade II (subluxation) injuries will cause increased pain and swelling with palpable anterior or posterior subluxation. Grade III (dislocation) injuries will cause severe pain with any ROM.

In Grade III injuries, the patient supports the injured arm across the trunk with the normal arm. In the supine position, pain increases and the involved shoulder does not lie flat on the table. It should be noted that with an anterior dislocation, the medial end of the clavicle is visibly prominent anterior to the sternum. In a posterior dislocation, the medial end of the clavicle is palpable and displaced posteriorly. Venus congestion may be present in the neck or upper extremity. Breathing difficulties, shortness of breath, swallowing difficulties, subcutaneous emphysema, and ipsilateral pulselessness, swelling, and discoloration can occur.

AP or posteroanterior x-ray views of the chest or sternoclavicular joint may suggest an abnormality as one clavicle appears displaced compared to the normal side. A 40° cephalic tilt view (Rockwood or Serendipity view) is recommended. CT scan or MRI can be used to evaluate anterior or posterior dislocation, fractures, great vessels, and trachea. The differential diagnosis should include evaluating for a fracture. Initial treatment consists of RICE, NSAIDs, or analgesics as needed plus sling immobilization. Continued management varies depending on injury severity. For Grade I, wean patient from immobilization at 5–10 days with a gradual return to use of the arm. For Grade II, reduction may be required; draw the shoulders back and hold them with a clavicle strap. Protection with a sling and/or clavicle strap for a period of 4–6 weeks is recommended. For grade III, if it is an anterior dislocation, have the patient supine on the edge of the table with a sandbag between the shoulders. With the upper extremity at 90° of abduction and extension, apply traction in line with the clavicle. Use a postreduction figure-eight dressing for 6 weeks. Operative repair is debatable. For posterior dislocations, have the patient supine with a sandbag between the shoulders. Apply lateral traction to the abducted arm, which is then gradually brought back into extension. Use a postreduction figure-eight dressing for 6 weeks. Because of potential damage to the posterior structures, some physicians prefer operative repair. Either way, reduction should be performed with extreme care for the posterior vasculature.[70] Complications from these injuries can include injury to the pulmonary vessels, trachea, superior vena cava, esophagus, and other mediastinal structures, especially with posterior dislocations. There is also risk of traumatic arthritis and chronic joint instability.

43.7.2 Acromioclavicular Sprain/Subluxation/Dislocation

The AC joint is commonly injured in contact sports and falls off bicycles. The mechanism of injury is a direct fall or blow to the point of the shoulder at the lateral edge of the acromion. Indirect force from a fall on an outstretched arm or blow to the upper back can also cause injury to the joint.[33] AC injuries are classified as Grades I through VI: Grade I, AC ligament and capsular stretching; Grade II, AC ligament complete disruption with slight upward migration of the clavicle and partial tearing of the coracoclavicular ligaments; Grade III, AC and coracoclavicular ligaments and intra-articular meniscus disruption (AC joint dislocation with the clavicle displaced upward relative to the acromion [Figure 43.14]); Grade IV, a Grade III injury with the clavicle anatomically displaced upward and posterior into or through the trapezius; Grade V, severe upward dislocation of the distal clavicle relative to the acromion with complete destruction of the AC and coracoclavicular ligaments and disruption of the deltoid and trapezius muscle attachments to the clavicle (clavicle may pierce the muscle and even the skin in some cases); and Grade VI, inferior dislocation of the clavicle underneath the coracoid with injury to the underlying neurovascular structures likely. Presentation of these injuries can differ depending on severity. With Grade I injuries, there may be mild swelling and along with tenderness over the AC ligament with no instability of the distal clavicle. The patient can perform the crossover test with minimal or no pain. With Grade II injuries, there can be snapping of the AC joint on shoulder motion with swelling and tenderness over the AC ligament and some lack of symmetry when compared to the normal side as well as tenderness and slight instability of the distal clavicle with downward pressure. The crossover test is painful, yet the patient can resist pressure when the examiner pushes the elbow downward. With Grades III to V injuries, there will be swelling and marked tenderness over the AC and coracoclavicular ligaments and marked asymmetry with high-riding clavicle. Marked instability of the distal clavicle is observed. The patient is unable to perform the crossover test. Bilateral AP views on plain radiographs allow for displacement comparison to contralateral side, and lateral views are also helpful to demonstrate widening of the AC joint and high-riding clavicle. The Zanca view provides better visualization of the AC joint.

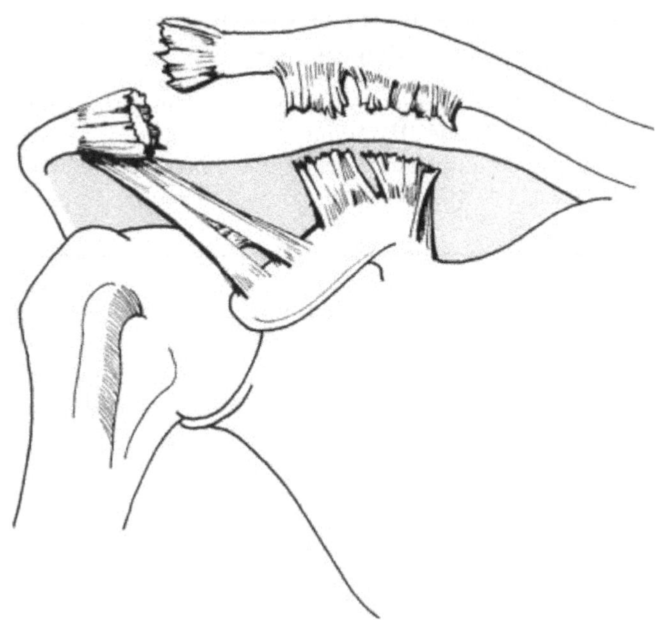

FIGURE 43.14 Grade III AC dislocation.

Clinical Pearl

Grade I and II AC joint sprains can be managed conservatively. Grade III sprains can be treated conservatively as well although it may need surgical intervention. All Grade IV–VI sprains should be referred for surgical management.

X-ray findings will vary depending on severity of injury with Grade I being normal, Grade II with asymmetry compared to contralateral side with less than 1.3 cm coracoacromial separation, and Grades III–V with greater than 1.3 cm separation or >50% increase in the distance when compared to the uninjured side. The differential diagnosis may include contusion, fracture, synovitis, and osteoarthritis. Initial treatment consists of RICE, NSAIDS, or analgesics as needed plus sling or shoulder immobilizer. Continued management for Grades I and II injuries consists of weaning out of immobilization as tolerated and beginning early physical therapy (ROM + PRE) for several weeks. For Grade III injuries, continued management includes the same as mentioned earlier followed by physical therapy for 6–8 weeks; surgery is occasionally indicated for the throwing arm of an athlete; however, in nonathletes, significant benefit from surgery is questionable as there have not been studies to show functional superiority of surgical versus conservative management.[52] For Grade IV, V, and VI injuries, operative treatment is recommended with reconstruction of the stabilizing structures.[7,38,52,64] Complications from these injuries consist of traumatic arthritis, persistent decreased ROM, and strength in addition to pain.

43.7.3 Glenohumeral Instability: Sprain/Subluxation/Dislocation

Instability and laxity are terms often applied to the shoulder. Laxity is the asymptomatic translation of the humeral head on the glenoid. It may be a normal variant and represent a necessary feature of the soft tissue about the shoulder required for glenohumeral rotation. Instability is the excessive translation of the humeral head on the glenoid occurring during active shoulder rotation in association with symptoms. It represents varying degrees of injuries to dynamic and static structures that function to contain the humeral head in the glenoid. A sprain occurs when there is sequential tearing of the glenohumeral ligaments and capsule with pain but no obvious displacement of the humeral head. Subluxation is the symptomatic increased humeral translation beyond that permitted by normal tissue laxity, but without complete separation of the articular surfaces. Dislocation is the complete separation of the articular surfaces of the glenoid and humeral head; 85% of dislocations detach the glenoid labrum (soft-tissue Bankart lesion).[40] Without the protection of the labrum, recurrent subluxations and dislocations can potentially lead to ectopic bone formation evident on radiographic images. In dislocations, 95% are anterior and inferior. Posterior injuries are uncommon, and pure superior and inferior injuries are very rare. Most cases of dislocation are anterior. Major trauma is usually involved, but the shoulder does not often dislocate as a result of a direct blow.[4] A combination of forces stress the abducted, extended, and externally rotated arm, which applies leverage to the anterior capsule, glenohumeral ligaments, and rotator cuff. The humeral head is forced anteriorly and out of the glenoid fossa. The most common type of anterior dislocation is the subcoracoid dislocation in which the humeral head is anterior to the glenoid and inferior to the coracoid process. The head of the humerus is anterior and below the glenoid fossa in subglenoid dislocation. The head of the humerus lies medial to the coracoid process at the inferior border of the clavicle in subclavicular dislocation. Significant trauma is associated with an intrathoracic dislocation where the head of the humerus lies between the ribs and thoracic cage.[49] A posterior shoulder dislocation can be caused by direct force such as a direct blow to the anterior aspect of the glenohumeral joint or can occur as a result of an indirect force such as a fall on an outstretched arm with the shoulder in internal rotation, adduction, and flexion. When blocking, as in football, a direct axial load applied to a flexed arm, adducted, and internally rotated may cause a posterior subluxation or dislocation of the humeral head. Seizure or electric shock can also produce a muscular contraction forceful enough to cause posterior displacement of the humeral head.[1] With chronic instability, glenohumeral translation is usually less than that detectable on physical examination but is sufficient enough to cause excessive edge loading or shearing stress to the labrum.[3] The result is the failure of the humeral head containment during motions such as throwing. Injuries can be classified as a sprain, which is sequential tearing of the glenohumeral ligaments and capsule; a subluxation, which is joint laxity causing more than 50% of the humeral head to passively translate over the glenoid rim without dislocation or causing the humeral head to actively translate more than 4 mm from the center of the glenoid; or a dislocation, which is joint instability with the humeral head losing contact with the glenoid and lodging beside the joint. With anterior dislocations, 85% detach the glenoid labrum (Bankart lesion), potentially leading to ectopic bone formation with recurrent dislocations.

Chronic injuries are less intense and have less localized pain; they get a sensation of instability or apprehension with overhead activities; they have a history of previous dislocations and progressively less trauma needed to sublux or dislocate shoulder.

With a sprain, the capsule is tender to palpation, there is no instability, but they will have a positive apprehension and relocation test (see Figure 43.15). With a subluxation, the patient may describe a sensation of the shoulder "popping" out and back into place with the pain sometimes be associated with paresthesias down the arm or a sensation of the arm "going dead," and the patient resists placing shoulder in abduction and external rotation and extension. The capsule is tender with mild swelling and a positive apprehension/relocation test. Brachial plexopathy commonly involves the axillary, musculocutaneous, or suprascapular nerves.[49] With an anterior dislocation, the patient will have acute severe pain with loss of ROM and possible numbness or weakness present before or after reduction.[11] Patient presents with arm slightly abducted and externally rotated and

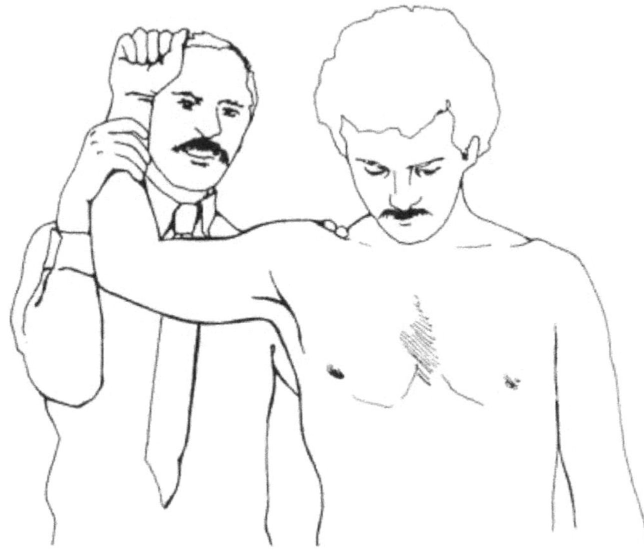

FIGURE 43.15 Apprehension test: testing for anterior stability.

held firmly by the other arm. A prominent acromion process and coracoid process may not be identified because of swelling but may be present on inspection and palpation in which the shoulder assumes a squared-off appearance with anterior shoulder fullness. Movement of the arm is painful and limited, especially with attempted adduction or internal rotation. With posterior shoulder dislocations, the arm is fixed in the adducted position and internally rotated and the coracoid process is more obvious. On the dislocated side, the anterior aspect of the shoulder is flat, and the posterior aspect of the shoulder is rounded and more pronounced than the normal shoulder. External rotation of the shoulder is blocked with severely limited abduction. Prereduction (if available) and postreduction plain radiographs reveal position of humerus and may demonstrate associated fractures or bony changes such as a bony Bankart lesion or Hill–Sachs deformity. Recommended views include AP views in internal and external rotation to evaluate overall bony structures with the axillary view and scapular Y view to evaluate humeral head position. If the patient's abduction is significantly limited and an axillary view cannot be obtained, a Velpeau view can be substituted to better evaluate humeral head position. A modified axillary lateral (west point) view is good for chip fractures of the anterior–inferior glenoid rim and labral tears (bony Bankart lesions). The Stryker notch view is a posterior view of the humeral head that helps check for a Hill–Sachs lesion. MRI is recommended for detailed assessment of the entire shoulder as it can identify bone bruising, muscle atrophy, neurovascular structures, and the extent of rotator cuff and biceps tears. It can also evaluate intra-articular pathology, such as the presence of ganglion cysts, glenoid labrum tears, and articular cartilage damage.[14] CT is useful for evaluating bony details especially with complicated fractures and for preoperative planning. The differential diagnosis may include a fracture (humerus, clavicle, scapula), AC joint sprain, rotator cuff injury, or atraumatic osteolysis of distal clavicle.

Initial treatment for shoulder dislocations includes successful reduction, then immobilization with a sling and swathe or shoulder immobilizer, RICE, NSAIDs, and analgesics as needed. For a *sprain* or *subluxation*, wean patient from immobilization in 5–10 days; the use of arm should return gradually. For a *dislocation*, the use of a sling and swathe or shoulder immobilizer can be used for 2–4 weeks especially for comfort, although recent studies do not support the use of the standard immobilization of the arm in adduction and internal rotation to reduce the risk of recurrence.[17] Several studies have supported immobilization in external rotation to improve the anatomical position of the displaced labrum on the glenoid rim to encourage healing although this practice has not been consistently shown to reduce rates or recurrent dislocations.[29] After immobilization, strengthening exercises should be initiated to determine if enough stability can be obtained to allow return to activities safely although the likelihood of recurrent instability is significant especially for younger, active individuals, and surgical intervention is usually necessary. In the acute setting, an attempt at reduction of a shoulder dislocation can be performed using a variety of techniques. There is no clear evidence that supports one method over another, and it mainly depends on clinician preference and the patient's condition. With all techniques, it is crucial for the patient to relax their shoulder muscles as much as possible for reduction to be successful, which can be a challenge due to pain causing involuntary muscle spasm. With regard to the pediatric population, traumatic glenohumeral dislocation in children with open physis can cause possible Salter–Harris fractures, which would therefore be a contraindication to attempt reduction, unless vascular compromise necessitates immediate treatment. The following are different reduction techniques for an anterior shoulder dislocation (Figure 43.16):

Clinical Pearl

There is no clear evidence to support one method over another regarding reduction of an anterior shoulder dislocation. With all techniques, it is crucial for the patient to relax their shoulder muscles as much as possible for reduction to be successful.

External rotation technique: The patient lies supine with the elbow flexed to 90°. Grasp the elbow with one hand to maintain the adducted position of the arm, and with the other hand, hold the patient's wrist and begin to slowly externally rotate the arm. Whenever pain or spasm is felt, the movement is stopped and the muscles are allowed to relax. Over 5–10 minutes, the arm can externally rotate to 70–100° to allow reduction. If external rotation approach does not result in reduction, the Milch technique can be added.

Milch technique: Keep the fully externally rotated arm in position while abducting it into an overhead position. Apply gentle traction in line with the humerus and use your thumb to apply direct pressure over the humeral head in the axilla to achieve reduction.

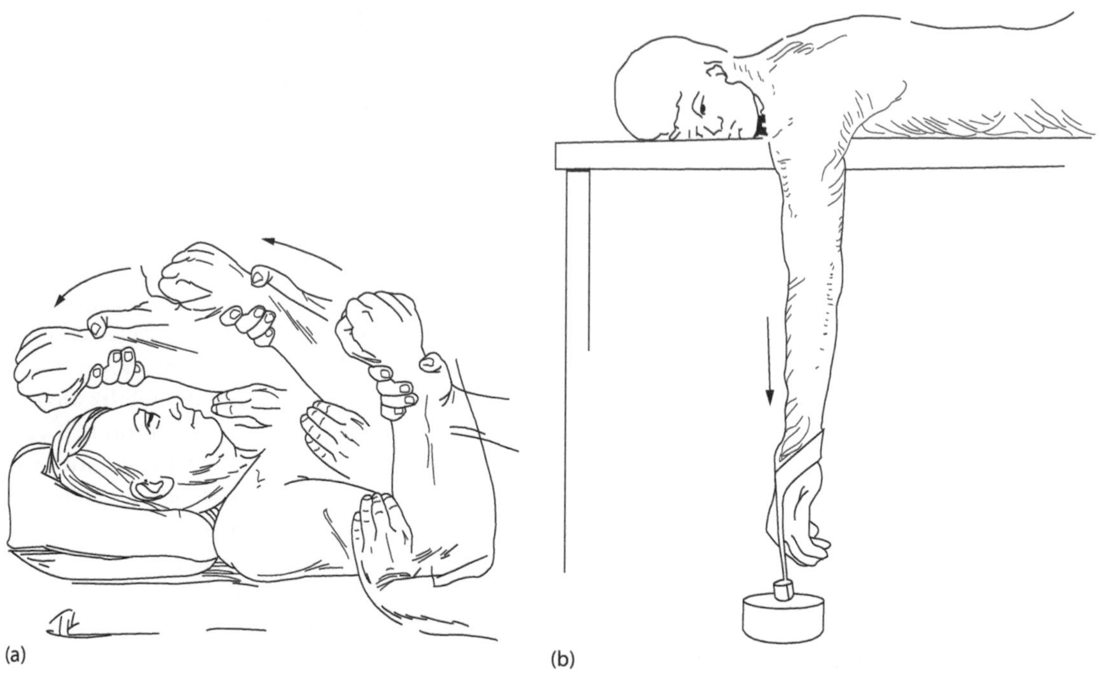

FIGURE 43.16 Shoulder reduction techniques. (a) External rotation technique combined with the Milch technique and (b) Stimson technique.

Scapular manipulation: Have the patient rest their unaffected shoulder against the upright portion of the bed. Locate the scapula and push the tip medially and the acromion inferiorly using the thumbs, thereby rotating the scapula. At the same time, an assistant provides gentle forward or downward traction on the arm.

Traction countertraction: One person provides continuous traction at the wrist/elbow (may use sheet wrapped around arm to help), while another person wraps a sheet under the patient's axilla to provide countertraction from the opposite side of the patient by pulling the sheet.

Stimson technique: Place the patient prone and hang the affected arm off the edge of the bed. Hang 10–15 pounds of weight from the wrist, and reduction is usually achieved within 30 minutes.

Spaso technique: Place the patient supine and provide gentle vertical traction and external rotation. Shoulder will reduce usually within 1–2 minutes.

Self-reduction technique: The patients clasp their hands together around the flexed ipsilateral knee from a seated position and slowly leans backward while also simultaneously extending the hip by sliding the foot forward.

Posterior reduction: With the patient supine, apply traction to the adducted, internally rotated, flexed arm in the line of deformity, along with a gentle lifting and internal rotation of the humeral head back into the glenoid fossa; open reduction is indicated following 1–2 unsuccessful trials.

After a dislocation event, immobilization for 2–4 weeks, depending on age and activity level, is recommended. The shoulder spica in the neutral position is preferred by some for posterior dislocations. ROM and isometric strengthening should be started early, followed by a resistive strengthening program. An exercise program should emphasize both internal and external rotators as well as large scapular muscles. Surgery is indicated for persistent instability.[10,37,66] The incidence of fractures associated with a dislocation event rises with age and include compression fracture of the humeral head (Hill–Sachs lesion), fracture of the glenoid lip (bony Bankart lesion), fracture of the greater or lesser tuberosity, and fracture of the acromion or coracoid, along with other complications including a rotator cuff tear or nerve injury (axillary [most common], brachial plexus, musculocutaneous) or vascular damage. Strengthening exercises of internal rotator muscles will improve anterior instability. There is a lack of evidence to support the use of shoulder harnesses to reduce further incidences of anterior shoulder dislocations but may serve a benefit due to proprioception and can be used if desired.

43.7.4 Clavicular Fractures

Clavicular fractures represent approximately 2.6% of all fractures and 44% of those in the shoulder. Most clavicular fractures occur in the middle third of the clavicle with the least common location being the proximal third.[54] The majority of these injuries occur in children or in collision/contact sports. Most clavicular fractures are caused by a fall onto the shoulder with less common mechanisms including a direct blow from an object or indirect trauma from a fall onto an outstretched hand. There has been no correlation found between the mechanism and location of clavicle fracture.[62] Clavicle fractures can be classified based on the location of the fracture. Group I comprises fractures of the middle third of the clavicle (most commonly fractured); Group II comprises fractures to the distal third; and Group III comprises fractures to the proximal third. Fractures of the distal third of the clavicle are subdivided again into three categories: nondisplaced fractures of the distal clavicle (Type I), displaced fractures (Type II), and articular fractures (Type III). When the fracture is displaced, the shoulder slumps downward and inward and the patient holds the arm against the chest to protect against shoulder movements. Pain may radiate to the trapezius. Direct and indirect tenderness, ecchymosis, and often a visible palpable deformity and crepitus at the fracture site are noted. Evaluation for evidence of skin tenting is important. Deformity may be absent in preadolescent greenstick fractures. Crepitus outside the fracture site suggests subcutaneous emphysema. Distal clavicular fractures may be initially confused with AC separations; the location of pain is similar and pain is worsened with cross arm testing; however, distal clavicle fractures will have maximal tenderness medial to the AC joint rather than directly over the AC joint as seen with a separation. For proximal clavicular fractures, pain, tenderness, and swelling at the area of the sternoclavicular joint are noted, as well as pain on hyperabduction of the shoulder. A neurovascular and pulmonary examination should be performed in the setting of a clavicle fracture to evaluate for other associated complications. Most clavicle fractures can be visualized with a single AP view; however, a 45° cephalic tilt view can be obtained for further evaluation. Stress views can be obtained to further evaluate distal clavicle fractures. Ultrasound may be a useful modality to evaluate clavicle fractures accurately at bedside.[20] The differential diagnosis may include an AC separation, sternoclavicular separation, or contusion. Emergent referral is necessary for any open fractures, tenting of the skin as there is a high risk for skin breakdown leading to an open fracture, neurovascular compromise, or suspected pulmonary injury. In general, conservative management involves pain control and limiting motion at the fracture site with a simple sling, which is preferable to a figure-eight immobilizer. ROM of the glenohumeral joint and elbow is encouraged to avoid stiffness and adhesive capsulitis. Follow-up care should include a 1- to 2-week postinjury evaluation with repeat of radiographic imaging if concern for further displacement or shortening. Otherwise, evaluation every 2–3 weeks is appropriate to determine clinical signs of union, which are no tenderness over the fracture site and full ROM with minimal to no pain. At this time, plain radiographs can be obtained to assess for evidence of bony healing in the form of callus formation although its absence should not prohibit beginning physical therapy for strengthening if there is clinical union.

Clinical Pearl

Conservative management of clavicle fractures involves pain control and limiting motion at the fracture site with a simple sling, which is preferable to a figure-eight immobilizer. Evaluations every couple of weeks are appropriate to determine clinical signs of union.

Nonemergent referral should be made for middle-third clavicle fractures if there is significant fracture displacement (greater than 1 bone width), comminution, or shortening. A significant risk of morbidity has been found with shortening greater than 18 mm in males and 14 mm in females.[39] Nondisplaced fractures of the middle third of the clavicle usually heal well with conservative management and rarely require surgery. As with all sports injuries and specifically with displaced middle-third clavicle fractures, it is important for the clinician to have a discussion with the patient and consider the fracture characteristics, patient's occupational and recreational needs, and patient's own preference as this will help guide surgical versus conservative management as there are risks and benefits to both. Orthopedic consultation may be useful in this setting. A case for conservative versus surgical management for distal clavicle fractures can be made in most instances except for Type I fractures confirmed with normal stress views, which can be managed conservatively. Treatment should be individualized and a discussion with the patient is necessary to guide the decision-making process. Fractures of the proximal clavicle are associated with more significant neurovascular and intrathoracic injuries in which thorough evaluation is necessary and possibly even emergent evaluation. Surgical intervention may be required if there is evidence of posterior displacement of the fracture fragment or posterior sternoclavicular dislocation. Conservative management is appropriate for nondisplaced fractures of the proximal clavicle. Complications associated with clavicle fractures include neurovascular injury, pneumothorax/hemothorax, and AC joint arthrosis.

43.7.5 Other Fractures

Fracture of the proximal humerus, acromion, glenoid fossa, coracoid, and scapular neck, spine, or body usually results from any violent force to the shoulder and should always be considered part of the differential diagnosis of acute painful shoulder injury. The trauma may follow a direct blow (e.g., fall on the upper arm) or indirect forces (e.g., fall on outstretched hand with an extended elbow or sudden contraction of arm flexors or rotators, such as occurs in throwing or wrestling). Fractures may be associated or confused with glenohumeral instability, AC separation, or a simple contusion. A limited ROM is usually noted, as well as significant disability, swelling and paresthesias around the shoulder, and, in the cases of coracoid and acromion fractures, point tenderness over these structures. Routine shoulder films will usually confirm the diagnosis; however, other views may be needed to further evaluate bony structures. Be aware of an unfused acromial epiphysis masquerading as a fracture in a prepubertal patient.

Treatment of stable coracoid, acromion, glenoid fossa, and scapular fractures is conservative. Open reduction is reserved for unstable fractures. Minimally displaced fractures of the proximal humerus (80% of cases) usually respond well to 3–4 weeks of a shoulder immobilizer or sling. Two-part fractures (10% of cases) are usually amenable to closed reduction and an immobilizer. Greater tuberosity fractures

(>1 cm displacement) and some shaft displacements require open reduction and internal fixation, as do three-part (30% of cases) and four-part (40% of cases) fractures, as well as articular surface fractures of more than 20%.

Humeral stress fracture has been reported in over-30 amateur baseball players. Treatment consists of a shoulder immobilizer or sling for 2–4 weeks.

Severe trauma (e.g., stock car racing, equestrian events, and pileup in rugby or football) is usually required to fracture the body of the scapula. Associated injuries include fractures of the vertebrae, sternum, and ribs, pneumothorax, brachial plexus injuries, and subcutaneous emphysema. Localized swelling and pain of the scapula and avoidance of all arm motion are noted. Conservative therapy including RICE, NSAIDs, analgesics, and a shoulder immobilizer usually suffices unless a displaced fracture is evident. CT or MRI is often necessary for evaluation. Early progressive rehabilitation emphasizing shoulder motion is essential for shoulder fractures.

43.8 PEDIATRIC INJURIES

43.8.1 Little League Shoulder

Ten percent of shoulder pain in the pediatric population can be attributed to overhead throwing activities, and 26% of these throwing injuries are related to overuse such as the case with little league shoulder, also known as a Salter–Harris Type I physeal injury of the proximal humeral growth plate.[47] It most commonly occurs in male baseball pitchers between the ages of 11 and 16 years; however, it can occur in other sports that involve overhead activity.[47] Overhead throwing can be divided into phases including the windup, stride, cocking, acceleration, deceleration, and follow-through.[8] The most mechanical stressful aspects of the throwing cycle on the shoulder are during the cocking phase and the deceleration phase. The cocking phase places an enormous amount of rotational torque on the physis of the proximal humerus, while the deceleration phase places a distraction force. Quantification of the relative stress across the shoulder estimates that the force across the physis from a rotational force during the cocking phase is equal to 400% of the force that the physeal cartilage can normally tolerate.[47] Therefore, the development of little league shoulder is believed to be mostly due to the rotational torque generated during throwing. Little league shoulder is an injury to the physis, or growth plate, or the proximal humerus. It is thought to be a stress fracture or Salter–Harris Type I injury in which the forces from throwing cause microfractures across the hypertrophic zone of the physis. This area is more susceptible to injury due to the vertically oriented collagen fibers found in this zone.[47]

Patients will typically present with a complaint of progressive shoulder pain localized to the proximal humerus during the act of throwing, and many will also report a recent increase in the amount of throwing prior to the onset of symptoms.[47] A large case series reported that physical examination revealed tenderness to palpation over the proximal humerus in 87% of the patients and 70% specifically had tenderness localized to the lateral aspect of the proximal humerus.[16] There may be swelling, weakness, atrophy, and loss of motion in the involved shoulder; however, these are not typical findings.[16] Plain radiographs of the shoulder including AP, scapular Y, and axillary views may reveal a widened proximal humeral physis and may be helpful to rule out other sources of shoulder pain. An AP view of the shoulder with the arm in external rotation is the best view to visualize widening of the proximal humeral physis.[47] It may be necessary to obtain plain radiographs of the contralateral shoulder for comparison as the widening may be subtle. Since little league shoulder can manifest within many stages of disease, radiographs should also be reviewed for other findings indicating severity, which include physeal irregularity, metaphyseal demineralization and fragmentation, and periosteal reaction.[47] If plain radiographs are negative and clinical suspicion is still high, MRI may be necessary to further evaluate for physeal injury.[47] It is important to note that radiographic findings should always be correlated with symptoms and clinical examination as changes in the proximal humerus growth plate have been noted in asymptomatic youth baseball pitchers.[47] The differential diagnosis may include glenohumeral instability or even neoplastic disease with pain that is progressing or not improving as expected with rest. Treatment of little league shoulder is predominantly nonoperative as the majority of cases will resolve with initial rest and activity modification for 3 months.[47] The initial rest period is followed by a progressive throwing program once the patient is no longer symptomatic. The throwing program consists of beginning with light tossing and then gradually increasing distance and velocity. If symptoms recur during this process, it is important to again implement a period of rest until asymptomatic before progressing.[47] During the treatment period, improper throwing mechanics and any ROM or strength deficits should also be addressed to aid recovery and prevent recurrence.

Prevention of little league shoulder involves assessing the athlete's throwing biomechanics and implementing guidelines to limit the frequency and volume of pitching as well as types of pitches thrown. Improper throwing mechanics can increase the amount of stress put on the throwing shoulder and thus can increase the risk for injury to the physis, which is why early recognition and correction of improper throwing mechanics is important. Additionally, the USA Baseball Medical and Safety Advisory Committee has established guidelines for youth baseball pitchers to prevent overuse injuries by limiting pitch counts, pitch types, and frequency of pitching.[47] Education reinforcing these guidelines is critical especially for players who are in multiple leagues or playing year-round baseball.[47]

43.9 MISCELLANEOUS SHOULDER INJURIES

43.9.1 Calcific Tendinitis

A different entity from impingement, calcific tendinitis occurs in up to 8% of the population over the age of 30 years with shoulder pain. Of asymptomatic patients, 30% demonstrate rotator cuff calcification, of which 35%–45% will eventually become symptomatic, possibly suddenly without any obvious trauma or overuse.

Clinical Pearl

The onset of severe shoulder pain with no evidence of infection should raise suspicion for calcific tendinitis in which calcium deposits can be visualized on plain radiographs.

The exact mechanism of calcific tendinitis is not well understood; however, it is believed to be multifactorial. A history of repetitive microtrauma, possibly in combination with hypoxic changes in the tendon, can lead to calcium deposition. The two types of deposits are amorphous deposits, which are characteristic of resorptive phase of healing but associated with exquisite pain, and well-circumscribed, sand-like deposits consistent with the asymptomatic, chronic phase. The calcification (calcium apatite) in the rotator cuff, particularly the supraspinatus, is typically seen 1–2 cm from the tendon insertion in the greater tuberosity. The presentation may consist of the patient holding their arm across the chest in the protected position. A key part of the history is that the onset of severe shoulder pain is sudden with symptoms present with activity and at rest. Patients experience difficulty in sleeping and any shoulder motion is extremely painful. Point tenderness over the area may be noted. Routine shoulder views reveal deposits, commonly seen in the area of the supraspinatus tendon at the point of insertion into the greater tuberosity, which are best visualized with the humerus externally rotated. The lateral scapula view is good for determining the precise location. No correlation exists between the size of the deposit and symptoms. MRI demonstrates soft-tissue calcification. Ultrasound demonstrates soft-tissue calcification and allows for simultaneous therapeutic intervention (e.g., injection, lavage). The differential diagnosis may include adhesive capsulitis, external impingement of the shoulder, rotator cuff tear, biceps tendinitis, or glenohumeral arthritis. Initial treatment consists of RICE, NSAIDs, and analgesics as needed. However, initial injection therapy can be helpful including injection of corticosteroids or in some cases using ultrasound guidance to break up deposit and aspirate. Shock wave therapy has been utilized with some reports of success. If conservative measures fail, surgical removal of calcium deposit can be utilized. Preventive measures can include modification of training program to improve biomechanics.

43.9.2 Adhesive Capsulitis (Frozen Shoulder)

CLINICAL PEARL

Inability to tolerate initial physical therapy for adhesive capsulitis is common. These patients should be treated with a corticosteroid injection into the glenohumeral joint followed by aggressive physical therapy.

Adhesive capsulitis (frozen shoulder) is a poorly defined syndrome in which both active and passive shoulder motion is lost because of soft-tissue contracture. An insidious onset of symptoms commonly occurs among individuals aged 40–60 years. Females are affected more than males. It is believed to be a benign self-limited disorder that tends to resolve over 1–2 years, although some patients are often left with some residual loss of motion. The etiology is unknown, but it is more common in patients with diabetes mellitus, for which it is frequently bilateral and resistant to treatment. The pathologic process is characterized by ROM limited initially by pain secondary to inflammation (capsulitis) and then mechanically from adhesions. Three stages have been defined. Stage 1 has pain with motion but no mechanical limitation in range. Stage 2 has pain with some functional limitations in ROM. Stage 3 is less painful, but the ROM is extremely limited mechanically by adhesions. It may be secondary to other pathologies such as impingement, fractures, cervical radiculopathy, coronary artery disease, reflex sympathetic dystrophy, and dislocations. It has been suggested that adhesive capsulitis is a predominantly fibrosing condition that follows subsequently after an inflammatory state because inflammatory cells are absent or scanty on histologic studies.[13]

Although clear pathophysiology is not fully understood, it is believed to be an initial synovial inflammatory stage followed by fibrosing of the shoulder capsule. Adhesive fibrosis and scarring occurs between the capsule, rotator cuff, subacromial bursa, and deltoid with the inferior glenohumeral ligament most commonly affected. The presenting signs and symptoms include onset of poorly localized pain that is insidious, frequently extending down the arm with nocturnal pain being common especially as it progresses. Shoulder stiffness and decreased active and, more notably, passive motion occur, particularly in external rotation and abduction. Palpable mechanical block to motion is with or without a tender end point. X-rays are usually negative. MRI may not reveal much evidence of the adhesions if resolution is poor and synovium thickness is less than 4 mm; however, improvements in image sequencing can demonstrate increased signal and capsular thickening specifically in the axillary pouch on coronal views.[22] The differential diagnosis may include a rotator cuff tear, calcific tendinitis, cervical radiculopathy, any fracture or dislocation of the shoulder, arthritis, and TOS. Initial treatment consists of NSAIDs with aggressive physical therapy to improve ROM. Many patients are unable to tolerate the physical therapy, which is the mainstay of treatment in which they can significantly benefit from an initial corticosteroid injection into the glenohumeral joint followed by aggressive physical therapy. It should be noted that physical therapy must be done carefully as to not increase symptoms by being too aggressive, which could cause a setback in recovery. If initial therapy fails, a second corticosteroid injection into the glenohumeral joint can be utilized. Otherwise, manipulation under anesthesia can help to restore ROM as well as a capsular release as a surgical option.[5,36] Complications can include prolonged disability although most cases are likely to resolve within 2 years regardless of treatment. Preventive measures include encouraging initiation of early physical therapy and ROM exercises after shoulder injuries and minimizing prolonged immobilization.

43.9.3 Thoracic Outlet Syndrome

Clinical Pearl

There are three recognized forms of thoracic outlet syndrome (TOS), which include arterial, venous, and neurogenic. Neurogenic TOS is the cause of more than 95% cases of TOS.

TOS is a condition that may be seen in racquet, throwing, and aquatic sports, and in such occupations as paper hanging, painting, and carpentry.[34,41] It occurs at a ratio of 6 females to 1 male, with an average age of occurrence of 36 years. Thirty percent of patients have a history of repetitive activity involving holding the arm over the head. There are three recognized forms of TOS, which include arterial, venous, and neurogenic. Neurogenic TOS is the cause of more than 95% cases of TOS. Symptoms are caused by compression of the subclavian artery, vein (effort thrombosis), or lower ramus of the brachial plexus in the interscalene, costoclavicular, or subcoracoid region from trauma, repetitive overhand/overhead movements, or poor posture.[57] Anatomical variations or conditions that may predispose someone to getting TOS include the presence of cervical or anomalous first rib, clavicular callus or malunion, shoulder droop, large transverse process (C7), and tumor. Presentation generally consists of vague, nonspecific ipsilateral upper extremity and neck pain, swelling, and paresthesias (C8 dermatome) that are noted with particular positions and activities with referred pain to ipsilateral breast or chest also sometimes being noted. Paresis, pallor, and cold in arm and hand with subclavian artery compression are observed, as are weakness of hypothenar and interossei muscles, hypalgesia, and hypesthesia in the region of the ulnar nerve (C8, T1). They may have difficulty when asked to spread the fingers apart against resistance or grip a test card between extended fingers. A positive Adson test is indicated by marked decrease of the radial pulse with abduction, extension, external rotation of the ipsilateral arm in association with a deep breath, and head turning to the same side. However, this maneuver must be interpreted with caution as it can be falsely positive in the normal patient. A positive Allen test is the same as the Adson test but with head turned toward the opposite side. The elevated arm test (Roos maneuver) is positive when pronounced arm weakness and pain are noted within 2 minutes when the arms are elevated to 90° in abduction, externally rotated with the shoulders and elbows braced back (i.e., military posture), and hands are opened and closed with moderate speed during a 3 minute period. The axial compression test, or Spurling's maneuver, should be negative. Rarely, a palpable mass or bruit is found in the supraclavicular area. AP, lateral, and oblique plain radiographs of cervical and upper thoracic spine and chest may demonstrate pathology or evidence of cervical ribs. Electrodiagnostic studies including nerve conduction velocity (NCV) and EMG may be helpful to support the diagnosis of TOS if symptoms are prolonged (>3 weeks at minimum) or if muscle atrophy is appreciated, but negative studies do not exclude the diagnosis given their lower sensitivities. Scalene muscle block can be used and may help predict response to surgical intervention. Cervical MRI can be used to exclude other diagnosis, and magnetic resonance neurography is a technique that injects dye around the plexus to evaluate anatomical course. Arteriography is only useful to evaluate for arterial TOS and venography is only useful to evaluate for suspected venous TOS.[57] The differential diagnosis may include cervical spine disease, shoulder pathology and tendon tears, pectoralis minor syndrome, and other peripheral nerve entrapments such as carpal and cubital tunnel syndromes. If arterial or venous TOS is present, surgical intervention should be implemented as initial treatment. For neurogenic TOS, the patient should avoid positions or activities that precipitate the symptoms and should begin physical therapy (ROM + PREs) to address poor posture. Conservative management should also include ergonomic correction of work sites, relaxation exercises, and stretching exercises for neck and shoulder. Advise patients to avoid sleeping with arms in an elevated position or folded under the pillow. At least a few months of conservative therapy should be pursued prior to considering surgical intervention. Surgical intervention for neurogenic TOS is intended to decompress the brachial plexus by either excising a cervical rib or scalene muscles.[6,57] Preventive measures include avoiding excessive overhead activity, maintain proper posture, and strengthening/flexibility exercises for shoulder girdle and neck muscles.

43.9.4 Vascular Injuries

Repetitive overhand activity (e.g., pitching) and violent abduction of the shoulder during repeated falls (e.g., wind surfing) have been reported to cause axillary artery occlusion. Symptoms include arm pain, numbness, and severe fatigability. Absent brachial, radial, and ulnar pulses, coolness of the extremity, and a positive arteriogram are diagnostic. Treatment is thrombectomy.

Compression of the posterior circumflex humeral artery and the axillary nerve within the area defined by the teres minor superiorly, glenohumeral joint capsule and humerus laterally, long head of the triceps medially, and fascia and adipose tissue inferiorly has produced the quadrilateral-space syndrome in throwers.[61] Overhead activity produces arm paresis, paresthesias, and shoulder pain and point tenderness at the space. Surgical decompression or modification of the overhead activity is recommended.

Primary or "effort" thrombosis of the axillary and subclavian veins is the most common vascular athletic problem and accounts for 2% of total venous thromboses. Vigorous repetitive activity (e.g., weightlifting, rowing, golf, swimming, volleyball, football, and baseball) generally precedes such symptoms as arm swelling, pain, paresthesias, and fatigability. This is known as Paget–Schroetter disease. It can also develop secondary to venous TOS when compression of the vein leads to clot formation. Examination reveals nonpitting edema, mottled skin, coolness, prominent superficial veins, and normal arterial and neurologic findings. A palpable axillary cord may be present. Venography confirms the diagnosis. Treatment options include rest, arm elevation, anticoagulation, thrombolytic therapy, and surgical thrombectomy.

43.9.5 Neural Injuries

Blunt trauma (e.g., a blow from a hockey stick) or a stretch injury (falling on the point of the shoulder) can damage the spinal accessory nerve (cranial nerve XI), a pure motor nerve.[43] Persistent aching of the shoulder girdle, loss of shoulder shrugging, rotary winging of the scapula, and trapezius atrophy follow paralysis. Conservative therapy includes NSAIDs, a sling, and physical therapy, but if recovery is not apparent after 6 weeks, exploration and neurolysis should follow.

Damage to the musculocutaneous nerve about the shoulder is rare but has been reported in competitive rowing, weightlifting, and model-airplane flying. Findings are weakness and wasting of the biceps and brachialis muscles and sensory impairment of the radial aspect of the forearm. The differential diagnosis includes a C5–C6 radiculopathy, brachial plexus injury, or rupture of the bicipital tendon at the elbow. EMG can help differentiate these entities. Conservative therapy, particularly cessation of the inciting activity, yields a favorable prognosis.

Injuries to the long thoracic nerve, causing paralysis of the serratus anterior muscle, have been reported in rope skipping, shooting, throwing and racquet sports, golf, gymnastics, wrestling, and weightlifting. Complaints include aching or burning around the shoulder that may radiate down the arm or over the scapula and weakness of shoulder flexion and abduction. Weakness of shoulder shrug and winging of the scapula are common findings. An EMG is confirmatory and helps distinguish the condition from other scapular and glenohumeral pathologies. The prognosis is good for cases due to excessive or repetitive microtrauma, although cessation of activity, braces, and physical therapy may be required for 1–2 years. Prognosis is less favorable for lesions resulting from acute closed trauma. The axillary nerve is acutely injured in at least 18% of anterior shoulder dislocations or following blunt trauma to the same area in such sports as football or wrestling. Chronic entrapment from repetitive microtrauma with overhead activities (e.g., racquet sports and gymnastics) occurs in association with the quadrilateral-space/tunnel syndrome. The tunnel is formed superiorly by the teres minor muscle; anteriorly by the glenohumeral ligament and subscapularis fascia; inferiorly by the teres major, venous plexus, and adipose tissue; laterally by the humerus and coracobrachialis and triceps tendons; and medially by the long head of the triceps and the inferior glenoid rim. Abduction, internal rotation, and dorsal projection stress the nerve by traction. Vague pain, paresthesias, and weakness (e.g., inability to screw in an overhead light bulb) can progress to pain and paresthesias radiating to the elbow and dorsal ulnar aspect of the hand, especially with abduction and external rotation (e.g., throwing or tennis serve), tenderness in the region of the posterior outlet of the tunnel (inferomedial humeral head between teres major and minor and long head of triceps), and eventual atrophy of the deltoid and teres minor.

Chronic microtrauma to the upper trunk of the brachial plexus may produce a severe and prolonged disability, particularly to the nondominant side in hikers, climbers, and campers who carry heavy backpacks (backpacker's palsy). Motor and sensory deficits occur in the distribution of musculocutaneous and radial nerves. Shoulder strengthening exercises without the backpack are important initially. Reduced weight loads are indicated when trekking resumes. The differential diagnosis should include injuries to the posterior cord of the brachial plexus and the thoracodorsal nerve. An EMG is helpful with chronic symptoms. Rest, avoidance of aggravating maneuvers, NSAIDs, and injection therapy suffice in 60%–80% of cases. Surgical decompression is indicated for refractory cases.

Suprascapular nerve injury is relatively common in athletes with a history of shoulder trauma causing traction on the nerve in the scapular notch (e.g., fall or dislocation). Poorly localized pain made worse while lying on the affected side (posterior subacromial position of the glenohumeral joint with radiation to the elbow), intact sensation, and insidious weakness of external rotation and abduction are typical. Atrophy of the supraspinatus and infraspinatus with normal deltoid function usually occurs. EMG and NCV confirm polyphasic motor activity, diminished amplitude, and increased conduction time between Erb's point and muscle. The differential diagnosis should include rotator cuff pathology and backpacker's palsy. Rest, analgesics, and injection therapy usually provide a favorable prognosis. Surgical exploration and decompression are indicated for refractory cases (20%), with 60%–70% showing improvement. Sometimes, this can also be caused by compression of the nerve by a labral ganglion cyst visualized with MRI, which can be treated by decompression via removal of the ganglion cyst to alleviate symptoms.

43.9.6 Others

Contusions commonly occur to the bones and muscles of the shoulder in collision/contact sports. A shoulder pointer represents a painful periosteal reaction following a contusive blow of the lateral clavicle or acromion. Myositis ossificans can occur 2–6 weeks after injury. The differential diagnosis includes cuff strain, AC separation, clavicular fracture, or subluxation/dislocation. Cumulative stress on the AC joint due to strength training, repeated contusions, increased training intensity, and the earlier entry of the athlete into certain sports (e.g., weightlifting, football, and swimming) can produce atraumatic osteolysis of the distal clavicle. The condition begins with insidious aching in the region of the AC joint several hours after exercise but progresses to earlier pain as the condition worsens. Eventually, performance is impaired. Dips, push-ups, and bench pressing especially aggravate the situation. The AC joint is tender and mildly prominent. Twenty percent of cases are bilateral. The differential diagnosis includes other AC and glenohumeral pathology. Conservative therapy (NSAIDs, analgesics, physical therapy) produces a favorable prognosis provided that relative rest utilizing a modified exercise prescription (e.g., cross-training) is mandated. Surgical resection of the distal clavicle is reserved for chronic cases—the end result of continued microtrauma. A snapping scapula is due to the forceful sliding of a prominent superomedial scapular border over the underlying ribs and muscles. Surgical resection may be indicated following a period of conservative therapy.

43.10 SUMMARY

Sacrificing structural integrity for functional capacity, the peculiar anatomy and complex motion of the shoulder make it susceptible to acute injury (in collision and contact sports) and, more commonly, to chronic overuse injuries (from throwing, swimming, and racquet sports, for example). The capable sports physician must be familiar with the diagnosis and management of acute shoulder trauma such as dislocation and AC sprains. Overuse problems such as the impingement of the shoulder and rotator cuff inflammation are particularly challenging, as a failure to adequately understand the mechanism of injury and natural history can result in a poor long-term outcome. Early recognition of injury patterns, aggressive nonoperative intervention, and an appreciation of therapeutic options are essential to successful resolution and return of the athlete to accustomed levels of performance (see Tables 43.2 and 43.3).

TABLE 43.2
Indications for Specialty Referral for Common Disorders of the Shoulder

Diagnosis	Primary Care Referral Considerations
Overuse	
External impingement of the shoulder	Consider referral for possible advanced injection therapies or for possible surgical decompression if symptoms not improving with conservative management.
Internal impingement of the shoulder	Consider referral for possible advanced injection therapies or for surgical consultation if symptoms not improving with conservative management.
Rotator cuff strain	Consider referral for possible advanced injection therapies or for surgical consultation if symptoms not improving with conservative management. If progression to full thickness tear, refer for surgical consultation.
Biceps tendon problems	Consider referral for possible advanced injection therapies or for surgical consultation if symptoms not improving with conservative management. Acute ruptures should be referred immediately for surgical consultation.
Glenoid labrum tears	Consider referral for possible advanced injection therapies or for surgical consultation if symptoms not improving with conservative management. Refer for surgical consultation if evidence of shoulder instability.
Scapulothoracic bursitis	Consider referral for possible advanced injection therapies. Surgical consultation should only be sought after failure to improve with extensive course of physical therapy and addressing posture.
Traumatic	
Sternoclavicular sprain/subluxation/dislocation	Referral should be if reduction necessary. All Grade III injuries should be referred for further evaluation. Referral should be made if suspicion for any injury to vasculature, trachea, esophagus, or mediastinal structures.
Acromioclavicular sprain/subluxation/dislocation	Referral should be made for Grade III injuries not responding to conservative management and for all Grades IV, V, and VI injuries.
Glenohumeral instability: sprain/subluxation/dislocation	Consider immediate referral to obtain imaging and successful reduction for acute dislocations. Consider referral if continued apprehension/instability with conservative management following instability episode. There should be a lower threshold to refer younger, active individuals for surgical consultation due to increased likelihood of recurrent instability without surgical intervention.
Clavicular fractures	Emergent referral is necessary for any open fractures, tenting of the skin as there is a high risk for skin breakdown leading to an open fracture, neurovascular compromise, or suspected pulmonary injury. Nonemergent referral should be made for middle-third clavicle fractures if there is significant fracture displacement, comminution, or shortening. More significant proximal and distal-third fractures should be referred for surgical consultation.
Other fractures	Referral should be made for unstable fractures, if there is significant displacement, or if lack of familiarity with criteria for managing conservatively.
Pediatric	
Little league shoulder	The large majority of cases will respond to relative rest and correction of improper biomechanics. Consider referral if not responding to conservative treatments.
Miscellaneous	
Calcific tendinitis	Consider referral for possible advanced injection therapies including aspiration/lavage. Consider referral for surgical consultation if not improving with conservative management.
Adhesive capsulitis (frozen shoulder)	Consider referral for possible advanced injection therapies. Consider referral for surgical consultation if not improving with conservative management.
Thoracic outlet syndrome	If arterial or venous TOS is present, referral should be made for surgical intervention. For neurogenic TOS, consider referral if not responding to adequate trial of conservative management or if identification of anatomical variant or abnormality causing the condition.
Vascular injuries	In general, referral should be made if there is identification of a vascular injury.
Neural injuries	Neural injuries that do not involve transection of the nerve usually can be treated with conservative management. Consider referral if concern for significant neural injury or if not responding to a trial of conservative management.

TABLE 43.3
SORT: Key Recommendations for Practice

Clinical Recommendations for Practice	Evidence Rating
All shoulder examinations should include a neurovascular assessment and a cervical spine evaluation to exclude cervical radiculopathy as the source of shoulder pain.	C
Plain radiographs (x-rays) are a useful initial screening of shoulder pathology. At least three views of the shoulder should be obtained. Magnetic resonance imaging is useful in evaluating the soft tissues or identifying occult fractures.	C
Physical therapy for external impingement of the shoulder should specifically focus on strengthening of the rotator cuff and scapular stabilizers.	C
There is no clear evidence to support one method over another regarding reduction of an anterior shoulder dislocation. With all techniques, it is crucial for the patient to relax their shoulder muscles as much as possible for reduction to be successful.	C
Inability to tolerate initial physical therapy for adhesive capsulitis is common. These patients should be treated with a corticosteroid injection into the glenohumeral joint followed by aggressive physical therapy.	C

REFERENCES

1. Ahlgren O, Lorentzon R, Larsson S. Posterior dislocation of the shoulder associated with general seizures. *Acta Orthopaedica Scandinavica*. 1981:694–695.
2. Altchek DW, Hatch JD. Rotator cuff injuries in overhead athletes. *Operative Techniques in Orthopaedics*. 2001:11(1):2–8.
3. Altchek DW, Warren RF, Wickiewicz TL et al. Arthroscopic labral debridement. A three-year follow-up study. *The American Journal of Sports Medicine*. 1992;6:702–706.
4. Aronen JG. Anterior shoulder dislocations in sports. *Sports Medicine*. 1986;3:224–234.
5. Arslan S, Celiker R. Comparison of the efficacy of local corticosteroid injection and physical therapy for the treatment of adhesive capsulitis. *Rheumatology International*. 2001;1:20–23.
6. Baker CL, Jr, Liu SH. Neurovascular injuries to the shoulder *Journal of Orthopaedic & Sports Physical Therapy*. 1993;1:360–364.
7. Bathis H, Tingart M, Bouillon B et al. Conservative or surgical therapy of acromioclavicular joint injury—What is reliable? A systematic analysis of the literature using "evidence-based medicine" criteria. *Chirurg*. 2000;9:1082–1089.
8. Bishop JY, Flatow EL. Pediatric shoulder trauma. *Clinical Orthopaedics and Related Research*. 2005;432:41–48.
9. Blasier RB, Guldberg RE, Rothman ED. Anterior shoulder stability: Contributions of rotator cuff forces and the capsular ligaments in a cadaver model. *Journal of Shoulder and Elbow Surgery*. 1992;3:140–150.
10. Bottoni CR, Wilckens JH, DeBerardino TM et al. A prospective, randomized evaluation of arthroscopic stabilization versus nonoperative treatment in patients with acute, traumatic, first-time shoulder dislocations. *The American Journal of Sports Medicine*. 2002;4:576–580.
11. Brown JT. nerve injuries complicating dislocation of the shoulder. *The Bone & Joint Journal (British Volume)*. 1952:34:526.
12. Brox JI, Gjengedal E, Uppheim G et al. Arthroscopic surgery versus supervised exercises in patients with rotator cuff disease (stage II impingement syndrome): A prospective, randomized, controlled study in 125 patients with a 2 1/2-year follow-up. *Journal of Shoulder and Elbow Surgery*. 1999;2:102–111.
13. Bunker TD, Reilly J, Baird KS et al. Expression of growth factors, cytokines and matrix metalloproteinases in frozen shoulder. *Journal of Bone and Joint Surgery*. 2000;5:768–773.
14. Burk DL, Jr, Karasick D, Mitchell DG et al. MR imaging of the shoulder: Correlation with plain radiography. *AJR American Journal of Roentgenology*. 1990;3:549–553.
15. Burkhart SS, Morgan CD, Kibler WB. The disabled throwing shoulder: Spectrum of pathology part I: Pathoanatomy and biomechanics. *Arthroscopy*. 2003;4:404–420.
16. Carson WG, Jr, Gasser SI. Little leaguer's shoulder. A report of 23 cases. *The American Journal of Sports Medicine*. 1998; 4:575–580.
17. Chalidis B, Sachinis N, Dimitriou C et al. Has the management of shoulder dislocation changed over time? *International Orthopaedics*. 2007;3:385–389.
18. Ciullo JV, Stevens GG. The prevention and treatment of injuries to the shoulder in swimming. *Sports Medicine*. 1989;3:182–204.
19. Cooper DE, Arnoczky SP, O'Brien SJ et al. Anatomy, histology, and vascularity of the glenoid labrum. An anatomical study. *Journal of Bone and Joint Surgery*. 1992;1:46–52.
20. Cross KP, Warkentine FH, Kim IK et al. Bedside ultrasound diagnosis of clavicle fractures in the pediatric emergency department. *Academic Emergency Medicine*. 2010;7:687–693.
21. Curtis AS, Snyder SJ. Evaluation and treatment of biceps tendon pathology. *Orthopedic Clinics of North America*. 1993;1:33–43.
22. Emig EW, Schweitzer ME, Karasick D et al. Adhesive capsulitis of the shoulder: MR diagnosis. *AJR American Journal of Roentgenology*. 1995;6:1457–1459.
23. Farin PU. Sonography of the biceps tendon of the shoulder: Normal and pathologic findings. *Journal of Clinical Ultrasound*. 1996;6:309–316.
24. Gill TJ, McIrvin E, Kocher MS et al. The relative importance of acromial morphology and age with respect to rotator cuff pathology. *Journal of Shoulder and Elbow Surgery*. 2002;4:327–330.
25. Hagberg M, Harms-Ringdahl K, Nisell R et al. Rehabilitation of neck-shoulder pain in women industrial workers: A randomized trial comparing isometric shoulder endurance training with isometric shoulder strength training. *Archives of Physical Medicine and Rehabilitation*. 2000;8:1051–1058.
26. Halpern B, Thompson N, Curl WW et al. High school football injuries: Identifying the risk factors. *The American Journal of Sports Medicine*. 1988:S113–S117.
27. Hawkins RJ, Hobeika PE. Impingement syndrome in the athletic shoulder. *Clinics in Sports Medicine*. 1983;2:391–405.
28. Heyworth BE, Williams RJ, 3rd. Internal impingement of the shoulder. *The American Journal of Sports Medicine*. 2009; 5:1024–1037.
29. Itoi E, Hatakeyama Y, Sato T et al. Immobilization in external rotation after shoulder dislocation reduces the risk of recurrence. A randomized controlled trial. *Journal of Bone and Joint Surgery*. 2007;10:2124–2131.
30. Jobe FW, Bradley JP. Rotator cuff injuries in baseball. Prevention and rehabilitation. *Sports Medicine*. 1988;6:378–387.
31. Jobe CM. Posterior superior glenoid impingement: Expanded spectrum. *Arthroscopy*. 1995;5:530–536.
32. Jobe CM. Superior glenoid impingement. *Orthopedic Clinics of North America*. 1997;2:137–143.

33. Jobe FW, Bradley JP. The diagnosis and nonoperative treatment of shoulder injuries in athletes. *Clinics in Sports Medicine.* 1989;3:419–438.
34. Karas SE. Thoracic outlet syndrome. *Clinics in Sports Medicine.* 1990;2:297–310.
35. Kirchhoff C, Imhoff AB. Posterosuperior and anterosuperior impingement of the shoulder in overhead athletes-evolving concepts. *International Orthopaedics.* 2010;7:1049–1058.
36. Kivimaki J, Pohjolainen T. Manipulation under anesthesia for frozen shoulder with and without steroid injection. *Archives of Physical Medicine and Rehabilitation.* 2001;9:1188–1190.
37. Kuhn JE. Treating the initial anterior shoulder dislocation—An evidence-based medicine approach. *Sports Medicine and Arthroscopy.* 2006;4:192–198.
38. Larsen E, Bjerg-Nielsen A, Christensen P. Conservative or surgical treatment of acromioclavicular dislocation. A prospective, controlled, randomized study. *Journal of Bone and Joint Surgery.* 1986;4:552–555.
39. Lazarides S, Zafiropoulos G. Conservative treatment of fractures at the middle third of the clavicle: The relevance of shortening and clinical outcome. *Journal of Shoulder and Elbow Surgery.* 2006;2:191–194.
40. Linter S, Speer K. Traumatic anterior glenohumeral instability: The role of arthroscopy. *Journal of the American Academy of Orthopaedic Surgeons.* October 1997;5:233–239.
41. Mackinnon SE, Novak CB. Thoracic outlet syndrome. *Current Problems in Surgery.* 2002;11:1070–1145.
42. Meister K, Buckley B, Batts J. The posterior impingement sign: Diagnosis of rotator cuff and posterior labral tears secondary to internal impingement in overhand athletes. *The American Journal of Orthopedics (Belle Mead, NJ).* 2004;8:412–415.
43. Mendoza FX, Main WK. Peripheral nerve injuries of the shoulder in the athlete. *Clinics in Sports Medicine.* 1990;2:331–342.
44. Nirschl RP. Prevention and treatment of elbow and shoulder injuries in the tennis player. *Clinics in Sports Medicine.* 1988;2:289–308.
45. O'Brien S, Newman A, Taylor S et al. The accurate diagnosis of biceps-labral complex lesions with MRI and "3-pack" physical examination: A retrospective analysis with prospective validation. *Orthopaedic Journal of Sports Medicine.* 2013;1(Suppl 4).
46. O'Brien SJ, Pagnani MJ, Fealy S et al. The active compression test: A new and effective test for diagnosing labral tears and acromioclavicular joint abnormality. *The American Journal of Sports Medicine.* 1998;5:610–613.
47. Osbahr DC, Kim HJ, Dugas JR. Little league shoulder. *Current Opinion in Pediatrics.* 2010;1:35–40.
48. Parentis MA, Mohr KJ, ElAttrache NS. Disorders of the superior labrum: Review and treatment guidelines. *Current Opinion in Pediatrics.* 2002;400:77–87.
49. Patel MR, Pardee ML, Singerman RC. Intrathoracic dislocation of the head of the humerus. *Journal of Bone and Joint Surgery.* 1963;1712–1714.
50. Patton WC, McCluskey GM, 3rd. Biceps tendinitis and subluxation. *Clinics in Sports Medicine.* 2001;3:505–529.
51. Petchprapa CN, Beltran LS, Jazrawi LM et al. The rotator interval: A review of anatomy, function, and normal and abnormal MRI appearance. *AJR American Journal of Roentgenology.* 2010;3:567–576.
52. Phillips AM, Smart C, Groom AF. Acromioclavicular dislocation. conservative or surgical therapy. *Clinical Orthopaedics and Related Research.* 1998;353:10–17.
53. Plafki C, Steffen R, Willburger RE et al. Local anaesthetic injection with and without corticosteroids for subacromial impingement syndrome. *International Orthopaedics.* 2000;1:40–42.
54. Postacchini F, Gumina S, De Santis P et al. Epidemiology of clavicle fractures. *Journal of Shoulder and Elbow Surgery.* 2002;5:452–456.
55. Rockwood C, Matsen F. Disorders of the sternoclavicular joint. In: *The Shoulder.* Eds. Philadelphia, PA: Saunders; 1990.
56. Rowe CR, Zarins B. Recurrent transient subluxation of the shoulder. *Journal of Bone and Joint Surgery.* 1981; 6:863–872.
57. Sanders RJ, Hammond SL, Rao NM. Thoracic outlet syndrome: A review. *Neurologist.* 2008;6:365–373.
58. Scheib JS. Diagnosis and rehabilitation of the shoulder impingement syndrome in the overhand and throwing athlete. *Rheumatic Disease Clinics of North America.* 1990;4:971–988.
59. Schenk TJ, Brems JJ. Multidirectional instability of the shoulder: Pathophysiology, diagnosis, and management. *Journal of the American Academy of Orthopaedic Surgeons.* 1998;1:65–72.
60. Shellock FG, Bert JM, Fritts HM et al. Evaluation of the rotator cuff and glenoid labrum using a 0.2-tesla extremity magnetic resonance (MR) system: MR results compared to surgical findings. *Journal of Magnetic Resonance Imaging.* 2001;6:763–770.
61. Sotta RP. Vascular problems in the proximal upper extremity. *Clinics in Sports Medicine.* 1990;2:379–388.
62. Stanley D, Trowbridge EA, Norris SH. The mechanism of clavicular fracture. A clinical and biomechanical analysis. *Journal of Bone and Joint Surgery.* 1988;3:461–464.
63. Taljanovic MS, Carlson KL, Kuhn JE et al. Sonography of the glenoid labrum: A cadaveric study with arthroscopic correlation. *AJR American Journal of Roentgenology.* 2000; 6:1717–1722.
64. Tauber M. Management of acute acromioclavicular joint dislocations: Current concepts. *Archives of Orthopaedic and Trauma Surgery.* 2013;7:985–995.
65. Tuckman GA. Abnormalities of the long head of the biceps tendon of the shoulder: MR imaging findings. *AJR American Journal of Roentgenology.* 1994;5:1183–1188.
66. Ufberg JW, Vilke GM, Chan TC et al. Anterior shoulder dislocations: Beyond traction-countertraction. *Journal of Emergency Medicine.* 2004;3:301–306.
67. van der Heijden GJ, van der Windt DA, de Winter AF. Physiotherapy for patients with soft tissue shoulder disorders: A systematic review of randomised clinical trials. *BMJ.* 1997;7099:25–30.
68. van der Heijden GJ, van der Windt DA, Kleijnen J et al. Steroid injections for shoulder disorders: A systematic review of randomized clinical trials. *British Journal of General Practice.* 1996;406:309–316.
69. Walch G, Boileau P, Noel E et al. Impingement of the deep surface of the supraspinatus tendon on the posterosuperior glenoid rim: An arthroscopic study. *Journal of Shoulder and Elbow Surgery.* 1992;5:238–245.
70. Wirth MA, Rockwood CA, Jr. Acute and chronic traumatic injuries of the sternoclavicular joint. *Journal of the American Academy of Orthopaedic Surgeons.* 1996;5:268–278.
71. Wise JN, Daffner RH, Weissman BN et al. ACR appropriateness criteria(R) on acute shoulder pain. *Journal of the American College of Radiology.* 2011;9:602–609.

44 Elbow and Forearm Injuries

Shawn F. Kane, James H. Lynch, and Francis G. O'Connor

CONTENTS

TABLE 44.1
Key Clinical Considerations

1. The differential diagnosis of elbow pain in primary care is conveniently approached from an anatomical perspective, with particular attention to mechanism of injury and age.
2. Tendinopathy is the most common adult elbow clinical presentation in the primary care setting; medial and lateral epicondylitis are the most common disorders and result in significant recreational and occupational disability.
3. Most overuse elbow disorders encountered in primary care respond to nonoperative therapy that largely consists of modification of the offending activity and restoring functional strength of the affected extremity.
4. Pediatric elbow disorders are additionally common in primary care, and principally the result of acute trauma from a fall on an outstretched hand or repetitive throwing activities.
5. Most pediatric elbow injuries are secondary to overuse, with overload to a growth site; initial treatment for pediatric athletes is to identify the inciting event and institute relative rest.

44.1 INTRODUCTION

Elbow disorders are commonly encountered in primary care; overuse and traumatic injuries present in all demographic age groups and can result in considerable recreational and occupational disability if not diagnosed and managed appropriately. Determining the underlying etiology of elbow and forearm pain can be challenging for the primary care provider secondary to the complex anatomy of the joint and the potential for referred pain from both the neck and the shoulder. As with other musculoskeletal complaints, the key to an accurate diagnosis is knowledge of functional anatomy in combination with a detailed history and physical and prudent utilization of diagnostic testing (see Chapters 17 through 21). As elbow injuries are commonly the result of activities unique to the individual, the patient's arm dominance, occupation, and recreational activities can additionally be important clues to the diagnosis. This chapter reviews the functional anatomy of the elbow and forearm and approaches diagnosis and management from a symptom-oriented and anatomical approach. The identification of evidence-based approaches are provided where applicable, as well as recommendations for referral to a consultant when clinically indicated (Table 44.1).

44.2 ELBOW FUNCTIONAL ANATOMY

The elbow joint is formed by three articulations that provide static and functional stability at this joint to allow for flexion, extension, supination, and pronation. Normal elbow motion includes 0°–135° of flexion and 75°–80° of pronation and supination. The bony anatomy includes the two condyles of the humerus, the trochlea and capitellum, which articulate with the proximal ends of the radius and ulna (see Figure 44.1).[10] The trochlea, or medial condyle, is grooved and articulates with the semilunar notch of the ulna to form the humeroulnar joint. This articulation forms a modified hinge that allows for flexion, extension, and stability. The capitellum, or spherical-shaped lateral condyle, articulates with the radial head to form a combination hinge and pivot joint called the humeroradial joint. This joint allows for flexion, extension, and axial rotation. Finally, the radial head articulates with the lesser sigmoid notch of the ulna to form the radioulnar joint, which also provides axial rotation.

Due to the relative instability of the osseous articulations at the elbow, ligaments are required to provide about 50% of elbow stability (see Figure 44.2). The medial collateral ligament complex, the strongest of the collateral ligaments, is formed by anterior, posterior, and transverse ligaments. The anterior ligament provides about 70% of valgus stability and remains tight throughout the entire range of elbow flexion, providing the majority of the stability of this ligament. The posterior ligament only becomes tight past 90° of flexion, providing minimal stability, and the transverse ligament does

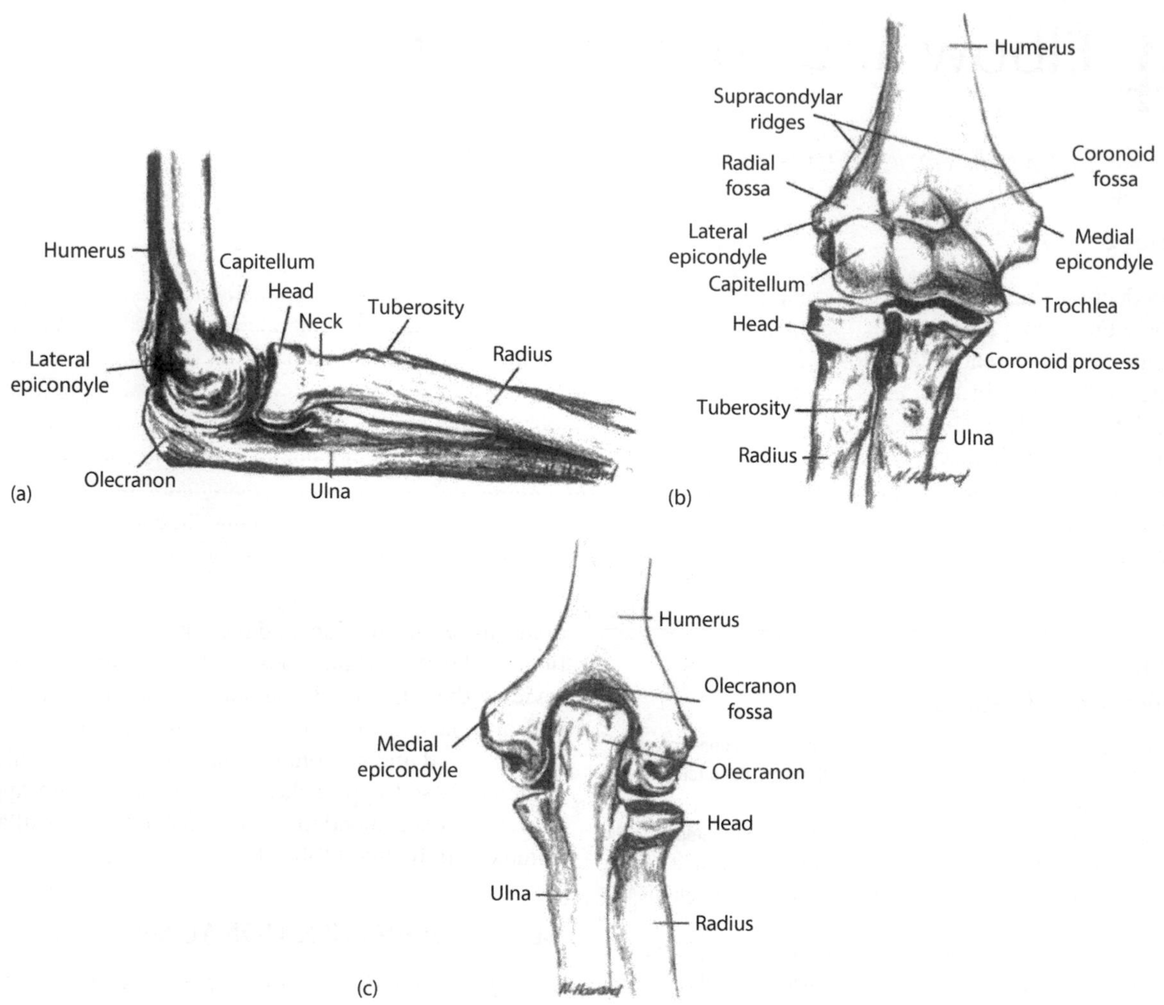

FIGURE 44.1 Bones of the elbow: (a) lateral, (b) anterior, and (c) posterior views. (From O'Connor, F.G. et al., in: *Handbook of Sports Medicine: A Symptom-Oriented Approach*, 2nd edn., Lillegard, W.A. et al., eds., Butterworth-Heinemann, Boston, MA, 1999, pp. 141–157. With permission.)

not appear to provide any significant stability. The lateral collateral ligament complex provides both rotational and varus elbow stability. This complex originates at the lateral epicondyle and inserts along the annular ligament. Four ligaments form this complex, with the radial collateral ligament providing the majority of varus stability, remaining tight throughout flexion and extension, and the lateral ulnar collateral ligament (UCL) providing inferior rotatory stability.

Separate muscle groups passing through the elbow joint control four major muscle activities. The biceps brachii, brachioradialis, and brachialis muscles perform flexion. The triceps and anconeus muscles control extension. The supinator and biceps brachii muscles control supination. Pronation involves the pronator quadratus, pronator teres, and flexor carpi radialis muscles. Also, the flexor pronator muscles of the wrist originate from the medial epicondyle, and the wrist extensors originate from the lateral epicondyle (see Table 44.2).

The three principal nerves that cross the elbow joint complex are the median, ulnar, and radial nerves. The median nerve crosses the anterior elbow medial to the biceps tendon and the brachial artery before entering the pronator teres. The median nerve is responsible for pronation. The ulnar nerve passes posterior to the medial epicondyle in the cubital tunnel before entering the flexor carpi ulnaris. The ulnar nerve provides sensation to the ulnar two digits and motor function to the flexor carpi ulnaris, dorsal and palmar interossei, and the flexor digitorum of the ulnar two digits. The radial nerve emerges from the radial groove behind the humerus to pass anterior to the lateral epicondyle before dividing into superficial (sensory component) and deep (motor component–posterior interosseous) branches. The radial nerve is responsible for the majority of the extensor muscles of the arm.

44.3 ANATOMICAL DIFFERENTIAL DIAGNOSIS

The differential diagnosis of elbow and forearm pain in primary care is optimally approached in a systematic fashion with focus on both mechanism of injury and location of pain (see Table 44.3). Subsequent chapter sections will cover specific adult and pediatric injuries to elbow and the forearm with a

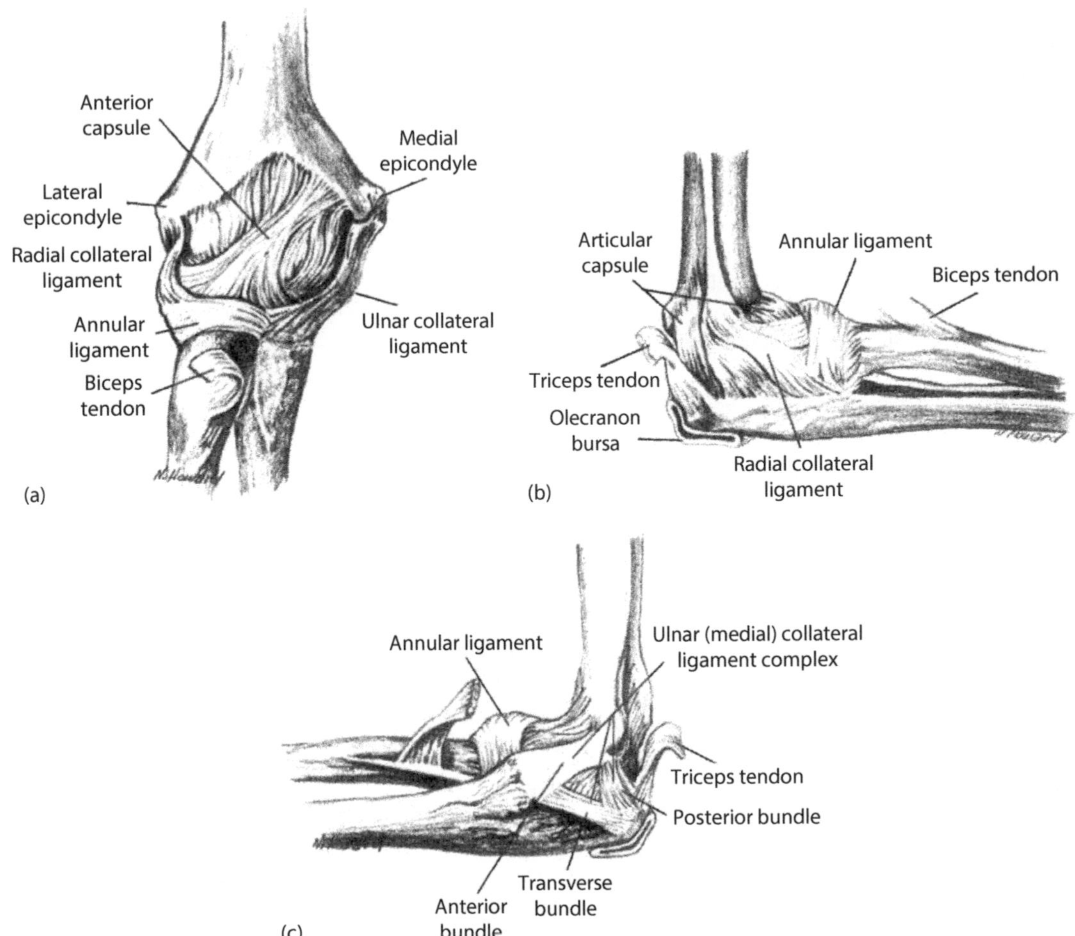

FIGURE 44.2 Ligaments of the elbow: (a) anterior, (b) lateral, and (c) medial views. (From O'Connor, F.G. et al., in: *Handbook of Sports Medicine: A Symptom-Oriented Approach*, 2nd edn., Lillegard, W.A. et al., eds., Butterworth-Heinemann, Boston, MA, 1999, pp. 141–157. With permission.)

symptom-oriented anatomical approach. The special tests that are referenced in the evaluation of a specific disorder are further described in Table 44.4. Indications for referral of common elbow and forearm disorders are summarized in Table 44.5.

44.4 ANTERIOR ELBOW PAIN

44.4.1 Overuse

44.4.1.1 Biceps Brachii Tendinopathy

The biceps tendon is the strongest supinator of the forearm, an important flexor of the elbow and a relatively common source of pain in the anterior elbow.[76] While distal biceps tendon ruptures are uncommon, composing approximately 3% of all tendon ruptures, distal biceps tendinopathy is more a frequent clinical presentation.[76] This condition presents with an insidious course with the complaint of vague anterior elbow pain. History often includes repeated elbow flexion with forearm supination/pronation such as maybe precipitated with repetitive dumbbell curls. On examination, with the elbow flexed to 90°, passive supination and pronation of the forearm should reveal a normal pistonlike movement of the biceps muscle belly. The absence of this motion may indicate a complete or partial tear. Resisted supination typically recreates pain deep in the antecubital fossa. The hook test, performed by hooking the biceps tendon with the examiner's fingertip, will confirm an intact tendon and may assist in localizing the pain generator (see Table 44.4). Magnetic resonance imaging (MRI) or ultrasound can be used to evaluate the biceps tendon and demonstrate continuity and changes in caliber and quality of the tendon.[5]

Not all anterior elbow pain is the result of biceps tendinopathy. Uncommon etiologies in the differential diagnosis include intra-articular processes such as osteoarthritis, rheumatoid arthritis, and gout. Initial treatment consists of relative rest, home exercise and/or physical therapy, and a short course of nonsteroidal anti-inflammatory drugs (NSAIDs) (see Chapter 28). If the pain fails to resolve, referral to a primary care sports medicine physician or an orthopedic surgeon for further diagnostic evaluation and/or secondary treatments and interventions, such as proliferative therapy or surgical intervention, should be considered (see Table 44.5).[26,45]

44.4.1.2 Pronator Syndrome

Pronator syndrome is an uncommon compression neuropathy of the median nerve as it crosses the elbow, seen in physically active people such as bicyclists and weight lifters.[60]

TABLE 44.2
Pertinent Muscles of the Elbow

Muscle	Function	Origin	Insertion
		Anterior	
Brachioradialis	Flexes the elbow	Lateral aspect of the humerus	Lateral aspect of the radial styloid
Biceps brachii			
Long head	Supinates and flexes elbow	Supraglenoid tubercle	Radial tuberosity (proximal radius)
Short head	Supinates and flexes elbow	Coracoid process	Radial tuberosity (proximal radius)
Brachialis	Flexes forearm	Distal anterior humerus	Ulnar tuberosity
		Medial	
Flexor carpi radialis	Flexes and abducts the wrist	Common flexor tendon from the medial epicondyle	Volar aspect base of the second and third metacarpals
Flexor carpi ulnaris	Flexes and adducts the wrist	Humeral head from the common flexor tendon; ulnar head from the olecranon and proximal ulna	Pisiform, hamate, and fifth metacarpal
Palmaris longus	Flexes the wrist	Common flexor tendon from the medical epicondyle	Flexor retinaculum
Pronator teres	Pronates the forearm	Humeral head medial epicondyle; ulnar head coronoid process	Lateral surface of the radius
		Lateral	
Extensor carpi radialis longus	Extends the wrist	Lateral supracondylar ridge	Base of the second metacarpal
Extensor carpi radialis brevis	Extends the wrist	Common extensor tendon from the lateral epicondyle of the humerus	Base of the third metacarpal
Extensor digitorum communis	Extends wrist and second through fifth metacarpophalangeal joints	Common extensor tendon from the lateral epicondyle of the humerus	Dorsum of the second through fifth digits
Extensor carpi ulnaris	Extends and adducts the wrist	Common extensor tendon from the lateral epicondyle of the humerus and the dorsal aspect of the mid ulna	Ulnar aspect of the fifth metacarpal
Extensor digiti minimi	Aids in wrist extension and extends proximal phalanx of the fifth digit at the metacarpophalangeal joint	Common extensor tendon from the lateral epicondyle of the humerus	Dorsal aspect of the fifth digit
Supinator	Supinates the forearm	Lateral epicondyle and lateral aspect of the olecranon	Lateral and anterior aspect of the proximal mid radius
		Posterior	
Triceps brachii			
Long head	Extends elbow	Infraglenoid tubercle	Olecranon
Lateral head	Extends elbow	Posterior, proximal humerus	Olecranon
Medial head	Extends elbow	Posterior, distal humerus	Olecranon

The compression commonly occurs in one of three locations: between the heads of the pronator teres, under the proximal edge of the pronator teres or the flexor digitorum superficialis, or under the ligament of Struthers or bicipital aponeurosis.[10] Compression is secondary to either hypertrophy of the muscles from repetitive use or from trauma to the median nerve.[45]

Patients with this condition will complain of the insidious onset of an achy pain in the anterior proximal forearm and have paresthesias in the hand consistent with a median nerve distribution.[54,56] Pronator syndrome can be a challenge to distinguish from carpal tunnel syndrome due to the hand complaints; unique features include forearm pain, the lack of nighttime pain, sensory loss over the thenar eminence, and the lack of a positive Tinel's or Phalen's sign at the wrist.[13,45] The diagnosis can be confirmed with electrodiagnostic testing, which will demonstrate slowed conduction velocity in the forearm and abnormalities in muscles innervated by the median nerve. Treatment typically includes rest, avoidance of inciting activities, and a short course of NSAIDs. Injections of corticosteroids and/or local anesthetics into tender sites in the pronator teres can be attempted and are described in numerous texts.[17] Ultrasound guidance may assist in a more targeted injection; however, there is no evidence at this time indicating a superior result.[56] Surgical decompression of the median

TABLE 44.3
Common Elbow and Forearm Disorders in Primary Care: An Anatomical and Symptom-Oriented Approach to Differential Diagnosis

Anterior	**Medial**
Overuse	Overuse
Biceps brachii tendinopathy	Golfer's elbow
Pronator syndrome	Cubital tunnel syndrome
	Valgus overload syndrome
Traumatic	Traumatic
Distal biceps rupture	Ulnar collateral ligament strain
Pediatric	Pediatric
Supracondylar fracture	Little league elbow
Lateral	**Posterior**
Overuse	Overuse
Tennis elbow	Triceps tendinopathy
Radial tunnel syndrome	Olecranon bursitis
Posterior interosseous nerve entrapment	Posterior impingement
Traumatic	Traumatic
Radial head fracture	Triceps rupture
	Posterior elbow dislocation
Pediatric	Pediatric
Panner's disease	Olecranon apophysitis
Osteochondritis dissecans	
Nursemaid's elbow	
Forearm	
Overuse	
Intersection syndrome	
Traumatic	
Compartment syndrome	
Nightstick fracture	
Galeazzi fracture	
Monteggia fracture	
Essex-Lopresti fracture	
Pediatric	
Forearm splints	

nerve at the site of compression is an option for those with a persistent disability (>6 months) despite previous treatments (Level of Evidence C: expert opinion).[56]

44.4.2 Traumatic

44.4.2.1 Distal Biceps Rupture

Ruptures of the biceps tendon account for a high percentage of traumatic tendon injuries; most of these injuries involve the proximal tendon with many treated nonoperatively. Distal biceps tendon ruptures, however, are less common (10%) and frequently require operative intervention. Distal tendon injuries occur, not commonly, in middle-aged men and are generally the result of an eccentric load resulting in a forced extension of the elbow tearing the distal biceps tendon at the radial tuberosity. The patient will complain of sudden onset anterior elbow pain with a tearing or popping sensation and immediate functional disability limiting flexion. The physical examination will reveal swelling and ecchymosis over the antecubital fossa.[76] Due to the bicep's role as the primary supinator and secondary flexor, weakness may be identified in ranges of motion. In the presence of a complete tendon rupture, the hook test will be positive as the examiner will not be able to hook their fingertip under the biceps tendon confirming the presence of a rupture.[45]

Diagnosis of a biceps tendon rupture is clinical; however, tendon rupture can be confirmed with either MRI or musculoskeletal ultrasound. Treatment can be conservative or operative depending on the degree of tear and the needs of the individual patient. Most active patients, however, will require operative treatment as nonsurgical treatment can result in a 40% and 30% decrease in supination and flexion strength, respectively, and an even more significant loss in endurance (Level of Evidence B: case series).[45,70,71]

44.4.3 Pediatric

44.4.3.1 Supracondylar Fracture

Supracondylar fractures are among the most common pediatric elbow traumatic injuries; these injuries account for nearly 60% of elbow fractures in the 5–10-year-old age group. The typical etiology is a fall on an outstretched arm with the nondominant arm being more commonly affected. The supracondylar region of the distal humerus consists of an area of thin, weak bone; fractures in this area can significantly injure associated soft tissue and vascular structures with resultant significant comorbidities.

Children typically present with a history of trauma and significant elbow pain, swelling, and a limited range of motion. Clinicians need to rapidly assess the skin for any evidence of open fracture, thoroughly assess the neurovascular status of the distal extremity, and monitor the compartments for any evidence of compartment syndrome. The neurovascular assessment, which must be frequently repeated, includes the radial and brachial arteries and the sensory and motor functions of the radial, ulnar, and median nerves. Radiographs, specifically a true lateral of the elbow, will be required to identify the specific fracture pattern. Forearm fractures are associated with these fractures; anterior–posterior and lateral views of the forearm should be obtained.

Supracondylar fractures should be splinted and urgently referred to a consultant for management and follow-up, as operative intervention with internal fixation may be required. The potential for complications may warrant hospitalization to monitor for the development of any neurovascular complications; again, consultation with an appropriate consultant is recommended.[61]

44.5 MEDIAL ELBOW PAIN

44.5.1 Overuse

44.5.1.1 Medial Epicondylitis (Golfer's Elbow)

Medial epicondylitis is clinically less common than lateral epicondylitis. This disorder is generally seen in athletes or workers who participate in activities that involve repetitive

TABLE 44.4
Elbow and Forearm Special Tests

Test	Performance	Positive Findings	Suggested Diagnosis
Elbow abduction stress test	Valgus stress applied against an elbow held in 20–30° of flexion.	Absence of a firm end point and movement of the articular surfaces of the medial epicondyle and ulna.	Ulna collateral ligament injury
Hook test	Shoulder abducted to 90° with the elbow in 90° of flexion. Examiners finger attempts to hook behind the distal biceps tendon.	Finger does not hook onto the biceps tendon.	Distal biceps tendon rupture
Resisted middle-finger test	With an outstretched arm, the patient attempts to extend the middle finger against resistance.	Weakness/inability to resist force.	Posterior interosseous nerve entrapment
Tennis elbow test	The examiner resists the patient's active wrist extension or flexion.	Pain isolated at the lateral epicondyle.	Lateral epicondylitis
Milking maneuver	Forearm supinated, shoulder extended, and elbow flexed to 90° with a valgus stress being put on the elbow by pulling on the thumb.	Apprehension, instability, and medial joint pain.	Ulna collateral ligament injury
Modified milking maneuver	Shoulder adducted and externally rotated.	Apprehension, instability, and medial joint pain.	Ulna collateral ligament injury
Moving valgus stress test	Shoulder is abducted and externally rotated, and while maintaining a constant valgus force, the elbow is quickly flexed and extended through a complete range of motion.	Pain between 70° and 120° is positive.	Ulna collateral ligament injury
Tinel's test	Gentle tapping over the course of a superficial nerve.	Tingling, paresthesias over the distal course of the nerve.	Cubital tunnel syndrome Radial tunnel syndrome

valgus stress and/or flexion activities at the elbow, as well as repetitive wrist flexion and pronation. Medial epicondylitis is thought to be the result of a tendinopathy of the common flexor tendon; most commonly the flexor carpi radialis and the pronator teres.[38,79]

Patients typically present with insidious onset of pain at the medial elbow with or without accompanying grip strength weakness. The point of maximal tenderness is usually at the insertion of the flexor–pronator mass, 5–10 mm distal and radial to the medial epicondyle.[81] Pain during resisted pronation has been reported to be the most sensitive physical finding. The pain can also typically be recreated with resisted wrist flexion.[30] Other conditions to consider in the differential diagnosis include cubital tunnel syndrome and possible valgus extension overload syndrome. Radiographs are rarely needed for the initial diagnosis or for developing a treatment plan; advanced imaging to include an MRI may be indicated in cases that fail to respond to initial conservative treatment and prior to referral.[79]

The natural history of medial epicondylitis is such that if left untreated, symptoms in the majority of patient will usually resolve spontaneously in 6 months to up to 2 years. A wait-and-see approach may be acceptable for patients who can adequately function. There exists, however, a wide range of treatment options for medial epicondylitis with varying degrees of evidence and success. A treatment plan that consists of activity modification, protection with a counter-force brace, short-term pain control, and rehabilitative exercise can be effective (see Chapters 28 and 31). Glucocorticoids are the mainstay injection therapy for epicondylitis and have been shown to have good short-term effect when utilized early in the clinical course but have not been demonstrated to have significant long-term impact (see Chapter 30).[16] Multiple other injection therapies have been used to treat both medial and lateral epicondylitis with varying degree of success; the role of platelet-rich plasma therapy remains undetermined.[50] Topical nitroglycerin patches are another treatment modality that has been used with some success for elbow tendinopathy; this therapy, however, requires a long-term commitment from the patient that may not provide long-term efficacy.[48] Ninety percent of cases of epicondylitis respond to typical treatments; those that fail to respond after 6 months should be referred for possible more advanced treatments of even possibly surgery (Level of Evidence C: consensus and expert opinion).[32,81]

44.5.1.2 Cubital Tunnel Syndrome

Cubital tunnel syndrome is a compressive or traction neuropathy of the ulnar nerve as it passes through the cubital tunnel of the medial elbow. It is the second most common compressive neuropathy of the upper extremity; carpal tunnel being the most common.[65] Approximately 60% of cases of medial epicondylitis may have a concomitant compressive ulnar neuropathy.[34]

TABLE 44.5
Indications for Specialty Referral for Common Disorders of the Elbow and Forearm

Diagnosis	Primary Care Referral Considerations
	Anterior
Biceps brachii tendinopathy	After failure of typical treatments may consider early referral for more advanced injection therapies if patient needs to return to a higher level of functioning quickly.
Biceps brachii rupture	High-grade or complete tears need to be referred immediately to allow for proper surgical decision making. Incomplete or low-grade tears should also be referred to get guidance on comanagement.
	Medial
Cubital tunnel syndrome	Recalcitrant cases that fail typical treatments should be referred after 4–6 months of treatment. High functioning, high-demand athletes may be referred sooner.
Medial epicondylitis "golfers' elbow"	Consider early referral for possible advanced injection therapies. Surgical referral indicated after a reasonable trial of all other conservative treatments.
Ulnar collateral ligament injury	High-demand athletes should be referred early to allow for proper surgical decision making. Low-grade, partial tears (grade 1 and 2) can be referred if still symptomatic after proper course of conservative treatment.
	Lateral
Lateral epicondylitis tennis elbow	Consider early referral for possible advanced injection therapies. Surgical referral indicated after a reasonable trial of all other conservative treatments.
Posterior interosseous nerve syndrome	Consider referral for surgical evaluation after failure of a reasonable course of conservative treatments.
Radial tunnel syndrome	Consider referral for surgical evaluation after failure of a reasonable course of conservative treatments.
	Posterior
Olecranon bursitis	Consider early referral for aspiration, cultures, and antibiotic treatment if warranted. Nonseptic cases should be referred after 2–3 if bursitis still exists despite proper treatment.
Posterior impingement	Refer in the presence of large osteophytes or abnormalities on radiographs and failure to respond to conservative treatment.
Triceps brachii tendinopathy	After failure of typical treatments, may consider early referral for more advanced injection therapies if patient needs to return to a higher level of functioning quickly.

Clinical Pearl

Consider the diagnosis of cubital tunnel syndrome in patients with medial epicondylitis that does not respond to typical treatment.

Patients clinically will complain of medial elbow pain with repetitive activity. The pain is usually associated with numbness and tingling in the ulnar border of the forearm and hand with extension to the ring and little fingers. If the condition exists for an extended period of time, weakness of the intrinsic muscles of the hand may develop.[34] Patients may also complain of nighttime pain due to sleeping with the elbow fully flexed. A thorough examination of the upper extremities and cervical spine is essential to rule out other compressive neuropathies and radiculopathies.[31,40]

A positive Tinel's sign at the cubital tunnel has a specificity of 48%–100% and a sensitivity from 44% to 75% for a compressive neuropathy (see Table 44.4).[66] Examination should focus on the flexor carpi ulnaris, flexor digitorum profundus, hypothenar eminence, and the hand intrinsics (muscles innervated by the ulnar nerve distal to the cubital tunnel). Other findings may include the inability to adduct the little finger (Wartenberg's sign) and flexion of the proximal interphalangeal joint and the distal interphalangeal joint of the ring and little fingers (claw hand deformity). The ulnar nerve should be palpated in the cubital tunnel during flexion and extension in order to detect any subluxation or dislocation of the nerve.[34]

Rest and removal from the offending activity, as well as consideration for a short course of an NSAID and physical therapy for nerve mobilization, are the mainstays of initial treatment. Educating patients to avoid positions that cause traction or compression of the cubital tunnel is effective for many with mild symptoms. For more extensive symptoms, addition of nighttime flexion-blocking splint may be helpful.[13] A corticosteroid injection in the area of the cubital tunnel can be considered but has not been shown to be more efficacious than physical therapy.[55] If after 4–6 months of treatment there is no improvement of symptoms, consider an EMG/NCV study and possible referral for ulnar nerve transposition.[23]

44.5.1.3 Valgus Extension Overload Syndrome

The dissipation of the forces created while throwing produces a shear force across the posterior compartment, which results in this syndrome. Patients complain of pain in the posteromedial elbow usually during the deceleration phases. Loose bodies, from osteophytes on the posteromedial tip of the olecranon, may result in the mechanical symptoms of locking or decreased range of motion.

Physical exam can recreate the pain with a "valgus extension overload" test—forcing the elbow into full extension while applying a valgus force. Radiographs are useful in identifying osteophytes, and MRI with contrast is recommended to identify loose bodies in the joint space or other concomitant injuries. The initial treatment is rest, but typically patients with osteophytes, loose bodies, concomitant injuries who wish to return to a high level of function will require surgery.[11,44]

44.5.2 Traumatic

44.5.2.1 Ulnar Collateral Ligament Strain

The anterior bundle of the UCL is the primary restraint to valgus stress during overhead throwing.[11] UCL injuries are commonly seen in athletes participating in sports that involve overhead throwing, such as baseball, javelin, and volleyball. UCL injuries are typically seen in year-round, taller and heavier baseball players.[19,26,47,50] Injury to the UCL results in significant valgus elbow instability and may predispose an athlete to other secondary injuries.[50]

Clinical Pearl

Injury to the UCL needs to be thoroughly assessed in throwing athletes with medial elbow pain. Delayed or missed diagnosis can have a significant impact on future performance.

The history should include questions about the onset of pain, what the patient was doing when the pain started, sports played, and the frequency of participation. Patients with an acute UCL injury usually report the sensation of a pop followed by the immediate onset of pain and bruising around the medial elbow. Tenderness over the UCL has an 81%–94% sensitivity but only 22% specificity for UCL tears.[22,36]

The most important examination for a possible UCL injury is assessing for medial joint space laxity or instability against valgus forces. The symptomatic medial joint space should be compared against the asymptomatic side for the amount of opening, the subjective quality of the end point while a valgus force is applied across the joint, and pain. A normal joint space will open less than 3 mm, and with a firm end point.[18,26,47]

The moving valgus stress test has a 100% sensitivity and a 75% specificity for diagnosing UCL injuries (see Table 44.4). This test is performed with the shoulder in 90° of abduction and external rotation. While maintaining constant valgus torque on the elbow, the elbow is quickly flexed and extended. A positive test is defined as pain between 70° and 120° of flexion.[38] The milking maneuver can also be done to provide additional information on the possible presence of a UCL injury. Patients with a UCL injury will complain of pain, instability, and apprehension.[37]

Athletes with low-grade partial tears to the UCL can be managed with rest, avoidance of inciting activities and bracing, and a gradual return to throwing when asymptomatic. Early referral is indicated for high-grade and complete tears, as well as management of high-demand athletes.[31]

44.5.3 Pediatric

44.5.3.1 Little League Elbow

Originally described as an avulsion injury to the medial epicondyle, Little League elbow is a term for a constellation of abnormalities of the medial elbow. This injury spectrum can include medial epicondylar apophysitis, medial epicondylar avulsion, and accelerated apophyseal growth with delayed closure of the epicondylar growth plate.[11] Studies have demonstrated that up to 50%–75% of adolescent baseball players report elbow pain and the most common etiology is repetitive valgus stresses and tension on the medial structures. Patients are typically less than 10 years old and complain of medial elbow pain, decreased throwing effectiveness, and decreased throwing distance.

Physical exam typically demonstrates mild medial swelling, tenderness over the medial epicondyle, and a loss of elbow extension and pain with valgus stress.[44] Plain films can be normal or they can show irregular ossification of the medial epicondyle or abnormalities in the apophasis; generally, radiographs of both elbows are required to distinguish subtle differences.

Rest from the inciting activity is the primary treatment along with NSAIDs and ice. If there is any separation of the apophysis >3 mm, early referral and/or consultation is indicated to ensure that surgery is not needed. After a period of rest, the athlete needs a stretching and strengthening program with a gradual return to throwing in about 6 weeks. Prevention for Little League elbow is the key. Pitch count and mechanics should be addressed and monitored in all young overhead athletes and especially those who have previously been diagnosed with Little League elbow. The provider should take this opportunity to educate the athlete and if needed their parents on the importance of adherence to pitch count recommendations (see www.usabaseball.com).

44.6 LATERAL ELBOW PAIN

44.6.1 Overuse

44.6.1.1 Lateral Epicondylitis (Tennis Elbow)

Lateral epicondylitis occurs in approximately 1%–3% of the population annually, and although commonly called tennis elbow, only 5%–10% of tennis players develop the condition. Most patients are in their 30s and 40s and develop this degenerative overuse tendinopathy in their dominant arm as a result of their occupation, and not their hobbies.[35] The lateral elbow is affected four to ten times more often than the medial side.[75]

The lateral epicondyle of the humerus serves as the common extensor origin for the active supinators and extensors of the forearm to include extensor carpi radialis brevis (ECRB). Physical exam reveals maximal tenderness approximately 1 cm distal and ulnar to the epicondyle at the origin of the ECRB. Pain and decreased strength with resisted gripping and with wrist supination and extension are often present.[75] Treatment for lateral epicondylitis is very similar to that of medial epicondylitis, which has previously been described. Particular to lateral epicondylitis, bracing of the wrist in extension should be considered along with commonly used with counterforce bracing.[16,27,74] Avoiding inciting activities, pain control, biomechanical correction, and stretching and strengthening program are the mainstays of treatment. Referral should be considered if symptoms persist after 6 months despite conservative therapy.

44.6.1.2 Radial Tunnel Syndrome and Posterior Interosseous Nerve Entrapment

When tennis elbow fails to improve, the primary care provider needs to include both radial tunnel syndrome (RTS) and posterior interosseous nerve (PIN) entrapment in the differential diagnosis. These are rare peripheral nerve entrapments making up only of 1%–2% of the total nerve entrapments.[40,43] There is some controversy over whether RTS and PIN are two separate entities or a continuum of the same condition. The critical clinical point is to recognize that a small percentage of patients who present with lateral elbow pain and are thought to have lateral epicondylitis on initial presentation actually have an entrapment neuropathy of the radial nerve.[13,43]

Patients typically present, in both syndromes, with a history of repetitive forearm supination and pronation (for example, carpenters or mechanics) and complain of insidious, poorly localized pain in the forearm. Physical exam typically reveals a positive Tinel's sign at the radial tunnel. The point of maximal tenderness usually resides distal to the lateral epicondyle and just ulnar to the radial head. The presence of weakness with resisted supination of the forearm and extension of the middle finger (middle finger test) is a common finding in PIN syndrome (see Table 44.4).[53] In contrast, RTS typically presents as a pure pain syndrome without any objective clinical muscular weakness.[12,34,44] Treatment consists of initially stopping the inciting activity and splinting the wrist in extension and the hand in supination. If unsure of the diagnosis or if the patient has not responded to treatment, an EMG/NCV should be considered prior to referral when surgical nerve decompression may be contemplated.[13,43] However, at this time, there is limited evidence to support the efficacy for either corticosteroid injections or surgical treatment for the management of these challenging nerve entrapments (Level of Evidence B: inconsistent patient-oriented evidence).[35,55]

44.6.2 Traumatic

44.6.2.1 Radial Head Fracture

The most common elbow fracture encountered in adults is that of the radial head, comprising 33%–50% of elbow fractures, with a slight male predominance.[62] The typical etiology is axial loading from a fall on an outstretched arm. Patients will complain of pain over the lateral aspect of the elbow, have point tenderness over the radial head, and will not be able to supinate or fully extend the joint without pain.[67] Plain radiographs are typically adequate for the diagnosis, but these fractures can be very subtle and diagnosis may be aided by identification of fat pads. A fat pad sign results from the distention of the joint capsule. A small anterior fat pad is a normal finding, but a prominent anterior sail-shaped lucency, as well as the presence of a posterior lucency, is always abnormal and indicative of an occult fracture.[26]

Initial treatment of a radial head fracture consists of a long arm splint with the elbow in 90° of flexion. If a significant hemarthrosis is present consider aspiration, which will provide immediate and significant pain relief. Radial head fractures are graded I–IV; I—nondisplaced fractures, II—<2 mm displacement, III—comminuted fractures, and IV—radial head fracture with associated dislocations.[69] Simple fractures, grades I and II, can be followed by primary care providers with a gradual increase in range of motion as pain decreases. Patients should be informed that pain and stiffness can be present for several weeks, with good function anticipated after 2–3 months of home rehabilitation. Grades III and IV fractures should be referred to an orthopedic surgeon for management (see Table 44.5).[26,58,62,67]

44.6.3 Pediatric

44.6.3.1 Panner's Disease and Osteochondritis Dissecans

Lateral compressive forces from repetitive valgus stress and compression increase the force across the radiocapitellar joint producing injury patterns unique to pediatric athletes. In children, the capitellum has a precarious blood supply and this contributes to a high incidence of injury in the dominant arm of throwing athletes and gymnasts. These athletes will complain of lateral elbow pain, locking, catching, or failure to fully extend the elbow.[67] The provider must differentiate between Panner's disease and an osteochondritis dissecans (OCDs) lesion as the sequelae for the latter may negatively alter the athlete's career.[14]

Panner's disease typically is a self-limiting condition occurring in children under 10 years of age. Athletes will typically complain of the acute onset of lateral elbow pain and rarely mechanical symptoms. Radiographs show a fragmentation of the capitellar (distal humeral) ossification nucleus.[3] Treatment for this condition is relative rest and rehabilitation and typically the capitellum will resume normal growth.[14,29,44]

Clinical Pearl

Determining the age of onset and the presence of mechanical symptoms is a great way to distinguish between Panner's disease and an OCD.

OCD lesions, most commonly seen in adolescent athletes older than 13, present with the insidious onset of lateral elbow pain, and with significant lesions patients will complain of decreased range of motion, locking, or catching.[3] Radiographs will show irregular ossification of the capitellum and sometimes the radial head, contralateral views may be helpful in identifying subtle lesions.[14] MRI is the preferred imaging modality and is more sensitive than plain radiographs in identifying chondral loose bodies. Stable lesions, those without mechanical symptoms, are initially treated conservatively with a period of rest followed by a gradual rehabilitative period. The offending activity must be stopped, and the athlete should be counseled that they may be out of competition for 6–12 months. Unstable lesions respond best to surgical intervention. An OCD lesion that is not properly treated can prevent an athlete's return to high-level activities; accordingly, early consultation is recommended.[44]

44.6.3.2 Nursemaid's Elbow

Nursemaid's elbow is a frequent pediatric injury seen most commonly in children aged between 6 months and 5 years. Previously described as a subluxation of the radial head, a more accurate pathological diagnosis is annular ligament displacement. The injury typically results from an axial traction force applied to the pronated arm; this force causes the annular ligament to slip over the radial head and come to rest in the radiocapitellar joint.

This injury should be suspected when a child resists moving their arm and holds it against their body in a semiflexed and pronated position.[59] If the physical examination does not identify any other areas of point tenderness, then the diagnosis of annular ligament displacement should be suspected and radiographs are not needed. Due to the frequency of the injury, reduction of the displaced ligament is an essential procedure for anyone who cares for pediatric patients. Classically, most providers have been trained to utilize the supination–flexion method to reduce the injury. Recent evidence suggests that the hyperpronation method may be more effective, with 95% successful first attempt rate (versus 77% with the supination–flexion method).[20] Both maneuvers allow the annular ligament to return to its normal anatomical position and the clinician will often, but not always, feel a click. It is recommended that providers know both techniques, and if one is unsuccessful, consider switching to the second technique. After the maneuver is complete, the child should quickly resume spontaneous movement of the arm. Recurrence is common, in up to one-third of patients, therefore anticipatory guidance needs to be provided to the caregivers.[9] Patients who do not regain full range of motion after treatment should have radiographs taken, splinted, and be referred for follow-up musculoskeletal care with an orthopedic consultant.

Clinical Pearl

After reducing a nursemaid's elbow, consider leaving the room, returning a few minutes later and "high-fiving" the patients' injured arm. If properly reduced, the patient will instinctively return the gesture.

44.7 POSTERIOR ELBOW PAIN

44.7.1 Overuse

44.7.1.1 Triceps Brachii Tendinopathy

The triceps tendon is the primary extensor of the elbow. Overall, an uncommon tendinopathy, but one that is occasionally seen in weight lifters or industrial workers where repetitive elbow extension against resistance is required.[6] Diagnosis is generally straightforward in the setting of a suggestive history. On examination, the patient reports pain at the posterior elbow with resisted extension and tenderness at the triceps insertion.[4,8] Treatment is similar to the other tendinopathies; rest, rehabilitative exercise, short courses of NSAIDs, and referral of refractory cases for more definitive treatment (see Chapter 28).[7,26]

44.7.1.2 Olecranon Bursitis

Olecranon bursitis is the most common superficial bursitis and a common cause of posterior elbow pain and swelling.[1] Bursitis can be differentiated from an elbow joint effusion by being able to extend the joint without significantly increasing pain.[3] Olecranon bursitis can be either septic or aseptic (trauma or inflammatory arthritis). Patients with septic olecranon bursitis present with pain, swelling, warmth, and erythema over the olecranon; roughly half have been demonstrated to have evidence of fever. Diagnosis of septic bursitis is confirmed by bursal fluid analysis; crystal analysis can rule out gout as an etiology.[67,73] By contrast, patients with aseptic olecranon bursitis may present with a history of minor trauma to the elbow and a boggy, nontender mass over the olecranon without redness, warmth, limited range of motion, or other signs of infection.[37]

Treatment for olecranon bursitis differs greatly dependent upon the etiology. Septic bursitis requires a high index of suspicion, with aspiration and subsequent directed antibiotic therapy and consideration for incision and drainage.[6] Patients with aseptic olecranon bursitis should be managed with joint protection. If not contraindicated, NSAIDs may be used to treat the pain and the swelling. In addition, intrabursal steroid injections can be useful in those cases that are documented to be nonseptic (Level of Evidence B: systematic review).[67] Aspiration of the bursa, however, can be associated with complications, such as introducing infection, and should only be undertaken with strict sterile technique; in addition, it is not uncommon for the fluid to reaccumulate unless the cause is addressed.[1] The use of a compressive dressing that does not impede range of motion is beneficial in preventing reaccumulation. Chronic, persistent bursitis may develop and if affects the patient enough will require surgical excision of the bursa.[32,33]

44.7.1.3 Posterior Impingement Syndrome

Hyperextension valgus overload syndrome is a condition that presents in younger athletes that are subjected to repetitive valgus stresses while in hyperextension (i.e., javelin throwers). This stress causes impingement of the olecranon tip in the olecranon fossa, which may cause osteophyte formation and a fixed flexion deformity over time. A similar condition exists in older patients with osteoarthritis. On exam, the patient will complain of posterior elbow pain when forced into full elbow extension.[2] Treatment consists of relative rest, protective bracing, and the minimization of inciting activities. If these initial interventions fail, consideration of advance imaging to rule out loose bodies and chondral injury, as well as referral for possible surgical intervention is indicated.[7]

44.7.2 Traumatic

44.7.2.1 Posterior Elbow Dislocation

Elbow dislocations are classified according to the direction of the olecranon in relation to the distal humerus, with posterior dislocations being most common.[66] Posterior elbow dislocations result from the discontinuity of the ulnohumeral articulation with an associated radiocapitellar joint disruption. Typically, the lateral ligaments tear first, followed by the anterior and posterior capsule. The medial ligaments usually remain intact but are unstable.[45] Patients present with a visible deformity and a significant amount of pain. A thorough neurovascular exam is necessary with emphasis on integrity of the median and ulnar nerve.

Plain radiographs are valuable in determining the direction and degree of dislocation and the presence of any concomitant fractures. In complex injuries or for preoperative planning, an MRI may be valuable for identifying ligamentous injuries; a CT scan assists in further defining the nature of the fracture. Treatment of simple dislocations is usually accomplished by a closed reduction with or without anesthesia primarily depending on the time since dislocation.[45] Elbows that are stable postreduction should be put in a sling for comfort with gradual increase in range of motion. Complex dislocations, unstable joints post reduction, or comorbid fractures will require consultation to consider an open operative reduction or fixation.

44.7.2.2 Triceps Brachii Rupture

A very uncommon injury, less than 1% of total tendon ruptures, occur in the triceps. When the triceps tendon does rupture, it occurs two to three times more commonly in men than women. The injury is usually common in those aged 30–50 years and occurs as a result of direct trauma, a fall on an outstretched hand, or weight lifting.[72] The rupture typically occurs at the insertion onto the olecranon. Patients present with acute pain, a tearing sensation, and immediate extensor weakness.

Radiographs will demonstrate a small avulsion fracture off the olecranon, or "flake sign," in 80% of cases, which is pathognomonic for triceps avulsions.[46] Radiographs do not adequately assess partial tendon tears, musculotendinous junction, and intramuscular injuries. MRI is the current standard diagnostic tool in the differentiation between complete and partial tears. Musculoskeletal ultrasound is becoming a more frequently utilized diagnostic tool, and multiple studies have shown ultrasound to be as accurate as MRI in diagnosing partial and complete triceps tendon tears.[72]

Complete tendon ruptures are managed operatively. The management of partial tears is not universally agreed upon, with recommendations varying from initial immobilization in 30° of flexion for 4–6 weeks to early surgery for those tears >50% tendon width. Multiple factors need to be taken into consideration when the patient and physician are deciding on treatment.[72]

44.7.3 Pediatric

44.7.3.1 Olecranon Apophysitis

Stress fracture of the olecranon results from overuse and repetitive tension on the proximal ulna that is usually seen in gymnastics or throwing athletes. It is also commonly seen in adolescents who will complain of insidious onset posterior and sometimes lateral elbow pain. Typically, there is focal tenderness to palpation over the olecranon without any tenderness over the triceps tendon.[45]

Plain films are typically negative; both elbows should be scrutinized for olecranon apophyseal asymmetries. If an occult fracture is suspected, a CT scan or an MRI is needed to definitively diagnose the injury. Treatment consists of immediately stopping the inciting activity. Conservative treatment consists of rest, rehabilitation, and a gradual return to activity. In those adolescents who present with an acute olecranon apophyseal separation, primary surgical repair with percutaneous screwing should be considered.[45]

44.8 FOREARM PAIN

44.8.1 Overuse

44.8.1.1 Intersection Syndrome

Intersection syndrome is an overuse syndrome of the distal dorsoradial forearm that is seen in patients involved in activities associated with repeated flexion–extension movements of the wrist. Patients complain of pain, swelling, crepitus, and edema proximal to Lister's tubercle in an area where the first extensor compartment tendons (abductor pollicis longus and the extensor pollicis brevis) intersect with the second extensor compartment tendons (extensor carpi radialis longus and brevis).[51,57] This condition can be diagnosed by musculoskeletal ultrasound, which will demonstrate peritendinous edema, and fluid-filled tendon sheaths at the point of intersection/pain.[21] Treatment is conservative, with splinting, stopping the offending activity, and possibly oral nonsteroidal anti-inflammatory medications or a selectively placed corticosteroid injection.[64] Surgery may be needed for recalcitrant cases that do not respond to conservative treatment.[24]

44.8.2 Traumatic

44.8.2.1 Nightstick Fracture

Nightstick fracture is an isolated fracture of the midshaft of the ulna that usually results from direct trauma (raising the arm in a defensive move against a blow from a nightstick). These fractures are usually stable and can be managed with immobilization in a long arm cast (see Chapters 32 and 33). Fractures that are greater than 50% displaced or greater than 15° of angulation warrant surgical reduction. Patients with middle and distal third fractures are at an increased risk of malunion and other complications, and these injuries warrant close follow-up and prolonged immobilization.[28]

44.8.2.2 Galeazzi Fracture

A fracture of the middle or distal third of the radius associated with instability of the distal radial ulnar joint (DRUJ), usually due to a fall on an outstretched pronated hand. These are unstable injuries and require operative intervention for definitive treatment.[28]

44.8.2.3 Monteggia Fracture

A fracture of the proximal third of the ulna with a concomitant dislocation of the radial head and radiocapitellar joint.[66] The mechanism of injury is usually a forced pronation of the forearm on an outstretched hand or direct trauma to the dorsal ulna. Like the Galeazzi fracture, these injuries require operative treatment.[28]

44.8.2.4 Essex-Lopresti Fracture

A rare and complex injury to the forearm that consists of a radial head fracture, rupture of the interosseous membrane, and disruption of the DRUJ.[66] The mechanism of injury is a significant longitudinal force that causes impact of the radial head into the capitellum with rupture of the interosseous membrane. These injuries are often initially missed, due to the focus on the significant radial head fracture. Like all complex forearm injuries, definitive treatment will be operative.[23,25,28]

44.8.2.5 Compartment Syndrome

Two form of compartment syndrome that can affect the forearm. Acute, which is a medical emergency, is commonly associated with significant acute trauma and must be addressed as soon as possible after onset. The second type is a chronic compartment syndrome, the result of overuse, which can be more challenging to diagnose and treat. Acute compartment syndrome (ACS) is a rare but serious condition that can be potentially devastating if not diagnosed and treated in a timely manner. ACS can result from fractures, crush injuries, infection, and even iatrogenic reasons such as IV infiltration and improper casting. Early identification and treatment is associated with a decreased incidence of complications. The early warning sign include swelling, paresthesias, and pain out of proportion to the injury. Late symptoms include diminished pulses, pallor, and progressive neurologic deficits. Children may demonstrate an increased analgesic requirements and difficulty being consoled.[39,42] Clinicians need to maintain a high index of suspicion for this condition and involve surgeons early as the treatment is early fasciotomy.

Chronic exertional compartment syndrome is an exercise-related condition secondary to increased pressure in the muscular compartments. The exact etiology is unclear, and the patient typically presents with pain, pressure, paresthesias, and weakness of the muscles in the affected compartment. Not as common as lower extremity exertional compartment syndrome, this syndrome can be seen in motocross riders, gymnasts, and laborers and should be considered in patients who present with exertionally associated symptoms of increased compartmental pressure.[67]

Clinical Pearl

A pressure greater than 30 mmHg is clinically significant and urgent surgical consultation for possible fasciotomy is required.

44.8.3 Pediatric

44.8.3.1 Forearm Splints

Forearm splints are unique forearm overuse injuries most commonly seen in male gymnasts and associated with pommel horse training. The mechanism of injury is similar to shin splints, but, in this case, due to repetitive wrist extension and excessive strain on the origin of the extensor carpi ulnaris. The patients will present most commonly with forearm pain that is exacerbated with wrist extension. Radiographs, if obtained, will most likely be normal. Treatment includes short-term decrease in the inciting event as well as ice before and after practice and taping or counterforce bracing of the forearm. Upon diagnosis, athletes should develop a long-term program to increase wrist extensor strength and improvement of technique (Table 44.6).[49,64]

TABLE 44.6
SORT: Key Recommendations for Practice

Clinical Recommendation	Evidence Rating	References
A positive Tinel's sign has a 44%–75% sensitivity and a 48%–100% specificity for the diagnosis of a compressive ulnar neuropathy at the cubital tunnel.	C	[18]
The moving valgus stress test has a 100% sensitivity and a 75% specificity for diagnosing an ulnar collateral ligament tear.	C	[30,31]
Tenderness over the ulnar collateral ligament has a 81%–94% sensitivity and a 22% specificity for a tear.	C	[30]
Musculoskeletal ultrasound has a sensitivity of 64%–82% compared to MRI's 90%–100% for diagnosing elbow tendinopathy.	C	[77]
In the diagnosis of olecranon bursitis, bursal fluid analysis of WBC count >100,000 WBC/μL is consistent with septic bursitis.	C	[1,6,33,67]
Multiple trials and systematic reviews have found that glucocorticoid injection for lateral epicondylitis improves many short-term (6 weeks) outcome measures but does not prevent recurrence and may lead to worse long-term outcomes.	B	[16,28,35,48,50]

REFERENCES

1. Aaron DL, Patel A, Kayiaros S et al. Four common types of bursitis: Diagnosis and management. *Journal of the American Academy of Orthopaedic Surgeons.* 2011;19(6):359–367.
2. Adla DN, Stanley D. Primary elbow osteoarthritis: An updated review. *Shoulder & Elbow.* 2011:3;41–48.
3. Anderson RJ, Todd DJ. Bursitis, An overview of clinical manifestations, diagnosis and management. www.uptodate.com. Accessed July 17, 2014.
4. Atanda A, Shah SA, O'Brien K. Osteochondrosis: Common causes of pain in growing bones. *American Family Physician.* 2011;83(3):285–291.
5. Bain GI, Durrant AW. Sports-related injuries of the biceps and triceps. *Clinics in Sports Medicine.* 2010;29(4):555–576.
6. Baumbach SF, Lobo CM, Badyine I et al. Prepatellar and olecranon bursitis: Literature review and development of a treatment algorithm. *Archives of Orthopaedic and Trauma Surgery.* 2014:134(3); 359–370.
7. Beaver C, Price DE, Jones RL. Triceps tendinitis. In: Bracker MD, ed., *The 5-Minute Sports Medicine Consult*, 2nd edn. Philadelphia, PA: Lippincott Williams & Wilkins; 2011.
8. Bell S. Elbow and arm pain. In: Brukner P and Khan K, eds. *Clinical Sports Medicine*, 3rd edn. Sydney, Australia: McGraw-Hill, 2006:302–303.
9. Browner EA. Nursemaid's elbow (annular ligament displacement). *Pediatrics in Review.* 2013;34:366–368.
10. Bryce CD, Armstrong AD. Anatomy and biomechanics of the elbow. *Orthopedic Clinics of North America.* 2008;39:141–154.
11. Cain EL, Dugas JR, Wolf RS et al. Elbow injuries in throwing athletes: A current concepts review. *The American Journal of Sports Medicine.* 2003:31;621–635.
12. Campbell WW, Landau ME. Controversial entrapment neuropathies. *Neurosurgery Clinics of North America.* 2008; 19:597–608.
13. Cass S. Upper extremity nerve entrapment syndromes in sports: An update. *Current Sports Medicine Reports.* 2014;13(1): 16–21.
14. Cheng CJ, Mackinnon-Patterson B, Beck JL et al. Scratch collapse test for evaluation of carpal and cubital tunnel syndrome. *Journal of Hand Surgery.* 2008;33A:1518–1524.
15. Christiani AK, Wallis D. Trigger point injection. In: Pfenninger JL, ed. *The Clinical Atlas of Office Procedures Joint Injection Techniques.* Philadelphia, PA: Saunders; 2002.
16. Coombes, BK, Blisset L, Vicenzino B. Efficacy and safety of corticosteroid injections and other injections for management of tendinopathy: A systemic review of randomized controlled trials. *Lancet.* 2010;376:1751–1767.
17. Crowther M. Elbow pain in pediatrics. *Current Reviews in Musculoskeletal Medicine.* 2009;2:83–87.
18. Cummines CA, Schneider DS. Peripheral nerve injuries in baseball players. *Neurologic Clinics.* 2008;26:195–215.
19. Delo M. Ulnar collateral ligament injuries of the elbow. In: Bracker MD, ed. *The 5-Minute Sports Medicine Consult*, 2nd edn. Philadelphia, PA: Kluwer, Wolter; 2011, pp. 616–617.
20. Dodds SD, Yeh PC, Slade JF. Essex-Lopresti injuries. *Hand Clinics.* 2008;24:125–137.
21. Draghi F, Bortolotto. Intersection syndrome: Ultrasound imaging. *Skeletal Radiology.* 2014;43:283–187.
22. Edwards H and Smith D. Sideline assessment and return-to-play decision making for an acute elbow ulnar collateral ligament sprain. *International Journal of Sports Physical Therapy.* 2013;8(2):212–215.
23. Eiff MP, Hatch RL, Calmbach WL. *Fracture Management for Primary Care*, 2nd edn. Philadelphia, PA: Saunders; 2003.
24. Ellenbecker TS, Pieczynski TE, and Davies GJ. Rehabilitation of the elbow following sports injury. *Clinics in Sports Medicine.* 2010;29(1):33–60.
25. Falcon-Chevere JL, Mathew D, Cabanas JG et al. Management and treatment of elbow and forearm injuries. *Emergency Medicine Clinics of North America.* 2010;28:756–787.
26. Freehill MT, Safran MR. Diagnosis and management of ulnar collateral ligament injuries in throwers. *Current Sports Medicine Reports.* 2011;10(5):271–278.
27. Garg R, Adamson GJ, Dawson PA et al. A prospective randomized study comparing a forearm strap braces versus a wrist splint for the treatment of lateral epicondylitis. *Journal of Shoulder and Elbow Surgery.* 2010;19:508–512.
28. Green S, Buchbinder R, Barnsley L et al. Nonsteroidal anti-inflammatory drugs (NSAIDs) for treating lateral elbow pain in adults. *Cochrane Database of Systematic Reviews.* 2001; (4):CD003686.
29. Greiwe RW, Saifi C, Ahmad CS. Pediatric sports elbow injuries. *Clinics in Sports Medicine.* 2010;29:677–703.
30. Hariri S and McAdams TR. Nerve injuries about the elbow. *Clinics in Sports Medicine.* 2010;29:655–675.
31. Hariri S, Safran MS. Ulnar collateral ligament injury to the overhead athlete. *Clinics in Sports Medicine.* 2010;29:619–644.
32. Hauser RA, Hauser MA, Baird NM. Evidence-based use of dextrose prolotherapy for musculoskeletal pain: A scientific literature review. *Journal of Prolotherapy.* 2011;3(4):765–789.
33. Herrera FA and Meals RA. Chronic olecranon bursitis. *Journal of Hand Surgery.* 2011;36(4):708–709; quiz 710.
34. Heuter CL, Giuffre BM. Overuse and Traumatic Injuries of the Elbow. *Magnetic Resonance Imaging Clinics of North America.* 2009;17:617–638.
35. Hong CZ, Long HA, Kanakamedala RV et al. Splinting and local steroid injection for the treatment of ulnar neuropathy at the elbow: Clinical and electrophysiological evaluation. *Archives of Physical Medicine and Rehabilitation.* 1996:77(6);573–577.
36. Howard TM, Shaw JL, Phillips J. Physical examination of the elbow. In: Seidenberg PH and Beutler AI, eds. *The Sports Medicine Resource Manual* Philadelphia, PA: Saunders, 2008.
37. Johnson GW, Cadwallader K, Scheffel SB. Treatment of lateral epicondylitis. *American Family Physician.* 2007;76:843–850.
38. Kane SF, Lynch JH, Taylor JC. Evaluation of elbow pain in adults *American Family Physician.* 2015;89(8):649–657.
39. Kanj WW, Gunderson MA, Carrigan RB et al. Acute compartment syndrome of the upper extremity in children; diagnosis, management, and outcomes. *Journal of Children's Orthopaedics.* 2013;7:225–233.
40. Kaw P, Deu R. Radial tunnel syndrome. In: Bracker MD, ed. *The 5-Minute Sports Medicine Consult*, 2nd edn. Philadelphia, PA: Kluwer, Wolter; 2011, pp. 502–503.
41. Kramer DE. Elbow Pain and injury in young athletes. *Journal of Pediatric Orthopaedics.* 2010;30:S7–S12.
42. Lavallee ME, Sears K, Corrigan A. The evaluation and treatment of elbow injuries. *Primary Care: Clinics in Office Practice.* 2013;40:407–429.
43. Lockman L. Treating nonseptic olecranon bursitis: A 3-step technique. *Canadian Family Physician.* 2010;56:1157.
44. Mariscalco MW, Salmon P. Upper extremity injuries in the adolescent athlete. *Sports Medicine and Arthroscopy Review.* 2011;19:17–26.

45. Mathison DJ, Agrewal D. General principles of fracture management: Fracture patterns and description in children. www.uptodate.com. Accessed July 17, 2014.
46. Maxwell DM. Nonseptic olecranon bursitis management. *Canadian Family Physician.* 2011;57:21.
47. McCall BR, Cain EL. Diagnosis, treatment, and rehabilitation of the thrower's elbow. *Current Sports Medicine Reports.* 2005;4:249–254.
48. McCallum SD, Paoloni JA, Murrell GA. Five-year prospective comparison study of topical glyceryl trinitrate treatment of chronic lateral epicondylosis at the elbow. *British Journal of Sports Medicine.* 2011:45(5):416–420.
49. Montechiarello S, Miozzi F, D'Amborosio I et al. The intersection syndrome: Ultrasound findings and their diagnostic value. *Journal of Ultrasound.* 2010:13;70–73.
50. Moraes VY, Lenza M, Tamaoki MJ et al. Platelet-rich therapies for musculoskeletal soft tissue injuries. *Cochrane Database of Systematic Reviews.* 2013;12:CD010071.
51. Neal SL, Fields KB. Peripheral nerve entrapment and injury in the upper extremity. *American Family Physician.* 2010;81:147–151.
52. O'Connor FG et al. In: Lillegard WA et al., eds. *Handbook of Sports Medicine: A Symptom-Oriented Approach*, 2nd ed. Boston, MA: Butterworth-Heinemann; 1999, pp. 141–157.
53. Presciutti A, Rodner CM. Pronator syndrome. *Journal of Hand Surgery.* 2011;36A:907–910.
54. Rahman RK, Leving WN, Ahmad CS. Elbow medial collateral ligament injuries. *Current Reviews in Musculoskeletal Medicine.* 2008;1:197–204.
55. Rinkel WD, Schreuders TA, Koes BW et al. Current evidence for effectiveness of interventions for cubital tunnel syndrome, radial tunnel syndrome, instability, or bursitis of the elbow: A systematic review. *The Clinical Journal of Pain.* 2013;29(12):1087–1096.
56. Rodner CM, Tinsley BA, O'Malley MP. Pronator syndrome and anterior interosseous nerve syndrome. *Journal of the American Academy of Orthopaedic Surgeons.* 2013; 21(5):268–275.
57. Rosenberg J, Phipps TA. Cubital tunnel syndrome. In: Bracker MD, ed. *The 5-Minute Sports Medicine Consult*, 2nd edn. Philadelphia, PA: Kluwer, Wolter; 2011, pp. 106–107.
58. Ruchelsman DE, Christoforou D, Jupiter JB. Fracture of the radial head and neck. *Journal of Bone and Joint Surgery.* 2013;95:469–478.
59. Rudloe TF, Schutzman S, Lee LK et al. No longer "Nursemaids's" elbow mechanisms, caregivers and prevention. *Pediatric Emergency Care.* 2012;28(8):771–774.
60. Rutkove SB. Overview of upper extremity peripheral nerve syndromes. www.uptodate.com. Accessed July 17, 2014.
61. Ryan LM. Evaluation and management of supracondylar fractures in children. www.uptpdate.com. Accessed July 17, 2014.
62. Schweich P. Distal forearm fractures in children: Initial management. www.uptodate.com. Accessed July 17, 2014.
63. Scott A, Ashe MC. Common tendonopathies in the upper and lower extremities. *Current Sports Medicine Reports.* 2006;5:233–241.
64. Servi JT. Wrist pain from overuse: Detecting and relieving intersection syndrome. *Physician and Sportsmedicine.* 1997:25(12):41–44.
65. Shapiro BE, Preston DC. Entrapment and compressive neuropathies. *Medical Clinics of North America.* 2009;93:285–315.
66. Sheehan SE, Dyer GS, Sodickson AD et al. Traumatic elbow injuries: What the orthopedic surgeon wants to know. *RadioGraphics* 2013;33:869–888.
67. Shell D, Perkins R, Cosgarea A. Septic olecranon bursitis: Recognition and treatment. *Journal of the American Board of Family Practice.* 1995;8(3):217–220.
68. Slabaugh MA. Radial head and neck fractures in adults. www.uptodate.com. Accessed July 18, 2014.
69. Slabaugh MA. Elbow injuries. In: Seidenberg PH and Beutler AI, eds. *The Sports Medicine Resource Manual.* Philadelphia, PA: Saunders; 2008, pp. 226–232.
70. Stevens KJ, McNally EG. Magnetic resonance imaging of the elbow in athletes. *Clinics in Sports Medicine.* 2010;29(4):521–553.
71. Sutton KM, Dodds SD, Ahmad CS et al. Surgical treatment of distal biceps rupture. *Journal of the American Academy of Orthopaedic Surgeons.* 2010;18(3):139–148.
72. Thompson JC. *Netter's Concise Orthopaedic Anatomy*, 2nd edn. Philadelphia, PA: Saunders; 2010, pp. 127–130.
73. Tom JA, Kumar NS, Cerynik DL et al. Diagnosis and treatment of triceps tendon injuries: A review of the literature. *Clinical Journal of Sport Medicine.* 2014;24:197–204.
74. Torralba KD, Quismorio FP. Soft tissue infections. *Rheumatic Disease Clinics of North America.* 2009;35(1):45–62.
75. Van Hofwegen C, Baker CL, Baker CL. Epicondylitis in the athlete's elbow. *Clinics in Sports Medicine.* 2010;29:577–597.
76. Vidal AF, Drakos MC, Allen AA. Biceps tendon and triceps tendon injuries. *Clinics in Sports Medicine.* 2004; 23(4):707–722,xi.
77. Walz DM, Newman JS, Konin GP et al. Epicondylitis: Pathogenesis, imaging, and treatment. *Radiographics* 2010; 30:167–184.
78. Wenzke DR. MR imaging of the elbow in the injured athlete. *Radiologic Clinics of North America.* 2013;51:195–213.
79. Willick SE, DeLuigi AJ, Taskaynatan M et al. Bilateral chronic exertional compartment syndrome of the forearm: A case report and review of the literature. *Current Sports Medicine Reports.* 2013;12(3):170–174.
80. Young CC, Porter E. Medial epicondylitis. In: Bracker MD, ed. *The 5-Minute Sports Medicine Consult*, 2nd edn. Philadelphia, PA: Kluwer Wolter, 2011:378–379.
81. Young CC, Walrod B. Lateral epicondylitis. In: Bracker MD, ed. *The 5-Minute Sports Medicine Consult*, 2nd edn. Philadelphia, PA: Kluwer Wolter; 2011, pp. 356–357.

45 Hand Injuries

Yaowen Eliot Hu, Fred H. Brennan, Jr., and Thomas Howard

CONTENTS

TABLE 45.1
Key Clinical Considerations

1. Flexor tendon injuries are usually treated surgically, while extensor tendon injuries are usually treated conservatively.
2. A high index of suspicion must be maintained for avulsion of the central slip as delayed diagnosis may lead to a boutonnière deformity.
3. Gamekeeper's thumb associated with a Stener lesion is at risk for poor healing and should be referred to orthopedics.
4. Flexor or extensor tendon lacerations should be referred to orthopedics within 48 hours.
5. If reduction of a dislocation is unsuccessful after two attempts, it should be splinted and referred to orthopedics.
6. Subungual hematomas involving >50% of the nail bed should be repaired surgically. Subungual hematomas involving <50% may be drained for comfort.
7. As a general rule, open reduction and internal fixation are generally considered if a fracture involves more than 25%–30% of an articular surface or if significant angulation, displacement, or rotation is present that cannot be reduced and maintained by closed manipulation and immobilization.

45.1 INTRODUCTION

Its high physical profile and large range of functional activities make the hand susceptible to a wide variety of sports-related trauma. The true incidence of hand injuries in athletes is difficult to determine because many athletes either ignore the injury or continue to play with a splint. McGrew et al.[15] reported that 11% of 1286 injuries in a primary care sports medicine setting were to the fingers and hand, but this statistic still underestimates the frequency of hand injuries in the pediatric population. Regardless of the patient's level of proficiency or age, all hand injuries require a careful medical evaluation, including appropriate x-rays. Even common abrasions and contusions should not be quickly dismissed as trivial. Local swelling, ecchymosis, and tenderness may indicate a more serious injury to underlying structures. Important treatment is delayed without early accurate assessment. A relatively simple problem requiring a splint or cast for a successful outcome may progress to a chronic condition requiring complicated surgery that may fail to restore normal strength and mobility. Nonetheless, the competent primary care provider should be able to appropriately manage the majority of hand injuries and understand what needs to be referred (Table 45.1).

45.2 FUNCTIONAL ANATOMY

The nine finger flexors and the median nerve pass into the hand through the carpal tunnel beneath the transverse carpal ligament. The five profundus tendons pass through the superficialis tendons to the distal phalanx of each finger and thumb, and four superficial flexors insert on the middle phalanx of each finger (Figure 45.1). The flexors pass beneath a series of ligaments between the distal palmar crease and the distal interphalangeal (DIP) joint. These annular ligaments (A) and cruciate ligaments (C) create "pulleys" (A1–A5 and C1–C3) and prevent the tendons from bowstringing. Tendon repair in this flexor area is therefore often unrewarding due to adhesions that form between the lacerated tendon ends and these ligaments.

The volar plate is a thickened portion of the joint capsule on the volar aspect and is a static stabilizer against hyperextension forces. Disruption will lead to chronic instabilities if it is not allowed to heal in its proper anatomic position. The collateral ligaments afford medial and lateral stability and are at maximal tautness at 70° flexion for the metacarpophalangeal (MCP), 30° for the proximal interphalangeal (PIP), and 15° for the DIP. When the hand is immobilized for any length of time, the collateral ligaments will contract; therefore, these joints should be immobilized, flexed at the above angles (collaterals maximally lengthened) to prevent permanent contractures. When describing these collaterals for orientation, one can describe them as the radial or ulnar collateral.

The extensor tendons enter the dorsal extensor hood at the distal end of the metacarpals (MCs) (Figure 45.2). Distal to the sagittal fibers of the hood enter the transverse and oblique fibers from the interosseous and lumbrical muscles. These blend into the sides of the extensor hood over the proximal phalanx and flex the MCP joint by pulling on the extensor hood. The central portion of this extensor complex travels distally over the PIP joint and inserts into the proximal dorsal aspect of the middle phalanx to extend the PIP. The lateral bands continue radially and ulnarly and insert onto the proximal dorsal aspect of the distal phalanx to extend the DIP.

45.3 ANATOMICAL DIFFERENTIAL DIAGNOSIS

The differential diagnosis of hand pain in primary care is best approached in a systematic fashion with focus on both mechanism of injury and location of pain (see Table 45.2). Subsequent chapter sections will cover specific adult and pediatric injuries to the hand with a symptom-oriented anatomical approach. The special tests that are referenced in the evaluation of a specific disorder are described in Table 45.3. Indications for referral are summarized in Table 45.4.

45.4 ANTERIOR HAND INJURIES

45.4.1 Overuse

45.4.1.1 Trigger Finger

Trigger finger occurs in rowing, rock climbing, or any activity requiring repetitive finger flexion and is due to nonspecific flexor tenosynovitis from overdemand. It is most common in the flexor tendons of the thumb and middle and long fingers and involves an inflammatory and degenerative nodule on the flexor digitorum profundus (FDP) catching on the A1 pulley. Symptoms include difficulty straightening of the involved finger (triggering) especially in the morning and variable degrees of pain. On physical exam, the patient will have variable amounts of tenderness over flexor tendon sheath aggravated by active finger flexion or passive extension. There may also be a palpable nodule in flexor tendon sheath just proximal to the head of the MC. X-rays are not indicated with this injury.[12] Ultrasound may be helpful with dynamic evaluation of trigger finger.

Differential diagnoses include infectious flexor tenosynovitis, and treatment depends on the amount and duration of triggering. For early or no triggering, the finger is splinted at night. For triggering, the flexor tendon sheath may be injected with corticosteroid through a midlateral approach over the distal one-third of the proximal phalanx while the patient resists with active flexion. Injections may be repeated within 6–8 weeks and night splinting continued. Resistant cases may ultimately require surgery, which should be a consideration after one to two injections. Complications include infection from a nonsterile injection, and prevention of injury involves education of proper technique.

45.4.1.2 Flexor Tendinopathy and Tenosynovitis

Flexor digitorum tendinitis is more common in sports requiring repetitive pulling (e.g., rowing) or prolonged pressure on the palms (cycling). Flexor tenosynovitis is commonly seen

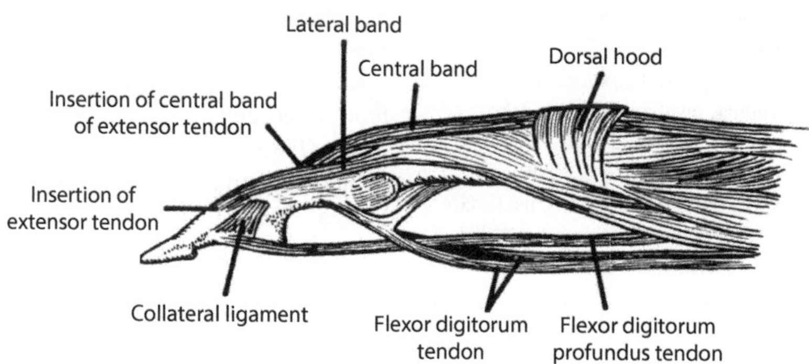

FIGURE 45.1 Lateral view of the flexor and extensor mechanism of the finger.

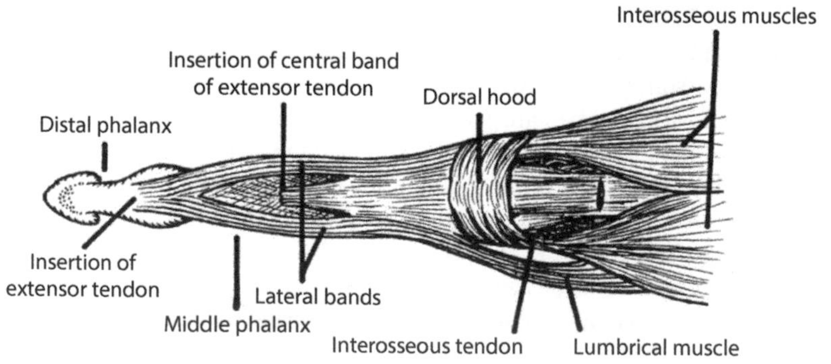

FIGURE 45.2 Dorsal view of the extensor mechanism of the finger.

TABLE 45.2
Common Hand Disorders in Primary Care: An Anatomical and Symptom-Oriented Approach to Differential Diagnosis

Anterior (Palmar)	Medial
Overuse	*Traumatic*
Trigger finger	Collateral ligament injury
Flexor tendinopathy and tenosynovitis	
Traumatic	
Jersey finger	
Flexor tendon laceration	
Subungual hematoma	
Distal phalangeal fracture	
Middle phalangeal fracture	
Proximal phalangeal fracture	
Metacarpal fracture	
Thumb carpometacarpal fracture dislocation	
Proximal interphalangeal volar dislocation	
Infectious flexor tenosynovitis	
Lateral	**Posterior (Dorsal)**
Traumatic	*Overuse*
Skier's/gamekeeper's thumb	Extensor tendinopathy and tenosynovitis
Collateral ligament injury	*Traumatic*
	Mallet finger
	Avulsion of the central slip
	Extensor tendon laceration
	Fingertip or nail laceration
	PIP fracture dislocation
	DIP joint dislocation
	PIP dorsal dislocation with volar plate rupture
	MCP dislocation
	Infectious extensor tenosynovitis

in overuse syndromes of the hand, and is frequently encountered in sports requiring repetitive gripping and pulling of the fingers. The mechanism of injury is the overuse (overdemand) or trauma of the tendons and their sheaths surrounding the hand. It is important to have a high suspicion in tenosynovitises that are not improving because flexor tenosynovitis may also have other causes such as psoriasis and atypical infections or may be idiopathic. In flexor digitorum tendonitis, the tendons pass through the carpal tunnel and can both mimic and cause carpal tunnel syndrome, including median nerve compression.

Symptoms include pain with active use or passive stretching of the involved tendon. Kanavel's four cardinal signs are helpful in diagnosing infectious flexor tenosynovitis. They include intense pain along the course of the tendon with any attempt to extend the partially flexed finger, flexion posturing of the finger for comfort, uniform swelling of the entire finger, and pain with percussion along the tendon sheath. Out of the four signs, the most important and the earliest sign is the pain along the tendon with extension. Tendinopathies can cause tendons to feel thickened or have a "rubbery" consistency when palpated. In flexor digitorum tendonitis, pain over the carpal tunnel is present, and limited mobility of the fingers and hypoesthesia in the median nerve distribution may be noted. Weakness of the thenar muscles and radial two lumbricals indicates motor damage to the median nerve.

X-rays are helpful and will rule out degenerative changes, avascular necrosis, and fracture. An oblique radiograph may reveal a calcific deposit along the tendon. Rheumatologic and infectious workup including blood tests may be required in flexor tenosynovitises that are resistant to treatment or recurrent despite multiple treatments. A three-phase bone scan can confirm active bony or soft-tissue inflammation of the involved tendon. Ultrasound or MRI may demonstrate edema of the tendon or fluid in the tendon sheaths.

Differential diagnoses include tendinitis, tenosynovitis, arthritis, chronic carpal instability, avascular necrosis, palmar space abscess, hematoma, or carpal tunnel syndrome. Treatment for flexor tendinitis is similar to that for flexor tenosynovitis. Initial treatment with rest, frequent icing, analgesics, ergonomic adjustments, and short-term splinting of the fingers is helpful in the acute setting for flexor tenosynovitises, but if flexor digitorum pain is resistant to conservative treatment or motor weakness is noted, a carpal tunnel release, synovectomy, or surgical debridement may be necessary. Treatment for flexor tendinitis or tenosynovitis may be augmented with a steroid injection directed into the calcific deposit or the tendon sheath. Complications include persistent pain with continued overdemand, and prevention of injury is through education of proper racquet holding and grip size, ergonomic assessment, and corrections.[1,14,16,18]

45.4.2 Traumatic

45.4.2.1 Jersey Finger (Football Finger)

Jersey finger is common in football, rugby, martial arts, or any sport where grabbing an opponent's clothing can occur. The mechanism of injury is a forced extension of the distal phalanx while actively flexing the DIP (e.g., athlete grabbing onto a jersey). It is caused by either a grade III tear or a bony avulsion fracture of the FDP tendon. An avulsion fracture of the volar lip of the distal phalanx limits retraction and enables repair by open reduction and internal fixation (ORIF). A large avulsion fragment will limit retraction to the A4 pulley (type III). Pure tendon avulsions may retract to the PIP at the A2 pulley (type II) or palm (typc III). If retracted to the palm, the blood supply via the vincula brevum and longum is compromised. Buscemi and Page[4] recommend the addition of a type VI injury in cases of tendon avulsion with a separate intra-articular fracture of the distal phalanx.[19] Symptoms include pain and swelling at the DIP, and the patient will be unable to flex the isolated DIP with localized tenderness at the level of retraction of the avulsed segment. The FDP is examined

TABLE 45.3
Hand Special Tests

Test	How It Is Performed	Positive Findings	Suggested Diagnosis
Tuning fork test	A vibrating tuning fork is placed over the affected bone.	Pain on the bony area.	Fracture of the bone
Trigger finger test	Active finger flexion or passive extension of the MCP joint.	Pain with possibly a palpable nodule in flexor tendon sheath just proximal to the head of the MC.	Trigger finger
Flexor tendon stress test	Resisted flexion of the finger flexor at the DIP, PIP, and MCP.	Pain and inability to flex the finger at the tested joint.	Jersey finger or flexor tendon laceration
Extensor tendon stress Test	Resisted extension of the finger extensor at the DIP, PIP, and MCP.	Pain and inability to extend the finger at the tested joint.	Mallet finger or extensor tendon laceration
Thumb UCL stress test	The first MC is stabilized with one hand and a valgus stress is placed on the MCP with the MCP in full flexion. Testing is done in full flexion because with extension or slight flexion, the normally taut volar plate gives the MCP stability.	Complete rupture (type 4) is suspected if angulation is 15° greater than the normal thumb or absolute angulation is greater than 35°. Angulation less than described previously is type 3 and considered stable.	Skier's or gamekeeper's thumb
Finger collateral ligament stress test	Valgus and varus stress is placed on the collateral ligaments of the finger at the DIP, PIP, and MCP.	Pain and laxity.	Finger collateral ligament sprain or tear

TABLE 45.4
Indications for Referral

Diagnosis	When to Refer
Anterior	
Trigger finger	Failure of conservative therapy with persistent pain and locking.
Jersey finger, flexor tendon laceration	Referral is needed within 48 hours for lacerated tendon and for long-term treatment of jersey finger especially with an avulsion fracture of the volar lip of the distal phalanx limiting retraction.
Subungual hematoma	If the hematoma involves >50% of the nail bed.
Distal phalangeal fracture, middle phalangeal fracture, proximal phalangeal fracture, MC fracture, PIP palmar dislocation	If a fracture involves more than 25%–30% of an articular surface or if significant angulation, displacement, or rotation is present that cannot be reduced and maintained by closed manipulation and immobilization.
Bennett's fracture	Long-term treatment is a referral to orthopedics because these are unstable.
Posterior	
Mallet finger, extensor tendon laceration	Refer for mallet finger if more than 30% of joint space is involved and within 48 hours for tendon laceration.
Central slip avulsion	If there is an avulsion fragment that involves >1/3 of the joint.
Fingertip and nail laceration	Larger amputations (>1 cm), bony amputations, or nail lacerations involving the nail bed.
PIP fracture dislocation, DIP joint dislocation, PIP dorsal dislocation with volar plate rupture, MCP dislocation	If a fracture involves more than 25%–30% of an articular surface; if there is significant angulation, displacement, or rotation is present that cannot be reduced and maintained by closed manipulation and immobilization; or if there is volar plate rupture.
Medial	
Skier's/gamekeeper's thumb	Type 2 injury, type 4 injury, a displaced fracture with >2 mm displacement or a rotated fracture, or evidence of a Stener lesion.
Lateral	
Collateral ligament injury	Unstable injury with active ROM or obvious angulation.

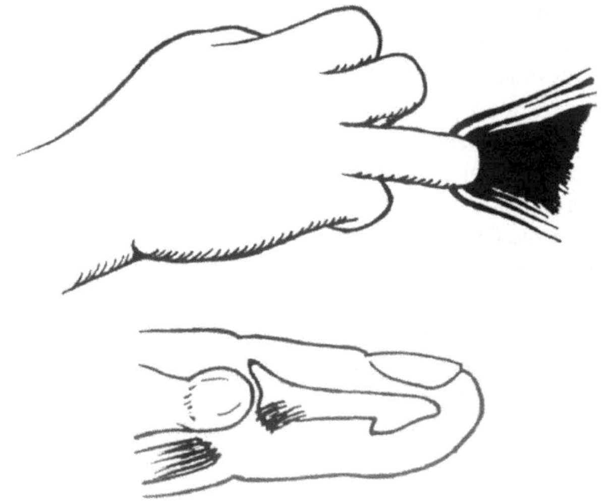

FIGURE 45.3 Mechanism of rupture of the flexor digitorum profundus tendon (jersey finger).

by holding the PIP straight and asking the athlete to flex the DIP. The superficialis is tested by holding the MCP straight and asking the athlete to flex the PIP. Imaging includes x-rays with posterior–anterior, lateral, and oblique views showing an avulsed fragment. This, along with ultrasound, may help to localize the level of retraction (see Figure 45.3).

Differential diagnoses include sprained DIP, collateral ligament tear, or a fracture of the distal phalanx. Initial treatment is RICE and analgesics as needed. For long-term treatment, a referral for surgical repair is advised. Type I injuries need a referral within 1 week, while types II and III require surgical referral within 3 weeks (beware that type II may convert to type III). If referral is delayed, reconstruction may be required rather than repair. Complications of the injury include permanent loss of flexion or reconstruction if the diagnosis is made late. Prevention of the injury is the education of proper technique.

45.4.2.2 Flexor Tendon Laceration

Flexor tendon lacerations occur in hockey, field hockey, lacrosse, or collision or contact sports. The flexor tendons course through an intricate system of pulleys and sheaths with the neurovascular bundle in close proximity. With this injury, there is bleeding, pain, and an inability to flex the affected finger. The patient presents with lacerations over flexor tendon. There is an inability to actively flex the DIP (profundus) or PIP (superficialis). Capillary refill may be delayed, and two-point discrimination will also be abnormal with concurrent neurovascular injury. X-rays may show an associated fracture.

Differential diagnoses include skin laceration, cellulitis, or flexor tenosynovitis. After thorough irrigation and debridement of wound, the skin may be closed loosely with interrupted 5–0 nylon and the wrist splinted dorsally in 45° flexion, with the MCPs 60°–80° and IPs slightly flexed. Patients should be referred to a hand surgeon within 48 hours. If diagnosis is delayed, the patient may require surgical reconstruction and the wound may become infected. Prevention of the injury is through education of proper technique and wearing protective gear.[16]

45.4.2.3 Subungual Hematoma

Subungual hematomas occur in collision or contact sports and are usually due to direct trauma. Crush injuries damage the nail and its underlying matrix and the resultant blood pools under the nail. Symptoms include bleeding and pain, and the patient will have bruising under the nail on physical exam. X-rays are important and will document any bone involvement because this injury may be associated with tuft fractures of the distal phalanx.[9]

Differential diagnosis includes a crush injury. Treatment depends on the percentage of hematoma involvement with the nail matrix. If there is <50% involvement of the nail bed, the hematoma may be drained using a heated paper clip, an 18 gauge needle, or an electrocautery device to create a hole in the nail to evacuate the hematoma. Anesthesia with a digital block may be needed prior to drainage. The finger should then be soaked in sterile water to facilitate drainage, and a sterile dressing should be applied. If there is an associated fracture, a stack splint should be applied. If the hematoma involves >50% of the nail bed, then the injury is presumed to be associated with an open fracture. Treatment involves x-rays, surgical removal of the nail, debridement of the wound, repair of the nail matrix, and replacement of the nail with splinting.[9,18] Complications usually involve cellulitis or deep space infections. Prevention of the injury is through education of proper technique and wearing protective equipment.

45.4.2.4 Distal Phalangeal Fracture

Distal phalangeal (DP) fractures occur in collision and contact sports, and the mechanism of injury is through compression or a crushing force. The fracture fragments of the DP are rarely displaced but result in extensive soft-tissue damage, including subungual hematomas and nail-bed injuries. Symptoms include pain and swelling of the distal phalanx, and patients will present with a subungual hematoma as the primary source of pain. Patients may also present with a disruption of the nail matrix. X-rays will generally show nondisplaced fracture fragments.

Differential diagnoses include soft-tissue injury or isolated subungual hematoma. Initial treatment is RICE and analgesics as needed. Long-term treatment includes using a protective splint for symptomatic relief rather than fracture stabilization. Subungual hematomas are drained. A disrupted nail matrix is repaired with 6-0 absorbable suture and the wound treated as a compound fracture.[3] Complications include a permanent nail deformity resulting from a disrupted nail matrix interposed between fracture fragments and delayed union of the fracture. Prevention of the injury involves wearing protective equipment and education of proper technique.

45.4.2.5 Middle Phalangeal Fracture

Middle phalanx fractures occur in collision or contact sports from direct trauma or twisting injuries. The fractures tend to be transverse, are generally angulated palmarily, and are often unstable due to the opposing forces of the dorsal extensor tendon and the flexor digitorum superficialis palmarily. Symptoms include pain and swelling, and the patient will present with tenderness and swelling over the middle phalanx with varying degrees of deformity. Rotational deformity should be evaluated on physical exam. X-rays are helpful in evaluating the degree of angulation or displacement.

Differential diagnoses include other soft-tissue injuries. Treatment initially is RICE and analgesics as needed. Long-term treatment depends on the stability, angulation, and displacement of the fracture. If the fracture is stable (reduction achieved and maintained), nondisplaced, and nonangulated, then buddy tape and use a thermoplastic splint for sport activity. For stable fractures with minimal angulation, these should be immobilized with the MCP flexed 70°, PIP flexed 45°, and DIP free, along with buddy taping to control rotation. The splint should be removed in 3–4 weeks and range-of-motion (ROM) exercises should be started; the splint should be worn during sporting activities for an additional 9–10 weeks. For unstable fractures (displaced, angulated, unable to hold reduction), referral to orthopedics is necessary.[3] Complications include rotational or angular deformity if mistreated initially. Prevention of the injury is through education of proper technique and wearing protective equipment.

45.4.2.6 Proximal Phalangeal Fractures

Fractures of the proximal phalanx usually occur in collision or contact sports and are due to direct trauma. Most fractures are spiral or oblique, tend to shorten, and are therefore unstable. These are difficult to treat due to the compact anatomy of extensor hood, lateral bands, and flexor tendons surrounding it. Scarring or displacement may disturb the tendon balance as well. Symptoms include pain, swelling, and variable degrees of deformity. On physical exam, the patient will have tenderness, swelling, and varying degrees of shortening, angulation, or rotation. A tuning fork test will also be positive. X-rays are useful and will reveal the type and extent of the injury.

Differential diagnoses include other soft-tissue injuries. Initial treatment includes RICE and analgesics as needed. Fracture stability and early ROM are critical to successful long-term treatment. For stable fractures, immobilize with the wrist in slight extension, MCP in 70° flexion, and PIP and DIP joints free, and buddy tape the injured finger to the adjacent finger for 3–4 weeks. Buddy taping is then continued until the patient is asymptomatic. For unstable (usual type) fractures, referral to orthopedics is necessary.[2,3] Complications include scarring, angulation, or shortening and result in poor tendon function. Prevention of injury is through education of proper technique and wearing protective equipment.

45.4.2.7 Metacarpal Fractures

Fifth MC neck fractures are common in boxing and martial arts, but MC fractures can occur in any contact or collision sport. The mechanism of injury is direct trauma from either an axial load or compressive forces. Neck fractures tend to angulate volarly to a significant degree. Shaft fractures are frequently stabilized by the intrinsic muscles; 60% are angulated >40°, and angulation up to 70° does not result in significant functional disability. The second and third digits are necessary for a power grip, and much less angulation (<10°) is acceptable here than for the fourth and fifth. Symptoms include pain and swelling, and there may be varying degrees of angular or rotational deformity on physical exam. X-rays confirm the fracture and are helpful in evaluating the degree of angulation and displacement.

Differential diagnoses include soft-tissue injuries and MCP dislocation. Initial treatment includes RICE and analgesics as needed. Long-term treatment requires reduction and splinting. For the reduction technique, the fracture site is anesthetized with hematoma block. The MCP is flexed 90°, and the direction and the force of the displacement and angulation are reversed. After reduction, the wrist is placed in a well-molded ulnar gutter splint incorporating the fourth and fifth fingers with the MCP flexed 70°. Postreduction x-rays should be obtained to confirm adequate reduction. The splint is worn for 4 weeks and early ROM exercises begun to prevent stiffness. Fifth MC neck fractures should be reduced to <30°, especially in boxers or baseball players who may have significant functional compromise with an angulation of 30°. Dorsal angulations <30° in fifth MC neck fractures demonstrate no significant loss in grip strength.[11] Second and third MC neck fractures should be reduced if angulated >10° and casted with the MCP at 70° for 4 weeks. MC shaft fractures should be immobilized with the adjacent finger, with the MCP flexed 70° and PIP slightly flexed. The splint is removed after 10 days and active ROM exercises begun. The splint is reapplied if the fracture site remains tender. Unstable fractures should be referred to orthopedics.[3] Complications include a higher risk of refracture in sports such as boxing or martial arts if the reduction is inadequate, cosmetic deformity with excess angulation, loss of power grip with second and third MC fracture angulation >20°, or pressure necrosis with "overtreatment" of fifth MC fractures. Prevention of the injury involves education of proper punching technique and wearing protective gear.

45.4.2.8 Thumb Carpometacarpal Fracture Dislocation (Bennett's Fracture)

Fracture dislocations of the first carpometacarpal (CMC) joint occur in collision or contact sports and are due to axial and abduction forces to the thumb. The anterior oblique CMC ligament holds the palmar fragment in its normal anatomic position. The abductor pollicis longus pulls the MC shaft fragment radially and dorsally. Symptoms include pain and swelling over the base of the thumb CMC, and the patient will have variable degrees of deformity over the thumb CMC on physical exam. X-rays with posterior–anterior, lateral, and oblique views will show the palmar fragment ranging in size from a small avulsion fracture to a large triangular fragment.

Differential diagnoses include scaphoid fracture, trapezium fracture, CMC dislocation, or soft-tissue injury. Initial treatment includes RICE and analgesics as needed. Long-term treatment is a referral to orthopedics because these are unstable. Complications include continued instability if the injury is not surgically reduced and fixed. Prevention of the injury includes education of proper technique and wearing protective gear.

45.4.2.9 PIP Palmar (Volar) Dislocation

Clinical Pearl

PIP palmar dislocation is associated with avulsion of the central slip.

Volar dislocations of the PIP joint occur in collision or contact sports and are caused by torsional or shearing stress applied to a semiflexed joint. The injury is often seen concurrently with an avulsion of the central slip. The torsional or shearing forces result in rupture of one collateral ligament from its proximal attachment and the central slip insertion, allowing the proximal phalangeal condyle to buttonhole through the torn extensor mechanism. The torn collateral ligament may become entrapped between the middle and proximal phalanges, preventing closed reduction. Symptoms include pain and swelling over the PIP, and the patient will have tenderness over the PIP, especially dorsally and on the side, along with varying degrees of angular or rotational deformity. X-rays with posterior–anterior, lateral, and oblique views will show volar displacement of the middle phalanx.

Differential diagnoses include collateral ligament tear, dorsal dislocation, volar plate rupture, or fracture. Initial treatment is RICE, splinting, and analgesics as needed. Long-term treatment involves reduction and splinting. Closed reduction may be attempted, but these injuries are frequently irreducible or unstable. If the reduction is successful and post-reduction films show normal congruence of joint surfaces, the treatment is the same as for central slip avulsions. Irreducible dislocations should be referred to orthopedics. Complications include an unstable joint due to soft-tissue interposition, and prevention of injury is through education of proper technique and wearing protective gear.

45.5 POSTERIOR HAND INJURIES

45.5.1 Traumatic

45.5.1.1 Mallet Finger

Mallet finger was originally described in baseball but can occur in any activity where the finger is subject to "jamming"; it is frequently missed initially, with subsequent deformity and medicolegal consequences. The mechanism of injury is an axial load against an actively extending finger. It can result in a dorsal bony avulsion or a grade III (complete disruption) injury to the extensor digitorum tendon. The patient may have pain at the DIP joint and exhibit an inability to extend the isolated DIP and tenderness over the dorsal proximal aspect of the distal phalanx. X-rays may show a bony avulsion from the dorsal proximal distal phalanx (seen in approximately 20%–30% of cases) (Figure 45.4).

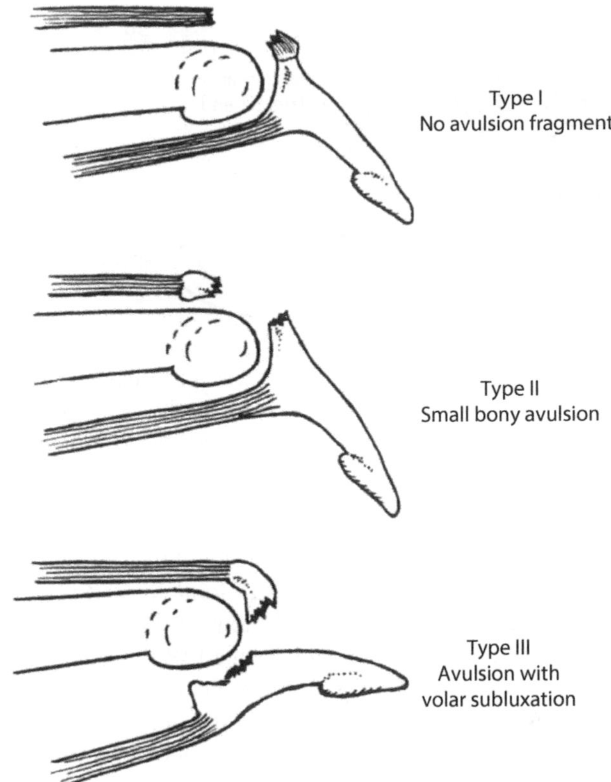

FIGURE 45.4 Types of rupture of extensor digitorum tendon at its insertion onto the proximal dorsal distal phalanx ("mallet" or "baseball" finger).

Differential diagnoses include finger sprain, DIP dislocation, collateral ligament tear, or fracture. Initial treatment includes RICE and analgesics as needed. Long-term treatment depends on whether or not there is an avulsion fracture. If there is no avulsion fracture, splint the DIP fully extended for 6–8 weeks straight and an additional 6–8 weeks if the patient is engaged in athletic activity; the splint should be worn 100% of the time, and, when removed for personal care, the DIP should be maintained in extension. If there is a bony avulsion, the dorsal finger splint should be worn in full extension for 4 weeks if less than 30% of joint space is involved; if more than 30% of joint space is involved, then refer for possible ORIF. Complications include permanent DIP extensor lag if untreated, and the patient may have pressure necrosis from the splint. Prevention of this injury is done with education of proper technique.[5]

Clinical Pearl

Flexor tendon injuries usually require surgery, but extensor tendon injuries are usually treated conservatively.

45.5.1.2 Central Slip Avulsion

Avulsion of the central slip commonly occurs in contact and collision sports. The mechanism of injury is a volar-directed force on the middle phalanx against a semiflexed finger

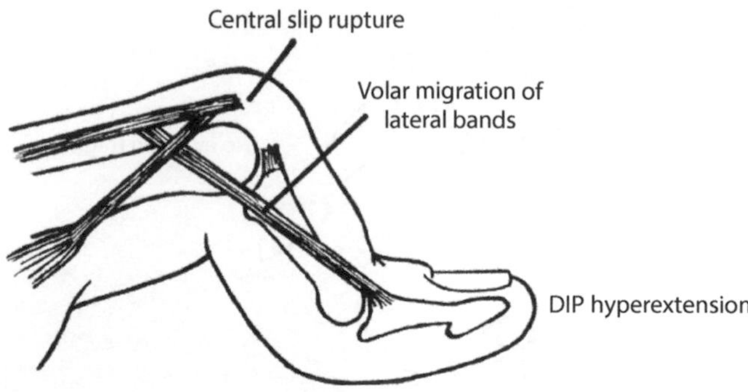

FIGURE 45.5 Central slip of the extensor mechanism rupture. Note the volar migration of the lateral bands leading to flexion of the proximal interphalangeal and extension of the distal interphalangeal ("boutonnière" deformity).

attempting to extend, and there may be volar dislocation of the PIP. The disruption of the central slip of the extensor digitorum communis tendon over the PIP joint allows for migration of the lateral bands volar to the axis of the joint. Patients present with pain and swelling over the PIP joint, and physical exam shows the PIP in 15°–30° of flexion with point tenderness over the dorsal lip of the middle phalanx. Early on, the patient may have limited extension, appearing stronger if extension is tested at 0° and weaker if tested at 30°. Later, there is an inability to actively extend the PIP with the DIP hyperextended ("boutonnière" deformity). X-rays may show an avulsion fracture at the dorsal base of the middle phalanx (see Figure 45.5).

Clinical Pearl

A high index of suspicion for avulsion of the central slip should be maintained as delayed diagnosis can lead to a boutonnière deformity.

Differential diagnoses include sprained finger, collateral ligament tear, and volar plate disruption, dislocation, or fracture. Treatment initially includes RICE and analgesics as needed. Long-term treatment includes splinting the PIP in full extension for 4–5 weeks and further protection during sporting activity for an additional 6–8 weeks. While splinted, the DIP should be allowed to flex to help relocate the lateral bands back to their normal position. If an avulsion fragment involves >1/3 of the joint, the patient should be referred for possible ORIF.[2,14] Complications include a "boutonnière" deformity if untreated. Prevention of this injury is through education of proper technique.[5]

45.5.1.3 Extensor Tendon Laceration

Lacerations of the extensor tendon occur in hockey, field hockey, lacrosse, or collision or contact sports. With this injury, PIP and DIP extension is still possible via the lumbricals and extensor juncturae tendinum if the MCP is flexed. Symptoms include bleeding, pain, and an inability to straighten finger. On physical exam, lacerations over the extensor tendon are observed (lacerated tendon edges may be visualized). There may be an inability to actively extend the PIP and DIP joints with the MCP in full extension. However, passive ROM is full. X-rays may show an associated fracture.

Differential diagnoses include superficial skin laceration and partial tendon laceration. Treatment for the injury involves debridement and irrigation of the wound. The wrist is splinted in extension with a volar splint to relax the tendon. Referral to surgery is required within 48 hours as these injuries may require surgical reconstruction with late diagnosis. Prevention of injury is through education of proper technique and wearing protective gear.

45.5.1.4 Fingertip or Nail Laceration

Fingertip or nail lacerations occur in collision or contact sports and are usually due to direct trauma. Lacerations may involve the nail and nail bed and include small avulsions of the pulp, larger pulp amputations, or bony amputations. Symptoms include bleeding and pain, and the patient will have lacerations, avulsions, or amputations on physical exam. X-rays are important and will document any bone involvement.

Differential diagnosis includes a crush injury. Treatment includes a protective dressing and analgesics as needed. Documentation of tetanus status is important, and dirty wounds may warrant coverage with a first-generation cephalosporin. For lacerations, irrigate and debride under digital nerve block, and close the wound with simple interrupted 5-0 nonabsorbable sutures. With small amputations (<1 cm), thoroughly irrigate and apply sterile dressing. Treatment of larger amputations is the same as small amputations but also requires immediate referral to a hand surgeon. In bony amputations, place the amputated part in a waterproof bag and then in ice water. Remember not to soak directly in ice water and refer immediately. With nail lacerations, trim or remove the nail. If the nail bed is involved, it must be repaired. The nail is removed and the nail bed is repaired using 5-0 or 6-0 absorbable sutures. Complications usually involve cellulitis or deep space infections. Prevention of the injury is through education of proper technique and wearing protective equipment.

45.5.1.5 PIP Fracture Dislocation

Fracture dislocations of the PIP occur in collision or contact sports and are caused by an axial load on a semiflexed finger. With the injury, the middle phalanx shears dorsally, impacting the palmar articular surface of the middle phalanx with the condyles of the proximal phalanx. Symptoms include pain and swelling over the PIP, and the patient will have a subtle dorsal prominence over the PIP with localized tenderness on physical exam. X-ray shows volar impaction fracture; the proximal aspect of the middle phalanx is dorsally displaced, and the palmar articular fragment is maintained palmarily.

Differential diagnoses include volar plate avulsion fracture, PIP dislocation, proximal or middle phalangeal fracture, or sprain. Initial treatment is RICE and analgesics as needed.

Long-term treatment if there is a small fragment without dislocation is to buddy tape. If there is a larger fragment but involves <40% of articular surface, then the treatment is closed reduction followed by extension block splint with the PIP in 30°–60° of flexion for 3 weeks. For fragments involving >40% of articular surface, surgical consultation for ORIF is required.[6,14] Complications include posttraumatic arthritis, and prevention is through education of proper technique and wearing protective equipment.

45.5.1.6 DIP Joint Dislocation

Dislocations of the DIP joint occur in collision or contact sports and are due to hyperextension, varus, or valgus forces. This is a rare injury due to the short lever arm of the distal phalanx and strong collateral ligaments. Often, dislocations are compound due to the dense cutaneous ligaments that anchor the overlying skin. Symptoms include pain and swelling over the DIP joint, and the patient will have dorsal or lateral angulation of the DIP joint on physical exam. X-rays will show the angulation and associated fractures.

Differential diagnoses include collateral ligament tear, DP fracture, sprain, mallet finger, or jersey finger. Initial treatment is RICE, splinting, and analgesics as needed. Long-term treatment involves reduction and splinting. The reduction technique is done after anesthesia with a digital block. The middle phalanx is stabilized with one hand, and the dorsal base of the distal phalanx is pushed into reduction. The finger postreduction should be splinted in slight flexion for 10–12 days. The rare irreducible dislocation should be referred for open reduction. Complications include joint stiffness if it is immobilized too long. Prevention of the injury involves education of proper technique.

45.5.1.7 PIP Dorsal Dislocation (Coach's Finger) with Volar Plate Rupture

Dorsal dislocation of the PIP joint occurs in collision or contact sports, and it is the most common dislocation of the hand and wrist.[15] Volar plate rupture at the PIP is common in volleyball, football, or any sport where the finger is subject to hyperextension and may be associated with a dorsal PIP dislocation. The mechanism of injury is a hyperextension injury with resultant disruption of the volar plate at its attachment to the middle phalanx, and there is loss of the volar stabilizing force, allowing the phalanx to ride dorsally on the proximal phalanx and producing a "bayonet" deformity while also allowing the extensor tendon to gradually pull the PIP into a hyperextension deformity (reverse or pseudo-boutonnière) over time. Symptoms include pain and swelling over the PIP, and patients will have a deformity and inability to move PIP on physical exam. With volar plate rupture, the PIP may present in varying degrees of hyperextension with maximal tenderness over the volar aspect; with active extension and flexion, the hyperextended PIP often "locks" in the extended position with an inability to initiate flexion. However, DIP ROM is normal. X-rays will reveal a dorsally displaced middle phalanx parallel to the proximal phalanx with some retraction, and in the case of volar plate rupture, x-rays may show an avulsion fragment at the base of the middle phalanx.

Differential diagnoses include collateral ligament tear, PIP fracture or dislocation, volar plate rupture, or sprain. Initial treatment is RICE, splinting, and analgesics as needed. If there is volar plate rupture, early active mobilization provides the best results. Long-term treatment requires reduction and splinting. The reduction technique is completed after anesthetizing the digit with an MC block. The middle phalanx is grasped with one hand, giving slight hyperextension of the PIP, and the other hand grasps the proximal phalanx and the thumb pushes the middle phalanx into reduction. Longitudinal traction of the middle phalanx may allow soft-tissue interposition into the PIP and should be avoided. The finger postreduction should be placed in a dorsal extension block splint with the PIP blocked at 20°–30° of flexion but allowed to flex for 3 weeks. The patient should be followed with buddy taping until symptoms resolve.[2,14] Surgery for volar plate rupture is indicated for PIP contracture. Complications include chronic dorsal instability if inadequately treated acutely and a hyperextension deformity with volar plate rupture (reverse boutonnière) if untreated. Prevention of the injury involves education of proper technique and wearing protective gear.

45.5.1.8 MCP Dislocation

Dislocations of the MCP occur in collision or contact sports and are due to torsional or shearing forces across the MCP. With simple dislocations, the volar plate remains attached and the proximal phalanx rests perpendicular to the MC. With complex dislocations, the MC head goes through the volar plate, creating a buttonhole effect, and rests between the lumbricals radially and long flexors ulnarly. Symptoms include pain, swelling, and stiffness at the MCP joint, and patients will exhibit variable degrees of deformity. In simple dislocations, the proximal phalanx is dorsally angulated 60°–90°, but complex dislocations are more subtle. The involved digit (usually the index finger) is slightly hyperextended and ulnar deviated, and there is dimpling on the palmar surface of the MCP. X-rays with lateral views will show a hyperextended MCP for simple dislocations. Posterior–anterior views for complex dislocation will show a widened joint space with asymmetric inclination of the proximal phalanx toward the more ulnar finger. Lateral views may show sesamoid interposition between the proximal phalanx and MC.

Differential diagnoses include traumatic dislocation of the extensor hood, fracture, or collateral ligament tear. Initial treatment is RICE, splinting, and analgesics as needed. For simple dislocations, the same technique as PIP dorsal dislocations is used. For complex dislocations, reduction may be attempted if injury is acute and if no swelling has occurred. If the deformity is exaggerated and the base of the proximal phalanx is pushed over the articular surface, no longitudinal traction is applied, as this will tighten the entrapment described previously. Once reduced, this dislocation is stable and the finger is buddy taped and early ROM begun. Complex dislocations are generally irreducible and should be referred to orthopedics. Complications include an unstable joint if not reduced, and prevention of injury is through education of proper technique and wearing protective gear.

Clinical Pearl

If after two attempts the reduction is unsuccessful, splint and refer to orthopedics.

45.6 MEDIAL AND LATERAL HAND INJURIES

45.6.1 Traumatic

45.6.1.1 Ulnar Collateral Ligament Tear/Strain ("Skier's" or "Gamekeeper's" Thumb)

Ulnar collateral ligament (UCL) rupture of the thumb, or "gamekeeper's thumb" or "skier's thumb," was initially observed in Scottish gamekeepers, who would kill hares by placing the thumb and index fingers around the neck to hyperextend it. This abduction force resulted in gradual weakening of the UCL and joint instability over time. The injury is now almost exclusively traumatically induced in sports such as skiing. The mechanism of injury is hyperabduction of the thumb MCP joint (e.g., the classic fall on a ski pole, causing the thumb to be held while the remainder of the hand plunges into the snow). There are four classes of UCL sprain. Type 1 is an avulsion fracture with no displacement. Type 2 is an avulsion fracture with displacement. Type 3 is a torn ligament that is stable in flexion. Type 4 is a torn ligament that is unstable in flexion.[13] Symptoms include pain over the UCL area, and patients may exhibit a weak and painful pinch (shown in Figure 45.6).

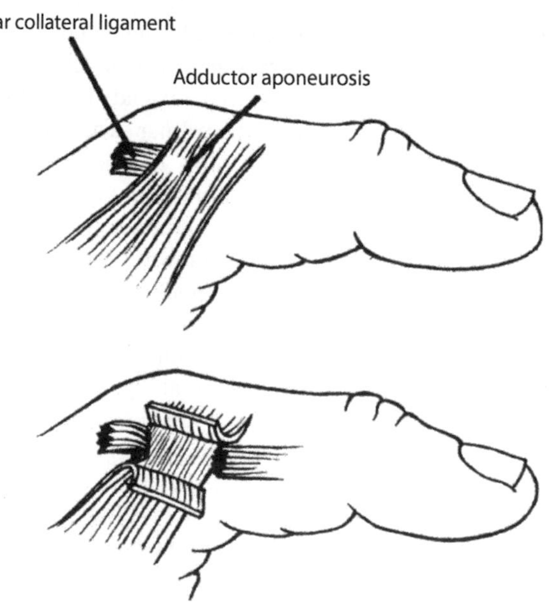

FIGURE 45.6 Ulnar collateral ligament (UCL) rupture, type 4. The free distal end of the UCL folds back on itself under or over the adductor aponeurosis, which prevents healing.

On physical exam, there is tenderness and swelling over the ulnar aspect of the thumb MCP. Stress testing should be performed if there is no evidence of avulsion fracture and is performed as follows:

1. The area is anesthetized with either a local block or median and radial nerve blocks at the wrist.
2. The thumb MC is stabilized with one hand and a valgus stress placed on the MCP with the MCP in full flexion. Testing is done in full flexion because with extension or slight flexion, the normally taut volar plate gives the MCP stability.
3. Complete rupture (type 4) is suspected if angulation is 15° greater than the normal thumb or absolute angulation is greater than 35°.
4. Angulation less than that described previously is type 3 and considered stable.

X-rays should be performed prior to any stress testing in order to reveal any avulsion fragment; if an avulsion fracture is evident, then stress testing should not be done. A displaced fracture with >2 mm displacement or a rotated fracture should be considered type 4. Ultrasound may be helpful with evaluation and MR arthrogram will show extravasation of dye in complete ruptures. MRI may be useful to diagnose Stener lesions or grade III tears. Sensitivities of 96% and specificity of 95% have been reported.[17]

Clinical Pearl

Stener lesions are at risk for delayed healing and should be referred to orthopedic surgery.

Differential diagnoses include dislocation, volar plate injury, sprain, or fracture. Initial treatment is RICE and analgesics as needed. Long-term treatment depends on the type of injury and is as follows:[8,10,18]

- Type 1—Thumb spica cast with MCP in full extension for 4 weeks
- Type 2—Refer for ORIF
- Type 3—Thumb spica cast with PIP free and MCP flexed 20° for 3 weeks
- Type 4—Refer for ORIF

Complications include loss of effective thumb apposition if inadequately treated. Prevention of injury involves proper technique and changing the grip of the ski pole into a sword-type grip.[7,8,10]

45.6.1.2 Collateral Ligament Tears

Collateral ligament tears occur often in collision and contact sports. These injuries result from valgus or varus stress to the PIP, DIP, or MCP and cause partial or complete tears of the ulnar or radial collateral ligaments. Symptoms include pain and swelling at the involved joint, and on physical exam, there is laxity with valgus or varus stress; the joint may be stable or unstable with active flexion and extension. X-rays may show avulsion fracture from capsular insertion, and ultrasound will show tears in the ligament.

Differential diagnoses include volar plate injury, flexor or extensor tendon strain, fracture, or dislocation. Initial treatment is RICE, splinting, and analgesics as needed. Long-term treatment if the injury is stable with active ROM is to buddy tape finger to finger adjacent to the side of the injury for 3 weeks. If the injury is unstable with active ROM or obvious angulation, then refer for possible surgical repair. Complications include an unstable joint if a complete tear is inadequately treated. Prevention of the injury involves education of proper technique.

45.7 SUMMARY OF THE HAND

The diverse function and complex structure of the hand and fingers make it a highly visible target in a wide variety of sports particularly basketball, football, wrestling, and gymnastics. The spectrum of trauma is vast, ranging from skin abrasions and contusions to displaced intra-articular fractures and complex ligamentous and tendon problems. Many of these injuries often appear trivial at the time of injury and yet may lead to considerable long-term impairment. The hand may also be prone to infections such as infectious flexor tenosynovitis, septic arthritis, and palmar space infections, requiring antibiotics and surgical interventions. A high degree of suspicion, clear understanding of anatomy and biomechanics, accurate evaluation, and early aggressive therapy including a comprehensive rehabilitation program will allow the competent primary care physician to maximize the functional outcome at the earliest possible time (Table 45.5).

TABLE 45.5
SORT: Key Recommendations for Practice

Clinical Recommendation	Evidence Rating	References
In a study of 190 patients with volar plate rupture, excellent or good results were achieved in 98% with early mobilization, independent of size or displacement of the volar fracture fragment.	B	[8]
For UCL injuries of the thumb, MRI may be useful to diagnose Stener lesions or grade III tears.	C	[17]
Dorsal angulations <30° in fifth MC neck fractures demonstrate no significant loss in grip strength.	B	[11]
X-rays are not required with trigger finger.	C	[12]

REFERENCES

1. Almekinders LC, Tao MA, Zarzour R. Playing hurt: Hand and wrist injuries and protected return to sport. *Sports Medicine and Arthroscopy Review*. 2014;22(1):66–70.
2. Bowers WH. Sprains and joint injuries in the hand. *Hand Clinics*. 1986;2:93.
3. Brunet ME, Haddad RJ. Fractures and dislocations of the metacarpals and phalanges. *Clinics in Sports Medicine*. 1986;5(4):773–781.
4. Buscemi MJ, Page BJ. Flexor digitorum profundus avulsions with associated distal phalanx fractures: A report of four cases and review of the literature. *The American Journal of Sports Medicine*. 1987;15(4):366–370.
5. Chauhan A, Jacobs B, Andoga A. et al. Extensor tendon injuries in athletes. *Sports Medicine and Arthroscopy Review*. 2014;22(1):45–55.
6. Culver JE, Anderson TE. Fractures of the hand and wrist in the athlete. *Clinics in Sports Medicine*. 1992;11(1):101–128.
7. Fassler PR. Fingertip injuries: Evaluation and treatment. *Journal of the American Academy of Orthopaedic Surgeons*. 1996;4(1):84–92.
8. Gaine WJ, Beardsmore J, Fahmy N. Early active mobilization of volar plate avulsion fractures. *Injury*. 1998; 29(8):589–591.
9. Idler RS, Manktelow RT, Lucas G et al. *The Hand Primary Care of Common Problems*. 2nd edn. New York: Churchill Livingstone; 1990.
10. Kahler DM, McCue FC. Metacarpophalangeal and proximal interphalangeal joint injuries of the hand including the thumb. *Clinics in Sports Medicine*. 1992;11(1):57–76.
11. Kanatli U, Kazimoglu C, Ugurlu M et al. Evaluation of functional results in conservatively treated boxer's fractures. *Acta Orthopaedica et Traumatologica Turcica*. 2002; 36(5):429–451.
12. Katzman BM, Steinberg DR, Bozentka DJ et al. Utility of obtaining radiographs in patients with trigger finger. *The American Journal of Orthopedics*. 1999;28(12):703–705.
13. Louis DS, Huebner JJ, Hankin FM. Rupture and displacement of the ulnar collateral ligament of the metacarpophalangeal joint of the thumb: preoperative diagnosis. *Journal of Bone and Joint Surgery*. 1986;68A(9):1320–1326.
14. McCue FC, Wooten L. Closed tendon injuries of the hand in athletics. *Clinics in Sports Medicine*. 1986;5:741–755.
15. McGrew C, Lillegard W, McKeag D et al. Profile of patient care in a primary care sports medicine fellowship. *Clinical Journal of Sport Medicine*. 1992;2:126–131.
16. Neumann JA, Leversedge FJ. Flexor tendon injuries in athletes. *Sports Medicine and Arthroscopy*. 2014;22(1):56–65.
17. Plancher KD, Ho CP, Cofield SS et al. Role of MR imaging in the management of "skier's thumb" injuries. *Magnetic Resonance Imaging Clinics of North America*. 1999; 7(1):73–84,viii.
18. Rettig AC. Closed tendon injuries of the hand and wrist in the athlete. *Clinics in Sports Medicine*. 1992;11(1):77–99.
19. Strickland JW. Management of flexor tendon injuries. *Orthopedic Clinics of North America*. 1983;14:827–846.

FURTHER READING

Almekinders, L.C. and Ruch, D., Hand and wrist injuries in sports medicine, *Sports Med Arthrosc.*, 22(1), 1, 2014.

Culver, J.E., Injuries of the hand and wrist, *Clin Sports Med.*, 11(1), 101–128, 1992.

Eiff, M.P., Hatch, R.L., and Calmbach, W.L., *Fracture Management for Primary Care*, Saunders, Philadelphia, PA, 1998, pp. 65–77.

Freiberg, M.R., Non-operative treatment of trigger fingers and thumbs, *J Hand Surg.*, 14A, 553–558, 1989.

Isani, A., Prevention and treatment of ligamentous sports injuries to the hand, *Sports Med.*, 9(1), 48–61, 1990.

McCue, F.C. and Meister, K., Common sports hand injuries: An overview of aetiology, management and prevention, *Sports Med.*, 15(4), 281–289, 1993.

Rettig, A.C., Ed., Hand and wrist injuries, *Clin Sports Med.*, 17(3), 401–406, 1998.

Szabo, R.M., Ed., Common hand problems, *Orthop Clin N Am.*, 23(1), 65–74, 1992.

46 Wrist Injuries

Yaowen Eliot Hu, Fred H. Brennan, Jr. and Thomas Howard

CONTENTS

TABLE 46.1
Key Clinical Considerations

1. De Quervain's syndrome has a high cure rate with a single corticosteroid injection.
2. A high index of suspicion must be maintained for scaphoid fractures as they may not be apparent on radiographs until weeks after the injury.
3. Electromyograms may be normal in 25% of patients with carpal tunnel syndrome.
4. A positive flick sign has the highest correlation to carpal tunnel syndrome.
5. Of all athletes, 9% of them under the age of 16 years sustained injuries of the wrist, and 90% of traumatic wrist injuries are secondary to falls where the wrist is dorsiflexed and resisting external forces or falling onto an outstretched hand.
6. MRI or MR arthrogram is the procedure of choice for carpal ligament tears.

46.1 INTRODUCTION

The wrist is a complex joint capable of motion in three planes. It provides the foundation for force transfer from the forearm and hand and postures the latter for fine motor activity and power grip. The wrist can sustain injury in a wide variety of sports and recreational activities in which weight bearing, twisting, throwing, and impact occur. Because of its diverse functional role, the wrist is particularly vulnerable to injury. Diagnosis and treatment of wrist trauma are especially complex due to its integrated multiple articulated anatomy. Nonetheless, a detailed understanding of anatomy, pathophysiology, and early diagnosis and treatment are crucial for the best possible outcome and maximal function. Long-term outcome is predicated on early diagnosis, treatment, and a sound rehabilitation program (Table 46.1).

46.2 FUNCTIONAL ANATOMY

Wrist motion is passive as no tendons originate from or insert into the carpal bones except for the sesamoid pisiform. The wrist bones are arranged in two rows, proximal and distal, with only the scaphoid bridging the two (Figure 46.1). Under compressive loads, this scaphoid bridge prevents the two rows from collapsing in a zigzag pattern. This same positioning also places the scaphoid and its surrounding ligaments at greatest risk of injury with compressive loads.

The volar aspect of the wrist is stabilized by a series of ligaments configured in a double inverted V pattern with the apices pointing toward the fingers (Figure 46.2). The more proximal V is formed by two intracapsular, extrinsic ligaments: the radiolunate and ulnolunate. The distal V is formed by two intracapsular and intrinsic ligaments: the capitoscaphoid ligament on the radial side and the capitotriquetral ligament on the ulnar side. A potential weak space exists between these two Vs and over the capitolunate articulation, called the "space of Poirier." This may be responsible for the perilunate instabilities in hyperextension injuries.

46.3 ANATOMICAL DIFFERENTIAL DIAGNOSIS

The differential diagnosis of wrist pain in primary care is best approached in a systematic fashion with focus on both mechanism of injury and location of pain (see Table 46.2). Subsequent chapter sections will cover specific adult and pediatric injuries to the wrist with a symptom-oriented anatomical approach. The special tests that are referenced in the evaluation of a specific disorder are described in Table 46.3. Indications for referral are summarized in Table 46.4.

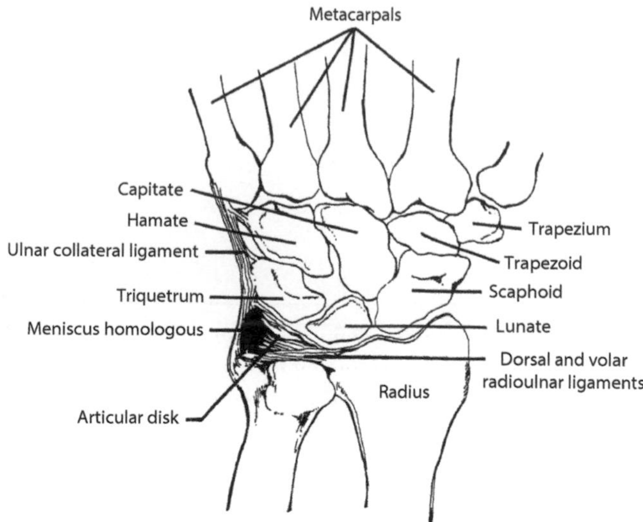

FIGURE 46.1 The carpal bones and the triangular fibrocartilage complex. The proximal row consists of the triquetrum, lunate, and scaphoid. The distal row comprises the hamate, capitate, trapezoid, and trapezium. The scaphoid bridges these two rows and is the only bone stabilizing the carpus; therefore, it is subject to injury.

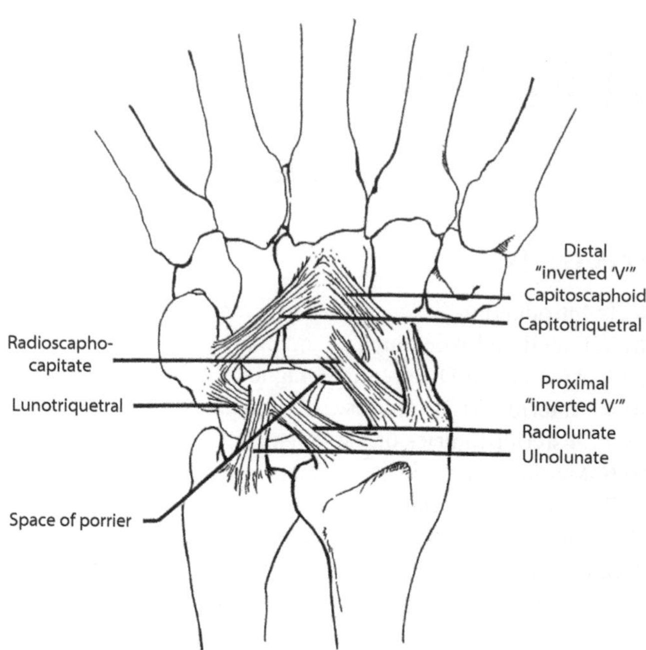

FIGURE 46.2 The stabilizing volar ligaments of the wrist.

46.4 ANTERIOR WRIST INJURIES

46.4.1 Overuse

46.4.1.1 Triangular Fibrocartilage Complex Injury

TFCC injuries occur in collision or contact sports, gymnastics, rodeo, parachuting, mountain climbing, or skiing and are due to dorsiflexion and rotation forces. The TFCC suspends the carpal bones from the radius, serves as a major stabilizer of the radio-ulnar joint, and functions as a cushion for ulnar axial loads (see Figure 46.1). It comprises a triangular fibrocartilage, a meniscus homolog, an articular disc, the ulnar collateral ligament, dorsal and volar radioulnar ligaments, and the extensor carpi ulnaris (ECU) sheath. Symptoms include pain with ulnar deviation of the wrist and variable amounts of swelling. Physical exam may reveal ulnar head instability manifested by dorsal subluxation of the ulna. Volar compression between the ulnar head and triquetrum may cause pain or crepitus. A painful clunk in the ulnar region may occur with passive supination or pronation of the wrist. The lift test involves having a patient lift himself or herself out of a chair by weight bearing with wrists extended. One study found this 100% sensitive for a TFCC tear.[14]

Plain radiographs in neutral position may show a fracture or ulnar subluxation (the ulnar styloid should be in the center of the ulnar head). Magnetic resonance imaging (MRI) is a reliable method for evaluating the TFCC because it obviates the need for a neutral wrist position. Arthrography is a good method to detect tears of the TFCC but can be difficult to interpret. An MR arthrogram may be the most sensitive noninvasive test to detect a TFCC injury. MR arthrogram is considered the most reliable and gold standard.[14]

Differential diagnoses include ulnar ligament instability, subluxation of ECU, fracture, or sprain. Initial treatment is

TABLE 46.2
Common Wrist Disorders in Primary Care: An Anatomical and Symptom-Oriented Approach to Differential Diagnosis

Anterior	**Medial**
Overuse	**Traumatic**
Triangular fibrocartilage complex tear	Ulnar collateral ligament injury
Flexor tendinopathy and tenosynovitis	Triquetrolunate dissociation
Carpal tunnel syndrome	Triquetrohamate dissociation
Guyon's canal syndrome	
Traumatic	
Scaphoid fracture	
Lunate fracture	
Hook of the hamate fracture	
Infectious flexor tenosynovitis	
Lateral	**Posterior**
Traumatic	**Overuse**
Radial collateral ligament injury	Extensor tendinopathy and tenosynovitis
Scapholunate dissociation	De Quervain's tenosynovitis
Perilunate dislocation	Intersection syndrome
Lunate dislocation	**Traumatic**
	Subluxation of the extensor carpi ulnaris
	Distal radioulnar joint instability
	Distal radius fracture
	Distal ulna fracture
	Infectious extensor tenosynovitis
	Pediatric
	Radial epiphysis injury

TABLE 46.3
Wrist Special Tests

Test	How It Is Performed	Positive Findings	Suggested Diagnosis
Lift test	Patient lifts himself or herself out of a chair by weight bearing with wrists extended.	Pain distal to the ulnar styloid on the volar side of the wrist	TFCC tear
TFCC grind test	Passive supination or pronation of the wrist with proximal loading force onto the ulna.	Pain distal to the ulnar styloid on the volar side of the wrist with possible painful clunk	TFCC tear
Flexor carpi radialis stress test	Resisted wrist flexion.	Volar radial wrist pain	Flexor carpi radialis tendinitis or tenosynovitis
Tinel's test	Tapping over the volar wrist over the carpal tunnel.	Wrist pain and numbness in radial 3.5 digits	CTS
Phalen's test	Shoulders abducted to 90°, elbow flexed to 90°, wrist flexed to 90° and pushing against the opposite wrist for 30–60 seconds.	Wrist pain and numbness in radial 3.5 digits	CTS
Finkelstein's test	The patient's thumb is grasped by the four fingers of the same hand, and a clenched fist is made. The patient then deviates the wrist ulnarly.	Significant pain over the radial aspect	De Quervain's syndrome
Watson's test	Patient's hand is placed in ulnar deviation and neutral. The examiner's thumb is on the scaphoid tuberosity pushing on the scaphoid in an attempt to keep it from becoming vertical as the patient radially deviates the hand.	Pain and/or a painful click over the scaphoid	Scapholunate dissociation
Lunotriquetral ballottement test	The lunate is stabilized with the examiner's thumb and index finger. With the other hand, the examiner grasps the patient's pisiform and triquetrum and moves them in a volar and dorsal direction.	Laxity, crepitus, and pain over the ulnar wrist	Triquetrolunate injury
Triquetrohamate stress test	With ulnar deviation and pronation of the wrist, palpate the triquetrum and the hamate.	Painful click over the ulnar wrist	Triquetrohamate instability

TABLE 46.4
Indications for Referral

Diagnosis	When to Refer
Anterior	
TFCC tear	Failure of conservative therapy with persistent pain
Flexor tendinitis and tenosynovitis	Failure of conservative therapy or motor weakness noted
Carpal tunnel syndrome	Failure of conservative therapy after 8–12 weeks or sooner if evidence of thenar muscle wasting is found
Guyon's canal syndrome	Failure of conservative therapy or motor loss noted
Scaphoid fracture	Fractures of the proximal third, displaced fractures, or those delayed in presentation (more than 2 weeks) due to high risk for AVN and nonunion
Lunate fracture	Displaced fracture
Hook of the hamate fracture	Displaced fragment
Posterior	
De Quervain's syndrome	After 4 months of symptoms and failure of two well-placed injections
Subluxation of the extensor carpi ulnaris	Failure of conservative treatment for 4 weeks
Medial	
Scapholunate dissociation and perilunate/lunate dislocations	Within 1 week of the injury
Lateral	
Triquetrohamate/triquetrolunate instability	Within 1–2 weeks of the injury

RICE, splinting, and analgesics as needed. Long-term treatment involves immobilizing for 6 weeks and reexamining. A corticosteroid injection may be attempted if pain persists after immobilization. Arthroscopy may be indicated if pain persists after these methods have failed. Depending on the location and extent of the tear, as well as the length of the ulnar, an ulnar shortening procedure may be advised.[14] Arthroscopic repair of 35 patients with TFCC injuries had a good outcome in 29 of 35 patients in a retrospective study.[12] Complications include persistent pain and clicking, and prevention of the injury involves education of proper technique.[14]

46.4.1.2 Flexor Tendinopathy and Tenosynovitis

Chronic tendon injuries or tendinopathies include tendinitis (inflammation of the tendon itself), tendinosis (degeneration of the tendon), and tenosynovitis (inflammation of the tendon sheath) and are caused by an overdemand of the involved tendon. The tendon responds first with inflammation and hemorrhage, followed by cellular invasion, collagen production, maturation, and strengthening. Tendinosis, with its degenerative tissue changes, occurs when chronic inflammation goes unresolved.[16] Furthermore, tendinosis causes pain that tends to only partially respond to conventional therapies.[4]

Flexor carpi radialis tendinitis is common in racquet sports. Flexor carpi ulnaris/pisiform tendinitis is the most common wrist flexor predisposed to tendinitis.[24] Flexor tenosynovitis is commonly seen in overuse syndromes of the wrist and is frequently encountered in sports requiring repetitive wrist acceleration and deceleration. The mechanism of injury is the overuse (overdemand) or trauma of the tendons and their sheaths surrounding the wrist. It is important to have a high suspicion in tenosynovitises that are not improving because flexor tenosynovitis may also have other causes such as psoriasis and atypical infections or may be idiopathic.

In flexor carpi radialis tendonitis, the flexor carpi radialis (FCR) tendon passes through a groove in the trapezium and passes near the scaphotrapezial and metacarpotrapezial joints as it approaches its insertion onto the volar surface of the second metacarpal. Inflammation in these joints may either cause or be caused by FCR inflammation. In flexor carpi ulnaris and pisiform tendonitis, the broad area of insertion into the pisiform and hypothenar fascia may cause vague pain anywhere from the forearm to the ulnar side of the hand, but it is usually well localized to the pisiform area. FCU tendon inflammation may irritate the nearby ulnar nerve, causing paresthesias.

Symptoms include pain with active use or passive stretching of the involved tendon. On physical exam, there will be volar radial wrist pain aggravated by resisted wrist flexion with flexor carpi radialis tendonitis. Moderate-to-marked swelling is observed over the pisiform in flexor carpi ulnaris tendinitis, with increased pain on medial and lateral movement of the pisiform. In flexor digitorum tendonitis, pain over the carpal tunnel is present, and limited mobility of the fingers and hypoesthesia in the median nerve distribution may be noted. Weakness of the thenar muscles and radial two lumbricals indicates motor damage to the median nerve. Tendinopathies can cause tendons to feel thickened or have a "rubbery" consistency when palpated. See Table 46.5 for more details.

X-rays are helpful and will rule out degenerative changes, avascular necrosis (AVN), and fracture. For flexor carpi ulnaris/pisiform tendinitis, an oblique radiograph may reveal a calcific deposit near the insertion of the FCU. Rheumatologic and infectious workup including blood tests may be required in flexor tenosynovitises that are resistant to treatment or recurrent despite multiple treatments. A three-phase bone scan can confirm active bony or soft tissue inflammation of the involved tendon. Ultrasound or MRI may demonstrate edema of the tendon or fluid in the tendon sheaths.

TABLE 46.5
Wrist Flexor and Extensor Tendinopathy and Tenosynovitis

Flexor carpi radialis	This is common in racquet sports due to overuse. Tenderness is noted over the scaphotrapezial and metacarpotrapezial joints and also along the tendon itself. The volar radial wrist pain is aggravated by resisted wrist flexion.
Flexor carpi ulnaris	This is the most common wrist flexor predisposed to tendinitis and results from overuse. Vague pain may be anywhere from the forearm to the ulnar side of the hand, but it is usually well localized to the pisiform area. Inflammation may also irritate the nearby ulnar nerve, causing paresthesias. Moderate-to-marked swelling is also observed over the pisiform with increased pain on medial and lateral movement of the pisiform.
De Quervain's syndrome	Tenderness and swelling are observed over the tendons lateral to the radial styloid. Finkelstein's test is positive and will result in significant pain over the radial aspect if the tendons are inflamed.
Intersection syndrome	Tenderness and swelling of the dorsolateral forearm are noted approximately 4–8 cm proximal to the wrist. There may be characteristic creaking of the wrist with extension of the wrist or palpable crepitus over the inflamed tendons.
Extensor carpi radialis brevis	Tenderness is localized over the second dorsal compartment on the dorsal radial aspect of the wrist.
EPL	Tenderness and swelling are noted over the EPL (third dorsal compartment).
Common extensor	Tender, erythematous "goosefoot" swelling can be observed over the middorsum of the wrist.
ECU	The close proximity of the ECU tendon to the TFCC makes differentiating between ECU tenosynovitis and old TFCC injuries as the source of pain more difficult. Local pain and tenderness may not be limited to the ECU tendon sheath in tenosynovitis.

Differential diagnoses include tendinitis, tenosynovitis, arthritis, chronic carpal instability, AVN, hematoma, or carpal tunnel syndrome (CTS). Treatment for flexor tendinitis is similar to that for flexor tenosynovitis. Initial treatment with rest, frequent icing, analgesics, ergonomic adjustments, and short-term splinting of the wrist is helpful in the acute setting for flexor tenosynovitises; but if the pain is resistant to conservative treatment or motor weakness is noted, surgical debridement may be necessary. Treatment for flexor carpi ulnaris/pisiform tendinitis may be augmented with a steroid injection directed into the calcific deposit or the tendon sheath. Complications include persistent pain with continued overdemand, and prevention of injury is through education of proper racquet holding and grip size, ergonomic assessment, and corrections.[3,15]

46.4.1.3 Median Nerve: Carpal Tunnel Syndrome

Clinical Pearl

The flick sign has 93% sensitivity and 96% specificity for ruling in CTS.

The median nerve at the level of the carpal tunnel contains the sensory branches to the radial 3.5 digits and a motor branch to the thenar eminence. CTS is more common with sports involving repetitive wrist motion, such as rowing and racquet sports. The mechanism of injury is swelling in the rigid tunnel compressing the median nerve, resulting in sensory and motor deficits. Symptoms include wrist pain and numbness in radial 3.5 digits, and on physical exam, Phalen's wrist flexion test reproduces symptoms, and Tinel's sign is positive in approximately 45% of cases. The flick sign where the patient feels the need to flick the wrist to relieve the pain has the highest correlation to CTS.[5] Decreased vibratory sensation in the radial 3.5 digits is the first neurologic finding, followed by decreased two-point discrimination. X-rays are usually not helpful; electromyograms may be normal in 25% of patients with CTS but are useful to exclude other etiologies of neurogenic wrist pain. Thyroid function tests including thyroid-stimulating hormone and diabetes screening should be done if indicated. Ultrasound or MRI of the carpal tunnel and median nerve has fair accuracy in assessing nerve health and degree of swelling.[9]

Differential diagnoses include median nerve entrapment at the elbow, CTS secondary to hypothyroidism or diabetes, flexor tendinitis, and double-crush injury associated with cervical radiculopathy. Treatment initially is conservative, consisting of splinting the wrist in 20°–30° of dorsiflexion (especially at night), NSAIDs, and relative rest of the wrist. For long-term treatment, a steroid injection may be given with persistent symptoms as follows. A long, 25-gauge needle is inserted just proximal to the distal flexion crease between the palmaris longus and flexor carpi radialis tendons, piercing the flexor retinaculum. If the needle insertion induces median nerve paresthesias, it must be withdrawn and redirected. Injections of 1 cc of 1% lidocaine and 1 cc of a steroid preparation are given. A single steroid injection of 15 mg of methylprednisolone acetate into the carpal tunnel was found to be more effective than a 10-day course of oral prednisolone up to 3 months after treatment.[23] Successful response to surgery may be predicted by positive response to injection.[6] Resistant cases should be referred for a possible carpal tunnel release if conservative measures have failed after 8–12 weeks or sooner if evidence of thenar muscle wasting is found. Complications include thenar atrophy and median nerve palsy. Prevention of the injury is through ergonomic assessment and correction of biomechanical factors.

46.4.1.4 Ulnar Nerve: Guyon's Canal Syndrome

The ulnar nerve traverses Guyon's canal between the pisiform and hamate and divides into a superficial terminal branch (supplying sensation to the ulnar palm, fifth digit, and ulnar side of the fourth digit) and a deep terminal branch (innervating the interossei, hypothenar muscles, lumbricals 3 and 4, adductor pollicis brevis, and the deep head of the flexor pollicis brevis). The deep terminal branch distal to the branch supplying the hypothenar muscles is most commonly affected. The second, less common, syndrome involves both the deep and superficial branches with compression proximal to Guyon's canal. The mechanism of injury involves chronic repetitive insults to the hypothenar area resulting in inflammation in Guyon's canal and ulnar nerve irritation. This injury is most common in cycling and weight lifting.

Symptoms include weakness of intrinsic muscles and/or paresthesias in ulnar 1.5 digits, and on physical exam, there is weakness in the interosseus, third and fourth lumbricals, adductor pollicis brevis, and flexor pollicis brevis with deep terminal ulnar nerve involvement (most common). The hypothenar muscles may be spared since the compression is usually distal to this nerve branch. Proximal Guyon's canal involvement results in weakness in all of the ulnar-innervated muscles plus numbness in the ulnar 1.5 digits. X-rays including carpal tunnel views should be done to assess for a hamate fracture or exostosis. Ultrasound and electrophysiologic studies help to localize the lesion.

Differential diagnoses include ulnar artery aneurysm and old hamate hook fracture. Treatment involves protective padding over the hypothenar area and NSAIDs. Resistant cases or cases with evidence of motor loss should be referred to an orthopedic surgeon. Complications include ulnar neuropathy with intrinsic muscle weakness, and prevention of the injury include wearing padded gloves while cycling or weight lifting and proper positioning of hands on the handlebars.[22]

46.4.2 Traumatic

46.4.2.1 Scaphoid Fracture

Of all carpal bone injuries, 70% are fractures of the scaphoid.[17] Scaphoid fractures are most common in contact and collision sports but can occur with any fall. The mechanism of injury is a forced dorsiflexion injury to the wrist, most commonly the result of a fall onto an outstretched hand (FOOSH). The scaphoid has a key stabilizing role as it bridges the proximal and distal carpal rows (see Figure 46.1). It is also vulnerable to AVN after a fracture due to its dependence on a single interosseous blood supply that enters distally and runs proximally. The more proximal the fracture, the more delayed the healing and the higher the risk of AVN. Fractures of the distal one-third average 8 weeks to heal, while waist fractures require 3 months. Fractures of the proximal one-third require 4 months or more to heal. Symptoms include pain, swelling, and limited range of motion. On physical exam, the patient will have tenderness and/or swelling in the anatomic "snuff box" formed by the tendons of the extensor pollicis brevis and abductor pollicis longus radially and the extensor pollicis longus (EPL) ulnarly. There is also limited range of motion and tenderness over the scaphoid tubercle.

X-rays are pivotal in the evaluation of a scaphoid fracture. A fracture line may be visualized with a scaphoid series done oblique with the wrist in ulnar deviation. If no fracture line is visualized on x-ray but clinical suspicion persists, the wrist should be immobilized in a thumb spica cast and repeat radiographs taken in 10 days to 2 weeks. Repeat x-rays may be needed at even 4 and 6 weeks if the patient remains symptomatic. However, if a more expedient diagnosis is desired, a bone scan will be positive within 72 hours of injury. A CT scan or MRI may also be used for immediate diagnosis if indicated.

Clinical Pearl

Scaphoid fractures may take weeks to appear on radiographs. A high index of suspicion must be maintained.

Differential diagnoses include scapholunate dissociation, lunate or perilunate dislocation, wrist sprain, or distal radius fracture. Treatment initially is RICE, thumb spica splinting, and analgesics as needed. For long-term treatment, nondisplaced scaphoid fractures can be treated in a long-arm thumb spica cast (with the metacarpal-phalangeal joints of the fingers included) for 6 weeks, followed by a short-arm thumb spica cast until radiographic evidence of healing is found.[7] Immobilization is then discontinued for activities of daily living and rehabilitation, but the wrist needs to be protected from impact loading for an additional 3 months.[7] An effective soft but rigid silastic cast as described by Bergfield is useful.[2] Fractures of the proximal third, displaced fractures, or those delayed in presentation (more than 2 weeks) are at high risk for AVN and nonunion and should be referred to an orthopedic surgeon. Complications include AVN with subsequent chronic pain and instability and nonunion. Prevention of injury is through education of proper technique and wearing protective equipment (e.g., wrist guards).

46.4.2.2 Lunate Fracture

The lunate is well protected in the radial fossa. Lunate fractures are rare and occur in contact and collision sports. The mechanism of injury is either a compressive force between the capitate and the distal radius causing a fracture through the lunate body or an avulsion injury resulting from traction of the ligaments at the extremes of motion.[13] Symptoms include pain, and on physical exam, the patient will have pain and swelling over the lunate in the dorsum of the wrist. X-rays may be helpful in evaluating lunate fractures, but a CT scan is needed for definitive diagnosis because the bony architecture of the lunate may be difficult to evaluate.

Differential diagnoses include scapholunate dissociation, carpal dislocation, distal radius or ulna fracture, tendinitis, tenosynovitis, or sprain. Treatment of nondisplaced fractures is immobilization for 6 weeks with a short-arm cast with the metacarpal-phalangeal (MCP) joints flexed to reduce the forces of gripping. Displaced fractures require open-reduction-internal-fixation in order to restore stability and to protect the blood supply. Immobilization after surgery is needed until healing is evident. Complications include fracture nonunion and development of AVN of the lunate (Kienbock's disease) if diagnosis is delayed.[1,13,18] Prevention of injury is through education of proper technique and wearing of a protective splint after healing.

46.4.2.3 Hook of the Hamate Fracture

Fractures of the hook of the hamate are more common in racquet sports and baseball and are due to trauma to the hypothenar area from a direct blow or from the proximal end of a racquet or baseball bat. The hook of the hamate forms the radial border of Guyon's canal and is vulnerable to fractures because of its perpendicular orientation to the rest of the carpal bones. Symptoms include pain and variable amounts of swelling over the hamate, and there will be tenderness over the palmar or dorsal hamate on physical exam. Routine views on x-ray are often normal, and supinated oblique and carpal tunnel views (Hart–Gaynor or supinated oblique projection) should be ordered to obtain the best views for evaluation. However, bone scans may be helpful if x-rays are negative, and a CT scan to better delineate the bony architecture should be ordered if the bone scan is positive.

Differential diagnoses include Guyon's canal syndrome, ulnar artery aneurysm, ulnar instability, and contusion. Initial treatment is RICE, splinting, and analgesics as needed. Long-term treatment for a stable, nondisplaced fracture includes initially immobilizing with the wrist in slight flexion, MCP of the ring and little finger flexed to 90°, and the base of thumb included.[17] Radiographic and/or tomographic surveillance should be done every 2 weeks to assure nondisplacement, anticipating 8–12 weeks of healing time. For a displaced fragment, referral to orthopedics is needed. Complications include nonunion for displaced fractures, and prevention of injury is through education of proper racquet handling technique and proper grips.

46.5 POSTERIOR INJURIES OF THE WRIST

46.5.1 Overuse

46.5.1.1 Extensor Tendinopathy and Tenosynovitis

Clinical Pearl

EPL rupture is associated with distal radius fractures.

Extensor tendinitis involves the extensor carpi radialis, ECU, extensor digitorum, extensor indices, or EPL and is common in racquet sports. De Quervain's syndrome is the most common of the tenosynovitises, and extensor carpi radialis brevis tenosynovitis is the second most common. Intersection syndrome is more common in athletes such as weight lifters and rowers. These injuries are commonly seen in overuse syndromes of the wrist and are frequently encountered in sports requiring repetitive wrist acceleration and deceleration. The mechanism of injury is the overuse (overdemand) or trauma of the tendons and their sheaths surrounding the wrist. It is important to have a high suspicion in tenosynovitises that are not improving because extensor tenosynovitis may also have other causes such as psoriasis and atypical infections or may be idiopathic.

In de Quervain's syndrome, the abductor pollicis longus and extensor pollicis brevis in the first dorsal compartment over the dorsal and radial aspect of the wrist are highly prone to tendinitis and tenosynovitis from repetitive wrist motion. Intersection syndrome is similar to de Quervain's disease but occurs more proximally, where the abductor pollicis longus and extensor pollicis brevis cross the radial wrist extensors.[24] Extensor carpi radialis brevis tenosynovitis involves inflammation of the second dorsal compartment on the dorsal radial aspect of the wrist. EPL tenosynovitis involves the third dorsal compartment. The EPL tendon passes through a narrow curved tunnel around Lister's tubercle at the middle of the radius. It is relatively thin there and is vulnerable to rupture if untreated, injected with a steroid, or associated with distal radius fracture. Common extensor tenosynovitis involves the extensor digitorum and extensor indicis tendons of the fourth compartment and ECU tenosynovitis involves the sixth dorsal compartment. Symptoms include pain with active use of involved tendon or passive stretching and variable degrees of swelling and erythema. Signs and findings on physical exam are as described in Table 46.5.

X-rays are helpful in ruling out underlying osseous pathology and may reveal soft tissue swelling. Rheumatologic and infectious workup including blood tests may be required in extensor tenosynovitises that are resistant to treatment or recurrent despite multiple treatments. For ECU tenosynovitis, an injection of the ECU tendon sheath with a local anesthetic may help differentiate tenosynovitis from TFCC pathology. Ultrasound is also helpful in evaluating the degree of swelling and inflammation in the tendon.

Differential diagnoses include tendinitis, tenosynovitis, cellulitis, TFCC tear, rheumatologic pathology, atypical infections, or impingement. Treatment with rest, frequent icing, analgesics, ergonomic adjustments, and short-term splinting of the wrist is helpful in the acute setting for extensor tenosynovitises. Early injection with corticosteroid may be helpful for de Quervain's and intersection syndromes. In a pooled qualitative literature evaluation, an 83% cure rate was achieved with injection alone for de Quervain's syndrome.[19] For EPL tenosynovitis, treatment is the same except steroid injections should not be given. De Quervain's disease may require surgical decompression for resistant cases. Surgical management is considered only after 4 months of symptoms and failure of two well-placed injections.[19] Persistent symptoms for other extensor tendinopathy or tenosynovitis may require surgical correction or debridement, and there are usually no complications. Prevention of injury includes ergonomic assessment of the workplace and avoidance of repetitive activities.[3]

Clinical Pearl

Tenosynovitis that is recurrent or resistant to treatment warrants a workup for rheumatologic and infectious causes.

46.5.2 Traumatic

46.5.2.1 Acute Subluxation of the Extensor Carpi Ulnaris Tendon

Subluxation of the ECU tendon occurs in collision or contact sports, gymnastics, rodeo, parachuting, mountain climbing, or skiing and is caused by an acute forceful supination of the wrist. The injury results in tears of the retinaculum over the sixth compartment, which allow the ECU tendon to snap out of the groove. Symptoms include painful "snapping" sensation over the dorsal ulnar aspect of the distal ulna with wrist supination and ulnar deviation. On physical exam, the patient will have tenderness over dorsal and ulnar aspect of distal ulna, with palpable tendon subluxation with wrist supination. X-rays are helpful in ruling out associated fracture. Dynamic evaluation with ultrasound may confirm subluxation of the tendon, tendonitis, or tendon rupture.

Differential diagnoses include triangular fibrocartilage complex (TFCC) tear, ulnar instability, fracture, and ECU tendinitis. The initial treatment is RICE, splinting, and analgesics as needed. Long-term treatment involves immobilization for 3–4 weeks. This allows the retinaculum to heal over but chronic injuries may require surgical correction. Complications include recurrent painful snapping if untreated and prevention of the injury is through education of proper technique.[2]

46.5.3 Pediatric

46.5.3.1 Radial Epiphyseal Injuries

Radial epiphyseal injury occurs in collision or contact sports and is one of the most common epiphyseal injuries. A study done at the Cleveland Clinic showed that 9% of all athletes under the age of 16 years sustained injuries of the wrist.[2] Ninety percent of traumatic wrist injuries are secondary to falls where the wrist is dorsiflexed and resisting external forces, but ligamentous injuries are uncommon in prepubertal children. This injury often is due to a FOOSH. The mechanism of injury is a dorsiflexion injury of the wrist such as with losing control of the weight bar in a military press and most commonly results in Salter–Harris type 1 or type 2 injuries. Symptoms include pain, swelling, and variable amounts of deformity at distal radius, and on physical exam, there is tenderness, swelling, and variable degrees of deformity at the distal radius. X-rays with posterior–anterior and lateral views will define the Salter–Harris type and the amount of angulation although initial films may look completely normal.

Differential diagnoses include scaphoid fracture, radial carpal instability, Bennett's fracture, or dislocation. Initial treatment is RICE, splinting, and analgesics as needed. For long-term treatment, closed reduction under hematoma block should be performed by a physician experienced in fracture reduction. Two thumbs are placed over the dorsum of the distal fracture, and a distal and downward pressure is applied. The amount of reduction depends on the age and maturity of the fracture. A long-arm cast is applied with the wrist flexed 25° and ulnarly deviated 15° with forearm supination, and the cast is molded over the dorsal carpus and volar concavity of the distal forearm. The cast is bivalved and tightened with tape for 3–5 days. Immediate postreduction x-rays should be done to confirm adequate reduction, and in 5 days, another x-ray should be obtained. The cast should be worn for a total of 5 weeks.[11] Manipulation after 1–2 weeks can damage the growth plate, and severe growth plate damage can result in significant future deformity. Prevention of injury is through education of proper technique and wearing protective gear (e.g., wrist guards).[2,11]

46.6 MEDIAL WRIST INJURIES

46.6.1 Traumatic

46.6.1.1 Radial Ligament Injuries

Radial ligament injuries of the wrist occur in collision or contact sports, gymnastics, rodeo, parachuting, mountain climbing, or skiing. However, sprains are uncommon in prepubertal children. The mechanism of injury is usually a traumatic hyperextension and/or rotational stress to the wrist. With scapholunate dissociation (rotatory subluxation of the scaphoid), the scaphoid normally palmar flexes (becoming more vertical) with radial deviation of the wrist. The intact scapholunate ligament will force the lunate to move with the scaphoid, resulting in the lunate also palmar flexing with radial deviation. With a ruptured scapholunate ligament, the scaphoid will still palmar flex with radial deviation, but the lunate will now dorsiflex, resulting in a vertical scaphoid (rotatory subluxation) and a dorsiflexed lunate. Because the lunate is essentially a passive, intercalated segment, this is called a dorsal intercalated segment instability (DISI) pattern (Figure 46.3).

In perilunate and lunate dislocations, a severe hyperextension injury to the wrist may result in tension rupture to the volar radioscaphoid and scapholunate ligaments, freeing the proximal pole of the scaphoid, while compressive forces wedge the capitate between the scaphoid and lunate. Continued dorsiflexion will cause the distal carpal row to "peel" away from the lunate and maintain a position dorsal to the lunate and radius, a perilunate dislocation. Further

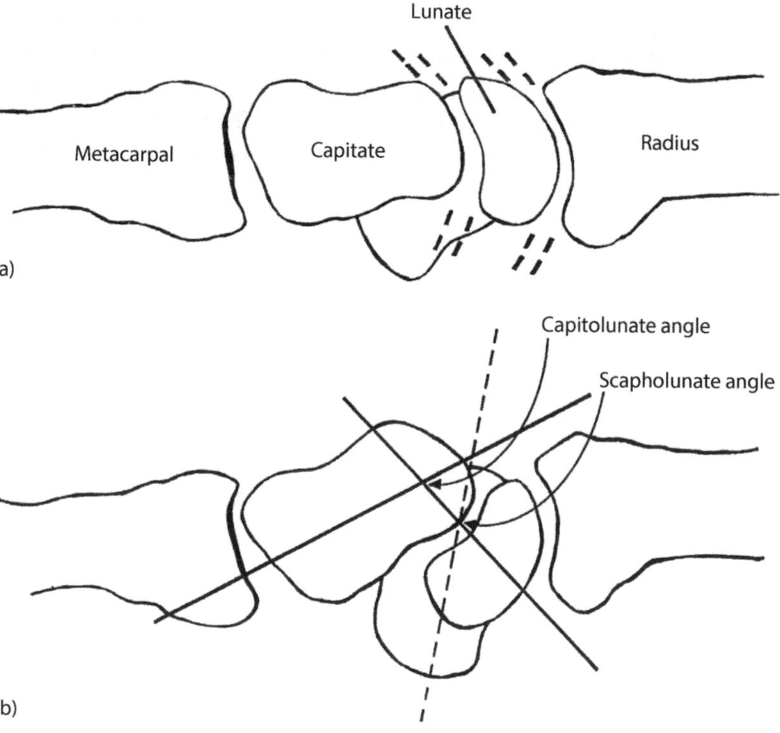

FIGURE 46.3 (a) The four Cs (distal radius, proximal lunate, distal lunate, proximal capitate) on a lateral radiograph should line up in a normal wrist. (b) The capitolunate angle is normally 0 ± 15, and the scapholunate angle should be 30°–60°. This example shows a dorsal intercalated segment instability pattern with an increase in both the scapholunate and capitolunate angles.

force will rupture the dorsal-restraining radiocarpal ligament, allowing the lunate to flip toward the palmar side (spilled teacup sign) as the distal carpal bones relocate, resulting in a lunate dislocation. Instabilities at the radial aspect of the wrist center around injuries to the ligaments surrounding the scaphoid. These include scapholunate dissociation (also called rotatory subluxation of the scaphoid), dorsal perilunate dislocation, and lunate dislocation and are graded 1–3. Symptoms include pain, swelling, and difficulty moving the wrist.

With scapholunate dissociation, the patient will have a tender and swollen wrist with limited range of motion on physical exam. Watson's scaphoid test may be positive and is performed as follows: The patient's hand is placed in ulnar deviation (making the scaphoid horizontal) and neutral. The examiner places his or her thumb on the scaphoid tuberosity and the four fingers of the same hand on the dorsal aspect of the distal radius. The thumb pushes on the scaphoid in an attempt to keep it from becoming vertical as the patient radially deviates the hand. With rupture of the scapholunate ligaments, the thumb will effectively prevent the scaphoid from palmar flexing and force the proximal pole to rotate dorsally, causing pain and/or a painful click.[10] For perilunate and lunate dislocations, the patient will have a tender and swollen wrist with marked limitation in range of motion on physical exam. Particular attention must be paid to median nerve function after this injury.

X-rays are useful in the evaluation of radial ligament injuries, resulting in scapholunate dissociation and perilunate and lunate dislocations (see Figure 46.3). For scapholunate dissociation, posterior–anterior radiographs (with and without a clenched fist) will show a scapholunate space >3 mm (Terry Thomas sign) or a space greater than that seen between the other carpal bones and a ring sign (the scaphoid appears short, and the end-on projection of the rotated scaphoid gives a ringed appearance). Lateral views show the lunate is dorsiflexed (DISI pattern) with a capitolunate angle of >15°. The scapholunate angle is >65° to 70°. If the plain posterior–anterior (PA) and lateral views are normal but suspicion remains, a full traumatic wrist series should be ordered. In perilunate and lunate dislocations, the lunate appears three-sided rather than its normal trapezoidal configuration on PA projections. A true lateral view shows the distal carpal row dorsal to the lunate and radius in a perilunate dislocation and shows a "spilled teacup" sign (the lunate faces toward the palm and rests volar to the radius and distal carpal row) with a lunate dislocation. MRI, arthrography, or diagnostic arthroscopy may be useful with suspected scapholunate injury with equivocal plain radiographic findings.[10]

Differential diagnoses include scaphoid fracture, wrist sprain, and ulnar instability. Treatment initially is RICE, splinting, and analgesics as needed.[10] Long-term treatment involves a referral to the hand surgeon for definitive treatment within 1 week of the injury. Complications may include chronic instability, pain, decreased range of motion, and arthritis with delayed diagnosis. Prevention of injury is through education of proper technique and appropriate equipment.[8,21]

46.7 LATERAL WRIST INJURIES

46.7.1 Traumatic

46.7.1.1 Ulnar Ligament Injuries

Ulnar ligament injuries of the wrist occur in collision or contact sports, gymnastics, rodeo, parachuting, mountain climbing, or skiing. Sprains are uncommon in prepubertal children. The mechanism of injury is a traumatic hyperextension or rotational injury of the wrist and instabilities on the medial aspect of the wrist center along with disruption of the stabilizing triquetrolunate or triquetrohamate ligaments.

The bony configuration of the carpal bones guides the triquetrum into dorsiflexion with ulnar deviation. Its ligamentous attachments to the rest of the proximal carpal row cause the lunate and scaphoid also to dorsiflex. With a triquetrolunate injury, there is rupture of the ligament connecting the triquetrum and lunate (triquetrolunate ligament). The triquetrum will still dorsiflex with ulnar deviation, but the lunate and scaphoid will now be volar flexed. This results in a volar intercalated segment instability (VISI). In triquetrohamate instability, the loss of the bony geometric influence of the hamate on the triquetrum allows for a VISI pattern with triquetrohamate ligament rupture. Symptoms include a swollen and painful joint with limited range of motion.

For triquetrolunate injuries, a painful click may occur on physical exam as the wrist is compressed and moved from ulnar to radial deviation. The lunotriquetral ballottement test may be positive and is performed as follows: The lunate is stabilized with the examiner's thumb and index finger. With the other hand, the examiner grasps the patient's pisiform and triquetrum and moves them in a volar and dorsal direction, assessing laxity, crepitus, and pain. In triquetrohamate instability, a painful click may occur on physical exam over the ulnar aspect of the wrist with ulnar deviation and pronation.

X-rays will be helpful in evaluating instability (see Figure 46.3). With triquetrolunate injury, plain PA and lateral radiographic views are often normal. PA views may show a break in the arc between the lunate and triquetrum, and lateral views may show a dorsiflexed triquetrum with a volar flexed scaphoid and lunate (VISI pattern). The scapholunate angle is >70° when positive. If clinical suspicion of triquetrolunate injury remains with negative plain films, fluoroscopy, an arthrogram, or arthroscopy may be necessary. An MRI or MR arthrogram may provide the most diagnostic information. In patients with triquetrohamate instability, lateral x-rays may show a volar flexed lunate (VISI pattern) with an acute unstable injury. Ulnar instabilities are often dynamic and not identified early on with plain static views. Video fluoroscopy is the most useful tool in evaluating dynamic instabilities, and if suspicion remains, these injuries should be referred to an orthopedic surgeon for further evaluation and treatment.

Differential diagnoses include radial ligament instability, fracture, or sprain. Initial treatment is RICE, splinting, and analgesics as needed. A referral to the hand surgeon is

TABLE 46.6
SORT: Key Recommendations for Practice

Clinical Recommendation	Evidence Rating	References
MR arthrogram is considered the most reliable and gold standard in evaluating TFCC injuries.	C	[14]
Arthroscopic repair of TFCC injuries has good outcome.	B	[12]
An 83% cure rate was achieved with a corticosteroid injection alone for de Quervain's syndrome.	B	[19]
Successful response to carpal tunnel surgery may be predicted by positive response to injection.	B	[6]
A positive flick sign has 93% sensitivity and 96% specificity in ruling in CTS.	C	[5]

needed for long-term definitive treatment. Complications include chronic instability, pain, decreased range of motion, and arthritis with delayed diagnosis. Prevention of the injury is through education of proper technique.[8,21]

46.8 SUMMARY OF THE WRIST

The injured wrist of an athlete deserves careful, thorough evaluation. Its central position to the transmission of forces and complex anatomy make it uniquely vulnerable to many modes of trauma. While many vague wrist injuries improve with temporary and conservative therapy, a wrist "sprain" should be a diagnosis of exclusion. A missed scaphoid fracture or undiagnosed ligamentous instability can lead to prolonged impairment and the need for protracted intervention. Other rheumatologic and infectious causes must be considered in recurrent and recalcitrant cases. The identification of a specific injury pattern will define a more precise treatment plan and, when appropriate, a more immediate and aggressive intervention permitting return to sport in a timely manner while avoiding unwanted chronic pain or impairment (Table 46.6).

REFERENCES

1. Beckenbaugh RD, Shiver TC, Dobyns JH et al. Kienbock's disease: The natural history of Kienbock's disease and consideration of lunate fractures. *Clinical Orthopaedics and Related Research.* 1980;149:98–106.
2. Bergfeld JA et al., Soft playing splint for protection of significant wrist injuries in sports. *American Journal of Sports Medicine.* 1982;10:293.
3. Chauhan A, Jacobs B, Andoga A et al. Extensor tendon injuries in athletes. *Sports Medicine and Arthroscopy Review.* 2014;22(1):45–55.
4. Childress MA, Beutler A. Management of chronic tendon injuries. *American Family Physician.* 2013;87(7):486–490.
5. D'Arcy CA, McGee S. The rational clinical examination: Does this patient have carpal tunnel syndrome? *Journal of the American Medical Association.* 2000;283(23):3110–3117.
6. Edgell SE, McCabe SJ, Breidenbach WC et al. Predicting the outcome of carpal tunnel release. *Journal of Hand Surgery.* 2003;28(2):255–261.
7. Geissler WB. Carpal fractures in athletes. *Clinics in Sports Medicine.* 2001;20(1):167–188.
8. Geissler WB, Burkett JL. Ligamentous sports injuries of the hand and wrist. *Sports Medicine and Arthroscopy Review.* 2014;22(1):39–44.
9. Jarvik JG. MR nerve imaging in a prospective cohort of patients with suspected carpal tunnel syndrome. *Neurology.* 2002;58(11):1597–1602.
10. Lewis DM. Scapholunate instability in athletes. *Clinics in Sports Medicine.* 2001;20(1):131–140.
11. Markiewitz AD, Andrish JT. Hand and wrist injuries in the preadolescent and adolescent athlete. *Clinics in Sports Medicine.* 1992;11(1):203–225.
12. Millants P, DeSmet L, Van Ransbeeck H. Outcome study of arthroscopic suturing of ulnar avulsions of the triangular fibrocartilage complex of the wrist. *Chirugie de la Main.* 2002;21(5):298–300.
13. Morgan WJ, Reardon TF. Carpal fractures of the wrist. In: Pappas, A.M., editor. *Upper Extremity Injuries in the Athlete.* New York: Churchill Livingstone; 1995, pp. 431–449.
14. Nagle DJ. Triangular fibrocartilage complex tears in athletes. *Clinics in Sports Medicine.* 2001;26(1):155–166.
15. Neumann JA, Leversedge FJ. Flexor tendon injuries in athletes. *Sports Medicine and Arthroscopy Review.* 2014;22(1):56–65.
16. Nirschl RP. Elbow and shoulder injuries in the tennis player. *Clinics in Sports Medicine.* 1988;7(2):289–308.
17. Perron AD. Orthopedic pitfalls in the ED: Scaphoid fracture. *American Journal of Emergency Medicine.* 2001;19(4):310–316.
18. Rettig ME, Dassa GL, Raskin KB et al. Wrist fractures in the athlete: Distal radius and carpal fractures. *Clinics in Sports Medicine.* 1998;17(3):469–89.
19. Richie CA, Briner WW. Corticosteroid injection treatment of DeQuervain's tenosynovitis: A pooled quantitative literature review. *JABFP.* 2003;16(2):102–106.
20. Ritchie JV. Emergency department evaluation and treatment of wrist injuries. *Emergency Medicine Clinics of North America.* 1999;17(4):823–842.
21. Slutsky DJ, Trevare J. Scapholunate and lunotriquetral injuries: Arthroscopic and open management. *Sports Medicine and Arthroscopy Review.* 2014;22(1):12–21.
22. Weinstein SM, Herring SA. Nerve problems and compartment syndromes in the hand, wrist, and forearm. *Clinics in Sports Medicine.* 1992;11(1):161–188.
23. Wong SM. Local versus systemic corticosteroids in the treatment of carpal tunnel syndrome. *Neurology.* 2001;56(11):1565–1567.
24. Wood MB, Dobyns JH. Sports related extraarticular wrist syndromes. *Clinical Orthopaedics and Related Research.* 1986;202:93.

FURTHER READING

Almekinders, L.C. and Ruch, D., Hand and wrist injuries in sports medicine. *Sports Med Arthrosc.* 22(1), 1, 2014.

Culver, J.E., Ed., Injuries of the hand and wrist. *Clin Sports Med.* 11(1), 101–128, 1992.

Eiff, M.P., Hatch, R.L., and Calmbach, W.L., *Fracture Management for Primary Care.* Saunders, Philadelphia, PA, 1998, pp. 65–77.

Howse, C., Wrist injuries in sport. *Sports Med.* 17(3), 163–175, 1994.

Rettig, A.C., Ed., Hand and wrist injuries. *Clin Sports Med.* 17(3), 401–406, 1998.

47 Lumbar Spine Injuries

Kenneth Bielak and Erik Berger

CONTENTS

TABLE 47.1
Key Clinical Considerations

1. More than 80% of Americans will have spine complaints in their lifetime.
2. In treating all low back pain, no matter what is done, 90% of all cases will improve in 6 weeks.
3. With the exception of trauma, radiographs are often not necessary in the acute phase of low back pain.
4. Persistent and unremitting pain unresponsive to conservative treatment or back pain with fever or unexplained weight loss, mechanical rest pain, history of cancer, or neurological deficits are indications for pursuing radiographs.
5. MRI is the preferred imaging modality for most lumbar disorders.
6. When MRI is contraindicated, CT is the modality of choice for most lumbar disorders.
7. Bone scans are highly sensitive in detection of stress fractures, infections, and most tumors but lack specificity.
8. Muscle spasm and strain account for the vast majority of acute back pain injuries and are typically related to specific events or improper lifting techniques. Imaging is not indicated but should be considered if there will be no improvement within 2–4 weeks.
9. Significant predictors of lumbar spine fractures are male sex, white race, enlisted ranks, service in the Army and Marines, age, and history of prior lumbar steroid injections.
10. Lumbar transverse process fractures typically occur with direct trauma to the spine and are generally considered stable.
11. A lack of posterior midline tenderness does not rule out a spinal fracture.
12. Plain radiographs can screen for fractures, but more extensive imaging with CT and MRI is useful to detect extent of bony lesions and soft-tissue and neural involvement.
13. Lumbar vertebral fractures are the result of high-energy trauma that generally requires further evaluation by a trauma surgical team.
14. Posterior herniations of disc material into the spinal canal occur with degeneration of the posterior longitudinal ligaments.
15. All patients should be asked about any difficulty with control of bowel or bladder functions to rule out cauda equina syndrome.
16. One meta-analysis demonstrated comparable outcomes between conservative management and microdiscectomies in athletes with lumbar herniations.
17. Spondylolysis is generally due to hyperextension stress fracture from extension activities prior to skeletal maturity.
18. Complaints of back pain in the pediatric patient should be the cause for more serious initial concern with infection and malignancy high on the preliminary differential.

47.1 INTRODUCTION

Spine complaints are a major cause of concern in both sports and industry. All age groups and body types sustain back injuries. Stars of some sports such as golf, tennis, and baseball have been incapacitated by low back pain. Other sports such as football, diving, and wrestling have their share of acute lumbar spine injuries.[31] High-velocity sports such as motor sports carry the highest risk for potentially life-threatening injuries to the spine. More than 80% of all Americans will have spine complaints in their lifetime.[31] Low back pain is the most common complaint and is seen typically in the third through sixth decades of life. It is the most common cause of disability in patients under 45 years of age. Significant risk factors for progressive disc degeneration in American high school football players included lineman position, the presence of Schmorl's nodes, and disc herniation.[22] In addition, playing football for more than 2 years of high school was a risk factor for the onset of LBP.[22] Backache is the second leading cause of work absenteeism after flu and colds, but it is unknown what percentage of this is truly discogenic back disease and how this really impacts on the sporting world. In a retrospective analysis of the 1996 portion of the Medical Expenditure Panel Survey, almost 9%, or 23 million, individuals experienced back pain, 4 million experienced work-related back pain, and approximately 2% or 5 million, experienced missed work days due to back pain. This incidence of back pain resulted in total expenditures of $23 billion just for the medical care, which represents just a fraction of the total economic cost (Table 47.1).[21]

47.2 ANATOMY

The axiom "form follows function" is most evident in the spine. The spine acts as a suspension mechanism when it is parallel to the cyclist's roadway, it acts as a high-tension spring coil when it is twisted in wrestling competition, and it acts as a tower with multiple levers for various resistance loads in the weight lifter hoisting a heavy load. The normal curves (cervical lordosis, thoracic or dorsal kyphosis, and lumbar lordosis) help facilitate the motion and support needed for that region. The vertebral body and facets are designed for stacking, while the bony canal protects the spinal cord. The appendages (the spinous and transverse processes) make natural lever arms for the dynamic (muscles) and static (ligaments) stabilizers (see Figure 47.1).

The disc comprises a central nucleus pulposus, which is circumferentially surrounded by the annulus fibrosus. Its water content is high (75%), and the connective tissue arrangement is designed to withstand repetitive loading. The annulus is arranged in concentric lamellae. Each layer has fibers oriented 120° to the adjacent layer, enhancing strength and durability. The interface of the disc and the vertebral body is tightly adherent tissue that dictates end points of motion such as torque and bending. The disc is located superior to the concomitant exiting nerve root. The vertebral body is composed of spongy trabecular bone that allows it to respond to different stresses. Vertical and oblique stress lines are evident in the vertebrae. The body of the vertebra and the discs comprise the anterior joint. The paired facets of the spine comprise the posterior joint. The bilateral facets, together with the vertebral body and discs, comprise a three-joint complex. The facet joints are oriented in different planes, depending on the spine segments. Motion at any one level is dictated by the surface area and inclination of the facets. The facets are positioned to give an interlocking effect that enhances stability and dissipates stress. The individual facet joint is a diarthrodial joint having a meniscoid interface, which includes a meniscal attachment. As in other joints, it can attrite from overuse. The triple-joint complex can bear up to one-half of the compressive loads delivered at each lumbar level.

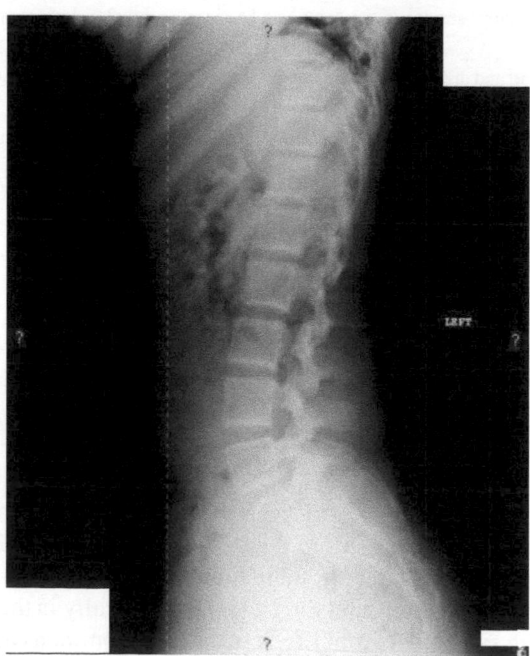

FIGURE 47.1 Lateral radiograph illustrating normal lumbar alignment and lordosis. (Courtesy of Ericka Garcia.)

The *hardware* of the spine is supported by the *software*. Motion is balanced with stability by the layered arrangement of the muscles. An imbalance produces either instability, when motion predominates, or stiffness, when stability dominates. Flexion balances extension. The extrinsic (i.e., rectus) and intrinsic (i.e., psoas and iliacus) flexors contract unilaterally, causing ipsilateral side bending, or they can contract bilaterally, causing forward flexion. Motion at the hip is responsible for more forward flexion than are the intrinsic flexors. Lumbar lordosis is maintained and sometimes increased during flexion (see Figure 47.2).

The lumbar extensors are divided into the superficial, intermediate, and deep groups. The superficial extensors are made up of the sacrospinalis or erector spinae muscle group—a large muscle mass in the sacroiliac (SI) area. Much like a suspension bridge cable system, the three columns of erector spinae muscles help keep the spine erect. The intermediate group (i.e., multifidus) is oriented obliquely so that unilateral contraction will cause theoretical pure side bending, although in actuality side bending occurs with some rotation. Bilateral contraction causes backward extension. The deepest layer of extensors is made up of two groups of muscles: rotators and intertransversarii. As with the other layers, unilateral and bilateral contractions work in concert with the contralateral unit to cause side bending or extension, respectively. Even with flexion, the extensor groups work in an eccentric fashion to control the primary movement.

Spinal motion is described as flexion or forward bending, extension or backward extension, side bending or lateral flexion, and rotation or twisting. Usually, rotation accompanies side bending as coupled motion. Motion is dictated by several variables: (1) orientation of the facets, (2) surface area of the facets, (3) disc resistance to motion,

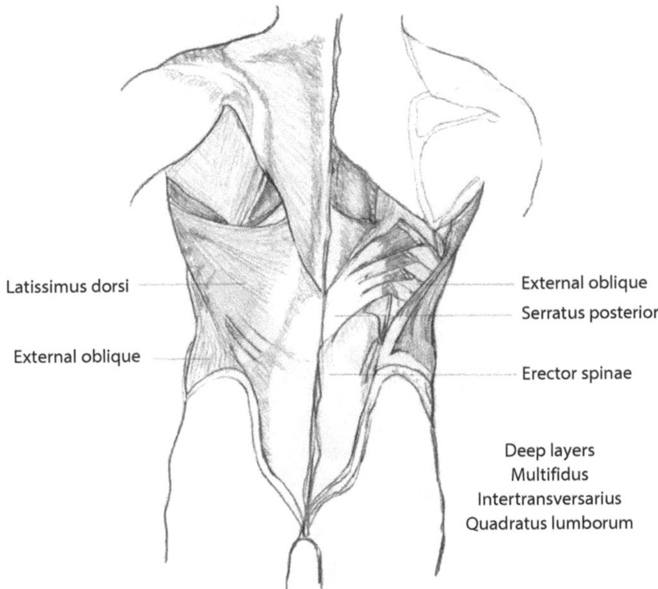

FIGURE 47.2 Superficial and intermediate layers of lumbar spine muscles. Deeper layers not illustrated, but noted in the margin. (Courtesy of Teagan Harris.)

(4) disc thickness, and (5) local soft-tissue attachments. In the normal lumbar spine, most flexion and extension occurs between L4–L5 and L5–S1.

The spine must balance several *moment arms* comprised of varying resistances or loads. The ligaments and muscles generate tension, and work must be done by the muscle to support the human chassis. The body's weight and any mass the body carries must be balanced by tensions generated by the ligament and muscle systems. The added mass of a gravid belly or the added mass of free weights must be balanced by increased work of the spine musculature. With overuse, this counterbalance mechanism weakens and its components will attrite, degenerate, tighten, inflame, or become unstable. In addition to the extremes of physiologic motion, compression and angular force can also be a mechanism of injury.

Lumbosacral nerve roots exit inferiorly to the vertebral body and disc with which they are associated. The sciatic nerve trunk lies adjacent to the lower one-third of the SI joint, separated only by the intervening capsule. Hypertrophic spurs and an inflamed SI joint can irritate the lumbosacral plexus enough to cause a radiculopathy similar to disc herniation. The conus medullaris is generally at the level of L1–L2 in the adult.

The posterior longitudinal ligament, posterior intervertebral disc, lateral and anterior aspects of the annulus fibrosus, posterior facet joints, and interspinous ligaments are also innervated (see Table 47.2).

47.3 EXAMINATION OF THE LUMBAR SPINE

The lumbar spine is inspected for signs of trauma such as ecchymosis and for stigmata such as café-au-lait spots or hairy patches that may herald underlying pathology. Exaggerated lumbar lordosis may result from weakened abdominal musculature. Loss of lordosis may be from paravertebral muscle spasm. Major body landmarks of the lumbosacral spine should be routinely identified and palpated, looking for underlying pathology. The lower extremities should be examined, as structural (anatomical short leg) and functional (pronated feet) problems are a frequent cause of back pain. Range of motion begins with observation of gait, then followed by testing back motion, including standing flexion, extension, lateral bending, and twisting (rotation), looking for limitations to motion or restrictions caused by pain and/or muscle spasm. Muscle testing allows the examiner to compare the relative strengths of the major muscle groups of the lower extremity, looking for weakness, atrophy, or asymmetry. The neurovascular exam is then completed by checking segmental areas for response to light touch, pinprick, temperature, and vibration and by checking the major pulses of the lower extremity. Finally, pelvic, rectal, and scrotal exams are an important part of the back evaluation.

47.3.1 Laboratory/Radiology Evaluation

With the exception of back trauma, radiographs (anteroposterior, lateral, obliques) are often not necessary in the acute phase. Persistent and unremitting pain unresponsive to conservative treatment, back pain with persistent fever or unexplained weight loss, nonmechanical rest pain, significant trauma, history of cancer, or neurological deficits are some indications for obtaining radiographs (Level of Evidence C: consensus opinion).[11,12,19] Radiographs may reveal fractures, infections, and tumors, as well as some pars defects but with quite limited sensitivity. Radiographs can demonstrate

TABLE 47.2
Commonly Tested Nerves and Nerve Roots

Disc Space	Nerve Root	Cutaneous Nerve	Motor	Sensory	Reflex
L1, L2	L2, L3	—	Cremaster, anal muscle	Anterior–lateral thigh	Cremaster, superficial anal muscle
L2, L3, L4	L2, L3	Femoral, obturator	Quadriceps, adductors	Anterior–lateral thigh, medial leg	Knee (patellar), adductor
L4, L5, S1, S2	L5–S3	—	—	Leg and foot	Plantar
		Sciatic	Hamstrings	Posterior thigh	Hamstring
S1,2	S2	Tibial	Gastrocnemius	Heel, lateral foot	Ankle (Achilles)

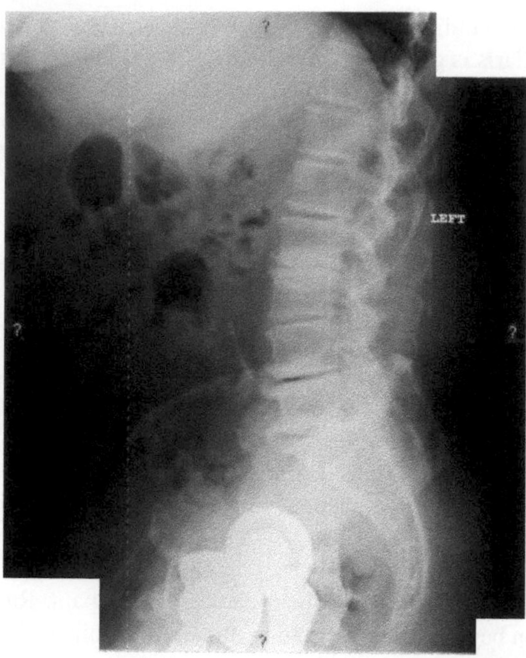

FIGURE 47.3 Lateral radiograph illustrating degenerative disc narrowing. Degenerative disc narrowing multiple levels. (Courtesy of Ericka Garcia.)

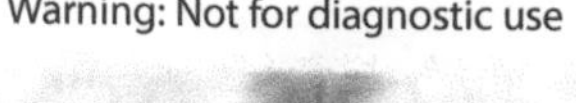

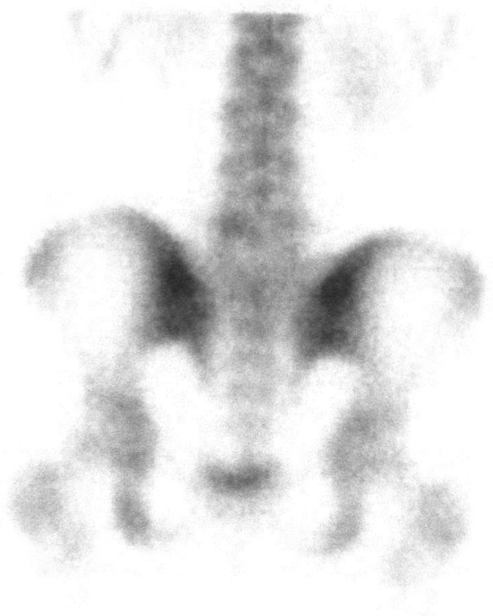

FIGURE 47.4 Bone scan illustrating positive stress injury, posterior view, L-5 on the left side. Posterior L-5 stress reaction, bone scan. (Courtesy Dr Anton Allen, University of Tennessee Medical Center, Knoxville, TN.)

degenerative disc narrowing but are unreliable for evaluation of disc herniation (see Figure 47.3).

Magnetic resonance imaging (MRI) is preferred in evaluation of most lumbar disorders, including disc diseases, radiculopathies, myelopathies, infections, and tumors. MRI is the procedure of choice in the diagnosis of cord abnormalities including edema and hemorrhage. Advantages of MRI include lack of radiation, superior soft-tissue contrast, multiplanar imaging, and ability to image large segments of the spine. Disadvantages of MRI include susceptibility to motion and other artifacts and evaluation of calcifications and dense cortices, as well as expense.

When MRI is contraindicated, computed tomography (CT) myelogram is the modality of choice for most spinal disorders. CT excels in evaluation of calcific or osseous processes (especially osseous processes involving the cortices). Thus, CT is the first-line modality for acute fracture evaluation and exquisitely defines facet joint disease, osseous foraminal narrowing, and pars defects. Advantages of CT include high resolution, speed, and multiplanar imaging potential. Disadvantages of CT scanning include a substantial radiation dose and less soft-tissue contrast relative to MRI. Myelography is almost never indicated as an isolated procedure, but in combination with CT, it remains very useful for evaluation of myelopathies and radiculopathies. This is an invasive procedure and is employed most often in settings where MRI is contraindicated or to further explore issues unanswered by MRI or CT.

The radionuclide three-phase bone scan is useful in the evaluation of suspected stress-related injuries, including lumbar pars interarticularis stress injuries. The bone scan typically becomes positive about the same time an overuse injury becomes symptomatic. Bone scans are highly sensitive in detection of stress fractures, infection, and most tumors but lack specificity. Anatomic localization is markedly improved if single-photon emission CT (SPECT) is employed. Electromyography (EMG) and nerve conduction velocity studies help localize herniated disc syndromes and root and peripheral nerve lesions; however, such testing requires 14–21 days for denervation changes to occur before these studies become positive (see Figure 47.4).

47.4 ACUTE LUMBAR SPINE INJURIES

47.4.1 Paraspinal Muscle Spasm and Strain

47.4.1.1 Epidemiology

Muscle spasm and strain accounts for the vast majority of acute back pain injuries.[28] These are acute in nature directly related to specific events and the result of poor posture and improper lifting mechanics. Lifting with the back instead of the legs is the usual cause. Unreasonable loads usually are not the culprit, but repetitions of near-maximal loads are dangerous. The most common mechanisms of injury include direct blunt trauma, indirect macrotrauma with sudden eccentric load, or overuse microtrauma. The muscles of the back that are the most commonly injured include the deep and superficial muscle groups that present with a constant, dull, vague ache poorly localized in the low back area, sometimes centrally located and sometimes on a particular side; usually, it does not radiate like a radiculopathy but can include posterior thigh pain.[2,24] The spasm can be brought on by improper posture even for just a moment, such as trying to push a refrigerator around to clean behind it, or by maintaining a seemingly innocuous posture, such as sitting in a car for a long trip. Patients generally feel better with rest, warmth, and aspirin. Usually, the patient has a history of a prior occurrence.

47.4.1.2 Clinical Examination

Clinical exam may show a widened stance and hobbling gait (antalgic) or patients may be observed sitting in a haunched, tri-podding posture while sitting on the table, or even standing and leaning against the exam table. They will show a markedly limited active range of motion in all planes, and large areas of tender, doughy muscle with some indiscrete areas of spasm are found. In addition, the examiner may find scoliosis and flattening of the lumbar lordosis due to muscle spasm with limited segmental passive range of motion when side bending with rotation. There should be no signs of neurovascular involvement but dysesthesias, hypesthesias, and inflammatory skin changes can be found overlying the affected muscle groups.

47.4.1.3 Imaging

Imaging is not indicated with acute strains but should be considered if no improvement occurs within 2–4 weeks. Images may show flattening of the normal lumbar lordosis and functional scoliosis, although an accentuated lumbosacral angle can be a normal variant or due to muscle spasm as well. Special studies are not indicated unless there is a question of an underlying pathology.

47.4.1.4 Diagnosis

Paraspinal strain (biomechanical back syndrome/lumbosacral strain). The differential diagnosis includes back pain to visceral disease (inflammatory bowel disease, diseases of the great vessels and pelvic viscera) and herniated nucleus pulposus (HNP).

47.4.1.5 Initial Treatment and Management

The initial treatment and management is focused on pain and spasm control. Simply advocating bed rest and judicious use of muscle relaxants (Level of Evidence C: consensus opinion) and analgesics such as NSAIDs can be effective for short-term symptomatic relief in patients with low back pain (Level of Evidence B: systematic review[29]). For longer-term treatment options, consider unloading the spine (e.g., walking in a swimming pool, inversion boots) and/or prescribing physical modalities such as ice, heat, galvanic stimulation, ultrasound, TENS, microwave applications, and cold low-power laser.[25] In addition, a prescription for therapy with back schools may have better short-term effects than other treatments for chronic low back pain. In an occupational setting, they are more effective compared to placebo or waiting list controls, but little is known about their cost-effectiveness (Level of Evidence B: systematic review).[30]

Lastly, modify the exercise prescription and activity profile by promoting a hardening program (attendance at a back school) and back exercises (e.g., Williams, McKenzie). The emphasis should be on achieving ideal weight, increasing aerobic power, strengthening abdominal muscles, and increasing hamstring flexibility. Physical conditioning programs that include cognitive-behavioral programs can be effective in reducing the number of sick days of workers with back pain, when compared to usual care, but no evidence of their efficacy for acute back pain has been reported.[27]

47.4.1.6 Complications and When to Refer

Recurrent pain/chronic disability and chronic dysfunction are considerations for referral to a specialist.

47.4.1.7 Prevention

Prevention should be focused on weight reduction, if overweight, aerobic power, hamstring flexibility, and abdominal muscle strength improvement as well as ergonomic issues such as proper sitting, lifting, and lying mechanics.

47.4.2 Lumbar Vertebral Fractures: Transverse and Spinous Processes, Compression, Burst, and Chance

47.4.2.1 Epidemiology

Lumbar vertebral fractures are rare in sports activities with most fractures occurring in high-velocity sports or the result of traumatic flexion injuries (i.e., jump from an excessive height). One long-term follow-up study of a small community found an annual incidence of 0.14 per 1000 adolescents between the ages of 16 and 18 years.[20] Between 2001 and 2010, the overall incidence of lumbar fractures was 0.38 per 1000 person-years in the U.S. military.[26] Male sex, white race, enlisted ranks, service in the Army and Marines, and age were found to be significant predictors of lumbar spine fracture. Service in the Army demonstrated the highest rate of lumbar fractures (0.48 per 1000 person-years). Risk factors include, but are not limited to, Asian/Caucasian females, low bone mineral density, and history of lumbar steroid injection.[14]

Lumbar vertebral fractures should be thought of in two distinct categories: *unstable* and *stable* depending on the location of the fracture. An unstable fracture is one from sufficient energy and force to compromise the spinal cord with fragments such as a fracture dislocation or significant burst fracture that results in compression of the spinal cord often with associated numbness, tingling, weakness, or bowel and bladder dysfunction. Lumbar burst fractures typically occur when the spine suffers axial loading with flexion and results in both anterior and posterior displacements of fracture elements, the most serious of which is the posterior displacement of fragments into the spinal cord. Lumbar transverse process fractures typically occur with direct trauma to the spine and are generally considered stable. These fractures are rarely associated with any neurologic injuries. However, intra-abdominal and retroperitoneal injuries can often be associated with these fractures and the clinician must not overlook this fact[18] (shown in Figure 47.5).

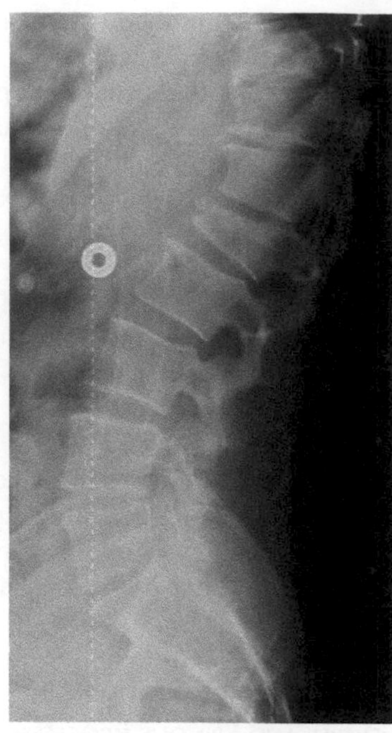

FIGURE 47.5 Lumbar vertebral burst fracture. L-1 burst fracture. (Courtesy of Dr Rong Zeng, University of Tennessee Medical Center, Knoxville, TN.)

47.4.2.2 Mechanism of Injury/History

Motor vehicle accident was the most common mechanism of injury (45%) in one 10-year prospective review with L1 being the most frequent level of fractured vertebra (24.4%).[5] Other common causes include diving accidents or falls from a significant height.

47.4.2.3 Signs and Symptoms

A significant history of high-velocity collision or fall from great height or pointed accelerated trauma to the spine should warrant complete examination of the spine with signs of localized pain and paraspinal tenderness. More serious injuries present with numbness, tingling, weakness, and loss of bladder and bowel control with the most serious symptoms extending to neurogenic shock (bradycardia and hypotension) and loss of spinal reflex activity. Of special note, the lack of posterior midline tenderness does not rule out a spinal fracture.[3]

47.4.2.4 Special Studies

As with any exam, a thorough history is always important to help narrow the differential diagnosis. The character and severity of the pain, including the location, duration, and aggravating/alleviating movements, should be ascertained. Mechanical back pain is typically located centrally, near the lower lumbar/sacral regions. Discogenic pain is usually exacerbated by flexion or the Valsalva maneuver. The clinical exam should begin with observing the patient for any skin changes or gross bony abnormalities that may signify the mechanism of injury. Palpation along the spinous processes for any step-offs or crepitus may elucidate critical injuries missed by observation alone. A component of that evaluation will likely include a complete blood analyses to evaluate for organ damage (kidney, spleen, liver, bladder) and hemorrhage from involved structures. Plain radiographs can screen for fractures, but more extensive imaging with CT and MRI is especially useful to detect extent of bony lesions and soft-tissue and neural involvement.

47.4.3 Management

Generally speaking, lumbar vertebral fractures are the result of such high-energy trauma that further evaluation by a trauma surgical team is warranted to explore the possibilities of abdominal trauma and spinal cord compromise.

47.4.3.1 Nonsurgical Fracture Management

Nonsurgical minor fractures or those with column stability are treated conservatively without surgery using various braces. Patients with spinal cord injuries or paraplegia require surgical stabilization through a number of approaches posteriorly or anteriorly to be determined by the surgical consultant. Spinal fusion and instrumentation in pediatric patients with unstable lumbar vertebral fractures with or without spinal cord injuries have favorable radiographic and functional outcomes. Lumbar vertebral fractures in late adolescence with no or minor neurological deficits have a predominantly favorable long-term outcome, even if no modelling capacity of the fractured vertebral body remains in late adolescence.[20]

47.5 CHRONIC AND SUBACUTE LUMBAR SPINE INJURIES

47.5.1 Herniated Nucleus Pulposus (Slipped, Herniated, Ruptured Disc)

HNP, together with a whole spectrum of degenerative disc disease, is a well-recognized cause of low back pain.

47.5.1.1 Epidemiology

The incidence of intervertebral disc disorders has been reported to be 0.2 per 1000 persons less than 18 years of age, 15.2 per 1000 persons aged 18–44 years, and 37.7 per 1000 persons aged 45–64 years. L5–S1 is the most common site, followed by L4–L5 and L3–L4.[25] Low back pain and discogenic disease are common in gymnastics, swimming, football, weight lifting, wrestling, track, bowling, and racket sports.[17,32]

47.5.1.2 Mechanism of Injury

Acute low back pain can result from sudden jarring insults to the spine such as a misstep on a field with a hole, pushing off the line in football, or twisting the torso against tension. During flexion and rotation, the disc material impacts against the weakest segment—the posterolateral annulus fibrosus. Repeated insults can result in herniation through this area. Other cases may be of slower onset, with increasing pain due to further activity or particular movements involving the back. A recent longitudinal study found that adolescent risk factors for future lumbar discectomy in males were daily smoking and participation in multiple sports clubs and being overweight in females.[13]

47.5.1.3 Anatomy

The disc is contained by intervertebral ligaments, the weakest of which is located posteriorly. Posterior herniations and extrusion of disc material into the spinal canal occur with degeneration of the posterior longitudinal ligaments. Desiccation of the disc will weaken its performance. The pain of the extruded disc is due to the mechanical action of pressure against a nearby nerve root, as well as to local inflammation due to chemical irritation from the substance of the nucleus. Thus, a laterally bulging disc is more likely to be symptomatic than a centrally bulging disc because of the proximity of the nerve root laterally.

47.5.1.4 Symptoms

Common symptoms of herniated disc pathology include pain that radiates from the SI and buttock area to lateral thigh and extends to the lower leg onto the dorsum of the foot in the first and second webs, occasional referred pain to hip and knee, paresthesia (*pins and needles*) along the dermatome, and radicular pain (electrical shock-like *zing*), usually unilateral but can be bilateral. Provocation of symptoms can occur when certain postures or activities are prolonged (such as riding in a car, standing, lifting, or physical exertion) or increased pain with coughing, sneezing, or straining. There may also be relief with resting in certain positions (e.g., lying on the back with hips and knees flexed, lying on the side or in fetal tuck position, or resting prone with belly supported). All patients should be asked about any difficulty with control of bowel (rectal sphincter disturbance) or bladder functions; the presence of either is an ominous sign (e.g., cauda equina syndrome).

47.5.1.5 Signs and Symptoms

The clinician looks for localized tenderness, paraspinal muscle spasm, unilateral plantar flexion weakness (difficulty with toe walking), decreased ankle jerk reflex, and diminished extension power of extensor hallucis longus (L5 nerve root). An increase in symptoms with the following tests is considered a positive sign. In general, true sciatic nerve compression or injury will elicit more than one of the following positive tests as noted in Table 47.3

Referred pain should be distinguished from radicular pain. As previously mentioned, pelvic, rectal, and scrotal exams also should be part of the back evaluation (see Table 47.4).

47.5.1.6 Imaging and Special Studies

For recurrent low back pain, complete blood count, erythrocyte sedimentation rate, liver and renal biochemistries, and blood sugar and serologic tests help rule out infections, kidney disease, diabetes, calcium deposits, and metabolic bone disease. The second tier of diagnostic tests includes the rheumatoid factor, antinuclear antibody, serum protein electrophoresis for multiple myeloma, acid phosphatase, prostatic-specific antigen prior to digital manipulation of the prostate, and thyroid function tests. Urinalysis with urine protein electrophoresis can be helpful to look for urinary tract infections or multiple myeloma. As a general rule, radiologic and other imaging studies should be done on patients over 50 and on younger patients whose low back pain lasts more than 6 weeks (see Table 47.5 for details in interpreting lumbar radiographs).

TABLE 47.3
Tests for Spinal Nerve Root Impingement

Tests for Spinal Nerve Root Impingement	How It Is Performed	Positive Findings
Straight-leg raise (SLR) (supine)	In the supine position, the extended leg is flexed passively at the hip to stretch the nerve root. A significant positive test is typically elicited from 10° to 60°.	Under 30 years of age, this test is very sensitive but not very specific (many false positives, usually related to paravertebral muscle spasm). Over 30 years of age, this test is very specific but not very sensitive (usually due to degenerative changes of the spine).
SLR (sitting)	Same as the aforementioned, except performed sitting.	discordant results may reveal secondary gain etiologies for back pain.
Contralateral SLR	SLR opposite leg to pain source.	Very sensitive and specific for all ages when pain is localized.
Lasegue's test	The hip and knee are both flexed to 90°; the knee is then further extended to the degree where pain occurs; additionally, the ankle can be dorsiflexed to determine whether symptoms increase.	
Bowstring test	During a SLR test, manual compression of the popliteal fossa will exacerbate the pain of the stretched sciatic nerve.	Sciatic nerve impingement.

TABLE 47.4
Test to Assess Sacroiliac Integrity

Tests to Assess SI Integrity	How It Is Performed	Positive Findings
Pelvic squeeze	The examiner's hands are placed over the anterior superior iliac spines (ASISs) of the pelvis and squeezed toward each other.	This maneuver opens the SI joint posteriorly, provoking pain.
Pelvic rock	The SI joint is stressed by placing a distraction or abduction force on the ASIS, which closes or pinches the SI joint.	
Direct sacral pressure	With patient lying prone, direct sacral pressure is applied in an anteroposterior direction, causing anterior displacement of the SI joint.	
Gaenslen's test	The supine patient flexes knees and hip, draws the legs up, and holds that position while the contralateral leg is allowed to actively hyperextend over the edge of the table.	Rotation of the hemipelvis occurs, increasing the contralateral SI torsion and SI joint pain (a positive test).
Patrick's (FABER) test	The hip is flexed, abducted, externally rotated, and extended, with the heel allowed to rest over the opposite knee. The examiner then presses the ipsilateral knee downward while securing the contralateral hip with the opposite hand.	A positive test suggests hip or SI joint pathology.

TABLE 47.5
Points to Remember When Interpreting Lumbar Radiographs

- Discs should normally be as wide or wider as one progresses distally in the lumbar spine. L5–S1 is the exception, often being narrower than L4–L5 as a normal variant in the absence of disc disease.
- Facet joints should not be narrowed and sclerotic as in osteoarthritis.
- The pars interarticularis should be intact (this can be viewed on lateral radiographs without the need for more radiation involved with oblique radiographs).
- No horizontal translation of one vertebral body on another should be evident, as in spondylolisthesis.
- No scoliosis or extremes of lordosis should be evident. Reversal of the normal lordotic curve may be a normal postural finding or due to muscle spasm.
- The interpedicular distance should not be focally widened, as can occur with fracture or canal tumor.
- No lytic compromise of cortices or blastic lesions should be present.
- No excessive demineralization should be present.
- No evidence of calcified abdominal aortic aneurysm anterior to the lumbar spine should be seen.

Note: The SI joints should be examined for gross abnormalities on the anteroposterior view.

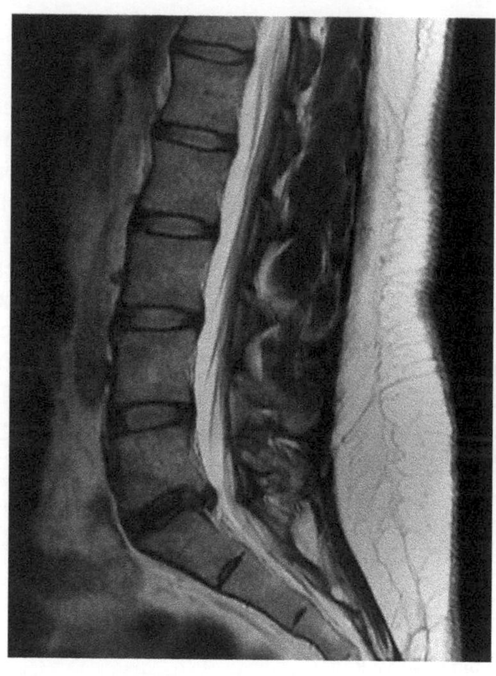

FIGURE 47.6 MRI of herniated disc. L-5/S-1 herniated disc. (Courtesy of Dr Rong Zeng, University of Tennessee Medical Center, Knoxville, TN.)

47.5.1.7 Additional Studies

EMG and nerve conduction velocities show 90% sensitivity, with 38% specificity. They are best for documenting motor lesions and poor for sensory disturbances; also, poor results are obtained with acute problems. MRI is the most sensitive for demonstrating extrusion of disc material into the spinal cord (see Figure 47.6).

Diagnosis

HNP level ________.

47.5.1.8 Differential Diagnosis

The differential diagnosis includes local infection, fracture, tumors (such as multiple myeloma, sarcoma, lymphoma, chordoma, and metastasis from breast, lung, thyroid, kidney, and prostate), benign bone tumors (e.g., osteochondromas, osteoid osteomas, aneurysmal bone cyst, osteoblastoma, and hemangioma), inflammatory causes (e.g., rheumatoid arthritis, ankylosing spondylitis, Reiter's syndrome, psoriatic arthritis), degenerative causes (e.g., disc degeneration without herniation, spinal stenosis, and osteoarthritis), osteoporosis, strains and sprains, and extraspondylitic diseases (e.g., piriformis syndrome, osteoarthritis of the hip, torsional deformities of the lower limb, peptic ulcer disease, cholecystitis, colitis and polyneuritis, aortic aneurysm, uterine myoma, and prostatitis).

Clinical Pearl

Muscle strains radiate to the thigh, usually stopping at the knee. Radicular pain is electric-like and extends into the leg and foot.

47.5.1.9 Initial Treatment and Management

In treating all low back pain, it is worthwhile to keep in mind that no matter what is done, 90% of all cases will probably improve in 6 weeks. The mainstays of treatment and when to refer are listed in Table 47.6.

47.5.1.10 Complications and When to Refer

Refractory cases may require surgical intervention (laminotomy, laminectomy, discectomy). Standard discectomy produces increased self-reported improvement at 1 year, but not at 4 and 10 years when compared to conservative treatment. No significant differences have been observed in clinical outcomes with standard discectomy versus microdiscectomy. Adverse effects are similar with both procedures.[10] However, one meta-analysis demonstrated comparable outcomes between conservative management and microdiscectomies in athletes with lumbar herniations.[9] Intensive multidisciplinary biopsychosocial rehabilitation with a functional restoration approach improves pain and function.[7] Further extrusion of the disc material with increased symptoms and progressive and permanent nerve damage results in the loss of bladder and bowel control and paralysis.

TABLE 47.6
Common Treatments and When to Refer for Herniated Disc Pathology

Relative bed rest—unload the spine for 3 or 4 days.
Pain management—minimize narcotics and maximize nonsteroidal agents and physical modalities such as ice and massage.
Spasm management—use ice, postural changes, manipulation, and proprioceptive neuromuscular facilitation (PNF).[28]
Flexion exercises can help maintain suppleness, but these aggravate disc disease so extension exercises are usually recommended.[28]
Hyperextension maneuvers can reduce symptoms.
Behavioral modification is helpful in reassessing expectations and in controlling drug-seeking behavior.
Immediate referrals include the diagnosis of *cauda equina syndrome* (bilateral neurological deficits associated with bowel or bladder function impairment), *progressive motor symptoms or paralysis, evidence of infection, abscess or epidural hematoma*, or patients with a *history of malignancy and new evidence of nerve entrapment.*
Epidural steroid injection is generally reserved for patients demonstrating limited response to conservative measures of oral medication, physical therapy, and other noninvasive measures (Level of Evidence C: consensus opinion).[23]

47.5.1.11 Prevention of Recurrence

To prevent recurrence, it is recommended for a consultation with a physical therapist or certified trainer to establish a program of exercises to promote strengthening of the *core* muscles including paraspinals, deep muscles of the pelvis, and the abdominals. In addition, increasing hamstring flexibility, reducing body fat below 25% range, and increasing aerobic conditioning can aid in preventing recurrence.

47.6 SPONDYLOLYSIS AND SPONDYLOLISTHESIS

47.6.1 Epidemiology

Spondylolysis is a bony defect in the pars interarticularis, once thought to be congenital but now taken to be an acquired defect or stress fracture to this inherently weak portion of the vertebra.[6,24] It may be multilevel and bilateral. Spondylolisthesis is the sliding of one vertebra over the top of another due to loss of the posterior locking mechanism. The incidence of spondylolysis is 63% in diving; 32%–36% in gymnastics, wrestling, and weight lifting; 23% in track and field; and 5% in the general population.[4,8]

Spondylolysis is generally due to a hyperextension stress fracture from extension activities prior to skeletal maturity. Spondylolysis is the most common cause of spondylolisthesis. The incidence of spondylolysis is 63% in diving; 32%–36% in gymnastics, wrestling, and weight lifting; 23% in track and field; and 5% in the general population.[6,24] A recent pediatric study out of New York found the most common sports associated with spondylolysis were soccer (19.3%), basketball (17.2%), and lacrosse (9.4%[13]). Internationally, fast bowlers in cricket appear to be at high risk.

47.6.2 Mechanism of Injury

Typical injuries occur with repetitive microtrauma from shear, longitudinal loading, and hyperextension of the vertebral column (e.g., gymnastics, swimming, rugby, American football, weight lifting, backpacking, and overhead lifting)

47.6.3 Anatomy, Signs, and Symptoms

Pathologically, spondylolisthesis may be isthmic (spondylolytic), dysplastic (congenital deficiency of the inferior fifth lumbar or superior sacral facets or both), degenerative, traumatic, or pathologic with 43.6% bilateral and 3.4% involving multiple levels.[13] Isthmic subtypes include acute fractures and repeated microfractures (most common) of

TABLE 47.7
Signs of Spondylolysis and Spondylolisthesis

Scoliosis and tenderness due to segmental muscle spasm are commonly seen.
Limited range of motion is noted, especially in backward extension and side bending to the affected side.
The pain is usually decreased by flattening the lumbosacral lordotic curve with a knee-to-chest maneuver.
The pain can be provoked by performing a stork leg stance, with very acute localization to the injured level.
Hyperesthesia over the affected level can also be found on examination of the skin; the neurovascular exam is usually normal.
A stepwise deformity between L5 and S1 indicates spondylolisthesis.
Marked hamstring tightness.[1]

the pars interarticularis. Spondylolisthesis usually involves L5 sliding over the sacral promontory. The most common complaint is that of a recurrent dull ache in the lumbar region with radiation to posterior thigh. The pain is usually localized, which can be provoked by extension activities such as one legged back extension and is accompanied by stiffness afterward. The stiffness is usually relieved by rest but may be worsened. An outstanding feature of spinal stenosis from slippage (spondylolisthesis) is neurogenic claudication (pseudoclaudication); pain is provoked by walking but relieved with sitting (see Table 47.7 for signs of spondylolysis and spondylolisthesis).

47.6.4 Imaging

At a minimum, a lateral radiograph should be taken in the upright position. The collar on the "scotty dog" (best seen in the oblique view) indicates spondylolysis; however, oblique lumbar views impart easily the largest radiation dose of any radiograph and are *not recommended on routine basis.* Anterior translation of the vertebral body on the lateral view indicates spondylolisthesis: grade 1, 0%–25% of the AP diameter of the vertebra; grade 2, 25%–50%; grade 3, 50%–75%; and grade 4, 75%–100%. There are additional special studies for imaging spondylolysis listed in Table 47.8 and shown in Figure 47.7.

Diagnosis

Spondylolysis level ________, spondylolisthesis level ________.

47.6.5 Differential Diagnosis

The differential diagnosis includes paraspinal muscle spasm, facet syndrome, HNP, and an intertransverse or interspinous ligament sprain (see Tables 47.9 and 47.10).

TABLE 47.8
Special Studies for Imaging Spondylolysis

The radionuclide bone scan is highly sensitive for acute or subacute lumbar spondylolysis. When SPECT tomographic imaging is employed, the abnormal activity can be localized to the pars region, improving specificity. High negative predictive value and sensitivity is obtained within 6 weeks of symptom onset.
Thin-slice CT imaging with sagittal and coronal reformations is sensitive and specific for diagnosis of pars defects. CT or bone scan is usually performed first when radiographs are inconclusive and symptomatic spondylolysis is suspected. Some diagnostic protocols recommend a 3-month follow-up CT in patients with a positive SPECT scan to answer questions about healing.[16] Thin-slice CT imaging with sagittal and coronal reformations is sensitive and specific for diagnosis of pars defects. CT or bone scan is usually performed first when radiographs are inconclusive and symptomatic spondylolysis is suspected. Some diagnostic protocols recommend a 3-month follow-up CT or MRI in patients with a positive SPECT scan to answer questions about healing.[15]
MRI may potentially detect early development of cancellous microfractures in the pars region before they are visible on CT and radiographs. MRI also excels at diagnosis of alternative causes for back pain; however, MRI is expensive, and bone scan or CT is usually ordered first to diagnose pars defects. MRI may be helpful in the setting of severe spondylolisthesis to define cord and nerve relationships.

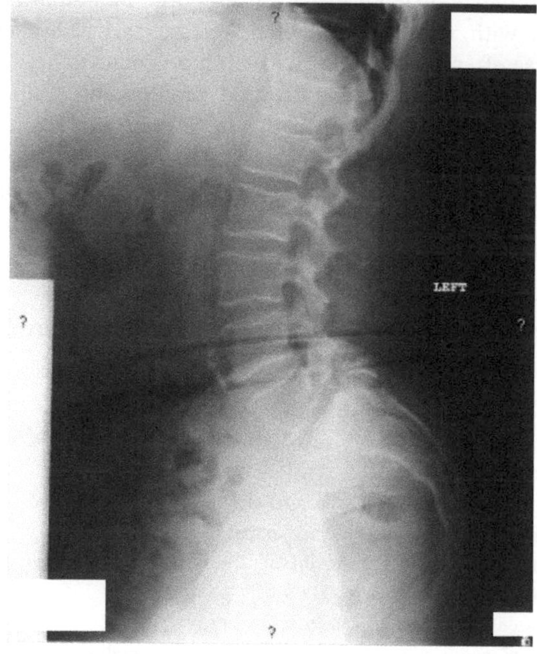

FIGURE 47.7 Lateral radiograph illustrating spondylolisthesis Grade I L-5 on S-1. (Courtesy of Ericka Garcia.)

47.6.6 Complications and When to Refer

Complications of *spondylolysis* can include a fibrous union, malunion, or nonunion that can progress to *spondylolisthesis* and occasionally spinal stenosis with neurogenic claudication. Any suspicion of progression should be immediately referred to an orthopedic specialist for more definitive treatment.

TABLE 47.9
Initial Treatment and Management of Spondylolysis

Acute injury (positive scan, negative radiograph): Rest, including avoidance of all activities placing loading forces on the spine for 8–12 weeks and the use of a modified Boston brace, may be required for up to 3–6 months and require comanagement with an orthopedic spine surgeon.
Semiacute injury (positive scan, positive radiograph): Rest, unloading, and immobilization with ambulatory antilordotic bracing (i.e., Boston) or body cast (e.g., one thigh pantaloon) for 12 weeks.
Brace advantages include continued participation to some degree in sport activity while under treatment and aesthetic consideration.
Gradual (over 3 months), progressive return to activity follows, beginning with flexibility and strengthening exercises and concentrating on lumbosacral stabilization program.
Return to play is allowed only after a symptom-free rehabilitation program is completed.
Chronic injury (negative scan, positive radiograph): Established nonunion unresponsive to immobilization; operative fusion of involved segments for symptomatic athlete who does not wish to forego aggravating activity.
Return to play 1 year following successful fusion.
Permanent avoidance of upright weight training (e.g., dead lifts, squats, snatch, and jerk). Surgical decompression or fusion appears to be no more effective than placebo or conservative treatment (Level of Evidence C: consensus opinion).[6]

TABLE 47.10
Initial Treatment and Management of Spondylolisthesis

Flexibility (hamstring) and strengthening exercises for grades 1 and 2
Surgical fusion for poorly controlled symptoms or symptomatic spinal stenosis due to high degrees of slippage (≥ grade 3)

47.7 FACET SYNDROME

47.7.1 Epidemiology

Facet syndrome usually occurs in people who use poor biomechanics or in people whose posture is held in one position for an inordinate period of time. Usually this occurs with some amount of muscle spasm. Facet syndrome is very common in sedentary people, truckers, and athletes involved in marksmanship, bowling, and golf.

47.7.2 Mechanism of Injury

The mechanism of injury can be from direct blunt trauma but more commonly from overuse microtrauma especially with axial loading and rotation (e.g., prolonged abnormal position such as hunched over a desk) or repetitive lumbar hyperextension.

47.7.3 Anatomy

Facet syndrome is localized over the facets and includes inflammation and immobility of one or more facet joints.

47.7.4 Signs and Symptoms

Typical signs and symptoms involve the loss or range of motion that can be more pronounced than the actual pain level and can also be somewhat painless if the patient is satisfied with staying in a fixed position. The pain is tolerable as a dull ache but can progress to a knifelike stabbing pain when the extremes of motion are approached. With lumbar etiology, the pain may be ill defined (sclerotomal) and may also radiate to the posterior thigh and occasionally below the knee mimicking radicular pain.

47.7.5 Clinical Examination

The clinical examination will show a bent over stance with a defensive gait, and there may be hyperesthesia and hyperemia overlying the dysfunctional segment, often with doughy, edematous paraspinal muscles. There will be marked limited range of motion specific to the level that is involved. The neurovascular exam is typically normal.

47.7.6 Imaging

See paraspinal spasm.

Diagnosis

Facet syndrome level ________.

47.7.7 Differential Diagnosis

The differential diagnosis includes pars interarticularis defects, intervertebral ligament sprain, paraspinal muscle strain, or any mechanical back etiology.

47.7.8 Initial Treatment and Management

See Table 47.11 for initial treatment and management of facet syndrome.

TABLE 47.11
Initial Treatment and Management of Facet Syndrome

Initial Treatment
Ice massage, analgesics, and NSAIDs.
Bed rest in the prone position with a small pillow under the umbilicus (lumbar facet); cervical collar (cervical facet).
Long Term
Focus on the surrounding soft tissue to increase the core strength, flexibility, and vascular supply.
The soft tissue is prepared and then, by effecting a passive range of motion, the joint usually falls into place.
Alternatively, osteopathic manual techniques such as high-velocity, low-amplitude maneuvers in a direction opposite to the fixed position can be effective. That is, if the facet is stuck in flexion, the movement should be toward extension.
PNF includes reciprocal innervation to relax tight supporting structures and allow normal motion.
Progressive resistance exercises can be used.

47.7.9 Complications and When to Refer

Referral is made when there is chronic pain/disability and ineffective treatment modalities.

47.7.10 Prevention

Prevention is best utilized by emphasizing proper body mechanics, maintaining proper body weight, and incorporating strengthening and flexibility exercises into the daily routine.

47.8 PEDIATRIC BACK PAIN

Complaints of back pain in the pediatric patient should be the cause for more serious initial concern when compared to the adult complaint of back pain. Although pediatric patients suffer from similar maladies as adults, infectious or malignant causes should be high on the preliminary differential. Degenerative causes of low back are typically less common. A CBC should be included in the evaluation. Complaints of night pain, radicular pain, or an abnormal neurologic exam should prompt the physician to investigate with advance imaging such as an MRI.

47.9 SUMMARY

With increasing levels of recreational activity and sports participation, the spine has joined the elbow, ankle, knee, shoulders, and other anatomic areas as a site for athletic-related trauma. Such injuries, while infrequent, are often severe, resulting in permanent disability or death. Spinal anatomy and biomechanics as well as a variety of pathologic conditions specific to the spine must be understood by the competent sports physician. High levels of fitness, young age, and lack of compensation considerations should not dissuade the wary physician from a thorough search for significant injury, underlying disease, training errors, and environmental factors. Finally, a comprehensive rehabilitative program emphasizing normal range of motion and strength and a preventive strategy including protective equipment are essential before return to full play should be prescribed (Tables 47.12 and 47.13).

TABLE 47.12
Indications for Specialty Referral for Lumbar Spine Injuries

Diagnosis	Primary Care Referral Considerations
Paraspinal spasm or strain	Acute spasm or strains that are recurrent or result in chronic dysfunction
Herniated discs	Refractory cases after comprehensive physical therapy
Spondylolysis or spondylolisthesis	Any suspicion of progression
Facet syndromes	Persistent chronic pain and disability

TABLE 47.13
SORT: Key Recommendations for Practice

Clinical Recommendation	Evidence Rating	References
The initial management of paraspinal muscle spasm and strain is focused on pain and spasm control with rest and judicious use of muscle relaxants.	C	[29]
Analgesics such as NSAIDs can be effective for short-term symptomatic relief in patients with low back pain.	B	[29]
In the occupational setting, a prescription for therapy with back schools is more effective compared to placebo or wait list controls.	B	[30]
Persistent and unremitting pain unresponsive to conservative treatment or back pain with fever or unexplained weight loss, mechanical rest pain history of cancer, or neurological deficits are indications for pursuing radiographs.	B	[19,11,12}
There are comparable outcomes between conservative management and microdiscectomies in athletes with lumbar herniations.	B	[9]

ACKNOWLEDGMENTS

Appreciation is extended to Cynthia Vaughn, National Library of Medicine Fellow at the Preston Medical Library of the University of Tennessee Graduate School of Medicine, and to Drs. Anton Allen and Rong Zeng for their pointed review of radiographic evidence supporting diagnostic evaluations.

REFERENCES

1. Auerbach JD, Ahn J, Zgonis MH et al. Streamling the evaluation of low back pain in children. *Clinical Orthopaedics and Related Research.* 2008;154:30–36.
2. Bernard TN and Kirkaldy-Willis WH. Recognizing specific characteristics of nonspecific low back pain. *Clinical Orthopaedics and Related Research.* 1987;217:266–280.
3. D'Costa HI, George G, Parry M et al. Pitfalls in the clinical diagnosis of vertebral fractures: A case series in which posterior midline tenderness was absent. *Emergency Medicine Journal.* 2005;22(5):330–332.
4. Dyment PG. Low back pain in adolescents. *Pediatric Annals.* 1991;20(4):170–178.
5. Erfani MA, Pourabbas B, Nouraie H et al. Results of fusion and instrumentation of thoracic and lumbar vertebral fractures in children: A prospective ten-year study. *Musculoskeletal Surgery.* 2014;98(2):107–114.
6. Gibson JNA, Waddell G, Grant IC. *Surgery for Degenerative Lumbar Spondylosis*, Issue 1. Middle Way, Oxford: Cochrane Review; 2003.
7. Guzman J, Esmail R, Karjalainien K et al. *Multidisciplinary Bio-Psycho-Social Rehabilitation for Chronic Low Back Pain.* Issue 1. Middle Way, Oxford: Cochrane Review; 2003.

8. Harvey J, Tanner S. Low back pain in young athletes. *Sports Medicine*. 1991;12(6):394–406.
9. Iwamoto J, Sato Y, Takeda T et al. The return to sports activity after conservative or surgical treatment in athletes with lumbar disc herniation. *American Journal of Physical Medicine & Rehabilitation*. 2010;89(12):1030–1035.
10. Jordan J, Morgan TS, Weinstein J. Herniated lumbar disease: Clinical evidence. *BMJ*. December (10), 1323–1335, 2003.
11. Kendrick D, Fielding K, Bentley E et al. Radiography of the lumbar spine in primary care patients with low back pain, randomized controlled trial. *BMJ*. 2001; 322(7283):400–405.
12. Kerry S, Hilton S, Dundas D et al. Radiography for low back pain: A randomised controlled trial and observational study in primary care. *British Journal of General Practice*. 2002;52(479):469–474.
13. Ladenhauf HN, Fabricant PD, Grossman E et al. Athletic participation in children with symptomatic spondylolysis in the New York area. *Medicine & Science in Sports & Exercise*. 2013;45(10):1971–1974.
14. Mandel S, Schilling J, Peterson E et al. A retrospective analysis of vertebral body fractures following epidural steroid injections. *Journal of Bone and Joint Surgery*. 2013;95(11):961–964.
15. Mattila VM, Saarni L, Parkkari J et al. Early risk factors for lumbar discectomy: An 11-year follow-up of 57,408 adolescents. *European Spine Journal*. 2008;17(10):1317–1323.
16. McCleary MD, Congeni JA. Current concepts in the diagnosis and treatment of Spondylolysis in young athletes. *Current Sports Medicine Reports*. 2007;6(1):62–66.
17. Micheli LJ. Back injuries in gymnastics. *Clinics in Sports Medicine*. 1985;4:85.
18. Miller CD, Blyth P, Civil ID. Lumbar transverse process fractures—A sentinel marker of abdominal organ injuries. *Injury*. 2000;31(10):773–776.
19. Miller P, Kendrick D, Bentley E et al. Cost effectiveness of lumbar spine radiography in primary care patients with low back pain. *Spine*. 2002;27(20):2291–2297.
20. Moller A1, Hasserius R, Besjakov J et al. Vertebral fractures in late adolescence: A 27 to 47-year follow-up. *European Spine Journal*. 2006;15(8):1247–1254.
21. Mychaskiw MA, Thomas J. Direct cost of back pain in the United States: A National Estimate. http://www.ispor.org/congresses/ne1102/present_pdf/poster/ PNP5.pdf. Accessed November 3–5, 2002.
22. Nagashima M, Abe H, Amaya K et al. Risk factors for lumbar disc degeneration in high school American football players: A prospective 2-year follow-up study. *The American Journal of Sports Medicine*. 2013;41(9):2059–2064.
23. Nelemans PF, deBie RA, deVet HCW et al. Injection therapy for subacute and chronic benign low back pain. *Spine*. 2001;26(5):501–515.
24. Porter RW. Mechanical disorders of the lumbar spine. *Annals of Medicine*. 1989;21(5):G361–G366.
25. Ross JS, Masaryk TJ. Degenerative disk disease. *Current Opinion in Radiology*. 1990;2(1):40–47.
26. Schoenfeld AJ, Romano D, Bader JO et al. Lumbar spine fractures within a complete American cohort: Epidemiology and risk factors among military service members. *Journal of Spinal Disorders & Techniques*. 2013;26(4):207–211.
27. Schonstein E, Kenny DT, Keating J et al. *Work Conditioning, Work Hardening and Functional Restoration for Workers with Back and Neck Pain*, Issue 1, Cochrane Review, Middle Way, Oxford; 2003.
28. Snyder-Mackler L. Rehabilitation of the athlete with low back dysfunction. *Clinics in Sports Medicine*. 1989; 8(4):717–729.
29. van Tulder MW, Scholten RJPM, Koes BW et al. *Non-Steroidal Anti-Inflammatory Drugs for Low Back Pain*, Issue 1, Cochrane Review, Middle Way, Oxford; 2003.
30. Van Tulder MW, Esmail R, Bombardier C et al. *Back Schools for Non-Specific Low Back Pain*, Issue 1, Cochrane Review, Middle Way, Oxford; 2003.
31. Vukmir RB. Low back pain: Review of diagnosis and therapy. *American Journal of Emergency Medicine*. 1991; 9(4):328–335.
32. Watkins RG, Dillin WH. Lumbar spine injury in the athlete. *Clinics in Sports Medicine*. 1990;9(2):419–448.

48 Hip and Pelvis

Peter H. Seidenberg and Michael A. Sirota

CONTENTS

TABLE 48.1
Key Clinical Consideration of the Hip and Pelvis

1. Dividing the hip into anterior, lateral, and posterior anatomic regions assists in guiding the differential diagnosis of hip/pelvis pathology.
2. Due to overlapping pain referral patterns, the differential diagnosis of hip and/or pelvis pain includes pathology from the low back and abdomen.
3. Skeletally immature individuals are more likely to suffer apophyseal injury than musculotendinous strain.
4. Adductor strains are the most common cause of hip and groin pain in athletes.
5. Asymptomatic cam lesions, pincer lesions and labral tears do not require surgical intervention.

48.1 INTRODUCTION

Hip and pelvis pain is often seen as the "black box" of sports medicine due to the complex anatomy, large differential diagnosis, and overlapping pain patterns that can present in this region (Tables 48.1 and 48.2). Additionally, individuals with chronic hip pain often have multiple simultaneous pathologies accounting for their symptoms. To further complicate matters, injury to surrounding anatomic structures can refer pain to the hip. Yet, despite the perceived difficulty in evaluating hip and pelvis disorders, they are fairly common, comprising 5%–6% of musculoskeletal complaints in adults and up to 24% in children.[11,35,41] They are frequently seen in sports with cutting activities, quick accelerations and decelerations, and repetitive rotational activity, as well as sports with contact and/or collision. These include soccer, hockey, rugby, dancing, running, and skating sports.[8,23,44]

48.2 FUNCTIONAL ANATOMY

The hip is a true ball and socket joint with the femoral head held snuggly within the acetabulum. Its stable design allows for excellent stability while maintaining motion in the frontal, sagittal, and transverse plains. The spherical shape of the femoral head is designed to distribute the forces experienced in activities of daily living, which during walking and running can equal three to five times body weight.[15] The socket is constructed from the ilium, ischium, and pubic bones, which join together to form the acetabulum. Like the shoulder, there is a fibrocartilage labrum surrounding the rim of the socket, which serves to deepen the acetabular recess and provides additional stability. It is analogous to the glenoid labrum of the shoulder. On the joint side, it attaches directly to the articular cartilage surface of the hip joint, and this chondrolabral junction is the common site of labral tears. On the exterior side, it attaches to a reflection of the joint capsule.

The labrum functions to increase the stability of the hip joint by resisting translation and distraction of the femur. It is believed to form a tight seal against the femoral head and neck, thereby creating a zone of constant pressure within the central compartment of the hip and leading to uniform distribution of compressive forces across the articular cartilage. Loss of this function is thought to lead to higher contact pressures, which eventually lead to cartilage injury and progression to osteoarthritis (OA).[7]

The joint contains four ligaments. The ligamentum teres attaches the femoral head to the acetabulum, while the remaining three (iliofemoral, ischiofemoral, and pubofemoral) comprise thickened fibers of the joint capsule. The innominate bones of the pelvis join anteriorly at the pubic symphysis, while the posterior pelvic ring is completed at the articulation of the ilium with the sacrum (sacroiliac joints [SIJ]). The pelvis joins the appendicular to the axial skeleton. As such, pathology in this region can have profound effects further up the kinetic chain.

The muscular anatomy is rather complex. To simplify visualization, the authors divide the hip into the medial adductor, anterior flexor, lateral abductor, and posterior extensor regions. This oversimplification does not account for the cardinal movements of internal and external rotation but serves as a convenient way to divide the hip and pelvis into regions when approaching the patient's presenting complaint. When evaluating for muscular pathology, it is important to realize that the muscles have origins as proximal as the lumbar spine and as distal as the tibia.[21]

48.2.1 History and Physical Examination

Armed with a systematic history and physical examination with targeted imaging modalities, the astute practitioner can accurately diagnose and then treat the individual who presents

TABLE 48.2
Differential Diagnosis of Hip and Pelvis Pain

Hip/Pelvis	Thigh	Low Back	Abdomen
Femoral neck stress fracture	Muscle strains	Sacroiliitis	Lower abdominal wall muscular strain (e.g., rectus abdominis)
Pubic ramus stress fracture	Adductors	Sacroiliac dysfunction	Inguinal hernia
Osteitis pubis	Rectus femoris	Sciatica	Ilioinguinal nerve entrapment
Snapping hip	Iliopsoas	Lumbar nerve root impingement	Sports hernia
Acetabular labral tear	Sartorius	Degenerative disk disease	Abdominal organ conditions
Bursitis (trochanteric, iliopsoas, ischial)	Tensor fascia lata	Lumbosacral strain	Abdominal aortic aneurysm
Avascular necrosis	Hamstring		Appendicitis
Osteoarthritis	Femoral hernia		Diverticulitis
Synovitis or capsulitis	Lymphadenopathy		Inflammatory bowel disease
Hip dislocation	Meralgia paresthetica		Pelvic inflammatory disease
Femoroacetabular impingement			Sexually transmitted infections
Gluteal strain/contusion			Ovarian cyst
Piriformis syndrome			Ectopic pregnancy
Coccygeal injury			
Iliac crest contusion			
Muscular strains			
Apophyseal injury			
Peripheral nerve entrapment			

Source: With kind permission from Springer Science+Business Media: *The Hip and Pelvis in Sports Medicine and Primary Care*, Adult hip and pelvis disorders, 2010, pp. 115–147, Seidenberg, P.H.

with musculoskeletal pathology of the hip or pelvis. The importance of a thorough history cannot be understated. This assists in narrowing the wide differential and will allow for a more efficient evaluation. As in other regions of the body, the age of the athlete is of upmost importance, as certain pathologies (e.g., Legg–Calve–Perthes disease, slipped capital femoral epiphysis [SCFE]) are much more common in certain age groups. The presence of open growth plates make injury to the apophysis more likely than the tendon, as the connective tissue strength within the tendon is greater than that of the apophysis. It is important to remember that several of the pelvic apophyses may remain open into young adulthood (Table 48.3).

That patient is asked to clarify the pain's location and character. Is it sharp, dull, or burning? Does it radiate? Is there pain in other areas, such as the back or knee? Is there a history of other joint problems, as is common with rheumatologic conditions? Is there clicking or catching? If so, can he or she reproduce it? Is there swelling, bruising, or redness? Are there constitutional, gastrointestinal, or genitourinary symptoms? Is the pain acute or chronic, abrupt or insidious in onset? Was there an antecedent mechanism of injury? Has there been a change to the training regimen? A nutritional history and menstrual history can also be helpful. Knowing the sport and position or the occupation and its physical requirements also provides essential diagnostic clues. Additionally, it is important to ask what the patient's activity goals are so that treatment success can be more easily defined.

Past medical, family, and medication histories are essential. A patient with osteoporosis treated with long-term bisphosphonates may be at risk for atypical femoral fracture, while the individual on recurrent corticosteroids is at risk of avascular necrosis of the femoral head. Furthermore, consideration must be made to the fact that the hip and pelvis are common sites of bony metastasis.

The physical examination can begin with observing the patient walking to the exam room. This will uncover abnormalities in gait, posture, and difficulties with transferring. Inspection continues with evaluation for muscle atrophy or fullness, pelvic obliquity, scoliosis, and abnormal lumbar

TABLE 48.3
Apophyses of the Hip and Pelvis

Apophysis	Appearance (Years)	Fusion (Years)	Muscle Attachment
Ischial	12–15	19–25	Hamstrings
ASIS	12–15	16–18	Sartorius
AIIS	12–15	16–18	Rectus femoris
Iliac crest	12–15	15–17	Abdominals
Lesser trochanter	8–12	16–18	Iliopsoas
Greater trochanter	2–5	16–18	Gluteals

Sources: Anderson SJ. Sports injuries. *Curr Probl Pediatr Adolesc Health Care* 2005; 35(4):110–164; Paletta GA Jr, Andrish JT. Injuries about the hip and pelvis in the young athlete. *Clin Sports Med* 1995; 14:591–628; Seidenberg PH, Childress MA. Physical examination of the hip and pelvis. In: Seidenberg PH and Beutler AI, eds. *The Sports Medicine Resource Manual*. New York: Saunders Publishing, 2008; 110–122.

Note: AIIS, anterior inferior iliac spine; ASIS, anterior superior iliac spine.

TABLE 48.4
Normal Values for Hip Range of Motion

Motion	Flexion	Extension	Abduction	Adduction	Internal Rotation	External Rotation
Range of motion in degrees	110–120	0–15	30–50	30	30–40	40–60

Source: Seidenberg, P.H. and Childress, M.A., *J. Musculoskel Med.*, 22(5), 246, 2005.

lordosis. Based on historical clues, lumbar, abdominal, and pelvic examination may also be required.

Palpation includes the bony prominences of the hip and pelvis, bursae, tendon origins and distal insertions, muscle groups, the sacral iliac joints, and the pubic symphysis. Range-of-motion (ROM) testing is an essential component of the evaluation and should be compared to the contralateral side. Normal values are shown in Table 48.4. Side-to-side asymmetries may be more important than the individual values. Attention should be paid to any snapping or clicking that occurs during the ROM. Next, strength testing of the individual muscle groups is performed and compared to the contralateral side. As lumbosacral pathology caused referred pain to the hip, it is also important to perform a lower extremity neurologic examination, to include distal strength testing, sensation, and lower extremity reflexes.

Special tests are then performed to further narrow the differential diagnosis. Several commonly used tests are listed in the succeeding text.

The *log roll test* is used to assess for the presence of a femoral neck fracture or an acetabular injury. The patient is supine, and the examiner gently rolls the tested leg in internal and external rotation. If the maneuver produces groin pain, it is considered positive.

The *Stinchfield test* is performed with the patient supine with the hips and knees in extension. The tested leg is then flexed to 20° while maintaining knee extension. The examiner then applies a downward force at the ankle. Anterior hip or groin pain suggests a femoral neck fracture, acetabular fracture, or OA.

The *fulcrum test* is used to assess for a femoral shaft stress fracture. The patient sits at the end of the exam table with the knees flexed and the feet off the ground. The examiner places his or her forearm under the patient's thigh and then uses the opposite hand to apply a downward force on the ipsilateral knee. Sharp pain or apprehension is considered a positive test.

The *Ober's test* is used to evaluate for iliotibial band (ITB) inflexibility. The patient is in the lateral decubitus position with the hips and knees flexed to 90°. The examiner then passively takes the top leg into further flexion followed by abduction and extension. The leg is then allowed to gently drift toward the exam table. Failure of the knee to adduct to the table or passive knee extension is considered a positive test.

The *lateral pelvic compression test* is also performed with the patient in the lateral decubitus position with the knees and hips flexed to 90°. The examiner then applies a downwardly directed force on the greater trochanter. Pain in the pubic symphysis signifies the presence of osteitis pubis.

The *Trendelenburg's sign* is used to evaluate for hip abductor weakness, specifically of the gluteus medius and minimus. The patient stands on the leg to be tested and then actively flexes the contralateral hip. If the contralateral pelvis dips downward, the test is considered positive.

The *flexion, abduction, and external rotation* (FABER) *test* evaluates for SIJ pathology. The patient is supine, and the examiner flexes, abducts, and external rotates the side to be tested, creating a figure 4. A positive test occurs if this maneuver produces ipsilateral SIJ pain.

The *flexion, adduction, and internal rotation* (FADIR) *test* is performed to evaluate for femoralacetabular impingement. The patient is supine, and the examiner passively flexes, adducts, and internally rotates the hip. Pain in the groin is considered a positive test.

The *scour* or *quadrant test* evaluates for labral pathology. With the patient supine and the knee flexed, the examiner passively flexes, axially loads, and then takes the hip from abduction to adduction and then back to abduction in an arc-like motion. Catching, pain, or apprehension with the maneuver is considered positive. This test is analogous to the modified crank test of the shoulder or the McMurray test of the knee.

To assess hamstring flexibility, the *popliteal angle* is performed. With the patient prone, the examiner passively takes the hip to 90° of flexion, while the knee is in flexion. The knee is then passively extended. The angle is then measured from complete extension to the patient's amount of extension. Normal is 0° in females and 10°–20° in males.

The *modified Thomas test* assesses for both iliopsoas and rectus femoris contracture. The patient sits on the far edge of the exam table with the knees flexed to 90°. He or she then pulls one knee to the chest and then lies supine while relaxing the other leg. If the thigh of the down leg rises off the table, an iliopsoas contracture is present. If the knee passively extends, the rectus femoris has a contracture. Both may be simultaneously positive.

The *Ely's test* also evaluates for quadriceps inflexibility. While stabilizing the pelvis, the prone patient's knee is passively flexed to its end ROM. Failure for the heel to touch the gluteus maximus is considered positive. Comparison should be made to the contralateral side. The test can be limited by concomitant knee pathology.

The *Weber–Barstow maneuver* is helpful in assessing for leg length discrepancy. The patient lies supine with both knees

TABLE 48.5
Hip and Pelvis Special Tests

Test	Performance	Positive Findings	Suggested Diagnosis
Log roll	Supine patient's hip is passively internally and externally rotated.	Groin pain.	Femoral neck fracture, femoral neck stress fracture, acetabular fracture
Stinchfield test	Supine patient's hip is actively flexed to 20° while maintaining knee in extension and resists examiner's downward force applied at the ankle.	Groin pain.	Femoral neck fracture or stress fracture, acetabular fracture, osteoarthritis
Fulcrum test	Patient sits on end of table with knee flexed and foot off the ground. Examiner places forearm under patient's thigh and uses the opposite hand to apply downward force on knee.	Sharp thigh pain.	Femoral shaft stress fracture
Ober's test	Patient in lateral decubitus position with knees and hips flexed to 90°. Top leg is passively further flexed followed by abduction and extension. Leg is allowed to gently fall toward the exam table.	Failure of knee to adduct to table or passive knee extension.	Iliotibial band inflexibility
Lateral pelvic compression test	Patient in lateral decubitus position with knees and hips flexed to 90°. Examiner pushes downward on greater trochanter.	Pain at pubic symphysis.	Osteitis pubis
Trendelenburg's sign	Standing patient stands on test leg and flexes contralateral hip.	Contralateral hip dips downward.	Hip abductor weakness
FABER test	Supine patient's hip is passively flexed, abducted, and externally rotated.	Ipsilateral SI joint pain.	SI dysfunction
FADIR test	Supine patient's hip is passively flexed, adducted, and internally rotated.	Groin pain.	Femoroacetabular impingement
Scour test	Supine patient with knee flexed. Hip is passively flexed, axially loaded, and taken from abduction to adduction and then back to abduction in an arc-like motion.	Catching, groin pain, or apprehension.	Labral tear
Popliteal angle	Supine patient's hip is flexed to 90°, and the knee is passively extended.	Angle is measured from true vertical.	Hamstring inflexibility
Modified Thomas test	Patient sits on edge of exam table, pulls opposite knee to chest, and lies supine.	1. Thigh rises off exam table. Knee passively extends.	1. Iliopsoas contracture Rectus femoris contracture
Ely's test	Prone patient's knee is passively maximally flexed.	Heel does not touch gluteus maximus.	Quadriceps inflexibility
Weber–Barstow maneuver	Supine patient with hips and knees flexed, with feet on table close together. Patient lifts pelvis off table and then gently sets pelvis back down. Knees and hips are then passively extended. Examiner places thumbs under each medial malleolus.	Unequal malleoli height.	Leg length discrepancy
Long-sit test	Following Weber–Barstow, with thumbs still under the medial malleoli, the patient sits up while maintaining knees in extension.	The leg that was longer on the Weber–Barstow maneuver now appears shorter.	Functional leg length inequality with pelvic obliquity

Note: SI, sacroiliac.

and hips flexed with the feet close together. To reset the pelvis, he or she then lifts the pelvis off the table and gently lowers it back down again. The knees and hips are then passively extended. The examiner then places his or her thumbs underneath the medial malleoli and compares their position. Differing thumb positions signify that a leg length inequality may be present. To assist in determining if this is functional in nature, the *long-sit test* is then performed. With the thumbs remaining under the medial malleoli, maintain the knees in extension and flex the hips to obtain a seated position. If the thumb that was at a higher level when the patient was supine becomes lower in position when the patient is seated, the test is positive and suggests a component of pelvic obliquity (Table 48.5).

48.2.2 Hip and Pelvis Injuries

To assist in the organization of the musculoskeletal etiologies of hip and pelvis pathology, it is helpful to divide disorders as causing anterior, lateral, or posterior pain. Although this is an oversimplification, it provides a good framework with which to approach patient complaints (Table 48.6).

TABLE 48.6
Indications for Specialty Referral for Common Disorders of the Hip and Pelvis

Diagnosis	Primary Care Referral Considerations
Femoral neck stress fracture	Tension-sided stress fractures should be referred for surgical intervention. Compression-sided stress fractures involving ≥50% of the femoral neck should also be referred.
Femoroacetabular impingement	Patients who fail to respond to conservative therapy should be considered for possible surgical correction of the impingement.
Labral tear	Patients who fail to respond to conservative therapy and who have been confirmed to have pain originating from the femoroacetabular joint should be considered for possible surgical intervention.
Osteoarthritis of the hip	Patients who fail to achieve adequate pain control with conservative therapy should be referred for possible hip arthroplasty.
Sports hernia	Patients who have not responded to conservative measures can be referred to general surgeon with expertise in sports hernia repair.

48.2.3 Anterior Hip and Pelvis Pain

48.2.3.1 Adductor Strain

Adductor strains are the most common cause of hip and groin pain in athletes. The adductor group includes the adductor longus, adductor magnus, adductor brevis, pectineus, and gracilis muscles. The adductor longus is the most commonly injured.[10] The injury is most common in the sports of soccer and ice hockey. The mechanisms of acute injury include sprinting, sudden cutting movements, force external rotation of an abducted leg, and a sudden, external abduction force on an actively adducted leg.[36] As is common with other musculotendinous injuries, acute or chronic pathology is likely. Overuse etiologies are common in skating sports.

Clinical Pearl

Adductor strains are the most common cause of hip and pelvis pain in athletes.

In the setting of acute injury, the patients will report the sudden onset of sharp groin pain, swelling, and possible bruising. Athletes often report an inability to continue the sporting activity. On examination, there will be tenderness over the pubic ramus and the injured muscle and/or tendon. Pain is reproduced with passive abduction or resisted active adduction. The diagnosis is clinical but can be confirmed with musculoskeletal ultrasound (MSKUS) or MRI if necessary.

Treatment includes rest from aggravating activity, ice, nonsteroidal anti-inflammatory drugs (NSAIDs) for pain control, and compression shorts. Physical therapy is instituted to restore ROM and regain strength, flexibility, and endurance. Early initiation of therapy is preferred to prevent muscle atrophy. When 80%–90% of strength is regained, a functional return to sport program is begun. Return can take up to 2 months for acute injuries and 6 months for chronic tendinopathy. Those that fail to respond to conservative therapy may respond to ultrasound-guided platelet-rich plasma (PRP) injection or surgical tenotomy. Avulsion injuries are rare and may require surgical repair. However, there is a paucity of evidenced-based research to support these interventions.

48.2.3.2 Quadriceps Strain

The quadriceps muscle group flexes the hip and extends the knee. It includes the rectus femoris, vastus medialis, vastus intermedius, and vastus lateralis. Of these, the rectus femoris is the most commonly injured in the hip region. Tendinosis is common in sports that involve running, jumping, skating, or cycling. The direct head of the rectus femoris originates from the anterior inferior iliac spine (AIIS), while the indirect head arises inferior to this on a brim above the acetabulum. Injuries in the skeletally mature usually occur from at the myotendinous junction from heavy eccentric load. However, in children and adolescents, apophyseal injury is more common as the growth plate is the weaker link in the kinetic chain.

Patients will present with pain with resisted hip flexion, passive hip extension, and direct palpation. In younger athletes, the tenderness will be at the AIIS, and an apophyseal avulsion is more likely. In this population, imaging with comparison views is recommended for further evaluation, whereas adults rarely require imaging. Depending on the severity of the injury, the treatment will include avoidance of painful activities to possibly include protected weight bearing. Rest, ice, compression, gentle ROM, and quad sets begin the rehabilitative process. Short-term NSAIDs are beneficial for pain control. The strengthening program then progresses from concentric to eccentric exercises. When strength is 80%–90% of the unaffected side, ROM is restored, and a functional sports progression is completed, return to sport can be considered. This may take up to 6 weeks. In patients who fail to respond to the conservative measures, advanced imaging (MSKUS or MRI) is recommended. Ultrasound-guided PRP injection can be utilized in these cases, but objective evidence of its efficacy has yet to be studied.

Clinical Pearl

Obtain contralateral radiographs for comparison to evaluate for subtle apophyseal injury.

In adults, injury can also occur within the quadriceps muscle belly, which presents with the abrupt onset of anterior thigh pain. There may be bruising and a palpable defect. Dynamic MSKUS is especially helpful in further evaluation of both the acute tear and to identify the later complication of myositis ossificans. This can occur as the initial tear induced hematoma calcifies. The complication is thought to be reduced by keeping the injured muscle in a lengthened position for the first 24 hours, thereby tamponading the bleeding.[4,42,43] This is then followed by early knee ROM, strengthening, and progression to weight bearing as tolerated. The subsequent rehabilitation course is similar to rectus femoris injury as described earlier.

48.2.3.3 Iliopsoas Strain

The iliopsoas is formed by the confluence of the iliacus and psoas muscles. They form a common tendon that inserts upon the lesser trochanter of the femur. Acute injury can occur when active hip flexion is prevented by a posteriorly directed force. A common scenario is the soccer player whose leg is blocked during an attempted kick. Overuse injury is also possible, especially during uphill running, weight training, sit-ups, and repetitive kicking.

The athlete will complain of deep groin pain, which increases with hip flexion. On physical examination, there will be weakness and pain with resisted hip flexion or passive hip extension or external rotation. There will be tenderness to deep palpation over the anterior hip. The Thomas test will be positive on the affected side. In the skeletally immature, the lesser trochanter may demonstrate point tenderness as apophyseal injury is more likely than tendon strain in this age group. In such cases, bilateral hip films are recommended to assist in the identification of subtle injury.

Treatment includes rest from aggravating activity, ice, NSAIDs for pain control, and compression shorts. Physical therapy is instituted to restore ROM and regain strength, flexibility, and endurance. When 80%–90% of strength is regained, a functional return to sport program begins. Return to sports participation typically takes 4–6 weeks. In the skeletally mature, imaging is often unnecessary. However, in those that fail to respond to the aforementioned conservative measures, MSKUS or MRI is obtained to evaluate for tendinopathy, partial or complete tears.[36] Some clinicians will perform PRP for recalcitrant tendinosis although efficacy has not been studied. Surgical tenotomy may also be considered.

48.2.3.4 Iliopsoas Bursitis

The iliopsoas bursa is a saclike cavity that lies between the anterior femoral acetabular joint and the iliopsoas tendon. It is the largest bursa in the body and communicates with the joint in approximately 15% of people.[12] It can become inflamed through friction or less commonly from direct trauma. It occurs most commonly in sports requiring heavy use of the hip flexors, such as soccer, hurdling, and dance. Patients will complain of anterior hip/groin pain that may radiate to the anterior thigh. It can result in a limp and a snapping sensation in the anterior hip when going from flexion to extension. Pain is often relieved with hip flexion and external rotation.[36] On exam, there will be pain with passive hip extension and with resisted hip flexion during a Stinchfield test.[2] MRI or MSKUS can be used to confirm the diagnosis. Conservative therapy with activity modification, physical therapy (PT), ice, and NSAIDs is typically helpful. In difficult cases, MSKUS is particularly useful as it can then be used to direct aspiration and injection of the bursa.

48.2.3.5 Rectus Abdominis Strain

The rectus abdominis inserts on the superior portion of the pubic ramus. As the adductor muscles originate adjacent to this,[27] strain or tendinopathy can be misinterpreted as originating from the adductor group. However, the astute clinician recognizes that the two pathologies can exist concomitantly, a possibility that impacts both evaluation and treatment. Athletes with rectus abdominis pathology will complain of deep groin pain that is worsened with sit-ups and/or weight training. On examination, the patient will have tenderness along the superior aspect of the pubic ramus. Pain will increase with resisted leg raises (bilateral hip flexion with knee extension). Treatment includes activity modification, ice, NSAIDs, core/pelvic stabilization,[36] and compression shorts. As will other tendinopathies, in recalcitrant cases, MSKUS can be used diagnostically and to guide injection therapy.

48.2.3.6 Sartorius Strain

The sartorius originates from the anterior superior iliac spine (ASIS) and inserts upon the anteromedial tibia as part of the pes anserine tendon group. Injury will typically occur during forceful contraction during hip extension with knee flexion (e.g., leg blocked at beginning of kicking motion). In the skeletally mature, injury will be at the myotendinous junction, while those with open growth plates will affect the apophysis.[23] On examination, there is tenderness to palpation at the ASIS, and resisted hip flexion with external rotation will reproduce the pain. Treatment is conceptually analogous to the previously mentioned tendon injuries.

48.2.3.7 Pubic Symphysis Dysfunction

Disruption of the pubic symphysis is typically the result of a high energy load to the pelvis and is easily recognized on trauma radiographs.[20] However, chronic groin pain from instability of the joint is an underappreciated etiology. Patients will often complain of groin pain and SIJ pain. Clicking may even be present on dynamic examination. Pain is worth with athletic activity and stair climbing. It can even affect walking and rolling over in bed in severe cases. The mechanism of injury is high-speed cutting activity, as seen in football, soccer, ice hockey, and rugby. The problem can also be seen in runners in the postpartum due to relaxation of the pelvic ligaments in preparation for delivery.

On examination, the patient will have tenderness over the pubic symphysis and one or both SIJ. The pubic rami may be unlevel when evaluated in the supine position. Lateral pelvic compression test is often positive. Positive FABER testing indicates SIJ involvement. Single-leg standing or flamingo radiographs have been suggested as methods to objectively measure the degree of instability.[39] Treatment is centered around pelvic stabilization exercises. Core compression shorts, sacroiliac belts, NSAIDs, and symphyseal injections may be considered for pain control.[36]

48.2.3.8 Osteitis Pubis

Osteitis pubis also causes deep groin pain originating from the pubic symphysis. It is a chronic inflammatory condition associated with sports requiring running, cutting, twisting, and side-to-side and multidirectional motion. The inflammation may affect the tendons that insert upon the pubic ramus, as such pain may radiate to the abdomen, proximal medial thigh, hip, scrotum, perineum, and suprapubic region. The pain is often described as sharp or burning. It is worsened by kicking, running, striding, twisting, leg raises, and stairs. Patients may report clicking with certain activities. Queries to systemic symptoms are very important as there infectious etiologies have been reported in the past.[45]

On examination, there will be tenderness directly over the pubic symphysis and possibly the proximal adductors or distal rectus abdominis. Pain is increased with passive hip abduction and active hip flexion or adduction. Other findings include a positive lateral compression test, a forward flexed gait, and pelvic obliquity due to associated muscle spasm.

Anteroposterior (AP) radiographs will show sclerosis and bony resorption of the pubic rami on both sides of the pubic symphysis in advanced disease. MRI will demonstrate symmetric inflammation of the pubic symphysis and rami. Various treatment methods have been reported in the literature to include activity modification, physical therapy with core/pelvic stabilization, ice, NSAIDs, corticosteroid injection, prolotherapy, and surgery. Unfortunately, no randomized controlled trials have been performed to compare the above in terms of efficacy or speed of return to sport.[9]

48.2.3.9 Femoral Neck Stress Fracture

Stress fractures are overuse injuries that result from an increased rate of bony resorption compared to buildup. They can occur throughout the skeleton but are most common in the lower extremity. Although relatively rare, untreated femoral neck stress fractures carry a high rate of morbidity (avascular necrosis) and, as such, require a high index of suspicion. The typical history is one of sudden increased activity, underrecovery, improper nutrition, and/or hormonal imbalance. The athlete will complain of groin pain that is worse with weight bearing. On examination, the patient will have a positive log roll, and the Stinchfield test will cause groin pain. The patient should be made nonweight bearing and sent immediately for radiographs. If these are negative, an urgent MRI should be obtained.

Clinical Pearl

In patients with suspected femoral neck stress fractures and normal radiographs, an urgent MRI should be obtained for further evaluation.

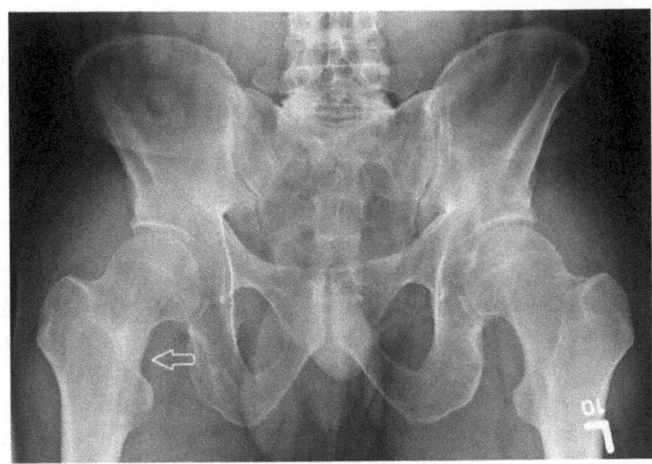

FIGURE 48.1 An anteroposterior pelvis film of a runner who had a prior history of right hip pain demonstrating callus formation from a prior compression-sided femoral neck stress fracture (arrow).

Femoral neck stress fractures are divided into two types: tension and compression side. The tension side is the superior aspect of the femoral neck, while the compression side is inferior (Figure 48.1). If the fracture is tension sided, or if it is compression sided but involves more than 50% of the femoral neck, the patient should be referred for surgical management. If it is a compression-sided stress fracture with less than 50% involvement, then it can be managed conservatively. Initial treatment involves nonweight bearing for 1–2 weeks, followed by partial weight bearing. The patient is slowly progressed to pain-free weight bearing. Gentle, pain-free ROM is initiated early with the gradual addition of strengthening. A slow, supervised return to activity program is then followed. The treatment should include nutritional and hormonal interventions if necessary.

48.2.3.10 Pubic Ramus Stress Fracture

Pubic ramus stress fractures are rarer than femoral stress fractures. They are more common in distance runners. The athlete will complain of groin pain that is worse with passive abduction or resisted adduction. There is tenderness with palpation of the inferior pubic ramus and single-leg stance on the affected leg. Diagnosis can be made on plain films but often requires MRI. If weight bearing is painful, the patient should be placed on crutches and gradually progressed to weight bearing as tolerated. Rehabilitation should work on hip ROM and strengthening, especially of the adductors. Nutritional, hormonal, and training imbalances should be identified and corrected. A gradual return to running program is begun once the athlete is pain-free with normal ROM and strength.

48.2.3.11 Tears of the Acetabular Labrum and Femoroacetabular Impingement

Labral pathology is a common and increasingly well-recognized source of hip pain in young, active individuals.[30] There is a growing body of evidence that ties damage to and loss of function of the labrum to the onset of OA. Labral injury can occur acutely as a result of a specific traumatic event.

More commonly, however, it is the culmination of a pattern of microtrauma in the setting of femoroacetabular impingement (FAI), which is defined as any movement pattern where hip flexion causes the proximal femur to abut (impinge) on the acetabulum, trapping and causing damage to the labral tissue. FAI, in turn, is typically due to one or more subtle predisposing anatomic variations and can be divided into two types: cam impingement, characterized by asphericity of the femoral head and proximal femoral neck, and pincer impingement, characterized by overcoverage of the femoral head by the anterior and anterolateral acetabulum. Both cam and pincer impingement can be present in the same individual.[14]

Cam-type deformity of the proximal femur can be defined as excess bone at the junction of the femoral head and femoral neck that impinges on the acetabulum when the hip flexes. It is typically located on the anterolateral aspect of the proximal femoral neck and is often described as a "pistol-grip" deformity as a result of its appearance on AP radiographs. It can be idiopathic, or it can be the consequence of various pediatric hip pathologies such as SCFE or Legg–Calve–Perthes disease.[30]

Pincer-type deformity can be defined as excess anterior and anterolateral coverage of the femoral head by the bony acetabulum. Like cam impingement, pincer impingement also leads to abnormal contact between the labrum and the proximal femur during hip flexion and likewise can be either idiopathic or secondary to other developmental hip pathologies, such as coxa profunda (overly deep socket) or acetabular retroversion.[31]

Labral tears are typically the consequence of FAI and, like most intra-articular hip pathology, will present as groin pain. Some patients will ascribe the injury to a specific event, whereas others will complain of an insidious onset. Pain is usually activity related, but can also be positional, with many patients finding prolonged sitting to be uncomfortable.[24,30] Since the differential diagnosis of groin pain is broad, physical examination to confirm an intra-articular source for the pain is of utmost importance. The hallmarks of hip joint pathology are pain with hip motion and a decreased ROM compared to the unaffected side. The examination is done with the patient supine and the hip flexed to 90°. Internal and external rotations are then assessed. Intra-articular hip pathology, whether FAI, labral tearing, or OA, will typically manifest as loss of internal rotation and pain with internal rotation, particularly when the hip is adducted as well as flexed. The combination of flexion, adduction, and internal rotation, termed the impingement test or FADIR test, is sensitive for both symptomatic FAI and OA, with reported sensitivity of 78%.[19,24,25]

Once an intra-articular source of pain is confirmed, radiographs are used to further characterize the pathology. OA will show the classic findings of joint space narrowing, osteophyte formation, and subchondral sclerosis. If these findings are not present, then FAI, with or without a labral tear, should be suspected. Radiographic findings suggestive of FAI are often more subtle than those of OA. For cam-type impingement, the classic finding is a pistol-grip deformity (Figure 48.2). This can be seen on an AP pelvic radiograph but is usually best visualized on either a frog-leg lateral or a modified Dunn view.[24,25] The degree of cam deformity can be quantified by measurement of the alpha angle, which is defined as the angle formed by the intersection of the long axis of the femoral neck with a line drawn between the center of the femoral head and the point at which the spherical femoral head ends and the neck (or cam deformity) begins. There is controversy regarding the cutoff value for a normal alpha angle, with various authors recommending anywhere from 42° to 63°. Once again, it is important to note that asymptomatic individuals can have alpha angles in the abnormal range.

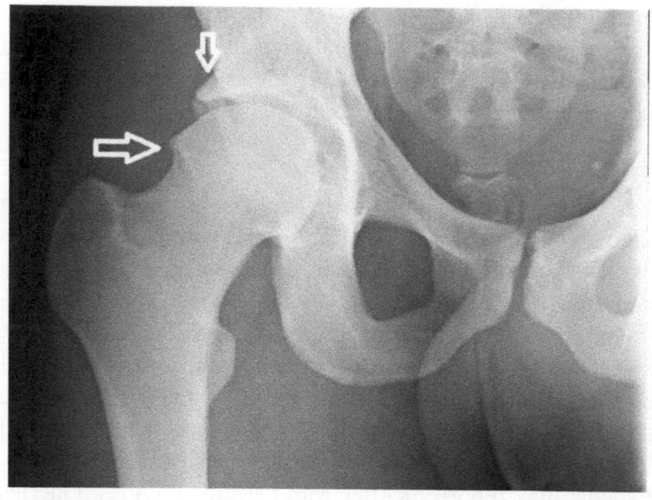

FIGURE 48.2 An anteroposterior radiograph of the right hip demonstrating both cam (horizontal arrow) and pincer lesions (vertical arrow). Adjacent to the pincer lesion is an os acetabuli, a finding associated with labral tears.

Pincer-type deformity can be recognized on AP radiographs by looking for a "crossover sign," which is defined as having the lateral portion of the anterior acetabular margin project laterally to the posterior acetabular margin. Such crossover is indicative of anterolateral overcoverage. It is also important to look for significant acetabular retroversion. A true measurement of version requires cross-sectional axial imaging such as CT or MRI, but a useful screening tool on an AP radiograph is the "posterior wall sign," which is defined as having the center of the femoral head lie lateral to the margin of the posterior wall. A positive posterior wall sign indicates deficiency of the posterior wall and, in combination with a crossover sign, suggests significant retroversion.[31]

While the anatomic characteristics of FAI can be seen on plain radiographs, imaging the labrum itself requires other modalities, typically MRI. Although MRI has good specificity for labral tears, the sensitivity is suboptimal. Magnetic resonance arthrography (MRA), in which contrast dye is injected into the hip joint under fluoroscopic or ultrasound guidance in order to enhance the quality of MRI data, increases the sensitivity of the test, but at the expense of significantly decreasing its specificity. A recent meta-analysis found the sensitivity of MRI and MRA to be 66% and 87%, respectively, with specificities of 79% and 64%. Additionally, MRA was found to have higher overall accuracy.[40] Therefore, it is of vital importance that any clinician ordering MRI studies of the hip, whether with contrast or without, have a working differential diagnosis based on a thorough history and physical exam. Otherwise, it is quite possible to either falsely rule out existing labral pathology or mistakenly diagnose it based on asymptomatic radiologic findings.[16]

The natural history of FAI and labral tears remains controversial. Biomechanical data show that labrum deficiency results in increased contact pressures of the acetabular and femoral cartilage surfaces; this is postulated to, in turn, lead to early onset of OA.[14] It is also well documented that up to 60% of patients who undergo hip arthroscopy and are found to have labral tears also have concomitant cartilage damage to some degree.[30] However, it remains to be definitively shown whether the labral tear is the initiating factor in hip joint deterioration, or whether it is a symptom of some other underlying process. Once again, it is important to note that many asymptomatic individuals have radiographic findings consistent with a diagnosis of FAI. Whether these individuals are at increased risk of sustaining labral injury is currently unknown. Therefore, no recommendation for treatment of asymptomatic cam and pincer lesions can currently be made.

The management of acetabular labral tears is driven by severity of symptoms and degree of functional impairment. Patients who are able to compensate for their injury through activity modification, or who become asymptomatic or minimally symptomatic with time, can be managed conservatively. However, patients who are high demand, including most athletes, generally fail conservative therapy and will progress to surgical management.[30] Currently, most acetabular labral tears and many cases of FAI are managed arthroscopically. The goal of surgical treatment is to debride any unstable tissue, resect any pincer and cam lesions such that impingement no longer occurs, and repair any viable labral tissue back to the acetabular rim.

Clinical Pearl

Asymptomatic labral tears do not require surgical intervention.

Postoperatively, those patients who undergo cam lesion resection are typically managed with protected weight bearing in order to minimize the risk of femoral neck stress fracture. Early postop rehab focuses on regaining muscle control and tone as well as ROM. Once these goals are achieved and sufficient time has progressed to allow healing of repaired labral tissue, focus turns to functional strength, endurance, and sport-specific conditioning. Return to play can occur once an athlete is pain-free and has regained their baseline strength and agility necessary for safe participation in their sport.[30]

48.2.3.12 Osteoarthritis

OA of the hip presents a significant burden to society and the health-care system. It is estimated that over 20 million adults in the United States were living with OA in 2006, and that number is estimated to rise to over 40 million by 2030.[17] It is also estimated that the direct medical costs of care for hip OA are in excess of $100 million per year.[26] Consequently, primary care physicians will frequently encounter patients living with hip OA and should be prepared to counsel them on initial nonoperative management and provide timely, but not unnecessary, orthopedic surgical referrals.

OA can be defined as the mechanical breakdown of the articular cartilage of a joint and spans the spectrum from mild to disabling. The classic symptom is pain in the involved joint, particularly with weight bearing. Radiographic features of OA include narrowing of the joint space on weight-bearing radiographs, the presence of marginal osteophytes, and the formation of subchondral cysts and areas of bony sclerosis.[22] Although, for most patients, the presence and progression of radiographic changes is a gradual and steady process that takes place over years, the clinical symptoms of pain and disability can fluctuate in severity and are often not directly proportional to the radiographic severity. Therefore, once the diagnosis of OA is made, it is more important to focus on the patient's clinical symptoms rather than on radiographic findings.

There are currently no formal clinical practice guidelines for treatment of hip OA. However, the American Academy of Orthopedic Surgeons has published a clinical practice guideline for the treatment of knee OA,[1] which may be of interest. Essentially, conservative management of OA revolves around pain control using nonnarcotic analgesics, with an emphasis on NSAIDs. Activity modification to avoid those activities that exacerbate a patient's symptoms is warranted, although maintaining a moderately active lifestyle with a focus on low-impact activities such as walking, swimming, or biking is generally felt to be beneficial. Physical therapy may be useful in order to address secondary gait disturbances such as a limp but is generally of limited utility in controlling pain. Assistive devices such as a cane, however, can be quite helpful, since they can offload the affected joint.

Another useful modality in OA treatment is intra-articular injections. Historically, cortisone or its derivatives, such as triamcinolone, have been used. In recent years, hyaluronic acid derivatives (synvisc, hyalgan, etc.) have been approved for use in OA of the knee; however, they have not been FDA approved for use in other joints, and consequently, their use in the hip is off-label. Additionally, one recent study found hyaluronic acid injections in the hip to be no more effective than placebo.[32] Consequently, steroid injections continue to be the main option for hip injections. Finally, since the hip is a deep structure, intra-articular injections require the use of imaging guidance, either with fluoroscopy or ultrasound. This adds a cost burden, since injections must typically be scheduled as a separate appointment rather than being done in conjunction with a routine office visit.

Ultimately, when conservative measures are no longer effective in providing satisfactory pain relief, surgical options should be considered. Surgery for hip OA consists of total hip arthroplasty and involves resection of the arthritic femoral head and neck as well as reaming of the arthritic acetabulum and replacement with a prosthetic acetabular component and a femoral head and stem. Various bearing surfaces are available, including metal-on-polyethylene, ceramic-on-polyethylene, ceramic-on-ceramic, and metal-on-metal. The choice of implants and bearing surfaces should be determined in conjunction between a patient and surgeon, taking into account the patient's age, activity level, and surgeon experience. It is important to note that the decision to proceed with surgery is based on patient symptoms rather than on radiographic severity and is entirely elective. Therefore, consultation with a joint replacement specialist is of limited utility unless a patient is medically, socially, and psychologically ready to consider surgery. Typically, hip replacement involves a two- to three-night stay in the hospital, followed by several months of physical therapy. Most patients are able to walk with assistance immediately after surgery, drive 4–6 weeks after surgery, and can resume full activities at 3–4 months after surgery. However, it can be 6 months to a year before maximum strength and endurance are achieved. Because of the lengthy and intensive rehabilitation process, it is important that patients be prepared in order to achieve the best possible outcome.

Clinical Pearl

Total hip arthroplasty is recommended for the treatment of osteoarthritis only after conservative treatment has failed to provide adequate pain relief.

48.2.3.13 Sports Hernia

Sports hernias are controversial hip injuries that involve a disruption of the posterior abdominal wall at the inguinal canal. Tears of the transverse abdominis muscle, conjoined tendon, internal oblique muscle, rectus abdominis muscle, adductor insertion, external oblique aponeurosis, and ilioinguinal nerve entrapment have all been implicated as possible etiologies. The injury is most common in sports that require fast cutting and twisting, such as soccer, ice hockey, football, and rugby. Athletes will complain of activity related unilateral groin pain. Pain is exacerbated by sudden movements, sit-ups, and Valsalva. In chronic cases, activities of daily living may also be affected. Unlike traditional hernias, no abdominal wall defect is outwardly palpable. However, there may be tenderness to palpation over the conjoined tendon, pubic tubercle, and/or midinguinal region. MRI or ultrasound can assist in confirming the diagnosis.[33] Initial treatment involves rest, NSAIDs, and ice. If conservative treatment fails, referral for surgical exploration and repair is recommended.

48.2.4 Lateral Hip and Pelvis Pain

48.2.4.1 Iliac Crest Contusion

Iliac crest contusions, also known as hip pointers, are the results of direct trauma to the iliac crest causing a periosteal hematoma. It is most commonly seen in contact–collision sports including football and ice hockey. The athlete will complain of pain with lateral side bending and/or rotation away from the affected side. There may also be the lateral aspect of the hip and thigh due to hematoma compression of the lateral femoral cutaneous nerve. On examination, there will be tenderness on and superior to the iliac crest with fullness over the hematoma. Radiographs are obtained if symptoms are prolonged to rule out avulsion fracture. Ice, compression, activity modification, and short-term NSAIDs are recommended for pain. MSKUS can readily demonstrate the hematoma and can assist in guidance of aspiration. In addition, it can demonstrate muscle disruption, signifying a tear. Anesthetic and corticosteroid injection has been suggested as a mode of speeding return to play; however, this controversial approach may actually slow the overall healing process.

48.2.4.2 Greater Trochanteric Bursitis

The greater trochanteric bursal complex overlies the greater trochanter and is actually made up of three separate bursae—gluteus maximus, gluteus medius, and gluteus minumus bursae. The bursa can become inflamed and painful from tightness of the ITB, snapping of the tensor fascia lata (TFL) over the greater trochanter, hip abductor weakness, and leg length discrepancy. The patient will complain of pain posterior to the greater trochanter, which may radiate to the gluteal region and/or down the lateral thigh. On physical exam, there will be tenderness over and posterior to the greater trochanter. The patient will complain of lateral hip pain during the FABER test, resisted abduction, and passive adduction. The Trendelenburg's and Ober's tests are typically positive.

Clinical Pearl

The greater trochanteric bursa is actually three separate bursae.

Treatment should consist of hip abductor strengthening, correction of functional leg length discrepancy, stretching of the ITB, and ice. NSAIDs can help with pain control. Individuals who have too much pain to do therapy may benefit from corticosteroid injection of the bursa.

48.2.4.3 Tensor Fascia Lata Strain

The TFL serves as a hip abductor and combines with fibers of the gluteus maximus to form the ITB. It is common in runners and cyclists, who often report a change in training program such as the addition of hills. In cyclists, improper bike fit has been implicated. Athletes will complain of the gradual onset of anterolateral hip pain that may progress to snapping as the TFL slides over the greater trochanter.

On exam, there will be tenderness of the TFL, tightness of the ITB, and snapping of the TFL over the greater trochanter when the hip is moved from flexion to extension. Therapy is similar to that of greater trochanteric bursitis. Additionally, adjustment of the training regimen and proper bike fit are beneficial.[6]

48.2.4.4 Meralgia Paresthetica

Meralgia paresthetica is caused by compression of the lateral femoral cutaneous nerve. It is most common with obesity, tight pants, belts, and girdles. In athletes, prolonged flexion, weight training, and compressive clothing are contributing factors.[12] The patient will complain of pain, burning, numbness, or tingling in the anterolateral thigh. On examination, there will be a positive Tinel's sign 1 cm medial and 1 cm inferior to the ASIS. The treatment includes adjustment of clothing, NSAIDs, PT, and local corticosteroid injection. If these measures are unsuccessful, nerve conduction study should be obtained to confirm the diagnosis prior to referral for surgical decompression.

48.2.5 Posterior Hip and Pelvis Pain

48.2.5.1 Hamstring Strain

The hamstring group originates from the ischial tuberosity. Going medially to laterally, the tendons are the semimembranosus, semitendinosus, and biceps femoris. Collectively, they function to extend the hip and flex the knee. As the muscle–tendon unit spans two joints, there is a high susceptibility to injury, with the biceps femoris most commonly affected. In adults, the injury is typically longitudinal through the muscle. However, in the skeletally immature, the ischial apophysis is more likely impacted. Injury typically occurs during sprinting or jumping and is more likely with concomitant hip girdle muscle imbalance, leg length discrepancy, inflexibility, and history of prior injury.[36]

Patients will report feeling an acute pop or pulling sensation in the posterior thigh. On examination, there will be swelling and, in large tears, a palpable defect. Bruising may be apparent if the injury is superficial. If there is tenderness at the ischial tuberosity, radiographs should be obtained to rule out ischial spine avulsion. There will be pain with passive hamstring stretch, resisted hip extension, and resisted knee flexion. In muscle belly injuries, imaging is unnecessary. However, for confirmation, MRI or MSKUS can confirm the injury. MSKUS is may be more beneficial in detecting more subtle defects with the addition of dynamic evaluation.

Initial treatment includes ice, compression, and if severe, crutches. Physical therapy to work on ROM with progression as pain resolves. Frequent hamstring flexibility exercises and correction of movement dysfunction have been shown to speed return to play and prevent recurrence in elite athletes.[18] There is preliminary evidence that eccentric programs are superior to those that emphasize concentric only.[5]

48.2.5.2 Ischial Bursitis

The ischial bursa is superficial to the hamstring origin on the ischial tuberosity. Inflammation can occur from a direct blow or from concomitant injury to the hamstring tendon. The athlete's primary complaint is pain with sitting. On exam, there is tenderness over the hamstring origin. Treatment includes offloading the area while sitting, NSAIDs, and hamstring rehabilitation. MRI or MSKUS can confirm the diagnosis, with the latter helpful to guide aspiration and injection if conservative measures are unsuccessful.

48.2.5.3 Piriformis Syndrome

The piriformis muscle is a hip external rotator that originates from the sacrum and inserts on the greater trochanter and upper femoral shaft. It lies deep to the gluteus maximus. The sciatic nerve is typically deep to the muscle, but it can bisect the muscle or even be superficial to it. Spasm of the piriformis can therefore cause compression of the sciatic nerve and produce neuropathic symptoms of classic sciatica. The piriformis can be injured through direct trauma and twisting of the hip during cutting movements. Spasm can occur from overuse and SIJ dysfunction.

Physical exam will demonstrate tenderness with palpation of the muscle, buttock pain with passive hip flexion with internal rotation pain, and piriformis testing. Treatment includes ice massage, deep tissue massage, stretching, physical therapy modalities, NSAIDs, and trigger point injections. Correction of underlying sacroiliac dysfunction is often helpful, while core and pelvic stabilization may help prevent recurrence.[36]

48.2.5.4 Sacroiliac Dysfunction/Sprain

Sacroiliac dysfunction or sprain can occur from direct blow to one side of the gluteal region when the hip is in flexion during a fall. Sudden, excessive contraction of the muscles that attach to the pelvis such as the hamstring or piriformis can also create acute injury to the joint. Sports with repetitive unilateral pelvic shear (skating, hockey, soccer, gymnastics) are at risk for overuse pathology. In addition, rheumatologic disease can cause inflammation of the SIJ, and these etiologies should be considered in the differential.

On physical examination, there will be tenderness to palpation of the affected SIJ and signs of SIJ dysfunction—positive FABER test, leg length inequality, and pelvic obliquity. Osteopathic manipulation can be utilized to reestablish a neutral pelvis, followed by physical therapy to correct any muscle imbalances that may have contributed to the pathology. NSAIDs, ice, and heat can assist with pain control. Sacroiliac belts may assist in patients with SIJ instability until the pelvic stabilizers are strengthened. Recalcitrant SIJ pain may benefit from corticosteroid injection, which should be performed under fluoroscopic or ultrasound guidance[13] (Table 48.7).

TABLE 48.7
SORT: Key Recommendations for Practice

Clinical Recommendation	Evidence Rating	References
Obtain bilateral radiographs to evaluate for subtle apophyseal injuries in skeletally immature athletes.	C	
Acute quadriceps contusions should be treated in the first 24 hours with immobilization with knee flexion to tamponade bleeding.	B	[4]
The FADIR test has a sensitivity of 78% in diagnosing femoroacetabular impingement.	A	[19,24,25]
Only symptomatic labral tears and/or femoroacetabular impingement require treatment. Surgery is considered after conservative measures fail.	B	[14,30]
Pain management and activity modification are the mainstays of conservative treatment for osteoarthritis of the hip.	C	[1]
Total hip arthroplasty is recommended for treatment of osteoarthritis only after conservative measures have failed.	C	[1]
Eccentric exercises should be included in the management of hamstring injuries.	B	[5]
Core and pelvic stabilization and correction of underlying sacroiliac joint dysfunction can help prevent recurrence of piriformis syndrome.	C	[36]

REFERENCES

1. AAOS. *Treatment of Osteoarthritis of the Knee: Evidence Based Guideline*, 2nd edn. American Academy of Orthopedic Surgeons, Rosemont, IL; 2013.
2. Anderson K, Strickland SM, Warren R. Hip and groin injuries in athletes. *The American Journal of Sports Medicine.* 2001;29(4):521–523.
3. Anderson SJ. Sports injuries. *Current Problems in Pediatric and Adolescent Health Care.* 2005;35(4):110–164.
4. Aronen JG, Garrick JG, Chronister RD et al. Quadriceps contusions: Clinical results of immediate immobilization in 120 degrees of knee flexion. *Clinical Journal of Sport Medicine.* 2006;16(5):383–387.
5. Askling CM, Tengvar M, Tarassova O et al. Acute hamstring injuries in Swedish elite sprinters and jumpers: A prospective randomized controlled clinical trial comparing two rehabilitation protocols. *British Journal of Sports Medicine.* 2014;48(7):532–539.
6. Asplund C, St Pierre P. Knee pain and bicycling: Fitting concepts for clinicians. *Physician and Sportsmedicine.* 2004;32(4):23–30.
7. Beck M, Kalhor M, Leunig M et al. Hip morphology influences the pattern of damage to the acetabular cartilage: Femoroacetabular impingement as a cause of early osteoarthritis of the hip. *Journal of Bone and Joint Surgery [Br]* 2005;87:1012–1018.
8. Bharam S, PHilippon MJ. Hip injuries. *Clinics in Sports Medicine.* 2006;25(2):xv–xvi.
9. Choi H, McCartney M, Best TM. Treatment of osteitis pubis and osteomyelitis of the pubic symphysis in athletes: A systematic review. *British Journal of Sports Medicine.* 2011;45(1):57–64.
10. Cunningham PM, Brennan D, O'Connell M et al. Patterns of bone and soft-tissue injury at the symphysis pubis in soccer players: Observations at MRI. *AJR American Journal of Roentgenology.* 2007;188(3):W291–W296.
11. DeAngelis NA, Busconi BD. Assessment and differential diagnosis of the painful hip. *Clinical Orthopaedics and Related Research.* 2003;406:11–18.
12. Farber AJ, Wilkens JH, Jarvis CG. Pelvic pain in the athlete. In: Seidenberg PH, Beutler AI, eds. *The Sports Medicine Resource Manual*, Philadelphia, PA: Saunders Elsevier; 2008, pp. 306–327.
13. Foley BS, Buschbacher RM. Sacroiliac joint pain: Anatomy, biomechanics, diagnosis, and treatment. *American Journal of Physical Medicine & Rehabilitation.* 2006; 85(12):997–1006.
14. Ganz R, Parvizi J, Beck M et al. Femoracetabular impingement: A cause of early osteoarthritis of the hip. *Clinical Orthopaedics and Related Research.* 2003;417:112–120.
15. Hurwitz DE, Foucher KC, Andriacchi TP. A new parametric approach for modeling hip forces during gait. *Journal of Biomechanics.* 2003;36(1):113–119.
16. Keeney JA, Peelle JW, Jackson J et al. Magnetic resonance arthrography versus arthroscopy in the evaluation of articular hip pathology. *Clinical Orthopaedics and Related Research.* 2004;429:163–169.
17. Leveille SG. Musculoskeletal aging. *Current Opinion in Rheumatology.* 2004;16:114–118.
18. Mason DL, Dickens VA, Vail. Rehabilitation for hamstring injuries. *Cochrane Database of Systematic Reviews.* 2012;12:CD004575.
19. Martin RL, Irrgang JJ, Sekiya JK. The diagnostic accuracy of a clinical examination in determining intra-articular hip pain for potential hip arthroscopy candidates. *Arthroscopy.* 2008;24(9):1013–1018.
20. Matta JM, Tornetta P. Internal fixation of unstable pelvic ring injuries. *Clinical Orthopaedics and Related Research.* 1996;329:129–140.
21. McFadden DP, Seidenberg PH. Physical examination of the hip and pelvis. In: Seidenberg PH and Bowen JD, eds. *The Hip and Pelvis in Sports Medicine and Primary Care.* New York: Springer Publishing; 2010, pp. 9–36.
22. Menkes CJ. Radiographic criteria for the classification of osteoarthritis. *Journal of Rheumatology.* 1991;27:13–15.
23. Morelli V, Weaver V. Groin injuries and groin pain in athletes: Part 1. *Prim Care* 2005;32(1):163–183.
24. Nepple J, Prather H, Trousdale R et al. Clinical diagnosis of femoroacetabular impingement. *JAAOS.* 2013;21:S16–S19.
25. Nepple J, Prather H, Trousdale R et al. Diagnostic imaging of femoroacetabular impingement. *JAAOS.* 2013;21:S20–S26.
26. Nho SJ, Kymes SM, Callaghan JJ et al. The burden of hip osteoarthritis in the United States: Epidemiologic and economic considerations. *JAAOS.* 2013;21:S1–S6.
27. Norton-Old KJ, Schache AG, Barker PJ et al. Anatomical and mechanical relationship between the proximal attachment of adductor longus and the distal rectus sheath. *Clinical Anatomy.* 2013;26(4):522–530.
28. Paletta GA Jr, Andrish JT. Injuries about the hip and pelvis in the young athlete. *Clinics in Sports Medicine.* 1995; 14:591–628.

29. Pakos EE, Pitouli EJ, Tsekeris PG et al. Prevention of heterotopic ossification in high-risk patients with total hip arthroplasty: The experience of a combined therapeutic protocol. *International Orthopaedics.* 2006;30(2):79–83.
30. Parvizi J, Leunig M, Ganz R. Femoroacetabular impingement. JAAOS. 2007;15(9):561–570.
31. Reynolds D, Lucas J, Klaue K. Retroversion of the acetabulum: A cause of hip pain. *Journal of Bone and Joint Surgery British Volume.* 1999;81:281–288.
32. Richette P, Ravaud P, Conrozier T et al. Effect of hyaluronic acid in symptomatic hip osteoarthritis: A multicenter, randomized, placebo-controlled trial. *Arthritis & Rheumatology.* 2009;60(3):824–830.
33. Robinson P, Bhat V, English B. Imaging in the assessment and management of athletic pubalgia. *Seminars in Musculoskeletal Radiology.* 2011;15(1):14–26.
34. Schasser KD, Disch AC, Stover JF et al. Prolonged superficial local cryotherapy attenuates microcirculatory impairment, regional inflammation, and muscle necrosis after closed soft tissue injury in rats. *The American Journal of Sports Medicine.* 2007;35(1):93–102.
35. Scoop M. The assessment of athletic hip injury. *Clinics in Sports Medicine.* 2001;20(4):647–659.
36. Seidenberg PH. Adult hip and pelvis disorders. In: Seidenberg PH and Bowen JD, eds. *The Hip and Pelvis in Sports Medicine and Primary Care.* New York: Springer Publishing; 2010, pp. 115–147.
37. Seidenberg PH, Childress MA. Evaluating hip pain in athletes. *Journal of Musculoskeletal Medicine.* 2005;22(5): 246–254.
38. Seidenberg PH, Childress MA. Physical examination of the hip and pelvis. In: Seidenberg PH and Beutler AI, eds. *The Sports Medicine Resource Manual.* New York: Saunders Publishing; 2008, pp. 110–122.
39. Siegel J, Templeman DC, Torentta P. Single-leg-stance radiographs in the diagnosis of pelvic instability. *Journal of Bone and Joint Surgery American Volume.* 2008;90(10): 2119–2125.
40. Smith TO, Hilton G, Toms AP et al. The diagnostic accuracy of acetabular labral tears using magnetic resonance imaging and magnetic resonance arthrography: A meta-analysis. *European Radiology.* 2011;21(4):863–874.
41. Spahn G, Schiele R, Langlotz A et al. Hip pain in adolescents: Results of a cross-sectional study in German pupils and review of the literature. *Acta Paediatrica.* 2005;94(5): 568–573.
42. Thorsson O, Lilja B, Nilsson P et al. Immediate external compression in the management of an acute muscle injury. *Scandinavian Journal of Medicine & Science in Sports.* 1997;7(3):182–190.
43. Trojian TH. Muscle contusion: Thigh. *Clinics in Sports Medicine.* 2013;32:317–324.
44. Watkins J, Peabody P. Sports injuries in children and adolescents treated at a sports injury clinic. *The Journal of Sports Medicine and Physical Fitness.* 1996;36(1):43–48.
45. Yusuf E, Hofer M, Steinrucken J et al. Septic arthritis of the pubic symphysis caused by *Streptococcus mitis. Acta Clinica Belgica.* 2014;69(6):454–455.

49 Thigh Injuries

Peter C. Wenger and Richard Levandowski

CONTENTS

TABLE 49.1
Key Clinical Considerations

1. The thigh is indistinguishable from the hip and pelvis from a biomechanical standpoint. The muscles that occupy the thigh provide the power and control of the pelvis and knee.
2. Skeletally immature patients are subjected to additional injuries at the enthesis, or bone–tendon interface. These injuries may occur at many entheses.
3. Most thigh injuries encountered in primary care respond well with nonoperative therapy including activity modification, anti-inflammatory medication, and targeted exercise therapy to correct biomechanical weakness.
4. The consequences of trauma to the thigh include compartment syndrome. If there is clinical suspicion of compartment syndrome, compartment pressures should be obtained as soon as possible.
5. Myositis ossificans is associated with quadriceps hematomas and is diagnosed as calcium deposition occurs in substance of muscle during healing. The athlete will complain of increasing or persistent pain and inhibition of the affected muscle.

Sources: Anderson, K. et al., *Am. J. Sports Med.*, 29, 521, 2001; Nau, T. et al., *Am. J. Sports Med.*, 28, 120, 2000; Rossi, F. and Dragoni, S., *Skeletal Radiol.*, 30, 127, 2001; Ryan, J.B. et al., *Am. J. Sports Med.*, 19, 299, 1991.

49.1 INTRODUCTION

The thigh is subjected to tremendous stress as part of athletic activity. As one of the proximal components of the kinetic chain, these structures are intimately related to athletes' power, endurance, and resistance to injury. Loads of up to eight times the athletes' body weight have been demonstrated across the hip joint during jogging with even greater loads observed during athletic competition.[4,14] The importance of thigh strength is stressed at all levels of competition, especially during preseason conditioning. Functional assessments of hip/core strength, agility, and proprioception have been studied as part of treatment after injury, return to sport clearance after ACL surgery, and injury prevention programs (Table 49.1).

Thigh injuries are common in athletes of all ages and are a known consequence of physical activity at any level. In a 2007 International Association of Athletics Foundation survey of sports-related injuries at the World Athletics Championships, thigh strains were found to be among the most common injuries.[3] In high school athletes, hip and thigh injuries comprise 5%–9% of all reported injuries.[4,21] Treatment of these injuries is challenging and symptom recurrence is common.[25] Because of the anatomic and biomechanical complexity of the thigh, rehabilitation times can be prolonged and early diagnosis essential.[4] The reinjury risk is significant. It has been estimated that the risk of sustaining a hamstring or a groin injury is almost doubled if the athlete experienced a previous injury.[25] These injuries lead to significant costs to society as well as the athlete, whether recreational or professional.

Clinical Pearl

Hip and core strength/flexibility deficits are important to identify. Addressing these issues puts athletes and patients at lower risk for overuse and injury.

Because of the prevalence and disability attributed to these injuries, exciting research is taking place in many fields including physiology, exercise science, nonoperative medicine, and surgery. A paradigm shift has occurred as newer conditioning programs are supplanting older but still widely implemented protocols that focus on traditional strengthening of the extremities. Only recently have programs been adopted that address the stability and athletic performance of the trunk, gluteal, thigh, and postural muscles.[4,29] These newer programs emphasize exercises that eccentrically load the muscles of the hip and thigh, and research suggests this conditioning has value in both treatment and prevention of hip and thigh injuries.[25,64]

As musculoskeletal imaging has advanced, so has the armamentarium of the clinician to accurately diagnose and treat these injuries. Imaging has shown to be prognostic in management of certain thigh conditions and useful as a tool for deciding the time until return to activity.[4] However, clinicians should use discretion in the utilization of imaging as a wide variety of radiographic abnormalities can be found, which carry minimal clinical consequence. Musculoskeletal imaging studies including x-ray, sonography, and magnetic resonance imaging (MRI) are most useful when selected on the basis of a thorough history and musculoskeletal physical examination.[4,47]

49.2 THIGH ANATOMY AND BIOMECHANICS

The thigh is indistinguishable from the hip and pelvis from a biomechanical standpoint. The muscles that occupy the thigh provide power and control of the pelvis.[4,36] The biomechanical relationship of the upper thigh and the lower abdominal musculature is an area of intense study.[4,28,36,46] Perturbations of normal muscle function in these regions have been implicated as a risk factor for injuries. A study in college female athletes has shown that strength and flexibility imbalances were associated with lower extremity injuries in general, but not specifically with the muscle group in which the imbalance was found.[28,55] Other studies suggest that decreased spinal mobility and trunk muscle strength need to be considered for its role in conditions that affect the pelvis and hip.[4,46] This complex interdependence of muscle groups leads to a variety of pathologic entities that may coexist simultaneously and present differently. Furthermore, evidence suggests that care has to be taken with which exercises should be prescribed as competing injuries can impede successful treatment.[27,40] This makes diagnosis difficult and treatment sublime.

Core stability and its role as a predisposing factor in injuries of the thigh are also being studied. Core stability is defined as the ability to control the position and motion of the trunk over the pelvis to allow optimum production, transfer, and control of force and motion to the terminal segment in athletic activities.[25,27] Injury of one structure will typically lead to compensatory adaptation in others. Muscular weakness and poor endurance alters the function of the hip/thigh, low back, and abdominal musculature, and thus change an individual's susceptibility to injury.[25]

Anatomically, the thigh is separated into three fascial compartments based on location and innervation (see Table 49.2). Mechanically, the hip and thigh functions in six planes of movement: flexion, extension, abduction, adduction, and internal and external rotations. The anterior muscles are involved with hip flexion and knee extension, the medial with hip adduction and internal rotation, and the posterior with hip extension and knee flexion. Abduction and internal hip rotation involve the anterior fascial compartment and gluteal muscles.

The quadriceps muscle, sartorius muscle, tensor fasciae latae muscle, femoral artery, vein, and nerve are contained in the anterior compartment. The iliopsoas is sometimes considered part of the anterior compartment.[30] The rectus femoris arises via two heads from the ilium: the direct and reflected heads. The direct head arises from the anterior inferior iliac spine (AIIS) just above the iliofemoral ligament. The reflected

TABLE 49.2
Pertinent Muscles of the Thigh

Muscle	Function	Origin	Insertion
Anterior			
Quadriceps	Flexes the hip and extends the knee	AIIS	Tibial tubercle
Sartorius	Flexes, abducts, and laterally rotates the hip; flexes the knee	ASIS	Pes anserine on medial tibia
Tensor fascia latae	Abducts, flexes, and internally rotates the hip	ASIS and the anterior portion the iliac crest	Iliotibial band
Iliopsoas	Flexes the hip	Iliac fossa, lumbar vertebra	Lesser trochanter
Medial			
Adductor longus	Adducts and externally rotates the hip	Pubis and pubic rami	Linea aspera of the femur
Adductor brevis	Adductors the hip	Pubis and inferior pubic rami	Linea aspera of the femur
Adductor magnus	Adducts and flexes the hip	Inferior rami of pubis and ischial tuberosity	Linea aspera of the femur
Gracilis	Adducts the hip and flexes the knee	Inferior rami of the pubis and the pubis	Pes anserine on medial tibia
Posterior			
Biceps femoris	Short head flexes the knee with the thigh extended; long head provides posterior stability to the pelvis and extends the femur at the hip	Short head, linea aspera and the lateral supracondylar line; long head, as part of the conjoint tendon from the ischial tuberosity	Short head; long head, the posterolateral capsule, the iliotibial tract, the fibular head, and the proximal lateral tibia
Semitendinosus	Flexes and internally rotates tibia at the knee and provides valgus stability to the knee	Part of the conjoint tendon from the ischial tuberosity	Pes anserine on medial tibia
Semimembranosus	Flexes and internally rotates the knee; extends, adducts, and internally rotates the hip	Deep and medial to conjoint tendon on ischium	Multiple insertions at the posteromedial corner of the knee

head arises from a shallow concavity just above the acetabulum. The muscle continues to its distal insertion as the patellar tendon on the tibial tubercle. The sartorius originates from the anterior superior iliac spine (ASIS). It runs obliquely in the upper and anterior parts of the thigh in an inferomedial direction. It descends to the medial aspect of the knee and passes behind the medial femoral condyle of the femur to end as part of the pes anserine. It attaches distal to the medial joint line on the tibia along with the gracilis and semitendinosus tendons. The tensor fasciae latae originates from the ASIS and the anterior portion the iliac crest. It attaches to the iliotibial band that then continues down the lateral aspect of the leg, crosses the knee, and inserts on the tubercle of Gerdy on the lateral aspect of the tibia. The tensor fascia latae functions by abducting, flexing, and internally rotating the hip.

The medial compartment contains the adductor longus, brevis, and magnus and the gracilis muscles as well as the sensory branch of the obturator nerve.[30] All muscles of this compartment are innervated by the obturator nerve. Adductor magnus is the largest muscle in the medial compartment. It is located posterior to the longus and brevis muscles. Functionally, the muscle can be divided into two parts: the adductor and the hamstring components. The adductor component originates from the inferior rami of pubis and the rami of ischium and attaches to the linea aspera of the femur. The hamstring portion (innervated by the tibial nerve) originates at the ischial tuberosity and attaches to the adductor tubercle on the distal/medial femur. Functionally, both muscles adduct the hip. Additionally, the adductor component flexes the thigh and the hamstring portion extends the thigh.

The adductor longus is a large, flat muscle. It lies between the brevis and magnus and partially covers both muscles. Adductor longus forms the medial border of the femoral triangle that contains the femoral vessels and nerve. It originates from the pubis and attaches broadly to the linea aspera of the femur and functions to adduct and externally rotate the hip. The adductor brevis is the shortest of the three adductors, lying superior and deep to the adductor longus. It is located between the anterior and posterior divisions of the obturator nerve. In musculoskeletal radiology especially ultrasound, this muscle used as an anatomical landmark to identify the nerve. It originates from the pubis and inferior pubic rami. Adductor brevis attaches to the linea aspera on the posterior surface of the femur, proximal to the attachment site of adductor longus, and functions as an adductor of the thigh. The gracilis is the most superficial and medial of the muscles in this compartment. It crosses both the hip and knee. It originates from the inferior rami of the pubis and the pubis. It attaches to the medial surface of the tibia as part of the pes anserine. It is sandwiched between the tendons of the sartorius (anteriorly) and the semitendinosus (posteriorly). Gracilis functions as an adductor of the thigh/hip and a flexor at the knee.

The posterior muscle group consists of the biceps femoris (long and short heads), the semitendinosus, and the semimembranosus. All three muscles, except for the short head of the biceps, originate from the ischial tuberosity. Studies have identified that at the ischial tuberosity, the conjoint tendon (the common origin of the semitendinosus and the long head of the biceps femoris) originates superficially and the semimembranosus originates separately, being located relatively lateral and deep.[1] The short head of the biceps femoris originates from the linea aspera and the lateral supracondylar line. The long head of the biceps femoris attaches to the fibular head and the lateral tibia.[52] The short head of the biceps femoris attaches into the long head of the biceps femoris and insertions to the posterolateral capsule, the iliotibial tract, the fibular head, and the proximal lateral tibia.[1] The short head of the biceps functions to flex the knee with the thigh extended, while the long head gives posterior stability to the pelvis and extends the femur at the hip.[1,2,12]

The semimembranosus has multiple insertions at the posteromedial corner of the knee.[61] The semitendinosus joins the sartorius and gracilis tendons to form the pes anserine on the medial aspect of the proximal tibia distal to the medial joint line.[1] The semimembranosus, semitendinosus, and long head of the biceps femoris are innervated by the tibial portion of the sciatic nerve, and the short head of the biceps is innervated by the peroneal portion of the sciatic nerve.[1] The semimembranosus adds stability to the knee and functions to flex and internally rotate the knee as well as extend, adduct, and internally rotate the hip.[2,12] The semitendinosus is a flexor and internal rotator of the tibia at the knee and provides valgus stability to the knee.[1,2,12]

It is also worth briefly discussing the posterior gluteal musculature as injuries and dysfunction in this anatomic location can manifest themselves as thigh pain. The gluteus medius, minimus, and maximus are considered the rotator cuff muscles of the hip joint.[15] They originate from the sacrum and attach to the lateral thigh at the greater trochanter. They are implicated in a variety of pathologic conditions of the thigh and are a focus of the rehabilitation protocol. The gluteal muscles along with many other smaller muscles including the quadratus femoris, piriformis, obturators, and gemelli function to balance the hip and pelvis as well as abduct and externally rotate the hip.

49.3 INJURIES

Clinical encounters with patients complaining of hip and thigh pain can be involved and complicated. When formulating a differential diagnosis, it is helpful to think both anatomically and functionally (see Table 49.3). The examination should include careful palpation and weight-bearing assessments of muscle strength and stability. Referred pain may also complicate the examination and these issues should be considered in the differential.

49.4 ANTERIOR

49.4.1 Thigh Contusion

Thigh contusions are one of the most common athletic injuries and are encountered in football and other contact sports.[4] The mechanism of injury involves the quadriceps muscle sustaining compressive force and functioning to

TABLE 49.3
Common Thigh Disorders in Primary Care: An Anatomical and Symptom-Oriented Approach to Differential Diagnosis

Anterior	Medial
Overuse	*Overuse*
Iliopsoas Tendonitis	Athletic Pubalgia
Femoral Shaft Stress Fracture	*Traumatic*
Internal Snapping Hip	Adductor Strain
Traumatic	*Pediatric*
Thigh Contusion	Growth Plate Avulsion- Adductor Origin
Compartment Syndrome	*Neurologic*
Pediatric	Obturator, Ilioinguinal, and Iliohypogastric nerve Compression
Growth Plate Avulsion- Anterior Inferior Iliac Spine	
Neurologic	
Meralgia Paresthetica	
Lateral	**Posterior**
Overuse	*Overuse*
Trochanteric Bursitis	Ischial tuberosity stress fracture
Greater Trochanteric Pain Syndrome	*Traumatic*
External Snapping Hip	Hamstring Strain
Traumatic	*Pediatric*
Hip Contusion	Growth Plate Avulsion- Ischial tuberosity
	Neurologic
	Sciatic Nerve/Hamstring Syndrome

diffuse the impact from the underlying bone. The compressive force generated can rupture blood vessels and shear stress may tear muscle fibers. Clinically, the patient often presents with significant hemorrhage and swelling. Physical examination will elicit tenderness to palpation in the involved muscles.[4] The initial treatment for an anterior thigh contusion involves rest, immobilization in knee flexion, ice, and compression. Initial measures attempt to preserve range of motion while minimizing hematoma formation. Knee flexion is usually recommended as knee flexion tightens the quadriceps, providing a compressive force to the hemorrhage. Weight bearing is limited until the patient has good quadriceps muscle control and 90° of pain-free knee motion.[4] Muscle atrophy can be substantial and studies have described the loss of up to 20%–30% of the preinjury muscle mass.[6] After initial range of motion goals have been achieved, a progressive strengthening program is initiated to regain strength, agility, and proprioceptive control of the hip and core.

Occasionally, injuries will cause a large hematoma.

Clinical Pearl

Early recognition and treatment of thigh contusions is important. Significant hemorrhage may occur and in extreme cases, compartment syndrome. This may result in hemodynamic compromise of the muscle.

The compressive force of the fluid collection can markedly limit range of motion and function of the leg. If an athlete struggles to regain motion, musculoskeletal imaging can be helpful in identifying the size and extent of the hematoma. Traditionally, MRI was the modality of choice to characterize these injuries, but more recently, point-of-care diagnostic musculoskeletal ultrasound has become helpful for diagnosis and treatment (see Figure 49.1). Evacuation or aspiration of the hematoma in these cases can be considered. Protection with padding over the involved area is important to avoid repeat injury. Nonsteroidal anti-inflammatory medications may be useful both for pain and for treatment of myositis ossificans.[35] Myositis ossificans is associated with large hematomas and is diagnosed as calcium deposition occurs in the hematoma and muscle during the healing process.

The athlete will complain of increasing or persistent pain, decreased range of motion, and inhibition of the affected muscle. Diagnosis is typically made with x-ray (see Figure 49.2). Risk factors include early use of heat in the treatment of quad contusion. Specific treatment protocols have been developed

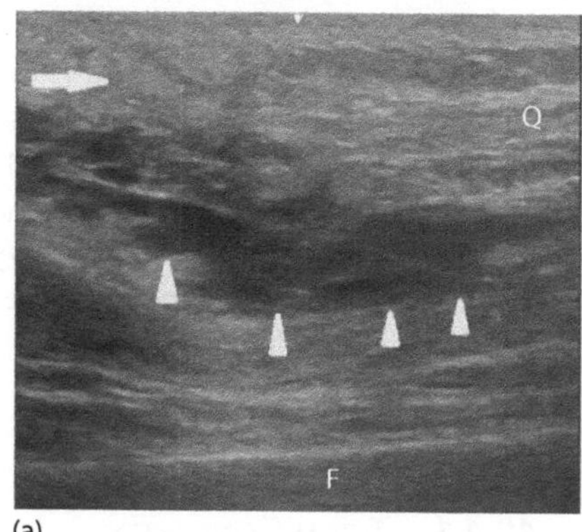

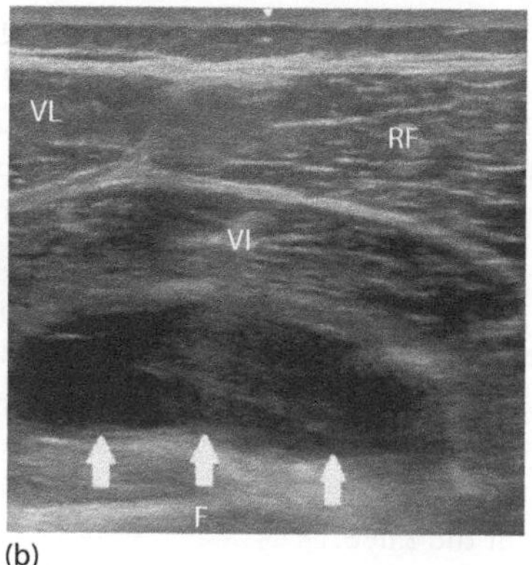

FIGURE 49.1 Long-axis ultrasound image (a) of quadriceps muscle (Q), quadriceps contusion (arrow), and hematoma formation (arrowheads). Note the loss of normal muscle echotexture in response to injury. The muscle swells and muscle fascicles may be obscured. (b) Short-axis view (right) of a vastus intermedius (VI) contusion and hematoma (arrows). RF, rectus femoris; VL, vastus lateralis. (Images courtesy of Peter Wenger, MD.)

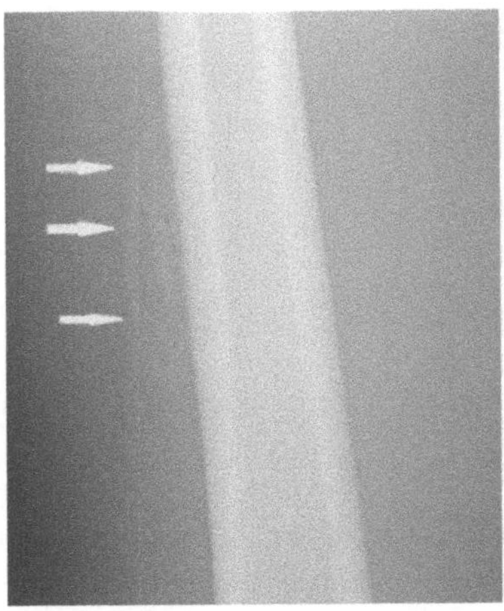

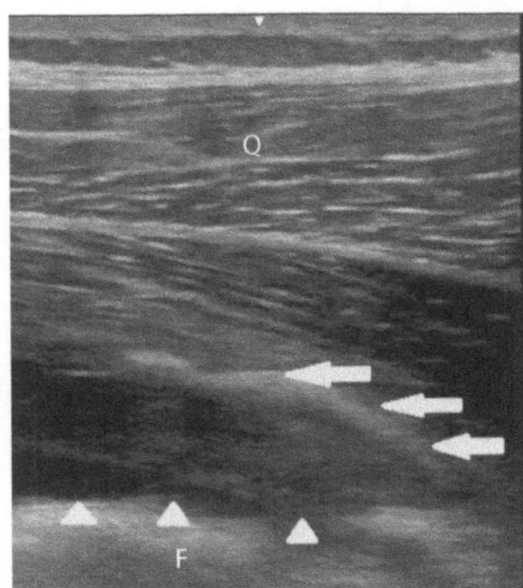

FIGURE 49.2 AP x-ray of the femur (left) showing lucency in an area of a previous quadriceps contusion (arrows). Ultrasound in long axis (right) to the femur in the same patient. Calcification is identified (arrows) along the margin of the hematoma (arrowheads). Q, quadriceps muscle; F, femur. (Images courtesy of Peter Wenger, MD.)

to minimize complications such as myositis ossificans or loss of motion and to improve functional outcome.[4,45] Treatment of myositis ossificans is generally nonoperative, but if a mature osseous mass interferes with function or range of motion, it may be excised.[4]

49.4.2 Thigh Strain

Injury surveillance studies identify strains of the hip and thigh as some of the most common injuries reported from athletic competition.[3,4,18] These injuries occur most frequently in muscles that cross two joints during an eccentric contraction in which the muscle is lengthened while actively contracted.[4,18] In athletics, these strains result from explosive hip flexion contractile forces generated in activities such as sprinting or kicking or jumping.[4] Strain or tear frequently occurs at the areas of highest force and structural weakness. The most common anatomic location of strain is at the musculotendinous junction approximately 8–10 cm below the ASIS. This injury can also occur in the muscle belly but this is less common.[4,18,54] On physical examination, strains of the rectus femoris muscle result in palpable swelling and tenderness in the anterior thigh. Soft tissue bruising can be substantial and acute treatment is similar to that of quad contusions. Initial treatment involves control of hemorrhage and edema with a compressive wrap, ice, and rest.

Once pain is reduced, gentle range of motion exercises should be started as soon as tolerated. Nonsteroidal anti-inflammatory medications should be used judiciously.[4] During the subacute phase, exercise therapy is recommended, which focuses on strength and flexibility. After full range of motion is achieved, progressive weight-bearing agility and proprioception may be initiated. Return to full activity should be closely monitored and advised only when the athlete has full range of motion and equal strength side to side and demonstrates the ability to perform functional drills. Unfortunately, recurrences are common. Often, recurrences may be more severe and require longer rehabilitation time than the initial injury.[4] Modifiable risk factors for recurrent thigh strain include deficits in strength, flexibility, and balance and tend to be an area of interest in sports conditioning programs.

49.4.3 Anterior Avulsion Injury

Skeletally immature patients are subjected to additional injuries at the enthesis or bone–tendon interface. Rectus femoris avulsions are commonly discussed in the pediatric and adolescent populations but seldom discussed in the adult athletic population.[18,44] The same mechanism that results in a muscle strain in an adult may cause an apophyseal avulsion in an adolescent.[4] Avulsion injuries represent the extreme end of a constellation of injuries that include enthesopathy, stress fracture, apophysitis, and true avulsion. These injuries may occur at every muscular origin of the thigh muscles and are common at numerous tendinous insertions.[4,18]

Athletes will typically present with acute or chronic anterior hip and thigh pain with the area of maximal tenderness at AIIS or ASIS. On physical examination, the patient may maintain a position that reduces tension on the involved area, usually hip flexion. Commonly, palpation will elicit localized tenderness or swelling at these locations. Ecchymosis is common with true avulsion. Contraction or stretch of the involved muscle will usually reproduce the pain during resisted manual muscle testing.[4,18]

Workup includes plain radiographs including comparison views of the contralateral side.[4] For true avulsion injury, x-rays can identify a bony fragment. In a study of 203 avulsion fractures seen on radiographs, the most commonly affected apophyses were the ischial tuberosity (origin of the hamstrings), the AIIS (origin of the direct head of the rectus femoris), the ASIS (origin of the sartorius and some fibers of the tensor fascia latae), and a portion of the pubic symphysis (origin of the adductor brevis and longus and the gracilis).[44] Avulsion may also occur at the lesser trochanter with vigorous contraction of the iliopsoas tendon as encountered in kicking.[4] If clinical suspicion is high, x-rays may be ordered to evaluate fore avulsion or fracture. In nondisplaced avulsion

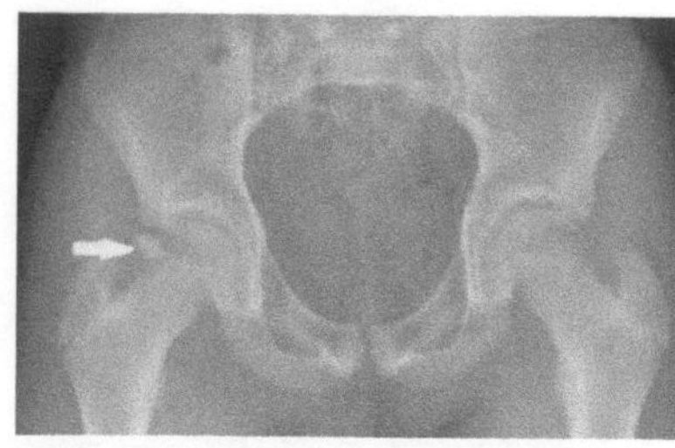
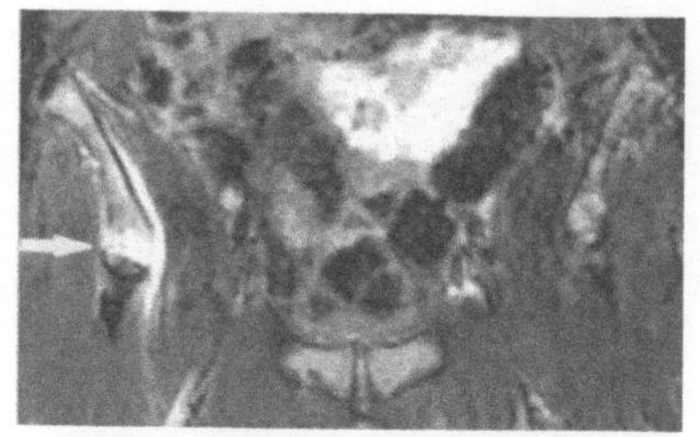

FIGURE 49.3 X-ray (left) and coronal T2-weighted MRI (right) of bony avulsion anterior inferior iliac spine (arrows) in a skeletally immature athlete. (Images courtesy of Peter Wenger, MD.)

injuries or cartilaginous avulsions in adolescents, radiographs are often interpreted as falsely negative.[4] In these circumstances, advanced imaging may be considered and MRI can be extremely useful (see Figure 49.3).[48]

In the case of avulsion, the bony periosteum and surrounding fascia typically limit severe displacement. For most injuries, initial treatment includes rest, activity modification, anti-inflammatories, and protected weight bearing with crutches. When the patient is able to tolerate weight bearing, exercise therapy becomes appropriate to restore normal range of motion.[32] Light stretching and strengthening exercises are appropriate and activities are advanced as symptoms allow. After full, pain-free range of motion is achieved and appropriate strength is demonstrated, patients can be advanced to a sport-specific conditioning program. Patients should not return to competition until equal bilateral strength, range of motion, agility, and proprioception are demonstrated.[4]

Nonoperative management of anterior hip avulsion fracture is successful in pediatric athletes as well as in adults. In a study conducted on 11 NFL players from 1997 to 2006, nonoperative treatment allowed faster return to sport with equal results on return to play statistics when compared to operative fixation.[18] There is an agreement that nonoperative management usually successfully restores function and the ability to return to high levels of athletics after hip avulsion injuries.[18] Newer treatments in skeletally mature athletes include proliferative therapy (prolotherapy), platelet-rich plasma (PRP) injection, and stem cell injection. Evidences of efficacy are mixed but studies are ongoing.

49.4.4 Compartment Syndrome

Compartment syndrome is a condition in which increased pressure within a defined space impedes the circulation and normal metabolic function of tissues.[39] The fascial compartments of the thigh are large and can accommodate a substantial amount of tissue edema and hemorrhage. If the compartment pressure alters the arteriovenous gradient, ischemia and tissue necrosis may occur.[39] In most reported cases, the pathology occurred in the anterior compartment and was attributed to direct trauma, fracture, or compression.[37,39] Anatomic studies have shown that the anterior compartment is surrounded by relatively stiff walls laterally and medially leading to a more limited ability to accommodate swelling.[39] Normal compartmental pressure ranges between 0 and 8 mmHg, and ischemia of muscle and nerves occurs at approximately 30 mmHg. This number is somewhat controversial as some studies suggest the pressure needed to cause tissue compromise is over 40 mmHg (see Chapter 23).[39]

History and physical exam attempt to elicit "the seven Ps,"[13] a constellation of symptoms used to identify prodromal symptoms of ischemic dysfunction in nerves and muscles (see Table 49.4).

These signs include (1) pain and the aggravation of (2) pain by passive stretching of the muscles in the compartment. One of the earliest objective findings of elevated compartment pressure is a (3) palpably tense compartment. Pulses (4) may be absent but are usually present until late in the course of the disease. Other findings include (5) paresthesia and (6) pallor. Paresis (7) may develop as another late complication indicative of ischemia or necrosis.[39]

Acute management of high-energy contusions includes close monitoring at the onset of injury as compartment syndrome will typically develop early. If there is clinical suspicion of compartment syndrome, compartment pressures should be obtained as soon as possible. Pressure criteria are similar to those of other anatomic regions, typically within 30 mmHg of the diastolic pressure.[26,39] Emergent fasciotomies are rarely necessary with quad contusion, but serial examinations are an absolute requirement.[4] If signs of tissue ischemia or necrosis is present, immediate fasciotomy is indicated. First aid measures include removal of all restrictive clothing, casts, dressings, or tape. The injured extremity should not be elevated but placed at heart level to optimize arterial pressure and venous drainage.[39] Despite the invasive nature of fasciotomy, studies show high levels of return to play are achieved by athletes after operative decompression of a compartment syndrome of the thigh.[30]

TABLE 49.4
Seven Ps of Compartment Syndrome

1. Pain
2. Passive stretch that increases pain
3. Palpable tense compartment
4. Pulseless (late finding)
5. Paresthesia
6. Pallor
7. Paresis (late finding)

Although exceedingly uncommon, exercise-induced compartment syndrome of the thigh can occur. Only a handful of cases are reported in the literature.[39] In these cases, the muscular swelling that occurs as a normal response to exercise causes a significant increase in pressure as to cause symptoms. Symptoms are similar to that of acute compartment syndrome but occur at a predictable level of exertion and improve with rest.

49.4.5 Femoral Shaft Stress Fracture

As the largest bone in the human body, the femur is relatively resistant to stress and strain. Acute fracture of the femur is uncommon and usually occurs after substantial trauma. In addition to acute injury, the femur is also at risk for pathology associated with overtraining. Many athletes subject the femur to repetitive stress as part of conditioning. Risk factors for stress fracture include genetic, hormonal, metabolic, biomechanical, musculoskeletal, form/training, and nutritional deficiencies.[7] If the resorptive activity of osteoclasts overcomes the osteoblasts ability to repair and remodel, bone stress injury may occur. The exact etiology for an athletes' stress fracture is complicated and requires thorough history taking and physical examination.[7] Many structural and biomechanical irregularities have been identified as risk factors for femoral shaft stress fracture including leg length discrepancy, pes planus/cavus, high Q-angle, foot varus or valgus, and hip weakness.[7] Functionally, these issues lead to increased load to the femur and can lead to an imbalanced distribution of force to bone. This increased load over time may increase the fracture risk.[7] If a diagnosis of femoral shaft stress fracture is made in a female athlete, it is important to evaluate for the female athlete triad. The female athlete triad includes amenorrhea, stress fracture, and negative calorie balance and represents an important diagnostic entity that needs to be considered in the differential.[7] Endurance athletes can burn thousands of additional calories daily secondary to athletics. If the athlete expends more calories than he or she consumes, the negative calorie balance will force the body into shunting calories to the most essential cellular processes. Shunting can lead bone resorption overtaking bone synthesis and microfractures develop. If the load is not modified, the microfactures can progress to stress injury.

Clinical Pearl

The fulcrum test and single-leg hop test will elicit pain and are helpful physical examination techniques in diagnosing femoral stress fracture.

Clinical Pearl

The female athlete triad consists of amenorrhea, stress injury/stress fracture, and negative calorie balance. Previous diagnostic criteria included anorexia; however, this diagnosis is no longer considered necessary for diagnosis of the triad.

Clinical presentation of femoral shaft stress fracture may include indolent and insidiously progressive thigh pain. Pain is usually worse with activity and improves with rest. If symptoms are ignored or the stress injury progresses, pain may be felt in activities of daily living including walking, sitting, and climbing/descending stairs. It is important to ascertain a history of night pain, weight loss, fatigue, and constitutional symptoms associated with malignancy or infection. Workup includes anterior/posterior (AP) and lateral radiographs of the femur. If the clinical suspicion is high and the radiographs are negative, it is appropriate to obtain advanced imaging with the MRI or CT scan (see Figure 49.4).

Treatment of femoral shaft stress fractures depends on the extent and location.[7] Displaced or bicortical fractures are usually referred for surgical evaluation. Fractures on the anterior aspect of the femur are more worrisome and treated more aggressively. Treatment includes nonweight bearing on crutches until pain-free with weight bearing. The patient is

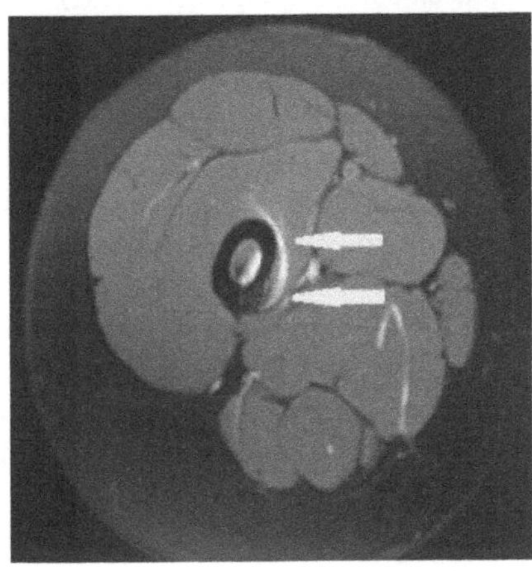

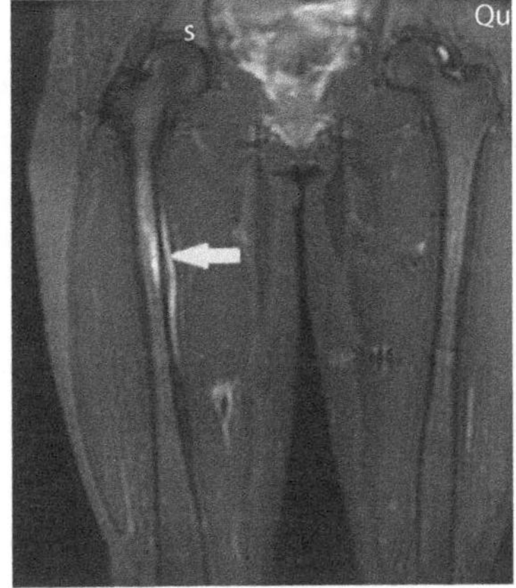

FIGURE 49.4 T2-weighted axial (left) and coronal (right) MRI images depicting femoral stress fracture. Note the periosteal swelling and edema seen on the axial image. (Images courtesy of Peter Wenger, MD.)

progressed to protected weight bearing and eventually to full weight bearing as symptoms allow. Weight-bearing restrictions are common for 4–6 weeks depending on clinical progress. Physical therapy and rehabilitation should be considered prior to return to sport as weakness and dysfunction are common after periods of altered weight bearing.

49.4.6 Iliopsoas Bursitis/Tendonitis and Internal Snapping Hip

The iliopsoas tendon and bursa have gaining interest for their roles as generators of hip and anterior thigh pain. Injury to the iliopsoas can occur acutely with strain or rupture. Tissue trauma can occur during resisted hip flexion or passive hyperextension during eccentric overload.[4,37] Soccer players are at risk for this injury as they attempt to kick against resistance, particularly during a 50–50 ball (see Figure 49.5).

Chronic and slowly progressive tendinopathy and bursal irritation may occur with overuse. Athletes may also complain of a snapping sensation in the anterior hip/thigh. Internal-type coxa saltans or "internal snapping hip syndrome" is the term used to describe snapping of the iliopsoas tendon over the iliopectineal eminence of the pelvis.[41] The relationship between the femoral head, the iliopectineal ridge, the iliopsoas bursa, and the iliofemoral ligament is implicated in the reproduction of pain and snapping with hip movement.[16,37,41] Overuse and repetitive snapping may lead to iliopsoas bursitis between the conjoined tendons of the psoas major and iliacus muscles and the pelvic brim.

Athletes will complain of pain with movement especially in the anterior hip and thigh that can present both acutely and chronically. Snapping may or may not be present. Snapping of the iliopsoas tendon is present in 10% of an active population as an incidental and asymptomatic finding.[10] If the athlete complains of snapping, the clinician must distinguish whether symptoms are emanating from the joint or soft tissue along with identifying if the snapping is symptomatic.[10]

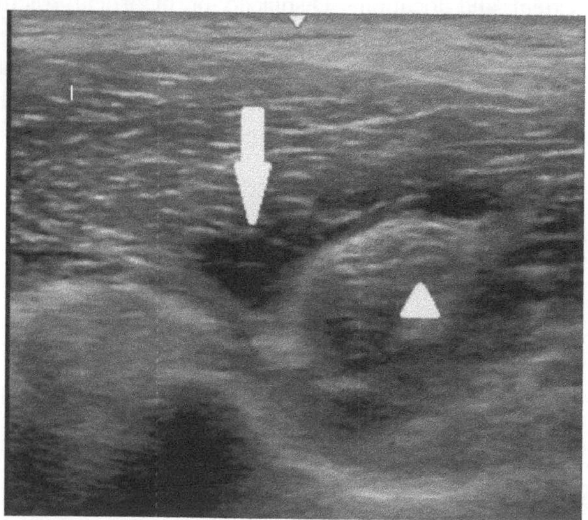

FIGURE 49.5 Short-axis ultrasound of an acute iliacus muscular strain with hemorrhage (arrow). Please note the proximal aspect of the iliopsoas tendon (arrowhead). This injury was sustained by a soccer player after a 50–50 ball. I, iliacus muscle. (Image courtesy of Peter Wenger, MD.)

On physical examination, the patient will point to the anterior hip, thigh, and groin as the area of maximal symptoms. Bruising and swelling is not typical but may occur as part of an avulsion injury. The anterior groin, anterior thigh, lower abdominal, and adductor areas must be carefully palpated to localize tenderness. Pain may be elicited with deep palpation of the iliopsoas especially at the iliopectineal eminence. Maximal flexion may be uncomfortable on range of motion testing. If pain is reproduced with hip flexion, adduction, and internal rotation, intra-articular hip pathology should be considered.[10] Resisted manual muscle testing of hip flexion should be performed and often elicits pain and weakness on the affected side. Functional tests such as rising from a squatting or seated position, leaping, cutting, or lateral hopping may elicit pain. Pain may also be reproduced with resisted sit-ups in hip flexion.[10] However, the force required to generate symptoms may not be reproduced in the office examination and may only occur with the rigors of actual sport.

In general, snapping of the iliopsoas tendon can usually be heard from across the room as an audible clunk or snap.[10] The patient should be asked to reproduce the snapping for the examiner. The clinician may be able to reproduce the snapping by bringing the hip from a flexed, abducted, and externally rotated position into extension with internal rotation. As the athlete attempts to compensate for the injury, he or she may develop symptoms associated with secondary dysfunction created by compensatory biomechanics. With iliopsoas injury, chronic gluteal discomfort, lateral thigh pain from trochanteric bursitis, hip abductor tendinopathy, and athletic pubalgia may be present. On examination, these secondary findings may be more evident and obscure the diagnosis of iliopsoas tendonitis and bursitis.[10]

Diagnosis is made with history and physical, but some imaging tests have been helpful with the diagnosis. Because of the overlap of symptoms with intra-articular hip problems, standard x-rays should be obtained of the hip and pelvis. The x-rays should be evaluated for degenerative changes, signs of femoroacetabular impingement (FAI), and sclerosis. Unfortunately, standard radiographs will often fail to show the cause of symptoms.[16] If intra-articular pathology is suspected, an MRI arthrogram can be helpful in diagnosing hip labral tears. Ultrasound is can be a useful tool for identifying iliopsoas tendonitis and bursitis and has also been helpful in diagnosing iliopsoas pathology after total hip replacement (see Figure 49.6).

If snapping is appreciated on physical examination, dynamic sonography can be performed. Snapping may be seen when the medial part of the iliac muscle is trapped between the iliopsoas tendon and the pubic bone during an abduction/flexion/external rotation movement.[16]

Initial treatments for iliopsoas tendinopathy, bursitis, and strain are rest, activity modification, stretching, oral anti-inflammatory medications, and exercise therapy.[10,16] Therapeutic modalities may be used including massage, iontophoresis, and therapeutic ultrasound. Studies of nonoperative

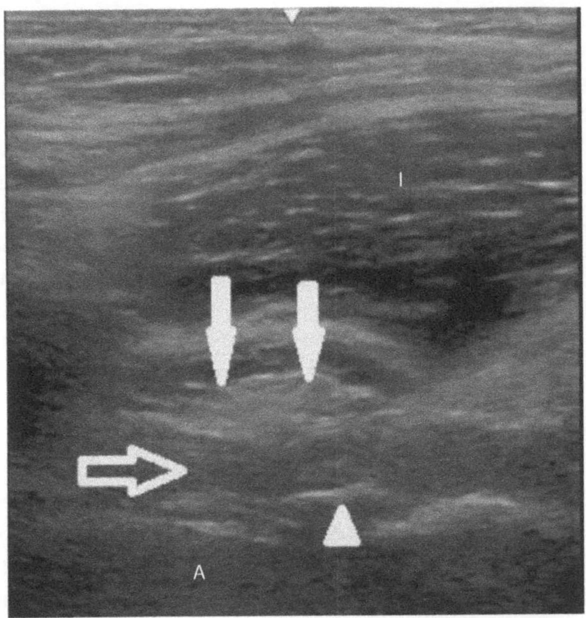

FIGURE 49.6 Short axis ultrasound of the iliopsoas tendon (arrows) in a patient with iliopsoas bursitis (open arrow). Note the anterior lip of the acetabular cup of the hip replacement (arrowhead). A, acetabulum; I, iliacus muscle. (Image courtesy of Peter Wenger, MD.)

treatment have shown exercise therapy for 6–8 weeks are generally successful in alleviating symptoms.[16] Therapeutic exercise regimens consist of concentric strengthening of the hip internal/external rotator and eccentric strengthening of the hip flexors and extensors. Sport-specific exercises may be helpful as part of the return to sport transition.

In cases that symptoms are recalcitrant to conservative care, injections of the iliopsoas bursa with an anesthetic and steroid can be considered. Studies have demonstrated symptomatic relief lasting from 2 to 8 months but symptom recurrence was common.[16] If nonoperative modalities fail, surgery should be considered. Surgical management may be appropriate for patients who are persistently symptomatic after three or more months of activity modification, physical therapy, and other conservative treatments. Surgical procedures include open and arthroscopic release of the tendon or a lengthening of the iliopsoas muscle–tendon unit.[4,5,16,24] Outcome studies of arthroscopic procedures demonstrate long-term relief from painful snapping of the tendon and can allow high school, college, and recreational athletes to return to full participation in their sport.[4,5]

49.5 MEDIAL

49.5.1 Adductor Strain

Adductor strains are common athletic injuries and can lead to significant time lost from sport. These injuries frequently recur and may lead to chronic disability. Athletic trainers and physicians have been interested in better methodology for diagnosis, treatment, and prevention of these injuries.[4] Sports identified as high risk for adductor strains include hockey, gymnastics, tennis, football, and soccer. These injuries usually occur early in the athletic season and often reflects poor preseason conditioning, prior injury, and strength/flexibility deficits.[4] Deconditioning or lack of appropriate conditioning has been implicated as a modifiable risk factor in these injuries. Playing sport tends to condition certain muscles but not lead to overall strength in all muscles important to sport. It has been recognized that training and playing of field sport does not induce a strength increase in the hip adductor muscles when compared with controls.[25,53] In other muscle groups, especially the hip abductors, playing sport leads to substantial strength gains, thus creating an imbalance of hip abductor to adductor strength.[7] Studies have demonstrated one of the best predictors of a future groin strain was an adductor-to-abductor muscle strength ratio of less than 80%.[55,56]

Patients present with complaints of groin or medial thigh pain. The pain can be acute in onset or insidious and progressive. Hip adductor injury can cause pain but also the sensation of weakness or tightness. This is a common complaint that athletes identify as a limiting factor in return to sport. Surveys of athletes with adductor injuries identify the sensation of hip adductor weakness or a "twinge" as prodromal for a more substantial injury.[22] Injuries can lead to bruising and swelling and a palpable defect may be present with a rupture or avulsion. Physical examination can elicit pain in the medial thigh, particularly when the patient is asked to adduct the leg against resistance.[4] This anatomic location has considerable muscular redundancy and objective weakness may be difficult to ascertain.[4]

Clinical Pearl

Athletes often complain of a *twinge* feeling prior to significant injury. Athletes should be counselled to identify this symptom and take appropriate next steps for diagnosis and management.

If history and physical is suspicious for substantial injury, x-ray and advanced imaging including musculoskeletal ultrasound and MRI may be utilized. Imaging can be both diagnostic and prognostic. In studies of profession athletes, MRI findings of greater than 50% cross-sectional area involvement of the affected muscle, fluid collections, and deep muscle tears were associated with longer recovery time.[4,42] Treatment includes activity modification, protected weight bearing, and modalities including electrical stimulation, therapeutic ultrasound, and progressive exercise rehabilitation. When tolerable, functional drills are initiated to improve proprioception and agility. Return to sport is considered when the athlete is able to perform functional drills without difficulty.

Adductor strain is an area of intense study and this research has provided practitioners an improved ability to detect and treat modifiable risk factors. Programs have been developed, which reduce the overall incidence of this injury, and if the injury is diagnosed, effectively treat the problem. In the NHL, studies have demonstrated that preseason hip strength testing of professional ice hockey players was helpful in identifying players at risk of developing adductor strains during the season.[55] Athletes with weaker adductor muscles were found to be more likely to sustain an adductor strain during the season.[55] Once risk factors are identified, adductor muscle-strengthening program can be instituted, which lower the athletes risk for injury. Specific training protocols for the adductor muscles vary from program to program. These protocols include static, concentric, and eccentric exercises.[25] In recent studies, strengthening with consideration to appropriate agonist and antagonist relationships, stretching, and appropriate warm-up have been identified as essential components to a conditioning program.[4]

49.5.2 Adductor Origin Injury

Similar to avulsion injuries of the anterior thigh, there are several apophyses in the medial compartment that may be injured in skeletally immature athletes. The adductor tendons are also at risk for tendonitis, avulsion, and rupture. Tendinous avulsions of the medial thigh most often occur at the origin of the adductor magnus and longus muscles. This injury may occur in a variety of sports including track and field, ice skating, gymnastics, and cheerleading.[59] The most common mechanism of injury is performing a straddle, or "the splits." Symptoms include pain in the groin and medial thigh and tenderness to palpation at the adductor origin and/or musculotendinous junction. Bruising or swelling may be present; and in the case of avulsion or rupture, a defect may be palpated. Treatment is similar to that for other types of avulsions that include protected weight bearing, pain management, activity modification, and progressive exercise therapy.[4] Many studies suggest excellent outcomes with nonoperative treatment. According to studies of NHL athletes, conservative management of adductor origin injuries often results in an excellent outcome when assessed by return-to-sport criteria.[59] Surgical referral is considered for complete tendon avulsions especially with retraction.

Considered as part of the continuum of adductor origin injuries, stress or fatigue fractures may occur at the origin of the adductor musculature. This injury is considered a consequence of muscular distraction forces applied to the bone as part of athletic conditioning. This mechanism is also implicated in the presence of pubic bone marrow edema in chronic groin injury as seen on MRI.[58,59] Signs and symptoms are similar to other adductor origin injuries including acute or chronic medial thigh pain that is exacerbated with athletic activity. Pain may be present with palpation of the adductor origin. The treatment is similar to that of other adductor origin injuries including modified weight bearing, activity modification, and exercise therapy when tolerable.[58,59]

49.5.3 Athletic Pubalgia

Athletic pubalgia is a diagnosis that refers to a variety of injuries associated with the abdominal and adductor musculature. Diagnoses include the "sports hernia," osteitis pubis, chronic musculotendinous strain/overuse, and obturator nerve entrapment.[34] The term "hernia" is a misnomer as *sports hernia* does not describe a true herniation of soft tissue but refers to chronic groin and abdominal muscle dysfunction. Differences of opinion exist regarding the exact cause of pain and pathophysiology.[34,54] Athletes engaging in rapid acceleration and deceleration movements and repetitive, high-speed twisting and cutting motions are especially vulnerable.[34] These injuries have been described in a variety of sports including ice hockey, soccer, tennis, and field hockey.[4] It has been proposed that increasingly rigorous, off-season conditioning programs have iatrogenically created an imbalance by focusing on strengthening the lower extremities while neglecting the abdominal musculature.[4] An aberrant ratio of adductor-to-core strength, adductor tightness, and tension from the adductor musculature against a fixed lower extremity causes significant shear forces across the pelvis.[4] This leads the overload of the inguinal wall musculature and ultimately leads to injury.[4] In the *sports hernia*, recently renamed to chronic abdominal and groin muscle injury, force leads to attenuation and tearing of the transversalis fascia or conjoined tendon.[4,23] Other studies have described abnormalities of the insertion of the rectus abdominis muscle on the pubis and avulsions of the internal oblique muscle fibers at the pubic tubercle.[4,33,50] Subtle contractures of the hip flexor or adductor muscles, or both, may develop.[4] These imbalances can further predispose an athlete to other lower extremity injuries.

Research shows that athletic pubalgia results as a consequence of several coexisting biomechanical abnormalities. This can complicate both history and physical examination and lead to treatment-resistant and prolonged symptoms.[4] Patients may present with progressive hip pain associated with athletic maneuvers. They may complain of anterior hip, medial thigh, or lower abdominal pain. Physical examination can yield a wide variety of findings. The rectus abdominis insertion on the mons and adductor muscle/musculotendinous junction/adductor tubercle should be palpated for tenderness. Adductor and core strength should be assessed with resisted manual muscle testing. Hip examination should be performed to evaluate for intra-articular pathology.

Clinical Pearl

Sports hernia is not a true herniation of tissue as would be seen in an inguinal hernia. Currently, sports hernia is referred to chronic abdominal and groin muscle injury and this nomenclature is more reflective of the true pathology.

Diagnosis is typically made by history and clinical findings but if appropriate radiographic studies can be helpful. AP and frog-leg x-rays can be useful for diagnosing FAI, developmental dysplasia of the hip, and degenerative conditions of the hip, spine, and sacroiliac joints.[34] X-rays can also be helpful in identifying sclerosis at muscular attachments or bony change at the mons pubis associated with osteitis pubis. Noncontrast MRI studies can show a variety of findings including subtle

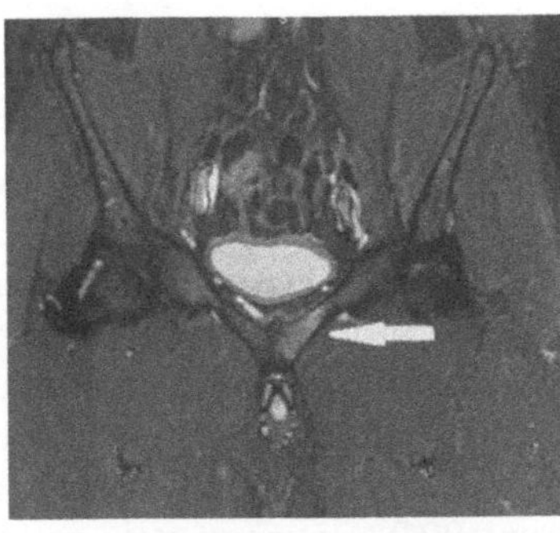

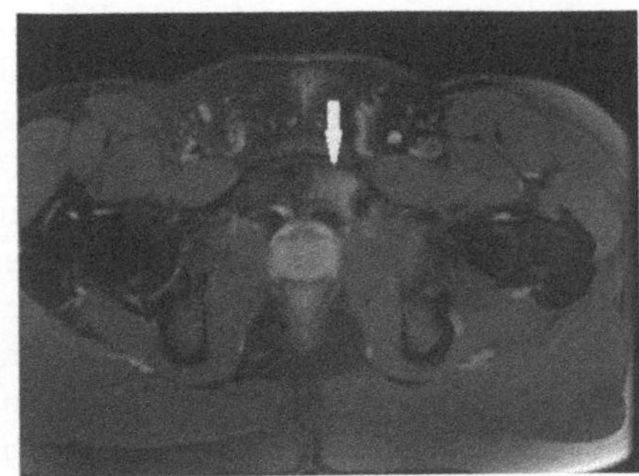

FIGURE 49.7 Coronal (left) and axial (right) T2-weighted MRI of the pelvis. Bone marrow edema of the pubic rami is observed (arrows) at the origin of the adductor musculature representing stress injury and early fatigue fracture. (Image courtesy of Peter Wenger, MD.)

abnormalities in the musculofascial layers of the abdominal and bone stress edema at the muscular insertions on the pubis (see Figure 49.7).[34] Scar tissue may be appreciated at the rectus abdominis insertion on the mons.

Abnormal fluid signal may also be seen in the pubic symphysis on T2-weighted images. However, the baseline prevalence of MRI changes appreciated in an at-risk population is uncertain. Moreover, studies have demonstrated that MRI findings may reflect the cumulative effect of chronic exercise and are not reflective of acute symptoms.[47] It is necessary to cautiously correlate the clinical presentation and physical examination with the findings detected by imaging.[47]

Nonoperative treatment is often effective for treatment of athletic pubalgia; but given the complicated pathophysiology, some athletes have a protracted clinical course. Exercise therapy is the mainstay of nonoperative treatment. Treatment of hip and core weakness and flexibility is emphasized. Once the athletes' symptoms improve and initial rehabilitation goals are met, a progressive, functional, and sport-specific exercise program can be helpful. Anti-inflammatories (nonsteroidal anti-inflammatory drugs [NSAIDs]) are often used for symptom management. Surgery can be considered if nonoperative treatment fails after 6–8 weeks, if the history and physical are typical, and particularly if the patient is a high-level athlete.[4,33] There is no consensus regarding the preferred surgical technique. The repairs are classified into three categories: primary pelvic floor repair without mesh, open anterior mesh repair, and laparoscopic mesh repair.[34] Return to play rates with surgery are high and have been validated by several studies.[4,33]

49.6 POSTERIOR

49.6.1 Hamstring Strain

Hamstring injuries are among the most common lower extremity injuries in athletes. They account for up to 29% of all injuries in sports and may lead to prolonged dysfunction.[1] Additionally, hamstring injuries carry a reinjury risk of 12%–31%.[1] Other studies have demonstrated that up to 30% of individuals with a history of hamstring strain sustain reinjury within 1 year of the initial injury.[31] These injuries are most common in sports requiring rapid acceleration such as running, hurdling, jumping, and kicking sports. Hamstring strains account for 50% of muscle injuries in sprinters and are the most common injury in hurdling.[1] A variety of risk factors have been proposed for hamstring injuries, including inadequate warm-up, strength imbalance, lower extremity flexibility, core stability, muscle weakness, fatigue, dehydration, and a history of previous injury.[1] Flexibility remains controversial as a risk factor in the pathogenesis of injury and its effectiveness as treatment is debated.[1]

The hamstring muscle group crosses both the hip and knee joints and physiologic loading has the potential for extreme force. The muscle must be tolerant of the stresses generated by rapid eccentric contractions.[1] The most common site of injury is musculotendinous junction and many studies have demonstrated that this location is subjected to the highest mechanical load.[1] Muscle belly injuries can occur with strain, direct trauma, or contusion. Complete ruptures are rare and tend to occur in athletes with history of previous injury and preexisting tendinopathy.[1] Chronic and subacute pain is common in endurance athletes and the location of maximal discomfort may vary.

Clinical Pearl

Hamstring strain recovery rates are incredible variable and may recur. This leads to frustration for both the patient and practitioner. This should be discussed to facilitate appropriate patient expectations.

History is important in the evaluation of hamstring injuries. In the case of a rupture or avulsion, the athlete may describe an audible pop. Commonly, an athlete with an acute strain will describe a burning pain that rapidly progressed with continued exertion. The history of chronic hamstring strain varies greatly. Most athletes will describe an ache or a *twinge* that can progress without activity modification and treatment.[1] On physical examination of an acute injury, the athlete may present with a *stiff-legged* gait pattern as the athlete tries to avoid simultaneous hip flexion and knee extension.[1] Bruising and edema can be identified especially if muscle fibers are torn. Substantial bruising swelling in the posterior thigh may indicate a high-grade musculotendinous or avulsion injury.[1] Palpation should include the hamstring from origin at the ischial tuberosity to the respective tendinous insertions at the knee. Tenderness may be elicited with palpation and with more substantial injury; a defect can be appreciated. The precise location of symptoms is often hard to elucidate, especially with chronic injury. Active and passive range of motion of both lower extremities should be assessed and a careful side-to-side comparison should be performed.[1] Resisted manual muscle strength testing can help identify weakness. If the athlete is able, functional testing can be performed.

Radiographic studies have a role in the evaluation of hamstring strain. X-rays can be useful in the case of a bony avulsion fracture but are often negative for pathology.[1] Dynamic ultrasonography is an excellent point-of-care modality that can provide high-resolution imaging. Typically, hamstring muscles and tendons are imaged using a linear probe in both the longitudinal and transverse planes with frequencies in the 7.5–13 MHz range. Higher frequencies provide better resolution, while lower frequencies provide better depth of penetration. Ultrasound can demonstrate fluid collections around and along the injured muscle and may reveal areas of echogenicity, representing edema and/or hemorrhage.[1] Ultrasonography can define tendon and muscle injury seen with proximal or distal avulsions and can allow clinicians to appreciate delayed soft tissue changes seen during the subacute phase of recovery. Ultrasound-directed procedures can be performed including aspiration along with a variety of injections.

Noncontrast MRI is the most commonly used advanced imaging modality to evaluate hamstring injuries. Axial, coronal, and sagittal T1- and T2-weighted images are obtained on a 1.5 T or higher unit. Proximal hamstring injuries are imaged through both ischial tuberosities and proximal thighs. Distal injuries are imaged from the midthigh through the distal tibiofibular joint.[1] MRI has the advantage of depicting bone stress injury that may be particularly useful in patients with open growth plates. Hamstring injuries can be classified with respect to their radiographic findings: grade 1, overstretching but minimal loss of the integrity of the muscle–tendon unit; grade 2, partial or incomplete tearing; and grade 3, complete rupture.[31] MRI and ultrasound have also been studied as tools to predict return to play. These studies showed that increased cross-sectional muscle involvement correlates to increased time to return to competition.[31] Athletes with normal imaging had a significantly faster return to competition and those with greater radiographic injury longer return to play.[31]

Initial nonoperative treatment includes activity modification, ice, compression, gentle stretching, early physical therapy, and NSAIDs. Sport-specific training can be utilized in the return to activity progression. Other modalities include massage, therapeutic ultrasound, electrical stimulation, and shock-wave therapy.[31] Intramuscular corticosteroid injection has been used in professional athletes as an early treatment to prevent prolonged disability and hasten return to play.[31] The proposed mechanism of action in acute injury is mediation of the painful inflammatory response triggered by the acute muscle strain.[31] In NFL studies, intramuscular corticosteroid injection decreased time to return to play without a risk of further injuries or complications in players with discrete injuries within the substance of the muscle.[31]

Unfortunately for some athletes, the result of conservative management is disappointing. Studies show that recovery from hamstring injuries is unpredictable. Athletes may experience protracted time lost from sport, high reinjury rates, persistent disability, and inability to return to previous level of play. Newer proliferative therapies are currently being investigated in hamstring injuries including prolotherapy, PRP treatment, stem cell therapy, and administration of growth factors.[31] The results of these early studies are mixed, and more information is needed before these treatments are fully endorsed.

In the case of proximal avulsion/tendon rupture, surgical management may be considered as initial treatment. For single-tendon avulsions and two-tendon tears with retraction less than 2 cm, nonoperative treatment is appropriate.[31] Generally, less active patients, those with medical comorbidities, and patients unable to comply with postoperative rehabilitation are also indications to nonoperative management.[31] Operative treatment for proximal hamstring tendon avulsions is recommended for two-tendon tears with retraction of >2 cm or for three-tendon avulsions.[31] Studies show that early surgery is indicated for rupture and yields superior results when compared to repair of chronic rupture.[31] Operative treatment has high success rates and is also considered for chronic injuries with complete or partial tears that fail nonoperative management.[31]

Prevention programs are a current area of interest in sports medicine. Few studies have investigated the effect of injury prevention programs on incidence of lower extremity injuries. The injury prevention program "The 11," developed with the support of FIFA, aims to reduce biomechanical risk factors in professional soccer and has been validated in this sport.[31] Currently, there is no consensus on the most effective hamstring injury prevention program.

49.6.2 Ischial Tuberosity Fracture

Ischial tuberosity fractures or *hurdler's fractures* occur as the result of hip flexion with knee extension, causing excessive hamstring muscle tension. These injuries are reported in both pediatric and athletes. These injuries have been seen with greater frequency in water skiing.[1] The mean age of patients with ischial tuberosity avulsions ranges from 18 to 40 years, and these patients will typically have a history of acute trauma.[4] Chronic fatigue fractures without acute injury have also been described in the athlete complaining of chronic pain (Figure 49.8).

The mechanism of injury often includes an eccentric contraction with the hip flexion and knee extension during ballistic activities like jumping. Athletes typically complain of posterior upper thigh pain and may hear an audible pop with injury. Bruising and swelling may occur and track down the posterior thigh. Tenderness may be elicited at the ischial tuberosity as well as midsubstance of the hamstring.

Generally, these injuries are managed nonoperatively. Avulsions can cause prolonged dysfunction and referred pain

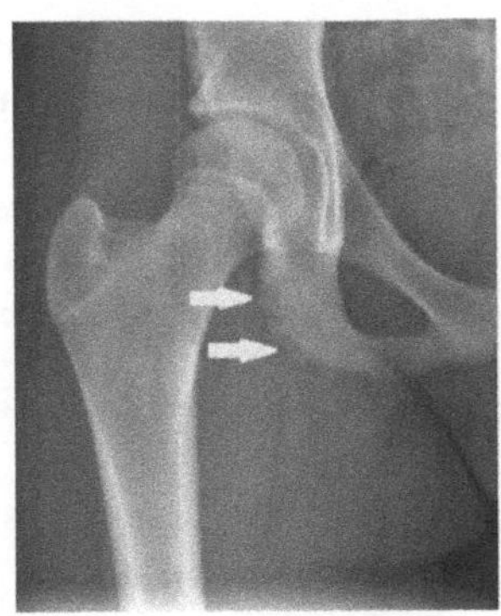
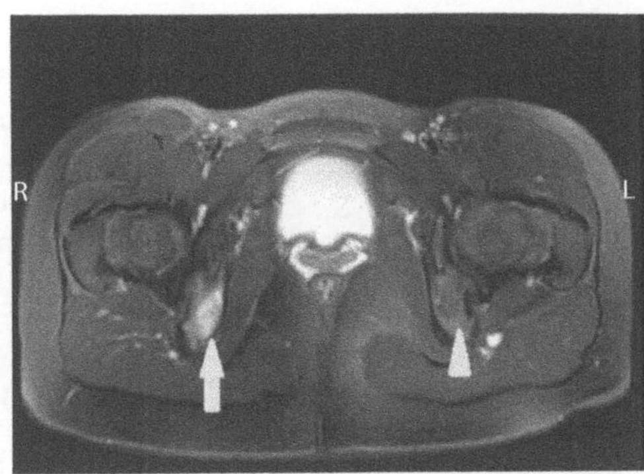

FIGURE 49.8 Ischial tuberosity stress fracture in a young dancer. Subtle lucency is observed at the hamstring origin in the x-ray on the left (arrow). T2 axial MRI imaging (right) shows increased signal in the ischial tuberosity at the hamstring origin (arrow). Note the difference between the effected and unaffected sides (arrowhead). (Images courtesy of Peter Wenger, MD.)

to the posterior parts of the thigh, rarely requiring operative intervention.[4] Late sciatic nerve palsy has been reported secondary to scar hypertrophy.[4] Nonoperative treatment includes activity modification, gentle stretching, physical therapy, and nonsteroidal anti-inflammatory medications (NSAIDs). For avulsions, patients may have difficulty tolerating activities of daily living including prolonged sitting. Weight distribution in the seated position may be addressed with donut pads to off-load the ischial tuberosity.

49.7 LATERAL

49.7.1 Trochanteric Bursitis and Greater Trochanteric Pain Syndrome

Pain in the lateral thigh is common among athletes and nonathletes alike. Greater trochanteric bursitis, which is specifically the pain and swelling of the gluteus maximus bursa, and greater trochanteric pain syndrome (GTPS), which is the constellation of findings including gluteus minimus and medius tendonitis, partial thickness tearing of these tendons, and bursitis, occur most frequently in sedentary individuals aged 40–60 years.[17] However, these findings have also been identified in younger age groups, particularly those involved in athletics.[17] Suspected predisposing factors include repetitive overuse injury, hip trauma, bone spurs, and calcium deposits.[43] Anatomically, the greater trochanter has three facets that represent the attachment sites of the of the gluteal muscles: the anterior facet is the attachment site of the gluteus minimus, the lateral facet is the primary attachment site of the gluteus medius muscle, and the posterior facet is the primary attachment site of the gluteus maximus muscle. These muscles act to abduct and externally rotate the hip. The anatomic relationship between three tendons/bursae, the hip muscles, the bony protuberances, and the overlying iliotibial band may predispose this area to biomechanical friction and irritation.[43] Newer studies on biomechanics of the hip and thigh have led to some authors to this consider this group of muscles as the rotator cuff of the hip.[60] Moreover, it has been proposed that tears of the hip abductor tendons may also occur through a progressive, degenerative process similar to rotator cuff tears in the shoulder.[15,60]

GTPS is commonly identified in runners and individuals who engage in sports requiring a climbing motion such as step aerobics, cross fit, martial arts, and performance arts.[4] Patients will typically present with subacute and progressive lateral hip and thigh pain. Pain may radiate into the gluteal muscles or laterally down the thigh. It is characterized by chronic intermittent or continuous discomfort at and around the greater trochanter. Pain may increase with physical activity and may get worse with transitioning from seated to standing and with stairs. Lying on the affected side may provoke pain, and the patient may complain of waking up at night secondary to symptoms. Physical examination may reveal tenderness to palpation of the greater trochanter, the gluteal bursae and tendons, and iliotibial band. Skin changes and bruising are not typical for GTPS. Provocative maneuvers may assist in diagnosis. Single-leg stance (Trendelenburg) and resisted hip rotation strength tests are helpful in identifying weakness, tendinopathy, and bursitis.[17,43]

Standard initial treatment of GTPS includes NSAIDs, activity modification, exercise therapy for hip and core weakness, and correction of training errors.[43] For athletes, agility and proprioceptive training may be helpful as part of their return to sport program. A local corticosteroid injection is regarded as standard of care if initial measures are unsuccessful or if symptoms are too great to begin more conservative measures.[43] There is no conclusive evidence that these injections are effective, although small observational studies suggest that injections with corticosteroids are effective in the short term.[43] Symptom recurrence and incomplete symptom relief are not uncommon after corticosteroid injection.[43] Other conservative modalities include stretching, massage, acupuncture, prolotherapy, PRP, and shock-wave therapy.[17,43]

Recalcitrant pain and lack of response to conservative measures with a presumed diagnosis of trochanteric bursitis may constitute a relative indication for imaging studies. X-rays include standard AP of the hips and findings include calcifications in the bursa or tendons. If initial conservative measures fail, advanced imaging may be appropriate including ultrasound and MRI (see Figure 49.9).[60] This may reveal a

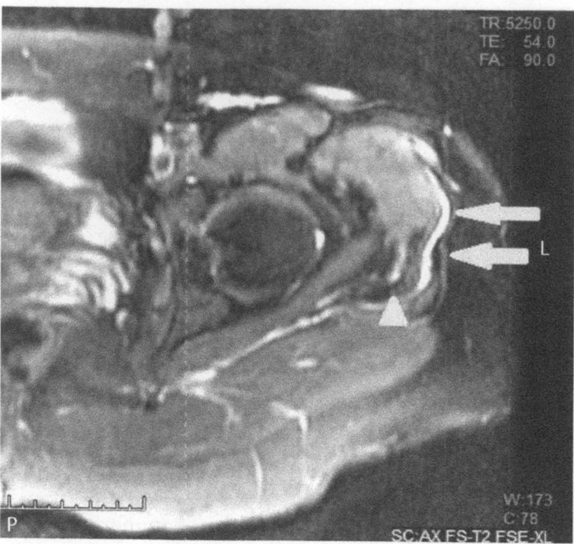

FIGURE 49.9 T2 axial image of the left lateral hip at the greater trochanter. Fluid is seen in the greater trochanteric bursa (arrows). Increased intrasubstance signal is identified in the gluteus maximus tendon indicating partial thickness tearing (arrowhead). (Image courtesy of Peter Wenger, MD.)

previously unappreciated tear of the gluteus medius or maximus, which has been well described as a cause of GTPS.[60]

However, studies have yet to determine the incidence of gluteus tears and their correlation with symptomatic pathology.[43,60] Surgical evaluation may be considered with recalcitrant pain and failure of conservative care. Surgical approaches include repair of tendon tear, debridement of tendinopathic regions, calcification debridement, bursectomy, and iliotibial release, among others.[43]

49.7.2 External Snapping Hip

Snapping of the iliotibial band, tensor fascia latae, and gluteus maximus tendon over the greater trochanter can lead to lateral hip and thigh pain. The most common anatomic etiology identified in external snapping hip is slipping of a thickened posterior border of the iliotibial band or anterior border of the gluteus maximus muscle over the greater trochanter.[11] On physical examination, snapping may elicited by passive movement from an adducted and internal rotation of the hip into flexion and external rotation. At about 15°–30° of hip flexion, the soft tissue subluxes abruptly and may reproduce pain.[11,62] The athlete can usually demonstrate the snapping to the examiner better than the examiner can detect on passive examination. The visual appearance may distress the patient and lead to self-reporting of *hip dislocation*. This appearance occurs as a result of soft tissue moving back and forth across the greater trochanter, and this snapping can be falsely interpreted as instability.[11,62] Dynamic evaluation should be performed with the patient standing on the contralateral leg and attempting to reproduce their snap. Standing more effectively reproduces the snap that would occur while standing or running.[11]

The treatment of external snapping hip syndrome includes conservative treatments such as rest, activity modification, foam rolling, stretching exercises, physical therapy, and anti-inflammatory medications. Local anesthetics and steroids may also be injected into the trochanteric bursa. Surgical procedures can be performed in cases refractory to conservative treatment.[11,62]

49.8 NEUROPATHIC

49.8.1 Compression Syndromes

There are two types of neuropathic pain described in the hip and thigh. First, the nerve can be impinged at the lumbar spine usually associated with herniated nucleus pulposus or spinal stenosis of the L1–L4 levels. Second, compression of nerve may occur peripherally as it crosses areas of potential entrapment. The patient's symptoms are dependent on the nerve root or peripheral nerve involved and the level of compression. Several types of peripheral nerve entrapment that present with thigh pain are described in the following sections.

49.8.2 Meralgia Paresthetica (Lateral Femoral Cutaneous Nerve Compression)

Meralgia paresthetica is a condition in which the lateral femoral cutaneous nerve is compressed by belts, pads, blunt trauma, or prolonged hip flexion.[4] More than 80 possible causes have been reported.[57] Idiopathic entrapment is the most likely etiology; however, direct trauma is implicated in the development of the nerve entrapments and posttraumatic neuritis. The nerve has several described anatomic variations that can predispose certain athletes to developing this disorder.[57]

Patients will complain of pain and paresthesia over the anterolateral thigh with the absence of motor findings.[4] Patients with meralgia paresthetica may also complain of secondary pain in the hip, knee, and calf. This constellation of symptoms may occur because of adaptive modification of muscle activation, gait pattern, and activities of daily living.[57] Sensory loss on the anterolateral thigh and a positive Tinel's sign over the nerve are diagnostic.[4] Treatment involves removal of the offending compressing agent, stretching, physical therapy, and anti-inflammatory medications. Occasionally, the local use of injected anti-inflammatory agents can be helpful. Ultrasound guidance is helpful for injections of lateral femoral cutaneous nerve, helping overcome the anatomic variability seen with this nerve.[49] The symptoms may be mild and may resolve spontaneously, or they may severely limit the patient for many years.[57] Surgical decompression is described and successful but is rarely necessary.[4]

49.8.3 Ilioinguinal, Iliohypogastric, and Obturator Nerve Compression

These entrapment syndromes occur as a result of injury affecting the external oblique aponeurosis, the conjoined tendon, the adductor tendons, or the inguinal ligament.[20] The resulting weakness of the pelvic musculature can lead to scar tissue, tendinopathy, and occult hernias.[20] Disruption of the external oblique aponeurosis also predisposes to entrapment and irritation of branches of ilioinguinal or iliohypogastric nerves.[20] Enthesopathy at the insertion of the abdominal and the adductor muscles to the pubic bone has been described as cause of groin pain secondary to obturator nerve entrapment.[20] Obturator nerve entrapment is also seen in skaters due to adductor muscle hypertrophy.[4]

Clinically, patients will complain of groin or thigh discomfort, tingling, or pain. Symptoms may be reproduced with running and may present as relapsing and remitting discomfort or as continuous irritation.[20] Rest may yield transient relief, but pain will typically return with activity. Physical examination may reveal a deficiency of the external inguinal ring, hernia, Tinel's sign at affected nerve, and aberrant hip and core biomechanics. The diagnosis is often made by exclusion.[20]

The initial treatment is conservative and includes activity modification, physical therapy, anti-inflammatory drugs, and corticosteroid injection.[20] Surgical exploration is an option if conservative treatment fails. Herniorrhaphy is appropriate for identified hernias.

49.8.4 Hamstring Syndrome

Injuries to the proximal hamstring origin are common in the athletic population. The most common mechanism of injury is eccentric loading of the muscle as it lengthens during activities involving rapid limb acceleration and deceleration.[8] These injuries can range from strain to complete avulsion of the tendon origin. A serious complication of proximal hamstring injuries is hamstring syndrome. This condition may develop after a single acute hamstring injury or develop slowly in the patient with chronic, recurrent hamstring tendinopathy.[8,63] Symptoms occur as a result of scarring, traction, compression, or irritation of the sciatic nerve by a fibrotic band between the proximal hamstring tendons at the lateral border of the semimembranosus muscle.[63] Symptoms include ill-defined pain in the high hamstring/buttock region that radiates into the posterior thigh and distally toward the popliteal fossa. Athletes report discomfort over the ischial tuberosity during sitting that may increase during stretching and exercises that target the hamstrings.[1] The pain occurs with exercise, mainly running, and there is often a report of associated weakness in the hamstring region.[63] Pain and symptom reproduction may result from resisted manual muscle testing of the hamstring and with sciatic nerve stretch. Hamstring weakness is common when strength is compared to the unaffected side.

Clinical Pearl

Hamstring syndrome often occurs after an untreated hamstring injury. Early identification and treatment of these injuries is essential.

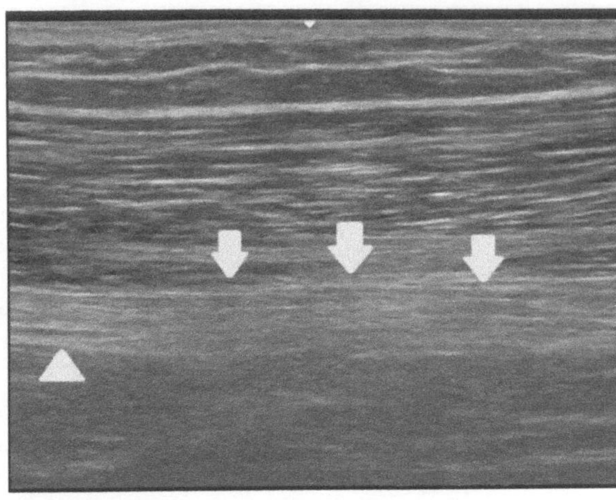

FIGURE 49.10 Long-axis ultrasound of sciatic nerve near an entrapment site near the proximal hamstring. The nerve is swollen and the nerve fascicles become less distinct proximal to the entrapment site (arrows). Normal nerve is depicted proximally (arrowhead). (Image courtesy of Peter Wenger, MD.)

When appropriate, MRI and ultrasound are the modalities of choice to evaluate the hamstring origin. Acute tears are characterized by a linear high T2 signal at the bone–tendon interface and evidence of fiber disruption, hypertrophy, and possible retraction on MRI.[8] On musculoskeletal sonography, the tendons may be dynamically evaluated during acute or chronic injury. Sonographic findings of hamstring syndrome include nerve swelling, entrapment, and tethering. These findings are usually identified in the chronic setting (see Figure 49.10).

Treatment options include activity modification, avoidance of aggravating factors, NSAIDS, and physical therapy. If symptoms persist, additional nonoperative treatment modalities include local injection with corticosteroids, prolotherapy, or PRP.[8] The evidence for proliferative therapy, including PRP and stem cell injection, are mixed, and currently these treatments are considered experimental. If conservative measures fail, continued nonoperative management of symptomatic partial tears and hamstring syndrome often results in patient frustration and a protracted clinical course. Successful operative repairs of hamstring tendon tear and decompression of the sciatic nerve have been described for these patients.[4,8]

49.9 MISCELLANEOUS

49.9.1 Hernia, Infection, and Malignancy

A thorough history and physical examination is essential for every clinical encounter. History should include information about weight loss, night pain, gastrointestinal distress, fever, and symptoms associated with sepsis. If clinical suspicion dictates, workup may include lab work, advanced imaging, and nuclear medicine studies (see Tables 49.5 and 49.6).

TABLE 49.5
Indications for Referral

Diagnosis	When to Refer
Anterior	
Quadriceps contusion	After failure of typical treatments. Consider early referral if there is clinical suspicion compartment syndrome or for advanced treatment modalities including aspiration and injection if patient needs to return to a high level of functioning quickly.
Compartment Syndrome	Early referral for surgical evaluation is critical if acute compartment syndrome is suspected. Compartment pressure measurements should be obtained.
Medial	
Adductor strain	Recalcitrant cases that fail typical treatments should be referred after 2–3 months of treatment. Highly competitive athletes may be referred earlier to sports medicine specialists.
Athletic pubalgia	Recalcitrant cases that fail typical treatments should be referred after 2–3 months of treatment. Highly competitive athletes may be referred earlier to sports medicine specialists. If extensive conservative measures fail, consider surgical referral.
Lateral	
GTPS	Recalcitrant cases that fail typical treatments may be referred after 2–3 months of treatment. Consider earlier referral to sports medicine specialists for advanced injection therapies. Surgical referral is indicated after a reasonable trial of all other conservative treatments.
Snapping hip	Consider sports medicine specialist referral after conservative treatments. Rarely, surgical referral is indicated.
Posterior	
Hamstring strain	Consider early referral to sports medicine for high-level or very active athletes. Complete ruptures (grade 3) should be referred early.
Hamstring origin injury	Consider early referral to sports medicine for proximal hamstring injuries. Two- or three-tendon tears should be referred for surgical evaluation. Avulsion injuries with greater than 1 cm of displacement should also be referred.
Ischial tuberosity stress fracture	Consider referral to sports medicine specialists for ischial tuberosity stress fractures especially early conservative measures are unsuccessful. Growth plate injuries in the skeletally immature may be referred early.

Sources: Ahmad, C. et al., *Am. J. Sports Med.*, 41, 2933, 2013; Anderson, K. et al., *Am. J. Sports Med.*, 29, 521, 2001; Arangio, G.A. et al., *J. Orthop. Sports Phys. Ther.*, 26, 238, 1997; Barrack, M. et al., *Am. J. Sports Med.*, 42, 949, 2014; Grote, K. et al., *Am. J. Sports Med.*, 32, 104, 2004; Holmich, P. et al., *Am. J. Sports Med.*, 39, 2447, 2011; Mozes, M. et al., *Br. J. Sports Med.*, 19, 168, 1985; Nau, T. et al., *Am. J. Sports Med.*, 28, 120, 2000; Rompe, J. et al., *Am. J. Sports Med.*, 37, 1981, 2009; Tyler, T.F. et al., *Am. J. Sports Med.*, 29, 124, 2001.

TABLE 49.6
SORT: Key Recommendations for Practice

Clinical Recommendation	Evidence Rating	References
The best predictor of a future groin strain was an adductor-to-abductor muscle strength ratio of less than 80% on physical exam.	C	[51,56]
For hamstring injuries, MRI and ultrasound can be used as tools to predict return to play. Increased cross-sectional muscle involvement correlates to increased time to return to competition.	C	[31]
For avulsion fractures of the hip and pelvis, nonoperative treatment allowed faster return to sport with equal results on return to play statistics when compared to operative fixation.	C	[18]
If compartment syndrome of the thigh is suspected, compartment pressures should be obtained. Normal pressure ranges between 0 and 8 mmHg and ischemia occurs at approximately 30 mmHg.	C	[39]
On physical exam, most common anatomic location of quadriceps strain is at the musculotendinous junction approximately 8–10 cm below the ASIS.	C	[4,18,54]
For proximal hamstring avulsions, single-tendon and two-tendon tears with retraction less than 2 cm can be managed nonoperatively.	C	[31]

REFERENCES

1. Ahmad C, Redler L, Ciccotti M, Maffulli N, Longo U, Bradley J. Evaluation and management of hamstring injuries. *The American Journal of Sports Medicine.* 2013;41:2933.
2. Åkermark C, Johansson C. Tenotomy of the adductor longus tendon in the treatment of chronic groin pain in athletes. *The American Journal of Sports Medicine.* 1992;20:640–643.
3. Alonso JM, Junge A, Renström P et al. Sports injuries surveillance during the 2007 IAAF World Athletics Championships. *Clinical Journal of Sport Medicine.* 2009;19(1):26–32.
4. Anderson K, Strickland S, Warren R. Current concepts: Hip and groin injuries in athletes. *The American Journal of Sports Medicine.* 2001;29(4):521–533.
5. Anderson S, Keene J. Results of arthroscopic iliopsoas tendon release in competitive and recreational athletes. *The American Journal of Sports Medicine.* 2008;36(12):2363–2371.
6. Arangio GA, Chen C, Kalady M et al. Thigh muscle size and strength after anterior cruciate ligament reconstruction and rehabilitation. *Journal of Orthopaedic & Sports Physical Therapy.* 1997;26(5):238–343.
7. Barrack M, Gibbs J, Nattiv A. Higher incidence of bone stress injuries with increasing female athlete triad-related risk factors: A prospective multisite study of exercising girls and women. *The American Journal of Sports Medicine.* 2014;42:949–958.
8. Bowman K, Cohen S, Bradley JP. Operative management of partial-thickness tears of the proximal hamstring muscles in athletes. *The American Journal of Sports Medicine.* 2013;41(1363).
9. Brubake CE, James SL. Injuries to runners. *Journal of Sports Medicine.* 1974;2(4):189–198.
10. Byrd, T. Femoroacetabular impingement in athletes: Current concepts. *The American Journal of Sports Medicine.* 2013; 42:737.
11. Choi Y, Lee S, Song B et al. Dynamic sonography of external snapping hip syndrome. *Journal of Ultrasound in Medicine.* 2002;21:753–758.
12. Clanton TO, Coupe KJ. Hamstring strains in athletes: Diagnosis and treatment. *Journal of the American Academy of Orthopaedic Surgeons.* 1998;6(4):237–248.
13. Colosimo AJ, Ireland ML. Thigh compartment syndrome in a football athlete: A case report and review of the literature. *Medicine & Science in Sports & Exercise.* 1992;24:958–963.
14. Crowninshield RD, Johnston RC, Andrews JG et al. A biomechanical investigation of the human hip. *Journal of Biomechanics.* 1978;11:75–85.
15. Del Buono A, Papalia R, Khanduja V et al. Management of the greater trochanteric pain syndrome: A systematic review. *British Medical Bulletin.* 2012;102:115–131.
16. Flanum M, Keene J, Blankenbaker D et al. Arthroscopic treatment of the painful "internal" snapping hip results of a new endoscopic technique and imaging protocol. *The American Journal of Sports Medicine.* 2007;35(5):770–779.
17. Furia J, Rompe J, Maffulli N. Low-energy extracorporeal shock wave therapy as a treatment for greater trochanteric pain syndrome. *The American Journal of Sports Medicine.* 2009;37:1806.
18. Gamradt S, Brophy R, Barnes R et al. Nonoperative treatment for proximal avulsion of the rectus femoris in professional American football. *The American Journal of Sports Medicine.* 2009;37(7):1370–1374.
19. Garrett WE Jr. Muscle strain injuries. *The American Journal of Sports Medicine.* 1996;24(6 (Suppl)):S2–S8.
20. Genitsaris M, Goulimaris L, Sikas N. Laparoscopic repair of groin pain in athletes. *The American Journal of Sports Medicine.* 2004;32(5):1238–1242.
21. Gomez E, DeLee JC, Farney WC. Incidence of injury in Texas girls' high school basketball. *The American Journal of Sports Medicine.* 1996;24:684–687.
22. Grote K, Lincoln T, Gamble J. Hip Adductor injury in competitive swimmers. *The American Journal of Sports Medicine.* 2004;32(1):104–108.
23. Hackney RG. The sports hernia: A cause of chronic groin pain. *British Journal of Sports Medicine.* 1993;27:58–62.
24. Hoskins JS, Burd TA, Allen WC. Surgical correction of internal coxa saltans: A 20-year consecutive study. *The American Journal of Sports Medicine.* 2004;32:998–1001.
25. Hölmich P, Nyvold P, Larsen K. Continued significant effect of physical training as treatment for overuse injury: 8- to 12-year outcome of a randomized clinical trial. *The American Journal of Sports Medicine.* 2011;39:2447.
26. Hutchinson MR, Ireland ML. Common compartment syndromes in athletes: Treatment and rehabilitation. *Sports Medicine.* 1994;17:200–208.
27. Kibler WB, Press J, Sciascia A. The role of core stability in athletic function. *Sports Medicine.* 2006;36:189–198.
28. Knapik JJ, Bauman CL, Jones BH et al. Preseason strength and flexibility imbalances associated with athletic injuries in female collegiate athletes. *The American Journal of Sports Medicine.* 1991;19:76–81.
29. Leinonen V, Kankaanpaa M, Airaksinen O et al. Back and hip extensor activities during trunk flexion/extension: Effects of low back pain and rehabilitation. *Archives of Physical Medicine and Rehabilitation.* 2000;81:32–37.
30. Machold W, Muellner T, Kwasny O. Is the return to high-level athletics possible after fasciotomy for a compartment syndrome of the thigh? A case report. *The American Journal of Sports Medicine.* 2000;28(3):407–410.
31. Malliaropoulos N, Papacostas E, Kiritsi O et al. Posterior thigh muscle injuries in elite track and field athletes. *The American Journal of Sports Medicine.* 2010;38:1813.
32. Metzmaker JN, Pappas AM. Avulsion fractures of the pelvis. *The American Journal of Sports Medicine.* 1985;13:349–358.
33. Meyers WC, Foley DP, Garrett WE et al. Management of severe lower abdominal or inguinal pain in high-performance athletes. *The American Journal of Sports Medicine.* 2000; 28:2–8.
34. Minnich JM, Hanks JB, Muschaweck U et al. Sports hernia: Diagnosis and treatment highlighting a minimal repair surgical technique. *The American Journal of Sports Medicine.* 2011;39(6):1341–1349.
35. Moed BR, Resnick RB, Fakhouri AJ et al. Effect of two nonsteroidal anti-inflammatory drugs on heterotopic bone formation in a rabbit model. *Journal of Arthroplasty.* 1994;9:81–87.
36. Montgomery WH III, Pink M, Perry J. Electromyographic analysis of hip and knee musculature during running. *The American Journal of Sports Medicine.* 1994;22:272–278.
37. Mozes M, Papa MZ, Zweig A et al. Iliopsoas injury in soccer players. *British Journal of Sports Medicine.* 1985;19:168–170.
38. Nakagawa TH, Muniz TB, Baldon Rde M et al. The effect of additional strengthening of hip abductor and lateral rotator muscles in patellofemoral pain syndrome: A randomized controlled pilot study. *Clinical Rehabilitation.* 2008;22:1051–1060.
39. Nau T, Menth-Chiari W, Seitz H et al. Acute compartment syndrome of the thigh associated with exercise. *The American Journal of Sports Medicine.* 2000;28(1):120–122.

40. Philippon M, Decker M, Giphart E et al. Rehabilitation exercise progression for the gluteus medius muscle with consideration for iliopsoas tendinitis: An in vivo electromyography study. *The American Journal of Sports Medicine.* 2011;39:1777.
41. Philippon M, Devitt BM, Campbell KJ et al. Anatomic variance of the iliopsoas tendon. *The American Journal of Sports Medicine.* 2014;42:807–811.
42. Pomeranz SJ, Heidt RS Jr. MR imaging in the prognostication of hamstring injury. *Radiology.* 1993;189:897–900.
43. Rompe J, Segal N, Cacchio C et al. Home training, local corticosteroid injection, or radial shock wave therapy for greater Trochanter pain syndrome. *The American Journal of Sports Medicine.* 2009;37:1981.
44. Rossi F, Dragoni S. Acute avulsion fractures of the pelvis in adolescent competitive athletes: Prevalence, location and sports distribution of 203 cases collected. *Skeletal Radiology.* 2001;30(3):127–131.
45. Ryan JB, Wheeler JH, Hopkinson WJ et al. Quadriceps contusions. West Point update. *The American Journal of Sports Medicine.* 1991;19:299–304.
46. Salminen JJ, Maki P, Oksanen A et al. Spinal mobility and trunk muscle strength in 15-year-old schoolchildren with and without low-back pain. *Spine.* 1992;17:405–411.
47. Silvis M, Mosher T, Smetana B et al. High prevalence of pelvic and hip magnetic resonance imaging findings in asymptomatic collegiate and professional hockey players. *The American Journal of Sports Medicine.* 2011;39:715.
48. Stevens MA, El-Khoury GY, Kathol MH et al. Imaging features of avulsion injuries. *Radiographics.* 1999;19(3):655–672.
49. Tagliafico A, Serafini G, Lacelli F et al. Ultrasound-guided treatment of meralgia paresthetica (lateral femoral cutaneous neuropathy) technical description and results of treatment in 20 consecutive patients. *Journal of Ultrasound in Medicine.* 2011;30:1341.
50. Taylor DC, Meyers WC, Moylan JA et al. Abdominal musculature abnormalities as a cause of groin pain in athletes. Inguinal hernias and pubalgia. *The American Journal of Sports Medicine.* 1991;19:239–242.
51. Temple T, Kuklo T, Sweet D et al. Rectus femoris muscle tear appearing as a pseudotumor. *The American Journal of Sports Medicine.* 1998;26(4):544–548.
52. Terry GC, LaPrade RF. The biceps femoris muscle complex at the knee: its anatomy and injury patterns associated with acute anterolateral–anteromedial rotatory instability. *The American Journal of Sports Medicine.* 1996;24:2–8.
53. Thorborg K, Couppe C, Petersen J et al. Eccentric hip adduction and abduction strength in elite soccer players and matched controls: A cross-sectional study. *British Journal of Sports Medicine.* 2011;45:10–13.
54. Tidball JG, Salem G, Zernicke R. Site and mechanical conditions for failure of skeletal muscle in experimental strain injuries. *Journal of Applied Physiology.* 1993;74:1280–1286.
55. Tyler TF, Nicholas S, Campbell R et al. The association of hip strength and flexibility with the incidence of adductor muscle strains in professional ice hockey players. *The American Journal of Sports Medicine.* 2001;29:124–128.
56. Tyler T, Nicholas S, Campbell R et al. The effectiveness of a preseason exercise program to prevent adductor muscle strains in professional ice hockey players. *The American Journal of Sports Medicine.* 2002;30(5):680–683.
57. Ulkar B, Yıldız Y, Kunduracıog˘lu B. Meralgia paresthetica: A long-standing performance-limiting cause of anterior thigh pain in a soccer player. *The American Journal of Sports Medicine.* 2003;31(5):787–789.
58. Verrall G, Slavotinek J, Fon G. Prevalence of pubic bone marrow edema in Australian Rules football players: relation to groin pain. *British Journal of Sports Medicine.* 2001;35:28–33.
59. Verrall G, Slavotinek J, Fon G et al. Outcome of conservative management of athletic chronic groin injury diagnosed as pubic bone stress injury. *The American Journal of Sports Medicine.* 2007;35(3):467–474.
60. Voos J, Shindle M, Pruett A et al. Endoscopic repair of gluteus medius tendon tears of the hip. *The American Journal of Sports Medicine.* 2009;37:743.
61. Warren LF, Marshall JL. The supporting structures and layers on the medial side of the knee: An anatomical analysis. *Journal of Bone and Joint Surgery.* 1979;61(1):56–62.
62. Winston P, Awan R, Cassidy JD et al. Clinical examination and ultrasound of self-reported snapping hip syndrome in elite ballet dancers. *The American Journal of Sports Medicine.* 2007;35(1):118–126.
63. Young I, van Riet R, Bell S. A surgical release for proximal hamstring syndrome. *The American Journal of Sports Medicine.* 2008;36(12):2372–2378.
64. Young MA, Cook JL, Purdam CR et al. Eccentric decline squat protocol offers superior results at 12 months compared with traditional eccentric protocol for patellar tendinopathy in volleyball players. *British Journal of Sports Medicine.* 2005;39:102–105.

50 Knee Injuries

Jesse DeLuca and Jillian Sylvester

CONTENTS

TABLE 50.1
Key Clinical Considerations

1. The differential diagnosis of knee pain in primary care may be approached in systematic form based on pain location, with particular attention to the clinical duration and mechanism of injury.
2. Osteoarthritis is the most common presentation of chronic knee pain in primary care setting, and nearly half of all adults may develop OA of the knee by age 85. Chronic overuse injuries such as PFP and medial tibial stress syndrome cause significant decrease of recreational ability in active, younger adults.
3. The overwhelming majority of pediatric knee injuries resolve once the patient reaches skeletal maturity. Treatment is supportive symptomatic care.
4. Many acute injuries affecting the knee involve either the ligaments or menisci. Partial tears are often managed conservatively. However, complete tears, complex injuries, and high-demand athletes often require early referral for surgical evaluation.
5. Fractures of the knee generally require orthopedic evaluation due to the demands on the joint. A straight-leg immobilizer and crutches are ideal while awaiting diagnosis and specialty evaluation. Fractures involving the patella are considered "high risk" and should be immediately referred for surgical evaluation.

50.1 INTRODUCTION

One of the most mobile joints in the body, the knee, is the focal point for sports that involve running, jumping, kicking, and changing direction. It is also essential to such everyday activities as standing, walking, and climbing stairs. Injuries to the knee occur in contact and noncontact sports and are the leading cause of long-term disability from athletics.[49]

One-third of musculoskeletal ailments presenting to outpatient primary care clinics involve the knee.[5] In 2010, providers documented more than 1.15 million outpatient encounters addressing knee pain as the chief complaint.[29] Several studies have found that, when evaluating all injuries of intercollegiate athletes, the knee is involved in 25% of cases.[9] In skiing, the relative frequency of knee injuries continues to increase despite an overall reduction in the number of skiing injuries.[49] The knee accounts for 20% of the injuries in football and 13% of those in long-distance running.[27] Football and other contact sports commonly produce traumatic injuries to the ligaments (9%) and menisci (7%), while the majority of knee injuries seen by the primary care physician fall into the overuse category—tendinitis (20%), apophysitis (10%), and chondropathy (10%).[27] Neurovascular injuries are rare. When they do occur, it is often the more superficial peroneal nerve on the lateral aspect of the knee near the fibular head that is injured (see Table 50.1).

50.2 KNEE FUNCTIONAL ANATOMY

The knee consists of four bones (femur, tibia, fibula, and patella) held together by strong ligaments, a capsule, and the muscle groups that transverse the joint (Table 50.2). The tibia and fibula have articular cartilage at their ends. Similarly, the patella has articular cartilage on the inner border, which tracks in the femoral groove. Between the tibial and femoral articular surfaces are the lateral and medial menisci, which are biconcave, C-shaped fibrocartilaginous disks (see Figure 50.1). Multiple interdigitating components make up their multilaminated structure. The blood supply comes from the periphery and only partially penetrates to the menisci.

As a result, the inner portions of the menisci do not repair when injured. The menisci are attached to the joint plateau by small coronary ligaments. They function in load bearing and absorb approximately 65% of the force transmitted across the knee. They also facilitate joint stability by maintaining the relative position of the femur on the tibia. An inability to absorb shock is linked to meniscal injury and degenerative joint disease. It has also been hypothesized that nutrition to the articular cartilage itself and joint lubrication may be aided by the menisci.

Support is given by the strong capsular ligaments, most notably the medial (tibial) collateral ligament, lateral (fibular) collateral ligament, and oblique (posterior and popliteal) and arcuate ligaments (see Figure 50.1). The medial collateral ligament (MCL) connects the femur and the tibia on the medial side of the knee and is intimately involved with the medial meniscus. The lateral collateral ligament (LCL) supports the knee laterally from the femur to the fibula. The proximal tibial–fibular ligament joins the tibia and fibula at the tibial plateau.

Internal stability is gained by the addition of the crisscrossing anterior and posterior cruciate ligaments (PCLs) (see Figure 50.1). Because of their role in maintaining the stability of the knee, the cruciate ligaments, particularly the anterior cruciate ligament (ACL), are often thought of as protectors of the meniscus. A high rate of meniscal injury is associated with tears of the ACL.

Anteriorly, the quadriceps muscles (vastus medialis, vastus lateralis, vastus intermedius, and rectus femoris) join to encase the patella and then become the infrapatellar tendon (see Figure 50.2). Posterior stability is enhanced by the hamstrings and the gastrocnemius/soleus/plantaris complex (see Figure 50.3). Medially, the adductors and the gracilis, sartorius, and semitendinosus (pes anserine muscles) give support. The popliteus, iliotibial tract, and biceps femoris aid in maintaining lateral stability of the knee (see Figure 50.4).

TABLE 50.2
Pertinent Muscles of the Knee

	Muscle	Function	Origin	Insertion
Anterior				
	Quadriceps femoris			
	Rectus femoris	Extends leg; flexes thigh	Anterior inferior iliac spine, rim of acetabulum	Patella and tibial tuberosity
	Vastus lateralis	Extends leg; flexes thigh	Linea aspera	Patella and lateral condyle of tibia
	Vastus medialis	Extends leg; flexes thigh	Linea aspera	Patella and medial condyle of tibia
	Vastus intermedius	Extends leg; flexes thigh	Anterior and lateral surfaces of femur	Tendon of rectus femoris
	Articularis genu	Elevates articular capsule of knee joint with extension	Anterior surface of femur above patella	Articular capsule of knee
Medial				
	Sartorius	Flexes thigh and leg		
	Gracilis	Adducts thigh, flexes and medially rotates thigh, flexes leg	Pubic symphysis and inferior pubic ramus	Medial surface of tibia (via pes anserine)
Lateral				
	Tensor fasciae lata	Flexes thigh, abducts thigh, medially rotates thigh	Anterior superior iliac spine	Iliotibial tract, ultimately inserting on lateral tibial tubercle (Gerdy's tubercle)
Posterior				
	Biceps femoris			
	Long head	Extends thigh and flexes leg	Ischial tuberosity	Fibular head
	Short head	Extends thigh and flexes leg	Linea aspera	Fibular head
	Semitendinosus	Extends thigh and flexes leg	Ischial tuberosity	Medial surface of tibia
	Semimembranosus	Extends thigh and flexes leg	Ischial tuberosity	Medial tibial condyle
	Gastrocnemius	Flexes leg, plantar flexes foot	Medial head: above medial femoral condyle lateral head: above lateral femoral condyle	Dorsum of calcaneus as Achilles tendon
	Plantaris	Flexes leg, plantar flexes food	Above lateral femoral condyle, superior to lateral head of gastrocnemius	Dorsum of calcaneus medial to calcaneal tendon
	Popliteus	Flexes and medially rotates leg	Lateral femoral condyle	Posterior surface of proximal tibia

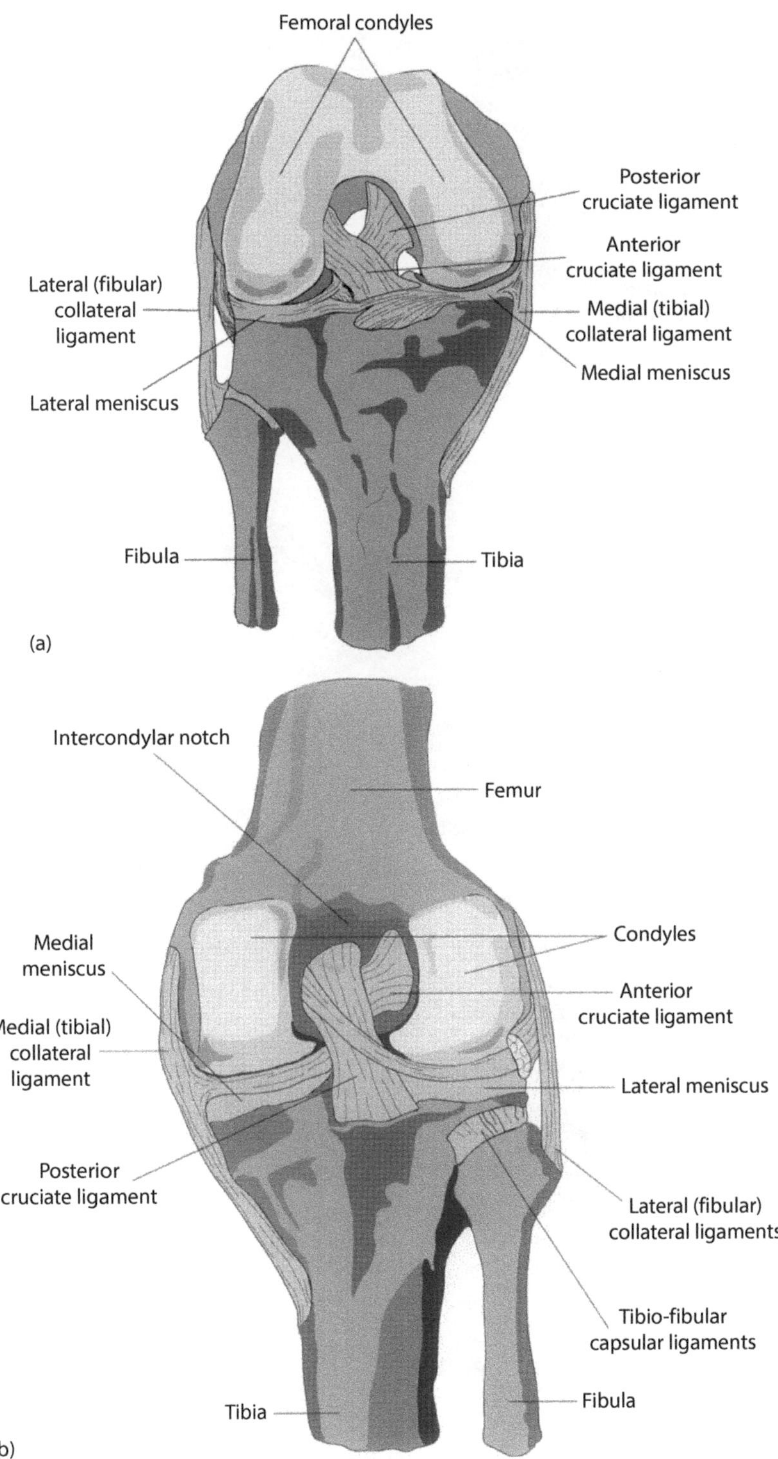

FIGURE 50.1 (a) Anterior view of right knee and (b) posterior view of right knee.

50.3 ANATOMICAL DIFFERENTIAL DIAGNOSIS

The differential diagnosis of knee pain in primary care is optimally approached in a systematic fashion with focus on both mechanism of injury and location of pain (see Table 50.3). Subsequent chapter sections will cover specific adult and pediatric injuries with a symptom-oriented anatomical approach. The special tests that are referenced in the evaluation of a specific disorder are further described in Table 50.4. Indications for referral of common knee injuries are summarized in Table 50.5. Some patients presenting to clinic with knee pain may warrant evaluation of the spine and hip, as certain derangements of these areas may also present with knee or thigh pain. These conditions are further explored in their respective chapters.

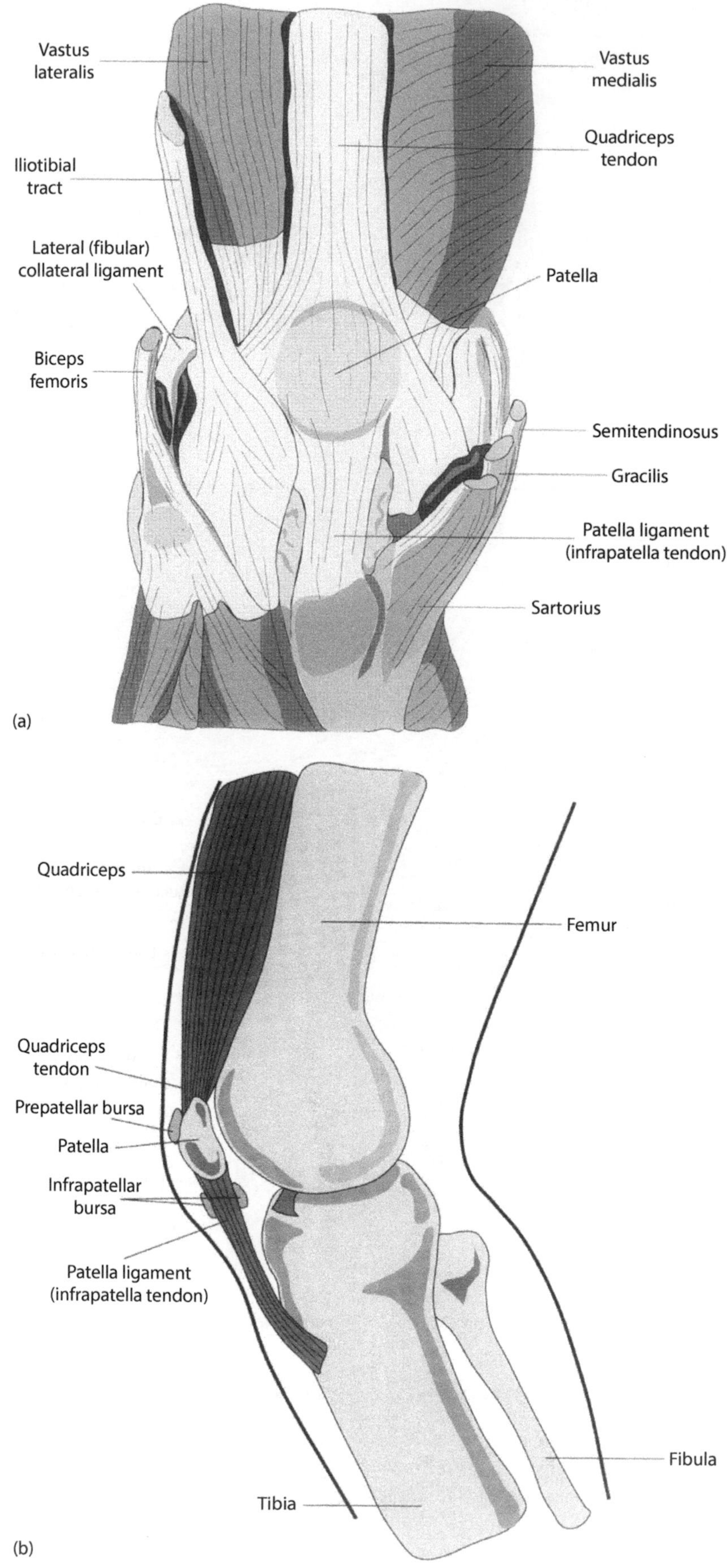

FIGURE 50.2 (a) Anterior view of the knee and (b) lateral view of the knee.

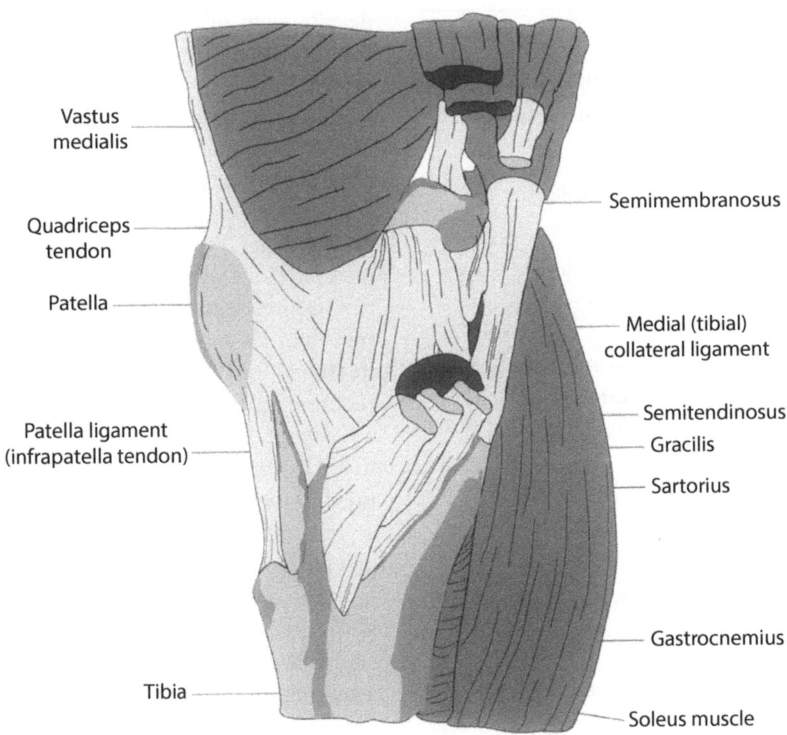

FIGURE 50.3 Medial view of the knee.

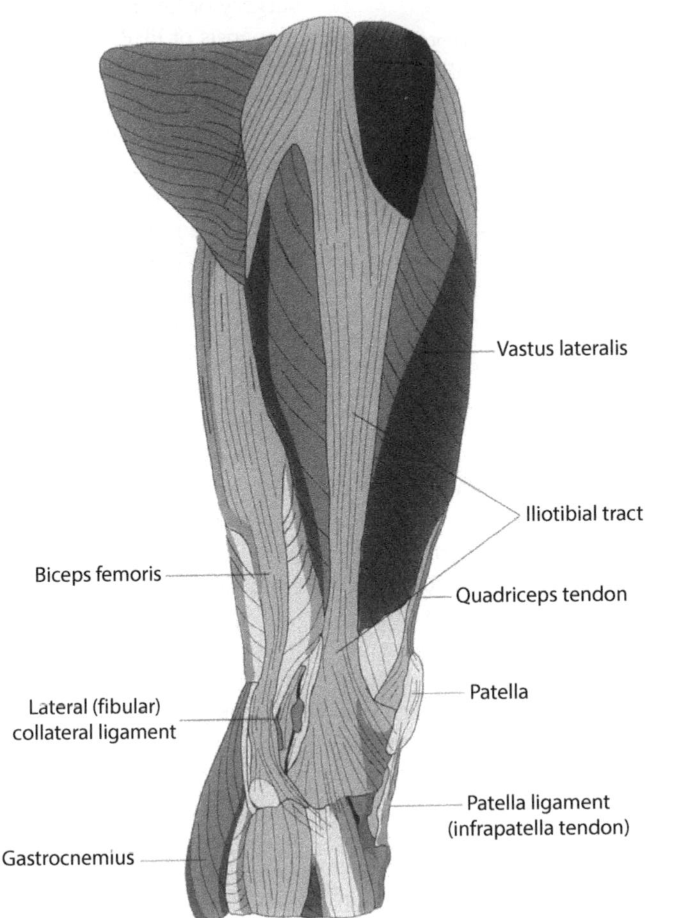

FIGURE 50.4 Lateral view of the knee and thigh.

TABLE 50.3
Common Knee Disorders in Primary Care: An Anatomical and Symptom-Oriented Approach to Differential Diagnosis

Anterior	Medial
Overuse	*Overuse*
Patellofemoral syndrome	Pes anserine tendinopathy/bursitis
Infrapatellar tendinopathy	Voshell's bursitis
Quadriceps tendinopathy	*Traumatic*
Prepatellar bursitis	Medial meniscus injury
Plica	Medial collateral ligament injury
Traumatic	Osteochondritis dissecans
Anterior cruciate ligament injury	
Subluxing or dislocating patella	
Osteochondritis dissecans	
Pediatric	
Osgood–Schlatter disease	
Sinding–Larsen–Johansson syndrome	
Lateral	**Posterior**
Overuse	*Overuse*
Iliotibial band syndrome	Popliteal (Baker's) cyst
Biceps femoris insertional tendinopathy/bursitis	Distal hamstring tendinopathy and MTJ injuries
Traumatic	*Traumatic*
Lateral meniscal injury	Meniscus injury (posterior horn)
Lateral collateral ligament injury	Posterior cruciate ligament injury
	Popliteus tendon injury
	Posterior capsule (posterior oblique, oblique popliteal, and arcuate ligament) injury

50.4 ANTERIOR KNEE PAIN

50.4.1 Overuse

50.4.1.1 Patellofemoral Pain Syndrome

Patellofemoral pain (PFP) syndrome is a common condition predominantly characterized by anterior knee pain.[42] PFP is the most common cause of knee pain presenting in the outpatient clinical setting,[7] accounting for up to 40% of all knee pain presenting to primary care clinics.[48] It is most commonly seen in adolescents aged 12–17 years, but can occur at any age. Predisposing factors include increased running mileage, especially with downhill running in individuals who have recently gone through a growth spurt or who are overweight. This condition is often incorrectly termed chondromalacia patella, which is a diagnosis that should be reserved for articular cartilage damage diagnosed by an arthroscopist or radiologist.

PFP is thought to be caused by abnormal alignment of the patellofemoral joint, which may result in both cartilage damage and repetitive microtrauma within the bone.[15,20,48] Though previously thought to be a risk factor, meta-analyses of studies have determined that Q angle does not play a role in the development of PFP. However, hip and trunk mechanics in running appear to play a role in gender-specific development of PFP.[48]

Currently, there is an ongoing debate on type of shoe wear and development of running injuries to mostly include PFP. Shoe selection appears to play a role in development of PFP, as shoes with a higher heel-to-toe drop increases stresses placed upon the patellofemoral joint.[4,17] Specific studies also examined barefoot versus shod running, determining that barefoot running resulted in less stress placed upon the patellofemoral joint.[4] However, evidence also supports foot orthosis as a treatment for PFP, specifically by improving dynamics of foot function in individuals with an overpronated foot.[2] Therefore, a thorough history of shoe wear and static and dynamic foot to hip exam should be achieved in order to individualize treatment of the PFP patient.

Patients present with complaints of poorly localized retropatellar and peripatellar pain with grating, grinding, or clicking. The onset may be insidious or acute. Pain is often worse with squatting or running or when walking on a slope or on stairs. Weakness, swelling (usually, mild if present at all), snapping, popping, pseudolocking, or giving way around the patella may all be present. When sitting in a cramped position for a prolonged period, the patient will need to shake out or flex and extend the knee ("theater sign"). Clinical history significant for recent increases in training or previous knee surgery or knee injuries may be important clues supporting a diagnosis of PFP.

The physical exam is best utilized to exclude other diagnosis and address findings that may inappropriately load the patellofemoral joint statically or dynamically. Observing the knees as they actively extend while the patient is in a seated position can reveal imbalanced excessive lateral tracking as the patella ascends above the femoral condyles known as the J sign. The popliteal angle, determined in supine with the hips at 90° while passively extending the knee and counting the remaining degrees left til full extension, is another sign resulting in increased load to the anterior knee.

Like the Q angle, some findings previously thought to be diagnostic are no longer utilized. For example, a positive PF compression test was once thought to be a good indicator of PFP; however, recent studies have called into question the sensitivity of this exam. Likewise, the patellar grind test—once frequently used in evaluation of PFP—is now considered a needlessly painful test. X-rays are generally unhelpful and findings do not correlate with disease severity.

Initial treatment for PFP is activity modification, ice, and NSAIDs. Once the pain begins to subside, physical therapy is recommended to address strength deficits in lower extremity and core musculature. However, specific treatment guidelines and exercise recommendations are controversial, as recent studies show that nearly 40% of those undergoing standard conservative care for PFP continue to experience symptoms 1 year after their initial presentation.[48] Other therapeutic modalities such as iontophoresis, electrical stimulation, laser, and therapeutic ultrasound have not been shown to offer any therapeutic effect when used alone.[24] Surgical intervention

TABLE 50.4
Knee Special Tests

Test	Performance	Positive Findings	Suggested Diagnosis
Abduction (valgus) stress at 0°	Place one hand on lateral knee and pull forefoot away from midline with the knee abducted and fully extended.	Medial joint motion or laxity.	PCL injury. Excessive laxity at 0° and 30° is indicative of a tear in both medial complex and PCL.
Abduction (valgus) stress at 30°	Place one hand on lateral knee and pull forefoot away from midline with the knee abducted and flexed to 30°.	Medial joint motion or laxity.	MCL injury. Excessive laxity at 0° and 30° is indicative of a tear in both medial complex and PCL.
Adduction (varus) stress at 0°	Place one hand on medial knee and pull forefoot toward midline with the knee abducted and fully extended.	Lateral joint motion or laxity.	PCL injury. Laxity at 0° and 30° is indicative of a tear in both LCL and PCL.
Adduction (varus) stress at 30°	Place one hand on medial knee and pull forefoot toward midline with the knee abducted and flexed to 30°.	Lateral joint motion or laxity.	LCL injury. Possible PCL injury. Laxity at 0° and 30° is indicative of a tear in both LCL and PCL.
Lachman	Knee flexed to 30°. Hands placed around distal thigh and proximal tibia with the thumb on the tibial crest. Attempt anterior translation.	Endpoint is not detected or excessive anterior translation occurs.	ACL injury. Acute ACL insufficiency.
Anterior drawer, neutral	Patient supine with hip at 45° and knee flexed to 90°. Foot in neutral position. Exert pressure on the posterior proximal tibia to attempt to translate the tibia forward.	Movement of the tibia on the femur suggests an ACL injury.	Patellar instability; *do not complete test in setting of possible acute dislocation due to risk of possibly worsening the injury.
Anterior drawer, internal rotation	Patient supine with hip at 45° and knee flexed to 90°. Foot internally rotated. Exert pressure on the posterior proximal tibia to attempt to translate the tibia forward.	Lateral tibial plateau moves anteriorly and rotates medially.	ACL injury + posterolateral capsule injury.
Anterior drawer, external rotation	Patient supine with hip at 45° and knee flexed to 90°. Foot externally rotated. Exert pressure on the posterior proximal tibia to attempt to translate the tibia forward.	Medial tibial plateau advances anteriorly, rotating from medial to lateral side.	ACL injury + medial capsular injury.
Posterior drawer	From position of neutral rotation, push the tibia posteriorly.	Excessive posterior translation.	Torn PCL.
Posterolateral drawer	Patient supine with hip at 45° and knee flexed to 90°. Foot externally rotated. Push tibia posteriorly.	Posterior rotation of the lateral tibial condyle.	Posterolateral corner injury.
Posterior sag/gravity	Patient supine with hip at 45° and knee flexed to 90°. Feet flat on floor. Observe from lateral side. For posterior displacement.	Posterior displacement or sagging of one tibial tuberosity compared with the other.	PCL injury.
Jerk	With patient supine with knee flexed to 90°, internally rotate the foot and leg. Knee is progressively extended while valgus force is applied.	At 20°–30° of flexion, the lateral tibial condyle subluxes anteriorly. Further extension causes sudden reduction.	ACL injury.
Pivot shift	Tibia and foot are internally rotated and the knee is hyperextended. Knee is flexed with valgus force applied.	At 20°–30° of flexion, patient feels a sudden shift as lateral tibial condyle rotates anteriorly on the femur.	Anterolateral rotatory instability.

(*Continued*)

TABLE 50.4 (*Continued*)
Knee Special Tests

Test	Performance	Positive Findings	Suggested Diagnosis
Reverse pivot shift	With patient supine with knee flexed to 90°, externally rotate the foot and leg. Knee is progressively extended while valgus force is applied.	Palpable "clunk" at 90° of flexion as lateral tibial condyle subluxes posteriorly.	Chronic lateral ligament injuries.
External rotation recurvatum	Lift the leg by the patient's great toe.	Varus, external rotation, and hyperextension.	LCL injury, posterolateral corner injury.
McMurray's test	Patient supine, knee in maximal flexion. Place fingers along joint line. With valgus stress, slowly extend the knee with the tibia externally rotated (medial meniscus) or internally rotated (lateral meniscus).	Painful clicking occurs at the medial joint line (medial meniscus) or lateral joint line (lateral meniscus).	Posterior meniscal injury.
Apley grind/compression	Patient is prone with the knee flexed to 90°. Push straight down on the foot while rotating the tibia and partially flexing and extending the knee.	Painful pop over the medial joint line during external tibial rotation (medial meniscus) or on lateral joint line during internal tibial rotation (lateral meniscus).	Medial meniscus or lateral meniscus injury.
Hypermobility/ apprehension	Patient is supine, relaxed quadriceps, knee flexed 30°–45°. Press against the medial border of the patella.	If the patella begins to sublux, the patient will show apprehension and will ask you to stop.	Patellar instability; *do not complete test in setting of possible acute dislocation.
Patellar inhibition test	Apply resistance to the superior pole of the patella. Ask the patient to contract the quadriceps forcefully.	Patient will be reluctant to do so or will have a painful crunching under the patella.	Patellofemoral pain syndrome.
Patellar compression	Compression of the patella against the femur longitudinally and/or transversely.	Pain and crepitation in knee.	Patellofemoral pain syndrome.
Ober's test	Patient is side lying with hips perpendicular to table. Tested leg is held at the lower leg and hip is extended keeping the ankle at the level of the hip.	Knee and thigh maintain parallel with table.	Tight ITB.
Noble's	Patient is supine and valgus stress applied to knee with hand over lateral knee. Knee is actively moved from 0° to 30° flexion.	Pain and snapping at the lateral femoral condyle.	ITB syndrome.
Malacrea's test	Patient lies on uninvolved side, affected leg abducted at the hip with the knee in extension. Apply resistance to abducted leg while patient fully flexes and extends at the knee.	Patient's pain is reproduced in the area of the lateral femoral epicondyle.	ITB syndrome.

TABLE 50.5
Indications for Specialty Referral for Common Disorders of the Knee

Diagnosis	Primary Care Referral Considerations
Anterior	
ACL injury	High-demand athletes should be referred early to allow for proper surgical decision making. Low-grade, partial tears (Grades 1 and 2) can be referred if still symptomatic after proper course of conservative treatment.
Patellofemoral syndrome	Consider referral for refractory cases that cause recurrent disability. In rare cases that fail conservative therapy, lateral release or extensor mechanism reconstruction may improve function.
Prepatellar bursitis	Consider early referral for aspiration, cultures, and antibiotic treatment if warranted. Nonseptic cases should be referred after 2–3 weeks if bursitis still exists despite proper treatment.
Patellar/quadriceps tendinopathy	Consider referral for injection-based therapies or surgery for refractory cases or findings of advanced tendon breakdown or tears.
Plica	Consider referral for surgical evaluation after failure of a reasonable course of conservative treatments.
Dislocating/subluxing patella	Recurrent dislocations or acute cases involving a VMO tear, fracture, or loose body warrant consultation.
Osteochondritis dissecans	Early consultation is recommended, as improperly treated OCD lesions can prevent an athlete's return to high-level activities.
Osgood–Schlatter disease	Consider referral for prolonged disability not responding to conservative therapy or if patient still experiences pain despite reaching skeletal maturity.
Medial	
MCL injury	High-demand athletes should be referred early to allow for proper surgical decision making. Low-grade, partial tears (Grades 1 and 2) can be referred if still symptomatic after proper course of conservative treatment.
Medial meniscal injury	Urgent referral for a "locked" joint. High-demand athletes should be referred early to allow for proper surgical decision making. Consider referral if extent of injury is unclear or if failed conservative treatment.
Pes anserine tendinopathy/bursitis	After failure of typical treatments, may consider early referral for more advanced injection therapies if patient needs to return to a higher level of functioning quickly.
Voshell's bursitis	After failure of typical treatments, may consider early referral for more advanced injection therapies if patient needs to return to a higher level of functioning quickly.
Lateral	
ITB syndrome	Consider referral for surgical evaluation after failure of a reasonable course of conservative treatments.
Lateral meniscal injury	Urgent referral for a "locked" joint. High-demand athletes should be referred early to allow for proper surgical decision making. Consider referral if extent of injury is unclear or if failed conservative treatment.
LCL injury	High-demand athletes should be referred early to allow for proper surgical decision making. Low-grade, partial tears (Grades 1 and 2) can be referred if still symptomatic after proper course of conservative treatment.
Posterior	
PCL injury	Obtain referral for Grade 3 injuries or if patient experiences recurrent instability. High-demand athletes should be referred early to allow for proper surgical decision making.
Popliteal (Baker) cyst	After failure of typical treatments, may consider early referral for surgical evaluation for cyst excision or more advanced injection therapies. Also consider referral for correction of underlying knee pathology.

should be considered a last resort, reserved only after failing 6–12 months of conservative treatment.

50.4.1.2 Infrapatellar Tendinitis

Infrapatellar tendinitis, or "jumper's knee," is a tendinopathy affecting the inferior pole of the patella. This condition is most commonly seen in athletes involved in jumping activities (e.g., volleyball, basketball, and track and field) and in those doing squats (e.g., powerlifting).[39] Repetitive microtrauma to the tendon occurs due to excessive jumping or other high-patellofemoral-stress activity. Patients present with infrapatellar pain; this pain is most severe at the onset of exercise, improves after warming-up, and then recurs later in activity. They may also report knee pain at rest. They typically report tenderness at inferior pole of patella and over the body of the patellar tendon. Extensor mechanism malalignment may be variably present (see Section 50.4.1.1), as well as tightness of hamstring, heel cord, and/or quadriceps muscles and ankle dorsiflexor weakness.

Routine x-rays are not indicated and are usually normal. Occasionally, irregularities at the inferior pole of patella or signs of malalignment (see Section 50.4.1.1) may be observed. Magnetic resonance imaging (MRI) may demonstrate degenerative changes within the tendon.

Initial treatment is supportive, including RICE, NSAIDs, and analgesia as needed. Physical therapy is an important mainstay of treatment, concentrating on hamstring, ankle dorsiflexors, heel cord, and quadriceps flexibility and strength. Counterforce bracing[18] has been shown to be beneficial by reducing stress on the tendon. Platelet-rich protein injections may be beneficial as an adjuvant therapy,[12] but more research must be done in this area. Steroid injection is very risky as it may promote rupture.[18]

50.4.1.3 Quadriceps Tendinitis

Quadriceps tendinitis occurs as a result of repetitive jumping (e.g., basketball and volleyball) with acceleration or deceleration. It is usually seen during a forceful contraction of the quads. This injury has become more common as the length of playing seasons and the frequency of daily participation have increased (Sommer). Tendinopathy arises from repetitive microtrauma of the quadriceps tendon at the superior pole attachment of the patella, causing inflammation and tendon injury. This inflammation may involve only vastus lateralis insertion into superolateral pole of patella or vastus medialis obliquus insertion into superomedial pole of patella. Patients typically present with suprapatellar pain, exacerbated by squatting or jumping. Physical exam reveals tenderness or swelling at superior pole of patella, hamstring, and heel cord, quadriceps muscle tightness, or signs of malalignment (see Section 50.4.1.1). Neither x-rays nor MRI is indicated for this condition, though MRI may show evidence of tendinopathy on imaging. Treatment is the same as treatment for infrapatellar tendinitis, focusing on RICE, NSAIDs, and physical therapy for improved muscle flexibility and strength (see Section 50.4.1.2).

50.4.1.4 Prepatellar Bursitis

Prepatellar bursitis, commonly known as "housemaid's knee," is an irritation of the bursa located immediately superficial to the patella. This inflammation may be induced by acute trauma to the distal patella or through repeated friction and irritation. In athletics, prepatellar bursitis is most commonly encountered in hockey, volleyball, and wrestling (Baumbach). Patients will present with anterior knee pain and swelling. The affected area may appear erythematous and swollen, with fluid collection palpable directly over the patella. The prepatellar bursa is tender to palpation, and patients may endorse pain with full knee flexion. Bursitis may best be imaged via ultrasound. X-ray films are not helpful. Bursal fluid aspiration may be necessary to differentiate septic from aseptic etiologies of bursitis.

As a superficial bursa, the prepatellar bursa is the common location of septic bursitis (Baumbach). Therefore, when evaluating a suspected case of prepatellar bursitis, it is important to differentiate between nonseptic and septic presentations of bursitis. Prepatellar pain and swelling accompanied by constitutional symptoms (temp >38°C, elevated WBC or CRP), significant warmth over affected bursa in comparison to contralateral side, skin lesions over affected bursa, or purulent bursal aspirate should raise suspicion for septic bursitis (Baumbach).

Nonseptic acute bursitis should be treated with compression bracing to decrease swelling, NSAIDs, and rest. Glucocorticoid injection into the affected bursa can provide significant relief for patients presenting with recurrent nonseptic or postinfectious bursitis. Septic bursitis should be treated with bursal aspiration and appropriate antibiotics based on results of bursal fluid culture. A good practice is to draw an ESR in concert with aspiration to monitor selection and route of antibiotics. Refractory bursitis that does not respond to conservative care may require surgical intervention and bursectomy.

50.4.1.5 Synovial Plica

A synovial plica is a congenital redundancy of synovial tissue that may manifest itself during overuse or after a direct blow to the medial patellofemoral joint (e.g., falling on turf or a dashboard injury). Synovial plica is common though not always symptomatic; painful plica is most commonly designated as being mediopatellar (most common), infrapatellar, or suprapatellar[18] in location. Overall, synovial plica is observed in 20%–60% of the population.[2] Repeated microtrauma from repetitive flexion and extension of the knee is thought to cause synovial thickening, sometimes progressing to fibrosis or even hemorrhage.[18]

Symptoms of plica include anterior knee pain and swelling, pain over suprapatellar or medial patellofemoral regions with long periods of knee flexion, snapping or popping sensation following knee extension, or painful pseudolocking over the medial knee joint. While often insidious in nature, some patients will report acute symptomatic onset following a marked increase in activity level. Tender plica may be palpable medially by passively flexing and extending the internally rotated tibia. Hamstring and heel cord tightness or other signs of extensor mechanism malalignment may be present. X-ray imaging is not indicated, while MRI may demonstrate cases of plica. Ultrasound is often useful, as the plica may be observed during dynamic movement of the joint. Recent studies have shown ultrasound to be a reliable method of identifying or confirming the diagnosis of plica.[30]

The mainstay of treatment is RICE, NSAIDs, and analgesics as needed. For long-term management, physical therapy and external patellar support have been shown to be beneficial. Recurrent or refractory cases may be treated by corticosteroid injection; patients with refractory or chronically fibrosed plica should be referred for arthroscopic removal as chronic cases may be complicated by degenerative articular changes in the knee.

50.4.2 Traumatic

50.4.2.1 Anterior Cruciate Ligament Injury

One of the most common knee injuries in sports, ACL tears have increased in incidence over the past several decades. From 1994 to 2006, the incidence of ACL reconstructions increased by approximately 50%.[26] ACL injuries are most commonly observed in soccer, skiing, football, and basketball.[14] Eighty percent of ski injuries involve the ACL. An estimated 100,000 ACL injuries per year result from skiing in the United States.[49] Despite an 83% return to some level of sports participation, only 63% return to their preinjury level of play.[1] The ACL is usually injured as part of a more complex injury through hyperextension, varus/internal rotation, extremes of valgus and external rotation, deceleration (usually noncontact), or the application of force that drives the tibia in an anterior direction when the knee is flexed at a right angle. ACL tears are most commonly seen in the midportion of the ligament, though they may occur at the femur or tibia. The injury usually involves damage to other knee structures, such as avulsion of the tibial spine in young athletes, damage to the middle third of the lateral capsular ligament or to the menisci, or often vertical longitudinal (circumferential) meniscal tears (so-called bucket-handle tears). In knee injuries caused by a noncontact, twisting event and result in acute effusion, more than 70% involve a tear in the ACL.[21,49]

Patients with acute ACL tears report hearing a loud pop at the time of injury with nearly immediate swelling. Other symptoms such as dizziness, sweating, faintness, and nausea can occur with severe swelling over the next several hours. Patient feels as though the knee is unstable, particularly in rotation. Full extension is difficult. Chronically, the patient reports often feeling a sensation of the knee "giving way" and has a history of a "knee sprain" or "trick knee," especially during pivoting and cutting. Following acute injury, large hemarthrosis and a positive Lachman test are observed on physical exam.[10] Chronic cases will also have a positive Lachman test and positive pivot shift or jerk test, suggesting functional instability. Anterior drawer signs are typically unreliable.

Routine films (anteroposterior [AP] and lateral) may reveal a lateral capsular sign (i.e., avulsion of midportion of lateral capsular ligament from the lateral tibial condyle also known as Segond fracture) and avulsion of tibial spine in young patients. MRI is sensitive and specific, especially with difficult cases. Arthroscopy is valuable in diagnosing associated intraarticular injuries (e.g., torn menisci or chondral fractures).[1,6] Arthrography has been supplanted by the aforementioned techniques.

The initial treatment of an acute ACL injury is RICE, NSAIDs, and analgesics as needed in conjunction with crutches and a limited motion brace or splint. Diagnostic or therapeutic aspiration is rarely indicated.

For Grades 1 and 2 sprains, orthotics, bracing, and/or taping may be used to prevent full extension during participation in contact sports; physical therapy (range-of-motion [ROM] and progressive resistance exercises) should concentrate on both quadriceps and hamstrings; resistive exercises between 0° and 45° of flexion during the first year following injury or reconstruction should be included (Level of Evidence A: randomized controlled trial).[19,43] Relative effectiveness of modalities remains to be established. A knee brace may be useful because it improves proprioception of the knee. For Grade 3 sprains, conservative therapy offers a prognosis of 33% improvement with minimal symptoms, 33% functional though still symptomatic, and 33% progressive functional disability requiring surgical reconstruction. Autografts have the highest success rate and lowest incidence of complications. A poor prognosis is associated with (1) age less than 30, (2) jumping and pivoting sports, (3) torn menisci, (4) marked anterior subluxation, and (5) generalized joint laxity.

Referral to orthopedics for Grade 3 sprains in active athletes and recurrent functional instability; in persons who do not participate in sports and who have had a full course of physical therapy; avulsion injuries or unclear associated intraarticular injuries.[18,31]

50.4.2.2 Patellar Subluxation or Dislocation

Patellar subluxation and dislocation are major causes of patient-reported knee instability. In patellar subluxation, there is disproportionate lateral movement of the patella, but the patella remains in the trochlear groove. Patellar subluxation may occur secondary to trauma or may be a result of congenital joint laxity. In patellar dislocations, the patella is dislodged from the trochlear groove. Lateral dislocation is most common.

Predisposing factors include (1) a dynamic imbalance with the lateral musculature overpowering the medial muscles, (2) hypoplastic patella, (3) patella alta, and (4) shallow femoral groove. Patellar dislocation commonly occurs as a noncontact injury, resulting from the force of contraction in the quadriceps combined with genu valgum. The injury can also occur in athletes with relatively normal lower extremity alignment and quadriceps mechanisms. Patellar subluxation may occur with less severe force than dislocation, or in normal, everyday activity.

Patients will commonly report patellar dislocation that spontaneously resolved prior to their initial presentation. They may have a chronic history of knee joint instability or pain. Following acute dislocation, patients typically report peripatellar and retropatellar pain; feelings of an unstable kneecap, deformity ("something coming out" medially or "something going back into place"); pain with rising from a seated position ("theater sign"); swelling within 2 hours of injury; or, rarely, locking and buckling. If the patella has reduced prior to presenting to clinic, signs include medial retinacular tenderness, anteversion of the femoral neck causing patellae to point inward, patella alta, increased Q angle, positive hypermobility and apprehension tests, and swelling. If the patella is still dislocated, signs include a deformity over the lateral femoral condyle with a prominence of uncovered medial femoral condyle and possible medial ligamentous instability.

Routine x-rays (AP and lateral) are usually normal as spontaneous relocation is typical. Infrapatellar views may show avulsion of the medial edge of the patella or large osteochondral fracture, lateral tilt, or subluxation. Lateral view may demonstrate a high riding patella (patella alta). Patella alta is most quickly determined by calculating the Insall–Salvati ratio in which the greatest diagonal length of the patella is compared to the posterior length of the patellar tendon. These measurements should be equal, and a patella to patellar tendon disparity of greater than 20% is considered abnormal. MRI may be useful in evaluating knee for further ligamentous injury in complex cases.

Treatment of acutely dislocated patella should begin with patellar reduction. Relocation is performed by knee flexion and then extension and gentle pressure along lateral patellar edge. Aspiration may be useful for diagnosis of associated fracture (fat in blood) and treatment. If it is the patient's first patellar dislocation, immobilize in extension with a foam pad over vastus medialis obliquus and lateral buttress for 4 weeks. The patient then progresses to physical therapy (ROM and progressive resistance exercise [PRE]) and functional patellar bracing that prevents subluxation but allows for increased flexion and extension.[43] In recurrent dislocations, temporary immobilization and crutches should be followed by physical therapy and bracing. Surgery is recommended for chronic cases or acute cases associated with a loose fracture fragment in the joint or Grade 3 strain of the VMO.

50.4.2.3 Osteochondritis Dissecans

Osteochondritis dissecans (OCDs) is a disorder in which a segment of bone and the overlying articular cartilage become separated from the rest of the bone. In patients under 15 years of age, it is generally not related to trauma, and patients typically heal with conservative management.[6] Patients over 15 are usually males who have experienced a traumatic incident (possibly a compression fracture). Other related factors are impairment of the blood supply to the affected area of the femur (avascular necrosis) and genetic predisposition. OCD lesions may result from dislocation of the patella, ACL tear, or other trauma to the joint surface (e.g., twisting or a direct blow). The majority of cases occur at the femoral condyles, but OCD may occur at the retropatellar surface as well. The lesion may be stable (still firmly attached) or unstable (only partially attached) or may be a loose body within the joint ("joint mouse").

Patients with OCD lesions typically report nonspecific knee pain, stiffness, or swelling. Symptoms usually worsen with activity, particularly high-impact activity, and improve with rest. Chronically, these patients may develop catching, locking, and buckling if loose bodies develop. Physical exam may reveal effusion, quadriceps atrophy, and tenderness in the anterior knee. MRI is the imaging modality of choice in these injuries, as they are excellent for defining stage of lesion and planning treatment. These lesions do not typically appear on x-rays, as cartilaginous fragments and very small, bony, loose bodies are not visible. Large lesions and significant bone fragments are usually visible.

For smaller or stable lesions, a trial of rest from pain-producing activities (possible enforced rest in an immobilizer) may provide symptomatic relief. Athletes who maintain full ROM, have full strength, have no effusion in the knee, and do not experience catching or locking in the knee may continue to play with close medical supervision.[6] Surgical debridement, internal fixation, or prolonged protected weight bearing may be necessary for large or unstable lesions. Defects may be treated in numerous ways. Unsalvageable OCD lesions are commonly treated with bone grafting or autologous chondrocyte implantation.[6] Microfracture is an alternative with reported faster return to play but may be less durable than other options.[22]

50.4.2.4 Pediatric

50.4.2.5 Osgood–Schlatter Disease

Osgood–Schlatter disease is a traction apophysitis of the tibial tubercle most commonly seen in children 10–15 years old.[11] It is most commonly associated with adolescent males who have recently experienced a growth spurt. This condition is thought to be a result of repetitive microtrauma at the secondary ossification center of the tibial tuberosity as the patellar tendon pulls against the apophysis during athletic activity.[11] Symptoms are characterized by pain, tenderness, and swelling at the tibial tuberosity. Patients will present with bilateral knee pain in 20%–30% of cases.[11]

Upon exam, the tibial tuberosity may appear enlarged and tender. Signs of patellar malalignment and inflexibility of the hamstrings, heel cords, and quadriceps may also be present.

Imaging of the knee often appears normal; however, more progressed cases may show enlarged, irregular tibial tuberosity, a loose ossicle separated from tuberosity, or patella alta. Loose ossicles may persist following apophyseal closure.

Treatment is supportive, with RICE, NSAIDs, and analgesics as needed. Patients with mild-to-moderate pain may exercise as tolerated using anti-inflammatories and knee pads. Those with more severe pain often benefit from active rest. Physical therapy is an important mainstay of treatment, as it works to improve flexibility, thereby alleviating traction on the apophysis.

This condition commonly recurs throughout adolescence, but generally subsides upon reaching skeletal maturity in 90%–95% of patients. For those who experience persistent knee pain despite closure of the apophysis, surgery is often indicated to excise any bony fragments. Stretching, bracing, and minimizing high-impact activities are helpful in preventing relapsing cases.

50.4.2.6 Sinding–Larsen–Johansson Syndrome

Similar to Osgood–Schlatter disease, Sinding–Larsen–Johansson syndrome is a traction apophysitis of the inferior pole of the patella. This condition often affects adolescents between ages 10 and 13 years, more commonly seen in active males.[18] Patients complain of anterior knee pain exacerbated by jumping, squatting, or running. Physical exam demonstrates tenderness over the inferior pole of the patella, at times accompanied by localized soft-tissue swelling. Pain or tenderness in the remainder of the knee and leg is absent. X-rays are generally not indicated, though they may show slight separation of the patellar apophysis at the inferior patellar pole. Treatment is conservative, and symptoms usually resolve with 2–3 weeks of rest, followed by a gradual return to activity.[18] Patellar bracing may be helpful in minimizing symptoms during activity, and physical therapy is effective in improving flexibility, minimizing stress on the patellar apophyses.[18] Symptoms often abate with closure of the patellar apophysis, and recurrence of pain past the age of skeletal maturity is rare. In the event of persistent pain or nonunion of the apophysis, surgical intervention may be considered.

50.5 MEDIAL KNEE PAIN

50.5.1 Overuse

50.5.1.1 Pes Anserine Tendinopathy and Bursitis

The pes anserine tendon is formed by the convergence of the medial hamstring tendons—sartorius, gracilis, and semitendinosus—as they insert upon the medial tibia. The tendon is separated from the medial tibial condyle by the pes anserine bursa. Both tendinopathy and bursitis may occur in this region secondary to overuse or acute trauma and occur both in isolation and in concert.[45] Studies have shown 2.5% of medial knee pain is due to pes anserine bursitis.[32]

Patients present to clinic with complaints of pain at the anteromedial proximal tibia, typically within 4–5 cm of the joint line. Pain is worsened by climbing stairs, rising to standing from a seated position, engaging the hamstring muscles, and getting in and out of a vehicle due to the added lateral motion. Patients may also report nocturnal pain.[45] Physical exam commonly reveals swelling and tenderness along the proximal medial tibia and medial joint line along with pain with valgus stress. Differentiation between this diagnosis and MCL strain can be determined by a keen palpation exam and understanding of the location of the underlying anatomy.

X-rays are generally not helpful, but ultrasound is useful in identifying both pes anserine bursitis and tendinopathy. MRI can be helpful in differentiating pes anserine pathologies from other causes of medial knee pain, though differentiation between tendinopathy and bursitis is difficult.[45]

Treatment of both bursitis and tendinopathy includes NSAIDs, RICE, and physical therapy. Local corticosteroid injection to the affected medial knee has also been shown to have symptomatic relief.[32,45]

50.5.1.2 Tibial Collateral Ligament (Voshell's) Bursitis

Tibial collateral ligament bursitis, known as Voshell's bursitis, is an uncommon cause of medial knee pain. Patients presenting with tibial collateral ligament bursitis often only complain of pain at the medial joint line, without mechanical symptoms.[20] Pain is insidious, and patients often deny any acute trauma to the knee. Physical exam is overall benign, with some tenderness over the medial joint line. Joint effusion is absent; McMurray's test and varus stress testing are negative. It is often considered a diagnosis of exclusion, as other pathologic entities such as MCL sprain, medial meniscal tear, and pes anserine tendinitis may produce identical patterns of pain.[20] Voshell's bursitis has also been noted to concomitantly occur with other overuse injuries of the knee, such as patellofemoral syndrome or infrapatellar tendinitis.

MRI may aid in diagnosis, as bursitis will demonstrate a characteristic *inverted U* pattern of fluid over the semimembranosus tendon. However, MRI is not necessary to diagnose bursitis.[33] The typical treatment for acute bursitis is localized corticosteroid injection. Voshell's bursitis responds well to such injections, as patients typically report pain cessation and return to previous activities.

50.5.2 Traumatic

50.5.2.1 Medial Ligament Injury

Injuries to the MCL and/or medial capsular ligament can occur in football from a tackle or block against the lateral aspect of the knee if the foot is planted. A skier can incur this injury if one ski becomes trapped in the snow and momentum carries the skier onward (see Figure 50.5). A swimmer can injure the medial ligament(s) when performing the whip kick with the breaststroke. In each of these examples, the mechanism of injury is a valgus force placed upon the lateral aspect of the knee with external tibial rotation.

Tearing of MCL may also involve peripheral detachment of medial meniscus and anterior cruciate ("unhappy triad") or injury to medial capsular ligament, tibial collateral ligament, and posterior oblique ligament. Patients with injuries to their MCL will present with medial knee pain and joint swelling. They may or may not present with limping or reports of joint instability ("giving way"). On physical exam, medial edema and tenderness are often present, as is a positive abduction stress test. With stress testing, there may be some valgus opening at 0° knee flexion, with marked opening of the joint at 30° knee flexion. Neutral anterior and posterior drawer tests are negative unless cruciate ligaments are involved. However, the anterior drawer test with external tibial rotation is often positive. A positive McMurray's test may be notable if the medial meniscus is involved.

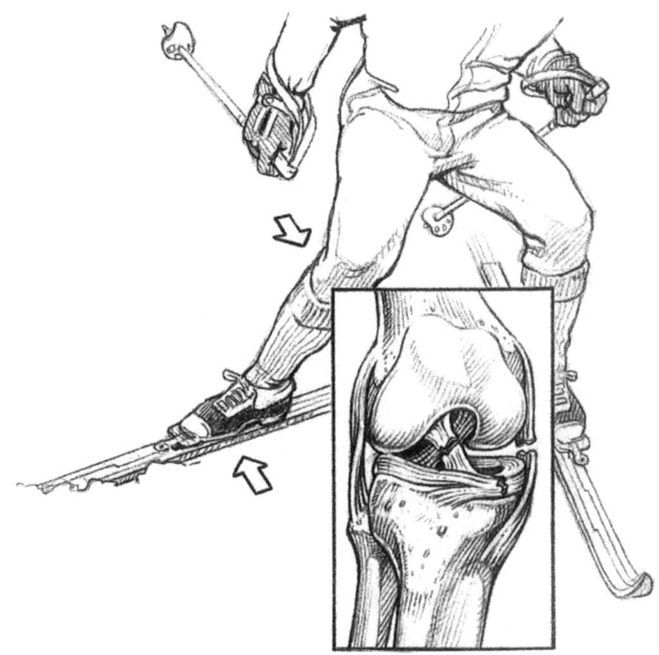

FIGURE 50.5 The "unhappy triad": medial meniscus, medial collateral, and anterior cruciate tears.

Routine films (AP, lateral) are negative. Abduction stress films are useful in distinguishing ligament injury from epiphyseal fracture in skeletally immature patients. In these images, the fracture opens at growth plate, while the ligamentous tear opens at the joint line. MRI has high sensitivity and specificity for MCL tears[15]; MRI cannot distinguish Grade 1 and 2 injuries (incomplete tears) but can separate them from Grade 3 (complete) tears.

Initial treatment of MCL injuries includes RICE, NSAIDs, and analgesics as needed. A posterior splint should be applied, followed by crutches with weight bearing. For incomplete (Grades 1 and 2) tears, treatment is symptomatic. For isolated complete tears, use a brace that allows for motion at the joint but prevents excess valgus stress and refer for physical therapy for ROM and progressive resistance exercises.[19,43] Surgery is recommended for complicated cases (e.g., ACL and MCL tears).[49]

50.5.2.2 Medial Meniscus Injuries

Meniscal tears occur less frequently in minor knee injuries, but most vertical longitudinal tears of the menisci occur in knees in which the ACL is torn.[49] These injuries are rare in preadolescents and often are not diagnosed in adolescents. Meniscal injuries commonly occur in soccer (rather than football), and many of these injuries occur at the time of medial collateral or ACL sprains but go unrecognized because of lack of symptoms and disability. The incidence of medial meniscal tears increases over time in ACL-deficient knees.[3] Medial meniscal tears are the result of a fixed-foot rotation injury while weight bearing with the knee flexed, which causes a combination of compression and rotational forces being exerted on the meniscus. The tibia rotates externally with respect to the femur. These forces cause disruption of the medial semilunar cartilage of the knee. In injuries with concomitant ACL tears, a circumferential ("bucket-handle") tear is common.

Patients with injury to their medial meniscus present with mild swelling; joint-line pain; reports of popping, slipping, or catching over joint line; recurrent locking in chronic setting; or buckling. Positive McMurray's test, positive Apley's test, joint-line tenderness, quadriceps atrophy, loud "clunk" during anterior drawer testing, and inability to squat and duck walk may be noted on exam. However, individual maneuvers may vary from exam to exam and have generally poor sensitivity and specificity (Level of Evidence B: prospective cohort; Level of Evidence A: quantitative systematic meta-analysis).

Routine x-ray films are usually unremarkable; if a tear has been present for a long time, possible joint-line spurring, narrowing of joint line, and cartilage calcification may be observed. MRI is the procedure of choice and offers high sensitivity, specificity, and accuracy. Arthroscopy has the additional advantage of being a treatment but has low sensitivity to tears in the posterior horn.

Initially, treatment of meniscal injury should include RICE, NSAIDs, and analgesics as needed. Physical therapy (ROM and PREs) should be employed for a stable tear without ligamentous instability.[43] Surgery should be considered in cases of persistent mechanical symptoms, continued pain and swelling, or injuries involving competitive athletes. During surgery, as much of the meniscus as possible should be saved to minimize the development of arthritic degeneration. Many tears, especially peripheral ones, can be repaired.

50.6 LATERAL KNEE PAIN

50.6.1 Overuse

50.6.1.1 Iliotibial Band Syndrome

Iliotibial band (ITB) syndrome is the most common cause of lateral knee pain. Predisposing factors include increasing running mileage to 20–40 miles/week and recent changes in the "S list" in training, especially hilly terrain.[41] Hard-surface running with increased speed is a common factor. ITB syndrome often occurs in athletes with neutral or varus knee alignment, particularly in the downside leg when the athlete is running on a sloping road. Men develop this condition more commonly than women because of lower body-fat percentages, alignment differences, and variations in bony morphology. If ITB syndrome occurs in a woman, it may be indicative of an eating disorder (e.g., anorexia nervosa). The ITB is pulled anteriorly by the tensor fascia lata in flexion and posteriorly by the gluteus maximus in extension. In ITB syndrome, the ITB becomes inflamed as excessive flexion and extension of the knee cause repetitive microtrauma and inflammation as it rubs back and forth over the lateral femoral epicondyle. Patients report lateral knee pain in activity, usually occurring at a fixed distance at a given pace, as well as stinging during deceleration when foot contacts the ground (footstrike). Inflexibility in the lower extremity and occasional popping in the knee are also common.

Upon exam, patients with ITB syndrome will endorse tenderness to palpation along distal ITB over lateral femoral epicondyle, commonly 3 cm proximal to lateral joint line. Malacrea's test will produce pain and tenderness. Renne's creak sign may be positive (lateral knee creaking sound when flexing or extending knee) as well as Noble's test. Intraarticular findings are negative. X-rays are not helpful, and MRI or ultrasound is typically not indicated for this condition.

Initial management of ITB syndrome is supportive, including RICE, NSAIDs, transverse friction, and ice massage. Physical therapy (ROM and PREs) should include stretching of hamstrings, gluteals, abductors, and iliotibial tract; lateral heel or sole wedge or orthotics may be beneficial. Stretching of the ITB, controlling abnormal foot motion or leg length discrepancy, running on softer surfaces, and minimizing downhill or sloped-road running may also be beneficial.

50.6.1.2 Lateral Collateral Ligament Injury

The lateral stabilizing complex is not as vulnerable to injury as the medial ligaments and is therefore injured less frequently. Injuries to these ligaments do occur in contact (e.g., wrestling and soccer) and noncontact (e.g., racquet sports and running) injuries. In these injuries, a varus force is applied with internal tibial rotation. Anterotibial trauma with hyperextension may also injure the posterolateral components. Severe injuries may also involve biceps tendon, ITB, peroneal nerve, popliteal tendon, and posterolateral corner of the lateral complex. Cruciate ligaments and meniscus are rarely involved.

Patients with Grade 1 or 2 strains typically present with pain over lateral ligament complex. Those with Grade 3 tears will also complain their knee giving way when twisting, cutting, and pivoting or with standing, walking, and backward running (with posterolateral injury). Acutely, patients will likely have an increased adduction stress test at 30° flexion and positive posterolateral drawer test. In chronic cases, a positive reverse pivot shift test and external rotation recurvatum test are often present; external rotation recurvatum may also be seen on standing.

Routine films (AP and lateral) of proximal lateral tibia are usually negative, though avulsion of midportion of lateral capsular ligament with small fragment of proximal lateral tibia (lateral capsular sign) or small avulsion fragment of proximal fibula with posterolateral ligament complex (arcuate sign) may be noted. As in the case of MCL injury, adduction stress films are useful in distinguishing ligament injury from epiphyseal fracture in skeletally immature patients. Likewise, MRI has a high specificity and sensitivity for identifying LCL tears.

Initial treatment of LCL injuries includes RICE, NSAIDs, and immobilization. For incomplete tears (Grades 1 and 2), treat with bracing, crutches with weight bearing, and physical therapy (ROM and PREs).[19,43] For Grade 3, surgical repair is recommended. Referral to orthopedics is warranted in patients with recurrent disability, fractures, Grade 3 injuries, large effusion, or abnormal x-rays.

50.6.1.3 Lateral Meniscal Injury

The lateral meniscus has greater mobility than its medial counterpart due to differences in tibial plateau topography, the interposition of the popliteus tendon between the LCL and the periphery of the meniscus, and its more narrowly spaced horns. As such, it is less likely to be torn over time in a chronically ACL-deficient knee or suffer an isolated tear; however, it is still susceptible to tears, especially during injuries causing acute ACL disruption. In fact, lateral meniscus tears are the most frequent injury associated with an acute ACL tear (Level of Evidence B: prospective cohort).[14,19] An increased incidence of lateral meniscus injuries may also be noted in wrestling and martial arts because of the frequently fixed attitude of the knee with the foot in external rotation. Injury may result from a single traumatic episode, degenerative processes, or a combination and may also be associated with abnormalities such as a congenital discoid meniscus.

In acute injury, compressive and rotational forces are exerted on a fixed foot and flexed knee, causing disruption of the lateral semilunar cartilage of the knee. Patients with injuries to their lateral meniscus present with mild swelling and joint-line pain, slipping or catching over joint line, recurrent locking in chronic setting, and knee buckling. Like the exam of the medial meniscus, individual maneuvers typically have poor sensitivity and specificity.[8,38] A positive McMurray's test, positive Apley's test, localized puffiness or distinct cystic lesion directly over lateral joint line, quadriceps atrophy, loud "clunk" during anterior drawer testing, and/or inability to squat and duck walk are indicative of a possible lateral meniscal tear.

MRI is the modality of choice as it has high sensitivity, specificity, and accuracy.[34] Arthroscopy is diagnostic and/or therapeutic. Routine x-rays are usually normal; chronic tears may show joint-line spurring, narrowing of the joint line, or calcification of cartilage. Widening of joint space may be noted in cases of congenital discoid lateral meniscus. Children with congenital discoid lateral menisci warrant orthopedic consultation. Treatment of a lateral meniscus injury is the same as treatment of medial meniscal injuries (see Section 50.5.2.2).

50.7 POSTERIOR KNEE PAIN

50.7.1 Overuse

50.7.1.1 Popliteal (Baker's) Cyst

A cyst is not a specific injury, but a fluid-filled lesion arising as a synovial outpouching, either into a normal bursal structure or into the soft tissue surrounding the knee. A popliteal (Baker's) cyst is the most common benign cysts in the knee, which can cause discomfort in the popliteal fossa along the posterior aspect of the knee. Patients typically experience swelling in the medial popliteal space or over the meniscus, as well as discomfort when running full speed. Examination will reveal cystic swelling in the medial popliteal space or over the midjoint line. X-rays may show soft-tissue swelling with a large popliteal cyst. MRI and ultrasonography are commonly employed to image Baker's cysts; in fact, popliteal cysts are commonly uncovered while patients are undergoing imaging for other knee complaints.[40] Popliteal cysts are typically classified as either primary or secondary; primary cysts are idiopathic, more common in children, and do not communicate with the knee joint, while secondary cysts are typically due to an internal derangement of the knee and may have appreciable communications with the joint.[40] Baker's cysts may increase in size with continued activity, causing worsening pain and restriction in ROM.[40] Complications may include claudication of the vasculature in the popliteal fossa, resulting in edema or claudication. Treatment methods vary depending on etiology of cyst formation and cyst size. In children, cysts typically regress without intervention. Likewise, asymptomatic cysts in adults are typically monitored as well. Cyst aspiration and injection with a corticosteroid have been shown to have moderate efficacy, while surgical excision of the cyst has a high recurrence rate. As secondary popliteal cysts are typically due to underlying knee pathology, identification and treatment of the knee disorders may aid in resolution of the cyst.[40]

50.7.1.2 Hamstring Injuries

Hamstring injuries can occur in all sports with a higher incidence of acute injuries in those associated with sprinting such as track, football, rugby, and soccer. Predominantly, the injuries are in the proximal hamstrings with the long head of the biceps femoris being the most common.[16] However, distal injuries can occur in the musculotendinous junction and distal muscle belly, which will present as posterior knee pain.

Acute injuries may present with the history of sudden audible pop with sharp pain and immediate cessation of activity, while overuse injuries will present with a tight or sore feeling that is worsened with activity but not always limiting. Inspection findings can be absent, but tenderness to palpation is found in the posterior knee at the musculotendinous junction, along the tendon, or at the insertions medially and laterally. Pain with resisted knee flexion is a hallmark. Passive straight leg raise pain can be associated with hamstring injury but should be differentiated from the classic neural tension findings of radicular pain with a straight leg raise with foot dorsiflexion. MRI and ultrasound have both been utilized to locate the exact muscle and tendon area of injury and may help guide the length of time to rehab but may not help determine risk of recurrence.[23]

Initial treatment is with cessation of activity, rest, and ice. Stretching to improve ROM can be done once pain-free walking and daily activities are achieved. Strengthening exercises that promote lengthening should be the initial strengthening exercises with gradual incorporation of eccentrics and sport-specific training.[16] Surgery is an option for complete tears.

50.7.2 Traumatic

50.7.2.1 Posterior Cruciate Ligament Injury

Injuries to the PCL often occur in sports when a player lands on the tibial tubercle with the knee flexed. This injury may occur on artificial turf in football or when skating into the boards in hockey. It usually occurs in conjunction with a lateral or medial ligament injury.

Injury may also occur with knee hyperextension, a direct blow to the anterior proximal tibia, valgus/varus or rotational stress placed on the knee while in full extension, rapid deceleration (e.g., hitting the dashboard in a motor vehicle accident), or falling on a flexed knee. Tears may be partial or complete and often involve the posteromedial and/or anterolateral bundles of PCL.

In acute PCL injury, the predominant symptom is swelling (less than in injury of ACL). Patients are often asymptomatic. The abduction or adduction stress test is positive with full extension in cases caused by varus or valgus trauma; the posterior drawer test is positive if injury was caused by blow to the anterior tibia. In chronic cases, patients may report feelings of femur sliding off the tibia, especially when decelerating or descending stairs or slopes. Secondary PFP symptoms may develop. In these cases, the posterior drawer test and gravity test are positive. Findings are of functional instability.

Routine films (AP and lateral) may show sag in tibia and bony avulsion with tibial attachment of PCL. Stress films assess posterior drawer sign while taking a cross table lateral view. Computed tomography is good for cases of bony involvement. MRI shows the PCL clearly and is effective in difficult diagnoses.

Initial treatment of acute injury includes RICE, NSAIDs, and analgesics as needed. For Grades 1 and 2 tears, treat with orthotics/bracing and physical therapy is warranted.[19,43] Many continue to recommend conservative treatment for isolated Grade 3 PCL injuries. Surgical repair/reconstruction using arthroscopy with autografts, allografts, or prosthetic ligaments has been attempted, but totally satisfactory surgical treatment has not yet been developed.[49]

50.7.2.2 Popliteus Tendon Injury

Injury to the popliteus tendon in the posterior knee can be a very difficult injury to diagnose. It is crucial that the provider maintain a high index of suspicion when assessing a patient with posterior knee pain. The typical described mechanism of injury is forced external rotation and extension on the knee while the patient is resisting the motion. Limited epidemiologic data exist for the popliteus tendon, but it has been described during skiing, martial arts, and daily activities such as stepping off a curb. The patient may have complaints of pain and possible feelings of instability on initial end range extension and initial flexion of the knee. On exam, the patient feels tenderness on the posterior lateral corner of the knee. Varus stress, McMurray's test, and posterior drawer should all be negative in isolated popliteus tendon injuries; however, LCL coinjuries are common. Pain with resisted internal tibial rotation and a positive dial test at 30° of flexion help narrow the diagnosis.

Initial treatment is with RICE and a brace with varus stabilization should be used for combined LCL and popliteus tendon injuries. Due to the low number of popliteus tendon injuries, there are sparse data to guide the practitioner on best treatment, but injection therapies and reconstructive surgeries have been described.

50.8 SUMMARY

The knee is a complex hinge joint, with a multitude of structures compiling to facilitate its high load demand. Injuries to any one of these structures can result in failure of the overall system. The astute physician must take into account a thorough history and execute a detailed exam with anatomical determinate palpation and supporting special test findings to make an accurate diagnosis. Correctly differentiating knee injuries that need surgery from those that can be managed conservatively is a critical function of the primary care physician (see Tables 50.5 through 50.7).

TABLE 50.6
High-Yield Criteria for Knee Radiography

Ottawa Knee Rules
Age >55 years
Isolated patellar tenderness
Tenderness at head of fibula
Inability to flex knee to 90°
Inability to walk four weight-bearing steps immediately after the injury and in clinical encounter
Pittsburgh Decision Rules
Age less than 12 years or greater than 50 years
Inability to walk four weight-bearing steps in clinical encounter

TABLE 50.7
SORT: Key Recommendations for Practice

Clinical Recommendation	Evidence Rating	References
Knee imaging guidelines such as the Ottawa and Pittsburgh knee rules should be used to guide the need for radiography in patients with trauma to the knee.	C	[13,44]
Evaluation of patients with suspected patellofemoral pain should consist of examination of the entire lower limb statically and dynamically.	B	[25]
The Lachman test is reliable and has good interater agreement in assessing for ACL deficient knees.	B	[28,37]
Redislocation rates are similar between conservative management compared to surgical management after patellar dislocation.	B	[36,46]
Osgood-Schlatter's Disease is typically treated conservatively, though surgical correction may be beneficial in patients with refractory symptoms who have achieved skeletal maturity.	C	[31,47]

REFERENCES

1. Ardern CL, Webster KE, Taylor NF, and Feller JA. Return to sport following anterior cruciate ligament reconstruction surgery: A systematic review and meta-analysis of the state of play. *British Journal of Sports Medicine.* 2011;45(7):596–606.
2. Barton CJ, Menz HB, Crossley KM. The immediate effects of foot orthoses on functional performance in individuals with patellofemoral pain syndrome. *British Journal of Sports Medicine.* 2011;45:193–197.
3. Bellabarba C, Bush-Joseph CA, Bach BR. Patterns of meniscal injury in the anterior cruciate-deficient knee: A review of the literature. *American Journal of Orthopedics.* 1997;26(1):18–23.
4. Bonacci J, Vincenzino B, Spratford W, Collins P. Take your shoes off to reduce patellofemoral joint stress during running. *British Journal of Sports Medicine.* 2014;48(6):425–428.
5. Calmbach WL, Hutchens M. Evaluation of patients presenting with knee pain. I. History, physical examination, radiographs, and laboratory tests. *American Academy of Family Physicians.* 2003;68:907–912.
6. Carey JL, Grimm NL. Treatment algorithm for osteochondritis dissecans of the knee. *Clinics in Sports Medicine.* 2014;33(2):375–382.
7. Dixit S, DiFiori JP, Burton M, Mines B. Management of patellofemoral pain syndrome. *American Family Physician.* 2007;75(2):194–202.
8. Fowler PJ, Lubliner JA. The predictive value of five clinical signs in the evaluation of meniscal pathology. *Arthroscopy.* 1989;5(3):184–186.
9. Fowler PJ. Injuries to university athletes: A challenge for all of us. Paper presented at FISU Sports Medicine Conference in Edmonton, AB, 1996.
10. Gersoff WK, Clancy WJ. Diagnosis of acute and chronic anterior cruciate ligament tears. *Clinics in Sports Medicine.* 1988;7(4):727–738.
11. Ghlove PA, Scher DM, Khakharia S, Widmann RF, Green DW. Osgood Schlatter syndrome. *Current Opinion in Pediatrics.* 2007;19(1):44–50.
12. Gosens T, Den Oudsten BL, Fievez E, van't Spijker P, Fievez A. Pain and activity levels before and after platelet-rich plasma injection treatment of patellar tendinopathy: A prospective cohort study and the influence of previous treatments. *International Orthopaedics.* 2012;36(9):1941–1946.
13. Gould SJ, Cardone DA, Munyak J, Underwood PJ, Gould SA. Sideline coverage: When to get radiographs? A review of clinical decision tools. *Sports Health.* May 2014;6(3): 274–278.
14. Granan LP et al. Sport-specific injury pattern recorded during anterior cruciate ligament reconstruction. *American Journal of Sports Medicine.* 2003;41(12):2814–2818.
15. Halinen J, Koivikko M, Lindahl J, Hirvensalo E. The efficacy of magnetic resonance imaging in acute multi-ligament injuries. *International Orthopaedics.* 2009;33(6):1733–1738.
16. Heiderscheit BC et al. Hamstring strain injuries: Recommendations for diagnosis, rehabilitation and injury prevention. *Journal of Orthopaedic & Sports Physical Therapy.* 2010;40(2):67–81.
17. Ho K, Blanchette MG, Powers CM. The influence of heel height on patellofemoral joint kinetics during walking. *Gait Posture.* 2012;36(2):271–275.
18. Hong E, Kraft MC. Evaluating anterior knee pain. *Medical Clinics of North America.* 2014;98(4):697–717.
19. Howell JR, Handoll HHG. Surgical treatment for meniscal injuries of the knee in adults. *Cochrane Review.* 2009;21(1).
20. Johar SK. Medial knee pain in a runner: A case report. *Sports Health.* 2010;2(4):318–320.
21. Karrasch G. The acutely injured knee. *Medical Clinics of North America.* 2014;98(4):719–736.
22. Kon E et al. Articular cartilage treatment in high-level male soccer players: A prospective comparative study of arthroscopic second-generation autologous chondrocyte implantation versus microfracture. *American Journal of Sports Medicine.* 2011;39(12):2549–2557.
23. Koulouris G et al. Magnetic resonance imaging parameters for assessing risk of recurrent hamstring injuries in elite athletes. *American Journal of Sports Medicine.* 2007;35(9): 1500–1506.
24. Lake DA, Wofford NH. Effect of therapeutic modalities on patients with patellofemoral pain syndrome: A systematic review. *Sports Health.* 2011;3(2):182–189.
25. Liporaci RF, Saad MC, Felício LR, Baffa Ado P, Grossi DB. Contribution of the evaluation of the clinical signals in patients with patellofemoral pain syndrome. *Acta Ortop Bras.* July 2013;21(4):198–201.
26. Mall NA et al. Incidence and trends of anterior cruciate ligament reconstruction in the United States. *American Journal of Sports Medicine.* 2014;42(10):2363–2370.
27. Montgomery DL, Koziris PL. The knee brace controversy. *Sports Medicine.* 1989;8(5):260–272.
28. Mulligan EP, McGuffie DQ, Coyner K, Khazzam M. The reliability and diagnostic accuracy of assessing the translation endpoint during the lachman test. *Int J Sports Phys Ther.* February 2015;10(1):52–61.
29. National Ambulatory Health Care Data. National Hospital Ambulatory Medical Care Survey: 2010 Outpatient Department Summary Tables. 26 pp. February 24, 2014.
30. Paczesny L, Kruczynski J. Medial plica syndrome of the knee: Diagnosis with dynamic sonography. *Radiology.* 2009; 251(2):439–446.

31. Pihlajamäki HK, Mattila VM, Parviainen M et al. Long-term outcome after surgical treatment of unresolved Osgood-Schlatter disease in young men. *J Bone Joint Surg Am.* 2009;91:23–50.
32. Rennie WJ, Saifuddin A. Pes anserine bursitis: Incidence in symptomatic knees and clinical presentation. *Skeletal Radiology.* 2005;34(7):395–398.
33. Rothstein CP, Laorr A, Helms CA, Tirman PF. Semimembranosus-tibial collateral ligament bursitis: MR imaging findings. *American Journal of Roentgenology.* 1996;166(4): 875–877.
34. Rubin DA. MR imaging of the knee menisci. *Radiologic Clinics of North America.* 1997;35(10):21–44.
35. Scholten RJPM, Opstelten W, van der Plas C, Bijl D, Deville WLJM, Bouter LM. Accuracy of physical diagnostic tests for assessing ruptures of the anterior cruciate ligament: A meta analysis. *Journal of Family Practice.* 2003;52(9): 689–695.
36. Smith TO, Donell S, Song F, Hing CB. Surgical versus non-surgical interventions for treating patellar dislocation. *Cochrane Database Syst Rev.* 2015, Issue 2. Art. No.: CD008106.
37. Solomon DH et al. The rational clinical examination. Does this patient have a torn meniscus or ligament of the knee? Value of the physical examination. *Journal of the American Medical Association.* 2001;286(13):1610–1620.
38. Solomon DH, Simel DL, Bates DW et al. Does this patient have a torn meniscus or ligament of the knee? Value of the physical exam. *Journal of the American Medical Association.* 2001;286(13):1610–1620.
39. Sommer HM. Patellar chondropathy and apicitis, and muscle imbalances of the lower extremities in competitive sports. *Sports Medicine.* 1988;5(6):386–394.
40. Stein D, Cantlon M, Mackay B, Hoelscher C. Cysts about the knee: Evaluation and management. *Journal of the American Academy of Orthopaedic Surgeons.* 2013;21(8):469–479.
41. Sutker AN, Barber FA, Jackson DW et al. Iliotibial band syndrome in distance runners. *Sports Medicine.* 1985;2(6):447–451.
42. Tandeter HB, Shvartzman P. Acute knee injuries: Use of decision rules for selective radiograph ordering. *American Family Physician.* 1999;60(9):2599–2608.
43. Thomson LC, Handoll HHG, Cunningham A, Shaw PC. Physiotherapist-LED Programmes and Interventions for Rehabilitation of Anterior Cruciate Ligament, medial collateral ligament and meniscal injuries of the knee in adults. *Cochrane Database of Systematic Reviews.* 2002;(2).
44. Tuite MJ, Daffner RH, Weissman BN et al. ACR appropriateness criteria: Acute trauma to the knee. *J Am Coll Radiol.* February 2012;9(2):96–103.
45. Valley VT, Shermer CD. Use of musculoskeletal ultrasonography in the diagnosis of pes anserine tendinitis: A case report. *Journal of Emergency Medicine.* 2001;20(1):43–45.
46. van Gemert JP, de Vree LM, Hessels RA, Gaakeer MI. Patellar dislocation: Cylinder cast, splint or brace? An evidence-based review of the literature. *Int J Emerg Med.* December 31, 2012;5(1):45.
47. Weiss JM, Jordan SS, Andersen JS et al. Surgical treatment of unresolved Osgood-Schlatter disease: Ossicle resection with tibial tubercleplasty. *J Pediatr Orthop.* 2007;27:844.
48. Witvrouw E, Callaghan MJ, Stefanik JJ et al. Patellofemoral pain: Consensus statement from the 3rd International Patellofemoral Pain Research Retreat held in Vancouver, September 2013. *British Journal of Sports Medicine.* 2014; 48(6):411–414.
49. Zarins B, Adams M. Knee injuries in sports. *New England Journal of Medicine.* 1988;318:950–961.

51 Lower Extremity Injuries: The Ankle

Richard B. Birrer and Jesse DeLuca

CONTENTS

TABLE 51.1
Key Clinical Considerations

1. Ankle sprains are the most common sports injury[4,5] accounting for 10%–15% of sport-related injuries,[6] and are responsible for 7%–10% of all emergency room visits.
2. The lateral complex is injured 85% of the time and involves the anterior talofibular ligament in 85% of cases.
3. The Ottawa ankle rules are the commonly used criteria for predicting which patients require radiographic images.
4. Sprains of the deltoid ligament, though uncommon, are almost always associated with other injuries, particularly fractures.
5. Subtalar and syndesmotic injuries must be ruled out in the setting of an ankle sprain as they are more serious and underreported.

51.1 INTRODUCTION

The ankle is a key focal point in the transmission of body weight, capable of the adjustments necessary for fine balance on a wide variety of terrain. The ankle is often involved in static and dynamic deformities that ordinarily do not affect other parts of the body because the joint is subject to the concentrated stresses of standing and movement. Ankle injuries are not always minor and may be associated with prolonged disability and recurrent instability in 25%–40% of patients for several months to several years. Therefore, a casual approach (e.g., "It is only a sprain") to the diagnosis and management of these injuries is inappropriate. The ubiquitous and unpredictable nature of ankle injuries mandates a precise understanding of the mechanism of injury, a thorough knowledge of the anatomy of the ankle joint, a clear ability to assess the degree of damage, and a solid understanding of appropriate treatment modalities in the acute and rehabilitative phases (Table 51.1).

51.2 INJURY EPIDEMIOLOGY

The majority of sports injuries (55%–90%) involve the lower extremity with the knee, ankle, and foot being the most common.[1,2] Ankle sprains are probably the most common (15%) generic sports injury with over 2 million annually and an incidence rate of 1/10,000 person-days.[58] While most ankle injuries follow acute trauma, 25%–30% of ankle injuries are of the "overuse" category. Low-velocity sports (or sports which are played with low velocity, or sports in which the individual is only propelled by oneself) (<20 mph) such as volleyball, baseball, basketball, football, tennis, racquetball, and others such as track and field events, swimming, and golf produce strains, sprains, and occasionally simple fractures such as nondisplaced fibular fractures of the ankle. These simple injuries are usually best dealt with nonoperatively. Simple bony injuries generally require 4–6 weeks of casting or bracing with weight-bearing during the last 2 weeks. Complex and severe fracture–dislocation problems are rare. Ligamentous injuries are rare in children and adolescents; trauma usually involves the growth plate in the form of fracture.

High-velocity sports like skydiving, skateboarding, ice hockey, in-line skating and downhill skiing, or sports that use machinery or animals (i.e., snowmobiling, horse racing, and motor racing) produce accelerations exceeding human capabilities. The resulting ankle injuries have a higher risk of being open and associated with other injuries. Such fractures may be quite comminuted, widely displaced, and may disrupt major portions of the tibial articular surface. Their management is complex and usually is handled through the consultative process. An intensive rehabilitation program must follow all ankle traumas.

51.3 ANKLE FUNCTIONAL ANATOMY

The mortise or hinge joint of the ankle (Figure 51.1) is formed by the distal articulation of the tibia, the fibula, and the dome of the talus.

Range of motion (ROM) occurs in one plane: plantar flexion and dorsiflexion. Dorsiflexion is somewhat restricted due to the anterior widening of the talar dome. The subtalar joint of the foot allows for the full range of inversion, eversion, supination, and pronation. The two joints often work together as a universal-type joint, with modification in one affecting the biomechanics and normal activity of the other. The medial malleolus (distal tibia) and the longer lateral malleolus (distal fibula) provide a significant amount of bony stability to the ankle joint through their downward extension along the talar dome. Functional integrity of the hinge joint is thus sacrificed to structural stability.

Ligaments are the second important element in ankle stability. The larger and stronger deltoid ligament is fan shaped, arises from the medial malleolus, and inserts on the navicular, calcaneal, and talar bones. The medial ligament has both superficial (anterior talotibial, calcaneotibial, and tibionavicular) and deep (posterior talotibial) components (Figure 51.2a). The ligament, particularly the latter component, stabilizes the joint during eversion and prevents subluxation.

There are three distinct lateral collateral ligaments (Figure 51.2b). The anterior talofibular ligament arises from the anterior tip of the fibula and attaches to the lateral neck of the talus. Its function is to prevent anterior and lateral subluxation of the talus during plantar flexion. Running from the fibular tip to the lateral aspect of the calcaneus in a posteroinferior direction is the calcaneal fibular ligament. This ligament functions to prevent lateral subluxation of the talus during strong adduction of the calcaneus. The posterior talofibular ligament arises from the posterior aspect of the lateral malleolus and inserts on the posterolateral margin of the talus as the strongest of the three lateral collateral ligaments. It is responsible for preventing posterior subluxation of the talus during forced dorsiflexion.

The interosseous membrane joins the tibia and fibula proximally, whereas distally the two bones are held together by a strong syndesmosis consisting of the anterior and posterior inferior tibiofibular ligaments, the inferior transverse

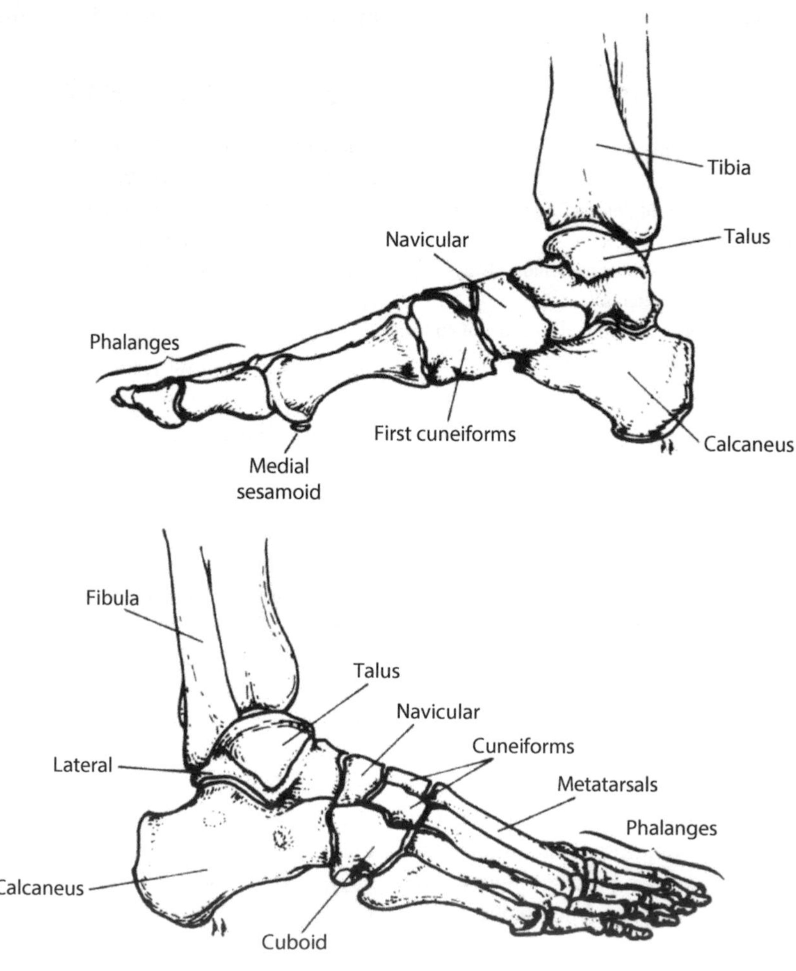

FIGURE 51.1 The bony structure of the ankle.

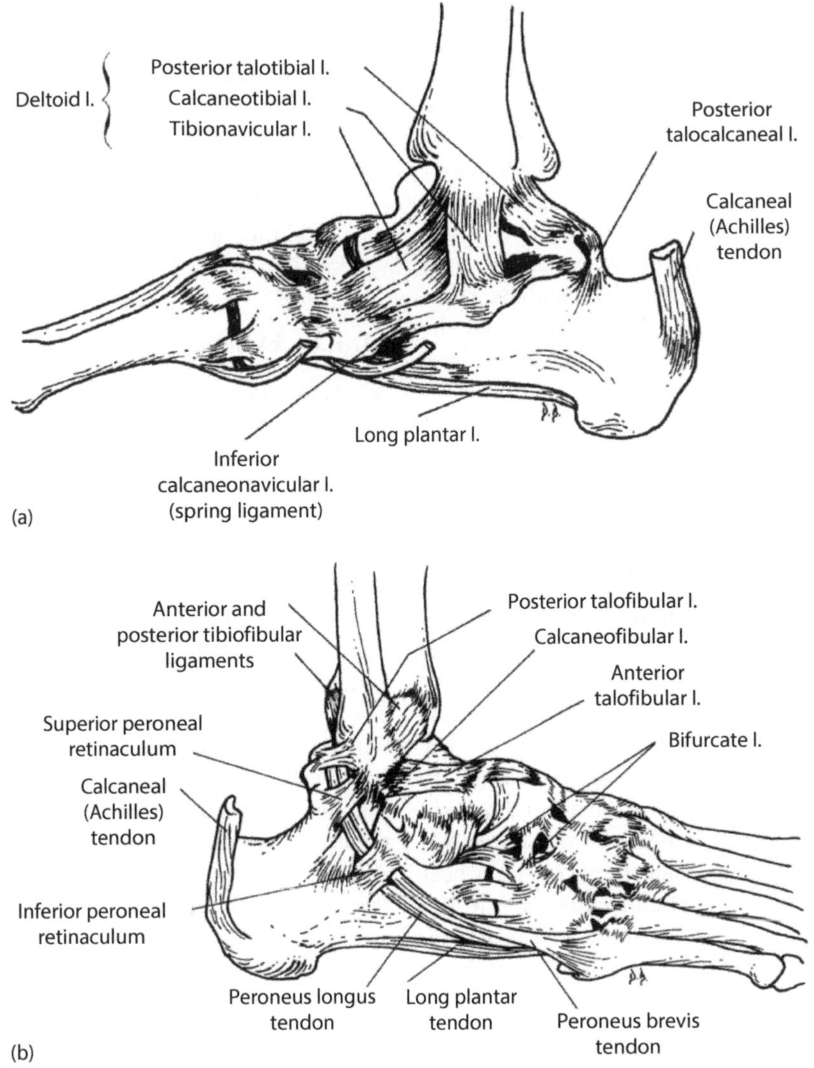

FIGURE 51.2 (a) The medial ligamentous complex of the ankle and (b) the lateral ligamentous complex of the ankle.

ligament, and the interosseus ligaments. The syndesmosis functions to maintain mortise stability, especially during dorsiflexion associated with weight-bearing or the exertion of upward or outward pressure.

The synovial joint capsule also provides additional support, since it encapsulates the entire joint. It is recessed and lax in its anterior and posterior aspects to permit joint motion, although in some individuals it may be thickened anteriorly. The capsule is taut in the medial and lateral aspects, thus contributing to associated ligamentous support.

Finally, a variety of tendons support the ankle, but these are secondary stabilizers because they transit the joint and have no firm attachments. Their superficial nature also makes them vulnerable to injury. The extensors are located anteriorly, whereas the flexors are situated posteriorly. The inverters are located medially and the evertors laterally (see Figure 51.2a and b). The Achilles tendon is the largest in the body. It connects the triceps surae (medial and lateral gastrocnemius plus soleus muscles) to the os calcis and transmits the forces necessary to propel the body in walking, jumping, and running. These forces range from two to three times body weight in walking to four to six times body weight in running and jumping.

Additionally, there are a number of important soft-tissue structures that are important for the functional integrity of the joint and the foot. The dorsal pedal artery lies on the anterior portion of the ankle and the foot between the extensor hallucis longus and the extensor digitorum longus tendons. In 10%–15% of cases, it is congenitally absent. It is a secondary source of blood supply to the foot. The long saphenous vein can be palpated medially and just anteriorly to the medial malleolus. The posterior tibial (PT) artery, the main blood supply to the foot and anatomical constant, is located between the tendons of the flexor digitorum longus and the flexor hallucis longus (FHL) muscles. It passes posterior and inferior to the medial malleolus and is not easily palpated unless the foot is nonweight-bearing and slightly plantar flexed. Immediately posterior and lateral to the PT artery lies the tibial nerve. Although difficult to palpate as an isolated structure, the neurovascular bundle is joined to the tibia by a ligament that creates the tarsal tunnel. The tibial nerve is the main nerve to the sole of the foot. Posteriorly, the calcaneal bursa lies between the Achilles tendon and the overlying skin. The retrocalcaneal bursa is located between the posterosuperior angle of the calcaneus and the anterior surface of the Achilles tendon. The deep peroneal nerve cannot be palpated. Sensation to the ankle is provided by L4 medially, L5 anteriorly, and the S1 dermatome laterally. The following peripheral nerves cover approximately the same area: medially, the long saphenous; anteriorly, the peroneals (deep supplies the first dorsal web space); and laterally, the sural nerve. Finally, lymphatic channels accompany the corresponding vascular bundles. There is a minimum amount of adipose tissue in and about the ankle, and a thin amount of elastic skin overlies all of these structures.

51.4 GENERAL MECHANISMS OF INJURY

Ankle mortise asymmetry creates inherent instability during inversion. The longer lateral malleolus provides a mechanical barrier to eversion ligamentous injury due to its greater surface contact with the talus. In addition, the dome of the talus is appreciably wider anteriorly than posteriorly. During inversion and plantar flexion, the narrow posterior aspect of the talus occupies proportionately less space within the mortise. As a result, there is increased ankle joint play, which, together with the inherent block to eversion, results in predominantly lateral stress forces. Finally, the lateral ligaments of the ankle are smaller and weaker (20%–50%) than the medial deltoid ligament. Additional complicating factors include tight heel cords and deficient proprioception. Many athletes, particularly females, have tight heel cords that force heel inversion. Regular walking on smooth, flat surfaces leads to a proprioceptive deficiency, which is aggravated on irregular, rough playing surfaces. Irregular surfaces, particularly those with holes, can produce obvious damage to the ankle. Less obvious circumstances, such as banked tracks, can lead to repetitive ankle trauma and long-term ankle disability. Defective, old, or inappropriately fitted footwear can result in inversion or eversion stress. All of these factors, when combined with a three-to-fivefold impact force placed on the joint during heel strike, put the ankle at risk for injury.

51.5 CLINICAL EVALUATION[3,4]

51.5.1 History

The following items should be carefully investigated in all ankle injuries:

1. What was the position of the foot and direction of stress when the injury occurred (e.g., eversion, inversion, flexion, extension, or a combination)?
2. Was there immediate disability or did symptoms occur at a later time? Was play continued?
3. At the time of injury were there any snaps, pops, or crunches noted?
4. What were the surface conditions at the time of injury?
5. When and to what degree were pain, swelling, and discoloration noted?
6. Were there any preexisting problems associated with the joint (i.e., previous injury or systemic disease)?
7. Was medical care sought out? What did the evaluation show? Was treatment initiated, and if so, what were the results?
8. Did the injury occur acutely or from overuse?
9. What is the functional capacity of the joint at present?

51.5.2 Examination

A careful exam, particularly during the "Golden Period," will usually identify the site of pathology and severity of tissue trauma. There are situations, however, where a misdiagnosis can result. The clinical examination begins with an inspection of the contour and alignment of the joint, particularly noting any swelling, abrasions, lacerations, or discoloration. In general, swelling is an unreliable sign since edema is mostly a function of how much time has gone by after the trauma and what has occurred in the interim. The patient should be asked to demonstrate the overall functional capacity, strength, ROM (20° dorsiflexion, 30° plantar flexion, 10° abduction/adduction, 17° internal/external rotation) and agility of the joint (i.e., while sitting, standing, walking, running, and at rest). The ankle should be carefully examined for painful trigger points, crepitus, temperature, passive ROM, and neurovascular status (e.g., sensation, strength, reflexes, and pulses). Begin palpation farthest from the suspected site of injury, since 30%–45% of patients will complain of tenderness in uninjured adjoining ligaments. The abnormal ankle should be compared with the normal ankle throughout the examination and should include the foot and footwear, leg, knee, hip, and lower back (Table 51.2).

Once the patient's confidence has been gained, the joint should be stressed.[4] The anterior drawer test is performed with the patient lying on the examination table with the ankle at 90° and consists of drawing the calcaneus and talus anteriorly while stabilizing the tibia (Figure 51.3).

The Gungor test is useful if the patient cannot relax due to pain. While lying prone, the heel of the extended ankle is pressed steadily downward. Capsule rupture leads to forward talar displacement and skin retraction on both sides of the Achilles tendon when compared to the normal side. Sliding of the talus anteriorly by more than 4 mm between ankles during either test is abnormal. A soft end point or the perception of a "clunk" may be appreciated and is considered a positive anterior draw sign.

The talar tilt test is performed by stressing the ankle laterally (inversion) and medially (eversion) while stabilizing the patient's leg (Figure 51.4).

A tear of the deep deltoid ligament will produce a palpable gap on the medial aspect of the ankle mortise. Gapping or rocking of the ankle mortise on the lateral side during lateral inversion stress indicates tears of both the anterior talofibular and the calcaneofibular ligaments. The normal angle of inversion talar tilt is up to 15°, although some individuals with

TABLE 51.2
Ankle Special Tests

Test	Performance	Positive Findings	Suggested Diagnosis
Anterior drawer	Anterior pull of the talus with hand on calcaneus against fixed tibia.	Pain and/or anterior translation of the talus	Anterior talofibular ligament injury
Gungor test	Patient lying prone with foot off table, downward pressure applied to the heel.	Pain, displacement toward the floor and skin retraction around the Achilles	Anterior talofibular ligament injury
Talar tilt	Inversion stress applied to the ankle while holding the calcaneus.	Pain and/or laxity by itself and with attention to contralateral ankle in degrees	Calcaneofibular ligament injury
Kleiger's test	With the ankle in passive dorsiflexion, externally rotate the foot.	Pain located at the syndesmosis and anterior tibiofibular ligament	Syndesmotic injury
Squeeze test	At the level of the midcalf, medial and lateral pressure is applied simultaneously, squeezing the tibia and fibula together and then relaxing.	Pain distal to the examiners hands in the area of the tibiofibular ligaments and syndesmosis	Syndesmosis injury
Passive flexion/ extension testing	Ankle is forcibly flexed and extended to end range passively.	Reproducible pain at end range of motion	Positive impingement
Thompson–Doherty test	Lying in prone, midthird of calf is squeezed.	Absence of plantar flexion	Complete or near complete rupture of the Achilles
Tinel's test	Gentle tapping over the course of a superficial nerve.	Tingling, paresthesias over the distal course of the nerve	Tarsal tunnel, superficial saphenous/ sural nerves

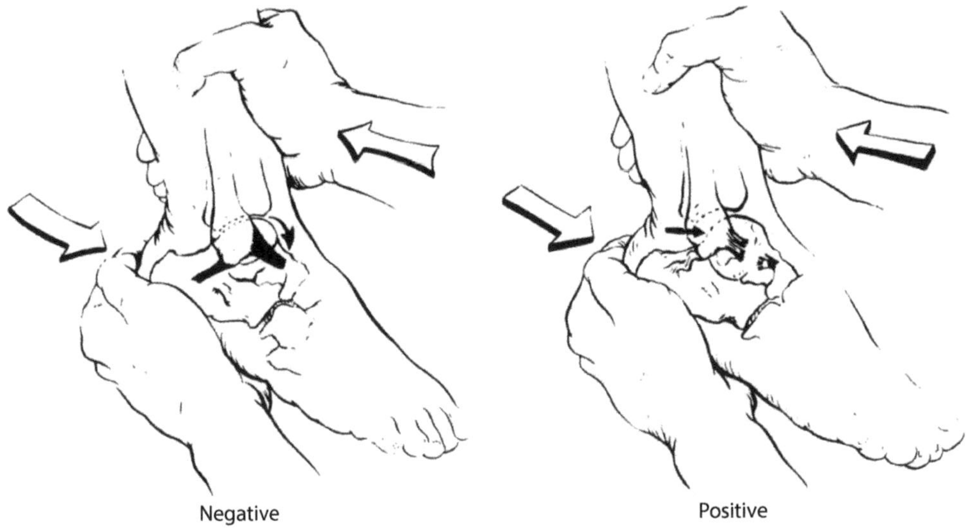

FIGURE 51.3 The anterior drawer test.

ligamentous laxity may tilt up to 20° without a tear. A difference of 10° between ankles is highly suggestive of a tear, and 15° is diagnostic. The fibular compression or squeeze test assesses the integrity of the syndesmotic ligaments. Distal ankle pain when the proximal tibia and fibula are squeezed suggests a syndesmotic sprain. Rotation of the foot while the tibia is stabilized produces similar pain and a sensation of talar motion if a diastasis is present. A joint block can facilitate stress tests. If necessary, 5–10 mL of 1% lidocaine are infiltrated into the joint opposite the side of injury and around the injured ligaments.

Routine x-rays include anterior, lateral, mortise (an AP with 10°–15° internal/external rotation). Oblique (45° of internal/external rotation) films are excellent for visualizing chip fractures and articular surfaces. It is occasionally advisable for the purpose of diagnostic accuracy, particularly in children, that radiographs be taken of the normal side for comparison. While 15% of ankle sprain adults have fractures, high-yield criteria have been identified (Table 51.3).

Soft tissue should be examined for swelling and foreign bodies, joint spaces for widening or narrowing, and bones for dislocation or fractures (avulsion or osteochondral). Syndesmotic injury is suggested by widening of the mortise (>4 mm) and the distal tibia–fibula clear space (>6 mm) and reduced overlap (<1 mm) of the tibia and fibula. Passive stress-test radiographs performed after the acute period are indicated when clinical findings are inconclusive or the lesion is chronic (Figure 51.5).

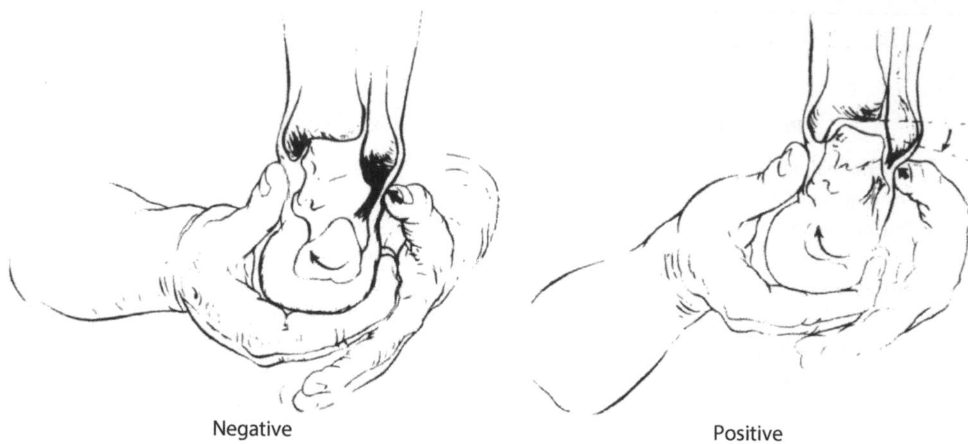

FIGURE 51.4 The talar tilt test.

TABLE 51.3
High-Yield Criteria for Ankle Radiographs (Ottawa Ankle Rules)

Pain in malleolar zone (distal 6 cm of tibia and fibula and talus) and any of the following:

- Bone tenderness at the posterior edge or tip of lateral malleolus
- Bone tenderness at the posterior edge or tip of medial malleolus
- Inability to bear weight immediately and in the emergency department using four steps

Sources: Bleakley, C.M. and Glasgow, P., *Br. J. Sports Med.*, 10, 1136, 2011; Colvin, A.C. et al., *Foot Ankle Int.*, 30(4), 292, 2009.

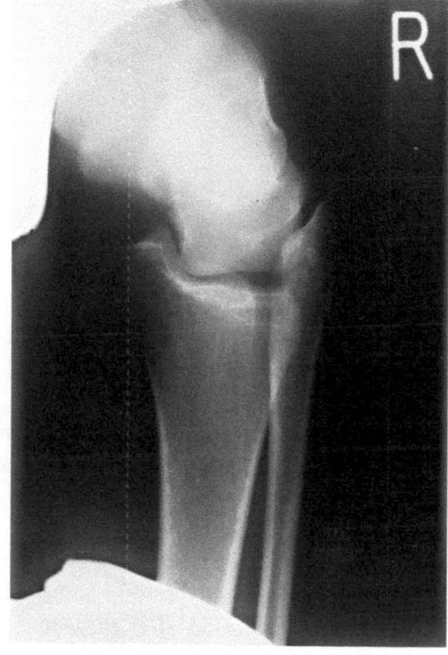

FIGURE 51.5 Normal stress film of the lateral right ankle.

Stress films are easy to perform and may be difficult to interpret unless a standardized stress device is used. They correlate well with both arthrographic and operative findings. If the stress films are positive, further evaluation is unnecessary. If stress films are inconclusive and there is a strong clinical suspicion of a complete tear, an arthrogram may be ordered. Dye appearing outside the joint capsule, particularly the anterolateral malleolus, or the peroneal tendon sheath is abnormal. False-positive results occur in 10%–25% of cases. The incidence of false negative examinations rises significantly due to postinjury healing. Also, the test is expensive, requires scheduling, and is associated with allergic reactions. Arthroscopy can also detect tears, defects, and debris. Isotopic bone scans are reserved for potential stress fractures.

Real-time ultrasound can be beneficial and relatively inexpensive in cases of tenosynovitis/tendinosis and partial and complete tears. Computerized tomography (CT) and magnetic resonance imaging (MRI) have been employed in diagnostic work-ups due to their high-resolution, multiplanar, thin-slice capabilities.[8] CT is excellent for tenosynovitis, complete and some partial ruptures, and associated fractures, particularly osteochondral lesions (OCLs), whereas MRI is useful in identifying soft-tissue, intraosseous, and neurovascular anatomy, particularly tenosynovitis, tendinosis, partial and complete tendon rupture, bone contusions, and large associated fractures. CT does not pick up bone contusions and the changes of tendinosis and other intratendinous abnormalities. Plain tomography is an inexpensive alternative to CT, although it is less sensitive. It is useful with the following criteria: ecchymoses or edema that covers two or more major stabilizing ligaments along with radiographic evidence of an effusion that distends the capsule by more than 5 mm. Thirty-five percent of such patients have occult fractures.[63]

While most ankle injuries are uncomplicated and can be treated in the office setting. However, the diligent primary care provider should know when to refer an injury to an orthopedic surgeon. Depending on the patient's progress and the physician's experience and clinical judgment, only difficult fractures (bi- and trimalleolar fractures), rare tendon injuries (peroneal or posterior tibialis), continuing pain

TABLE 51.4
Common Ankle Disorders in Primary Care: An Anatomical and Symptom-Oriented Approach to Differential Diagnosis

Anterior	Medial
Overuse	*Overuse*
Tibialis anterior tendinopathy	Posterior tibial tendinopathy
Extensor hallicus longus tendinopathy	Flexor hallicus longus tendinopathy
Anterior impingement	*Traumatic*
Traumatic	Posterior tibial tendon
Osteochondral defect (OCD) of the talar dome (OLT)	Subluxation/dislocation
Anterior tibiofibular ligament and syndesmosis injury	Deltoid ligament tear
	Anteromedial capsule tear
	Anterior tibiofibular ligament tear
	Interosseous membrane
	Tibia fracture (Maisonneuve)
	OLT
	Pediatric
	Tibial avulsion fracture
	Medial malleolus accessory ossicle[a]
Lateral	**Posterior**
Overuse	*Overuse*
Peroneal tendinopathy	Achilles tendinopathy (distal 2–6 cm from insertion/myotendinous junction)
Sinus tarsi syndrome[b]	
Traumatic	Insertional Achilles tendinopathy (d/w Haglund's/Sever's)[b]
Lateral ligament sprains	
Peroneal tendon subluxation/dislocation	Posterior impingement
Distal fibular fracture	Os trigonum
Lateral talus fracture (snowboarder's fracture)[b]	*Traumatic*
	Achilles rupture
Pediatric	Posterior talar process fracture
Tillaux and triplane fractures	Stieda's fracture
Fibular physeal and avulsion fractures	Trimalleolar fracture

[a] Add to chapter for rare end components of ankle pain (Reference 1)—may be helpful if going into coalition as part of the foot chapter to differentiate development anomalies.
[b] Possible crossover from the foot chapter.

5–7 days postinjury, failure to recover as expected, or general discomfort treating an injury should prompt a referral (see Tables 51.4 and 51.5).

51.6 LATERAL ANKLE PAIN

51.6.1 Traumatic

51.6.1.1 Lateral Collateral Injury

The lateral ankle is the most frequently injured structure in sports (25% of all sports injuries) where running and jumping are important, particularly basketball (70%–80% of players have had one sprain, 60%–80% have had multiple sprains, 50% have had residual symptoms, 15% have compromised performance), volleyball, football, soccer, field hockey, and racquetball. There are 1.6 (male) and 2.2 (female) significant sprains per 1000 person-days of sports; 85% of ankle injuries are sprains; 85% involve the lateral compartment; 85% involve the anterior talofibular ligament; 25% involve the anterior talofibular and calcaneofibular ligaments; 1% involve the posterior talofibular ligament; 30%–40% have a history of previous injury; and 25% result in recurrent instability.[8–13] Fifty to 60 percent do not seek professional treatment. Risk factors include tibial varum and calcaneal eversion in females and increased talar tilt in males, postural instability, and lower proprioception.[10,11] For both genders, a history of ankle injury increases the risk of repeat trauma fivefold, shoes with air cells in the heel 4.3-fold and lack of stretching 2.2 times.[13]

Clinical Pearl

Eighty-five percent of ankle injuries are sprains; 85% of ankle injuries involve inversion; and 85% tear the anterior talofibular ligament.

TABLE 51.5
Indications for Specialty Referral for Common Disorders of the Ankle

Diagnosis	Primary Care Referral Considerations
	Anterior
Syndesmosis injury	Grade 3 injuries and Grade 2 with failed conservative management require surgical management with open reduction internal fixation utilizing a syndesmotic screw.
Anterior tibialis rupture	Surgical repair recommended depending on individuals level of function.
Anterior impingement	Consider surgical referral if conservative managements fail and radiographic evidence of osteophytes or divot sign. Corticosteroid injection to the area may be helpful in diagnostic differentiation as well as therapeutic in the case of soft tissue impingement.
	Medial
Osteochondral lesion of the talus	Continued pain in the medial or anterior ankle or mechanical symptoms after appropriate rehab may be a consideration for further imaging and/or referral for diagnosis of lesions of the cartilage and subchondral bone following inversion injury.
Posterior tibialis tendinopathy	Consider referral for surgical evaluation or injection-based therapies after failure of a reasonable course of conservative therapy.
	Lateral
Lateral ligament injuries	Grade 3 injuries and repeat Grade 2 injuries especially with objective findings of ligament laxity should be referred for evaluation for surgical or injection-based therapies.
Peroneal tendinopathy	Consider referral for surgical evaluation or injection-based therapies after failure of a reasonable course of conservative therapy.
	Posterior
Achilles tendinopathy	Consider early referral for injection-based therapies and nonweight-bearing status for palpable defect or worsening symptoms after start of eccentric exercise rehabilitation.
Posterior impingement	Refer in the presence of large osteophytes or abnormalities on radiographs and failure to respond to conservative treatment.

Inversion in plantar flexion and adduction (supination) (Figure 51.6), especially during landing is the culprit.

There is sequential tearing of anterior talofibular, calcaneofibular, and posterior talofibular ligaments (see Figure 51.2b).

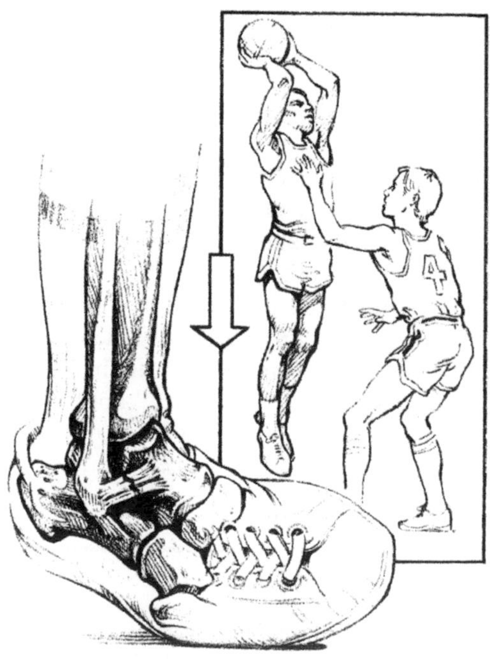

FIGURE 51.6 Spraining of the anterior talofibular ligament following forced plantar flexion and inversion.

There are three grades: Grade 1—minimal pain and disability but weight-bearing not impaired; Grade 2—moderate pain and disability and weight-bearing difficult; Grade 3—severe swelling, pain, discoloration and no weight-bearing possible and significant functional loss. Signs[8] found are Grade 1—slight tenderness and swelling over ligament with no laxity. The anterior drawer test and talar tilt (see Figures 51.3 and 51.4) are negative; Grade 2—moderate tenderness and edema, hemarthrosis (40%–50%), ecchymosis (30%–40%), positive talar tilt of 5°–10° difference, and a positive anterior drawer 4–14 mm; Grade 3—pronounced edema, loss of function, severe pain typical but may be painless, hemarthrosis (80%–90%), ecchymosis (60%–70%), positive talar tilt >10° difference, and anterior drawer >15 mm. Radiographs may see localized tissue swelling, lateral clear space >2 mm (Figure 51.2 AP, lateral, mortise). The interpretation of stress films (Figures 51.7 and 51.8) may be difficult; a mechanical stress device is recommended.

Grade 1 injuries are negative; Grade 2 shows a 5°–10° tilt difference with 3–14 mm anterior displacement of talus; and Grade 3 reveals a >20° tilt difference with >15 mm anterior displacement of talus. Arthrograms may show extravasation of dye with calcaneofibular tears but are infrequently used. MRI allows direct visualization of the anterior talofibular and calcaneofibular ligaments in acute and chronic injuries; 27% show bone contusions.[7] The diagnosis should include grading of the injury based on clinical finings. Posterior compartment osteochondral fracture, peroneal tendon subluxation/dislocation, peroneal quartus strain, physeal injury

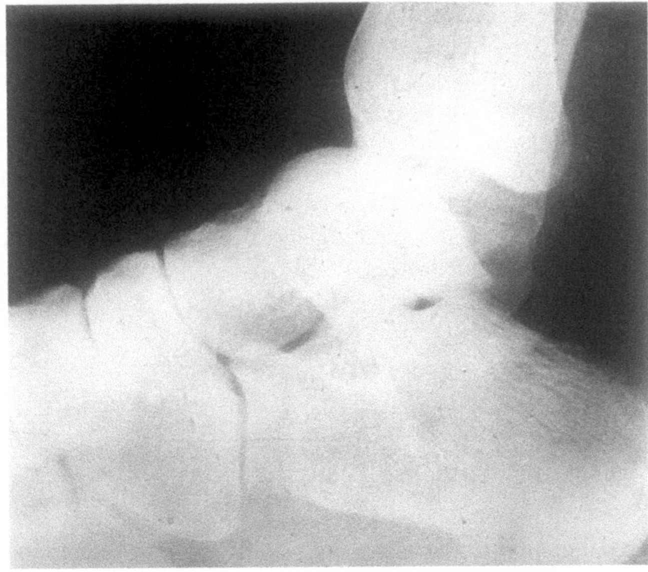

FIGURE 51.7 Stress film of the ankle.

of the distal fibula in skeletally immature patients, interosseus membrane tear, tibiofibular ligament sprain, Achilles tendon rupture, subtalar and Lisfranc joint sprain, avulsion fracture of fibula, or break of os calcis are differential considerations.

The initial treatment is protection, optimal loading, ice, compression, and elevation (POLICE), posterior plaster or air splint, no weight-bearing, NSAIDs, and analgesics as needed.[5,14–19] Homeopathic ointment for 10 days has been found to significantly improve pain control versus placebo. Long-term management focuses on functional treatment when compared to immobilization. There is limited evidence of improved outcome (earlier return to work and sports activity and higher levels of satisfaction) with functional treatment compared to minimal treatment.[16] There is no good evidence that surgery is superior to immobilization and the evidence comparing surgical versus functional treatment is conflicting.[19] Associated bone contusions have little clinical significance. Current management approach by injury grade is

1. *Grade 1*: Weight-bearing brace or strapping for 2–3 weeks.
2. *Grade 2*: Walking, well-padded dorsiflexion cast, Unna® boot weight-bearing brace or air stirrup for 2–4 weeks, followed by strapping at 90° for 2–4 weeks. Avoid casting severely swollen limbs.
3. *Grade 3*: Dorsiflexion cast or weight-bearing brace for 3–6 weeks, followed by orthotic or strapping for 3–6 weeks; surgical repair. Best approach is unresolved, although aged <40 and athletic competition favor surgical repair.

Sports physical therapy emphasizes isometrics while cast is on, then ROM, PRE (progressive resistance exercises), and proprioceptive exercises (balance/wobble board), plus functional activity (Grade 1 [2 weeks], Grade 2 [4 weeks], Grade 3 [6 weeks]). Injection therapy can be used in a stable ankle that is chronically inflamed, preventing progression in a rehabilitative program.[20] Ultrasound, hyperbaric oxygen, and cold packs have been found to offer no significant benefit over placebo, and the benefit for diathermy over sham therapy is conflicting.

51.6.1.1.1 Consultation: Grade 3 and Recurrent Injuries

Complications include recurrent sprains (10%–30%), osteochondral fracture (6%–7%) instability (10%), peroneal and/or tibial nerve injury, and peroneal tendon subluxation/dislocation.[21,22]

Clinical Pearl

All significant sprains should be reexamined 4–6 weeks post injury for instability.

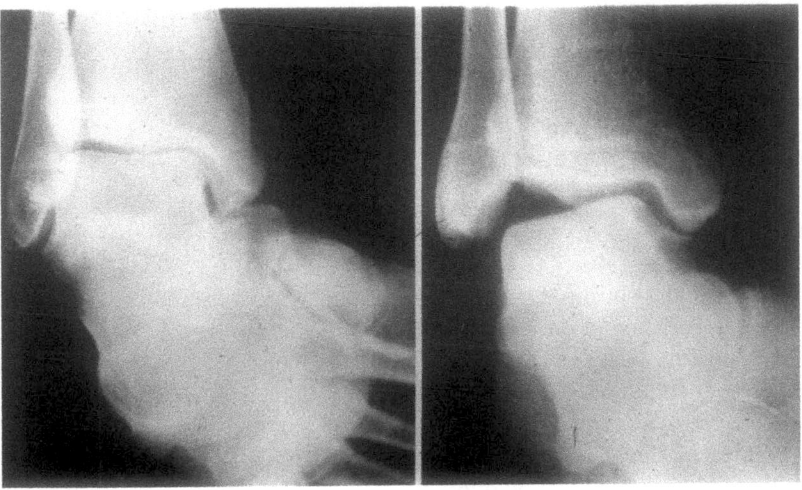

FIGURE 51.8 Stress film of the ankle.

The prevention of lateral ankle injuries includes[23–27] a peroneal muscle conditioning program, teaching players to land with a relatively wide-based stance, supporting with tape or an orthotic brace (semirigid or air cast) for previously injured ankles as well as uninjured ones, particularly in high-risk sporting activities (e.g., basketball and soccer). An ankle brace/stabilizer may be superior to taping in reducing the incidence but not the severity of injury,[25,28–30,47,55,56] using an outer heel wedge, coordination training on a balance board,[20,31] and using high-top, flexible shoes with cushioned midsoles and adequate toe box.

Clinical Pearl

It is best to err on the conservative side for diagnosis and on the liberal side for treatment and rehabilitation of a sprain.

51.6.1.2 Peroneal Tendon Injury

Other injuries that produce lateral ankle pain are peroneal tendon subluxation and dislocation. The structure is injured most commonly in sports with significant dynamic forces applied to the foot, as in cutting, turning, and falling forward (e.g., wrestling, football, skiing, ice skating, basketball, and soccer). The mechanism of injury involves sudden forceful passive dorsiflexion of everted foot or inversion stress with violent reflex contraction of peroneals and plantar flexors: direct blow to posterior lateral malleolus.[35,36] There is disruption of the peroneal retinaculum (see Figure 51.2b) from its periosteal attachment at the lateral malleolus often in association with an absent or flat peroneal groove or flat or convex distal fibula. Peroneal brevis tears have occurred without prior subluxation/dislocation.[49]

Classification is Grade 1: Retinaculum with periosteum is stripped off the lateral malleolus; Grade 2: Distal 1–2 cm of dense fibrous lip is elevated along with retinaculum; Grade 3: Retinaculum avulses a thin fragment of bone along with the fibrous lip.

Acutely, there is a painful snap, crepitus, swelling, and discoloration posterior to the lateral malleolus. Chronically, there may be an unpleasant snapping or clicking sensation and instability on ankle rotation, particularly during resisted active dorsiflexion, pronation, and eversion with the patient prone and the knee flexed 90° or by anterior/posterior directed motion.

Radiographs are normally negative but may reveal associated distal avulsion fracture of fibula (15%–50% of cases). MRI/CT scans specific to peroneals—positive, but rarely required—should be used for confirmation or doubtful cases. Dynamic ultrasound is usually positive but rarely necessary.

The differential should consider sprain of lateral compartment ligaments, peroneal tenosynovitis (occurs as it passes around the cuboid [e.g., in modern dancers]) or retrofibular sulcus, contusion, and rupture of the peroneal tendon (rare) in association with compartment syndrome.

Acutely, a posterior splint with no weight-bearing is important. Long-term, well-molded weight-bearing cast in slight plantar flexion and pronation for 4–8 weeks with dynamic ankle brace or strapping plus horseshoe- or J-shaped pad is useful, although referral for surgical repair of the retinaculum or rupture in acute unstable or chronic injuries (Jones or Du Vries methods), particularly in the competitive athlete is recommended. Corticosteroid injections should not be used. Rehabilitation emphasizes ROM, PRE, and proprioceptive exercises (2 months).

51.7 MEDIAL ANKLE PAIN

51.7.1 Trauma

51.7.1.1 Medial Collateral Injury

Five to ten percentage of all ankle injuries involve the medial compartment. They are usually more serious than a lateral injury.[57] Eversion, dorsiflexion, and abduction (pronation) are the usual pathogenesis with sequential tearing of the superficial deltoid ligament (tibionavicular), anteromedial capsule, anterior deep deltoid component, anterior tibiofibular ligaments, interosseus membrane, and remaining superficial and deep components (see Figure 51.2a). Classification by exam and imaging studies is similar to lateral sprains except that the findings are in eversion. The differential diagnosis should consider avulsion fracture of medial malleolus (15%), sprain of the interosseous membranes, injury to the tibialis posterior or FHL tendons, and osteochondral and Tillaux fractures.

Treatment[13,16,17] and sports physical therapy is similar to lateral ankle sprains but is more aggressive: Grade 1: Weight-bearing cast for 2–3 weeks, followed by brace/strapping; Grades 2 and 3: Weight-bearing cast for 5–6 weeks, followed by brace/strapping. Operative repair is reserved for unstable injuries and competitive athletes.

Complications are chronic ankle instability and recurrent injury. Preventive strategies include strengthening of the posteromedial muscles, taping/strapping/bracing (a brace/stabilizer may be superior to taping), inner heel wedge, and balance board training.[21–23]

51.7.1.2 Posterior Tibial Injury

Isolated dislocation of the PT is rare but is common with severe ankle fractures. It follows inversion with dorsal flexion (i.e., stumbling over a fixed object and running on an uneven surface). The flexor retinaculum is torn with dislocation of the PT tendon from its groove to above the medial malleolus.

Medial ankle pain, particularly on inversion, may be associated with a locking sensation. There is full ROM of the ankle and foot but crepitus may be present over the groove to tibialis posterior tendon. Unless associated with a fracture, radiographs are normal. MRI shows displacement of tendon and edema (superior to CT).

Treatment consists of surgical repair of the flexor retinaculum followed by 5–6 weeks of casting and then rehabilitation.

51.7.2 Overuse

PT tendinitis occurs in sports requiring a quick change of direction (tennis, dancing, soccer, basketball, ice hockey, football), dancing on point; more common with hypermobile flat feet and in individuals with navicular accessory.[46] Repetitive microtrauma during the pronation phase of running/cutting/jumping, etc., is etiologic. There is inflammation and degeneration of the tendon/sheath posterior and inferior to the medial malleolus or adjacent to its partial insertion on the navicular tubercle.

Findings include diffuse swelling and pain with edema and tenderness behind medial malleolus or proximal to its insertion on navicular tubercle. Pain is worsened by inversion and plantar flexion against resistance. Imaging studies are usually unnecessary.

After acute modalities, long-term management should include a nonweight-bearing short leg cast with foot in inversion for 2–4 weeks. A medial posted orthosis is then fashioned. Tenolysis is reserved for refractory cases. The regular use of orthotics while reducing the training program (i.e., distance, intensity) may be preventive.

Rupture of the PT usually involves 40–60-year-old females but also marathon athletes who have had cortisone injections for tendinitis. Repetitive microtrauma in a setting of degenerative chronic tendinitis is typical although a traumatic blow rarely is the culprit. There is transverse rupture of the PT tendon in its avascular zone just posterior to the medial malleolus or rupture at its insertion into the navicular and first cuneiform.

Chronic pain and swelling occurs from the midposterior medial shaft of the tibia to the insertion of the tendon at the navicular, which is worse in the pronated foot. There may be instability on ambulation. Findings include erythematous swelling occurs slightly over or inferior to the medial malleolus; tenderness occurring 2–3 in. above the medial malleolus to the navicular and, in some cases, loss of foot supination to the inferior aspect of the first and second cuneiforms; loss in height of medial longitudinal arch; palpable gap in the tendon and weakness during resisted inversion in complete tears; inability to raise the heel more than 1–2 in. while standing on one foot in complete tears; valgus position with compensatory adduction of the forefoot; and "more toes sign"—abduction of the forepart of the foot at Chopart's joint.

Comparison radiographs show increase in the talocalcaneal angle (axial view), a talonavicular break (i.e., decreased longitudinal arch) sagittally (lateral view), and a decrease in the talonavicular articulation transversely in the injured foot (AP view). The MRI is positive.

Following standard acute treatment,[46] nonoperative repair for incomplete lesions consists in nonweight-bearing cast in slight inversion for 6–8 weeks, walking cast for 4–6 weeks, followed by shoe modification (medial sole and heel wedge and longitudinal arch support). Surgical repair is reserved for complete tears; followed by 6–8 weeks of nonweight-bearing cast in inversion and plantar flexion; walking cast for 4–6 weeks. ROM and PRE exercises follow with orthotic and strapping to decrease unwanted pronation during running, jumping, skiing, or similar activities.

Injury to the FHL is common in dancers (dancer's tendinitis)[48] due to repetitive push-offs, and use of en pointe or demi-pointe positions.

Irritation and edema of the FHL tendon in the fibroosseous tunnel occur behind the medial malleolus or between the sesamoids at the base of the first metatarsal (Henry's knot). Findings include pain with toe flexion in association with tenderness and swelling over the tendon behind the medial malleolus; crepitus, especially with active and passive motion of the hallux, decreased ROM, triggering and clawing of the big toe (hallux saltans); and decreased first toe flexion at the interphalangeal joint. Imaging studies are usually not necessary.

Routine treatment may require tenolysis for severe cases of chronic recurrent tenosynovitis.[45] Steroid injections are not recommended. Preventive strategies include stretching and the use of a rigid shoe.

51.8 ANTERIOR ANKLE PAIN

51.8.1 Traumatic

51.8.1.1 Syndesmotic Injury

Syndesmotic sprains are not rare (10% of sprains), more common among males and competitive events, follow forced external rotation or hyperdorsiflexion and eversion of the joint with internal tibial rotation (collision sports), and are frequently incomplete.[32–34] There may be difficulty noted running uphill, an inability to "push off" especially to the opposite side and a preference to walk on the toes. The complaints are usually greater than the findings (i.e., less swelling compared to medial or lateral ankle injuries). Tenderness is located over the syndesmosis and anterior and posterior tibiofibular ligaments especially with external foot rotation and dorsiflexion (Kleiger's test). The squeeze test is positive when done at midcalf. The crossed-leg test (i.e., the injured leg resting at midcalf on the knee) is used to detect a high (syndesmotic) ankle sprain. Pain in the syndesmotic area (just above the ankle) occurs when pressure is applied to the lateral side of the proximal lower leg. Standard films during the acute period show a >6 mm tibiofibular "clear space" and widening of the mortise and demonstrate avulsion fractures of the anterior or PT tubercle in 20%–50% of cases. Tears of the distal tibiofibular syndesmosis and the interosseous membrane are associated with Maisonneuve fracture, a spiral fracture of the proximal third of the fibula (see Section 51.10). There is an associated fracture of the medial malleolus or rupture of the deep deltoid ligament, an injury that can be difficult to detect. There may be a fracture of the anterolateral distal tibial epiphysis noted in adolescent population. Films taken 3–5 weeks postinjury may demonstrate calcification of the syndesmosis or adjacent deltoid ligament. Grade 1 injuries are managed with an aggressive functional rehabilitation program. Cast immobilization with progressive weight-bearing over 3–6 weeks followed by a vigorous rehabilitation program is appropriate for Grade 2 injuries. The prognosis for these injuries is usually excellent with recurrence and residual instability uncommon. Grade 3 injuries are managed with open reduction and internal fixation with a syndesmotic screw. Recovery is prolonged.

51.8.2 Overuse

51.8.2.1 Impingement Syndrome

Impingement is a rare condition affecting high-arched athlete, loose lateral ligaments secondary to prior ankle sprain; jumping (jumper's ankle), football, running, dancing, gymnastics, rugby (footballer's or English ankle).[42] Hitting bottom in the plié (deep knee bend, with the "bravura" technique) or explosive "drive off" from the planted foot leads to anterior impingement.[43] Proliferative bony spur formation on the anterior marginal lip of the tibia and sulcus of the talus (talotibial exostoses) develops.

Vague anterolateral pain with extreme dorsiflexion during running, cutting, or pushing off at full speed; weakness/loss of "drive" occurs in association with point tenderness and edema over anterior ankle and decreased painful dorsiflexion. Radiographs demonstrate spurring in the talar sulcus, a normal joint line, and positive divot sign (localized wedge in the talar neck accepting the tibial osteophyte during dorsiflexion). The differential diagnosis should include tibiotalar or talonavicular degenerative disease and osteoid osteoma of tarsal navicular. Treatment should focus on modification of technique/activities (especially "drive-off technique"), appropriate stretching, injection of a long- and short-acting corticosteroid after confirmation with lidocaine, and surgical excision if conservative therapy fails.

51.8.3 Tendon Injuries

Factors that contribute to tendon injury include poor sports technique, increased patient's age, improper conditioning, malalignment, and excessive intensity or duration of activity.[48–50] MRI, CT, and ultrasound are reliable diagnostic modalities. Trauma, training on hills, downhill hiking, direct shoe compression (ski boots), overuse, and rheumatologic disorders lead to tibialis anterior tendinitis. Its relatively straight course under the retinaculum causes minimal mechanical irritation. Modifications of training gear and program in conjunction with rest, ice, compression, and elevation (RICE), anti-inflammatory agents, and stretching are remedial for most overuse injuries.

Ruptures of the anterior tibialis have been reported but are very rare. Such injuries have been associated with multiple intratendinal steroid injections and age over 50 years. Rupture of the tibialis anterior causes a drop-foot gait and difficulty in walking on the heels. Treatment options include surgical repair (younger or competitive patients) or casting and orthotic devices with a 90% dorsiflexion brace for 6–8 weeks. A posterior leaf spring brace may aid ambulation, particularly in the older patient.

51.9 POSTERIOR ANKLE PAIN

51.9.1 Overuse

Achilles tendinitis constitutes 9%–18% of running injuries (from hills, uneven surfaces, increased mileage or intensity of training, or recommencement of training after prolonged inactivity) but is also seen in jumping, skiing, basketball, gymnastics, dancing, and cycling. There may be a background of tight heel cord, congenitally small or thin tendon, tibia vara, pronated or cavus foot, or history of injected or oral steroids.[37,38] Repetitive overloads, particularly with faulty technique, use of rigid-soled shoes, landing hard upon the heels, or hyperpronation in association with weakness and inflexibility of the gastrocsoleus complex are the usual cause.[37] Microscopic tears of collagen fibers on the surface or in the substance of the tendon, pseudosheath thickening at its relatively avascular isthmus (3–4 cm above insertion into os calcis), and chronically, nodule and adhesion formation occur.

Pain on walking that gradually worsens with the degree of injury. Tenderness, thickening, erythema, crepitus, edema, and nodules of the tendon in association with dorsiflexion weakness are characteristics. Imaging studies are usually not indicated. The differential diagnosis should include calcaneal/retrocalcaneal bursitis, tendon rupture, calcaneal contusion or stress fracture, gastrocnemius strain, and arthropathies.

In addition to acute modalities ROM + PRE before and after activities (1–3 weeks) with full eccentric strengthening of the gastrocsoleus complex, heel lifts and cross training are indicated.[37,39] Tenolysis and debridement with 3–6 weeks of a short leg cast is reserved for refractory cases. Steroid injection is contraindicated.

Chronic tendinopathy, weakness, and rupture are potential complications. Preventive strategies are shoes with a soft-flared heel counter, adequate heel wedge (10–15 mm) and molded Achilles pad, heel cord stretching exercises (i.e., wall "push-ups") and the avoidance of hill running, sudden increases in training intensity, or running on uneven/hard surfaces.

Poorly conditioned 30- to 45-year-old male patients, particularly weekend athletes, are subject to rupture.[37,38] The incidence is 1 per 1000 athlete-years. There is often a background of tendinitis/degenerative changes and history of oral/injected steroids. The cause is sudden dorsiflexion of a plantar-flexed foot, sudden unexpected dorsiflexion of the ankle, pushing off the weight-bearing foot with the knee locked, and extended or a direct blow. Anatomically, there is rupture of the tendon 2–6 cm proximal to insertion, secondary to poor vascular supply, or rarely, avulsion fracture of the calcaneus. Sudden calf pain associated with audible snap, followed by antalgia, and difficulty tiptoeing and climbing is characteristic, but pain may be inconsistent. With the patient prone or kneeling, there is loss of plantar flexion when midthird of calf is squeezed (i.e., positive Thompson–Doherty test). It may be falsely negative due to sympathetic activity of peroneal and PT tendons in combination with lateral collateral ligaments (Figure 51.9).

Additionally, there is a positive heel resistance test: easy dorsiflexion of the heel and foot against plantar flexion.

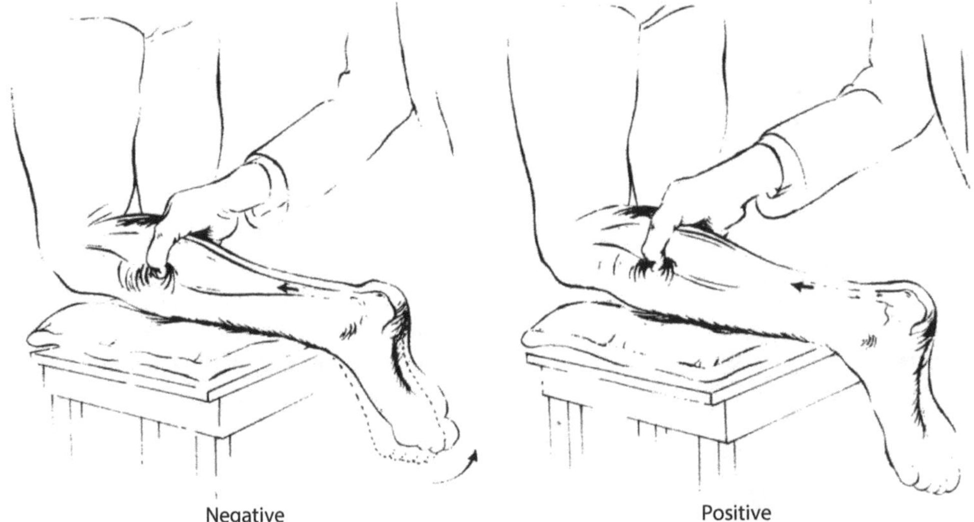

FIGURE 51.9 Thompson–Doherty squeeze test.

There may be a palpable gap in tendon (may be absent if edema is significant). Radiographs may show a loss of radiolucency or distortion of Kager's triangle on lateral view, usually negative. The ultrasound, CT, and MRI are positive. The differential should include an acute strain of medial gastrocnemius, plantaris rupture, lateral collateral sprain, and bursitis.[60]

Treatment varies with severity of injury, length of time between diagnosis and treatment, and age and caliber of athlete.[39–41] Nonoperative options are nonweight-bearing, long-leg, gravity equinus cast for 6 weeks, followed by short-leg equinus cast for 2 weeks, and then a short-leg walker for 2 weeks. The result is a return of 75%–85% normal function—good for recreational athletes.[39,40] Operative repair produces improved strength and endurance and decreased risk of rerupture (<5%) but significant complications (15%–25%). It is preferred for professional athletes (75%–90% function).[41]

> **Clinical Pearl**
>
> Nonoperative treatment for Achilles tendon rupture is usually preferred for the recreational athlete with surgical repair reserved for the professional athlete.

ROM + PRE (6 months) and a 2 cm heel orthotic for 3 months are part of the sports physical therapy program. Complications include recurrent rupture (approximately 10%).[60]

51.9.2 Impingement Syndrome

Full weight-bearing in maximum plantar flexion (demipointe or full pointe) can lead to os trigonum irritation (ununited lateral tubercle on posterior talus present in 15% of population) and eventual impingement. Posterolateral ankle pain on leaving the ground in a jump or during such dance maneuvers as the tendu, frappé, and relevé in association with posterolateral tenderness and tenderness with forced passive plantar flexion and relief of pain following 1 cc 1% lidocaine injection into posterior capsule of ankle behind peroneal tendons is diagnostic. An os trigonum on lateral radiograph view in full plantar flexion is positive. MRI shows bone contusions of the lateral talar tubercle and os trigonum.[43,44] The differential diagnosis should consider marsupial meniscus, peroneal tendinitis, FHL/Achilles tendinitis, calcaneal apophysitis, and retrocalcaneal bursitis.

Treatment consists of the usual acute modalities, followed by long-term modification of technique/activities ("push off"), appropriate stretching, injection of a long- and short-acting corticosteroid after confirmation with lidocaine, and surgical excision if conservative therapy fails.[42]

51.10 FRACTURES

51.10.1 Trauma

These injuries are seen most commonly in high-velocity, high-impact sports (e.g., football, soccer, skiing, hockey, and automobile racing); stress fractures occur in running, gymnastics, dancing; Salter type I and II fractures of the fibula are the most common ankle injuries in children. Classification is based on the mechanism of injury (Figure 51.10):

1. *Type A*: Lateral displacement of the talus
   a. Eversion force + supinated ankle—50% of all fractures
   b. Eversion force + pronated ankle
   c. Abduction force + pronated ankle
2. *Type B*: Medial displacement of the talus
   a. Adduction force + supinated ankle
   b. Adduction force + dorsiflexed/plantar-flexed ankle
3. *Type C*: Axial compression of the talus
4. *Type D*: Repetitive microtrauma

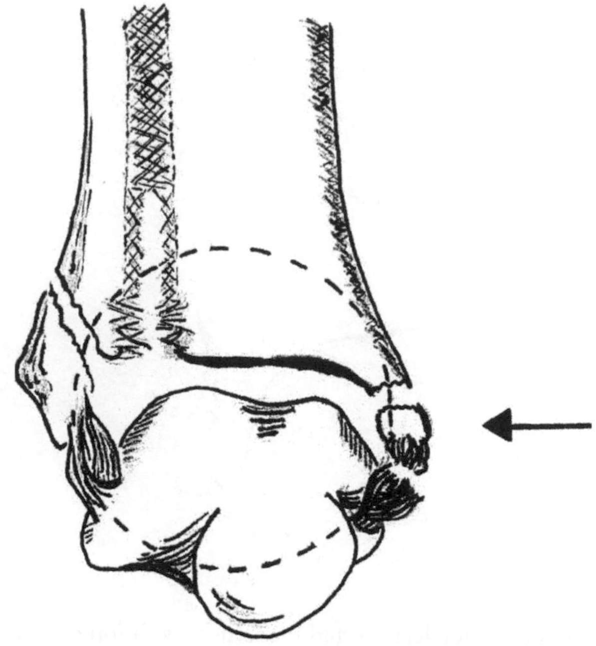

FIGURE 51.10 Type A fracture. Lateral displacement force (eversion) with rupture of the mortise ring: spiral/vertical fracture of fibula, rupture of the anterior inferior tibiofibular ligament, transverse fracture of medial malleolus, deltoid ligament rupture, and interosseus membrane tear.

Associated anatomic injuries are as follows:

- A1. Rupture of anterior inferior tibiofibular ligament → spiral oblique fracture of fibula → posterior malleolar fracture → medial malleolar fracture or deltoid ligament rupture
- A2. Rupture of deltoid ligament or fracture of medial malleolus → rupture of anterior inferior tibiofibular ligament → tear of interosseous membrane → spiral fracture of fibula (Maisonneuve) → rupture of posterior inferior tibiofibular ligament or avulsion fracture of posterior malleolus; in children, Type II or VI Salter fracture of tibia
- A3. Fracture of medial malleolus or rupture of deltoid ligament → rupture of anterior inferior ligament → oblique fracture of distal fibula → posterior malleolar fracture
- B1. Avulsion of the lateral malleolus or rupture of the talofibular ligament → vertical fracture of the medial malleolus; in children, Type I or II Salter fracture of fibula → Type III (Tillaux) or IV fracture of medial malleolus
- B2. Medial malleolar fracture or tibiofibular diastases; medial or lateral osteochondral fractures
- C. Impaction fracture → marginal fractures → tibiofibular diastases
- D. Medial osteochondral fractures or distal fibular stress fractures

Acutely, there may be an audible pop or crack, abrupt moderate-to-severe pain and swelling, or immediate disability and discoloration. Findings include localized/point tenderness, edema, possible crepitus, ecchymosis, and positive osteophony with certain fractures. Chronically, there is often a history of a *sprained* ankle resistant to all treatment, dull ache with slight swelling after excessive walking, increased pain with activity, and complete relief with rest. Physical findings are usually negative except point tenderness on talar dome with ankle plantar flexed (osteochondral fracture) or on distal fibula (stress fracture).

Mortise and oblique radiographic views good for osteochondral fragments (OCL); routine films negative for stress fractures for first 2–3 weeks following injury. Stress films may suggest associated ligamentous injury and joint instability. Arthrograms may show leakage of dye. CT arthrography is useful in the evaluation of articular cartilage integrity (osteochondritis dissecans and osteochondral fracture) and in the diagnosis of intra-articular loose bodies.[52] MRI is good for defining location of larger fragments and percentage of involved joint surface. Bone scans are reliable for stress fractures.

1. A fibular spiral fracture 2–3 in. proximal to the mortise is associated with a rupture of the deltoid ligament and/or a medial malleolar fracture and a rupture of the anterior inferior tibiofibular ligament.
2. A distal fibular fracture at the joint line should suggest a deltoid ligament injury. Displacement of the lateral malleolus is often accompanied by a medial malleolar fracture and/or deltoid ligament rupture.
3. A vertical medial malleolar fracture is associated with either a rupture of the lateral ligament or a lateral malleolar fracture.
4. Transverse malleolar fractures are ligamentous avulsion injuries.
5. Vertical, comminuted, spiral malleolar fractures follow talar compression (check spine and calcaneus).
6. Displaced fractures are usually associated with ligament injuries.
7. There may be potentially serious ligamentous injury despite negative x-ray findings.
8. Stable injuries consist of one break in the mortise ring; unstable injuries consist of two or more breaks. The breaks may be any combination of fractures and ligament ruptures (see Figure 51.11).
9. A nondisplaced physeal injury (Salter–Harris I or II) must be considered in any child with normal radiography, well-documented trauma, and ankle pain.
10. Chronic or subacute pain and ankle effusion in association with running activities suggest stress fracture of the malleoli.

The differential diagnosis should include sprains of either compartment, tenosynovitis, or contusion.

Following acute management that includes a nonweight-bearing posterior splint definitive care depends on stability. A neutral-positioned walking cast for 4–6 weeks is indicated

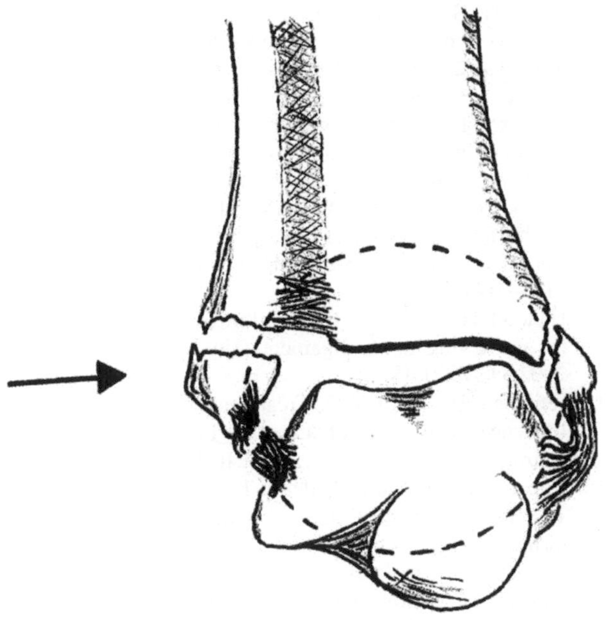

FIGURE 51.11 Type B fracture. Medial displacement force (inversion) with rupture of the mortise ring: vertical fracture of medial malleolus, transverse fracture of fibula, and rupture of the talofibular ligament.

for a stable fracture. Reduction (closed/open) followed by immobilization for 4–8 weeks is indicated for unstable lesions. Hinge cast provides early ROM and minimizes harmful effects of immobilization. Outcome is directly related to the degree of anatomical reduction. For epiphyseal injuries,

- Type I and II fibular fractures: Precise anatomic reduction by closed manipulation, 2–4 weeks short-leg weight-bearing cast; additional 2–3 weeks if region still tender. Open reduction rarely necessary.
- Type II tibial fracture: Long-leg cast for 6 weeks with precise anatomic reduction by closed manipulation. Open reduction rarely necessary.
- Types III and IV tibial fracture: Open reduction and internal fixation for displacements >2 mm.
- Type IV medial malleolar fracture: 3–4 weeks of midadduction/inversion casting.
- Tillaux fracture: 3 weeks in a long-leg nonweight-bearing cast plus 3 weeks in a short-leg walking cast following closed reduction for undisplaced fragments or open reduction plus internal fixation for displaced fractures.

All growth-plate injuries should be followed up regularly for at least 2 years or to skeletal maturity.

Medial OCLs require 12–24 weeks nonweight-bearing cast and lateral injuries arthroscopic repair and pinning.[52]

All fractures should receive ROM, PRE, and proprioceptive and functional exercises after healing.

- Ankle injuries/diagnosis/physiopathology/rehabilitation*
- Athletic injuries/rehabilitation
- Foot injuries/diagnosis/physiopathology/rehabilitation*
- Achilles tendon/physiopathology
- Biomechanics
- Fasciitis, plantar
- Humans
- Patient education as topic
- Sprains and strains/physiopathology/rehabilitation

Foot and ankle injuries are extremely common among athletes and other physically active individuals. Rehabilitation programs that emphasize the use of therapeutic exercise to restore joint range of motion, muscle strength, neuromuscular coordination, and gait mechanics have been shown to have clinical success for patients suffering various foot and ankle pathologies. Rehabilitation programs are discussed for ankle sprains, plantar fasciitis, Achilles tendonitis, and turf toe.

Clinical Pearl

Predictors of return to sporting activities at 1 year include younger age, male gender, no or mild systemic disease, and a less severe ankle fracture. Negative predictors include older age, female gender, and the presence of severe medical comorbidities.[53,54]

Complications, seen mostly after unstable fractures, include traumatic arthritis (20%–40%), particularly with lateral osteochondral fracture, persistent talar instability, Sudeck's atrophy, and interosseous membrane ossification. With epiphyseal injuries, chronic epiphysiolysis, premature closure, deformity, and early arthritis can occur. Prognosis for growth-arrest-induced deformities is worse for children under 10 years.

Preventive interventions include the regular use of properly fitted protective equipment, the application of approved and supervised techniques, and the avoidance of overtraining.[51–54]

51.11 SUMMARY

Sacrificing structure for function, the dynamic ankle is the most frequently injured area of the body in sports and recreational activities. Underestimation of morbidity is common. The generic sprain is probably the most frequent sports injury and can be associated with a significant amount of morbidity. A solid understanding of pathomechanics and good clinical acumen are essential in distinguishing bony, ligamentous, and muscle–tendon pathology. The majority of low-velocity ankle

* Consultations advised for unstable, epiphyseal, and osteochondral fractures and continuing pain 5–7 days postinjury.

TABLE 51.6
SORT: Key Recommendations for Practice

Clinical Recommendation	Evidence Rating	References
The Ottawa ankle rules should be used to rule out fractures and prevent unnecessary radiography in patients with suspected ankle sprain.	A	[5,6]
Cryotherapy should be applied for the first 3–7 days to reduce pain and improve recovery time in patients with ankle sprain.	C	[1,15]
An air stirrup brace combined with an elastic compression wrap, or a lace-up support alone, reduces pain and recovery time after an ankle sprain and allows early mobilization.	B	[12,16–18]
Early mobilization and focused range-of-motion exercises reduce pain and recovery time after an ankle sprain and are preferred to prolonged rest.	B	[16]
Patients at risk of reinjury after an ankle sprain should participate in a neuromuscular training program.	C	[11,53]
Air stirrup braces, lace-up supports, and athletic taping can reduce the risk of ankle sprains during sports.	A	[25,28–30]

injuries, including stable fractures, can be quickly identified and successfully managed by the knowledgeable primary care physician. High-velocity injuries invariably require surgical consultation due to their complexity and potential poor prognosis (Table 51.6).

REFERENCES

1. Anandacoomarasamy A, Barnsley L. Long term outcomes of inversion ankle injuries. *British Journal of Sports Medicine.* 2005;39(3):e14.
2. Berglund CL, Philipps LE, Ojofeitimi S. Flexor hallucis longus tendinitis among dancers. *Orthopaedic Practice.* 2006;18(3):26–31.
3. Beynnon B. The use of taping and bracing in treatment of ankle injury. *ISAKOS—FIMS World Consensus Conference on Ankle Instability*, Stockholm, Sweden; 2005: pp. 38–39.
4. Beynnon BD, Renstrom PA, Alosa DM et al. Ankle ligament injury risk factors: A prospective study of college athletes. *Journal of Orthopaedic Research.* 2001;19(2):213–20.
5. Bleakley CM, Glasgow P. POLICE: An improved alternative over RICE. *British Journal of Sports Medicine.* 2011;10:1136.
6. Colvin AC, Walsh M, Koval KJ, McLaurin T, Tejwani N, Egol K. Return to sports following operatively treated ankle fractures. *Foot & Ankle International.* 2009;30(4):292–296.
7. Deland JT, Hamilton WG. Posterior tibial tendon tears in dancers. *Clinics in Sports Medicine.* 2008;27:289–294.
8. Del Buono A, Smith R, Coco M, Woolley L, Denaro V, Maffulli N. Return to sports after ankle fractures: A systematic review. *British Medical Bulletin.* 2013;106:179–191.
9. Donatto KC. Ankle fractures and syndesmosis injuries. *Clin Orthopedics.* 2001;32(1):91–103.
10. Elbeshbeshy BR, Koval KJ, Zuckerman JD. Avoiding pitfalls in the treatment of ankle fractures. *Journal of Musculoskeletal Medicine.* 2000;17(2):86–92.
11. Fong DT, Hong Y, Chan LK, Yung PS, Chan KM. A systematic review on ankle injury and ankle sprain in sports. *Sports Medicine.* 2007;37(1):73–94.
12. Foster AP, Thompson NW, Crone MD, Charlwood AP. Rupture of the tibialis posterior tendon: An important differential in the assessment of ankle injuries. *Emergency Medicine Journal.* 2005;22(12):915–916.
13. Gluck GS, Heckman DS, Parekh SG. Tendon disorders of the foot and ankle, Part 3: The posterior tibial tendon. *American Journal of Sports Medicine.* October 2010;38(10): 2133–2144.
14. Handoll HHG, Rowe BH, Quinn KM et al. Interventions for preventing ankle ligament injuries. *Cochrane Library.* 2002;3:CD000018.
15. Heijnders IL, Lin CWC. Treatment of acute ankle sprains: Evidence on the use of an ankle brace is unclear. *British Journal of Sports Medicine.* 2012;46(12):852–853.
16. Hopper D, Samsson K, Hulenik T, Ng C, Hall T, Robinson K. The influence of Mulligan ankle taping during balance performance in subjects with unilateral chronic ankle instability. *Physical Therapy in Sport.* 2009;10(4):125–130.
17. Hosea TM, Carey CC, Harrer MF. The gender issue: Epidemiology of ankle injuries in athletes who participate in basketball. *Clinical Orthopaedics.* 2000;372:45–49.
18. Hubbard TJ, Hertel J. Mechanical contributions to chronic lateral ankle instability. *Sports Medicine.* 2006;36(3): 263–277.
19. Jenkin M, Sitler MR, Kelly JD. Clinical usefulness of the Ottawa ankle rules for detecting fractures of the ankle and midfoot. *Journal of Athletic Training.* 2010;45(5):480–482.
20. Kaminski TW, Hertel J, Amendola N, Docherty CL, Dolan MG, Hopkins JT, Nussbaum E, Poppy W, Richie D. National Athletic Trainers' Association: National Athletic Trainers' Association position statement: Conservative management and prevention of ankle sprains in athletes. *Journal of Athletic Training.* 2013;48(4):528–545.
21. Kerkhoffs GMMJ, Handoll HHG, de Bie R, Rowe BH, Struijs PAA. Surgery versus conservative treatment for acute ankle sprains in adults. *Cochrane Database of Systematic Reviews.* 2007;2:CD000380.
22. Kerkhoffs GMMJ, Rowe BH, Assendelft WJJ, Kelly KD, Struijs PAA, van Dijk CN. Immobilisation and functional treatment for acute lateral ankle ligament injuries in adults. *Cochrane Database of Systematic Reviews.* 2002;3:CD003762.
23. Khoury V, Guillin R, Dhanju J, Cardinal E. Ultrasound of ankle and foot: Overuse and sports injuries. *Seminars in Musculoskeletal Radiology.* 2007;11(2):149–161.
24. Kolt GS. Research on the ankle in sport. *Journal of Science and Medicine in Sport.* 2013;16(5):387.
25. Lamb SE, Marsh JL, Hutton JL, Nakash R, Cooke MW. On behalf of The Collaborative Ankle Support Trial (CAST Group): Mechanical supports for acute, severe ankle sprain: A pragmatic, multicentre, randomised controlled trial. *Lancet.* 2009;373:575–581.
26. Linklater J. Ligamentous, chondral, and osteochondral ankle injuries in athletes. *Seminars in Musculoskeletal Radiology.* 2004;8(1):81–98.
27. Mabee J, Mabee C. Acute lateral sprained ankle syndrome. *International Journal of Family Practice.* 2009;7:1.
28. Maffulli N. The foot and ankle in sport: Modern perspectives (part II). *Sports Medicine and Arthroscopy Review.* 2009;17(3):148.
29. Mazzone MF, McCue T. Common conditions of the Achilles tendon. *American Family Physician.* 2002;65:1805–1810.

30. McGuine TA, Hetzel S, Wilson J, Brooks A. The effect of lace-up ankle braces on injury rates in high school football players. *American Journal of Sports Medicine*. 2012;40(1):49–57.
31. McGuine TA, Brooks A, Hetzel S. The effect of lace-up ankle braces on injury rates in high school basketball players. *American Journal of Sports Medicine*. 2011;39(9): 1840–1848.
32. McKay GD, Goldie PA, Payne WR et al. Ankle injuries in basketball: Injury rate and risk factors. *British Journal of Sports Medicine*. 2001;35(2):103–108.
33. Minoyama O, Uchiyama E, Iwaso H et al. Two cases of peroneus brevis tendon tear. *British Journal of Sports Medicine*. 2002;36(1):65–66.
34. Mulligan EP. Evaluation and management of ankle syndesmosis injuries. *Physical Therapy in Sport*. 2011;12(2):57–69.
35. Nilsson-Helander KS, Silbernagel KG, Thomee R et al. Acute Achilles tendon rupture: A randomized, controlled study comparing surgical and nonsurgical treatments using validated outcome measures. *American Journal of Sports Medicine*. 2010;38(11):2186–2193.
36. Nugent PJ. Ottawa ankle rules accurately assess injuries and reduce reliance on radiographs. *Journal of Family Practice*. 2004;53:785–788.
37. O'Loughlin PF, Heyworth BE, Kennedy JG. Current concepts in the diagnosis and treatment of osteochondral lesions of the ankle. *American Journal of Sports Medicine*. 2010;38:392–404.
38. Osborne MD, Rizzo TD Jr. Prevention and treatment of ankle sprain in athletes. *Sports Medicine*. 2003;33:1145–1150.
39. Pedowitz D, Tjoumakaris FP, Bernstein J. Eminence-based medicine versus evidence-based medicine: When can the athlete with a sprained ankle return to play? *Physician and Sports Medicine*. 2013;41(3):110–114.
40. Raikin SM, Elias I, Nazarian LN. Intrasheath subluxation of the peroneal tendons. *Journal of Bone and Joint Surgery*. 2008;90(5):992–999.
41. Robinson P. Impingement syndromes of the ankle. *European Radiology*. 2007;17(12):3056–3065.
42. Roth JA, Taylor WC, Whalen J. Peroneal tendon subluxation: The other lateral ankle injury. *British Journal of Sports Medicine*. 2010;44:1047–1053.
43. Sanders TG, Rathur SK. Impingement syndromes of the ankle. *Magnetic Resonance Imaging Clinics of North America*. 2008;16(1):29–38.
44. Schon LC. Assessment of the foot and ankle in elite athletes. *Sports Medicine and Arthroscopy Review*. 2009;17(2):82–86.
45. Silbernagel KG, Brorsson A, Lundberg M. The majority of patients with Achilles tendinopathy recover fully when treated with exercise alone. *American Journal of Sports Medicine*. 2011;39(3):607–613.
46. Sman AD, Hiller CE, Refshauge KM. Diagnostic accuracy of clinical tests for diagnosis of ankle syndesmosis injury: A systematic review. *British Journal of Sports Medicine*. 2013;47(10):620–628.
47. Stoffel KK, Nicholls RL, Winata AR, Dempsey AR, Boyle JJ, Lloyd DG. Effect of ankle taping on knee and ankle joint biomechanics in sporting tasks. *Medicine & Science in Sports & Exercise*. 2010;42(11):2089–2097.
48. Strauss JE, Fornberg JA, Lippert FG. Chronic lateral ankle instability and associated conditions: A rationale for treatment. *Foot and Ankle International*. 2007;28:1041–1044.
49. Struijs P, Kerkhoffs G. Ankle sprain. *Clinical Evidence*. 2001;6:798–806.
50. Tang YM, Wu ZH, Liao WH, Chan KM. A study of semi-rigid support on ankle supination sprain kinematics. *Scandinavian Journal of Medicine & Science in Sports*. 2010;20(6):822–826.
51. Umans HR, Cerezal L. Anterior ankle impingement syndromes. *Seminars in Musculoskeletal Radiology*. 2008;12(2):146–153.
52. Van Dijk CN. Diagnosis of ankle sprain: History and physical examination. *ISAKOS—FIMS World Consensus Conference on Ankle Instability,* Hollywood, FL; 2005: pp. 21–22.
53. Van Rijn RM, van Os AG, Bernsen RM et al. What is the clinical course of acute ankle sprains? A systematic literature review. *American Journal of Medicine*. 2008;121: 324–331.
54. Verhagen EALM, Bay K. Optimising ankle sprain prevention: A critical review and practical appraisal of the literature. *British Journal of Sports Medicine*. 2010;44:1082–1088.
55. Verhagen E, van der Beek A, Twisk J, Bouter L, Bahr R, van Mechelen W. The effect of a proprioceptive balance board training program for the prevention of ankle sprains: A prospective controlled trial. *American Journal of Sports Medicine*. 2004;32:1385–1393.
56. Verhagen EA, van Mechelen W, de Vente W. The effect of preventive measures on the incidence of ankle sprains. *Clinical Journal of Sport Medicine*. 2000;10(4):291–296.
57. Waterman BR, Belmont PJ, Cameron KL et al. Risk factors for syndesmotic and medial ankle sprain: Role of sex, sport, and level of competition. *American Journal of Sports Medicine*. 2011;20(10): 992–998.
58. Waterman BR, Owens BD, Davey S, Zacchilli MA, Belmont Jr PJ. The epidemiology of ankle sprains in the United States. *Journal of Bone and Joint Surgery*. 2010;92(13): 2279–2284.
59. Werd MB. Achilles tendon sports injuries: A review of classification and treatment. *Journal of the American Podiatric Medical Association*. 2007;97(1):37–48.
60. Wilkins R, Bisson LJ. Operative versus nonoperative management of acute Achilles tendon ruptures. A quantitative systematic review of randomized controlled trials. *American Journal of Sports Medicine*. 2012;40(9):2154–2160.
61. Witchalls J, Blanch P, Waddington G, Adams R. Intrinsic functional deficits associated with increased risk of ankle injuries: A systematic review with meta-analysis. *British Journal of Sports Medicine*. 2012;46(7):515–523.
62. Wolfe MW, Uhl TL, Mattacola CG et al. Management of ankle sprains. *American Family Physician*. 2001;63(1):93–103.
63. Zoga AC, Schweitzer ME. Imaging sports injuries of the foot and ankle. *Magnetic Resonance Imaging Clinics of North America*. 2003;11(2):295–310.

GENERAL REFERENCES

Chinn L, Hertel J. Rehabilitation of ankle and foot injuries in athletes. *Clinics in Sports Medicine*. 2010;29(1):157–167.

Kerkhoffs GM, van den Bekerom M, Elders LAM et al. Consensus statement: Diagnosis, treatment and prevention of ankle sprains: An evidence-based clinical guideline. *British Journal of Sports Medicine*. 2012;46(12):854–860.

Saluta J, Nunley JA. Managing foot and ankle injuries in athletes. *Journal of Musculoskeletal Medicine*. 2010;27(9):355–363.

Veenema KR. Ankle sprain: Primary care evaluation and rehabilitation. *Journal of Musculoskeletal Medicine*. 2000;17:563–574.

Verhagen E. Acute lateral ankle ligament injuries. *British Journal of Sports Medicine*. 2010;44(5):305.

52 Foot Injuries

Jeffrey B. Roberts, David Rupp, and Michael J. Petrizzi

CONTENTS

TABLE 52.1
Key Clinical Considerations

1. Overuse injuries of the foot are common. Identifying the type of footwear, discussing training regimen and identifying potential errors in training, and examining foot anatomy should be included in the evaluation.
2. Apophysitis overuse injuries are common in the pediatric and adolescent population. These issues are often associated with growth spurts and are affected by the type of activity.
3. The diagnosis of foot pain should begin with history, mechanism of injury, involved anatomy, and age of patient.
4. Plantar fasciitis is a common presentation of foot pain and can affect exercise and daily activities. Plantar fasciitis usually responds well to conservative management.
5. Treatment of fractures at the base of the fifth metatarsal is determined by the location within the three zones. There is potential for delayed healing in zones 2 and 3, which should be referred for specialty care.
6. Midfoot injuries can be difficult to treat and have potential for delayed diagnosis and long-term complications. The Lisfranc joint should be carefully evaluated on radiographs after an acute injury to the midfoot.
7. Bilateral radiographs can be helpful when the diagnosis is in question (i.e., physis versus fracture, comparison of the Lisfranc joint for widening, and os bones).

52.1 INTRODUCTION

The foot is a combination of bones—tarsals (7), metatarsals (15), phalanges (14), and sesamoids (2)—ligaments, and muscles and their tendons. It must be strong enough to support our body weight and propel us forward, yet flexible enough to absorb the impact of running or jumping. While performing these varied functions, the foot can easily be traumatized or subjected to overuse. An injury to the foot may be disabling; however even when it is not, it predisposes other links in the kinetic chain to significant injury (Table 52.1 and Figures 52.1 and 52.2).

The two main normal motions of the foot are pronation and supination. When pronating, the foot uses the longitudinal arch, which is supported by the plantar fascia, to help absorb contact forces. When supinating, the foot becomes more rigid, helping it to act as a stable lever to push off. Many foot problems are associated with excessive degrees of these two normal functions. Injuries can result from either abnormal stresses on a normal structure, such as increased running mileage, or normal stress placed onto an abnormal structure, such as a high arch.[81]

Using gait analysis, the interplay between these motions becomes clear (see Chapter 26). When preparing for heel strike, the foot begins to supinate because the muscles that are responsible for ensuring that the foot descends in a slow, controlled fashion also invert the foot, causing the heel to be supinated. Thus, the bones of the foot are tightly bound together during heel strike. Moving into pronation (or rolling in), the bones of the foot become looser, allowing the arches to absorb some of the shock of contact, which can be five to seven times an individual's body weight while running. At toe-off, the foot moves back into supination creating a rigid lever for propulsion.[81]

52.2 APPROACH TO THE PATIENT

52.2.1 History

Important questions include inquiries about previous injury, whether the athlete has started playing a new sport, purchased new shoes, or suddenly increased mileage or rate of training or whether relatively no change has occurred, thus implying constant overuse of the same portion of the foot over the course of many weeks, months, or years.[59,81]

52.2.2 Examination

Look at the foot both statically and dynamically while comparing the involved with the uninvolved side. Have the athlete bring in his or her shoes to observe for any abnormal wear patterns, again comparing both shoes. All shoes have some wear on the lateral portion of the heel, as this is the location of heel strike in most individuals. Callus formation at the bottom of the foot indicates stress patterns to which that the foot is subjected. It is often helpful to observe the patient's foot while standing, particularly from behind, to determine the height of the longitudinal arch, angulation of the Achilles tendon, and degree of pronation of the foot at rest. Observe the individual

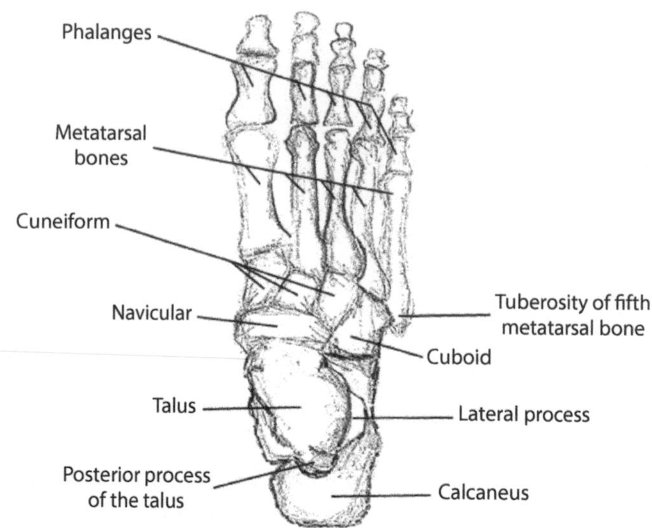

FIGURE 52.1 Anatomy: AP view.

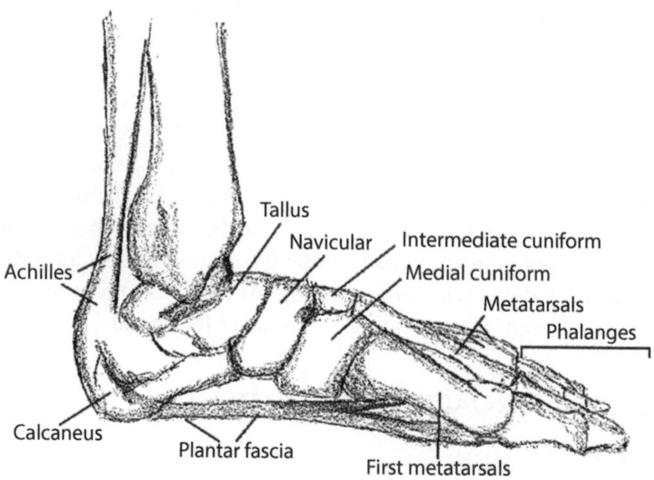

FIGURE 52.2 Anatomy: medial view.

walking, jogging, and cutting. Skillful palpation, beginning in nontraumatized areas, should assess trigger points, range of motion, foot flexibility, and neurovascular status. The injured foot should always be compared to the uninjured foot.[81] When indicated, x-rays are often invaluable but may not initially show any findings in the case of a stress fracture. Additionally, the practitioner must order the appropriate x-ray for the injury (e.g., weight bearing, on toes, and navicular). A bone scan may be indicated. The use of hematologic analysis (e.g., complete blood count and erythrocyte sedimentation rate) is often not necessary in the acute injury setting.

52.2.3 Treatment

General guidelines include the rest, ice, compression, elevation (RICE) + progressive resistance exercise (PRE) regimen (see Chapter 27). The use of orthotics or better-constructed athletic footwear to resist abnormal motion is a critical part of the treatment and prevention of injuries; however, the high-arched foot may require a more cushioned design as opposed to motion control. Sometimes, the use of taping, strapping, or casting may be necessary. Surgery should always be a last resort.

52.3 FOOT ANATOMY

52.3.1 Hindfoot

52.3.1.1 Overuse

52.3.1.1.1 Os Trigonum

The os trigonum is the name for an unfused ossicle of the lateral process of the posterior tubercle of the talus. It stems from an ossification center that appears between the 8th and 11th years of life.[11] Prevalence is varied and has been reported in 1.7%–50% of the population.[11] Injury to the os trigonum is primarily caused by a forced plantar flexion, which causes the os trigonum to contact the posterior tibial plafond. Football kickers, soccer players, and ballet dancers are at risk for developing this condition.

Patients present with posterior ankle pain that is worse with plantar flexion. They may report a plantar flexion injury. Examination revels tenderness over the posterior talus, and forced plantar flexion may worsen the pain. The differential diagnosis includes stress fracture of the lateral tubercle, Haglund's deformity, and Achilles tendinopathy. Radiographic examination should include AP, lateral, and oblique views. In addition, a 30° subtalar view can aid in differentiating between an acute posterior talar process fracture and a symptomatic os trigonum.[11] Symptomatic os trigonum or os trigonum syndrome is treated with activity modification that avoids plantar flexion. Anti-inflammatory medication and analgesics can assist with pain control. Ankle bracing to limit plantar flexion may be beneficial. Surgical treatment to remove the os trigonum is reserved for cases that fail to respond to conservative measures. Complications include posterior ankle impingement syndrome and persistent pain.

52.3.1.2 Tarsal Tunnel Syndrome

Tarsal tunnel syndrome is a peripheral neuropathy that involves the entrapment of the posterior tibial nerve or one of its three main branches: medial plantar, lateral plantar, or calcaneal nerve. The affected nerve is entrapped within the tarsal tunnel. The tibial nerve is the terminal branch of the sciatic nerve and initiates from the L4-S2 roots. The affected nerve is entrapped within the tarsal tunnel which a fibro-osseous space located on the medial side of the ankle, inferior and posterior to the medial malleolus. The floor of the tarsal tunnel consists of the medial wall of the talus, calcaneus, and the medial wall of the distal tibia. The flexor retinaculum creates the roof for the structure. In addition to containing the previously mentioned nerves, the tarsal tunnel also contains the tibialis posterior tendon, flexor digitorum longus tendon, posterior tibial artery, posterior tibial vein, and flexor halluces longus tendon.

Tarsal tunnel syndrome occurs due to compression of the posterior tibial nerve, or one of its branches, as it courses through the tarsal tunnel. Compression of the nerve can be caused by numerous etiologies. It can be caused by direct trauma, constrictive foot wear, lower extremity edema, valgus hindfoot, varus hindfoot, systemic arthropathies, osteophytes, hypertrophic retinaculum, tendinopathy, lipomas, tumors, neuromas, and ganglion cysts.[9,29] Patients will present with pain located posterior to the medial malleolus that may radiate into the heel. They may also complain of paresthesia and neuropathic pain in the heel, plantar aspect of the foot, and into the toes. The pain may be worsened with activities such as running or jogging and may be relieved with rest or wearing loose-fitting shoes. Physical exam will have tenderness to deep palpation over the tarsal tunnel, a positive Tinel's sign, and positive provocative testing (either dorsiflexion and eversion or plantar flexion and inversion).[9]

The differential diagnosis for tarsal tunnel syndrome includes plantar fasciitis, posterior tibialis tendinopathy, and medial ankle sprain. Radiographs of the ankle are used to investigate anatomic structural abnormalities. Magnetic resonance imaging (MRI) can be used for investigating possible space-occupying lesion as an etiology. Nerve conduction studies along with electromyography (EMG) can help differentiate tarsal tunnel syndrome from other causes of neuropathic pain.[9,29] Musculoskeletal ultrasound can aid in the diagnosis of tarsal tunnel syndrome by identifying ganglion cysts, tenosynovitis, mass lesions, and talocalcaneal coalitions.

Treatment for tarsal tunnel syndrome is conservative. Activity modification, proper foot wear, and orthotics are the mainstays of treatment. If medications are needed, nonsteroidal anti-inflammatory drugs are recommended. Neuroleptic medication such as tricyclic antidepressants and antiepileptics may also be used. Other, more invasive, treatment depends on the etiology of pain. Ganglion cysts can be aspirated. Corticosteroids can be injected into the tarsal tunnel. Resistant cases of tarsal tunnel syndrome should be referred for possible surgical intervention.

52.3.1.2.1 Medial Plantar Nerve Compression

Medial plantar nerve compression is also known as jogger's foot. The medial plantar nerve is a branch of the tibial nerve which divides into the medial and lateral plantar nerves in the tarsal tunnel. Once the medial plantar nerve exits the tarsal tunnel, it courses in a plantar direction before dividing into medial and lateral terminal branches at the base of the first metatarsal. The terminal branches of the medial plantar nerve further divide into digital nerves and innervate the medial three and a half toes. The medial plantar nerve can become compressed either distal to the tarsal tunnel or by compression from the abductor halluces muscle. Other causes of compression include space-occupying lesions such as tumors and osteophytes, eversion injuries, and high-arched orthotics. This neuropathy is rare but can be found in runners, ballet dancers, and gymnasts. Patients will present with pain or dysesthesia on the medial sole, medial heel, and medial toes.[9] Pain is usually worse with activity or exercise and relieved with rest. The patient may report onset of symptoms after new orthotic use. Examination of the patient will show pain along the medial longitudinal arch. The patient may have a positive Tinel's sign. Forced eversion or plantar flexion may provoke symptoms. It may also be beneficial to have patient run or exercise prior to the examination, as the exam can be normal after periods of rest or inactivity. Radiographs, which are typically normal, are usually ordered to exclude other pathologic etiologies. EMG and nerve conduction studies may help delineate the etiology of patient's symptoms. Musculoskeletal ultrasound may be useful to detect space-occupying lesions. Other etiologies in the differential diagnosis are tarsal tunnel syndrome and flexor hallucis tendinopathy. Treatment is conservative in nature and includes rest, footwear modification, anti-inflammatory medications, analgesics, and physical therapy to strengthen the medial longitudinal arch. Corticosteroid injections may be diagnostic and therapeutic in difficult cases. Orthotics that prevents hyperpronation of the hindfoot or a medial heel wedge to prevent eversion may also be beneficial. Surgical release of the nerve is performed only for resistant cases. Compression of the medial plantar nerve may lead to muscle atrophy if left untreated.

52.3.1.2.2 Lateral Plantar Nerve Compression

Compression of the lateral plantar nerve is a rare cause of neuropathy in the foot. Gymnasts are one athletic population that have had reported cases of lateral plantar nerve compression.[26] The lateral plantar nerve is a branch of the tibial nerve which divides into the medial and lateral plantar nerves in the tarsal tunnel. The lateral plantar nerve courses beneath the abductor hallucis muscle and then courses between the flexor digitorum brevis and quadratus plantae muscles.[53] Its first branch is also known as Baxter's nerve or the first branch of the lateral plantar nerve. The lateral plantar nerve divides into interdigital nerves near the metatarsal bases. The lateral plantar nerves supplies sensation to the plantar aspect of the lateral one and half toes and motor function to the interossei and lateral lumbricals. Injury and trauma have been the reported etiologies for this condition. The nerve is typically compressed in the abductor tunnel in the medial aspect of the foot. Patients will present with heel pain and dysesthesia of the lateral foot. Exam may show decreased sensation over the lateral foot and lateral one and a half toes. Tinel's sign may be positive over the tarsal tunnel. Radiographs are obtained to rule out other causes of heel pain. The differential diagnosis includes tarsal tunnel syndrome, calcaneal fracture, and stress fracture. Treatment is conservative and incorporates rest, ice, analgesics, and anti-inflammatory medications.

52.3.1.2.2.1 First Branch of the Lateral Plantar Nerve Compression (Baxter's Neuropathy) Compression of the first branch of the lateral plantar nerve is the most common cause of neurologic heel pain and is a leading cause of chronic heel pain. The first branch of the lateral plantar nerve is also known as the inferior calcaneal nerve or Baxter's nerve. It branches off the lateral plantar nerve at the tarsal tunnel. It courses deep to the abductor hallucis longus muscle before turning laterally through the flexor digitorum brevis and quadratus plantae muscles. It innervates the adductor digiti minimi muscle.[9] While the nerve typically branches off the lateral plantar nerve, it can be a branch directly off the tibial nerve. Runners form the bulk of the patient population suffering with Baxter's neuropathy. Compression of the nerve can occur at three locations: in the tarsal tunnel, at the medial calcaneal tuberosity, or at the abductor hallucis longus mucle. Compression at these sites occurs from muscle hypertrophy, calcaneal spurs, space-occupying lesions, scar tissue, and peripheral edema.

Patients will present with medial heel pain that may be chronic in nature. Activity may worsen the symptoms. On examination, patients will have medial heel pain with palpation. Radiographs are used to rule out other etiologies of heel pain. Ultrasound may be useful to identify sites of entrapment. The differential diagnosis includes plantar fasciitis, heel pad syndrome, and fat pad atrophy. Treatment is conservative and includes: activity modification, anti-inflammatories, and physical therapy. Orthotics can also be used as a first line therapy. Corticosteroid injections can be used in difficult cases, and surgical release can be considered for symptoms that last[6–12] months despite conservative measures.

Clinical Pearl

Baxter's neuropathy presentation is similar to plantar fasciitis and should be considered in resistant plantar fasciitis. If the patient has a clinical presentation of plantar fasciitis with the combination neurological findings (numbness, positive Tinel's sign, etc.), then consider the diagnosis of Baxter's neuropathy.

52.3.1.3 Sural Nerve Entrapment

Sural nerve entrapment affects runners or track athletes. Sural nerve entrapment is a rare cause of foot pain. The S1 and S2 nerve roots supply the sural nerve with its pure sensory function. It is formed from portions of the tibial and peroneal nerves. It runs laterally along the Achilles tendon with the small saphenous vein. At 2 cm proximal to the lateral malleolus, the sural nerve divides into a lateral branch that courses behind the lateral malleolus to the base of the fifth metatarsal and a medial branch that innervates the fifth digit and fourth interdigital space.[24] The sural nerve supplies sensory innervation for the posterior calf, ankle joint, lateral heel and foot, fifth digit, and fourth interdigital space.

Entrapment of the nerve can be caused by direct trauma, space-occupying lesions, recurrent lateral ankle sprains, and fractures of the talus and calcaneus.[24,40] There are three areas where entrapment typically occurs. The first is along the Achilles tendon. The second area is the base of the fifth metatarsal, and the last one is the calcaneus–cuboid joint.

Patients present with sharp shooting lateral foot pain that can radiate to the knee. Patients may also complain that the pain is worse at night. Past medical history may reveal a pattern of ankle inversion injuries. Physical exam will have a positive Tinel's sign. Symptoms may be provoked with passive plantar flexion and inversion. Radiographs are obtained to rule out other etiologies and investigate associated fractures. Ultrasound can be used to evaluate entrapment. MRI is used to investigate potential etiologies but is less useful in examining the nerve itself. Nerve conduction studies and EMG may aid in the diagnosis. Lateral ankle sprains, chronic exertional compartment syndrome, popliteal artery entrapment syndrome, and lumbar nerve root impingement are part of the differential diagnosis.[40]

Treatment of sural nerve entrapment includes wearing proper footwear to lessen the pressure on the sural nerve, ankle physical therapy, and if needed edema management and corticosteroid injections. Surgical release of the nerve is indicated for persistent symptoms.

52.3.1.4 Medial Calcaneal Branch of the Tibial Nerve

Compression of the medial calcaneal nerve is an uncommon source of heel pain in athletes. Runners and gymnasts are two athletic populations at risk for developing this condition. The medial calcaneal nerve is typically a branch of the tibial nerve; however, it can branch from the lateral plantar nerve.[29] It arises from the tibial nerve in the tarsal tunnel. It courses superficially through the flexor retinaculum to provide sensory function to the posterior, medial, and plantar cutaneous aspects of the heel. The mechanism of injury is believed to include direct compression, excessive pronation, and repetitive microtrauma of hard heel strikes. The typical site of compression is the flexor retinaculum as the nerves exits the tarsal tunnel. Patients present with neuropathic pain symptoms and dysesthesia of the heel that increase with activity. On exam, patients will have a tender heel. Strength testing will be normal. Compressing the nerve at the flexor retinaculum may provoke symptoms. Radiographs are used to rule out other etiologies of heel pain. Treatment includes rest, ice, shoe wear modification, heel cups, and anti-inflammatory medications. If pain persists, surgical intervention may be beneficial.

52.3.1.5 Superficial Peroneal Nerve

Superficial peroneal nerve entrapment has affected athletes who are runners, jockeys, dancers, competitive weight lifters, soccer players, tennis players, and hockey players.[53] The superficial peroneal nerve is one of two terminal branches of the common peroneal nerve, and it innervates the peroneus longus and brevis muscles. The common peroneal nerve divides into the superficial and deep peroneal nerves at the fibula. The superficial peroneal nerve runs deep in the anterolateral compartment of the lower leg until it pierces the fascia 10–12 cm proximal to the lateral malleolus. The nerve exits the fascia at 6–7 cm proximal to the lateral malleolus and is subcutaneous as it courses distally and transitions into the intermediate and lateral dorsal cutaneous nerves. The superficial peroneal nerve can be entrapped in the fascia in dancers due to peroneal muscle hypertrophy. Dancers may also compress the nerve with ballet shoe ribbon placement.[46] The usual mechanism of injury is stretching of the nerve due to chronic ankle instability or repetitive lateral ankle sprains.

Patients present with lateral leg pain and dorsum of the foot pain. The athlete may complain of paresthesia on the dorsum of the foot. The symptoms are typically worsened by activity and improved with rest. Physical exam may show lateral lower leg pain, dorsum of the foot pain, and paresthesia over the dorsum of the foot. Symptoms may be provoked either by resisted dorsiflexion and eversion of the foot or by passive stretching of the foot into plantar flexion and inversion. A positive Tinel's sign may be present where the nerve exits the deep fascia. Radiographs are used to exclude other etiologies. Nerve conduction studies and EMG can help delineate superficial peroneal nerve entrapment from chronic ankle instability. MRI is useful to detect entrapment in the deep fascia. The differential diagnosis includes lateral ankle sprain, chronic exertional compartment syndrome, proximal peroneal nerve entrapment, and lumbar disc herniation.

Treatment is conservative and aims to treat the cause. Physical therapy with proprioception training, orthotics, lateral heel wedges, and avoiding excess valgus and varus foot positions are examples of focused noninvasive treatment modalities.[40] Corticosteroid injections can be therapeutic and diagnostic. Surgeries to release the nerve from the fascia or lateral compartment fasciotomy are two surgical options for persistent symptoms despite exhausting conservative treatment.

52.3.1.6 Deep Peroneal Nerve

Entrapment of the deep peroneal nerve is also known as anterior tarsal tunnel syndrome or ski boot syndrome. The entrapment occurs in soccer players, skiers, and runners. The deep peroneal nerve is a continuation of the common peroneal nerve. It courses distally in the anterior compartment of the lower leg, along with the anterior tibial artery, between the tibialis anterior and the extensor digitorum longus and innervates these two muscles as well as the extensor hallucis longus. It travels under both the superior extensor retinaculum and inferior extensor retinaculum. Approximately 1 cm proximal to the ankle joint, the deep peroneal nerve divides into a lateral mixed nerve that both innervates extensor digitorum brevis and supplies the lateral tarsal joints with sensory function and a medial sensory branch nerve that innervates the first interdigital space. The inferior extensor retinaculum is a Y-shaped structure comprising two bands, the superomedial and inferomedial bands. The inferomedial band of the inferior extensor retinaculum forms the roof of the anterior tarsal tunnel. At the distal portion of the inferomedial band, the medial sensory branch of the deep peroneal nerve can be become entrapped. In soccer players, it occurs from direct trauma to the dorsum of the foot. In skiers, it occurs from ski boots that are too tight. In runners, it occurs from chronic exertional compartment syndrome, improper-fitting shoes, or sequela of recurrent ankle sprains. Dancers can have symptoms caused by tight ribbon placement of their ballet shoes.[46] The syndrome can also be caused by space-occupying lesions such as osteophytes, tumors, edema, and neuromas.[40]

Patients will present with complaints of dysesthesia over the dorsum of the foot and numbness in the first web space. Patients may also have a sensation of achy pain over the talonavicular joint. The pain typically worsens with activity and improves with rest. Night symptoms may occur due to stretching of the nerve over the talonavicular joint while plantarflexing the foot. Exam will show paresthesia over the dorsum of the foot and first web space. A positive Tinel's sign is common over the location of the entrapment. Placing the foot in plantarflexion and inversion may provoke symptoms. Other diagnoses in the differential include lumbar nerve entrapment, proximal common peroneal nerve entrapment, Morton's neuroma, peripheral neuropathy, chronic ankle instability, and anterior compartment syndrome.[40] Radiographs of the foot are used to exclude fractures from the differential and to evaluate for osteophyte formation. MRI is not useful due to the small size of the nerve. Ultrasound may identify any space-occupying lesions. Exercise testing can assist if compartment syndrome is suspected. EMG and nerve conduction studies may be of benefit.

Treatment consists of conservative measures. Proper-fitting shoes, anti-inflammatories, ankle stability rehab programs, and orthotics are typical first-line treatments. Corticosteroid injections can be considered in difficult cases. Surgical release of the deep peroneal nerve at the site of entrapment is used in cases resistant to treatment. Other surgical approaches focus on treating the etiology of the entrapment (see Table 52.2).

52.3.1.7 Plantar Fasciitis

Plantar fasciitis is the most common cause of plantar heel paint that can affect up to 10% of the population and accounts for up to 600,000 outpatient visits per year.[14,73] It affects men and women at equal rates. The plantar fascia is broad aponeurosis that originates on the medial tuberosity of the calcaneus and distally divides into five bands that insert on the proximal phalanges.[73] Plantar fasciitis was believed to be an inflammatory condition, but recent studies have shown the possibility of a noninflammatory degenerative process as a result of repetitive microtrauma. While the exact etiology is unknown, obesity, pes planus, overtraining, and improper footwear are risk factors for plantar fasciitis.[14,43]

Patients with plantar fasciitis present with heel pain that is worse with the first few steps of the morning or after periods of prolonged sitting or rest. The pain may improve with continued ambulation before worsening again with extended periods of activity. On exam, the patient will have tenderness over the medial calcaneal tuberosity and plantar fascia. Dorsiflexion of the foot may elicit pain by stretching the plantar fascia. Radiographs are not necessary to make the diagnosis of plantar fasciitis. X-rays may be performed to rule out other etiologies of heel pain. X-rays may show an incidental finding of heel spurs in up to 50% of cases, but the heel spur is usually not the pain generator in plantar fasciitis.[43,64,89] No additional imaging is needed to make the diagnosis; however, ultrasound may show a thickened aponeurosis of greater than 5 mm.[75,89] The differential diagnosis of plantar heel pain includes heel pain syndrome, talar fractures, calcaneal fractures, tarsal tunnel syndrome, and insertional Achilles tendinopathy.

TABLE 52.2
Common Nerve Entrapments of the Foot

Nerve	Location of Entrapment	Etiologies	Symptoms	Treatment
Posterior tibial nerve	Tarsal tunnel	Trauma Constrictive footwear Edema Tendinopathy Osteophytes Tumors	Pain posterior to medial malleolus; paresthesia of heel, plantar aspect of the foot; worse with activity	Activity modification Proper footwear Orthotics Tricyclic antidepressants Corticosteroid injections
Medial plantar nerve	Distal to tarsal tunnel or abductor halluces muscle	Eversion injury Osteophytes High arched orthotics Tumors	Dysesthesia of medial heel, medial arch, and medial 3.5 toes Improve with rest	Activity modification Footwear modification Orthotics/medial heel wedge NSAIDs Corticosteroid injections
Lateral plantar nerve	Abductor tunnel	Injury Trauma	Dysesthesia of lateral 1.5 toes; heel pain; weakness in interossei muscles and lateral lumbricals	Rest Ice Analgesia NSAIDs
First branch of the lateral plantar nerve	Tarsal tunnel Medial calcaneal tuberosity Abductor hallucis longus	Muscle hypertrophy Calcaneal spurs Space-occupying lesions Scar tissue Edema	Heel pain	Activity modification Analgesia NSAIDs Physical therapy Orthotics Corticosteroid injection
Medial calcaneal branch of the tibial nerve	As it exits the tarsal tunnel	Direct compression Excessive pronation Repetitive microtrauma	Heel pain and dysesthesia of the heel that worsen with activity	Rest, ice, NSAIDs Shoe wear modification Orthotics; heel cups Analgesia
Sural nerve	Along Achilles tendon Base of the fifth metatarsal Calcaneal–cuboid joint	Direct compression Recurrent lateral ankle sprains Compressive lesions Calcaneal or talar fractures	Sharp shooting lateral foot pain that can radiate to the knee and is worse at night	Rest, ice, NSAIDs Physical therapy Proper footwear Corticosteroid injection
Superficial peroneal nerve	Lateral lower leg fascia	Stretching of the nerve from recurrent inversion injuries Muscle hypertrophy	Pain in lateral lower leg and dorsum of foot Pain is worse with activity	Proprioception therapy Rest, ice, NSAIDs Orthotics Lateral heel wedge
Deep peroneal nerve	Anterior tarsal tunnel	Trauma Tight ski boots Exertional compartment syndrome Recurrent ankle sprains Improper footwear	Dysesthesia over the dorsum of the foot Numbness in the first web space Pain is worse with activity	Proper-fitting shoes NSAIDs Analgesia Physical therapy Orthotics Corticosteroids

Sources: Flanigan, R.M. and DiGiovanni, B.F., *Foot Ankle Clin.*, 16(2), 255, 2011; Fredericson, M. et al., *Clin. J. Sport Med.*, 11(2), 111, 2001; Gould, J.S., *Foot Ankle Clin.*, 16(2), 275, 2011; Hirose, C.B. and McGarvey, W.C., *Foot Ankle Clin.*, 9(2), 255, 2004; Kennedy, J.G. and Baxter, D.E., *Clin Sports Med.*, 27(2), 329, 2008; McCrory, P. et al., *Sports Med.*, 32(6), 371, 2002.

Treatment generally begins with conservative noninvasive methods. Analgesics, anti-inflammatory medications, stretching, heel cups, proper footwear, and ice bottle rolls are typically first-line therapies. Night splints and custom orthotics may be of benefit in the compliant patient. Physical therapy may be useful in difficult cases. Corticosteroid injections have shown efficacy as a second-line treatment. Extracorporeal shock wave therapy has shown some promising results and could be a potential modality for resistant cases. If the patient's pain persists for 6–12 months despite exhausting all conservative measures, referral for endoscopic plantar fascia release is warranted.

Clinical Pearl

Conservative management of plantar fasciitis including proper footwear, rehab exercise (home or with PT), heel cups, and night splints are very effective and should be first-line management of plantar fasciitis.

52.3.1.8 Insertional Achilles Tendinopathy

Achilles tendinopathy is a broad definition of disorders affecting the Achilles tendon. It can be further subdivided into insertional and non-insertional Achilles tendinopathy. The former makes up 20% of Achilles tendon disorders, while the latter comprises the other 80%.[51] Insertional Achilles tendinopathy occurs within 2 cm of the calcaneal insertion. Insertional Achilles tendinopathy is more common in older athletes. Other risk factors include obesity, diabetes, hypertension, corticosteroid use, and inflammatory arthropathies.[72] Abruptly increasing workout duration, intensity, or both as well as changing training surfaces and poor foot wear also increase risk of developing insertional tendinopathy.[58] Anatomically, the Achilles tendon is the distal continuation of both the gastrocnemius and soleus muscle. It attaches on the calcaneal tuberosity. It is bordered anteriorly by the retrocalcaneal bursa and is buffered from overlying skin by the retroachilles (superficial calcaneal) bursa.

Patients will complain of posterior heel pain over the insertion of the Achilles. On exam, the patient may have pain with passive dorsiflexion of the ankle. X-rays are ordered to investigate potential coexisting Haglund deformity. X-rays may also show calcification of the tendon insertion. Additional imaging by MRI and ultrasound can provide information on the health of the tendon, degree of bursa inflammation, and potential bony abnormalities.[82,93] The differential diagnosis for insertional Achilles tendinopathy includes noninsertional Achilles tendinopathy, retrocalcaneal bursitis, Haglund syndrome, Reiter syndrome, rheumatoid arthritis, and calcaneal stress fracture.

Most insertional Achilles tendinopathies respond to conservative treatment strategies. Initial options include rest, activity modification, and analgesics. Eccentric exercises, which are the hallmark treatment of noninsertional Achilles tendinopathy, may improve insertional Achilles tendinopathy if performed at floor level and dorsiflexion is avoided.[42,72] Heels lifts may reduce symptoms by reducing dorsiflexion. Nonsteroidal anti-inflammatory drugs may have initial analgesic effects, but their benefits may be limited by the lack of an inflammatory mechanism of pain. Immobilization may aid in pain reduction but should be limited. Weight bearing has been shown to aid in the reorganization of tendon fibers. Corticosteroid injections should be avoided due to increased risk of Achilles tendon rupture, but nitro patches have shown potential benefit for insertional Achilles tendinopathy.[65] Extracorporeal shockwave therapy is an emerging treatment modality.[72] A referral to a sports medicine specialist or orthopedist for prolotherapy, PRP injection, or sclerosing therapy may be beneficial in patients wishing to avoid surgery.[30,51,72] Surgical intervention is reserved for cases that fail to respond to conservative measures for 6 months at minimum.

52.3.1.9 Haglund Deformity

Haglund deformity was first described in 1928, and it is commonly known as a pump bump. A Haglund deformity is commonly found in women who wear high heels and hockey players whose skates have a rigid heel counter.[79,89] It can be an individual etiology of heel pain but can occur with retrocalcaneal bursitis or insertional Achilles tendinopathy. Other risk factors include high-arched feet, rear foot varus, rear foot equinus, and trauma to the apophysis.[79] A Haglund deformity is a bony prominence on the superior lateral posterior calcaneus. The bony prominence is irritated by friction from ill-fitted footwear. The local irritation can cause inflammation of the retroachilles bursa, which produces pain.

The patient will complain of posterior heel pain worse when wearing shoes. On exam, the patient will have a tender erythematous lateral prominence. Radiographs evaluate the presence of an enlarged superior posterior calcaneal process and rule out other etiologies of posterior heel pain. Ultrasound can evaluate the posterior calcaneus in addition to soft tissue structures such as the retrocalcaneal bursa and retroachilles bursa. Other etiologies to consider include Reiter syndrome, rheumatoid arthritis, retrocalcaneal bursitis, and insertional Achilles tendinopathy.

Treatment starts with rest, ice, NSAIDs, and shoe modifications. Heel lifts are used to elevate the Haglund deformity above the heel counter. Wearing open back shoes will also alleviate symptoms. Patients may benefit from orthotics to reduce excessive rear foot motion and stress on the Achilles tendon. Corticosteroids may be beneficial if there is coexisting retrocalcaneal bursitis, but extreme care must be shown to avoid injection into the Achilles tendon. Surgical treatment for difficult cases involves removing the Haglund deformity and possible bursectomy.

52.3.1.10 Retrocalcaneal Bursitis

Retrocalcaneal bursitis is an etiology of posterior heel pain that is common in runners who train on inclines. The dorsiflexion that occurs while running on an incline causes compression of the retrocalcaneal bursa.[79] The retrocalcaneal bursa is positioned between the Achilles tendon and the calcaneus. Anteriorly, it comprises fibrocartilage and posteriorly it is continuous with the Achilles tendon. The patient will present with posterior heel pain typically worse with dorsiflexion. Athletes may report the pain is worse at the beginning of exercising and improves with activity before worsening again. The pain is located anterior to the Achilles tendon and superior to the Achilles insertion.[79] On exam, the patient will have tenderness with palpation bilaterally anterior to the Achilles tendon. This is also known as the two-finger squeeze test. X-rays are useful to rule out other etiologies of posterior heel pain and to investigate possible Haglund deformities. Ultrasound may be used to find a fluid-filled bursa. Treatment for this condition is conservative. Ice, rest, analgesia, and activity modification are common initial therapies. NSAIDs are used due to the inflammatory nature of the problem. Orthotics to limit rear foot motion and Achilles tendon stress may improve pain symptoms. Corticosteroid injections should generally be avoided but may be of benefit in select cases and should be performed under ultrasound guidance to insure accurate injection. The relative proximity of the retrocalcaneal bursa to the Achilles tendon creates the possibility of tendon rupture from erroneously placed injection.[90,93]

Surgery is recommended for those who fail to respond to conservative treatment. Surgery removes the bursa and any offending bony prominences such as Haglund deformity.

52.3.1.11 Stress Fracture of the Talus

Talar stress fractures are a rare condition. Repetitive overloading of the talus causes the stress fracture. The talar head is the most common site of talar stress fractures, although the lateral process, body, and posterior tubercle can also have stress fractures. Ballet dancers are one group of at-risk athletes for talar stress fractures. Patients present with lateral ankle pain or sinus tarsi pain.[6] Physical examination reveals a tender heel. Pain may be provoked with passive extremes range of motion depending on the location of the stress fracture. Radiographs are typically negative. MRI or CT is used to confirm diagnosis. The differential diagnosis includes chronic ankle sprain. Treatment is nonoperative and patients are encouraged to be non–weight bearing (NWB) for 6 weeks and are immobilized in a CAM walker or short leg cast with a posttreatment rehabilitation period.[6,94] The risk of avascular necrosis is low after talar stress fracture. Despite this, there is evidence that pain with activity can continue to occur and that talar stress fractures may not be as low risk as previously believed.[83]

52.3.1.12 Calcaneal Stress Fractures

Stress fractures of the calcaneus are the result of repetitive overload.[89] Patients may report having recently increased their workout load, switched to a harder running surface, or drastically changed their footwear. Dancers, runners, and patients participating in high-impact aerobics are populations at risk for stress fractures. Patients present with heel pain. The pain can be reported to be worse during the first steps of the day. If symptoms have been occurring for quite some time, then pain may be more persistent. The clinician may be able to elicit pain by squeezing the medial and lateral walls of the calcaneus simultaneously. Physical exam may also reveal a positive tuning fork test. Radiographs may show the fracture but are often negative. MRI is a sensitive test and can be used when the diagnosis is unclear. The differential diagnosis includes plantar fasciitis and Achilles tendinopathy. Calcaneal stress fractures typically respond to conservative treatment. Treatment consists of reducing and modifying activities. Crutches and NWB are used when patients have pain with ambulation. Orthotics and heel cups may be beneficial in relieving pain. Anti-inflammatory medications and analgesics are recommended for pain control if needed. Once symptoms have resolved, patients can slowly progress to resuming full normal activities over 4–6 weeks. High-level athletes may benefit for doing NWB activities such as pool running to maintain cardiovascular fitness while the stress fracture heals.

52.3.1.13 Traumatic

52.3.1.13.1 Contusion: Stone Bruise

A contusion or stone bruise is a common running sport injury that affects men and women equally. It can occur in athletes of all ages. The injury occurs from striking the foot on either the ground or a stone without appropriate padding. The calcaneus and head of the first metatarsal are the most frequently injured bones but any weight-bearing bone may be injured. The patient will have pain over the affected area and likely can remember the exact moment of injury. Physical exam will reveal erythema and point tenderness. X-rays are obtained to rule out other etiologies of pain. Special studies such as MRI or bone scans are necessary only when suspicion of stress fracture remain high. The differential diagnosis includes stress fracture. The initial treatment entails rest, ice, elevation, compression, and analgesia. Additional treatment, including metatarsal pads, heel cups, and felt donuts, may alleviate symptoms and allow for a quicker return to play. Prevention can be achieved through proper footwear, shoe wear with steel shanks, and rock guard shoes.

52.3.1.13.2 Talus Fractures

The talus is an important bony structure. It is involved in the transmission of weight and force from the leg to the foot. It is a dense bone that can with stand great force. The superior surface of the talus bears a greater load per unit area than any other structure in the body. Fractures of the talus account for less than 1% of all fractures and are usually the result of high-energy impact such as motor vehicle accidents or falls from height.[25] The talus is divided into three areas: the head, neck, and body. The body articulates with the tibia, fibula, and calcaneus. The head articulates with the navicular bone. Within the body of talus, there are two landmarks of note: the lateral process and the posterior tubercle. The lateral process forms a portion of the subtalar joint. The posterior tubercle has lateral and medial processes. Sixty percent of the talus is covered with articular cartilage, which limits its blood supply and makes the talus susceptible to osteonecrosis after injury. While the talus has a high proportion of articular cartilage, it has no musculotendinous attachments (Figure 52.3).

52.3.1.13.2.1 Talar Head Fractures of the talar head make up less than 10% of all fractures of the talus.[20] The mechanism of injury is a forceful axial load applied to a plantar flexed foot forcing the foot into dorsiflexion and inversion.[50] This will typically create an intra-articular talar fracture. Fracture of the talar head can lead to disruption of the talonavicular

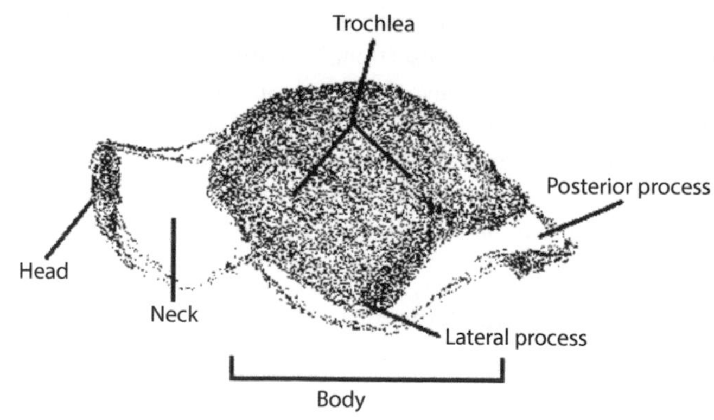

FIGURE 52.3 Talus anatomy: lateral view.

joint, which can result in either subluxation or dislocation of the talus. Talar head fractures commonly occur with other injuries because of the high-energy impact, which can result in the talar head fracture being missed. Due to the nature of blood supply to the talar head, the risk of avascular necrosis following a talar head fracture is 5%–10%.

The patient will present with pain, inability to ambulate, and swelling with a history of a high-energy impact. On physical exam, the patient will be tender to palpation over the talonavicular joint. There will be ecchymosis in the medial midfoot or medial hindfoot. This ecchymotic pattern should raise suspicion that the injury is more than just an ankle sprain. A Canale view radiograph of the ankle should be ordered in addition to the standard three views of the ankle and foot. If a talar head fracture is seen on the radiographs or is suspected clinically, a CT scan of the foot should be obtained for better definition of the fracture.[25] Nondisplaced fractures involving less than 5 mm of the talonavicular joint and that do not extend into the anterior subtalar joint may be treated with an NWB short leg cast. The fracture is followed closely with repeat imaging performed every 2–3 weeks. Casting may be discontinued at 6–8 weeks or sooner if the patient's pain has resolved and the radiographs show evidence of bone healing.[25] After the cast is discontinued, the patient is transitioned into a longitudinal arch support for 2–3 months. All displaced fractures and nondisplaced fractures involving more than 5 mm of the talonavicular joint should be referred to an orthopedist for potential surgical intervention. While the risk for avascular necrosis for talar neck fracture is relatively low when compared to the other types of talar fractures, there is a significant risk of developing osteoarthritis of the talonavicular joint.

52.3.1.13.2.2 Talar Neck Mechanism of injury is forced dorsiflexion caused by either high-energy collision or fall from height. The fracture occurs when the talar neck collides with the anterior tibial crest.[25] The talocalcaneal ligament may be disrupted by the injury leading to subluxation or dislocation.[25] Talar neck fractures account for 5%–50% of all fractures of the Talus.[25,69] They typically occur more frequently in males than females. Isolated talar neck fractures are rare.

Vertical fractures through the talar neck can be grouped by the Hawkins classification system. This system stratifies the risk of avascular necrosis by initial displacement of the fracture.[32,91] Type I are minimally displaced fractures. Type II fractures have subluxation or dislocation of the subtalar joint. Type III have displacement of the talar body from the subtalar and ankle joints. Type IV fractures have displacement of the talar body from the subtalar, ankle joints, and the talonavicular joints.[25,69]

Patients present with swelling and pain of the hindfoot and ankle after a motor vehicle accident or a fall from height. They may report a forced dorsiflexion injury. They may be unable to bear weight. Exam may show edema, ecchymosis, gross deformity, and tenderness to palpation. Evaluation should include thorough neurovascular exam. In addition to anteroposterior, lateral, and oblique views of the ankle, a Canale view may represent the best view to visualize talar neck fractures. There is a strong association of thoracolumbar fractures occurring with talar neck fractures. X-rays of the spine may be warranted to rule out fractures of the spine. CT scan of the ankle and foot will aid in the classification of the talar neck fracture, evaluating other potential coexisting fractures of the foot, and preoperative planning.

Using the Hawkins classification system, only Type I are amenable to nonoperative treatment. All other types should be referred to orthopedics for possible ORIF. The goal of treatment is anatomic reduction. This is necessary to prevent foot instability. Type I fractures are treated with immobilization and NWB for 6–8 weeks. Close follow-up with serial radiographs is necessary to monitor potential displacement. The other three types should have reduction attempted to reduce skin necrosis and then referred promptly. Complications from talar neck fractures include avascular necrosis of the talar body, posttraumatic arthritis, and nonunion. Talar neck fractures account for 90% of all traumatic AVN.[2]

52.3.1.13.2.3 Medial Posterior Tubercle of Talus Fractures of the medial posterior tubercle (Cedell fracture) are very rare.[44] They occur due to high-speed injury that dorsiflexes and pronates the foot and ankle. The fracture is typically an avulsion injury because the deltoid ligament attaches to the medial posterior tubercle.[44] The mechanism of injury usually results in medial subtalar dislocation in addition to the medial posterior tubercle fracture.

Patients present with medial posterior ankle pain and swelling. On exam, the patient will exhibit tenderness posterior to the medial malleolus and anterior to the Achilles tendon.[44] The fracture may be difficult to detect on the standard anteroposterior and lateral views of the ankle. An oblique view with the foot and ankle rotated externally 40° and the x-ray beam centered to an area 1 cm posterior and 1 cm inferior to the medial malleolus may improve diagnosis. MRI and CT may be beneficial if the diagnosis is unclear. Medial subtalar dislocations are associated with the injury. The patient may also have tarsal tunnel syndrome due to either the presence of a hematoma or localized swelling. Treatment of nondisplaced or minimally displaced fractures is immobilization in a short leg NWB cast for 4–6 weeks. Weight bearing is permitted after the initial period of immobilization. However if pain symptoms persist, an additional period of immobilization of 4–6 weeks is recommended. Large fractures, significantly displaced fractures, or high-end athletes with persistent symptoms should be referred for surgical intervention.

52.3.1.13.2.4 Lateral Posterior Tubercle of Talus The lateral posterior tubercle is also known by the name Stieda process. It serves as the insertion for the posterior talofibular ligament. If present, the os trigonum is located just posterior to the lateral posterior tubercle. Fractures of the lateral posterior tubercle occur by either of two mechanisms. The first is hyperplantarflexion, which causes compression fractures. The other is forced inversion, which typically results in an avulsion injury (Shepherd fracture). Both mechanisms of injury have been associated with kicking injuries in American football and rugby. The ankle is plantar flexed in both sporting activities.

The patient will present with pain and swelling of the posterolateral ankle. Activities that cause plantar flexion may exacerbate the pain. On exam, the patient may have swelling. Deep palpation anterior to the Achilles tendon will cause pain. Dorsiflexion of the great toe may also trigger pain because the tension on the flexor hallucis longus tendon, which runs between the medial and lateral posterior tubercles, will compress the fracture site.

The differential diagnosis includes lateral ankle sprain, high ankle sprain, and os trigonum. Lateral foot x-rays are the test of choice in diagnosing lateral posterior tubercle fractures. MRI or CT may be beneficial if the diagnosis is unclear or if the injury is not acute. MRI and CT can help distinguish between an os trigonum and old lateral posterior tubercle fracture. Treatment of nondisplaced or minimally displaced fractures is immobilization in short leg NWB cast for 4–6 weeks. Weight bearing is permitted after the initial period of immobilization. However, if pain symptoms persist, an additional period of immobilization of 4–6 weeks is recommended. If pain persists after 6 months for a nondisplaced or minimally displaced fracture, surgical excision of the fracture fragment may be beneficial. Displaced fractures are referred for surgical intervention.

52.3.1.13.2.5 Lateral Process (Snowboarder's Fracture)

Lateral process fractures are normally rare. They account for only 10% of all talus fractures. However in the snowboarding population, they are much more common. They account for 32% of all ankle fractures and 15% of all ankle injuries in the snowboarding population.[7] This increase in rate is believed to be related to the fixed position of the boots onto the snowboard that places the ankle in a rigid dorsiflexed and rotated position.[20] When the athlete lands a jump, the axial load is then applied to the fixed ankle position. The lateral process makes up a large section of the lateral wall of the talus. It plays an important role in the motion at both the talocrural and subtalar joints. The mechanism of injury falls into one of three categories: falls from significant height, motor vehicle accidents, or snowboarding injuries. The injury pattern involves an axial force applied to a rapidly dorsiflexed, inverted, and externally rotated foot.[7,20]

The patient presents with symptoms closely resembling a lateral ankle sprain. This often leads to misdiagnosis. The patient will have pain, swelling, ecchymosis, and typically an inability to bear weight. On exam, the patient will have point tenderness over the lateral process. The area of tenderness is found just anterior and inferior to the lateral malleolus between the ATFL and CFL. The patient will also have pain with dorsiflexion and plantarflexion. The talar tilt test will also elicit pain. A radiographical series of anteroposterior, lateral, and mortise views will show the fracture. Lateral views may show a posterior subtalar effusion that can be indicative of occult lateral process fractures. A CT scan can confirm diagnosis and better classify the fracture.[20]

Treatment of lateral process fractures is dependent on its classification. The system is based on the McCrory–Bladin classification.[7] Type I is a small chip fracture of the process that does not involve the articular surfaces. Type II is a fracture that involves both the ankle and subtalar joints. Type III is a comminuted fracture. Nondisplaced type I fractures can be treated nonoperatively. Treatment includes 4 weeks in short leg NWB cast followed by 2 weeks in walking cast or removable boot.[20] A physical therapy program can be initiated once the patient is pain-free. If pain persists, a repeat CT should be ordered to assess for nonunion. The patient should be referred if a lack of healing evidence exists at 3 months. Type I fractures that are displaced more than 2 mm, type II, and type III fractures should all be referred to orthopedics for potential open reduction and internal fixation. Complications of lateral process fractures include nonunion, malunion, persistent pain, avascular necrosis, and posttraumatic arthritis.

52.3.1.13.3 Osteochondral Lesions of the Talus

Osteochondral fractures of the talus affect the articular cartilage and underlying bone. They have also been called OCD lesions or osteochondritis dissecans. Previously, these lesions were thought to be related to ischemic events but now are known to be a sequla of a previous injury or trauma.[78] The talar dome is the location of most of the osteochondral lesions in the talus. Berndt and Harty have proposed two mechanisms of injury. The first is an axial load applied to a dorsiflexed and inverted foot that can produce a compressive injury. The second is a plantar flexed foot that is forcibly inverted and externally rotated.[78]

Patients may present with either an acute ankle injury or chronic ankle pain following a previous ankle injury. Physical examination will reveal a painful swollen ankle in the case of an acute injury. The patient with chronic ankle pain may not have swelling. Palpation of the anterior joint line may reveal tenderness. The talar dome should be palpated with the ankle in both dorsiflexion and plantarflexion.[86] Exam may show decreased range of motion when compared to the contralateral ankle. Examination of the lateral ligaments of the ankle should be performed to look for coexisting injuries. In the patient with chronic ankle pain, the ligamentous exam should be negative. AP, lateral, and mortise radiographic views of the ankle should be obtained.[86] If the radiographs are negative but suspicion is high for osteochondral injury, further imaging is warranted. CT scans, bone scintigraphy, and MRI have all been used with MRI emerging as the modality of choice. MRI can detect early nondisplaced lesion and also assess articular cartilage injury.

Treatment is nonoperative for low-grade lesions. Progressive weight bearing and mobilization follow immobilization and NWB. Full recovery time to full ambulation is 12–16 weeks. Surgical intervention is performed on advanced lesions or those patients who fail conservative treatment.[78]

52.3.1.13.4 *Calcaneal Fractures*

While calcaneal fractures are an uncommon fracture accounting for 1–2% of all fractures, the calcaneus is the most common tarsal bone fractured, accounting for 60% of all tarsal bone fractures.[49] The calcaneus, the largest tarsal bone, has three facets: the anterior, middle, and posterior facets. The three facets are on the superior surface of the calcaneus forming the subtalar joint. Other bony landmarks include the anterior surface of the calcaneus which articulates with the cuboid bone and the calcaneal tuberosity serves as the insertion site for the Achilles tendon. Additionally, the calcaneal tuberosity has additional landmarks which are the medial and lateral processes.

The typical mechanism of injury is a high-energy trauma that results in an axial load after a fall or jump from height. Ski jumpers, skiers, climbers, and gymnasts are athletic populations at risk for calcaneal fractures.[49] They are classified as intra-articular or extra-articular with intra-articular being more prevalent. Extra-articular fractures have a better prognosis and rarely require surgical intervention. Extra-articular calcaneal fractures include fractures of the anterior process, medial, and lateral process, tuberosity, sustentaculum tali, and extra-articular body fractures. Intra-articular fractures are more difficult to evaluate, diagnosis, and treat. Due to the nature of the mechanism of injury, it is important to evaluate each patient carefully for coexisting injuries. There is a strong correlation between calcaneal fractures and vertebral fractures with up to a 10% concominance.[92] Radiographic examination should include lateral and axial views. Lateral x-rays are used to calculate Bohler's angle and the angle of Gissane, which are used to assess calcaneal height, joint depression, and proper alignment.[31] Advanced imaging with CT is used to assess suspected intra-articular fractures. MRI is useful for diagnosing stress fractures and fractures that CT fails to identify.[49] Complications of calcaneal fractures include acute compartment syndrome, skin necrosis, persistent pain, malunion, nerve entrapment, and posttraumatic arthritis.

52.3.1.13.4.1 *Calcaneal Anterior Process Fracture*

Fractures of the anterior process account for 15% of calcaneal fractures and are often misdiagnosed.[44] The anterior process has two mechanisms of injury that produce distinct injury patterns. An avulsion injury can occur when the foot is forced into adduction and plantarflexion causing the bifurcate ligament to avulse the anterior process.[44] The second mechanism is foot abduction, which creates a compression injury by compressing the anterior process against the cuboid.[44] Patients present with lateral ankle pain and swelling. Examination will reveal tenderness to palpation anterior to the lateral malleolus over the calcaneocuboid joint.[44] Oblique radiographic views of the foot should be obtained for avulsion fractures. These fractures are subtle and typically nondisplaced or minimally displaced. Compression fractures are best visualized with lateral radiographs. These fractures are more challenging to treat even when not displaced therefore surgical referral is recommended. CT scans are needed to assess total calcaneocuboid joint involvement. If greater than 25% of the joint is involved, surgical referral is indicated.[76] See Figure 52.4.

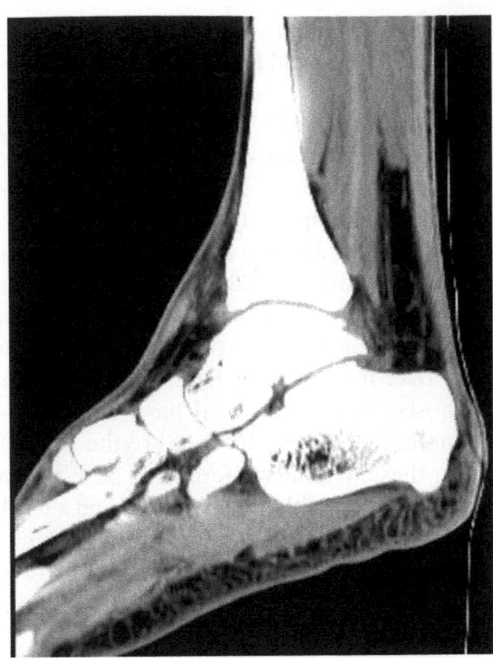

FIGURE 52.4 CT of calcaneal anterior process fracture.

Nondisplaced or minimally displaced avulsion fractures involving less than 25% of the calcaneocuboid joint can be treated with conservative treatment.[76] Initial treatment includes NWB, splinting, elevation, ice, and analgesia. Once the swelling has decreased, a short leg NWB cast is appropriate. Casting is continued for 4–6 weeks. Range of motion and strengthening can be gradually increased after cast removal. Cutting sports or activities that have a potential for reinjury should be avoided for up to 4 weeks after cast removal.[21] Full recovery may take up to 1 year.

52.3.1.13.4.2 Calcaneal Medial and Lateral Process Fracture The medial and lateral process fractures usually occur from an axial load applied to an inverted or everted foot. This mechanism of injury sheers a fragment from either the medial process or lateral process. Patients present with swelling and heel pain that may localize to the lateral or medial aspect of the posterior heel. The overlying skin may have bruising. Physical examination will reveal tenderness to palpation, edema, and ecchymosis. Axial radiographs are the ideal view to evaluate for medial and lateral process fractures.[76] Treatment starts with NWB of the injured heel along with splinting, ice, elevations, and analgesia. Once the acute swelling has subsided, the patient is placed in either a short leg walking cast or fracture boot. The duration of immobilization is 8–10 weeks. NWB is the ambulatory status of choice for minimally displaced fractures. Once the cast is removed, patients can gradually increase activity level as long as cutting sports or activities that pose a high risk of reinjury are avoided for up to 4 weeks after cast/boot removal.[21] Fractures that are displaced more than 1.5 cm or fail closed reduction should be treated surgically.[76]

52.3.1.13.4.3 Calcaneal Extra-Articular Tuberosity Fracture The mechanism of injury for an extra-articular tuberosity fracture is an avulsion injury involving the triceps surae complex (gastrocnemius and soleus). The injury occurs when an axial load is placed on plantar flexed foot creating forced dorsiflexion. Patients will present with posterior heel pain, swelling, and bruising. Physical examination of the patient will reveal tenderness to palpation over the posterior heel. There may be edema and ecchymosis. The patient will have decreased plantar flexion strength. Lateral radiographs are the view of choice for detecting these avulsion fractures. These fractures are commonly associated with displacement and subtalar joint involvement. Radiographs must be examined closely to detect these associations. If there is concern for subtalar joint extension of the avulsion fracture, a CT scan should be ordered for clarification. Fractures that are displaced <1 cm can be treated with a short leg NWB cast once the immediate swelling has subsided. Duration of casting is 6 weeks, and the foot should be placed in mild plantar flexion within the cast.[21] Follow-up imaging is performed at 7–10 days to insure nondisplacement of fracture. Fractures displaced >1 cm and any fracture with associated skin tenting should be referred for potential surgical intervention. Other indications for surgical referral include potential posterior skin compromise (the posterior portion of the bone will affect shoe wear), incompetent gastrocnemius–soleus complex, and articular surface involvement.[76] The recovery period is slightly longer for these fractures due to the involvement of the gastrocnemius and soleus muscles. Physical therapy for a strengthening and stretching program may be necessary.

52.3.1.13.4.4 Calcaneal Sustentaculum Tali Fracture Sustentaculum tali fractures are the result of high-energy trauma and are rarely seen in isolation. A fall from height onto an inverted ankle is the typical mechanism of injury. These fractures commonly extend into the subtalar joint. Patients present with medial heel pain, swelling, and discoloration. Inverting the ankle or passively dorsiflexing the great toe may provoke pain symptoms during the physical exam. These fractures are best seen in the axial view of radiographs and a CT scan is beneficial in excluding subtalar joint involvement. Isolated sustentaculum tali fractures rarely proceed to surgery, but they also rarely occur in isolation. Treatment of an isolated fracture is a short leg NWB cast for 6–8 weeks.[21] Once the cast is removed, a gradual return to preinjury activities is accomplished over 3–4 weeks. Formal physical therapy may be of benefit in this stage.

52.3.1.13.4.5 Calcaneal Body Fractures Calcaneal body fractures are fractures that do not involve the subtalar joint and account for 20% of calcaneal fractures.[76] These patients land on their heel after a fall from height. The fracture line occurs posterior to the subtalar joint. Patients present with heel pain, swelling, and inability to ambulate. Physical examination will reveal a painful swollen heel. The level of pain and swelling is usually greater than the other extra-articular fractures. The patient will be NWB. While radiographs may detect the fracture, CT scans are usually ordered as well to exclude intra-articular extension. Calculating Bohler's angle can assist the clinician in detecting potential fracture displacement. Nondisplaced fractures are treated with NWB and then progression to toe touch weight bearing when tolerated and finally to partial weight bearing for 6–12 weeks.[21] Repeat radiographs are obtained at 10–12 weeks to insure healing.[76]

52.3.1.13.4.6 Calcaneal Intra-articular Fractures Intra-articular fractures are more complicated than extra-articular fractures and account for 65% of all calcaneal fractures.[56] These fractures occur after landing on the heel after a fall from height or a high-energy trauma. Patients will have a more pronounced deformity of the ankle, greater pain, and greater swelling. The increase in swelling leads to increase risk of fracture blisters and increases the risk of compartment syndrome. Anteroposterior, lateral, and oblique radiographs may show fracture. CT scans better characterize the fracture pattern and aid in treatment decision-making. With the high risk of complications from intra-articular fractures, the overwhelming majority of these fractures should be referred to a surgical specialist. Minimally displaced fractures (2 mm or less) can be treated conservatively with immobilization for 4–6 weeks in a removable splint, while fractures displaced more than 2 mm usually require surgical repair.[49] Ågren et al. showed that at 1 year operative and nonoperative treatment yielded similar results, but surgical management had better results at follow-up 8–12 years after treatment.[3]

52.3.1.14 Pediatric

52.3.1.14.1 Sever's Disease (Traction Apophysitis of Calcaneus Insertion of Achilles Tendon)

Patients complain of pain in the posterior heel at the insertion of the Achilles onto the calcaneus. It commonly occurs during growth spurts in preadolescent athletes (8–15 years old) and can affect athletes of all sports but most commonly those requiring a lot of running and jumping (soccer, basketball, tennis, etc.). An activated Achilles tendon applies tension across the apophysis, which results in pain. Treatment includes RICE, heel lifts, activity modification, and a stretching program.[81,87]

52.3.2 Midfoot

52.3.2.1 Overuse

52.3.2.1.1 Os Navicular (Accessory Navicular)

The navicular bone can have a separate ossification center located on the medial aspect of the navicular.[60] There is either a cartilaginous attachment to the navicular, or it is completely separated and can be divided into three types: Type 1 is contained within the posterior tibialis tendon, Type 2 has a fibrocartilaginous attachment, and Type 3 has a bony fusion and produces a prominent protrusion referred to as a cornuate navicular. The posterior tibialis tendon attachment is in the same location, but the os navicular usually only involves a small portion of the insertion of the posterior tibialis tendon. Pain can develop over the os navicular, which is related to improper footwear causing compression over the bony prominence or overuse related to constant tension from the posterior tibialis. Athletes that participate in sports that require constant change in direction and repetitive jumping (soccer, basketball, etc.) are more likely to develop symptoms. Activities where tight shoes are often worn (soccer, ballet, etc.) can also predispose to a symptomatic os navicular. On physical exam, the patient will have pain over the medial plantar navicular and will often have a prominence. Forced dorsiflexion and eversion can sometimes elicit pain as this puts the posterior tibialis tendon under tension. The os is usually seen on radiographs and can often be confused for an avulsion fracture. The absence of an acute injury during the history taking makes an avulsion fracture less likely. If the diagnosis is still in question, then advanced imaging with CT or MRI can differentiate os versus avulsion fracture. MRI offers the advantage of better evaluation of soft tissues such as the posterior tibialis tendon, evaluation of the presence of fibrocartilaginous attachment, and evaluation of bone anatomy for fracture and/or bone marrow edema to suggest acute injury. Initial treatment involves NSAIDs, activity modification, wider shoes, shoe insert to decrease pronation, ice, and physical therapy.[60] Persistent symptoms sometimes require immobilization, and if still painful, surgical excision or percutaneous drilling is an option.[60]

52.3.2.1.2 Os Peroneum

Os peroneum is a small accessory bone located within the peroneus longus tendon as it passes along the cuboid bone.[37,63] It can be found in 4%–30% of normal feet and is usually asymptomatic.[63] The os can be intact or multipartite. Injury to the os peroneum can result in painful os peroneum syndrome and is common after an inversion injury and with prolonged or repetitive activities.[63] Symptoms are common in runners and ballet dancers. Injury to the os peroneum can result in lateral ankle pain due to fracture of the os or injury to the fibrocartilaginous union resulting in diastasis of a multipartite os peroneum.[37,63] Pain can also be located in this area due to peroneus longus tendonitis, cuboid subluxation, or fracture to surrounding bones.[37] Symptoms can also be due to chronic overuse that can be seen with repetitive directional changes and plantar flexion. On exam, there is tenderness located over the lateral foot in the region of the cuboid bone.[37] Pain can be elicited with resisted plantar flexion and eversion. Radiographs can demonstrate os peroneum, but it is sometimes difficult to determine fracture versus bipartite or multipartite os peroneum. Ultrasound can demonstrate tendinosis and can often detect cortical irregularities associated with fracture.[37] Ultrasound is also helpful in evaluating for split peroneal tendon that results in lateral foot pain.[63] MRI is excellent at determining tendinosis, presence of fracture, and injury to the tendon. Treatment for acute injury is usually conservative with immobilization, NSAIDs, and icing, followed by rehab.[37] If symptoms are chronic, then a trial of immobilization is recommended. If conservative measures have failed, then surgical excision and tendon repair is indicated.[37,63] Treatment with a biologic agent such as PRP or prolotherapy can be beneficial and can be used as an alternative to surgery.

52.3.2.1.3 Cuboid Syndrome (Subluxation)

Cuboid subluxation results from laxity of the ligamentous supports that are congenital, as a result of acute injury such as cuboid fracture or repetitive microtrauma that can be seen with dancing, particularly ballet. Subluxation causes pain with plantar flexion or toe-off such as seen with running and ballet. The diagnosis is usually made primarily from the history. Radiographs can sometimes show subluxation. Ultrasound can be useful in demonstrating subluxation. For atraumatic subluxation, the treatment begins with supporting the cuboid with taping, bracing, or orthotics. Manipulation techniques can often be helpful. Subluxation resulting from acute trauma is treated with immobilization and then transitioning to bracing. Rarely is surgery required.

52.3.2.1.4 Navicular Stress Fracture

Navicular stress fractures can occur in any sport with a high demand for running and repetitive jumping.[67] As with any stress fracture abrupt increases in exercise duration or intensity are risk factors for injury. Pain is in the midfoot over the navicular, and there is tenderness on exam in the "N" spot located directly over the dorsal aspect of the navicular.[34,67] Diagnosis is usually delayed with an average time to diagnosis of 4 months.[34] Athletes will usually self-treat with rest and activity modification, which leads to improvement of symptoms only to have symptoms return with full resumption of activity. This leads to a delay in presentation of these athletes for medical treatment. The exam can often be normal as patients have often been resting prior to the office visit and symptoms have abated. Radiographs are usually normal. MRI can demonstrate stress fracture and is helpful in grading stress reaction to complete fracture.[10] CT scan is recommended in differentiating the type of fracture, as this is critical in determining treatment.[10,34,67] The navicular blood supply is from branches of the dorsalis pedis artery and medial plantar artery and creates a watershed region in the central part of the bone making this region at risk for delayed healing and nonunion. Most navicular stress fractures occur in the central third of the navicular in the sagittal plane. Stress reaction without disruption of the cortex and Type 1 stress fracture, which involves one cortex only, can proceed with a trial of conservative treatment with casting or walking boot with NWB for 6–8 weeks followed by progressive weight bearing and advancement of activities.[34,67,77,87] If conservative treatment fails or quick return to play for high-level athletes is desired, then the athlete should proceed with surgical intervention. Type 2 fractures extend into the body of the navicular and type 3 fractures are complete fractures propagating through the entire body.[67]

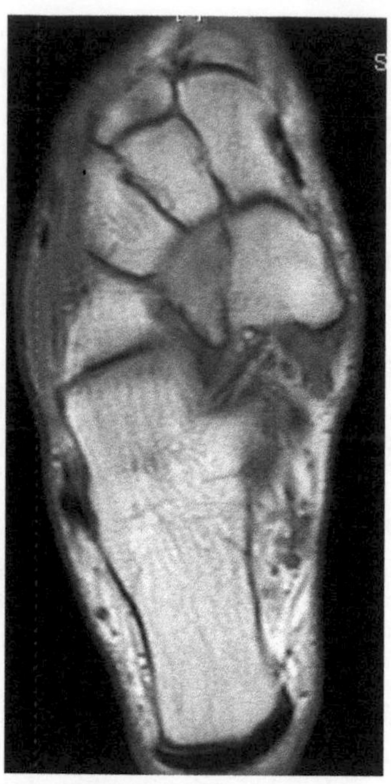

FIGURE 52.5 Navicular fracture—Type 3.

Type 2 and type 3 fractures should be referred for ORIF as these fractures have a high rate of nonunion.[10,34,67] Any fracture with associated sclerosis or avascular necrosis should also be referred for ORIF. See Figure 52.5.

Clinical Pearl

Treatment of navicular fractures depends on the depth of the fracture. CT scan is the current gold standard to identify the anatomy of a navicular fracture.

52.3.2.1.5 Cuboid Stress Fracture

Stress fractures of the cuboid are associated with change in training program or related to footwear (old shoes, abrupt transition to minimalist shoes). Pain is over the lateral foot proximal to the base of the fifth metatarsal over the cuboid. Clinically, there can be tenderness over the cuboid. Radiographs are often negative. MRI can confirm the diagnosis. Cuboid stress fractures are low risk and will heal well with conservative management.

52.3.2.2 Traumatic

52.3.2.2.1 Midfoot Sprain

The midfoot is a stable structure that comprises the navicular, cuboid, and cuneiform bones (medial, middle, and lateral). The interlocking effect of the bones and ligamentous structures make these joints relatively rigid and immobile. The midfoot joins the metatarsals at the tarsal metatarsal joints also referred to as the Lisfranc joint. The second metatarsal is connected to the medial cuneiform by the strong plantar ligament called the Lisfranc ligament. The Lisfranc ligament as well as the bony alignment of the second metatarsal and cuneiform joint supports the arch structure of the midfoot with the second metatarsal cuneiform joint serving as the keystone. The arch-like structure of the midfoot serves to protect the neurovascular structures on the plantar aspect of the foot during weight bearing. The rigidity of the midfoot from the bony configuration and strong ligamentous supports makes a sprain of the midfoot uncommon. When sprains occur, the ligaments supporting the Lisfranc joint are the most common ligaments involved, and the majority of the injuries are located at the base of the first and second metatarsals and involve the Lisfranc ligament.

52.3.2.2.2 Lisfranc Injury

Lisfranc injuries can either be high-velocity or low-velocity injuries.[52,61] Most athletic injuries fall into the low-velocity category, while high-velocity injuries involve excessive forces such as seen in motor vehicle accidents. High-velocity injuries can have multiple complications including compartment syndrome, neurovascular compromise, poor healing, and chronic pain. This discussion will focus on low-velocity injuries that usually occur in athletics.[52,61]

Athletes can incur Lisfranc ligament injuries by hyperplantarflexion of the foot or by an axial load to the foot directed through the heel while the foot is plantarflexed and the metatarsophalangeal joints are dorsiflexed[52] (Figure 52.6). Hyperplantarflexion injuries usually occur when the foot is strapped in place such as windsurfing and horseback riding. This was the original description of the injury by Dr. Jacques Lisfranc as he recognized this injury in Calvary men who fell off the horse but their foot remained in the stirrup.[52] The latter mechanisms of injury can be seen in American football players as they are falling or being tackled and have another player fall on the heel while the foot is plantarflexed. On exam, the athlete will have tenderness over the junction of the medial and middle cuneiform to the base of the first and second

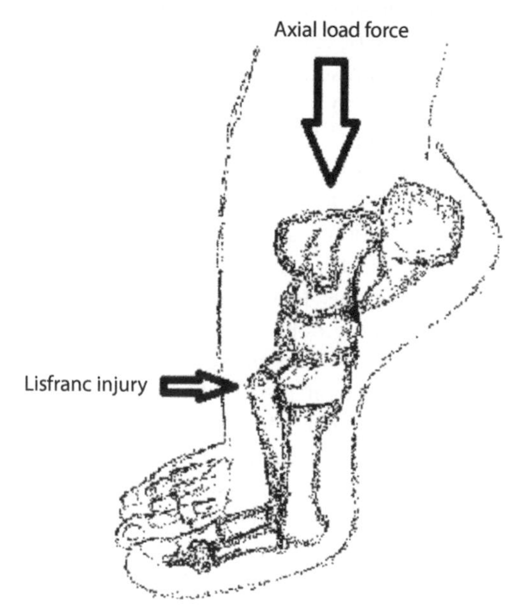

FIGURE 52.6 Mechanism for Lisfranc injury.

metatarsals. In the event of a severe Lisfranc injury, there can be a deformity over the dorsal aspect of the foot where the second metatarsal has subluxed.[52] Compression across the MTP joints as well as moving the forefoot in and out supination and pronation will cause pain with Lisfranc injury.[52] The athlete will have pain with toe rise and will often not be able to complete the task due to pain. Imaging should begin with three views of the foot (AP, lateral, and oblique). Radiographs should be done weight bearing if the patient can tolerate. Weight bearing, bilateral AP views can be very helpful in the diagnosis of Lisfranc injury as it offers a comparison view of the uninjured contralateral foot.[4,52,61] On the AP view, attention should be made to any widening of the space between the base of the first and second metatarsal. Normal spacing is usually 1–2 mm but should also be compared to the contralateral side especially if there is questionable widening.[52] The lateral view should be evaluated for collapse of the midfoot as well as subluxation of the tarsometatarsal joint at the base of the first metatarsal and medial cuneiform that occurs in severe Lisfranc injury. MRI is useful if the diagnosis is unclear from exam and radiographs.[61] Treatment depends on severity of injury, which is classified by the Nunley Classification.[4,52,61] Nunley Stage 1 is stable and can be treated conservatively with cast or walking boot for 6 weeks. The athlete should be NWB for the first 2 weeks and repeat radiographs should be done at 2 weeks to ensure stability of the Lisfranc joint and no increased diastasis. If radiographs demonstrate stability and there is no point tenderness on exam, then weight bearing as tolerated can begin while in a walking boot. If there is point tenderness on exam, then continue with NWB for the remaining 4 weeks. After 6 weeks, the athlete should transition to a well molded orthotic for the next 3–4 months. If the patient falls conservative treatment or has displacement greater than 2 mm or there is a fracture present at the Lisfranc joint, then the patient should be referred to an orthopedic surgeon for operative reduction and fixation (Figure 52.7).[52,61]

52.3.2.2.3 Spring Ligament

The spring ligament, also called the calcaneonavicular ligament, is an important static stabilizer of the medial longitudinal arch and a key to the stability of the hindfoot.[8,88] The spring ligament comprises the inferior calcaneonavicular and superomedial calcaneonavicular ligaments.[8] The spring ligament connects on the plantar surface of the calcaneus and navicular and the body of the ligament supports the head of the talus.[88] Rupture of the spring ligament results in loss of the arch causing flatfoot.[8,33] Rupture is usually seen in degenerative or acquired flat foot in association with posterior tibialis tendon dysfunction.[33] Acute rupture of the spring ligament is uncommon, but when it occurs is usually associated with an eversion injury. Patients will present with pain in the midfoot and pes planus. Degenerative failure of the spring ligament usually presents with bilateral acquired pes planus where as an acute rupture of the spring ligament will have asymmetric pes planus occurring in the affected foot. Additional exam finding might include a valgus heel deformity and "too many toes" sign on the affected foot. Testing of the Achilles and posterior tibialis demonstrates normal strength but the patient is unable to perform a single toe rise. MRI and ultrasound can be used to identify a torn spring ligament.[33,88] Surgical reconstruction is recommended for acute ruptures.[8]

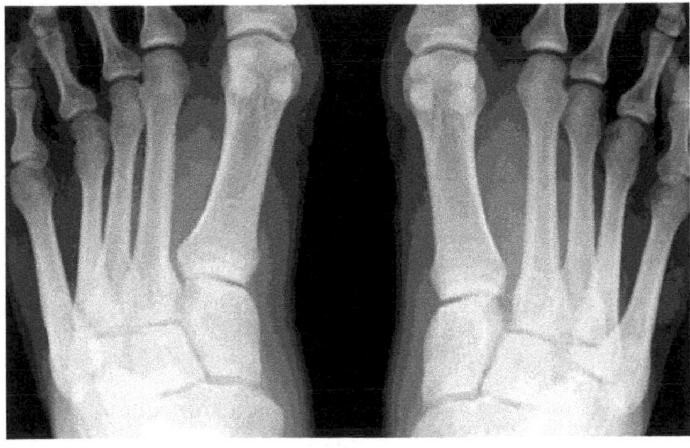

FIGURE 52.7 Lisfranc injury—widening of the right Lisfranc joint.

52.3.2.2.4 Navicular Fractures

The navicular plays an important role in supporting the medial arch of the foot and functions as a keystone. It has cartilage on three sides and articulates with the talus proximally, cuneiforms distally, and cuboid laterally. The distal attachments to the cuneiforms are rigid and are responsible for creating the midfoot arch as discussed earlier (Section 52.3.2.2.2). The proximal talonavicular joint is more mobile and allows for the majority of hindfoot motion. The blood supply is from the dorsalis pedis artery and medial plantar artery. There is a watershed zone in the central third of the bone that can lead to nonunion and avascular necrosis for fracture present in this area. Stress fractures are related to overuse and training errors and are more common in athletics. Avulsion injuries can also be seen in athletics. Other navicular fractures are related to high-velocity injuries (motor vehicle accidents), crush injuries, or falls from heights and are rarely seen in athletics.

52.3.2.2.5 Navicular Avulsion Fracture

Avulsion fractures occur when the foot is forcefully plantar flexed or everted causing stress over the tibionavicular portion of the deltoid ligament or tibialis posterior tendon, respectively. An eversion force with or without dorsiflexion can result in a plantar avulsion fracture from tension placed on the navicular from the spring ligament; however, this is rare. Imaging begins with three views of the foot. A navicular accessory bone can be confused for a fracture. This can be differentiated by sharp margins associated with a fracture versus smooth rounded margins of an accessory bone. Comparison views can also be helpful as accessory bones are often bilateral. Avulsion fractures are usually treated conservatively with casting or walking boot. If conservative treatment fails, there is significant displacement of the avulsed bone, there is a large bone fragment extending into the body of the navicular, or the patient is a high-level athlete, then a referral should be made to orthopedics for evaluation of ORIF.

52.3.2.2.6 Navicular Body Fracture

Acute fractures of the body of the navicular are rare in athletics as these fractures usually result from high-velocity axial load injuries such as motor vehicle accidents or from a crush injury. Navicular body fractures are divided into three types. Type 1 fractures are transversely oriented and divide the navicular into dorsal and plantar portions. Type 2 fractures are obliquely oriented and run dorsolateral to plantarmedial. Type 2 fractures are the most common body fracture and result from an axial load. The talonavicular joint is often injured concurrently with a Type 2 fracture. Type 3 fractures are comminuted and displaced and result from a laterally directed force. Associated injuries include naviculocuneiform and calcaneocuboid joint disruption as well as cuboid and anterior calcaneal fractures. Navicular body fractures often have other associated fractures or ligament injury that can lead to an unstable midfoot. Due to the importance of the navicular and the ligamentous attachments to the structural integrity of the midfoot and proper hindfoot mobility, it is imperative for proper alignment and healing. There is also risk of nonunion from poor blood supply and malunion from the high-velocity injury that is associated with these fractures. It is recommended that acute fractures of the body of the navicular be referred for evaluation of ORIF.

52.3.2.2.7 Navicular Tuberosity Fracture

Tuberosity fractures usually occur from an eversion or rotational force on the ankle and with forced dorsiflexion, which puts tension on the tibialis posterior attachment. Treatment of a tuberosity fracture depends on the size and displacement of the fracture fragment. Small fractures that are non-displaced (<2–3 mm), and no other associated injury can be treated conservatively with casting or short leg walking boot for 6–8 weeks. Larger fractures that extend into the body or are significantly displaced (>2–3 mm) should be referred for evaluation of ORIF.

52.3.2.2.8 Cuboid Fracture

Cuboid fractures caused by a compressive force are often associated with other midfoot injuries such as tarsal metatarsal fracture dislocation, subtalar fracture dislocation, navicular fractures, and Chopart's fracture dislocation. This is due to the lateral and medial columns of the foot functioning in concert and transmitting force throughout the mid-foot from a compressive force. Isolated cuboid fractures usually result from a nutcracker effect generated by force applied from the fourth and fifth metatarsal and calcaneus when the foot is forcefully plantar flexed and everted.[21] Fractures are often detected on radiographs of the foot but usually require CT for better appreciation of anatomy and for determining appropriate treatment. Nondisplaced extra-articular fractures are usually treated with cast or walking boot immobilization and transitioning to post-op shoe or hard sole walking shoe as symptoms improve. Displaced and intra-articular fracture should be referred for evaluation of open reduction and internal fixation.[21]

52.3.2.2.9 Cuneiform Fracture

The cuneiform bones (medial, middle, and lateral) have various ligamentous attachments that help form the arch of the midfoot and give the foot structural stability. Cuneiform fractures are usually the result of direct trauma, but stress fractures can occur. Isolated fractures of the cuneiform bones are rare as there is usually a ligament injury (i.e., Section 52.3.2.2.2 as discussed earlier).[1] Patients have swelling in the midfoot and tenderness over the affected cuneiform. Foot radiographs including AP, lateral, and oblique views are the standard first-line imaging studies followed by MRI if there is concern for occult fracture, stress injury, or ligament injury. Isolated fractures of the cuneiforms can be managed conservatively with walking boot or cast for 4–6 weeks with weight bearing as tolerated. Immobilization can be followed with orthotics to support the arch for the next 4–6 months during rehab and gradual return to sports. Comminuted and displaced fractures as well as fractures associated with dislocation and ligament injury should be splinted and referred to an orthopedic foot specialist.[21]

52.3.2.3 Pediatric

52.3.2.3.1 Kohler Disease

Kohler bone disease is an osteochondrosis of the navicular bone. It typically affects young patients between the ages of 2 and 9 years.[28] Kohler disease affects male children more commonly than female children.[5] The exact etiology is unknown but several risk factors have been proposed: trauma with disruption of the blood supply, poor nutrition, endocrine dysfunction, infection, and inflammation. The dorsalis pedis and medial plantar arteries constitute the bulk of the navicular bone's blood supply.[48] Typically the pain is unilateral, but there have been reports of bilateral disease. The child presents with a complaint of midfoot pain with or without a limp. Many patients will deny a history of trauma to the area. Physical exam will show tenderness over the navicular bone and possible swelling.[5] Range of motion is normal. Radiographs of the foot will show navicular sclerosis, fragmentation, or flattening.[5,28] MRI can be useful if there is a question as to the diagnosis. Bone scintigraphy can be useful in diagnosis as it can show a photopenic area early in the disease prior to radiographic changes and can show increase uptake later in the disease process indicating revascularization.[48] Other diagnoses in the differential include ankle sprain, fracture, infection, and reactive arthritis. Treatment methods vary, but all patients experience full recovery. Casting with a short leg cast for 6–8 weeks has been shown to decrease the time to full recovery considerably.[5,48] Since all patients experience full recovery, there are no long-term sequela, but persistent pain can be a complication if the patient is noncompliant with activity restrictions.[95]

52.3.2.3.2 Traction Apophysitis of the Navicular

Symptoms consist of pain located over the medial portion of the navicular at the insertion of the tibialis posterior tendon. Risks include growth spurts and sports that require a lot of running, jumping, and change of direction. The accessory navicular and associated physis usually forms around age 9. Younger patients are treated with RICE, heel lifts, activity modification, and a stretching program. Older patients are treated as per recommendations for Os Navicular.

52.3.2.3.3 *Tarsal Coalition*

Tarsal coalitions are abnormal bony or fibrocartilaginous unions between two tarsal bones most commonly between the calcaneus and navicular or talus and calcaneus. Although many patients are born with these unions, they do not typically become symptomatic until adolescence. Symptoms usually develop between the ages of 8 and 16 years when the coalition starts to ossify. Patients have a painful, stiff, flat foot, and about half the time symptoms are bilateral. Patients can suffer from recurrent ankle sprains as the ankle is under more stress due to a rigid foot. Bony coalitions can be seen on radiographs. MRI can be used if there is suspicion and radiographs are normal as an MRI will demonstrate both bony and fibrocartilaginous unions.[81] Treatment involves RICE, orthotics, and activity modification. If symptoms persist and are interfering with activities, then the patient can proceed with surgical resection of the coalition.

52.3.3 Fore Foot

52.3.3.1 Overuse

52.3.3.1.1 *Morton's Neuroma*

Morton's neuroma is also known as Morton's neuralgia, Morton's metatarsalgia, plantar neuroma, and intermetatarsal neuroma.[66] It is commonly found in individuals who participate in running, dancing, and aerobics. It is most commonly found in middle-aged females.[41,45] It can be precipitated by wearing narrow toed shoes and high heels. The exact mechanism of injury is still unclear, but several theories have been proposed: compression of the nerve by an enlarged intermetatarsal bursa, repeated trauma to the interdigital nerve at the transverse metatarsal ligament, ischemia of the plantar digital artery, entrapment of the interdigital nerve by the transverse metatarsal ligament during ambulation, and compression of the third intermetatarsal space during ambulation with an over pronated foot.[41,45,66] Although it is called a neuroma, histologic evaluation has shown demyelination, perineural fibrosis, epineural fibrosis, and degenerative vascular changes.[45]

Patients often present with pain in the third web space, between the third and fourth metatarsals.[41,45] The pain is typically worse when wearing narrow toed shoes. The pain may be associated with paresthesia of the third and fourth toes. The patient may have the sensation of walking on a pebble or something is their shoe. On exam, the patient may have tenderness to direct palpation of the plantar aspect of the third web space. Swelling may be palpable. Compressing all the metatarsals with lateral force may elicit pain. A positive Mulder's click may be present with medial to lateral compression.[41] While typically located in the third intermetatarsal space, Morton's neuroma can be present in other web spaces or in multiple web spaces. Radiographs are obtained to rule out other etiologies. Advanced imaging such as ultrasound and MRI are useful if the diagnosis is unclear or multiple neuromas are suspected.[41] The differential diagnosis includes metatarsal stress fractures. Treatment of Morton's neuroma begins with footwear modification, lower heels, metatarsal pads, anti-inflammatory medication, and orthotics.[41] Corticosteroid injections directly into the web space have been beneficial. Surgical intervention focuses on decompression or excision.[45] While typically used in persistent cases, some researchers advocate operative treatment as first-line therapy.[41] Complications of surgery are rare and include persistent pain, incomplete surgical excision, and recurrence.[45]

52.3.3.1.2 *Hallux Rigidus*

Hallux rigidus is degenerative arthritis of the first metatarsophalangeal joint.[54,55,62] It typically occurs in the sixth decade of life and is more common in females than males. It is characterized by pain at the first MTP joint with associated limited range of motion especially limited dorsiflexion.[54,55] The osteoarthritis begins dorsally with associated osteophyte formation.[17,55] The osteophytes on the head of the first metatarsal restrict the motion of the first proximal phalanx. Patients will present with pain and swelling of the first MTP joint. They may complain of pain with toeing off or decreased range of motion. On exam, the patient will have a painful swollen joint. They may have a dorsal bony prominence. This bony prominence may be erythematous caused by irritation from their shoe wear. They will have limited dorsiflexion. Anterior–posterior, lateral, and oblique x-rays should be obtained. The radiographs will show decreased joint space between the proximal phalanx and metatarsal with osteophyte formation. Advanced imaging is not necessary to make the diagnosis. Treatment is conservative with nonsteroidal anti-inflammatories, ice, and activity modification as first-line treatments.[55] Patients can be advised to switch to a hard soled shoe, rocker bottom shoes, or firm orthotics to limit dorsiflexion of the first MTP joint and thereby decrease pain symptoms.[54,55] Corticosteroid injections can be administered in difficult cases.[55] Surgical intervention for cases that fail conservative measures includes cheilectomy, osteotomy, arthroplasty, or arthrodesis.[54,55,62] Cheilectomy and osteotomy are performed on mild cases of osteoarthritis, while arthroplasty and arthrodesis are typically performed on moderate-to-severe cases.[16,54,55,62]

52.3.3.1.3 *Hallux Valgus*

Hallux valgus is a rare condition in athletes but has been reported to be the most common forefoot problem in adults.[36] It is associated with high heel use, narrow toed shoes, and constricting footwear. Other risk factors include pes planus, hindfoot pronation, Achilles tendon contracture, and genetic predisposition. It is much more common in adult females than males. It is a progressive deformity characterized by lateral deviation of the great toe with medial deviation of the first metatarsal. Advanced cases can have subluxation of the first metatarsophalangeal joint.[36] Medial deviation of the first metatarsal creates pressure on the head of the metatarsal. This pressure causes local irritation, erythema, and pain of the overlying tissues. The body may respond by forming an exostosis, which produces the characteristic "bunion" associated with this condition.

Patients will present with painful red first metatarsal head. The pain is usually worse with footwear or with activity. On exam, the patient will have a laterally deviated great toe that may become more deviated with standing. The head of the first metatarsal may have a bony prominence and the overlying tissue may be erythematous. There may be hyperkeratosis of the overlying skin. The first ray may be hypermobile at the metatarsocuneiform joint.[19] The patient's feet should be examined in both the sitting and standing positions to evaluate for pes planus and hyperpronation. The patient's footwear should be examined for wear patterns. Weight-bearing radiographs should be obtained, which help rule out other diagnoses as well as classify the severity of the hallux valgus deformity. The severity is gauged by two angle measurements. The intersecting lines of the proximal phalanx and the first metatarsal create the hallux valgus angle. The other measurement is the intermetatarsal angle, which is the angle between the first and second metatarsals. Advanced imaging is not required to make the diagnosis. The differential includes turf toe and stress fracture. Initial treatment is nonoperative and includes shoe wear modification, anti-inflammatory medication, analgesics, orthotics, physical therapy, and bunion pads. Patients should wear shoes with wider toe boxes. Orthotics may help correct hyperpronation and pes planus, but have not been shown to prevent progression of hallux valgus deformity. Physical therapy helps with Achilles tendon contractures. Corticosteroid injections may be helpful in tough cases. Due to the unpredictable nature of surgical treatment, high-level athletes should exhaust all conservative measure before proceeding with surgical intervention. Surgical intervention for athletes may consist of a distal chevron osteotomy with or without a closing wedge osteotomy of the proximal phalanx. Arthrodesis, arthroplasty, and proximal osteotomies are more extensive surgical procedures and should be avoided in athletes due to the risk of decreased range of motion, impaired foot function, and prolonged healing times. Surgery can lead to over correction of the deformity in those who are skeletally immature. There is also a risk of persistent pain, activity intolerance, and continued need for orthotics and shoe wear modifications. Complications of hallux valgus include persistent pain, sesamoid subluxation, great toe proximal phalanx stress fractures, and lateral foot pain.[96] Proper-fitting shoes are one method of prevention as well as correcting pes planus and hindfoot pronation.[70]

52.3.3.1.4 Metatarsalgia

Metatarsalgia refers to pain under the plantar aspects of the metatarsal heads of the second, third, and fourth toes. It is a common overuse injury from repetitive microtrauma. Runners and individuals who participate in high-impact aerobics are patient populations at risk for developing metatarsalgia.[18] Young adult females are most likely to be affected. There is an association of metatarsalgia and high heel use, hypermobile first ray, posteriorly displaced sesamoids, hallux valgus, and short great toe or first metatarsal. The mechanism of injury is altered gait mechanics with increased repetitive stress applied to the metatarsal heads of the lesser toes.

Patients will present with forefoot pain and swelling. The pain is typically worsened by activity. On exam, the patient will have tenderness to palpation of one or more of the metatarsal heads on the plantar aspect of the foot. Clinicians should evaluate for callus formation under the metatarsals and check for cavus deformity or hallux valgus.[23] The patient's footwear should be examined for any abnormal wear pattern. Radiographs are necessary to evaluate for other causes of forefoot pain such as stress fractures, Freiberg's disease, posterior sesamoid displacement, or short first metatarsals. Treatment is conservative and incorporates proper-fitting shoes, avoidance of high heels, analgesia, metatarsal pads, orthotics, and anti-inflammatory medications. If a patient has significant callus formation, then paring down the callus may be necessary.[23] Most patients respond to conservative measures; but if a patient has exhausted all modalities, then referral is warranted. By wearing appropriate footwear and gradual increasing exercise and training regimens, most patients can avoid developing metatarsalgia.

52.3.3.1.5 Morton's Toe

Morton's toe is a metatarsalgia of the second metatarsal caused by a short first metatarsal or elongated second metatarsal. This changes the mechanics of the foot and puts additional pressure on the second metatarsal head. Additionally, patients may size their shoes off the first digit and not the longer second toe. This creates impact on the longest toe and increases pressure on the metatarsal. Patients who participate in high-impact aerobics or running may experience pain with repetitive overloading of the second metatarsal head from plantarflexing the foot and extending the toes. Patients will present with forefoot pain that is worse with activity. On exam, the patient will be tender to palpation at the second metatarsal head. There may be callus formation. The second toe may be visibly longer than the first toe. Radiographs are obtained to rule out other pathology such as stress fracture. Treatment consists of shoe wear modification, metatarsal pads, and analgesia. Rocker bottom shoes or shoes that limit flexion of the forefoot may be beneficial. If patients fail conservative treatment or have persistent pain, surgical referral is warranted.

52.3.3.2 Traumatic

52.3.3.2.1 Turf Toe

First described in 1976 by researchers at West Virginia University, turf toe is a strain or tear of the capsular ligaments of the first metatarsophalangeal joint.[15,27] It is a common injury among football players.[27] The mechanism of injury is an axial load applied to an equinus foot with the great toe in extension[15] (Figure 52.8). The great toe is then forced into hyperextension disrupting the capsular structures.[4,15,27] There is an increased risk of injury on artificial surfaces compared

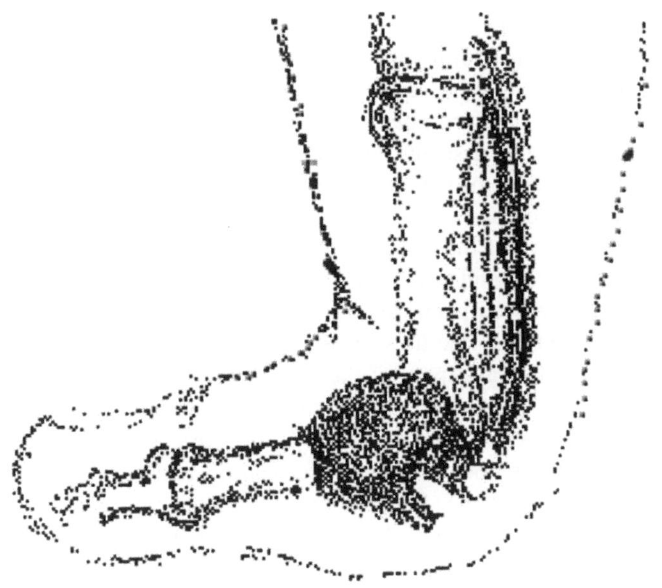

FIGURE 52.8 Mechanism for turf toe injury.

to natural grass.[27] Patients will present with great toe pain. On exam, the athlete may have swelling and ecchymosis of the first MTP joint. There will be tenderness to palpation at the first MTP joint. Pain may be provoked by extension. Valgus and varus stresses should be applied to the joint to evaluate stability. AP and lateral radiographs are obtained and are usually negative but may show avulsion injuries. A lateral radiograph with the great toe dorsiflexed may show distal migration of the sesamoids, which can indicate a more serious injury. MRI investigation is needed for suspected partial or complete ligamentous tears.[4,15] Treatment is based on the classification of the injury.[4] Grade I injuries are mild injuries that have minimal ecchymosis and localized swelling. The capsular structures are intact. Treatment is to reduce pain symptoms and athletes can return to play as pain allows. Grade II injuries involve a partial tear of the plantar capsular structures with restricted motion.[15] Treatment involves walking boot and weight bearing as tolerated as well as rest, ice, elevation, and analgesia. It may take up to 14 days for athletes to resume full athletic participation. Grade III injuries involve the complete tear of the plantar ligamentous complex. These injuries are treated with long-term immobilization in either a cast or walking boot and NWB for 8 weeks. Afterward, there is a slow progression of activity with full recovery taking up to 6 months. Surgical intervention may be needed in some cases of grade III injuries.

52.3.3.2.2 Toe Dislocation

Toe dislocations result from hyperextension or hyperflexion after the toe is axially loaded as can occur during kicking. Most occur with hyperextension and the dislocation is usually dorsal. Dislocations can occur at the interphalangeal or metatarsophalangeal joint. Examination demonstrates a malaligned toe, and three-view radiographs (AP, lateral, and oblique) of the toe can confirm the diagnosis. Radiographs are important to rule out associated fractures, and postreduction

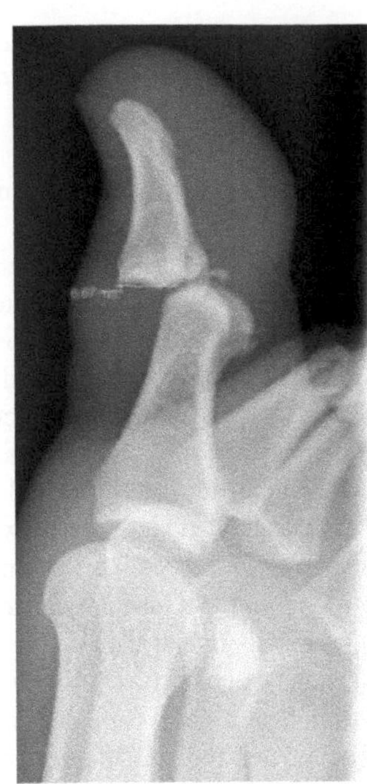

FIGURE 52.9 Great toe IP joint dislocation.

radiographs should be obtained to verify alignment and evaluate for injury associated with reduction. A ring block (digital nerve block) can be performed prior to reduction for comfort. Reduction is obtained with traction in the longitudinal plane with hyperflexion (for the most common dorsal dislocation) just prior to the application of traction. After reduction, the toes are buddy taped for 3–4 weeks.[21] Entrapment of soft tissue can cause closed reduction to be unsuccessful and open reduction is required. After reduction, the joint should be examined to evaluate for ligament stability (shown in Figure 52.9).

52.3.3.3 Toenail Injury

52.3.3.3.1 Subungual Hematoma

Subungual hematoma is a collection of blood under the nail. Toe subungual hematomas can occur as a result of direct trauma to the toe (i.e., dumbbell falling on toe) or from a constant shear force of the nail and nail plate due to long periods of running in tight shoes (i.e., marathon). Subungual hematomas are painful and the hematomas related to direct trauma tend to be more painful than those due to shear forces. Some authors recommend treating subungual hematomas that involve less than 50% of the nail with simple trephination and those involving greater than 50% of the nail with removing the nail, extensive irrigation, and repair of the nail plate if present and then replacement of the nail. There are several studies that have compared nail removal, irrigation and repair to simple triphenation regardless of size of the subungual hematoma and there was no difference between treatment groups as far as healing and cosmesis as long as the nail margins are intact.[74,80] Nail removal, irrigation, and repair have also been recommended when associated with a fracture as well as antibiotics for infection prophylaxis. There is a double-blind, randomized placebo-controlled trial by Stevenson et al. that showed no difference in infections with the addition of antibiotics versus standard wound care.[84]

52.3.3.3.2 Ingrown Toenail

Ingrown toenail or onychocryptosis is a common soft tissue problem of the foot and predominantly affects the great toe.[38,97] Risk factors include improper trimming of the nail, tight-fitting footwear, trauma, and obesity.[38] These risk factors lead to irritation along the nail border and cause the nail to fit poorly within the nail groove. Inflammation of the nail fold and subsequent hypertrophy of the soft tissue results from the constant irritation and trauma.[97] The improper fit of the nail in the nail fold allows for foreign material to be introduced to the nail groove, which is often followed by infection. Patients present with swelling and pain along the nail border and often have drainage. Gait can be affected due to pain and patients have tenderness along the nail border.[38] Treatment depends on severity of the ingrown toenail. Mild-to-moderate lesions that have no signs of infection, minimal erythema, and minimal pain can be treated with gutter splint, cotton wisps applied under the nail edge, warm water soaks (with mild soap or sitz salts), and topical antibiotic ointment.[38,97] If conservative therapies fail, then the patient should proceed with partial nail removal, which involves removing 25% of the affected nail edge.[38,97] Caution should be taken to make sure the entire portion of the nail edge is removed as remnants can lead to a nail spicule and continued symptoms.[97] Antibiotics are not necessary in most cases although they are commonly prescribed as infections are usually contained to the nail groove, which is effectively drained with partial nail removal. Antibiotics should be prescribed if soft tissue infection is suspected. The patient should be instructed on proper nail maintenance including cutting the nail straight without rounded edges and appropriately fitting foot wear to prevent recurrence.[97] If there is recurrence, then the matrix can be destroyed along with the removal of the nail edge with agents such as phenol or silver nitrate.[38]

52.3.3.3.3 Toenail Avulsion

Toenail avulsion can occur with a crush injury or direct trauma to the nail that lifts the nail off the toe, which can occur during an axial load injury. Avulsions can occur on any nail border. The nail and nail bed should be gently but thoroughly irrigated. The nail matrix should be repaired if damaged, and the nail is then placed back in position and anchored with sutures. If the avulsion involves the proximal nail, the repair of the germinal matrix is imperative to ensure continued nail growth. Chronic nail avulsions can be seen in runners and associated with old, large subungual hematomas and should not be anchored. Proper trimming of the nail and bandaging of the toe during competition can prevent an acute chronic avulsion.

52.3.3.4 Metatarsal Fractures (Metatarsals 1–4)

52.3.3.4.1 Metatarsal Shaft Fracture 1–4

Most metatarsal shaft fractures result from a direct blow to the dorsal foot (i.e., dumbbell dropped on foot), and some are due to a twisting mechanism. First metatarsal shaft fractures require excessive force due to girth and strength. Alignment of the first metatarsal is important as it plays a significant role in the structural support of the arch of the foot and has a significant role in weight bearing. Fractures of the shaft of metatarsals 2–4 are able to tolerate slightly more misalignment than the first and tend to be more stable due to the splinting effect of the adjacent metatarsal. The tension from the intrinsic muscle and flexor tendons of the toes can cause displacement of the fracture. Displacement is more common of metatarsal head fracture where the metatarsal head is commonly displaced plantarly. Arterial injury is a concern with first metatarsal fractures as the dorsalis pedis artery runs along the lateral aspect of the first metatarsal and branches at the base of the first metatarsal into the arcuate artery and later branches to form the deep plantar artery.[21] Injuries to these arteries could compromise healing and lead to compartment syndrome. Patients usually present with a swollen foot and difficulty with bearing weight or they cannot bear weight. Patient is tender over the metatarsal and has pain with axial loading. Pain with axial loading is more indicative of a fracture instead of soft tissue injury alone. Radiographs of the foot (AP, lateral, and oblique) are usually sufficient in identifying the fracture. Nondisplaced fractures are placed in a posterior ankle splint with follow-up in 7–10 days for repeat radiographs for assess for stability. Fractures that are stable are treated with a short leg walking boot (or cast) for 3–4 weeks followed by an additional 2–4 weeks of a post-op shoe or firm-soled shoe.[21] Fractures with more than 10° of dorsal/plantar angulation should be reduced or referred for reduction. Comminuted fractures, fractures displaced more than 3 mm and fractures that are rotated should be referred to an orthopedist. The skin over the dorsal foot is thin and very close to the metatarsal, which makes the skin susceptible to injury. Open fracture should be emergently referred and fractures associated with skin injury that could lead to necrosis should be urgently referred.[21]

52.3.3.4.2 Metatarsal Stress Fracture

Metatarsal stress fractures are a common problem in athletics and can affect any of the metatarsals.[13] The fifth metatarsal will be discussed separately in the following text. The most common metatarsal stress fracture involves the second and third metatarsals.[13] The second is the most common and is often referred to as a "marcher's fracture" due to the high incidence in military recruits.[13] It is also seen in athletes, especially runners, who change their activities or training regimen abruptly. Symptoms usually begin as mild pain with activities that steadily progress unless modifications are made in the athletes' training.[13] Patients usually have tenderness over the affected metatarsal and can have pain when a vibrating tuning fork is placed over the affected metatarsal (tuning fork test). As with most stress fractures, radiographs are often normal with early stress injury and MRI may be required for diagnosis. These fractures usually heal well with activity modification.[13] Patient's activity should be reduced to a level that is nonpainful. Patients decrease activity to walking only. If there is pain with walking, then the patients are to be NWB in a boot or cast. After 1–2 weeks of NWB, the

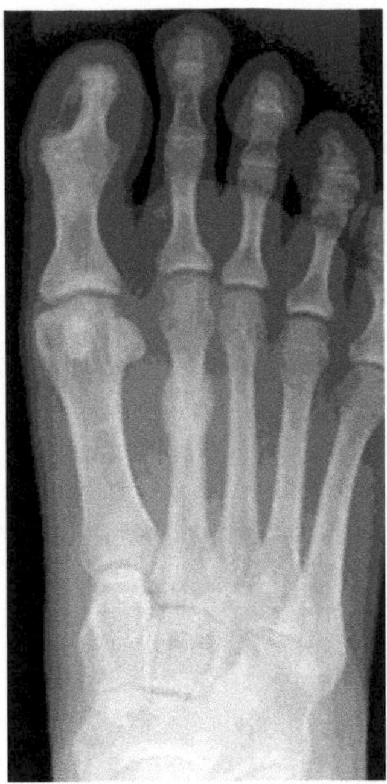

FIGURE 52.10 Second metatarsal stress fracture.

patient can gradually increase weight bearing as long as there is no pain. After 1–2 weeks of pain-free walking in a boot or cast, gradual increase in activity can be started. Care must be taken to not resume activities too quickly as this can lead in recurrence. Pool exercises are an excellent way to maintain cardiovascular conditioning while maintaining NWB status (i.e., swimming or running in the deep end of the pool with a life vest). The base of the second metatarsal stress fractures, also called dancer's fracture due to its high incidence in ballet from en pointe stance, can require more care as there is a higher risk for delayed union and nonunion.[13] Symptoms can last 3 months or more and require longer period of immobilization and a prolonged return to activities.[13] The base of the fourth metatarsal can be equally as challenging due to delayed healing and prolonged symptoms. Initial treatment involves NWB immobilization with walking boot or cast with gradual progression to weight bearing.[39] See Figure 52.10.

52.3.3.5 Fifth Metatarsal Fracture

52.3.3.5.1 Distal Fifth Metatarsal Fracture

Metatarsal neck fractures are usually the result of direct trauma. Nondisplaced fractures heal well with a walking boot or post-op shoe for 4 weeks and then transitioning to a firm-soled shoe. Displaced fracture should be reduced as this can lead to pain with weight bearing if the fracture heals angulated. Closed reduction or surgery should be performed for displaced fractures.

52.3.3.5.2 Shaft Fracture of the Fifth Metatarsal

Shaft fractures of the fifth metatarsal are also known as dancer's fracture. Some author's refer to avulsion fractures (discussed in the following paragraphs) as a dancer's fracture as there is a high incidence of this injury in the performing arts; however, for the discussion of fifth metatarsal fractures, the terminology "dancer's fracture" will be reserved for the fifth metatarsal shaft fractures (dancer's fracture has also been used to refer to stress fractures of the proximal second metatarsal). The mechanism of the fracture is an inversion injury while the ankle in plantarflexed. This is common in ballet when the injury occurs while the dancer is en pointe. The injury results in a spiral fracture of the shaft of the fifth metatarsal. Patients have difficulty bearing weight and have tenderness over the midportion of the fifth metatarsal. The injury is usually accompanied by swelling and ecchymosis. Fractures are initially treated with splinting and RICE. Nondisplaced fractures are followed up in 1 week for repeat radiographs. Stable fractures are treated with a walking boot or casting for 4 weeks with weight bearing as tolerated and then transitioned to a post-op shoe or firm-soled shoe for an additional 4 weeks. Radiographs should be repeated at 4–6 weeks to evaluated healing. Closed reduction can be attempted on displaced fractures. If reduction is obtained, then the patient is placed in a walking boot or cast and is NWB for 4 weeks followed by 4 weeks of protected weight bearing in a walking boot or cast.[21] Reduced fractures should have repeat radiographs at 1 week to evaluate stability and again at 4–6 weeks to evaluate healing. Unstable displaced fracture and nonunion will require ORIF. Open fractures and fractures associated with neurovascular injury need acute surgical evaluation.

52.3.3.5.3 Base of the Fifth Fracture

Fractures of the proximal fifth metatarsal can be difficult to treat.[22] The level of activity of the patient as well as the location of the fracture should be considered when determining the treatment for fifth metatarsal fractures.[47] Fractures can occur with acute injury usually involving an inversion injury of the ankle. Fractures can also be the result of repetitive microtrauma that results in the formation of a stress reaction.[22] The blood supply to the base of the fifth metatarsal involves several small metaphyseal arteries that enter at the tuberosity and a nutrient vessel that enters at the proximal diaphysis. This creates a watershed region in the metaphyseal–diaphyseal junction, and as a result, fractures in this area have a tendency for poor healing. The base of the fifth metatarsal is broken down into three zones: Zone 1 involves the tuberosity, zone 2 is located at the fourth and fifth metatarsal intersection (approximately 1.5 cm distal from the tuberosity), and zone 3 is in the proximal diaphysis just past the fourth and fifth metatarsal junction[47,71] (Figure 52.11). The diagnosis can be delayed, as patients do not immediately present for medical evaluation because they believe they have only sprained their ankle.

52.3.3.5.4 Avulsion Fractures of the Fifth Metatarsal (Zone 1)

Avulsion fractures involve the tuberosity of the fifth metatarsal.[22,71] The peroneus brevis and lateral band of the plantar fascia inserts on the tuberosity. With forced inversion of the foot, the lateral band of the plantar fascia can create tension to the tuberosity resulting in an avulsion fracture.[71] Patients will have pain with ambulation and have tenderness at the base of the fifth

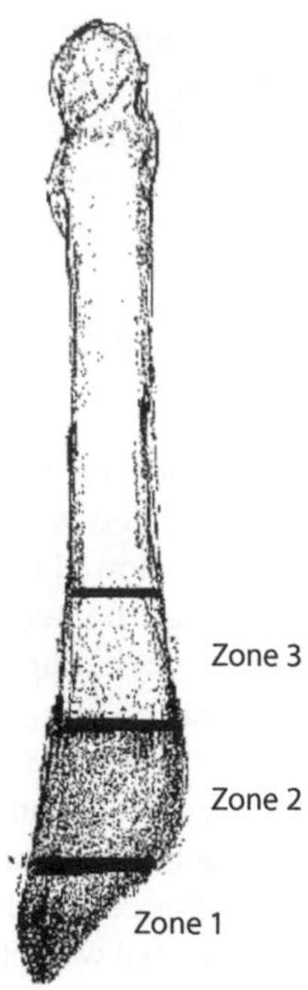

FIGURE 52.11 Base of the fifth metatarsal zones.

metatarsal. Imaging studies include AP, lateral, and oblique radiographs. Advanced imaging is rarely required. This fracture is usually minimally displaced, and there is good blood supply to the tuberosity, which allows for good healing with conservative treatment.[47,71] Treatments can vary from a post-op shoe to a walking boot for 4–8 weeks with weight bearing as tolerated.[71] Crutches are used to assist ambulation until the patient can bear weight without pain. Average time for bone union is 6–8 weeks and return to play can be 8–12 weeks. If the fracture is displaced more than 3 mm or nonunion at 12 weeks, then the patient should be considered for ORIF[47,71] (see Figure 52.12).

52.3.3.5.5 Fractures at the Metaphyseal–Diaphyseal Junction: Jones Fracture (Zone 2)

Fractures at the base of the fifth metatarsal in the metaphyseal–diaphyseal junction are known as Jones fractures as Sir Robert Jones first described this fracture in 1902.[47,57,68] The fracture results from an inversion ankle injury typically when the foot is adducted and inverted while the ankle is in plantar flexion.[68] Stress fractures can also occur in this area.[68] A varus hindfoot can be a predisposing risk factor to Jones fracture.[68] This injury occurs at the junction of the fourth and fifth metatarsal, which is a vascular watershed area, and due to this poor blood supply, Jones fractures are associated with delayed healing and nonunion.[22,57,68] Patients are tender over the base of the fifth metatarsal and often have a focal point of tenderness approximately 1.5 cm distal to the tuberosity. Nonoperative management of Jones fractures is an option, but conservative treatment is associated with delayed healing and a high rate of nonunion; some studies suggest failed conservative treatment in 44% of patients.[22,47,57] Conservative management varies based on expert opinion but usually consists of 4–6 weeks of NWB in a cast or walking boot followed by 4–8 weeks of immobilization with gradual increase in weight bearing as tolerated.[22,47] Nonoperative management is associated with delayed union and a high risk of nonunion; therefore, ORIF is recommend for most Jones fractures.[22,47,57,68] Nonoperative management should be reserved for those patients that are not good surgical candidates. ORIF typically consists of an intramedullary screw; however if this is not possible, then tension wire is a viable alternative[22,47] (depicted in Figure 52.13).

52.3.3.5.6 Proximal Diaphysis (Zone 3)

Fractures in the proximal diaphysis of the fifth metatarsal are often associated with stress fracture. These fractures are

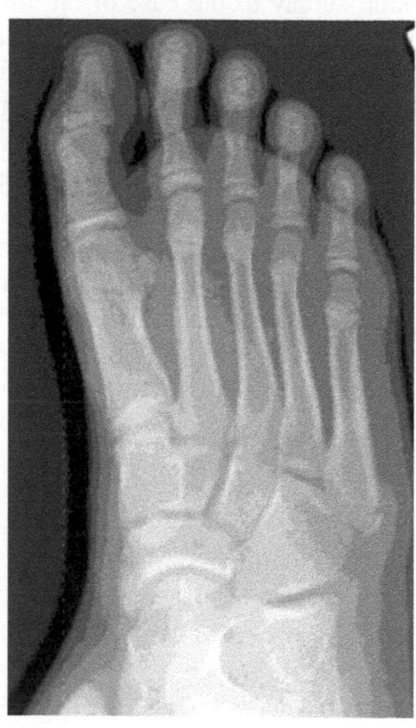

FIGURE 52.12 Avulsion fracture at the base of the fifth metatarsal.

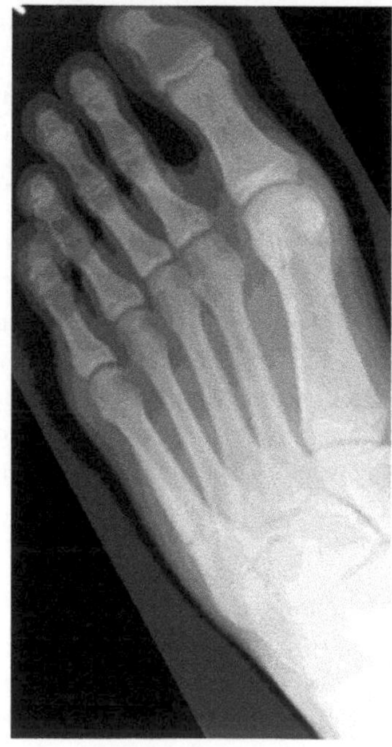

FIGURE 52.13 Jones fracture of the base of the fifth metatarsal.

associated with abrupt changes in training, footwear, mechanics of running, and nutritional status. These fractures can present after an acute injury such as an inversion ankle sprain.[22,85] The fractures often present as prodromal pain in the lateral foot. The injury can be on a gradient of stress reaction to complete fracture. The patient will have tenderness at the base of the fifth metatarsal. A vibrating tuning fork placed over the base of the fifth metatarsal will illicit pain if there is a stress injury present. Imaging studies begin with radiographs and include AP, lateral, and oblique views of the foot. Early stress fractures and stress reactions sometimes are not seen on plain films and an MRI is needed for further evaluation. Reviews are mixed regarding treatment options for fractures in the proximal diaphysis.[47] The nutrient vessel is usually distal to the fracture site and blood supply can be poor in this region as is the case for Jones fracture. As with any fracture that is located in an area of poor blood supply, there can be delayed union and nonunion, and many studies suggest similar healing rates as a Jones fracture.[22] It is becoming more common to address these fractures with ORIF similar to Jones fractures due to the high rate of nonunion and delayed healing associated with conservative management.[22,47] Early stress fractures and stress reactions are treated with casting or walking boot.[47] If they have pain with protected weight bearing, then a period of NWB for 4–6 weeks followed by gradual weight bearing as tolerated for an additional 4–8 weeks is recommended. If the patient is still symptomatic or no radiographic evidence of healing is seen at 12 weeks, then the patient should be considered for ORIF.[47] Athletes with complete fractures should be referred for ORIF.[22] Nonathletes who have good functional status should also be considered for ORIF due to high failure rates of nonoperative management; however, the discussion regarding conservative management should still be discussed with the patient.[47] Patients with poor functional status or poor surgical candidates should receive conservative management. ORIF typically consists of an intramedullary screw; however if this is not possible, then tension wire is a viable alternative.[22]

Clinical Pearl

Zones 2 and 3 fractures of the fifth metatarsal are in a watershed area and are susceptible to delayed healing and nonunion. These fractures should be referred to an orthopedic surgeon for evaluation of ORIF.

52.3.3.5.7 *Phalangeal Fracture*

Toe fractures are very common with the first and fifth toe being the most common toes injured due to their vulnerable positions along the medial and lateral foot.[35] Most fractures occur by an axial load (stubbing the toe) or a crush injury.[35] Patients will have a painful toe that is usually ecchymotic and swollen. Patients can bear weight but have an antalgic gait. Almost all toe fractures will heal well with conservative management. Displaced fractures can be reduced with axial traction.[35] Buddy taping the toe and firm-soled shoes for 3–4 weeks (until nontender) is often all that is required for management.[35] Patients can bear weight as tolerated. Great toe fractures can potentially be problematic due to the importance of the great toe in balance, weight bearing, and ambulation.[35] Nondisplaced phalanx fractures of the great toe can be managed conservatively with buddy taping and post-op shoe or firm-soled shoe. Surgical evaluation is advised if there is angulation, displacement, or the fracture involves more than 25% of the articular surface.[35,37]

52.3.3.5.8 *Sesamoid Injury*

The sesamoid bones of the foot are located just plantar to the first metatarsal head. There are the medial (tibial) and lateral (fibula) sesamoids which are incorporated within the flexor hallucis brevis tendon and serve to increase the mechanical advantage of the tendon. The abductor hallucis and adductor hallucis tendons have fibrous insertions to the medial and lateral sesamoids, respectively, and this fibrous tendon complex forms portions of the plantar plate and helps to stabilize the first MTP joint. The medial sesamoid is exposed to greater impact forces during running and jumping and thus is more likely to be injured than the lateral sesamoid. Sesamoid injuries are often seen in sports requiring significant running (cross country) and jumping (basketball and dance). Overpronation during running and jumping is also a risk facture for developing a sesamoid injury. Sesamoiditis is an inflammatory response around the sesamoid bone and usually responds well to rest, ice, NSAIDs, activity modification, and proper footwear. Occasionally, corticosteroid injections can be used to treat acute sesamoiditis. Sesamoid fractures are most commonly in the category of stress fracture related to overuse, poor footwear, or abrupt changes in the athlete's training regimen. As with most stress fractures, there is a prodromal phase of waxing and waning symptoms that worsens over time. Acute fractures are less common and are associated with direct trauma or hyperdorsiflexion of the great toe. Patients have pain with weight-bearing activities and will be tender over the sesamoid (most commonly the medial sesamoid). Patients will also have pain and weakness with resisted great toe flexion (plantarflexion) as well as pain with passive great toe extension (dorsiflexion). Radiographs including the sesamoid view and three views of the foot (AP, lateral, and oblique) are the initial imaging modality.[12] Bipartite sesamoids occur in about 25% of the population and can be confused for a fracture. Bipartite sesamoids are present bilaterally 85% of the time so a radiograph of the contralateral foot can be helpful in distinguishing bipartite sesamoid and fracture. It is recommended that the AP foot be done as a bilateral radiograph on the same film for evaluation of the presence of bipartite sesamoids. This prevents additional radiographs of the contralateral foot when a bipartite sesamoid is detected and decreases radiographs and radiation exposure. Bipartite sesamoids have rounded smooth edges versus the irregular and sharp margins of a fracture. Stress fractures are often not seen on plain films and MRI is required for diagnosis. MRI can also stage the stress injury from stress reaction to stress fracture and can differentiate bipartite sesamoid from fracture if this cannot be determined on radiographs. Bone scan is a less favorable option in identifying stress injury and differentiating between a bipartite sesamoid and acute fracture as the bone scan can be positive due to inflammation associated with sesamoiditis. Regardless of the mechanism of injury, most fractures respond well to conservative management with post-op shoe or walking boot.[12] Symptomatic nonunions are treated with surgical excision.

52.3.3.6 Pediatric

52.3.3.6.1 Freiberg's Disease

First described in 1914, Freiberg's disease is osteonecrosis of the metatarsal head. It is most commonly associated with osteonecrosis of the second metatarsal head.[81] Adolescent females are the population typically affected by Freiberg's disease.[5,81] Vascular compromise and trauma are the precipitating etiologies.[5] Patients will present with foot pain that is worse with activity or simple weight bearing. On physical exam, the patient may have swelling in the forefoot. The patient will have tenderness to palpation over the affected metatarsal head. Patients may also have a positive tuning fork test. Initial radiographs may be negative, but x-rays taken after a couple of weeks may demonstrate the typical pattern of metatarsal head flattening. Advanced imaging is usually unnecessary, but MRI or bone scan may be useful to rule out other etiologies such as stress fracture. Initial treatment involves activity modification, off-loading the affected foot, metatarsal pads, and analgesics.[81] Surgical consultation is needed in the event of failing conservative treatment. Of note, reossification of the metatarsal head may take 2 or 3 years to appear on x-rays.[28]

52.3.3.6.2 Iselin's Disease (Traction Apophysitis of the Base of the Fifth Insertion of Peroneus Brevis)

Patients complain of pain at the base of the fifth metatarsal where the peroneus brevis inserts. Risks include growth spurts and sports that require a lot of running, jumping, and change of direction. The apophysis runs parallel to the fifth metatarsal and should not be confused with an avulsion fracture or Jones fracture, which run perpendicular to the metatarsal. Treatment includes RICE, heel lifts, activity modification, and a stretching program (see Tables 52.3 through 52.5).

Clinical Pearl

The major physis of the first metatarsal is located proximal instead of distal as for 2–5 (except for the fifth metatarsal that has small physis that runs parallel to the bone). This should be taken into account when evaluating young patients with potential metatarsal fractures.

TABLE 52.3
Common Foot Disorders in Primary Care: An Anatomical and Symptom-Oriented Approach to Differential Diagnosis

Hindfoot		
Overuse	Posterior	Os trigonum, Achilles tendonitis (insertion), retrocalcaneal bursitis, Haglund deformity
	Medial	Tarsal tunnel syndrome,
	Lateral	Sural nerve entrapment
	Plantar	Plantar fasciitis, medial, and lateral plantar nerve entrapment
Traumatic	Posterior	Talus fracture (medial and lateral posterior tubercle, stress fracture)
	Medial	Talus fracture (medial posterior tubercle)
	Lateral	Talus fracture (lateral process, lateral posterior tubercle)
	Plantar	Contusion (stone bruise), plantar fasciitis, calcaneal fracture
Pediatric	Posterior	Sever's disease
Midfoot		
Overuse	Medial	Os navicular,
	Lateral	Os peroneum, cuboid stress fracture
	Central	Navicular stress fracture
Traumatic	Medial	Navicular fracture, cuneiform fracture
	Lateral	Cuboid fracture
	Central	Midfoot sprain, Lisfranc injury, spring ligament injury, navicular fracture, cuneiform fracture
Pediatric	Medial	Kohler disease, traction apophysitis of the navicular
	Central	Tarsal coalition
Fore Foot		
Overuse	Medial	Hallux rigidus, hallux valgus, metatarsalgia, sesamoiditis, ingrown toenail
	Lateral	Fifth metatarsal stress fracture
	Central	Morton's neuroma, Morton's toe, metatarsalgia metatarsal stress fracture
Traumatic	Medial	Turf toe, toe dislocation, nail hematoma, nail avulsion, first metatarsal fracture, toe fracture
	Lateral	Fifth metatarsal fracture and toe fracture
	Central	Second–fourth metatarsal fracture and toe fracture
Pediatric	Lateral	Iselin's disease
	Central	Freiberg's disease

TABLE 52.4
Indications for Referral

General	Open fracture and/or dislocation
	Fracture involving a joint space
	Neurovascular compromise
Hindfoot	Achilles tendonitis not responding after 12 weeks' conservative treatment
	Talus and calcaneal fractures
	Plantar fasciitis not responding after 12 weeks' conservative treatment
Midfoot	Navicular fracture
	Lisfranc injury
	Symptomatic tarsal coalition
Fore Foot	Morton's neuroma not responding to conservative management
	Great toe fracture
	Base of the fifth metatarsal fracture

TABLE 52.5
SORT: Key Recommendations for Practice

Clinical Recommendations	Evidence Rating	References
Musculoskeletal ultrasound has a sensitivity of 80% for diagnosing plantar fasciitis.	B	[75]
X-rays may show an incidental finding of heel spurs in up to 50% of plantar fasciitis.	B	[64]
Eccentric exercises may improve insertional Achilles tendinopathy if performed at floor level and dorsiflexion is avoided.	B	[42]
Intermittent midfoot pain with exercise associated with tenderness over the navicular (N-spot) was associated with a navicular stress fracture 81% of patients.	C	[34]
Fifth metatarsal fractures in zones 2 and 3 have a nonunion rate of up to 44% and should be referred to an orthopedic surgeon for evaluation of ORIF.	A	[22,47,57,85]

REFERENCES

1. Abell BE, Evanson JRL. Foot and Ankle Fractures. In: O'connor, Francis G, *ACSM's Sports Medicine: A Comprehensive Review.* Lippincott Williams & Wilkins; 2012: pp. 455–463.
2. Adelaar RS, Madrian JR. Avascular necrosis of the talus. *Orthopedic Clinics of North America.* 2004;35(3):383–395.
3. Ågren P, Wretenberg P, Sayed-Noor AS. Operative versus non-operative treatment of displaced intra-articular calcaneal fractures: A prospective, randomized, controlled multicenter trial. *Journal of Bone and Joint Surgery.* 2013;95(15):1351–1357.
4. Anderson RB, Hunt KJ, McCormick JJ. Management of common sports-related injuries about the foot and ankle. *Journal of the American Academy of Orthopaedic.* 2010;18(9):546–556.
5. Atanda A Jr, Shah SA, O'Brien K. Osteochondrosis: Common causes of pain in growing bones. *American Family Physician.* 2011;83(3):285–291.
6. Boden BP, Osbahr DC. High-risk stress fractures: Evaluation and treatment. *Journal of the American Academy of Orthopaedic Surgeons.* 2000;8(6):344–353.
7. Boon AJ, Smith J, Zobitz ME, Amrami KM. Snowboarder's talus fracture: Mechanism of injury. *American Journal of Sports Medicine.* 2001;29(3):333–338.
8. Borton DC, Saxby TS. Tear of the plantar calcaneonavicular (spring) ligament causing flatfoot: A case report. *Journal of Bone & Joint Surgery, British Volume.* 1997;79(4): 641–643.
9. Bouche P. Compression and entrapment neuropathies. *Handbook of Clinical Neurology.* 2013;115:311–316.
10. Burne SG, Mahoney CM, Forster BB, Koehle MS, Taunton JE, Khan KM. Tarsal navicular stress injury: Long-term outcome and clinicoradiological correlation using both computed tomography and magnetic resonance imaging. *American Journal of Sports Medicine.* 2005;33(12):1875–1881.
11. Chao W. Os trigonum. *Foot and Ankle Clinics.* 2004; 9(4):787–796.
12. Christensen SE, Cetti R, Niebuhr-Jorgensen U. Fracture of the fibular sesamoid of the hallux. *British Journal of Sports Medicine.* 1983;17(3):177–179.
13. Chuckpaiwong B, Cook C, Pietrobon R, Nunley JA. Second metatarsal stress fracture in sport: Comparative risk factors between proximal and non-proximal locations. *British Journal of Sports Medicine.* 2007;41(8):510–514.
14. Covey CJ, Mulder MD. Plantar fasciitis: How best to treat? *The Journal of Family Practice.* 2013;62(9):466–471.
15. Crain JM, Phancao J, Stidham K. MR imaging of turf toe. *Magnetic Resonance Imaging Clinics of North America.* 2008; 16(1):93–103.
16. Deland JT, Williams BR. Surgical management of hallux rigidus. *Journal of the American Academy of Orthopaedic Surgeons.* 2012;20(6):347–358.
17. Dellenbaugh SG, Bustillo J. Arthritides of the foot. *Medical Clinics of North America.* 2014;98(2):253–265.
18. DiPreta JA. Metatarsalgia, lesser toe deformities, and associated disorders of the forefoot. *Medical Clinics of North America.* 2014;98(2):233–251.
19. Doty JF, Coughlin MJ. Hallux valgus and hypermobility of the first ray: Facts and fiction. *International Orthopaedics.* 2013;37(9):1655–1660.
20. Early JS. Talus fracture management. *Foot and Ankle Clinics.* 2008;13(4):635–657.
21. Eiff PM, Hatch R. Calcaneus and other tarsal fractures. In: Eiff PM, Hatch RL (eds.). *Fracture Management for Primary Care.* Saunders/Elsevier, Philadelphia, PA; 2012: pp. 276–298.
22. Ekstrand J, van Dijk CN. Fifth metatarsal fractures among male professional footballers: A potential career-ending disease. *British Journal of Sports Medicine.* 2013;47(12): 754–758.
23. Espinosa N, Brodsky JW, Maceira E. Metatarsalgia. *Journal of the American Academy of Orthopaedic Surgeons.* 2010;18(8):474–485.
24. Flanigan RM, DiGiovanni BF. Peripheral nerve entrapments of the lower leg, ankle, and foot. *Foot and Ankle Clinics.* 2011;16(2):255–274.
25. Fortin PT, Balazsy JE. Talus fractures: Evaluation and treatment. *Journal of the American Academy of Orthopaedic Surgeons.* 2001;9(2):114–127.
26. Fredericson M, Standage S, Chou L, Matheson G. Lateral plantar nerve entrapment in a competitive gymnast. *Clinical Journal of Sport Medicine.* 2001;11(2):111–114.

27. George E, Harris AH, Dragoo JL, Hunt KJ. Incidence and risk factors for turf toe injuries in intercollegiate football: Data from the national collegiate athletic association injury surveillance system. *Foot and Ankle Internation*. 2014;35(2):108–115.
28. Gillespie H. Osteochondroses and apophyseal injuries of the foot in the young athlete. *Current Sports Medicine Reports*. 2010;9(5):265–268.
29. Gould JS. Tarsal tunnel syndrome. *Foot and Ankle Clinics*. 2011;16(2):275–286.
30. Gross CE, Hsu AR, Chahal J, Holmes GB Jr. Injectable treatments for noninsertional achilles tendinosis: A systematic review. *Foot and Ankle International*. 2013;34(5):619–628.
31. Guerado E, Bertrand ML, Cano JR. Management of calcaneal fractures: What have we learnt over the years? *Injury*. 2012;43(10):1640–1650.
32. Halvorson JJ, Winter SB, Teasdall RD, Scott AT. Talar neck fractures: A systematic review of the literature. *Journal of Foot and Ankle Surgery*. 2013;52(1):56–61.
33. Harish S, Kumbhare D, O'Neill J, Popowich T. Comparison of sonography and magnetic resonance imaging for spring ligament abnormalities: Preliminary study. *Journal of Ultrasound in Medicine*. 2008;27(8):1145–1152.
34. Harmon KG. Lower extremity stress fractures. *Clinical Journal of Sport Medicine*. 2003;13(6):358–364.
35. Hatch RL, Hacking S. Evaluation and management of toe fractures. *American Family Physician*. 2003;68(12):2413–2418.
36. Hecht PJ, Lin TJ. Hallux valgus. *Medical Clinics of North America*. 2014;98(2):227–232.
37. Heckman DS, Gluck GS, Parekh SG. Tendon disorders of the foot and ankle, part 1: Peroneal tendon disorders. *American Journal of Sports Medicine*. 2009;37(3):614–625.
38. Heidelbaugh JJ, Lee H. Management of the ingrown toenail. *American Family Physician*. 2009;79(4):303–308.
39. Hetsroni I, Mann G, Dolev E, Morgenstern D, Nyska M. Base of fourth metatarsal stress fracture: Tendency for prolonged healing. *Clinical Journal of Sport Medicine*. 2005;15(3):186–188.
40. Hirose CB, McGarvey WC. Peripheral nerve entrapments. *Foot and Ankle Clinics*. 2004;9(2):255–269.
41. Jain S, Mannan K. The diagnosis and management of morton's neuroma: A literature review. *Foot and Ankle Specialists*. 2013;6(4):307–317.
42. Jonsson P, Alfredson H, Sunding K, Fahlstrom M, Cook J. New regimen for eccentric calf-muscle training in patients with chronic insertional achilles tendinopathy: Results of a pilot study. *British Journal of Sports Medicine*. 2008;42(9): 746–749.
43. Joong MA, El-Khoury GY. Radiologic evaluation of chronic foot pain. *American Family Physician*. 2007;76(7):975–983.
44. Judd DB, Kim DH. Foot fractures frequently misdiagnosed as ankle sprains. *American Family Physician*. 2002; 66(5):785–794.
45. Kasparek M, Schneider W. Surgical treatment of morton's neuroma: Clinical results after open excision. *International Orthopaedics*. 2013;37(9):1857–1861.
46. Kennedy JG, Baxter DE. Nerve disorders in dancers. *Clinics in Sports Medicine*. 2008;27(2):329–334.
47. Kerkhoffs GM, Versteegh VE, Sierevelt IN, Kloen P, van Dijk CN. Treatment of proximal metatarsal V fractures in athletes and non-athletes. *British Journal of Sports Medicine*. 2012;46(9):644–648.
48. Khoury J, Jerushalmi J, Loberant N, Shtarker H, Militianu D, Keidar Z. Kohler disease: Diagnoses and assessment by bone scintigraphy. *Clinical Nuclear Medicine*. 2007;32(3):179–181.
49. Kolodziejski P, Czarnocki L, Wojdasiewicz P, Brylka K, Kuropatwa K, Deszczynski J. Intra-articular fractures of calcaneus—Current concepts of treatment. *Polish Orthopedics and Traumatology*. 2014;79:102–111.
50. Kou JX, Fortin PT. Commonly missed peritalar injuries. *Journal of the American Academy of Orthopaedic Surgeons*. 2009;17(12):775–786.
51. Krishna Sayana M, Maffulli N. Insertional achilles tendinopathy. *Foot and Ankle Clinics*. 2005;10(2):309–320.
52. Lattermann C, Goldstein JL, Wukich DK, Lee S, Bach BR Jr. Practical management of lisfranc injuries in athletes. *Clinical Journal of Sport Medicine*. 2007;17(4):311–315.
53. McCrory P, Bell S, Bradshaw C. Nerve entrapments of the lower leg, ankle and foot in sport. *Sports Medicine*. 2002; 32(6):371–391.
54. McNeil DS, Baumhauer JF, Glazebrook MA. Evidence-based analysis of the efficacy for operative treatment of hallux rigidus. *Foot and Ankle International*. 2013;34(1):15–32.
55. Migues A, Slullitel G. Joint-preserving procedure for moderate hallux rigidus. *Foot and Ankle Clinics*. 2012;17(3):459–471.
56. Mitchell M, McKinley J, Robinson C. The epidemiology of calcaneal fractures. *Foot*. 2009;19(4):197–200.
57. Mologne TS, Lundeen JM, Clapper MF, O'Brien TJ. Early screw fixation versus casting in the treatment of acute jones fractures. *American Journal of Sports Medicine*. 2005;33(7):970–975.
58. Morelli V, James E. Achilles tendinopathy and tendon rupture: Conservative versus surgical management. *Primary Care: Clinics in Office Practice*. 2004;31(4):1039–1054.
59. Murphy DF, Connolly DA, Beynnon BD. Risk factors for lower extremity injury: A review of the literature. *British Journal of Sports Medicine*. 2003;37(1):13–29.
60. Nakayama S, Sugimoto K, Takakura Y, Tanaka Y, Kasanami R. Percutaneous drilling of symptomatic accessory navicular in young athletes. *American Journal of Sports Medicine*. 2005;33(4):531–535.
61. Nunley JA, Vertullo CJ. Classification, investigation, and management of midfoot sprains: Lisfranc injuries in the athlete. *American Journal of Sports Medicine*. 2002;30(6):871–878.
62. O'Malley MJ, Basran HS, Gu Y, Sayres S, Deland JT. Treatment of advanced stages of hallux rigidus with cheilectomy and phalangeal osteotomy. *Journal of Bone and Joint Surgery*. 2013;95(7):606–610.
63. Oh SJ, Kim YH, Kim SK, Kim MW. Painful os peroneum syndrome presenting as lateral plantar foot pain. *Annals of Rehabilitation Medicine*. 2012;36(1):163–166.
64. Osborne H, Breidahl W, Allison G. Critical differences in lateral X-rays with and without a diagnosis of plantar fasciitis. *Journal of Science and Medicine in Sport*. 2006;9(3):231–237.
65. Paoloni JA, Appleyard RC, Nelson J, Murrell GA. Topical glyceryl trinitrate treatment of chronic noninsertional achilles tendinopathy. A randomized, double-blind, placebo-controlled trial. *Journal of Bone and Joint Surgery*. 2004;86(5):916–922.
66. Pastides P, El-Sallakh S, Charalambides C. Morton's neuroma: A clinical versus radiological diagnosis. *Foot and Ankle Surgery*. 2012;18(1):22–24.
67. Potter NJ, Brukner PD, Makdissi M, Crossley K, Kiss ZS, Bradshaw C. Navicular stress fractures: Outcomes of surgical and conservative management. *British Journal of Sports Medicine*. 2006;40(8):692–695; discussion 695.
68. Raikin SM, Slenker N, Ratigan B. The association of a varus hindfoot and fracture of the fifth metatarsal metaphyseal-diaphyseal junction: The jones fracture. *American Journal of Sports Medicine*. 2008;36(7):1367–1372.

69. Rammelt S, Zwipp H. Talar neck and body fractures. *Injury.* 2009;40(2):120–135.
70. Rietveld AB. Dancers' and musicians' injuries. *Clinical Rheumatology.* 2013;32(4):425–434.
71. Ritchie JD, Shaver JC, Anderson RB, Lawrence SJ, Mair SD. Excision of symptomatic nonunions of proximal fifth metatarsal avulsion fractures in elite athletes. *American Journal of Sports Medicine.* 2011;39(11):2466–2469.
72. Roche A, Calder J. Achilles tendinopathy. *The Bone & Joint Journal.* 2013;95-B:1299–1302.
73. Rosenbaum AJ, DiPreta JA, Misener D. Plantar heel pain. *Medical Clinics of North America.* 2014;98(2):339–352.
74. Roser SE, Gellman H. Comparison of nail bed repair versus nail trephination for subungual hematomas in children. *Journal of Hand Surgery.* 1999;24(6):1166–1170.
75. Sabir N, Demirlenk S, Yagci B, Karabulut N, Cubukcu S. Clinical utility of sonography in diagnosing plantar fasciitis. *Journal of Ultrasound in Medicine.* 2005;24(8):1041–1048.
76. Sanders RW, Clare MP. Calcaneus fractures. In: Bucholz RW, Heckman JD et al. *Rockwood and Green's Fractures in Adults,* 7th edn. Lippincott Williams & Wilkins, Philadelphia, PA; 2010.
77. Saxena A, Fullem B. Comment on torg et al, "management of tarsal navicular stress fractures: Conservative versus surgical treatment". *American Journal of Sports Medicine.* 2010;38(10):NP3–NP5; author reply NP5.
78. Schachter AK, Chen AL, Reddy PD, Tejwani NC. Osteochondral lesions of the talus. *Journal of the American Academy of Orthopaedic Surgeons.* 2005;13(3):152–158.
79. Schepsis AA, Jones H, Haas AL. Achilles tendon disorders in athletes. *American Journal of Sports Medicine.* 2002;30(2):287–305.
80. Seaberg DC, Angelos WJ, Paris PM. Treatment of subungual hematomas with nail trephination: A prospective study. *American Journal of Emergency Medicine.* 1991;9(3):209–210.
81. Sherman KP. The foot in sport. *British Journal of Sports Medicine.* 1999;33(1):6–13.
82. Simpson MR, Howard TM. Tendinopathies of the foot and ankle. *American Academy of Family Physicians.* 2009;80(10):1107–1114.
83. Sormaala MJ, Niva MH, Kiuru MJ, Mattila VM, Pihlajamaki HK. Outcomes of stress fractures of the talus. *American Journal of Sports Medicine.* 2006;34(11):1809–1814.
84. Stevenson J, McNaughton G, Riley J. The use of prophylactic flucloxacillin in treatment of open fractures of the distal phalanx within an accident and emergency department: A double-blind randomized placebo-controlled trial. *Journal of Hand Surgery.* 2003;28(5):388–394.
85. Strayer SM, Reece SG, Petrizzi MJ. Fractures of the proximal fifth metatarsal. *American Family Physician.* 1999;59(9):2516–2522.
86. Talusan PG, Milewski MD, Toy JO, Wall EJ. Osteochondritis dissecans of the talus: Diagnosis and treatment in athletes. *Clinics in Sports Medicine.* 2014;33(2):267–284.
87. Torg JS, Moyer J, Gaughan JP, Boden BP. Management of tarsal navicular stress fractures: Conservative versus surgical treatment: A meta-analysis. *American Journal of Sports Medicine.* 2010;38(5):1048–1053.
88. Toye LR, Helms CA, Hoffman BD, Easley M, Nunley JA. MRI of spring ligament tears. *American Journal of Roentgenology.* 2005;184(5):1475–1480.
89. Tu P, Bytomski JR. Diagnosis of heel pain. *American Family Physician.* 2011;84(8):909–916.
90. Turmo-Garuz A, Rodas G, Balius R et al. Can local corticosteroid injection in the retrocalcaneal bursa lead to rupture of the achilles tendon and the medial head of the gastrocnemius muscle? *Musculoskeletal Surgery.* 2013:1–6.
91. Vallier HA, Reichard SG, Boyd AJ, Moore TA. A new look at the Hawkins classification for talar neck fractures: Which features of injury and treatment are predictive of osteonecrosis? *Journal of Bone and Joint Surgery.* 2014;96(3):192–197.
92. Walters JL, Gangopadhyay P, Malay DS. Association of calcaneal and spinal fractures. *Journal of Foot and Ankle Surgery.* 2014;53(3):279–281.
93. Weinfeld SB. Achilles tendon disorders. *Medical Clinics of North America.* 2014;98(2):331–338.
94. Wilder RP, Sethi S. Overuse injuries: Tendinopathies, stress fractures, compartment syndrome, and shin splints. *Clinics in Sports Medicine.* 2004;23(1):55–81.
95. Williams GA, Cowell HR. Kohler's disease of the tarsal navicular. *Clinical Orthopaedics.* 1981;158:53–58.
96. Yokoe K, Kameyama Y. Relationship between stress fractures of the proximal phalanx of the great toe and hallux valgus. *American Journal of Sports Medicine.* 2004;32(4):1032–1034.
97. Zuber TJ. Ingrown toenail removal. *American Family Physician.* 2002;65(12):2547–2552, 2554.

Section VI

Medical Issues in Sports Medicine

53 Cardiovascular Considerations in the Athlete

Francis G. O'Connor and Ralph P. Oriscello

CONTENTS

TABLE 53.1
Key Clinical Considerations

1. Cardiovascular disease is the leading cause of exertional sudden death in athletes; coronary artery disease accounts for the majority of deaths in older athletes (>35), while hypertrophic cardiomyopathy is the leading culprit in younger athletes.
2. Regular aerobic exercise has not only been consistently demonstrated to confer substantial long-term health benefits upon the individual but also been associated with a transient increase in risk for cardiovascular morbidity and mortality.
3. Hypertension is the most common cardiovascular disorder encountered in athletes; the hallmark of therapy is exercise.
4. Exertional syncope is a potentially ominous symptom that warrants careful evaluation prior to clearance for athletic participation.
5. The clinician should approach the patient with atherosclerotic cardiovascular disease with the intent to identify exercise that can be permitted rather than looking for exercise restrictions.

53.1 INTRODUCTION

Enhanced cardiovascular health is one of the key benefits of most forms of consistent athletic endeavors throughout life. Regular physical activity promotes cardiovascular fitness and has been demonstrated to lower the risk of disease. While there is generally a net cardiovascular benefit from athletic activity, there is also an increased cardiovascular risk for certain susceptible individuals. These individuals may be known with identified cardiovascular disorders, or they may be unrecognized until the adverse event occurs. This chapter will initially review the benefits and risk of exercise in the child and adult in order to provide a framework that will allow clinicians to make recommendations for their patients participating in all levels of athletic activity. The chapter will then detail the principal cardiovascular issues of athletic activity for the primary care provider, in an evidence-based and problem-oriented approach (Table 53.1).

53.2 CARDIOVASCULAR BENEFITS OF EXERCISE

Numerous studies have clearly identified physical inactivity and sedentary lifestyle as significant risk factors for the development and progression of coronary heart disease and for the incidence of adverse cardiovascular events, including death.[16,29,30,33,42] Moreover, studies have consistently confirmed the cardiovascular benefit of aerobic exercise with a reduction in the number of adverse events and a reduction in mortality.[2,30,41] While there is a definite increased risk for certain susceptible individuals, particularly middle-aged persons with coronary artery disease (CAD) and a sedentary lifestyle who begin a sudden intensive exercise program or young athletes with congenital or genetic cardiovascular disorders, there is abundant evidence of net cardiovascular benefits from consistent vigorous exercise as a primary-prevention recommendation for coronary disease in asymptomatic middle-aged and older persons.[2] The individuals at increased risk need to be identified, stratified, counseled, and guided to an appropriate activity level. Most others need to be encouraged, motivated, and supported in their efforts to achieve a vigorous lifestyle that will reduce cardiovascular risk and promote optimal physical functioning throughout life.

53.3 CARDIOVASCULAR RISKS OF EXERCISE

As mentioned earlier, while there is considerable net cardiovascular benefit to exercise, there is also a clear risk for susceptible individuals. Indeed, as Barry J. Maron has clearly shown, there is a "paradox of exercise" that requires a clinical assessment of risk prior to the initiation of a vigorous program.[18]

Overall risk of sudden death during exercise is low. Estimates from various studies range from 1:15,000 joggers per year to 1:50,000 marathon participants.[22,35,36,39] For high school and college-aged athletes, the range is estimated at 1:83,000 to 1:300,000 per academic year.[20,25,40] Of course, the risk of sudden death with exercise increases with age. As the demographics of the population continue to shift and more middle-aged and elderly heed the advice to exercise, it should certainly be expected to see an increase in the prevalence of sudden death. In the older athlete, CAD is the most common etiology. In the younger athlete, multiple etiologies, including congenital abnormalities can also lead to malignant arrhythmias during intense activity. Generally, it is the combination of underlying cardiac disease (recognized or unrecognized) with intense exercise that leads to the fatal arrhythmia in both age groups.[15] For young athletes, basketball, football, track, and soccer have the highest incidence of sudden deaths. Cardiovascular etiologies outnumber traumatic etiologies nearly 2 to 1 for sports-related fatalities in high school and college.[3]

Clinical Pearl

The most common cause of nontraumatic exertional sudden death in athletes ≥ 35 is atherosclerotic heart disease; in younger athletes, hypertrophic cardiomyopathy is the leading killer.

The specific etiologies contributing to sudden cardiac death are most closely related to age; generally, the dividing age is 35.[1] This primarily stems from the observation that for sudden deaths over 35 years of age, >75% are associated with CAD. The high prevalence of atherosclerosis in this age group clearly predominates as an etiology. In younger athletes, hypertrophic cardiomyopathy (HCM) is the most common etiology. Coronary artery anomalies, premature atherosclerotic disease, myocarditis, and dilated cardiomyopathy are next most common, at least in the United States. In European studies, arrhythmogenic right ventricular dysplasia is more commonly recognized as an etiology than it is in the United States.[9,34,37] Other less common etiologies include aortic rupture from Marfan's syndrome, genetic conduction system abnormalities, idiopathic left ventricular (LV) hypertrophy, substance abuse (cocaine and/or steroids), aortic stenosis, mitral valve prolapse, sickle-cell trait, and blunt chest trauma (commotio cordis).

53.4 PREPARTICIPATION CLEARANCE OF THE YOUNG ADULT

As alluded to the aforementioned, screening for the risk factors associated with sudden death requires attention to the subtle details of personal and family history, a careful cardiovascular exam, and directed ancillary studies. The American Heart Association (AHA) Science and Advisory Committee published consensus guidelines for preparticipation cardiovascular screening for high school and college athletes in 2007, which were amended in 2014.[23,25] It is recommended that a complete personal and family history and physical examination be done for all athletes (see Figure 53.1). It should focus on identifying those cardiovascular conditions known to cause sudden death. It should be done every 2 years with an interim history between exams. The 36th Bethesda Conference specifies participation guidelines for different conditions[24] (see Table 53.2).

It is the primary care provider's responsibility to attempt to identify and assess those conditions through a thorough history and physical examination and to promptly refer suspected cases to the cardiology consultant for definitive diagnosis and specific exercise recommendations and limitations when required. Family history should include a specific inquiry for a premature CAD, diabetes mellitus, hypertension, sudden death, syncope, and significant disability from cardiovascular disease in relatives younger than age 50, HCM, arrhythmogenic right ventricular dysplasia (ARVD), Marfan's syndrome, prolonged QT syndrome, or significant arrhythmias. Personal past history should include specific inquiries on the detection of heart murmur, diabetes mellitus, hypertension, hyperlipidemia, or smoking, or on the presence of HCM, ARVC, Marfan's syndrome, prolonged QT syndrome, or significant arrhythmias. Recent history inquiries must include a history of syncope, near syncope, profound exercise intolerance, exertional chest discomfort, dyspnea, or excessive fatigue.

Clinical Pearl

Critical review of systems *red flag* questions for the young athlete include syncope, near syncope, profound exercise intolerance, exertional chest discomfort, dyspnea, or excessive fatigue.

Physical exam should specifically address hypertension, heart rhythm, cardiac murmur, and the findings of unusual facies or body habitus associated with a congenital cardiovascular defect, especially Marfan's syndrome.[12,17] Cardiac auscultation should be performed in the supine and standing positions, and murmurs should be assessed with Valsalva and position maneuvers when indicated. Femoral pulses should be assessed and blood pressure (BP) measured with the appropriately sized cuff in the sitting position.

Clinical Pearl

Murmurs in athletes that meet the following criteria should warrant referral for echocardiography: ≥ grade III, holosystolic, diastolic, continuous, fixed or paradoxical S2 splitting, or an increase in intensity with Valsalva maneuver or squat to stand.

Electrocardiograms (EKGs) and echocardiograms are not currently recommended as screening tools; however, this is

TABLE 53.2
Fourteen-Element AHA Recommendations for Preparticipation Cardiovascular Screening of Competitive Athletes[a]

Personal History

1. Exertional chest pain/discomfort
2. Unexplained syncope/near syncope[b]
3. Excessive exertional and unexplained dyspnea/fatigue, associated with exercise
4. Prior recognition of a heart murmur
5. Elevated systemic blood pressure
6. Prior restriction from participation in sports
7. Prior testing for the heart, ordered by a physician

Family history

8. Premature death (sudden and unexpected, or otherwise) before age 50 years due to heart disease, in first-degree relative
9. Disability from heart disease in a close relative <50 years of age
10. Specific knowledge of certain cardiac conditions in family members: hypertrophic cardiomyopathy, long QT syndrome, or other ion channelopathies, Marfan's syndrome, or clinically important arrhythmias

Physical Examination

11. Heart murmur[c]
12. Femoral arterial pulses to exclude aortic coarctation
13. Physical stigmata of Marfan's syndrome
14. Brachial blood pressure (sitting position)[d]

Sources: Reproduced with permission from Maron, BJ, PD Thompson, MJ Ackerman, G Balady, S Berger, D Cohen, R Dimeff, PS Douglas, DW Glover, AM Hutter, Jr., MD Krauss, MS Maron, MJ Mitten, WO Roberts, and JC Puffer. Recommendations and considerations related to preparticipation screening for cardiovascular abnormalities in competitive athletes: 2007 update: a scientific statement from the American Heart Association Council on Nutrition, Physical Activity, and Metabolism: endorsed by the American College of Cardiology Foundation. *Circulation*. 2007, 115:1643–1455; O'Connor, F. G. et al., *Clin. J. Sport Med.*, 19, 429, 2009.

[a] Parental verification is recommended for high school and middle school athletes.
[b] Judged not to be neurocardiogenic (vasovagal), of particular concern when related to exertion.
[c] Auscultation should be performed in both supine and standing positions (or with Valsalva maneuver), specifically to identify murmurs of dynamic left ventricular outflow tract obstruction.
[d] Preferably taken in both arms.

a controversial area of active debate.[7,21,23,32] As mentioned earlier, the normal adaptations of the "athletic heart" make interpretation of the routine EKG and echocardiogram problematic.[30] The role for these modalities lies in the hands of the cardiology consultant who must interpret the findings in the setting of the individual patient who has been referred for questionable symptoms or physical findings. At this point, the state of the technology does not allow for significant sensitivity to cost-effectively case-find true positives and reliably exclude true negatives. The primary care physician should not rely on these tools to "find" patients. High rates of false positivity, high relative costs, limited availability, and low prevalence of disease make these modalities impractical as screening devices, at this point in time. That being stated, emerging strategies assist in identifying abnormal from normal variants among the athletic population[5,6,8] (see Table 53.3).

53.5 PREPARTICIPATION CLEARANCE OF THE ADULT

Ancillary testing should be directed by the patient's history, physical examination results, and age. Lipid profiles should be checked in the older athlete and should be considered in athletes of any age. Exercise stress testing is not routinely recommended as a routine screening device for the detection of early CAD because of low predictive value and high rates of false-positive and false-negative results. However, a recent AHA Science Advisory recommends stress testing on those older athletes with a moderate to high cardiovascular risk profile for CAD.[19] Specifically, this includes men > 40–45 years old or women >50–55 years old (or postmenopausal) with one or more independent coronary risk factors. The risk factors are as follows: (1) total cholesterol >200, (2) LDL >130, (3) HDL <35 for men and <45 for women, (4) systolic BP> 140 or diastolic BP >90, (5) current or recent smoking, (6) diabetes mellitus, and (7) history of MI or sudden death in first-degree relative <60 years old. In addition, stress testing is recommended for athletes of any age with suggestive symptoms of CAD or for those >64 years of age regardless of risk factors or symptoms. Recently published guidelines from the ACSM assist the provider in risk stratifying and assessing patients for both a medical examination and treadmill stress testing prior to beginning a moderate or vigorous exercise program (see Table 53.4 and Figure 53.1).

TABLE 53.3
Classification of Abnormalities of the Athlete's Electrocardiogram

Group1: Common and Training-Related ECG Changes
Sinus bradycardia
First-degree AV block
Incomplete RBBB
Early repolarization
Isolated QRS voltage criteria for left ventricular hypertrophy
Group 2: Uncommon and Training-Unrelated ECG Changes
T-wave inversion
ST-segment depression
Pathological Q waves
Left atrial enlargement
Left-axis deviation/left anterior hemiblock
Right-axis deviation/left posterior hemiblock
Right ventricular hypertrophy
Ventricular preexcitation
Complete LBBB or RBBB
Long or short QT interval
Brugada-like early repolarization

RBBB, right bundle branch block; LBBB, left bundle branch block

Source: Reproduced with permission from Corrado, D. et al., *Eur. Heart J.*, 31, 243, 2010.

TABLE 53.4
ACSM Guidelines for Exercise Testing: Atherosclerotic Cardiovascular Disease Risk Factors and Defining Criteria

Risk Factor	Defining Criteria
Age	Men ≥ 45; women ≥ 55.
Family history	Myocardial infarction, coronary revascularization, or sudden death before 55 years in father or other male first-degree relative or before 65 years in mother or other female first-degree relative.
Cigarette smoking	Current cigarette smoker or those who quit within the previous 6 months or exposure to environmental tobacco smoke.
Sedentary lifestyle	Not participating in at least 30 minutes of moderate intensity, physical activity (40%–60% VO2R) on at least 3 days of the week for at least 3 months.
Obesity	Body mass index of 30 kg/m^2 or waist girth >102 cm (40 in.) for men and >88 cm (35 in.) for women.
Hypertension	Systolic blood pressure ≥ 140 mmHg and/or diastolic ≥ 90 mmHg, confirmed by measurements on at least two separate occasions or on antihypertensive medication.
Dyslipidemia	LDL cholesterol ≥ 130 mg/dL or HDL cholesterol < 40 mg/dL or on lipid-lowering medication. If total serum cholesterol is all that is available, use ≥ 200 mg/dL.
Prediabetes	Impaired fasting glucose (fasting plasma glucose ≥ 100 and 125 mg/dL) or impaired glucose tolerance test (2 hours values ≥ 140 and 199) confirmed by measurements on at least two separate occasions.
Negative Risk Factor	**Defining Criteria**
HDL	≥ 60mg/dL

Source: Adapted from Pescatello, L., senior ed., *ACSM's Guidelines for Exercise Testing and Prescription*, Ninth ed., ACSM 2013, Wolters Kluwer/Lippincott Williams and Wilkins.

53.6 SYNCOPE IN THE ATHLETE

Syncope is most often defined as a sudden loss of consciousness for a brief duration, not secondary to head trauma but usually secondary to a sudden drop in cerebral blood flow or metabolic change (e.g., hypoglycemia, hypoxia). Exercise-associated collapse (EAC) refers to athletes who are unable to stand or walk unaided because of lightheadedness, faintness, dizziness, or outright syncope. The potential differential diagnosis is extensive and includes multiple cardiovascular and neurologic etiologies.[14,26] Athletes who present with a history of "passing out with exercise" require a careful history and physical examination to differentiate benign from life-threatening etiologies.[27]

The first step involves determining if the event was a brief, true syncopal episode versus the more common and generally benign EAC event that involves a longer time period of "being out of it" even in the supine position with normal vital signs. The second step is to differentiate between syncope that occurs during the event (suggesting a more ominous arrhythmic etiology) and syncope that occurs following the event, usually associated with orthostatic hypotension upon exercise cessation (suggesting a less ominous etiology). It is also critical to identify prodromal symptoms that may have occurred during exercise such as palpitations (arrhythmia), chest pain (ischemia or aortic dissection), nausea (ischemia or vagal activity), wheezing, or pruritus (anaphylaxis).

Clinical Pearl

Exertional syncope that occurs during an event tends to be more ominous than syncope that occurs after an activity. Both, however, require a prudent history and physical examination.

The physical exam should include a careful assessment of orthostatic vital signs, precordial auscultation especially focusing on ruling out the murmurs of aortic stenosis and HCM, and a careful search for the morphologic features of Marfan's syndrome.[17]

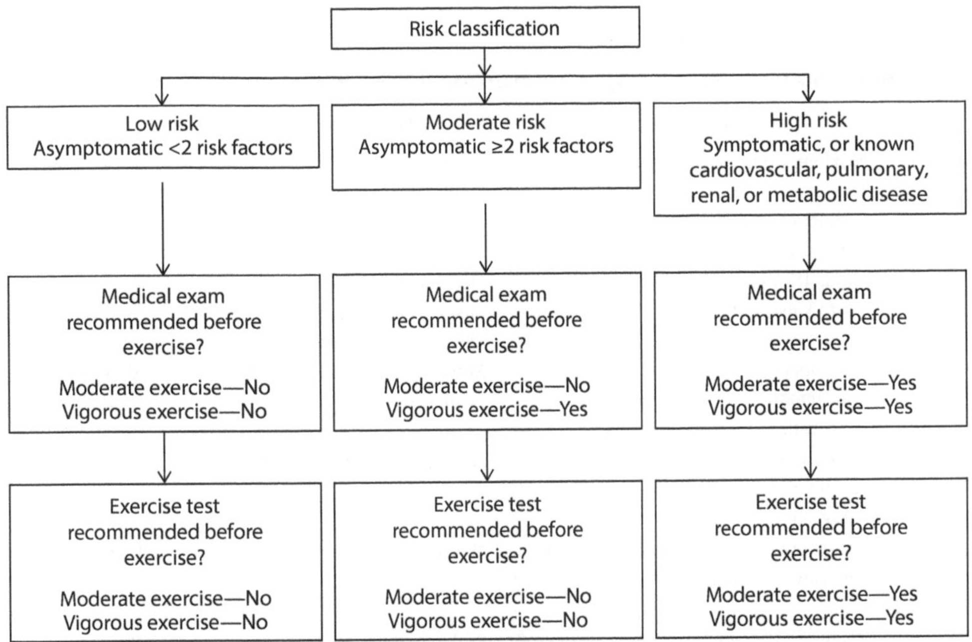

FIGURE 53.1 ACSM guidelines for exercise testing. *Risk factors*: Determined from Table 53.4. *Moderate exercise*: An intensity that causes substantial increases in heart rate and breathing; 40% to ≤60 VO2R; <6 METs. *Vigorous exercise*: An intensity that causes substantial increases in heart rate and breathing; ≥60% VO2R; ≥6 METs. (Adapted from Pescatello, L., senior ed., *ACSM's Guidelines for Exercise Testing and Prescription*, Ninth edn., ACSM. 2013, Wolters Kluwer/Lippincott Williams and Wilkins.)

An EKG should be ordered in most cases and should be evaluated closely for rate, rhythm, QT interval, repolarization abnormalities, left or right hypertrophy, preexcitation evidence, and complications of ischemic heart disease. Further testing, including blood work, echocardiogram, and stress testing, may be done depending on whether a diagnosis has been made or suggested or remains unexplained. Table 53.5 highlights clinical clues to conditions that present with exertional syncope.

If the etiology is diagnosed or strongly suggested, then the athlete may be reassured, restricted, or referred for further testing depending on the etiology. If the event remains unexplained, then the athlete must remain restricted and undergo further testing with echocardiography, stress testing, and cardiac consultation. See Figure 53.2 for a suggested algorithm for the primary care evaluation of exertional syncope in the young athlete.[26]

53.7 HYPERTENSION IN THE ATHLETE

Systemic hypertension remains one of the most common life-threatening cardiovascular disorders in the United States and affects athletes of all ages and sports. The primary care physician will frequently encounter opportunities to newly diagnose the condition in young athletes during the preparticipation examination process and to manage established hypertensives of all ages engaged in various sporting activities. The diagnosis, workup, and initial nonpharmacologic approach to treatment do not differ between athletes and nonathletes. This approach is well described in the Joint National Commission (JNC-VIII) recommendations.[13] Care must be taken not to overdiagnose the condition in young athletes and to utilize proper fitting cuffs with three different measures on three different days, adjusting for norms for age, gender, and height.[11] An appropriate search for secondary etiologies and target organ damage assessment should guide the history, physical, and laboratory evaluation. History should include an inquiry about performance-enhancing substances (e.g., anabolic steroids), and lab should include EKG, urinalysis, CBC, electrolytes, fasting glucose, lipid profile, BUN, creatinine, and uric acid. It often includes a chest x-ray and echocardiogram to assess for LV hypertrophy as well as a stress test to assist in determining the intensity level of activity participation.[10]

Clinical Pearl

Hypertension is the most common cardiovascular disorder diagnosed in young athletes; normal values are based on age, gender, and *height*.

Nonpharmacologic treatment should be properly initiated with enthusiastic physician endorsement.[10,27] It includes engagement in moderate physical activity, maintenance of ideal body weight, limitation of alcohol, reduction in sodium intake, maintenance of adequate potassium intake, and consumption of a diet high in fruit and vegetables and low in total and saturated fat. When indicated, pharmacologic treatment should be initiated. Generally, ACE inhibitors, calcium channel blockers, and angiotensin II receptor blockers are excellent choices for athletes with hypertension. Their low side-effect profile and

TABLE 53.5
Clinical Clues to Common Etiologies Presenting with Exertional Syncope

Diagnosis	Clinical Clues	Electrocardiogram	Suggested Diagnostic Testing
Neurocardiogenic syncope	Noxious stimulus, prolonged, upright position	Normal	Exercise testing
Supraventricular tachyarrhythmias	Palpitations, response to carotid, sinus pressure	Preexcitation	Electrophysiologic study and definitive therapy
Hypertrophic cardiomyopathy	Grade III/VI systolic murmur, louder with Valsalva maneuver (when present)	Deep inverted T waves, Q waves, pseudoinfarction pattern, left ventricular hypertrophy with strain	Echocardiography with Doppler (consider cardiac MRI with gadolinium)
Myocarditis	Prior upper respiratory tract infection, pneumonia, exertional fatigue, shortness of breath, recreational drug use	Simulating a myocardial infarction with ectopy	Viral studies, echocardiogram, drug screening
Aortic stenosis	Exertional syncope, grade III/VI harsh systolic crescendo–decrescendo murmur	Left ventricular hypertrophy	Echocardiography with Doppler
Mitral valve prolapse	Thumping heart, midsystolic click with or without a murmur	Normal	Echocardiography with Doppler
Prolonged QT syndrome	Recurrent syncope with family history of sudden death	Prolonged corrected QT interval (>0.47 males, >0.48 females)	Family history, exercise stress test with EKG after exercise
Coronary anomalies	Syncope, exertional chest pain	Normal resting electrocardiogram	Cardiac MRI or CT angiography
Acquired coronary artery diseases	Acute coronary syndrome (chest pain), family history	Ischemia, may be normal	Exercise testing with or without perfusion or contractile imaging
Arrhythmogenic right ventricular cardiomyopathy	Syncope, tachyarrhythmias	T-wave inversion v1-v3 PVCs with LBBB configuration	Echocardiography with Doppler study, cardiac MRI

favorable physiologic hemodynamics make them generally safe and effective. It is preferable to avoid diuretics and beta-blockers in young athletes. Volume and potassium balance issues limit diuretic use, and beta-blockers adversely impact the cardiovascular training effect of exercise. Both substances and a number of other antihypertensives are banned by the National Collegiate Athletic Association and the U.S. Olympic Committee.[27]

Restriction of activity for athletes with hypertension depends on the degree of target organ damage and on the overall control of the BP.[10,13] Most patients who have controlled BP (<140/90 at rest for adults) and are mild-to-moderate hypertensives with no target organ damage can have unrestricted participation. Adult patients with target organ damage or uncontrolled BP or have severe but controlled hypertension should be restricted to lower-intensity sports. In children and adolescents, the presence of severe hypertension or target organ disease warrants restriction until hypertension is under adequate control. Its presence should not limit a person's eligibility for competitive athletics.

53.8 CORONARY ARTERY DISEASE IN THE ATHLETE

As discussed in some detail earlier in the chapter, vigorous exercise represents a dangerous "paradox" for cardiovascular disease.[18] While it may be a potent preventive tool, it can also represent substantial risk for the susceptible individual. This is particularly poignant for the athlete with an established diagnosis of CAD. These individuals will absolutely require careful risk stratification prior to returning to their active lifestyle. They will require procedures for LV assessment, maximal treadmill testing to determine functional capacity, and testing for inducible ischemia. Patients should be tested on their medications. The 36th Bethesda Conference defines clear stratification criteria (Table 53.6) accompanied by activity recommendations (Table 53.7).[38] This provides a general and conservative approach to the individual in regard to competitive sports.

Clinical Pearl

Exercise in the adult with coronary artery disease represents a potentially dangerous paradox; the long-term benefit of mitigating risk with regular exercise is accompanied by the short-term transient risk increase in cardiac events with an increase in activity.

The recommendations, however, are particularly restrictive and do not address the "casual" participant and the individual jogger. This puts the primary responsibility on the primary care physician. It requires an individualized activity, risk

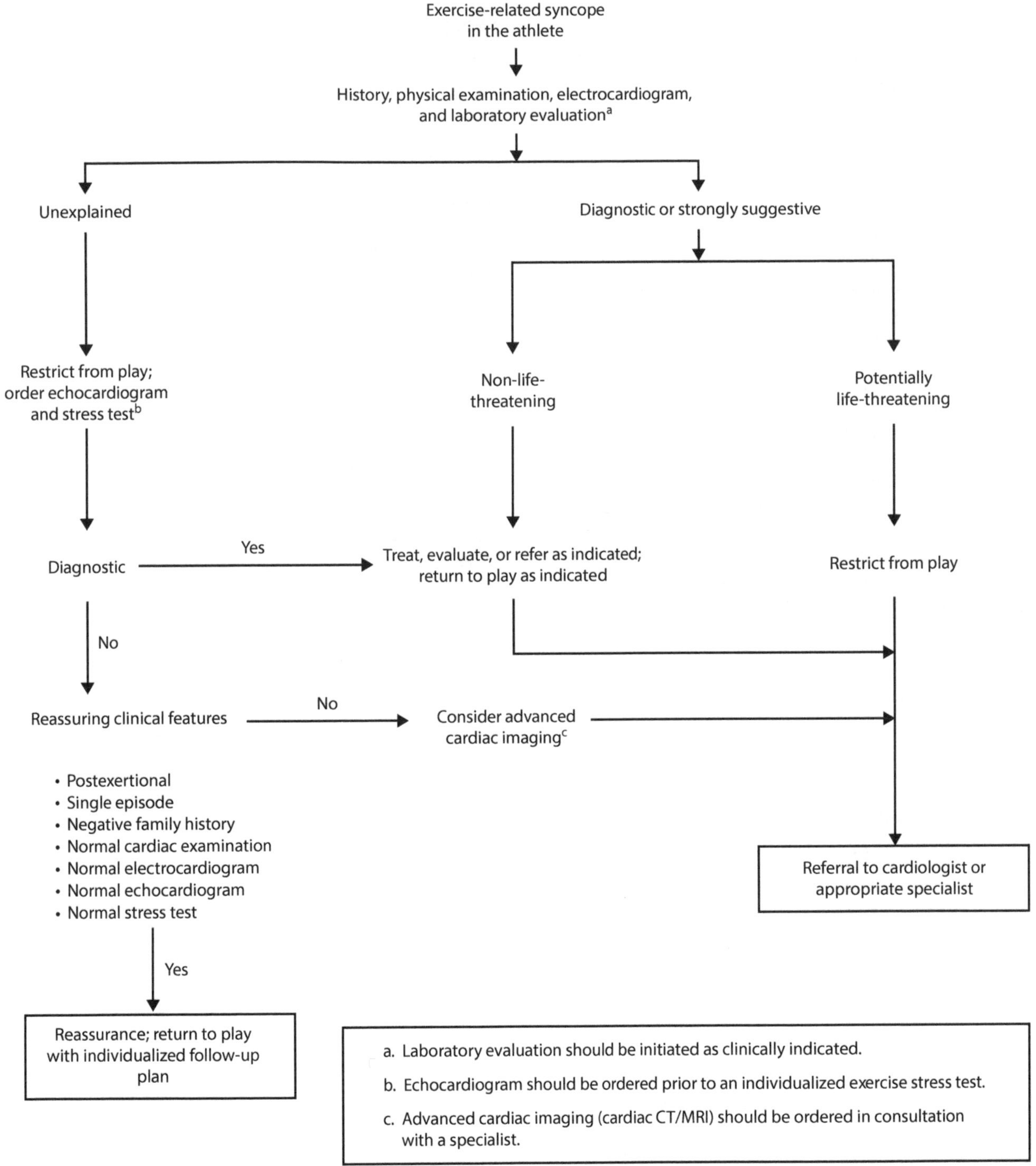

FIGURE 53.2 Algorithm for the evaluation of exercise-related syncope in the athlete. (Reproduced with permission from O'Connor, F.G. et al., *Clin. J. Sport Med.*, 19, 429, 2009.)

factor modification, and rehabilitation program that are monitored by the primary care physician in close consultation with a cardiologist in order to safely reintegrate these patients back into a reasonable and active lifestyle. The American College of Sports Medicine has recently published guidelines that assist the primary care physician in guiding the level of aerobic intensity.[11]

53.9 ARRHYTHMIAS IN THE ATHLETE

As mentioned earlier, lethal cardiac arrhythmias represent the most serious risk for sudden death in athletes. It is absolutely essential that the symptoms of a potential arrhythmia are taken seriously and thoroughly evaluated. These include the symptoms of syncope, near syncope, palpitations, exertional chest discomfort, severe dyspnea, or uncommon exertional

TABLE 53.6
Stratification Categories for Coronary Artery Disease Patients by the 36th Bethesda Conference

Mildly Increased Risk

- Left ventricular ejection fraction (LVEF) >50%
- Normal exercise tolerance for age
  - >10 METS if aged <50
  - >9 METS if aged 50–59
  - >8 METS if aged 60–69
  - >7 METS if aged >70
- Absence of exercise-induced ischemia and exercise-induced or postexercise complex ventricular arrhythmias
- Absence of hemodynamically significant stenosis (generally regarded as 50% or more luminal diameter narrowing) in any major coronary artery by coronary angiography
- Successful myocardial revascularization by surgical or percutaneous techniques if such revascularization was performed

Substantially Increased Risk

- Impaired LV systolic function at rest (LVEF less than 50%)
- Evidence of exercise-induced myocardial ischemia or complex ventricular arrhythmias
- Hemodynamically significant stenosis (generally regarded as 50% or more luminal diameter narrowing) of a major coronary artery if coronary angiography was performed

Source: Adapted from Thompson, P.D. et al., *J. Am. Coll. Cardiol.*, 45, 1348, 2005.

TABLE 53.7
Summary of 36th Bethesda Conference Recommendations for Patients with Coronary Artery Disease

- Athletes in the mildly increased risk group can participate in low dynamic and low/moderate static competitive sports but should avoid intensely competitive situations. Selected athletes with mildly increased risk may be permitted to compete in sports of higher levels of intensity when their overall clinical profile suggests very low exercise risk.
- All athletes should understand that the risk of a cardiac event with exertion is probably increased once coronary atherosclerosis of any severity is present.
- Athletes with mildly increased risk engaging in competitive sports should undergo reevaluation of their risk stratification at least annually.
- Athletes in the substantially increased risk category should generally be restricted to low-intensity competitive sports.
- Athletes should be informed of the nature of prodromal symptoms (such as chest, arm, jaw, and shoulder discomfort, unusual dyspnea) and should be instructed to cease their sports activity promptly and to contact their physician if symptoms appear.
- Those with a recent MI or myocardial revascularization should cease their athletic training and competition until recovery is deemed complete.
- All athletes with atherosclerotic CAD should have their atherosclerotic risk factors aggressively treated as studies suggest that comprehensive risk reduction is likely to stabilize coronary lesions and may reduce the risk of exercise-related events.

Source: Adapted from Thompson, P.D. et al., *J. Am. Coll. Cardiol.*, 45, 1348, 2005.

TABLE 53.8
SORT: Key Recommendations for Practice

Clinical Recommendation	Evidence Rating	References
A careful personal and family history and physical examination designed to identify cardiovascular conditions in young athletes should be included in preparticipation examinations.	C	[19,22]
Athletes with a murmur that becomes softer with squatting or louder or longer with standing or during a Valsalva maneuver should be evaluated for hypertrophic cardiomyopathy and mitral valve prolapse.	C	[19,22,23]
Routine screening with noninvasive tests, such as echocardiography, exercise stress testing, and electrocardiography, is not recommended.	C	[19,22,23]
Athletes with suspicious cardiovascular examination findings or a history of unexplained exercise-related symptoms (e.g., syncope, presyncope, and chest pain) after initial testing should be restricted from athletic participation pending further cardiologic evaluation.	C	[19,22,23]
Athletes with stage 2 hypertension (i.e., blood pressure above the 99th percentile [based on age, sex, and height] plus 5 mm Hg or blood pressure more than 160/100 mm Hg for athletes older than 18 years) should be restricted from participation until hypertension is controlled.	C	[5,11]

fatigue. Structural heart disease must be ruled out before the athlete is allowed to return to sports.[43] This will include a meticulous history, physical examination, and EKG and may be followed by chest x-ray, echocardiogram, stress test, Holter monitoring, electrolytes, and other laboratory testing. It may very well include early referral to a cardiologist for electrophysiologic study and/or ongoing management.

Various arrhythmias are compatible with competitive sports once they are diagnosed and controlled. Other conditions may be clearly incompatible with vigorous activity. Symptomatic dysrhythmias require evaluation and consultation with a cardiologist. The 36th Bethesda Conference provides recommendations for participation for common dysrhythmias.[43] The Committee on Sports Medicine and Fitness of the American Academy of Pediatrics specifically recommends that the presence of a symptomatic dysrhythmia requires exclusion from physical activity until this problem can be adequately evaluated by a cardiologist and controlled (Table 53.8).[41]

REFERENCES

1. Basilico FC. Cardiovascular disease in athletes. *The American Journal of Sports Medicine.* January–February 1999;27(1):108–121.
2. Blair SN, Kohl HW 3rd, Barlow CE, Paffenbarger RS Jr, Gibbons LW, Macera CA. Changes in physical fitness and all-cause mortality. A prospective study of healthy and unhealthy men. *Journal of the American Medical Association.* April 1995;273(14):1093–1098.

3. Cantu RC. Congenital cardiovascular disease—The major cause of athletic death in high school and college. *Medicine & Science in Sports & Exercise*. March 1992;24(3):279–280.
4. Cardiac Dysrhythmias and Sports. American Academy of Pediatrics Committee on Sports Medicine and Fitness. *Pediatrics*. May 1995;95(5):786–788.
5. Corrado D, Pelliccia A, Heidbuchel H, Sharma S, Link M, Basso C, Biffi A et al. Recommendations for interpretation of 12-lead electrocardiogram in the athlete. *European Heart Journal*. January 2010;31(2):243–259.
6. Drezner JA, Ackerman MJ, Anderson J, Ashley E, Asplund CA, Baggish AL, Borjesson M et al. Electrocardiographic interpretation in athletes: The 'Seattle Criteria'. *British Journal of Sports Medicine*. February 2013;47(3):122–124.
7. Drezner J, Berger S, Campbell R. Current controversies in the cardiovascular screening of athletes. *Current Sports Medicine Reports*. March–April 2010;9(2):86–92.
8. Drezner J, Corrado D. Is there evidence for recommending Ecg as part of the pre-participation examination?. *Clinical Journal of Sport Medicine*. 2010.
9. Firoozi S, Sharma S, Hamid MS, McKenna WJ. Sudden death in young athletes: Hcm or Arvc? *Cardiovascular Drugs and Therapy*. January 2002;16(1):11–17.
10. The fourth report on the diagnosis, evaluation, and treatment of high blood pressure in children and adolescents. *Pediatrics*. August 2004;114(2) Suppl 4th Report:555–576.
11. Garber CE, Blissmer B, Deschenes MR, Franklin BA, Lamonte MJ, Lee IM, Nieman DC, Swain DP. American College of Sports Medicine Position Stand. Quantity and Quality of Exercise for Developing and Maintaining Cardiorespiratory, Musculoskeletal, and Neuromotor Fitness in Apparently Healthy Adults: Guidance for Prescribing Exercise. *Medicine & Science in Sports & Exercise*. July 2011;43(7):1334–1359.
12. Giese EA, O'Connor FG, Brennan FH, Depenbrock PJ, Oriscello RG. The athletic preparticipation evaluation: Cardiovascular assessment. *American Family Physician*. April 2007;75(7):1008–1014.
13. James PA, Oparil S, Carter BL, Cushman WC, Dennison-Himmelfarb C, Handler J, Lackland DT et al. 2014 evidence-based guideline for the management of high blood pressure in adults: Report from the panel members appointed to the Eighth Joint National Committee (JNC 8). *Journal of the American Medical Association*. February 2014;311(5):507–520.
14. Kapoor WN. Current evaluation and management of syncope. *Circulation*. September 2002;106(13):1606–1609.
15. Kohl HW 3rd, Powell KE, Gordon NF, Blair SN, Paffenbarger RS Jr. Physical activity, physical fitness, and sudden cardiac death. *Epidemiologic Reviews*. 1992;14:37–58.
16. Leon AS, Connett J, Jacobs DR Jr, Rauramaa R. Leisure-time physical activity levels and risk of coronary heart disease and death. The multiple risk factor intervention trial. *Journal of the American Medical Association*. November 1987;258(17):2388–2395.
17. Loeys BL, Dietz HC, Braverman AC, Callewaert BL, De Backer J, Devereux RB, Hilhorst-Hofstee Y et al. The revised Ghent Nosology for the Marfan syndrome. *Journal of Medical Genetics*. July 2010;47(7):476–485.
18. Maron BJ. The paradox of exercise. *New England Journal of Medicine*. November 2000;343(19):1409–1411.
19. Maron BJ, Araujo CG, Thompson PD, Fletcher GF, de Luna AB, Fleg JL, Pelliccia A et al. Recommendations for preparticipation screening and the assessment of cardiovascular disease in masters athletes: An Advisory for Healthcare Professionals from the Working Groups of the World Heart Federation, the International Federation of Sports Medicine, and the American Heart Association Committee on Exercise, Cardiac Rehabilitation, and Prevention." *Circulation*. January 2001;103(2):327–34.
20. Maron BJ, Doerer JJ, Haas TS, Tierney DM, Mueller FO. Sudden deaths in young competitive athletes: Analysis of 1866 deaths in the United States, 1980–2006. *Circulation*. March 2009;119(8):1085–1092.
21. Maron BJ, Friedman RA, Kligfield P, Levine BD, Viskin S, Chaitman BR, Okin PM et al. Assessment of the 12-lead electrocardiogram as a Screening Test for Detection of Cardiovascular Disease in Healthy General Populations of Young People (12–25 Years of Age): A Scientific Statement from the American Heart Association and the American College of Cardiology." *Journal of the American College of Cardiology*. October 2014;64(14):1479–1514.
22. Maron BJ, Poliac LC, Roberts WO. Risk for sudden cardiac death associated with Marathon running. *Journal of the American College of Cardiology*. August 1996;28(2):428–431.
23. Maron BJ, Thompson PD, Ackerman MJ, Balady G, Berger S, Cohen D, Dimeff R et al. Recommendations and considerations related to preparticipation screening for cardiovascular abnormalities in competitive athletes: 2007 update: A Scientific Statement from the American Heart Association Council on Nutrition, Physical Activity, and Metabolism: Endorsed by the American College of Cardiology Foundation. *Circulation*. March 2007;115(12):1643–1455.
24. Maron BJ, Zipes DP. Introduction: Eligibility recommendations for competitive athletes with cardiovascular abnormalities-general considerations. *Journal of the American College of Cardiology*. April 2005;45(8):1318–1321.
25. Maron BJ, Friedman RA, Kligfield P, Levine BD, Viskin S, Chaitman BR, Okin PM et al. Assessment of the 12-lead ECG as a screening test for detection of cardiovascular disease in healthy general populations of young people (12–25 Years of Age): a scientific statement from the American Heart Association and the American College of Cardiology. *Circulation*. October 2014;130(15):1303–1334.
26. O'Connor FG, Levine BD, Childress MA, Asplundh CA, Oriscello RG. Practical management: A systematic approach to the evaluation of exercise-related syncope in athletes. *Clinical Journal of Sport Medicine*. September 2009;19(5):429–434.
27. O'Connor FG, Meyering CD, Patel R, Oriscello RP. Hypertension, athletes, and the sports physician: Implications of Jnc Vii, the Fourth Report, and the 36th Bethesda Conference Guidelines. *Current Sports Medicine Reports*. April 2007;6(2):80–84.
28. O'Connor FG, Oriscello RG, Levine BD. Exercise-related syncope in the young athlete: Reassurance, restriction or referral?" *American Family Physician*. November 1999;60(7):2001–2008.
29. Paffenbarger RS Jr, Hyde RT, Wing AL, Lee IM, Jung DL, Kampert JB. "The Association of changes in physical-activity level and other lifestyle characteristics with mortality among men." *New England Journal of Medicine*. February 1993;328(8):538–545.
30. Pate RR, Pratt M, Blair SN, Haskell WL, Macera CA, Bouchard C, Buchner D et al. Physical activity and public health. A Recommendation from the Centers for Disease Control and Prevention and the American College of Sports Medicine. *Journal of the American Medical Association*. February 1995;273(5):402–407.
31. Pelliccia A, Maron BJ, Culasso F, Di Paolo FM, Spataro A, Biffi A, Caselli G, Piovano P. Clinical significance of abnormal electrocardiographic patterns in trained athletes. *Circulation*. July 2000;102(3):278–284.

32. Pelliccia A, Zipes DP, Maron BJ. Bethesda Conference #36 and the European Society of Cardiology Consensus Recommendations Revisited a Comparison of U.S. and European Criteria for Eligibility and Disqualification of Competitive Athletes with Cardiovascular Abnormalities. *Journal of the American College of Cardiology*. December 2008;52(24):1990–1996.
33. Powell KE, Thompson PD, Caspersen CJ, Kendrick JS. Physical activity and the incidence of coronary heart disease. *Annual Review of Public Health*. 1987;8:253–287.
34. Priori SG, Aliot E, Blomstrom-Lundqvist C, Bossaert L, Breithardt G, Brugada P, Camm JA et al. Task force on sudden cardiac death, European Society of Cardiology. Summary of Recommendations. *Italian Heart Journal*. October 2002;(10) Suppl 3:1051–1065.
35. Ragosta M, Crabtree J, Sturner WQ, Thompson PD. Death during recreational exercise in the State of Rhode Island. *Medicine & Science in Sports & Exercise*. August 1984;16(4):339–342.
36. Siscovick DS, Weiss NS, Fletcher RH, Lasky T. The incidence of primary cardiac arrest during vigorous exercise. *New England Journal of Medicine*. October 1984;311(14):874–877.
37. Tabib A, Miras A, Taniere P, Loire R. Undetected cardiac lesions cause unexpected sudden cardiac death during occasional sport activity. A report of 80 cases. *European Heart Journal*. June 1999;20(12):900–903.
38. Thompson PD, Balady GJ, Chaitman BR, Clark LT, Levine BD, Myerburg RJ. Task force 6: Coronary artery disease. *Journal of the American College of Cardiology*. April 2005;45(8):1348–1353.
39. Thompson PD, Funk EJ, Carleton RA, Sturner WQ. Incidence of death during jogging in Rhode Island from 1975 through 1980. *Journal of the American Medical Association*. May 1982;247(18):2535–2538.
40. Van Camp SP, Bloor CM, Mueller FO, Cantu RC, Olson HG. Nontraumatic sports death in high school and college athletes. *Medicine & Science in Sports & Exercise*. May 1995;27(5):641–647.
41. Villeneuve PJ, Morrison HI, Craig CL, Schaubel DE. Physical activity, physical fitness, and risk of dying. *Epidemiology*. November 1998;9(6):626–631.
42. Williams PT. Physical fitness and activity as separate heart disease risk factors: A meta-analysis. *Medicine & Science in Sports & Exercise*. May 2001;33(5):754–761.
43. Zipes DP, Ackerman MJ, Estes NA 3rd, Grant AO, Myerburg RJ, Van Hare G. Task force 7: Arrhythmias. *Journal of the American College of Cardiology*. April 2005;45(8):1354–1363.

54 Pulmonary Considerations in the Athlete

Carrie A. Jaworski and Scott Repa

CONTENTS

TABLE 54.1
Key Clinical Considerations

1. Athletes with pulmonary conditions can safely exercise if they are educated on proper management of their disease process, which may include behavioral and medication-type therapies.
2. Regular exercise has been shown to decrease the number of asthma exacerbations, reduce the need for medication use, and decrease the number of days missed from school or work.
3. EIB can occur in athletes either with or without the diagnosis of asthma.
4. The diagnosis of EIB requires careful consideration of the athlete's conditioning, sport, and level of competition in order to most closely replicate the scenario in which they exercise when performing diagnostic testing.
5. Clinicians should include appropriate amounts of exercise in the management of patients with chronic lung diseases such as COPD or CF in order to help maximize their lung capacities and provide emotional and physical benefits.

54.1 INTRODUCTION

Pulmonary conditions can influence safe participation in activities in a number of ways and can affect patients of all ages. Proper education and management of the medical and environmental factors influencing these pulmonary disorders are necessary to ensure maximum benefit and enjoyment of activity. The focus of this chapter is to highlight the most common and pertinent pulmonary conditions affecting both recreational and elite athletes and review the current understanding, diagnosis, and treatment considerations relevant to these populations (Table 54.1).

54.2 ASTHMA

54.2.1 Definition

Asthma is a complex pulmonary disorder characterized by acute and chronic inflammatory processes that produce varying degrees of decreased airflow, bronchial hyperresponsiveness, and resulting respiratory symptoms.[24] Several cell types and cell mediators, as well as immunoglobulin E (IgE) antibodies, facilitate and perpetuate inflammation. Persistent asthma can lead to remodeling of the airway, characterized by mucus hypersecretion, epithelial injury, smooth muscle hypertrophy, angiogenesis, and underlying fibrosis. Atopy and gene-by-environment interactions are two of the strongest influences on the development of asthma.[24]

54.2.2 Prevalence

Approximately 22 million adults and 6 million children in the United States have asthma, accounting for approximately 1 in 11 persons in the United States today.[1,24] Research suggests that athletes have a higher prevalence of asthma, up to 15% versus 9% in the general population.[35] Exposure to allergens, irritants, and viruses, along with increased ventilation rates over longer periods, is one of the factors influencing the higher prevalence.

Clinical Pearl

The highest rates of asthma have been observed in elite athletes and those participating in endurance activities, such as cross-country skiers, swimmers, cyclists, and distance runners.[35]

54.2.3 History, Physical Assessment, and Diagnosis

The clinician's initial focus should concentrate on a detailed personal and family medical history, as well as a thorough examination of the upper respiratory tracts, chest, and skin. The classic clinical symptoms of airflow obstruction caused by asthma, which include a history or presence of episodic wheezing, chest tightness, shortness of breath, or cough, are important for establishing a diagnosis.

Hallmarks of physical exam findings in asthmatics may include thoracic hyperexpansion, use of accessory muscles, increase in nasal secretions, edema of mucous membranes, the presence of nasal polyps, and signs of atopy. However, the absence of these symptoms at the time of examination does not exclude the diagnosis, nor is the presence of the symptoms alone sufficient to establish the diagnosis.

Also necessary for diagnosis is demonstration that the patient's airflow obstruction is at least partially reversible, through the use of Pulmonary Function Testing (PFT). To achieve this, clinicians must first establish that airflow obstruction exists.

Clinical Pearl

Interpreting Spirometry Results to Establish a Diagnosis of Asthma:

Confirm an FEV_1 <80% of predicted *and* FEV_1/FVC <65% or below the lower limit of normal. FEV_1 = forced expiratory volume in 1 second, and FVC = forced vital capacity.

Establish Reversibility with an FEV_1 increase of ≥12% from baseline or ≥10% of predicted FEV_1 after using a short-acting inhaled β2-agonist.[24]

If spirometry is normal, clinicians should consider alternative diagnoses, taking into consideration age, physical exam, and results of diagnostic testing. Once a diagnosis of asthma is established, classification of severity is based on history, symptoms, risk, and spirometry results (see Figure 54.1).

Components of Severity		Classification of Asthma Severity ≥12 years of age			
			Persistent		
		Intermittent	Mild	Moderate	Severe
Impairment Normal FEV_1/FVC: 8–19 yr 85% 20–39 yr 80% 40–59 yr 75% 60–80 yr 70%	Symptoms	≤2 days/week	>2 days/week but not daily	Daily	Throughout the day
	Nighttime awakenings	≤2x/month	3–4x/month	>1x/week but not nightly	Often 7x/week
	Short-acting $beta_2$-agonist use for symptom control (not prevention of EIB)	≤2 days/week	>2 days/week but not daily, and not more than 1x on any day	Daily	Several times per day
	Interference with normal activity	None	Minor limitation	Some limitation	Extremely limited
	Lung function	• Normal FEV_1 between exacerbations • FEV_1>80% predicted • FEV_1/FVC normal	• FEV_1>80% predicted • FEV_1/FVC normal	• FEV_1>60% but <80% predicted • FEV_1/FVC reduced 5%	• FEV_1>60% predicted • FEV_1/FVC reduced >5%
Risk	Exacerbations requiring oral systemic corticosteroids	0–1/year (see note)	≥2/year (see note) →		
		← Consider severity and interval since last exacerbation. → Frequency and severity may fluctuate over time for patients in any severity category. Relative annual risk of exacerbations may be related to FEV_1.			
Recommended Step for Initiating Treatment		Step 1	Step 2	Step 3	Step 4 or 5
				and consider short course of oral systemic corticosteroids	
(See figure 4–5 for treatment steps.)		In 2–6 weeks, evaluate level of asthma control that is achieved and adjust therapy accordingly.			

Key: FEV_1, forced expiratory volume in second; FVC, forced vital capacity; ICU, intensive care unit

FIGURE 54.1 Reference tool for classifying asthma severity and initiating treatment in youth > 12 years of age and adults. (From National Heart, Lung, and Blood Institute; National Institutes of Health; U.S. Department of Health and Human Services.)

54.2.4 Management

Management of the athlete with asthma should focus on a stepwise approach based on disease severity, as well as identifying and moderating environmental triggers and comorbid conditions. Patient education and objective monitoring are equally important, and clinicians must assess each athlete's ability to manage their asthma.

The primary goals of management are to decrease symptoms and impairment, moderate risk, and establish periodic assessments of asthma control both by the clinician and through self-monitoring[24] (see Figure 54.2).

There are two main classes of asthma medications: long-term control medications that are used to treat and control the persistent symptoms of asthma and short-acting agents that provide immediate relief. Long-term controller medications for asthma have an established history of effectiveness.[15,24,25,38,39] The most common medications and their uses are summarized in Table 54.2. Each of these medications can have a potential role, but inhaled corticosteroids (ICSs) are considered to be the most consistently effective long-term controller asthma medication.[24,39]

Short-term controller medications can provide prompt relief of acute asthma symptoms and include short-acting β2-agonists (SABAs) and the anticholinergic medication ipratropium bromide. Ipratropium bromide reduces vagal tone in the airway and can be useful in moderate-to-severe exacerbations due to cholinergic-mediated bronchospasm, but is generally not used alone unless there is an intolerance to SABAs or concurrent chronic obstructive pulmonary disease (COPD). SABAs, such as albuterol and levalbuterol, relax smooth muscle in airways and cause bronchodilation, similar to the effect of long-acting β2-agonists (LABAs). They are the treatment of choice to provide rapid relief from symptoms related to an acute exacerbation and are generally considered safe. Long-term daily use is discouraged because it can lead to decreased effectiveness and should be viewed as a sign of poor disease control.

Systemic corticosteroids are effective adjuncts in managing moderate-to-severe asthma exacerbations. They do not act as quickly as the short-term medications but can help to speed recovery and prevent relapse. Conversely, they are not to be used long term, and even short-term use carries risk. Abnormal glucose metabolism, weight gain, hypertension, peptic ulcer, mood alteration, decreased immune function, and rarely aseptic necrosis are all known side effects to using these medications.

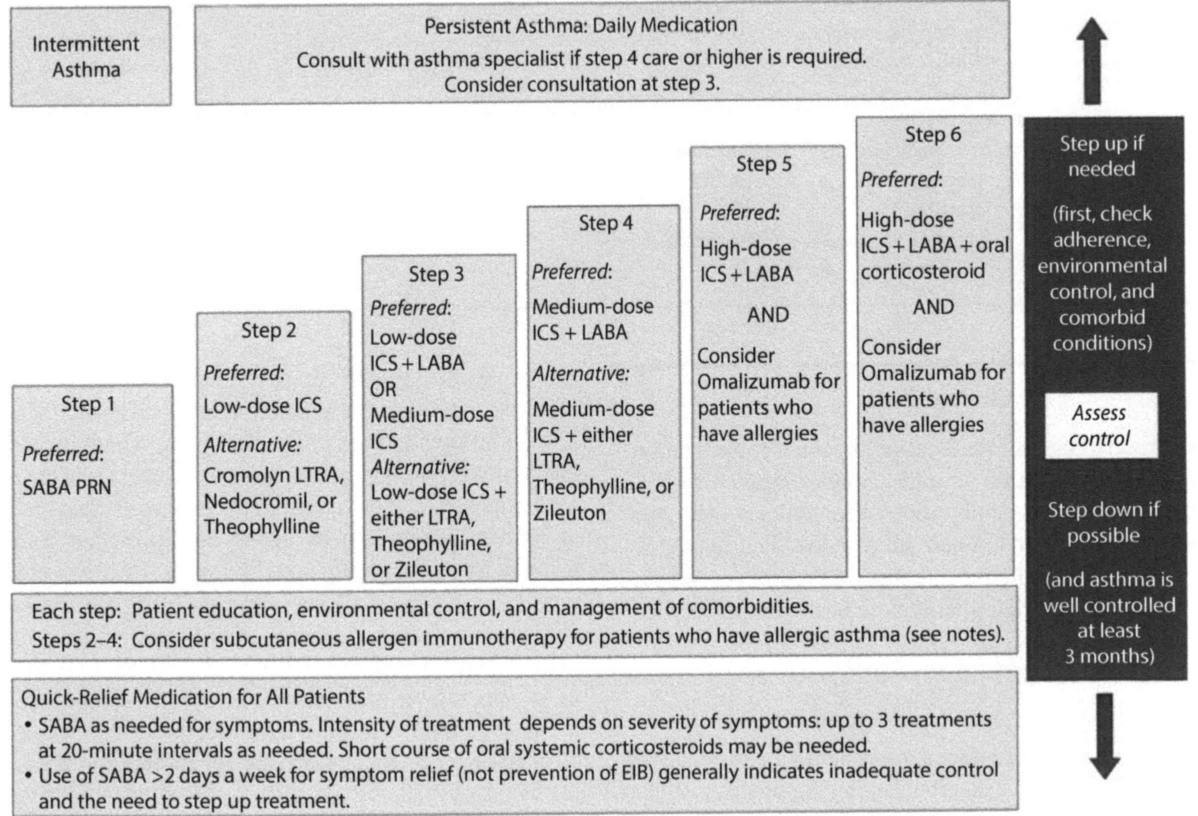

FIGURE 54.2 Sample stepwise approach for managing asthma in youth >12 years of age and adults. (From National Heart, Lung, and Blood Institute; National Institutes of Health; U.S. Department of Health and Human Services.)

TABLE 54.2
Long-Acting Asthma Controller Medications

	Mechanism of Action	Effects	Route and Usage	Safety Profile
Inhaled corticosteroids	• Inhibit reactivity to allergens • Inhibit inflammatory cells • Decrease airway hyperresponsiveness	• Anti-inflammatory, most effective and common first-line therapy	• Daily • Inhaled • Not useful as a rescue medication	• Generally safe and well tolerated. • Side effects: • irritation/bronchospasm, dysphonia, oral candidiasis • Side effects can be mitigated with use of a spacer/MDI and by rinsing mouth after treatment
Khellin derivatives	• Stabilize mast cells, though exact MOA preventing release of inflammatory mediators is unknown	• Anti-inflammatory, not as effective in outcome measures compared to ICS	• Daily • Inhaled • Alternative to ICS, not preferred	• Excellent safety profile. • Cromolyn sodium—approved for all ages • Nedocromil sodium—approved over age 6
Leukotriene modifiers	• LTRA 9 (zafirlukast or montelukast) or 5-lipo-oxygenase inhibitor (zileuton)	• Anti-inflammatory—blocks the effects of formed leukotrienes	• Daily • Oral • Alternative or supplement to ICS • Zileuton not recommended	• Generally safe • Side effects include headache, sore throat, drowsiness, GI upset, hypersensitivity reactions, sleep, and mood disorders
Long-acting β2-agonists	• Smooth muscle relaxation	• Bronchodilation • Lasts up to 12 hours, but decreases to 5 hours with chronic use	• Daily • Usually combined with ICS • Discouraged as monotherapy	• *Black box warming* increase in asthma exacerbations and death • Consensus opinion suggests weighing benefit vs. likely minor risk
Immune modulators	• Monoclonal antibody • Prevents the binding of IgE to basophils	• Anti-inflammatory	• Daily • Oral • Supplement to high-dose ICS and LABA • For patients 12 years and older	• Consider only for severe, persistent asthma not controlled on maximal therapy • Generally safe and well tolerated, rare anaphylaxis
Methylxanthines	• Bronchodilation via smooth muscle relaxation • Inhibits TNF-α and leukotriene synthesis	• Also mild anti-inflammatory and immunomodulator	• Daily • Oral • Alternative adjunctive therapy with ICS, though not preferred	• Theophylline requires monitoring of blood levels

Clinical Pearl

When prescribing any medication, special consideration and appropriate caution should always be given to collegiate, professional, and other elite athletes who are subject to testing for banned substances. The appropriate governing body should be consulted whenever there is concern and appropriate therapeutic use exemptions filed if necessary.

SABAs remain the hallmark of treatment in asthmatic athletes who have an acute exacerbation during practice or competition. Consideration should be made for transfer to an emergency department if frequent doses of inhaled SABAs fail to provide relief of symptoms.

An essential way to combine education, empowerment, and effective management with all patients suffering from asthma is with an updated asthma action plan, which provides clear and simple actions to take in an exacerbation and defines each medicine's role. The asthma action plan is also transferable and easily interpreted by health-care providers and athletic trainers who often evaluate athletes during travel or competition. For athletes of all ages, proper use of a peak flow meter is also necessary for periodic monitoring and for maximum benefit from an asthma action plan.

In general, regular exercise should be encouraged for all asthmatics whose disease is under good control. An FEV_1 of at least 80% of the expected levels should be a signal for initiation of exercise, with the goal of eventually achieving 20–30 minutes of exercise per day on most days of the week, consistent with the recommendations of the American College of Sports Medicine.[14]

Clinical Pearl

Exercise has been shown to decrease the number of asthma exacerbations, reduce the need for medication use, and decrease the number of days missed from school or work.[9,24]

54.3 EXERCISE-INDUCED BRONCHOSPASM

54.3.1 Introduction

Exercise-induced bronchospasm (EIB) is an asthma-like event characterized by airway narrowing and is thought to be caused by exposure of the lower respiratory tract to air that is cooler and/or drier than the ambient environment of the lungs.[10,29] During exercise, increased ventilation rates result in increased exposure and reaction to the ambient conditions. The presence of existing mucus plugs, mucosal edema, exposure to airborne irritants, and intensity of exercise represent potential additive triggers.

EIB can be seen in up to 90% of athletes who have been previously diagnosed with asthma.[1] These patients could rightfully carry the often-synonymous diagnosis of exercise-induced asthma (EIA). However, nonasthmatics can have EIB. The presence of allergic rhinitis or atopic dermatitis without underlying asthma predicts a 40% chance of EIB. The same inflammatory mediators and cells are usually involved regardless of asthma status, and therefore the treatments are the same. With an established diagnosis of asthma, the presence of EIB suggests inadequate control of underlying asthma. EIB in athletes without a previous diagnosis should raise suspicion for potentially undiagnosed asthma. This highlights the theoretical difference between EIB and EIA, which is the presence of underlying chronic inflammation.

54.3.2 History

A classic story for EIB is cough, wheezing, shortness of breath, chest tightness, or endurance problems associated with exercise. The symptoms occur during or just after exercise, usually worsen in the 5–10 minutes after stopping exercise, and resolve over 20–30 minutes.

Clinical Pearl

After an EIB episode, there is often a refractory period of 1–2 hours during which ~50% of athletes will feel essentially symptom-free. This refractory period is important to identify for its diagnostic value, but is also a useful focus for management.

54.3.3 Diagnosis

Because relying only on history or self-reported symptoms can lead to both overdiagnosis and underdiagnosis of EIB, it is important to utilize more objective testing to guide appropriate treatment. The use of a direct or indirect challenge tests can help to confirm a diagnosis of EIB or asthma and also help to differentiate them from masqueraders like vocal cord dysfunction (VCD).

Direct pharmacologic testing is often performed with a methacholine challenge, while indirect testing is usually in the form of an exercise challenge. Methacholine and other direct challenge tests are highly sensitive, but are far less specific without an already high pretest probability for asthma. They are useful for ruling in asthma as a possible cause of symptoms. These are called direct tests because they directly cause contraction in the smooth muscle of the airway to achieve the bronchospasm. By contrast, indirect challenge tests focus on stimulating the release of an athlete's endogenous mediators of bronchospasm. Indirect tests are more specific for ruling in asthma or EIB and are usually the test of choice for evaluating EIB.

Indirect testing often involves an exercise protocol, such as recording serial peak expiratory flow (PEF) or FEV measurements at 5 minute intervals for 20–30 minutes before exercise and then exercising to achieve and sustain 80% of maximum heart rate for 4–8 minutes, followed by additional PEF or FEV_1 measurements at 5 minute intervals for another 20–30 minutes. This testing can be done in both formal and informal settings. The diagnosis of EIB requires a drop in PEF or FEV_1 testing by at least 15%.[24] Normal testing and inspiratory wheezing should raise suspicion for VCD as a possible diagnosis. Gastroesophageal reflux disease and cardiac disorders may also produce symptoms with normal challenge testing and should remain on a differential diagnosis, along with respiratory infection and hyperventilation syndromes.

Both forms of indirect exercise challenge testing have advantages and disadvantages, which help to account for the significant difference in prevalence estimates for EIB.[24,28] PEF testing is convenient and reliable for highly symptomatic individuals, but does not correct for effort and has decreased sensitivity in detecting subtler forms of EIB, especially in elite athletes. Spirometry is able to detect and account for changes in effort, and so is more accurate, but ambient laboratory conditions often do not adequately reproduce the crucial decreases in air temperature, humidity, or airborne/chemical irritants. Level of fitness can also complicate the decision of what effort protocol to utilize in a challenge test, regardless of the testing instrument. Submaximal work rates that keep an athlete below their individual lactate threshold may not provoke EIB, and the exact level of the threshold is likewise variable among athletes.

Because of these difficulties, while EIB in the general population is estimated between 10% and 15%, estimates for athletes vary widely, from 10% to 50%.[8,10,20,24,29] Not, surprisingly, cold-weather athletes have higher rates, estimated between 25% and 75%, as well as sports that involve higher minute ventilations or expose the participant to higher levels of airborne pollutants.[8,17,22,29]

Clinical Pearl

- Choosing an appropriate test and protocol for evaluation of EIB is an individualized process requiring careful consideration of the athlete's sport, conditioning, environment, and level of competition.[8]
- Indirect tests are more specific for ruling in asthma or EIB and are usually the test of choice for evaluating EIB.

For any potential or current Olympic athlete, the United States Olympic Committee requires an indirect test known as eucapnic voluntary hyperventilation (EVH) testing to confirm a diagnosis of EIB. Permission to use long-term or rescue medications for EIB will not currently be granted without it.[3,11] EVH testing utilizes controlled hyperventilation of a "dry" gas mixture to provoke bronchospasm. A decrease of FEV_1 by 20% with documented reversibility through use of a SABA establishes the diagnosis of EIB.

54.3.4 Management

There is strong evidence for the use of SABAs as the primary intervention in EIB. When administered 15 minutes before exercise, they typically provide relief from EIB lasting 2–3 hours.[24] However, a chronic requirement of SABA before exercise warrants consideration of adjunctive medication and consideration of poorly controlled or undiagnosed asthma. If appropriate, use of a long-acting medication such as an ICS should be considered.[18] In cases of previously diagnosed asthma, increasing the dosage of daily control medicines should also be considered.

LABAs, leukotriene-receptor antagonists (LTRAs), and cromolyn can also be considered as adjuncts, but should not be used alone and are not first-line agents unless SABAs are not tolerated. The use of LABAs can provide relief for up to 12 hours in EIB; however, chronic use can reduce the effectiveness to only 5 hours.[24,30,32] LTRAs have shown some promise as well in the attenuation of EIB in up to 50% of those who use them.[24]

An appropriate warm-up before exercise may reduce EIB symptom severity in subsequent competition or even induce a refractory period in the athlete.[13] Maximizing the recognition and use of the refractory period promotes the development of self-awareness about EIB and can improve symptom management, but shouldn't take the place of prescribed medications. Items such as scarves or masks can help to mitigate the effects of cold-induced EIB.

As is the case with asthma medications, athletes and those prescribing the medications should be aware of any governing bodies relevant to their sport and their related medication guidelines, regulations, or bans. The U.S. Anti-Doping Agency has many resources available to the public.

Clinical Pearl

- SABAs are the hallmark of treatment for athletes with acute exacerbation during competition and for prevention of exacerbations once a diagnosis is made.
- Disclosure of medication use is often necessary, and some athletes will require a therapeutic use exemption for medication use.

54.4 COPD

54.4.1 Introduction

COPD is a progressive lung disorder that makes breathing difficult. COPD comes in two distinct forms, chronic bronchitis and emphysema. While they develop as separate processes, both conditions can occur at the same time, and most people with COPD have some measure of each.[23]

Chronic bronchitis results from long-term irritation and inflammation in the airway. The lining of the airways becomes thickened from increases in viscous mucus and airway hyperreactivity, resulting in obstructions that can lead to the dyspnea and hypoxemia associated with COPD. Chronic air trapping and increased accessory muscle from these obstructions also lead to deconditioning, and this state further perpetuates respiratory decline. By contrast, emphysema results from damage to the walls and membranes lining the airways and especially in the alveolar air sacs where air exchange occurs. The destruction of the airway and alveolar linings not only impairs gas exchange but also compromises the elasticity of the system. Elastic compliance is vital to generate the negative pressure needed to inhale properly and effectively. Without stretch or structural integrity, dyspnea and hypoxemia follow.

54.4.2 Prevalence

COPD is common. While prevalence estimates range from 6% to 19%, the condition is thought to be underdiagnosed.[16] COPD is most commonly caused by cigarette smoking, though other causes, such as alpha-1 antitrypsin deficiency, do exist. Environmental irritants such as air pollution, dust, and fumes also play a role, especially with long-term exposures.

54.4.3 Evaluation and Management

The most common symptoms of COPD are congested or productive cough, wheezing, shortness of breath, and chest tightness. Concern for COPD should prompt a comprehensive examination, as well as PFT to assess respiratory status. Once a diagnosis has been established, treatment of COPD focuses on maintaining and maximizing the remaining functional capacity of the lungs using a multidisciplinary approach.[16]

Clinical Pearls

- Multidisciplinary treatment of COPD focuses on maintaining and maximizing the remaining functional capacity of the lungs,[16] and safe exercise should be part of that plan if possible.
- Though exercise does not seem to reverse COPD or increase life expectancy, it can still provide sizable physical and emotional benefits.[5,23]

Assessment should start with determination of cardiac risk and exercise capacity in all patients with COPD.[16] A treadmill or stationary cycle exercise test can follow several established protocols and will help determine what level of exercise is safe to avoid serious complications, what medications might be helpful to facilitate participation, and what amount of supplemental oxygen may be needed during activity. Those with more serious diseases should consider enrolling in a pulmonary rehabilitation program to increase their activity level safely.[5,16,23,26,36] Most patients with COPD should strive to exercise 3 days per week at 60%–80% of maximal heart rate for 20–30 minutes.[16,19,23]

Both medications and supplemental oxygen can help COPD patients be active. Bronchodilators and anticholinergic medications should be deployed as needed to promote and enable exercise.[16,26,27,36] In addition, ICSs can be used to decrease inflammation, and mucolytics can thin obstructive secretions, helping to facilitate secretion clearance. Oral steroids are usually reserved for severe exacerbations and are not routinely part of an exercise protocol.[16] Preventative medical therapies have an important role in COPD as well. Remaining current with recommended vaccinations, particularly influenza and pneumococcal immunizations, is vital to mitigating unnecessary risk and potential complications.[16,26,27] Mechanical measures such as use of bronchopulmonary toilet and pursed lip breathing can also help patients advance safely and comfortably toward their goals.

54.5 CYSTIC FIBROSIS

54.5.1 Introduction

Cystic fibrosis (CF) is an autosomal recessive disorder that affects the secretory glands in the pulmonary, gastrointestinal (GI), reproductive, skeletal, and integumentary systems. Clinical complications of CF relate to the thick, sticky mucus that is abnormally produced in place of normal thin mucus. The increased viscosity of the mucus and increased salt in sweat follow from abnormal CTFR protein production, which results in poor regulation of water and salt balance within and between cells. Location and severity of the genetic defects causing CF impact the severity of the disease, and there is some evidence that other genes may also play a role. The chronic pulmonary manifestations of CF represent the most significant burden from CF and account for the most morbidity and mortality overall. Persistent mucus production leads to obstruction in the lungs, impairing proper lung function and oxygenation as well as increasing opportunities to harbor and incubate infectious organisms.

54.5.2 Prevalence and Diagnosis

CF can affect both males and females and persons of any ethnic background. It is most common in Northern European Caucasians, but is common also in Latino and certain Native American groups. Current estimates suggest that about 10 million people in the United States today carry an abnormal CF gene.[7] While many carriers are asymptomatic and unaware that they have CF gene, CF testing is now in standard in every State's newborn screening panels, which is increasing awareness and early diagnosis. Prenatal screening is also available and can be considered for couples who may be at increased risk. Positive screening tests undergo confirmatory sweat chloride testing.

54.5.3 Management

CF has no "cure" at this time, so the goal for the management includes the prevention and prompt management of upper and lower respiratory infections, adequate thinning and clearing of secretions, and prevention of dehydration and malnutrition.[7] Disease severity varies between individuals and also often waxes and wanes, which warrants the inclusion of providers experienced with CF as part of the health-care team.[7] Respiratory complications are mainly treated with the use of medications, chest physiotherapy, and exercise.

Inhaled steroids, bronchodilators, oxygen, and antibiotics are often used in the management of CF.[12,37] These can be used prophylactically or symptomatically based on clinical context. The principal aims of these medicines are the same as in other lung disorders and include maintenance of a patent airway and respiratory tree by reducing inflammation, relaxing smooth muscle, thinning secretions, and facilitating their clearance. Oral steroids, oxygen therapy, and lung transplantation are more serious interventions usually reserved for more advanced disease.

Chest physical therapy, or chest percussion, can help to facilitate loosening and clearance of respiratory secretions.[34] It can be performed alone or with a therapist, and several techniques and devices have been developed. Exercise, in addition to being an important part of overall physical conditioning, also helps to improve secretion clearance due to increased ventilatory rate and effort.[12,37] These effects can be additive when complemented by chest therapy.[34] However, increased salt content in the sweat makes exercise potentially dangerous for CF patients, especially as ambient temperature rises. Dehydration, weakness, fatigue, tachycardia, hypotension, and even death can result from sweating in active CF patients.

TABLE 54.3
SORT: Key Recommendations for Practice

Clinical Recommendation	Evidence Rating	References
Use of ICSs is an effective controller therapy in the management of EIB in an athlete with underlying asthma.	A	[13,18,24]
Athletes with EIB can attenuate symptoms through the use of a SABA prior to exercise.	A	[13,24]
Self-reported symptoms should not be the sole method to diagnose EIB.	C	[13,24]
Warming up prior to exercise may induce a refractory period and reduce the degree of EIB.	C	[13,24]
Patients with COPD who participate in pulmonary rehabilitation show improved exercise capacity and health-related quality of life.	A	[19,26,27,36]

Digestive manifestations of CF often result from decreased nutrient absorption and can affect multiple organ systems function as well as exercise capacity. Increased mucus can block the delivery of pancreatic enzymes to the GI tract, which are essential for digestive processing of fat and protein. In young patients, nutritional deficiencies can affect growth and development, and CF patients of all ages can experience decreases in exercise capacity that correlate with the decreased energy availability (Table 54.3).[31]

Clinical Pearl

- With milder forms of CF, patients can usually be encouraged to exercise as tolerated. With more severe CF, exercise can be guided in a pulmonary rehabilitation program.
- Proper education about salt and fluid maintenance is essential for safe participation in exercise.
- Exercise can help to combat osteoporosis and diabetes, which are common in CF patients.[31]

REFERENCES

1. Akinbami LJ, Moorman JE, Liu X. Asthma prevalence, health care use, and mortality: United States, 2005–2009. National health statistics reports; no 32. Hyattsville, MD: National Center for Health Statistics; 2011.
2. American College of Sports Medicine. Physical Activity and Public Health: Updated Recommendation for Adults from the American College of Sports Medicine and the American Heart Association. *Medicine & Science in Sports & Exercise.* 2007;39(8):1423–1434.
3. Anderson SD, Fitch K, Perry CP et al. Responses to bronchial challenge submitted for approval to use inhaled beta2-agonists before an event at the 2002 Winter Olympics. *Journal of Allergy and Clinical Immunology.* 2003;111(1):45–50.
4. Bundgaard A. Exercise and the asthmatic. *Sport Medicine.* 1985;2(4):254–266.
5. Casaburi R. Exercise training in chronic obstructive lung disease. In: Casaburi R, Petty TL (eds.). *Principles and Practice of Pulmonary Rehabilitation.* Philadelphia, PA: Saunders. pp. 204–224.
6. Centers for Disease Control and Prevention. Chronic obstructive pulmonary disease among adults—United States, 2011. *Morbidity and Mortality Weekly Report.* 2012;61(46):938–943.
7. Cystic Fibrosis Foundation. About cystic fibrosis: Overview, frequently asked questions, testing for cystic fibrosis. Available at http://www.cff.org/AboutCF/. Accessed March 30, 2014.
8. Dickinson JW, Whyte GP, McConnell AK et al. Screening elite winter athletes for exercise induced asthma: A comparison of three challenge methods. *British Journal of Sports Medicine.* 2006;40:179–182.
9. Disabella V, Sherman C. Exercise for asthma patients: Little risk, big rewards. *Physician and Sportsmedicine.* 1998; 26(6):75–85.
10. Feinstein RA, LaRussa J, Wang-Dohlman A et al. Screening adolescent athletes for exercise-induced asthma. *Clinical Journal of Sport Medicine.* 1996;6(2):119–123.
11. Fitch KD, Sue-Chu M, Anderson SD et al. Asthma and the elite athlete: Summary of the International Olympic Committee's Consensus Conference, Lausanne, Switzerland, January 22–24, 2008. *Journal of Allergy and Clinical Immunology.* Available at http://www.ncbi.nlm.nih.gov/pubmed/18678340. Accessed February 16, 2014.
12. Flume PA, Robinson KA, O'Sullivan BP et al. Clinical Practice Guidelines for Pulmonary Therapies Committee. Cystic fibrosis pulmonary guidelines: Airway clearance therapies. *Respiratory Care.* 2009;54(4):522–537.
13. Dryden DM, Spooner CH, Stickland MK et al. Exercise-induced bronchoconstriction and asthma. Evidence Reports/Technology Assessments, no. 189. AHRQ publication no. 10-E001. Rockville, MD: Agency for Healthcare Research and Quality; January 2010.
14. Garber CE, Blissmer B, Deschenes MR. Quantity and quality of exercise for developing and maintaining cardiorespiratory, musculoskeletal, and neuromotor fitness in apparently healthy adults: Guidance for prescribing exercise. *Medicine & Science in Sports & Exercise.* 2011;43(7):1334–1359.
15. Garcia-Garcia ML, Wahn U, Gilles L et al. Montelukast, compared with fluticasone, for control of asthma among 6- to 14-year-old patients with mild asthma: the MOSAIC study. *Pediatrics.* 2005;116(2):360–369.
16. Global Strategy for the Diagnosis, Management and Prevention of COPD, Global Initiative for Chronic Obstructive Lung Disease (GOLD) 2014. Available from http://www.goldcopd.org/. Accessed February 18, 2014.
17. Helenius IJ, Tikkanen HO, Haahtela T. Association between type of training and risk of asthma in elite athletes. *Thorax.* 1997;52:157–160.
18. Koh MS, Tee A, Lasserson TJ, Irving LB. Inhaled corticosteroids compared to placebo for prevention of exercise induced bronchoconstriction. *Cochrane Database of Systematic Reviews.* 2007;(3):CD002739.
19. Lacasse Y, Goldstein R, Lasserson TJ, Martin S. Pulmonary rehabilitation for chronic obstructive pulmonary disease. *Cochrane Database of Systematic Reviews.* 2006;(4):CD003793.
20. Langdeau JB, Boulet LP. Prevalence and mechanism of development of asthma and airway hyperresponsiveness in athletes. *Sports Medicine.* 2001;31:601–616.

21. LeGrys VA, Yankaskas JR, Quittell LM et al. Diagnostic sweat testing: The Cystic Fibrosis Foundation guidelines. *Journal of Pediatrics*. 2007;151(1):85–89.
22. Mayers LB, Rundell KW. Exercise-induced asthma. ACSM Current Comment. Available at http://www.acsm.org. Accessed February 16, 2014.
23. Mink BD. Exercise and chronic obstructive pulmonary disease: Modest fitness gains pay big dividends. *Physician and Sportsmedicine*. 1997;25(11):43–52.
24. National Asthma Education and Prevention Program, Third Expert Panel on the Diagnosis and Management of Asthma. Expert Panel Report 3: Guidelines for the Diagnosis and Management of Asthma. Bethesda (MD): National Heart, Lung, and Blood Institute (US); August 2007. Available at http://www.ncbi.nlm.nih.gov/books/NBK7232/. Accessed January 20, 2014.
25. Ostrom NK, Decotiis BA, Lincourt WR et al. Comparative efficacy and safety of low-dose fluticasone propionate and montelukast in children with persistent asthma. *Journal of Pediatrics*. 2005;147(2):213–220.
26. Qaseem A, Wilt TJ, Weinberger SE et al. Diagnosis and management of stable chronic obstructive pulmonary disease: A clinical practice guideline update from the American College of Physicians, American College of Chest Physicians, American Thoracic Society, and European Respiratory Society. *Annals of Internal Medicine*. 2011;155:179–191.
27. Ries AL, Bauldoff GS, Carlin BW et al. Pulmonary rehabilitation: Joint ACCP/AACVPR evidence-based clinical practice guidelines. *Chest*. 2007;131(5 Suppl):4S–42S.
28. Rundell KW, Wilber RL, Szmedra L et al. Exercise-induced asthma screening of elite athletes: Field versus laboratory exercise challenge. *Medicine & Science in Sports & Exercise*. 2000;32(2):309–316.
29. Schumacher YO, Pottgeiser T, Dickhuth H-H. Exercise-induced bronchoconstriction: Asthma in athletes. *International Sportmed Journal Impact Factor*. 2011;12(4):145–149.
30. Simons FE, Gerstner TV, Cheang MS. Tolerance to the bronchoprotective effect of salmeterol in adolescents with exercise-induced asthma using concurrent inhaled glucocorticoid treatment. *Pediatrics*. 1997;99(5):655–659.
31. Sinaasappel M, Stern M, Littlewood J et al. Nutrition in patients with cystic fibrosis: A European Consensus. *Journal of Cystic Fibrosis*. 2002;1(2):51–75.
32. Storms WW. Exercise-induced asthma: Diagnosis and treatment for the recreational or elite athlete. *Medicine & Science in Sports & Exercise*. 1999;31(Suppl 1):S33–S38.
33. Storms WW, Joyner DM. Update on exercise-induced asthma: A report of the Olympic Exercise Asthma Summit Conference. *Physician and Sportsmedicine*. 1997;25(3):45–55.
34. Thomas J, Cook DJ, Brooks D. Chest physical therapy management of patients with cystic fibrosis: A meta-analysis. *American Journal of Respiratory and Critical Care Medicine*. 1995;151:846.
35. Thomas S, Wolfarth B, Wittmer C et al. Self-reported asthma and allergies in top athletes compared to the general population—Results of the German part of the GALEN-Olympic study 2008. *Allergy, Asthma & Clinical Immunology*. 2010;6(31). http://www.aacijournal.com/content/6/1/3. Accessed February 12, 2014.
36. Wilt TJ, Niewoehner D, MacDonald R, Kane RL. Management of stable chronic obstructive pulmonary disease: A systematic review for a clinical practice guideline. *Annals of Internal Medicine*. 2007;147(9):639–653.
37. Yankaskas JR, Marshall BC, Sufian B et al. Cystic fibrosis adult care: Consensus conference report. *Chest*. 2004;125(Suppl 1):1S–39S.
38. Zeffer SJ, Phillips BR, Martinez FD et al. Characterization of within-subject responses to fluticasone and montelukast in childhood asthma. *Journal of Allergy and Clinical Immunology*. 2005;115(2):233–242.
39. Zeiger RS, Szefler SJ, Phillips BR et al. Childhood Asthma Research and Education Network of the National Heart, Lung, and Blood Institute. Response profiles to fluticasone and montelukast in mild-to-moderate persistent childhood asthma. *Journal of Allergy and Clinical Immunology*. 2006;117(1):45–52.

55 Dermatology

Rodney L. Thompson and Kenneth B. Batts

CONTENTS

TABLE 55.1
Key Clinical Considerations

1. Diagnosing dermatoses is achieved by a thorough history and meticulous physical exam. Ancillary testing is rarely necessary.
2. The majority of dermatological disorders arising from athletic participation are self-limited and preventable with good hygiene, properly fitted equipment and clothing, and acclimatization to the environment.
3. Treatment regimens for dermatoses must be individualized to account for presenting symptoms and history, level of competition, necessity to return to participation, and risk to fellow participants.
4. The intensity, duration, and level of participation within an activity or sport commonly predispose an athlete to certain dermatoses. Certain dermatoses tend to be sport specific.
5. The health-care team must be familiar with the regulations and restrictions at all levels governing participation and return to play for athletes who have acquired an infectious dermatological condition.

55.1 INTRODUCTION

The skin offers protection from our harsh environment while we exercise for fitness and compete for victory. At times, we take this pliable, protective barrier for granted, potentially leading to our inability to participate. Athletes and clinicians need to be aware of the most common dermatological conditions that may arise within certain sports and types of exercise. Early recognition and treatment of these dermatological disorders can prevent degradation in performance, speed recovery for earlier return to play, and obviate further spread to a team member or an opposing athlete. The chapter is divided into four main sections: mechanical, environmental, infectious, and miscellaneous dermatological conditions. In-depth descriptions of the most common skin disorders in athletes, along with treatment regimens and primary prevention strategies, are provided (Table 55.1).

55.2 MECHANICAL CONDITIONS

55.2.1 Abrasions

Abrasions are superficial skin wounds stemming from friction forces that strip the epidermis from the underlying dermal layer. Abrasions are commonly referred to as rug burn, strawberries, turf burn, mat burn, and road rash. Treatment is focused on promoting rapid healing and prevention of infection and "tattooing" or scarring.[57] Abrasions should be cleaned with potable tap water, not saline. For heavily contaminated wounds, high-pressure irrigation should be performed using a small syringe and a splatter shield. All foreign material and debris should be removed. Topical antibiotics are unnecessary for uncomplicated wounds.[44] Abrasions should be covered with an occlusive hydrogel or hydrocolloid dressings in order to facilitate healing and prevent transmission of potential blood-borne pathogens. Athletes may be advised to wear more protective equipment on high-risk areas, such as boney prominences of the hands, elbows, and knees. If active bleeding exists, athletes must be removed from the competition to apply a dressing that covers the injury, prevents seepage of blood, and withstands the rigors of the competition.[18]

55.2.2 Friction Blisters

Blisters are one of the most frequent injuries of endurance athletes, occurring in up to 39% of marathon runners.[39] They form when repetitive friction shears the dermoepidermal junction, leading to separated layers filled with blood or transudate. Moisture, heat, ill-fitting shoes, and overtraining contribute to developing blisters. They occur on tips of the toes, balls of the feet, and the posterior heel but also may be seen on the palms or fingers. Small blisters resolve spontaneously if left alone. Larger bullae (greater than 2 cm) are usually more painful and may interfere with activity. Draining the bulla alleviates the pain and can be achieved by lancing the lesion at the periphery with a needle or scalpel blade, leaving the blister roof intact to minimize chance of infection and to aid in healing. This process may be performed up to three times within 24 hours.[39] Once drained, moleskin padding may also be used to minimize additional trauma to the blister and to relieve discomfort. Hydrocolloid dressings and silvadene cream can alleviate discomfort, help prevent infection, and aid in healing.[12] Prevention is aimed at decreasing friction by wearing properly fitted shoes and averting moisture with dry, wicking socks. Antiperspirants, absorbent talc powders, and 10% tannic acid soaks can also help inhibit moisture.

55.2.3 Chafing

Clinical Pearl

When managing a friction blister in an athlete, leaving the skin roof intact can decrease the risk of infection, alleviate pain of the underlying tissue, and speed healing.

Chafing is an irritant dermatitis caused by repetitive friction of the skin by another body part, clothing, or piece of equipment. This injury commonly presents as "jogger's nipples" in long-distance runners, especially those who participate in marathons or triathlons. Jogger's nipples are painful and erythematous and have crusted erosions of the nipple and areola caused by repetitive friction of the runner's shirt over the areola and nipple regions. They are sometimes caused by shirts with rubberized logos that participants wear during races.[25] Jogger's nipples occur more commonly in male athletes but also occur in female athletes who run without bras. Prevention is the basis of treatment, but petroleum jelly can be applied to the affected nipples for relief. Running without a shirt or wearing a semisynthetic bra is beneficial.[39] In addition, covering the area with tape or bandages removes the source of friction.

55.2.4 Corns and Calluses

A corn is a discrete, dry, horny, hyperkeratotic papule with a central conical deposit of keratin that is produced in response to recurrent mechanical trauma over a bony prominence. Hard corns are the most common type and develop on the dorsolateral aspect of the fifth toe or the dorsum of the interphalangeal joints of the lesser toes. Soft corns are characterized by a white, macerated appearance and found between the fourth and fifth toes.[55] Calluses, or callosities, are painless, broad hyperkeratotic plaques that arise under the metatarsal heads. Calluses are protective but are more susceptible to human papillomavirus (HPV) and therefore require periodic examination to ensure they do not harbor warts.[39] Paring calluses with a scalpel blade reveals smooth translucent skin, in contrast to plantar warts that demonstrate small black dots representing thrombosed capillaries.

Active treatment of corns and calluses is the same and consists of paring the lesions or applying keratolytics. Though enucleation of corns temporarily reduces pain, multiple treatments can cause damage to surrounding tissues and increase the risk of intractable pain. Corticosteroid injections and applications of silver nitrate or 50% pyrogallic acid are not helpful. For paring, the area is soaked in warm water followed by debulking with a scalpel blade or debriding with a pumice stone or file. Keratolytic therapy consists of the application of creams with high concentrations of urea or salicylic acid.[55] A 1% cantharidin, 30% salicylic acid, and 5% podophyllin topical solution can be used as an adjunct to paring to decrease the chance of recurrence.[2] Corns and calluses are prevented by the use of weight-lifting gloves, fitted footwear with wide toe boxes, and orthotic devices. Orthotic silicone splints or insoles lined with felt will minimize friction and distribute weight more evenly.[12,55] Synthetic socks can be used to reduce friction.

55.2.5 Auricular Hematoma

Auricular hematomas are collections of blood induced by trauma between the skin and cartilage of the pinna. If left untreated, these injuries can evolve into "cauliflower ear," also known as "wrestler's ear." The resultant deformity is common in athletes who compete in combat sports. Cauliflower ears were noted as far back as the ancient Greek Olympics, and many coaches and athletes still today consider this a "badge of courage."[12]

Initial treatment involves analgesia, compression, and ice. Needle aspiration can help alleviate accumulation of blood in the acute phase. If the blood has not clotted, large hematomas can be drained and combined with bolsters (pressure dressings) to prevent reaccumulation.[53] The bolster technique has a high rate of reoccurrence due to lack of adherence. Another technique involves incision and drainage of large hematomas followed by mattress sutures. This method is highly successful with low reaccumulation risk and permits immediate return to play for athletes.[49] If a cauliflower ear has already formed, then reconstructive plastic surgery can restore normal ear shape. The wearing of head gear prevents auricular hematomas, but most professional athletes do not wear protective headgear.

55.2.6 Talon Noir

Talon noir, also known as "black heel" or calcaneal petechiae, is caused by intraepidermal bleeding from shearing forces applied to the skin surface. Talon noir is characterized by discrete brown or blue-black macules on the posterior, medial, and lateral sides of the heel, just above the thick plantar skin where blood vessels are minimally protected by fatty tissue. Repeated stop-and-start motions, changes in direction, and constant pounding on hard surfaces cause injury of the heel against the back of the shoe. Running, basketball, soccer, gymnastics, and hockey participants are susceptible to injury.[1] These macules may be confused with melanoma; however, the diagnosis is confirmed by "scratch testing," by paring the lesion with a scalpel blade to scrape away the old hemorrhages. Suspicion of melanoma demands a biopsy. Dermatoscopy can be an informative tool to help differentiate the injuries by visualizing a reddish-black homogeneous pattern of pigmentation, often bordered by isolated red-black globules.

Tennis players, gymnasts, and weight lifters can have similar lesions on the thenar eminence called "tache noir," which is also known as black palm or palmar petechiae. The petechiae usually resolve with 2–3 weeks of rest. Skin lubrication, heel cups, changing footwear, and wearing two pairs of thick socks can reduce the incidence of the lesions.[55]

55.2.7 Jogger's Toe

Jogger's toe refers to dystrophic changes to the nail caused by repetitive trauma. It is characterized by subungual hematomas and hyperkeratosis. Thickened nails and hemorrhage of the nail matrix frequently occur from repetitive thrusting of the nail into the toe box or start–stop maneuvers by athletes. Associated callosities may develop in the hyponychium. Soccer players sometimes experience complete nail plate avulsion caused by the forces of kicking. Jogger's toe is fairly common and occurs in up to 14% of marathon runners, as well as ice skaters and tennis players.[39] If onychomycosis or melanoma is suspected, a culture or biopsy should be performed.

Jogger's toe is self-resolving; however, the nail changes may persist for several months before complete resolution. Evacuation of blood with portable cautery probes may prevent spread of the hemorrhage and loss of the nail in acute injuries.[39] Prevention is vital. Properly fitted footwear with a snug midfoot and adequate toe box can prevent the foot from sliding forward and, in combination with properly trimmed (straight cut, not curved cut) nails, ensures equal distribution of forces and reduces the incidence of nail dystrophies.[1]

55.2.8 Ingrown Toenail

Ingrown toenails (onychocryptosis) form when the nail plate punctures the related nail fold. The first (great) toe is frequently affected. Signs and symptoms include edema, pain, and localized tenderness with exudates and granulation at the nail fold–plate junction. The diagnosis is made by exam. Poorly fitting shoes, inappropriate trimming of the lateral nail plate, pincer nail deformity, and trauma all contribute to its incidence.

Mild-to-moderate onychocryptosis may be treated conservatively with warm, soapy water soaks for 10 minutes three times daily (TID) and pushing the lateral nail fold away from the nail plate, for 1 to 2 weeks. Alternatively, cotton wicks or dental floss elevation of the affected nail plate can be used.[55] Topical corticosteroid ointment can be applied to reduce inflammation. Moderate to severe lesions are regularly associated with infection (paronychia) and are treated with nail border resection. Recurrent ingrown nails require avulsion of the lateral nail plate combined with lateral matricectomy.[14] Nail bed ablation can be achieved using phenol (88%), sodium hydroxide (10%), laser ablation, or electrocautery.[14] Preventative measures include cutting toenails straight across to allow for a more equal distribution of forces across the toe box.

55.2.9 Runner's Rump

Runner's rump is a condition in which ecchymoses develop on the superior portion of the gluteal cleft. It affects long-distance runners and results from perpetual friction between the gluteal folds during running. Properly applied skin lubricants in either creams or ointments can reduce the incidence. It is completely asymptomatic and spontaneously resolves with decreased training.[39]

55.2.10 Acne Mechanica

Acne mechanica is an occlusive process that produces comedones, papules, and pustules. It is caused by mechanical stresses on the skin, such as pressure and repeated friction from overlying sports gear or equipment, combined with heat and perspiration. Athletes with a history of acne vulgaris are predisposed to developing acne mechanica. Football and hockey players typically present with the rash under their pads, helmet, or chinstrap. Golfers or caddies typically present with the rash over the shoulder in a golf bag strap pattern. Equestrians have a chinstrap pattern.[47] Eruptions usually cover the forehead, cheeks, and chin, but the shoulders, back, and hips can also be affected.

Acne mechanica can be responded by reducing friction on the skin. Washing the affected areas immediately after a game or practice may decrease the severity of the rash. Acne therapy, such as benzoyl peroxide, topical retinoids such as tretinoin cream, and topical and systemic antibiotics, may be helpful. However, if the acne is severe and refractory, systemic isotretinoin may be indicated, but the risk of myopathy and tendinitis with these treatments may limit their use.[47] Undergarments made of cotton and sweat-wicking materials reduce skin irritation. Fitting pieces of soft fabric between the skin and equipment can attenuate friction and heat. Appropriate hygiene and washing equipment with soap and water or an alcohol solution can help decrease bacteria.

55.2.11 Keloids

Keloids are benign, hyperproliferative growths of dermal collagen that result in smooth, shiny, and firm plaques. They usually result from excessive tissue response to skin trauma. There is a higher incidence in dark-skinned athletes.[34] The condition is usually painless, but can be accompanied by pruritus, pain, and hypersensitivity. Common locations are the forehead, cheeks, and posterior neck where the headgear contacts the skin or where the undergarment pads cover the thighs, knees, or shoulders.[29]

The most effective treatment is intralesional steroids. Other beneficial treatments include silicone gel sheeting, intralesional bleomycin, 5-fluorouracil, electrical stimulation, and pulsed-dye laser. Surgery, in and of itself, can lead to even larger keloid formation, but when combined with intralesional steroids has a high success rate.[58]

55.2.12 Piezogenic Papules

Piezogenic papules are herniations of fat typically on the medial and lateral aspects of the heel. The lesions, which may or may not be painful, are 2–5 mm yellow or white papules found on the medial or posterolateral heel of long-distance runners. In some cases, the discomfort of painful piezogenic pedal papules can be dramatic and temporarily sideline athletes. However, the pain and papules disappear after the feet are elevated for a few minutes. Treatment is merely symptomatic and entails using heel cups and compressive stockings and reducing prolonged standing. A combination of steroid and anesthetic injection (betamethasone and bupivacaine) has been effective in some patients.[55]

55.2.13 Athlete Nodules

Athlete nodules refer to benign fibrotic lesion over various parts of the body due to recurrent trauma from repetitive friction and pressure. Boxers develop athlete nodules on the knuckles ("knuckle pads"), and hockey players develop lesions on the ankles ("skate bite"). Surfer nodules can occur on the knee, tibial prominence, or dorsal aspects of the feet.[1] Runner nodules develop over the dorsum of the feet from tightly laced shoes. The diagnosis of athlete nodules is based on history and physical examination. Some cases may be unclear, and biopsy may be necessary to distinguish from gout, ganglion cyst, epidermoid cyst, or elastoma. These lesions are less common as protective clothing and gear continue to improve. For example, wet suits allow surfers in cold water to lie prone on the board thus obviating surfer nodule of the knee.[1] Treatment includes intralesional steroids or excision; but most of the time, these lesions are self-limited and resolve upon cessation of activity.

55.3 ENVIRONMENTAL CONDITIONS

55.3.1 Sunburn

Sunburn is caused by thermal damage to the skin from prolonged ultraviolet (UV) light exposure. Most of the damage is inflicted by UVB; however, UVA can potentiate the effects. Outdoor sports significantly increase UV exposure, and some athletes can experience erythema from UV radiation only after a few minutes. However, it usually takes a few hours for symptoms to develop. The erythema from sunburn usually lasts for several days and can be associated with pain, edema, and blisters. Skin desquamation occurs within 1 week of onset. Winter athletes, such as skiers, are at increased risk due to higher altitudes and the reflective properties of snow. Water sports also carry a greater risk of developing sunburn, as water is highly reflective. Athletes with lightly pigmented skin are at greater risk, but sunburn can occur in athletes with darker complexions as well.[25]

Treatment for sunburn is symptomatic and includes cool compresses, emollients (aloe vera), and oatmeal soaks. Nonsteroidal anti-inflammatory drugs (NSAIDs) can be used to alleviate pain and may relieve some erythema.[43] Topical corticosteroids and antihistamines are ineffective.[25] Repeated and prolonged UV exposure can lead to photodamage and skin cancer. Athletes tend not to adequately protect themselves, as a study by the National Collegiate Athletic Association (NCAA) reveals that only 6% of athletes use sunscreen at least 3 days per week and 85% had not used sunscreen.[22] Prevention involves wearing protective clothing, applying sunscreens judiciously, and avoiding sun exposure during peak hours (between 10 am and 2 pm standard time). Tanning should be strictly discouraged.

55.3.2 Miliaria

Miliaria, or heat rash, is a pruritic, erythematous, fine vesiculopapular exanthem that develops during exposure to high heat and humidity. The rash may be accompanied by a prickling or stinging sensation. It is caused by occlusion of eccrine sweat glands when the skin is covered by clothing. It commonly occurs around the waistline or over the trunk or groin. The palms and soles are always spared due to lack of eccrine sweat glands.[51]

Treatment consists of cooling and drying the skin to avoid further perspiration that exacerbates the condition. Pruritus can be treated with calamine lotion, anhydrous lanolin, wet compresses, mild topical corticosteroids, and/or oral antihistamines. The eruption is self-limited and resolves once the patient is removed from the source of excessive heat. As acclimatization occurs, the lesions may reoccur less, but take up to 10 days to fully resolve.[51]

55.3.3 Chilblains

Chilblains, or pernio, are localized bluish-red vesicles, bullae, or plaques that develop after prolonged exposure to a cold, damp environment that induces vasoconstriction. Symptoms include intense pruritus and/or burning. The lesions are erythematous and can become cyanotic in color. The lesions typically occur on the hands, feet, legs, and thighs. They can occur at freezing temperatures but can also occur at temperatures up to 20°C. Chilblains can have a quick onset, within an hour, but often develop within a few hours of exposure.[41] Individuals at particular risk include those who participate in outdoor activities, such as kayaking, winter horseback riding, and hiking. Chilblains are self-limited and are almost always benign.

Treatment is achieved by removing the individual from the cold, wet environment drying off and gently massaging the affected skin. Active rewarming above 30°C significantly worsens the pain and should be avoided.[41] In extreme cases, basic wound care with dry bandages may be necessary. Nifedipine (20 mg, TID) is effective at reducing pain and duration of lesions.[3] Prophylactic measures to prevent chilblains include minimizing cold exposure, wearing protective clothing and gear when outdoors, and maintaining adequate warmth indoors.[56]

55.3.4 Frostnip

Frostnip is the most common injury related to cold weather exposure at temperatures below 10°C. It is characterized by cooling of the superficial skin and associated vasoconstriction that results in blue-purple discoloration. Frostnip typically affects the face, nose, cheeks, chin, and ears and is associated with pain, burning, and/or numbness. Frostnip is at the beginning of the cold-induced skin injury spectrum and precedes frostbite.

The treatment of frostnip is simple rewarming. There is no permanent skin damage associated with frostnip. Emollient skin creams can help to maintain higher skin temperatures.[56]

Clinical Pearl

The wearing of moisture-wicking garments in multiple layers is key to primary prevention of cold injuries by transferring moisture away from the body, providing warmth to regulate body temperature and offering protection from wind and rain.

55.3.5 Frostbite

Frostbite is a freezing injury of the skin that is similar to thermal injury and can be classified in four phases (degrees), depending upon the depth of tissue damage. First-degree injury manifests as firm plaques with surrounding erythema and edema. Second-degree injury results in superficial vesicles and bullae filled with clear or milky fluid and surrounded by erythema and edema. Third-degree injury develops deeper, hemorrhagic blisters. Fourth-degree injury is the most profound and represents damage extending through the dermis, down to the muscle or even bone. These injuries are necrotic and can produce mummification. A simpler, two-tier system can be used to indicate either mild/superficial tissue loss or severe/deep tissue loss.[3] Injuries can only be classified after rewarming, due to most frostbite appearing the same on initial evaluation.[3] The prevention and management of frostbite is detailed in Chapter 63, Environmental Illness.

55.4 INFECTIOUS CONDITIONS

55.4.1 Cellulitis and Erysipelas

Cellulitis and erysipelas arise from bacteria that invade the skin and cause dermatitis. Clinical manifestations classically include erythema, edema, and warmth within the affected area of the skin. The most common bacteria causing cellulitis and erysipelas are group A streptococcus (GAS) and *Staphylococcus aureus* (SA). These dermatoses are common in contact sports but can also occur in soccer players, weight lifters, and volleyball players.[12] Cellulitis involves the deeper dermis and subcutaneous fat, whereas erysipelas involves the superficial lymphatics and upper dermis. Therefore, erysipelas raises the skin and forms well-demarcated lesions. Erysipelas is acute in onset and associated with fever and chills. Cellulitis has less distinct borders and is more indolent in nature. Disruptions in the skin barrier from toe web intertrigo, trauma, eczema, or tinea pedis are major risk factors for the formation of cellulitis. Diagnosis is made by history and physical exam. Cultures of the site can improve diagnostic accuracy and decrease the duration of treatment.

Antibiotics, dicloxacillin or cephalexin, are the mainstay of treatment with the aim to cover both GAS and SA. Macrolides can be effective but should be used with caution due to increasing rates of resistance. Purulent lesions are more likely to be caused by community-acquired methicillin-resistant *Staphylococcus aureus* (CA-MRSA). Appropriate antibiotic regimens should include coverage for both methicillin-sensitive SA and MRSA. Local antibiograms are valuable in guiding appropriate antibiotic choice. Trimethoprim–sulfamethoxazole and tetracycline are also cheap and effective.[37] Clindamycin is a second-line agent and should be used with caution due to increasing resistance.[28] Duration of antibiotic therapy depends on response. If the cellulitis or erysipelas involves the upper or lower extremities, elevation of the infected extremity alleviates edema and accelerates recovery. Severe infections with systemic symptoms, or in patients with comorbidities, may require intravenous antibiotics and hospital admission.

Prevention of cellulitis hinges upon hygiene, immediate showering after practice, and not sharing towels. In addition, limiting contact with the infected individual is important once the diagnosis is made. Athletes must have no new skin lesions for 48 hours, have no moist draining lesions, and have completed 72 hours of antibiotic therapy prior to participating in an event.[17] Lesions can be properly covered to allow participation, as long as they are not active.[17] The National Federation of State High School Associations (NFHS) require 48 hours of therapy before an athlete can return to play.[28]

Clinical Pearl

The health-care team must be very cautious in returning an athlete to full participation or competition with infectious skin conditions. Governing high school and collegiate associations have very specific guidelines and regulations to safeguard play.

55.4.2 Impetigo

Impetigo is a prevalent bacterial infection caused by SA in the majority of cases, though GAS can cause a significant number of infections. CA-MRSA is a very rare cause of impetigo.[38] Lesions present as papules and pustules surrounded by erythema and serosanguineous discharge and form honey-colored crusts. Topical antibiotics can be used to treat impetigo effectively, and agents include mupirocin and retapamulin. If topical agents fail, then oral agents should be instituted with a penicillinase-resistant beta-lactam (dicloxacillin) or a first-generation cephalosporin (cephalexin).[33] Athletes with impetigo are highly contagious, thus limiting their participation in practice and competition until all lesions have resolved. Guidelines for returning to play are the same as those for cellulitis/erysipelas.

55.4.3 Folliculitis

Bacterial folliculitis is a superficial infection limited to the epidermis with purulent material located around the hair follicles. It appears as an erythematous exanthem with clusters of small pustulopapular lesions and is often pruritic and/or painful. Folliculitis is common in wrestlers, swimmers, and triathletes.[12] Staphylococcal folliculitis can occur in areas of the body with occlusive protective padding or tightly fitted sportswear. Pseudomonas folliculitis ("hot tub folliculitis") occurs from contaminated whirlpools and hot tubs. The diagnosis and type of folliculitis are made by history and clinical manifestations. Bacterial cultures may be helpful in determining the type of folliculitis.

Folliculitis is typically a self-limited process and resolves without intervention in 5–10 days. If necessary, treatment of localized folliculitis can be accomplished with topical mupirocin. Diffuse infections or the development of systemic symptoms requires oral antibiotic. The prevalence of CA-MRSA can guide antibiotic choice.[28] Fluoroquinolones are beneficial in cases that do not spontaneously resolve. Prevention of infection includes ensuring hot tubs and whirlpools are properly maintained and disinfected regularly. Occlusive dressings can be used to cover open wounds, but athletes should not share towels or soap. Preventive measures include decreasing frequent shaving in areas of high friction and discussing shaving precautions with athletes who have had previous infections.[47] Protocols for return to play are the same for folliculitis as mentioned in cellulitis.

55.4.4 Furunculosis

Furuncles (boils) are abscesses that form within the dermis and deeper skin tissues, originating from infected hair follicles. A carbuncle is simply a cluster of furuncles. In athletes, abscesses most typically form in places of friction and perspiration, such as the back of the neck, axilla, groin, and buttocks. Furunculosis is spread by skin-to-skin transmission, putting athletes who participate in contact sports, such as wrestling, at higher risk. Up to a 25% of football players and 20% of basketball players develop furunculosis.[1] The vast majority of cases are caused by SA, and almost 60% are caused by CA-MRSA. However, perianal abscesses may involve gram-negative rods.[37] Abscesses present as erythematous, tender, fluctuant nodules with surrounding pustules and erythema. Diagnosis is made by clinical manifestations.

Small lesions do not necessarily warrant antibiotic therapy. Successful treatment can be provided by applying warm compresses and performing incision and drainage of larger lesions. Cellulitis requires antibiotic therapy targeted at CA-MRSA. Clindamycin 300–600 mg TID per day and trimethoprim–sulfamethoxazole DS twice a day are commonly recommended for oral therapy. Wound culture results can help guide therapy in resistant cases. For prevention, stringent hygiene measures must be followed. Recurrent cases or ongoing transmission among team members calls for decolonization. Strategies include combination of nasal decolonization (with mupirocin twice daily [BID] for 5–10 days) and topical body decolonization regimens (with chlorhexidine or dilute bleach baths for 5–14 days).[37] Athletes can typically return to sports once the lesion is dry; but if a lesion is still draining or moist, the athlete cannot return to participation, even if the site is covered.[47]

55.4.5 Erythrasma

Erythrasma is characterized by patchy, erythematous or brown, plaques usually affecting the intertriginous areas. It is caused by *Corynebacterium minutissimum*, the most common bacterial infection of the foot. Up to 30% of patients affected by erythrasma also have concomitant candidiasis.[50] Erythrasma should be considered in athletes with presumed tinea who are not improving with topical antifungal therapy. Obesity, hyperhidrosis, and poor hygiene are risk factors for acquiring the disease. Diagnosis is made by physical exam, and Wood's lamp (black light) examination aids in confirmation. Under a Wood's lamp, the lesions appear a fluorescent coral-red; in contrast, tinea does not fluoresce.[50]

For athletes with localized disease, topical therapy includes macrolides (1% clindamycin) or 5% benzoyl peroxide.[50,59] Lesions at multiple sites require systemic therapy with an oral macrolide. Whitfield's ointment (combination of salicylic and benzoic acids) is effective. Oral tetracycline can be used but is not as effective as other therapies.[24] Athletes with asymptomatic infections should be treated.[50] Athletes need to keep intertriginous areas and interdigital lesions on the feet dry and isolated from communal showers until clear. There are no return-to-play guidelines. It is prudent for athletes to receive treatment for 72 hours before resuming participation since erythrasma is contagious. Lesions should be covered prior to team practice or competition.[50]

55.4.6 Pitted Keratolysis

Pitted keratolysis, also known as "sweaty sock syndrome," is a bacterial infection of the plantar surface of the feet, likely to occur in runners and tennis and basketball players. Eruptions are caused by infection with *Corynebacterium*, *Micrococcus* (*Kytococcus*), or *Dermatophilus* species and are characterized by "pits," circular or longitudinal punched-out depressions, on the skin surface. Hyperhidrosis with foul odor and skin maceration are typical signs. Pitted keratolysis is often misdiagnosed as tinea pedis. If the diagnosis is in question, a shave biopsy of the stratum corneum demonstrates filamentous and coccoid microorganisms on hematoxylin and eosin staining.[12]

Topical treatment includes clindamycin (with or without 5% benzoyl peroxide), erythromycin, or mupirocin. Topical 20% aluminum chloride can be used as an antiperspirant and reduces hyperhidrosis, decreasing the risk of infection. Preventative measures include the use of synthetic socks and avoidance of prolonged occlusive footwear.[12] Athletes do not have to be restricted from play.

55.4.7 Onychomycosis

Onychomycosis (tinea unguium) is a fungal infection of the toenails, primarily caused by dermatophytes but occasionally by yeast. Nails become discolored and thickened, and often the nail plate spontaneously avulses. Occlusive footwear, history of tinea pedis, and being in close contact with someone who has onychomycosis are risk factors for developing the disease. Swimmers have a predisposition for developing onychomycosis, and nearly all cases of pedal onychomycosis are associated with tinea pedis.[56] The primary criteria for diagnosis consists of white/yellow or orange/brown patches or streaks of the nail, whereas the secondary criteria include onycholysis, subungual hyperkeratosis/debris, and nail plate thickening. Microscopy or culture confirms the diagnosis.

Topical antifungals are ineffective. The mainstay of therapy is oral antifungals. Terbinafine is the most effective and has a relatively uncomplicated side effect profile. A 12-week, daily dose of 250 mg is usually necessary. Itraconazole can also be successful, in a pulsed dose of 200 mg BID for 1 week for three consecutive months. Pulsed dose is more effective than daily dosing of itraconazole. Overall, itraconazole is not as effective as terbinafine.[56] Fluconazole is effective against candida species but not dermatophytes.[56] Hepatic transaminases require monitoring during therapy. A normal nail may not reappear for 18 months, and some nails may indefinitely remain dystrophic in appearance, even after completion of therapy.

55.4.8 Tinea Corporis

Tinea corporis is a dermatophyte infection on the torso, extremities, head, and face. Tinea corporis presents as well-defined, erythematous, scaling papules and plaques. Lesions are annular in shape with a raised leading edge and central clearing, thus the common name "ringworm." Most reported cases are caused by *Trichophyton tonsurans*. Tinea corporis is also known as tinea corporis gladiatorum or simply tinea gladiatorum, due to the high prevalence (up to 77%) in wrestlers.[1] Wrestling is conducive to transmission from frequent skin-to-skin contact in conjunction with moisture, traumatized skin, and hot environments.[12] Tinea capitis, or ringworm of the scalp, is associated with alopecia. Diagnosis is clinical but can be confirmed with potassium hydroxide (KOH) slide.

Treatment consists of either a topical azole, allylamine, or ciclopirox. Athletes who fail topical therapy or who have extensive disease require systemic therapy with an oral azole or allylamine antifungal. Regimens include terbinafine 250 mg daily for 1–2 weeks, fluconazole 150 mg once weekly for 2–4 weeks, and itraconazole 200 mg daily for 1–2 weeks.[28] Tinea capitis requires oral therapy with griseofulvin, but azoles and allylamines are therapeutic options.[30,10] Preventative measures include showering, washing uniforms, and disinfecting mats daily. Teams should also have strict surveillance by athletic trainers who promptly refer athletes to team physicians. Infected individuals must keep lesions covered with bandages when practicing or competing. The NCAA and the NFHS require athletes to have been treated with topical therapy for at least 72 hours prior to competition, and active lesions must be covered with an occlusive or semiocclusive dressing.[36] Scalp lesions necessitate a minimum of 2 weeks of oral therapy before return to play.[36]

55.4.9 Tinea Cruris

Tinea cruris, or "jock itch," is a dermatophytic eruption in the area of the groin (crural folds). It is primarily caused by *Trichophyton rubrum*, but infrequently caused by *Epidermophyton floccosum* and *Trichophyton mentagrophytes*. Lesions present as pruritic erythematous plaques with well-demarcated, scaly borders that spread to the groin, upper thighs, and perineum but spare the scrotum. Many cases of tinea cruris are due to autoinoculation from an athlete's infection with tinea pedis. Tinea cruris can be confused with psoriasis, erythrasma, seborrheic dermatitis, and candidal intertrigo.[29] Microscopy with a KOH slide demonstrating fungal hyphae can confirm the diagnosis. Sparing of the scrotum differentiates tinea from candidal infections. Erythematous patches with satellite papules and pustules are characteristic of candidiasis.

Clinical Pearl

An easy way to remember the difference between tinea and candida infections in the groin is the appearance of erythematous patches on the scrotum, indicating candida. Tinea cruris does not usually colonize the scrotum.

Topical antifungal treatment with azoles (clotrimazole) or allylamines (terbinafine) is sufficient. Resistant infections can be treated with oral antifungals (griseofulvin, terbinafine). Mild topical corticosteroids can assuage inflammation. Applying desiccant powders (talcum), emphasizing personal hygiene, and disinfecting fomites help prevent recurrences. Itching can be alleviated by anti-itch lotions, but powders and lotions applied to inflamed or excoriated skin can exacerbate the condition.[19]

55.4.10 Tinea Pedis

Tinea pedis, "athlete's foot," is the most common dermatophyte infection, caused by *T. mentagrophytes* or *T. rubrum*.[56] It mainly affects the interdigital spaces, but sometimes will extend to the arch of the foot. Lesions are characterized by erythematous erosions and scales, though some subtypes present with a moccasin or vesiculobullous pattern that involves the plantar surface. The dorsum of the foot is typically spared. Interdigital lesions cause the skin to become macerated and to fissure, making the area more susceptible to superinfection with bacteria, such as *Staphylococcus* or *Streptococcus*. Diagnosis should be confirmed by KOH slide.

First-line treatment of mild tinea pedis consists of topical antifungals, such as azoles, thiocarbamates (tolnaftate) or allylamines (terbinafine).[6] Duration of therapy depends on resolution of the infection. Soaks in aluminum acetate solution may be helpful as an adjunct if maceration is present. Keratolytics and humectants, such as salicylic acid, lactic acid, and urea, help remove or soften scale and enhance absorption of topical antifungal therapy. Bacterial superinfection warrants treatment with appropriate antibiotics, though antifungals, such as azoles or ciclopirox, have some antibacterial effect.[56] The use of a moderately potent topical glucocorticosteroid can relieve pruritus and inflammation. Recalcitrant cases require systemic therapy with azoles or allylamines, and nail involvement necessitates oral therapy.[56] Prevention of tinea pedis infections, both primary and recurrent, is best achieved by keeping feet dry, wearing moisture-wicking socks, changing socks on a regular basis, wearing well-ventilated shoes, and using of footwear in showers and locker rooms. Antifungal powder on the feet and in shoes can help prevent recurrence. Education, prompt diagnosis, and treatment are all crucial in preventing outbreaks among athletes.

55.4.11 Tinea Versicolor

Tinea versicolor, also known as pityriasis versicolor, is an infection caused by *Malassezia furfur* that is not a dermatophyte. It is a chronic condition that presents as either hypo- or hyperpigmented scaly macules and patches. Lesions occur on the chest and back, but can be present on the upper arms, neck, abdomen, groin, and thighs. The lesions become more prominent after sun exposure. Formal diagnosis is made with KOH microscopy revealing a "spaghetti-and-meatballs" appearance. Wood's lamp examination reveals yellow-green fluorescence. The infection is often self-limiting and does not require medical therapy. However, selenium sulfide 2.5% scrub (15 minutes daily for three consecutive days) or topical antifungal medications are available to treat tinea versicolor successfully.[36] Oral griseofulvin and terbinafine are not effective.[19] Athletes with tinea versicolor are not contagious and therefore have no participation restrictions.

55.4.12 Herpes Simplex

Herpes simplex virus 1 (HSV-1) is a prevalent infection, common among wrestlers and rugby players. Infections in wrestlers and rugby players have been dubbed herpes gladiatorum, herpes rugbeiorum, or scrum pox. The virus is spread by skin-to-skin contact and is highly contagious. Up to 47% of cutaneous infections are caused by HSV-1 in athletes.[52] The typical infection is characterized by grouped vesicles on an erythematous base, associated with pain, burning and tingling sensation, and pruritus. Lesions usually resolve without intervention in 10–14 days, taking on a scabbed appearance once healed. Primary infection can be associated with fever, malaise, and myalgias, but systemic symptoms are rare in recurrent infections. Diagnosis is made on clinical appearance of the lesions, but a Tzanck smear can confirm the diagnosis. A viral culture may provide definitive diagnosis but takes several days for results.

The purpose of antiviral therapy is to reduce the duration of symptoms. Treatment is most effective during the prodromal phase or within the first 24 hours of symptom onset. New-onset HSV-1 requires 7–10 days of the following antivirals: acyclovir, 400 mg TID; famciclovir, 250 mg BID; or valacyclovir, 1 g BID. Recurrent infections require shorter therapeutic courses: acyclovir, 800 mg TID for 2 days; famciclovir, 1000 mg BID for 1 day; or valacyclovir, 500 mg BID for 3 days.[60] Suppressive therapy is a reasonable option for prophylaxis during the season and can be achieved with valacyclovir, 500 mg daily or 1 g in individuals who have a high recurrence rate.[52,60] The prevention of herpes gladiatorum includes instituting good personal hygiene, cleaning of shared equipment, and performing daily skin checks.[28] For return to play, the NCAA requires an athlete be free of systemic symptoms, have developed no new blisters for 72 hours before the examination, have all lesions dried with a firm crust, and have been on antivirals for at least 120 hours prior to competition.[52] Active lesions cannot be covered to allow for participation. The NFHS also requires athletes to be free of systemic symptoms but requires no new lesions 48 hours before competition and athletes to have been on antivirals for 10–14 days.[52]

55.4.13 Molluscum Contagiosum

Molluscum contagiosum is a Poxviridae skin infection that manifests as skin-colored, dome-shaped papules with umbilicated centers. Lesions are mostly found on the face, neck, and torso and are generally asymptomatic. Transmission is by direct skin-to-skin contact with an infected person but can also be spread by autoinoculation, swimming in contaminated swimming pools, or contact with fomites.[48] Athletes involved in contact sports have a predilection for developing and spreading the virus, but anyone who plays sports or uses gym equipment is at risk.

Lesions usually resolve within 6–9 months, but many athletes find this an unreasonable time to wait. There are multiple effective treatments, including curettage, cryosurgery, and electrodessication. Topical treatments are effective and include cantharidin, silver nitrate, and imiquimod cream.[48] Other efficacious treatments include sodium nitrite coapplied with salicylic acid, Australian lemon myrtle oil, topical KOH, tretinoin, and tea tree oil with iodine.[26] The NCAA dictates that lesions must be curetted or removed before clearance for competition.[17] Lesions on the trunk or upper thighs can be covered with uniform/clothing. Solitary lesions or localized clusters may be covered with a gas-impermeable dressing and then covered with tape.[17] The NFHS suggests holding a wrestler out of competition for 24 hours following curettage.[48]

55.4.14 Verrucae

Verrucae (warts) are gray-brown, hyperkeratotic growths with black dots on the skin surface but begin as smooth, flesh-colored papules. They are caused by infection with the HPV. In general, warts are few in number, but it is not unusual for common warts to become so numerous that they become confluent and obscure large areas of normal skin. Plantar warts occur on the hands and feet, often forming at points of maximum pressure, such as over the heads of the metatarsal bones or on the heels. These warts are usually caused by HPV types 1, 2, 4, and 63.[56] Plantar warts on the foot can be particularly detrimental to athletes, producing pain that hinders running, jumping, or skating. Diagnosis is made by exam but can be confirmed by paring with a scalpel blade, revealing thrombosed capillaries that appear as punctate black dots.

Plantar warts do not require treatment unless painful. There are multiple nonsurgical treatments, but debridement in conjunction with keratolytic therapy (salicylic acid) and cryoablation (liquid nitrogen) are the most common and effective methods. Many other methods (duct tape, imiquimod, intralesional immunotherapy with mumps or candida antigens, cantharidin, laser ablation, and electrocautery) exist but have no clear proven benefit.[16,35] Topical dinitrochlorobenzene patches can be applied to refractory lesions.[16] Since HPV may remain viable on surfaces in training facilities, athletes are advised to wear sandals in the shower and locker room areas. Athletes in contact sports with multiple digitate verrucae on their face must be covered with a mask in order to compete.[17] Solitary or scattered lesions can be curetted away before participating. Competitors with multiple lesions must have them adequately covered.[17]

55.5 MISCELLANEOUS CONDITIONS

55.5.1 Contact Dermatitis

Contact dermatitis may be either irritant or allergic and can range from acute to chronic. Recognition that these processes can occur with brief or prolonged exposure to numerous irritants or allergens, including many substances in common sports equipment and paraphernalia, is key to prompt treatment and further prevention.

Irritant contact dermatitis (ICD), the most common contact dermatitis, is a localized inflammatory skin response from direct exposure to an irritant. The athlete will exhibit erythema, edema, vesicles, or bullae with a burning or stinging sensation. Common symptoms occur after exposure to prolonged water immersion, detergents, and soaps, adhesive pretape sprays, sunscreens, and fiberglass.[1] Exposure to sports-specific clothing and equipment can cause ICD.

Allergic contact dermatitis (ACD) is an immune-mediated process that develops after repeated exposures to an offending agent. A reaction usually occurs within 12–48 hours after repeat exposure. The affected area is characterized by pruritic patches of erythema, edema, and vesicles. Chronic ACD can present with lichenification. The eruption may be localized to areas of contact; but majority of the time, this is not the case, as allergens can be spread to other sites by incidental contact. Rubber products, and many of the chemicals used in manufacturing these products, are often the offending agents. These include coverings on golf clubs, padding on swimming goggles, swim caps, basketballs, knee guards, tennis racquets, wetsuit linings, and insoles of running shoes.[32] Other offending items include face masks, shin guards, neoprene braces, latex products, iodine preparations, topical antibiotics ointments, topical anesthetic creams, adhesive tapes, metals (nickel), and poison ivy, oak, and sumac.

After a careful sports-directed history and a high index of suspicion, treatment involves avoidance of the offending agent, treating active inflammation and skin restoration and protection. There are many rubber-free sports products that have been made and can be used by athletes to avoid future flares. For skin inflammation, topical corticosteroid ointments are first-line agents. Other topical treatments (aluminum acetate compresses, calamine lotion, oatmeal baths) can provide symptomatic relief. Oral corticosteroids are first-line treatments for contact dermatitis greater than 20% of body surface or for sensitive skin (the face and intertriginous areas). Mild potency topical steroids or topical calcineurin inhibitors may also be used for sensitive skin areas.[11] Skin restoration is achieved with emollient moisturizers. These products should not contain lanolin or fragrances.[61] Barrier creams can be helpful in the prevention of future eruptions.[5] Patch testing can often help identify an allergen triggering ACD.

55.5.2 Swimmer's Itch (Cercarial Dermatitis)

Swimmer's itch, or cercarial dermatitis, is a transient, pruritic rash that occurs predominantly after swimming in freshwater lakes. There are rare cases associated with swimming in the ocean.[9] The rash is characterized by small 1–2 mm erythematous maculopapules that may progress into pustules, localized overexposed areas. It is caused by blood flukes, most notably avian schistosomes that penetrate the skin while in their cercarial (larval) form. The disease is self-limited, as the larvae die within a few hours of skin penetration. Symptoms are usually mild and last from 1 to 2 weeks.

Treatment is symptomatic and usually achieved with antihistamines, cool compresses, and calamine lotion. For more intense symptoms, topical corticosteroids can be used. Immediately toweling off can prevent the larvae from penetrating the skin.[20]

55.5.3 Seabather's Eruption

Seabather's eruption is an urticarial maculopapular rash found on areas of the body covered by bathing suits. It is caused by sea thimble larvae found in Atlantic waters from New York to Brazil.[20,31] Upon immediately exiting the water, the nematocysts are activated and inject toxin into the skin. Further activation can be brought on by strenuous exercise, wearing a contaminated bathing suit or wet suit, showers or exposure to freshwater. The rash can appear while the athlete is in the water or up to 36 hours later. The rash can last anywhere from 2 to 28 days, with most reactions resolving in 2 weeks.[31]

Initial treatment involves combatting the inflammatory response with topical applications of ice packs, warm compress, and/or vinegar. Further treatment is symptomatic and may include topical corticosteroids and/or oral antihistamines. If symptoms persist despite initial therapy, oral steroids may be necessary. BID topical application of 1.5 g of thiabendazole can also be used for two days. Thoroughly cleaning or discarding affected swimsuits removes persistent larvae, thereby preventing recurrent rashes.[54] Preventive measures include avoiding water known to contain larvae and avoiding excessive clothing when swimming in seawater. Some barrier lotions such as Safe Sea™ are effective for prevention.[8]

55.5.4 Green Hair

Green hair (chlorotrichosis) is a green discoloration that occurs due to copper ion uptake into the outer hair sheath. It occurs almost exclusively in athletes with blond, gray, or white hair, either naturally colored or dyed, and it is a purely cosmetic disorder.[23] Swimmers, divers, and water polo players are at risk for developing green hair. Copper concentration in pool water is usually increased by being leached from copper fittings or copper-containing algicides in acidic water. Treatment of hair can be achieved with bleaching with 3% hydrogen peroxide for 2–3 hours or washing with the chelating shampoos for about 30 minutes. These shampoos generally contain either EDTA or penacillamine.[15] Wearing a cap during water sports can help prevent green hair.

55.5.5 Envenomation

Athletes can encounter a variety of bites and stings, causing simple local dermatologic reactions, or more severe systemic symptoms. Insects, particularly hymenoptera (bees, wasps, hornets, fire ants), are ubiquitous and are of concern because of the potential to cause allergic reactions, and possibly anaphylaxis, from the venom.[20] Injection of the venom causes painful red wheals and papules. These symptoms usually resolve within hours.

For stings localized to the skin, treatment is symptomatic, but the first step is removal of the stinger. Ice packs, cool compresses, or topical lidocaine can relieve the discomfort. Meat tenderizer or baking soda can neutralize the toxin.[54] Itching can be relieved with antihistamines or topical corticosteroids. For anaphylactic reactions, epinephrine should be administered. Patients with a history of insect sting anaphylaxis and/or positive skin test results should have epinephrine available, in the form of an injectable kit (EpiPen®).

Coelenterates, such as the true jellyfish and Portuguese man of war, can also sting and cause injuries. These animals are also cnidarians and as such have venom-filled nematocysts that inject their toxins subcutaneously in response to either chemical or mechanical stimuli. Local symptoms of nematocyst envenomation include burning pain, erythema, edema, urticaria, and bullae formation. Initial treatment involves removing any remaining source of toxins and also deactivating the nematocysts. Ice packs, warm compresses, or vinegar can be effective treatment. Pain can be treated with oral analgesics. Avoiding areas with high concentrations of these species and wearing wet suits may help prevent some envenomations.

55.5.6 Infestations

Scabies is a highly contagious, pruritic infestation by the mite *Sarcoptes scabiei*. The mites burrow into the superficial skin layers producing tortuous erythematous tracks predominantly in the finger webs and wrists. Scabies cause discrete vesicles and papules. These lesions typically involve the extensor surfaces of the elbows and knees, sides of the hands and feet, axillae, buttocks, waist area, and ankle area. More sensitive areas, such as the penis and scrotum or breasts, may be involved as well. Diagnosis is mainly based on history but can be confirmed with testing, either by skin scraping, dermoscopy, or the adhesive tape test. Treatment includes permethrin, lindane, malathion, or ivermectin. A sulfur solution can also be used for treatment, by mixing 5%–10% sulfur in a petrolatum base and applying to entire body once daily for 3 days.[20] Decontamination of equipment, clothing, and bedding is crucial.[36] Athletes are restricted from contact sports until complete resolution. NFHS guidelines allow return to play 24 hours after completion of treatment.[45] NCAA requires negative scabies testing.[17]

Pediculosis is an infestation with lice and is usually asymptomatic. Diagnosis is clinical, identifying nits confirmed with microscopy. Treatment includes permethrin, lindane, malathion, benzyl alcohol, or spinosad. Decontamination prevents spread of fomites.[36,42,40] Athletes should be restricted from contact and team sports until nits are eradicated. NFHS allows return to play 24 hours after completion of treatment; NCAA requires treatment and reexamination to ensure resolution.[17,45]

55.5.7 Physical Urticaria

Urticaria (hives) are well-defined, edematous, erythematous pruritic plaques of varying size that appear rapidly, usually within minutes, and resolve within 24 hours. They result from mast cell activation and release of histamine. There are many different classifications of urticaria, including cholinergic, cold, solar, aquagenic, and exercise induced.

55.5.8 Cholinergic Urticaria

Cholinergic is the most common form of physical urticarias. These lesions result from increasing body temperature and sweat gland activation. Lesions present as small wheals with surrounding flares, usually spreading distally on the neck and trunk.[12] Triggers are exercise, hot water immersion, and spicy foods. Onset is within half an hour, and lesions can last up to several hours. The diagnosis is made by history but can be confirmed by exercise testing. A positive exercise test reproduces lesions after onset of perspiration. Hot water immersion in a bath at 43°C can raise the patient's oral temperature by 1°C–1.5°C. The immersion is safer, as it does not produce symptoms in patients with exercise-induced anaphylaxis (EIA). Intradermal injection of methacholine can also be diagnostic in some patients.[21]

Treatment is aimed at avoiding symptoms by limiting strenuous exercise and other triggers. Showering with hot water the night before an event can be effective by inducing a refractory period by temporarily depleting histamine. Immediate cooling after sweating with a cool shower or application of ice packs can abort attacks. Antihistamines, such as cetirizine, 10 mg BID, can be effective in providing relief. Hydroxyzine, 10 mg, taken 1 hour before exercise helps prevent urticaria. Severely affected patients may respond to stanozolol or beta-blockers, but these substances are prohibited in competitive athletes.[12]

55.5.9 Cold Urticaria

Cold urticarias are incited by mast cell activation and degranulation in response to cold exposure and can result in hives, angioedema, and even anaphylaxis. The lesions are usually larger in cold-exposed areas but can rapidly spread to other parts of the body. Cold urticaria occur in athletes participating in winter sports but can also occur in susceptible athletes with simple cold exposure, such as contact with ice or cold water. The diagnosis is confirmed by a positive cold-stimulation test or "ice cube test," in which ice is applied to the skin for 15 minutes. If urticarias develop within 3 minutes during a cold test, this is associated with a higher risk of serious reactions.[56]

Avoidance of cold environments is the only complete preventative measure. However, wearing protective clothing can be beneficial if cold climates cannot be avoided. Second-generation antihistamines, such as cetirizine, can be used for treatment and prevention, but some patients will require up to four times the daily recommended dose to achieve an adequate response.[21] Acute treatment with more traditional first-generation antihistamines, diphenhydramine and hydroxyzine, is limited due to sedation. Those with anaphylaxis should carry an epinephrine injectable kit (EpiPen®).[13]

55.5.10 Solar Urticaria

Solar urticarias are rare. Lesions occur after exposure to UV and visible light. Athletes are usually sensitive to a specific wavelength. They appear within minutes on unexposed skin and can spread to exposed areas as well. Lesions usually disappear in 1–2 hours. Eruptions are typical pruritic hives and wheals, but intensity and duration of symptoms vary with length and time of exposure. These lesions are thought to be caused by an IgE reaction due to a photoallergen in the skin. Diagnosis is made on history, but phototesting can help if the diagnosis is uncertain.[21]

Sunscreen can be effective at preventing eruptions. Antihistamines can be used to treat pruritus associated with eruptions. For those who do not respond to antihistamines, desensitization by various hardening techniques (UV therapy) is effective and can have long-lasting results.[7]

55.5.11 Aquagenic Urticaria

Aquagenic urticarias are rare. This condition is associated with direct contact with water of any temperature and of any source. The lesions formed are very similar to those of cholinergic urticaria and occur on all parts of the body. The pathogenesis is poorly understood, and many instances have a genetic component. Diagnosis is made by history and water challenge test.[46] Keeping water at 35°C distinguishes aquagenic urticaria from cold or cholinergic urticarial. [46] The ice cube test can be used to differentiate aquagenic from cold urticaria if the diagnosis is unclear.

Complete control of symptoms can be achieved with antihistamines. For patients in whom adequate relief cannot be obtained by antihistamines alone, treatment with psoralen and phototherapy can be successful. Prevention can sometimes be managed with barrier creams (dimethicone–petrolatum).[46]

55.5.12 Exercise-Induced Urticaria

Exercise-induced urticarias are physical urticaria that can be either cholinergic or anaphylactic. The cholinergic urticaria can develop in athletes participating in a variety of sports but is most commonly associated with running. A more serious etiology that has been associated with urticaria is EIA. The diagnosis is clinical and is based upon a history of anaphylactic symptoms associated with exercise. Development of cutaneous and systemic symptoms indicates EIA, and symptoms may include urticaria, angioedema, and/or flushing in combination with hypotension, dyspnea, stridor, wheezing, nausea, dyspepsia, or diarrhea.[1] EIA is idiopathic but can also be associated with ingestion of food allergens (most commonly), cold exposure, ingestion of NSAIDs, or exposure to contact allergens. Not all episodes of EIA result in cardiovascular collapse, but signs and symptoms should be recognized and appropriately addressed.

Clinical Pearl

Antihistamines are the first-line therapy in all environmental urticarial skin dermatoses. Steroids may be added in more severe cases to speed recovery. The health-care team must be keenly aware of regulations in the use of steroids.

Treatment of urticaria primarily includes administration of antihistamines and topical corticosteroids. If symptoms of anaphylaxis manifest, then acute physical exertion should be immediately terminated. Pharmacotherapy for EIA includes epinephrine, antihistamines, and systemic corticosteroids.[4] Prevention is the primary target. Avoiding specific food triggers 4–6 hours before exertion and avoiding NSAIDs and heat and excessive sun exposure and layering of clothes decreases occurrences. Pretreatment with antihistamines or leukotriene inhibitors can be effective for prevention. Omalizumab can be an effective treatment but is very expensive.[27]

55.6 CONCLUSION

As a natural barrier, the skin offers a resilient covering from our environment and a mechanism for our bodies to dissipate heat as we exercise. Minor changes to our protective covering not only can degrade an athlete's training but may also ultimately prevent him or her from either achieving their maximum performance or having the ability to compete. Team trainers and clinicians play a cohesive role in education, early identification, and proper treatment of skin disorders (Table 55.2).

TABLE 55.2
SORT: Key Recommendations for Practice

Clinical Recommendations	Evidence Rating	References
Diagnosing dermatoses is achieved by a thorough history and meticulous physical exam. Ancillary testing is rarely necessary.	C	[1,3,12,20–22, 30,48,49,51,52,56,57]
The majority of dermatological disorders arising from athletic participation are self-limited and preventable with good hygiene, properly fitted equipment and clothing, and acclimatization to the environment.	C	[1,12,30,40,56,57]
Treatment regimens for dermatoses must be individualized to account for presenting symptoms and history, level of competition, necessity to return to participation, and risk to fellow participants.	B C	[5,6,8,10,14,17,34,36,41,43,59,60] [1,30,56,57]
The intensity, duration, and level of participation within an activity or sport commonly predispose an athlete to certain dermatoses. Certain dermatoses tend to be sport specific.	C	[1,12,30,40,56,57]
The health-care team must be familiar with the regulations and restrictions at all levels governing participation and return to play for athletes who have acquired an infectious dermatological condition.	C	[18,19,46]

REFERENCES

1. Adams BB. Dermatologic disorders of the athlete. *Sports Medicine.* 2002;32(5):309–321.
2. Akdemir O, Bilkay U, Tiftikcioglu YO et al. New alternative in treatment of callus. *Journal of Dermatology.* February 2011;38(2):146–150.
3. Auerbach PS. *Wilderness Medicine*, 6th edn. Philadelphia, PA: Elsevier Health Sciences, ch 8; 2011: pp. 181–201.
4. Barg W, Medrala W, Wolanczyk-Medrala A. Exercise-induced anaphylaxis: An update on diagnosis and treatment. *Current Allergy and Asthma Reports.* February 2011;11(1):45–51.
5. Bauer A, Schmitt J, Bennett C et al. Interventions for preventing occupational irritant hand dermatitis. *Cochrane Database of Systematic Reviews.* 2010;(6);Art. No. 10:CD0034414.
6. Bell-Syer SE, Khan SM, Torgerson DJ. Oral treatments for fungal infections of the skin of the foot. *Cochrane Database of Systematic Reviews.* October 2012;Art. No: 10:CD003584.
7. Botto NC, Warshaw EM. Solar urticarial. *Journal of the American Academy of Dermatology.* December 2008:59(6); 909–922.
8. Boulware DR. A randomized, controlled field trial for the prevention of jellyfish stings with a topical sting inhibitor. *Journal of Travel Medicine.* May–June 2006;13(3):166–171.
9. Brant SV, Cohen AN, James D et al. Cercarial dermatitis transmitted by exotic marine snail. *Emerging Infectious Diseases.* September 2010;16(9):1357–1365.
10. Caceres-Rios H, Rueda M, Ballona R, Bustamante B. Comparison of terbinafine and griseofulvin in the treatment of tinea capitis. *Journal of the American Academy of Dermatology.* 2000;42(1):80–84.
11. Clark SC, Zirwas MJ. Management of occupational dermatitis. *Dermatologic Clinics.* 2009;27(3):365–383.
12. De Luca JF, Adams BB, Yosipovitich G. Skin manifestations of athletes competing in the summer Olympics: What a sports medicine physician should know. *Sports Medicine.* May 2012;42(5):399–413.
13. Dover G, Borsa PA, McDonald DJ. Cold urticarial following an ice application: A case study. *Clinical Journal of Sport Medicine.* November 2004;14(6):362–364.
14. Eekhof JA, Van Wijk B, Knuistingh NA, Van der Wouden JC. Interventions for ingrowing toenails. *Cochrane Database of Systematic Reviews.* April 2012;Art No. 4:CD001541.
15. Fisher AA. Green hair: Causes and management. *Cutis.* June 1999;63(6):317.
16. Focht DR, Spicer C, Fairchok MP. The efficacy of duct tape vs cryotherapy in the treatment of verruca vulgaris (the common wart). *Archives of Pediatrics and Adolescent Medicine.* October 2002;156(10):971–974.
17. Guideline 2j: Skin infections in athletics. *National Collegiate Athletic Association Sports Medicine Handbook*, 24th edn. Indianapolis. In: National Association of Intercollegiate Athletics; 2008: pp. 67–73.
18. Guideline 2l: Blood-borne pathogens. *National Collegiate Athletic Association Sports Medicine Handbook*, 24th edn. Indianapolis. In: National Association of Intercollegiate Athletics; 2008: 78 p.
19. Habif TP. *Clinical Dermatology: A Color Guide to Diagnosis and Therapy*, 5th edn. St Louis, MO: Mosby; 2009:ch 13, pp. 491–540.
20. Habif TP. *Clinical Dermatology: A Color Guide to Diagnosis and Therapy*, 5th edn. St Louis, MO: Mosby; 2009:ch 15, pp. 581–634.
21. Habif TP. *Clinical Dermatology: A Color Guide to Diagnosis and Therapy*, 5th edn. St Louis: Mosby; 2009:ch 6, pp. 181–216.
22. Harmant ES. Sunscreen use among collegiate athletes. *Journal of the American Academy of Dermatology.* 2005; 53(2):237–241.
23. Hinz T, Klingmuller K, Bieber T, Schmid-Wendtner MH. The mystery of green hair. *European Journal of Dermatology.* July–August 2009;19(4):409–410.
24. Holdiness MR. Management of cutaneous erythrasma. *Drugs.* 2002;62(8):1131–1141.
25. Honsik KA, Romeo MW, Hawley CJ, Romeo SJ, Romeo JP. Sideline skin and wound care for acute injuries. *Current Sports Medicine Reports.* June 2007;6(3):147–154.
26. Huffer P. Martonffy AI. What is the most effective treatment for molluscum contagiosum? *Evidence-Based Practice.* September 2013;16(9):6.

27. Jaqua NT, Peterson MR, Davis KL. Exercise-induced anaphylaxis: A case report and review of the diagnosis and treatment of a rare but potentially life-threatening syndrome. *Case Reports in Medicine.* 2013;6(10):726.
28. Jaworski CA, Donohue B, Kluetz J. Infectious disease. *Clinics in Sports Medicine.* July 2011;30(3):575–590.
29. Jeffords MD, Batts KB. *Dermatology, ACSM Sports Medicine: A Comprehensive Review.* O'Connor FG, Casa DJ, Davis BA et al. (eds.). Philadelphia: Lippincott, Williams & Wilkins; 2013;28:181–186.
30. Kakourou T, Uksal U. European Society for Pediatric Dermatology. Guidelines for the management of tinea capitis in children. *Pediatric Dermatology.* 2010;27:226–228.
31. Khachemoune A, Yalamanchili R, Rodriquez C. What is your diagnosis? Seabather's eruption. *Cutis.* March 2006;77(3):148, 151–152.
32. Kockentiet B, Adams BB. Contact dermatitis in athletes. *Journal of the American Academy of Dermatology.* June 2007;56(6):1048–1055.
33. Koning S, Van der Sande R, Verhagen AP et al. Interventions for impetigo. *Cochrane Database of Systematic Reviews.* January 2012;18(1):CD003261.
34. Kundu RV, Patterson, S. Dermatologic conditions in skin of color: Part II. Disorders occurring predominantly in skin of color. *American Family Physician.* June 2013;87(12):859–865.
35. Kwok CS, Gibbs S, Bennett C et al. Topical treatments for cutaneous warts. *Cochrane Database of Systematic Reviews.* September 2012;9:CD001781.
36. Likness LP. Common dermatologic infections in athletes and return-to-play guidelines. *Journal of the American Osteopathic Association.* June 2011;111(6):373–379.
37. Liu C, Bayer A, Cosgrove SE et al. Clinical practice guidelines by the infectious diseases society of America for the treatment of methicillin-resistant *Staphylococcus aureus* infections in adults and children. *Clinical Infectious Diseases.* 52(3), February 2011: 285–292.
38. Liu Y, Kong F, Zhang X et al. Antimicrobial susceptibility of *Staphylococcus aureus* isolated from children in China from 2003 to 2007 shows community-associated methicillin-resistant *Staphylococcus aureus* to be uncommon and heterogeneous. *British Journal of Dermatology.* 2009;161:1347.
39. Mailler-Savage EA, Adams BB. Skin manifestations of running. *Journal of the American Academy of Dermatology.* August 2006;55(2):290–301.
40. McCormack PL. Spinosad: In pediculosis capitis. *American Journal of Clinical Dermatology.* 2011;12(5):349.
41. McMahon JA, Howe A. Cold weather issues in sideline and event management. *Current Sports Medicine Reports.* May–June 2012:11(3);135–141.
42. Meinking TL, Villar ME, Vicaria M et al. The clinical trials supporting benzyl alcohol lotion 5% (Ulesfia): A safe and effective topical treatment for head lice (*Pediculus humanus* capitis). *Pediatric Dermatology.* 2010;27(1):19–24.
43. Miners AL. The diagnosis and emergency care of heat related illness and sunburn in athletes: A retrospective case series. *Journal of the Canadian Chiropractic Association.* 201;54(2):107–117.
44. Morton LM, Phillips TJ. Wound healing update. *Seminars in Cutaneous Medicine and Surgery.* March 2012;31(1):33–37.
45. NFHS Medical Release Form for Wrestler to Participate with Skin Lesions. Available at: https://www.nfhs.org/media/869160/wrestling_skin_lesion_form_2014-15.pdf. Accessed June 12, 2014.
46. Park H, Kim HS, Yoo DS et al. Aquagenic urticaria: A report of two cases. *Annals of Dermatology.* December 2011;23(Suppl 3): S371–S374.
47. Pecci M, Comeau D, Chawla V. Skin conditions in the athlete. *American Journal of Sports Medicine.* February 2009;37(2):406–418.
48. Pleacher MD, Dexter WW. Cutaneous fungal and viral infections in athletes. *Clinics in Sports Medicine.* July 2007; 26(3):397–411.
49. Roy S, Smith LP. A novel technique for treating auricular hematomas in mixed martial artists (ultimate fighters). *American Journal of Otolaryngology.* January–February 2010;31(1):21–24.
50. Sedgewick PE, Dexter WW, Smith CT. Bacterial dermatoses in sports. *Clinics in Sports Medicine.* July 2007;26(3): 383–396.
51. Seto CK, Way D, O'Connor N. Environmental illness in athletes. *Clinics in Sports Medicine.* July 2005;24(3):695–718.
52. Shah N, Cain G, Naji O, Goff J. Skin infections in athletes: Treating the patient, protecting the team. *Journal of Family Practice.* June 2013;62(6):284–291.
53. Summers A. Managing auricular haematoma to prevent 'cauliflower ear'. *Emergency Nurse.* September 2012;20(5): 28–90.
54. Taylor KS, Zoltan TB, Archer AS. Medical illnesses and injuries encountered during surfing. *Current Sports Medicine Reports.* September 2006;5(5):262–267.
55. Tlougan BE, Mancini AJ, Mandell JA et al. Skin conditions in figure skaters, ice-hockey players and speed skaters: Part I-mechanical dermatoses. *Sports Medicine.* September 2011;41(9):709–719.
56. Tlougan BE, Mancini AJ, Mandell JA et al. Skin conditions in figure skaters, ice-hockey players and speed skaters: Part II-cold-induced, infectious and inflammatory dermatoses. *Sports Medicine.* November 2011;41(11):967–984.
57. Trott A. *Wounds and Lacerations: Emergency Care and Closure*, 4th edn. Philadelphia, PA: Saunders; 2012:ch.16, pp. 220–235.
58. Ud-Din S, Bayat A. Strategic management of keloid disease in ethnic skin: A structured approach supported by the emerging literature. *British Journal of Dermatology.* October 2013;169(Suppl 3):71–81.
59. Wolff K, Goldsmith LA, Katz SI et al. *Fitzpatrick's Dermatology in General Medicine*, 7th edn. New York: McGraw Hill; 2007: 1694 p.
60. Workowski KA, Berman SM. Centers for Disease Control and Prevention. Sexually transmitted diseases treatment guidelines, 2010. *MMWR Recommendations and Reports.* 2010;59:21–22.
61. Yokota M, Maibach HI. Moisturizer effect on irritant dermatitis: An overview. *Contact Dermatitis.* August 2006; 55(2):65–72.

56 Gastrointestinal Problems in Training and Competition

David L. Brown and Alain Michael P. Abellada

CONTENTS

TABLE 56.1
Key Clinical Considerations

1. GI symptoms are common in athletes and increase with demanding endurance activities. Symptom patterns follow the type of exercise performed: lower GI symptoms predominating in runners, upper and lower GI symptoms occurring with equal frequency in triathletes, and upper GI symptoms predominating in weight lifters.
2. GI symptoms should be correlated with the athlete's pretraining and precompetition diet as well as their sporting activity, training mode, and transitions in training volume/intensity.
3. Prior to initiating long-term traditional NSAID therapy, testing for *H. pylori* should be considered. If a patient is *H. pylori positive*, treatment with eradication therapy is indicated.
4. Classic runner's diarrhea typically responds to a temporary reduction in training intensity for 1–2 weeks. A full return to high-intensity exercise can usually be achieved by gradually increasing training as symptoms tolerate.
5. Red flags for the upper GI tract (dysphagia, odynophagia, hematemesis, melena, and early satiety) and lower GI tract (diminution of stool caliber, hematochezia, and unremitting abdominal pain) should prompt an immediate gastroenterology consultation.

56.1 INTRODUCTION

The athlete in training and competition is no stranger to disorders of the gastrointestinal (GI) system. There are factors that impact GI function. Knowledge of these factors will help the primary care physician understand and manage their active patients (Table 56.1).

56.2 EPIDEMIOLOGY

GI symptoms are highly prevalent in athletes, particularly those involved in demanding endurance activities. Upper GI symptoms include nausea, vomiting, belching, heartburn, and abdominal pain. Lower GI symptoms reported include bloating, cramps, fecal urgency, diarrhea, and fecal incontinence. In addition to subjective symptoms, abnormalities on laboratory evaluation have been observed, including elevations in liver-associated enzymes. Long-distance runners have been the most studied group from a GI perspective; however, recent studies have also looked at long-distance walkers, cyclists, triathletes, and weight lifters. In a study of 606 athletes, 36% of runners, 67% of cyclists, and 52%–54% of triathletes reported some of these symptoms.[33] Upper and lower GI tract symptoms occur with equal prevalence in cyclists (67% and 64%, respectively). Lower GI symptoms predominate over upper GI symptoms in endurance runners (71% vs. 36%). Whether running or riding, these same patterns also hold true among triathletes. In low-intensity, long-distance walking, the overall occurrence of GI symptoms has been found to be much lower than in other sports studied. During one event, only 24% of walkers surveyed reported symptoms. The most common symptoms were flatulence and nausea, each of which occurred in only 5% of walkers.[34]

Symptomatic gastroesophageal reflux is extremely common in athletes. Collings et al.,[10] using esophageal pH monitoring, found that cyclists had the lowest esophageal acid exposure, followed closely by runners. In their study, weight lifters had the highest rates of reflux, occurring for over 18% of their exercise period. All groups had increased reflux when exercising in the postprandial period. Cyclists had a modest increase in reflux after eating; however, weight lifters nearly doubled their amount of reflux to 35% and runners tripled their reflux (from 8% to 26%).

When peptic ulcer disease (PUD) is observed, it is associated with the primary risk factors of *Helicobacter pylori* infection and, of particular importance in athletes, use of nonsteroidal anti-inflammatory drugs (NSAIDs). The prevalence of *H. pylori* infection varies by location. One study in China, for example, showed the prevalence of *H. pylori* was 93%[23] among patients with peptic ulcers, while the rates have decreased to 50%–75% in the United States.[8,9,18,30] In Western countries, NSAIDs, less commonly cyclooxygenase-2 inhibitors (COX-2) and ASA, are the most common causes of PUD. A meta-analysis revealed that the risk of uncomplicated ulcer increased 4-fold in *H. pylori*–positive patients compared to *H. pylori*–negative patients and 17-fold in *H. pylori*–positive NSAID users compared to *H. pylori*–negative nonusers.[30]

Clinical Pearl

Runners are most commonly afflicted by lower GI symptoms (diarrhea), while weight lifters are more commonly affected by upper GI symptoms (reflux).

Lower GI tract symptoms affecting athletes, which include lower abdominal cramping, urge to defecate, increased bowel frequency, and diarrhea, have been reported with varying prevalences, occurring in 37%–71% of runners either during or following a run.[38] Running is not typically associated with GI bleeding. However, incidence figures for GI bleeding range from 7.4% up to 85% in athletes running ultramarathon distances.[15]

56.3 GASTROINTESTINAL HISTORY AND PHYSICAL

56.3.1 History

The organized evaluation of any GI complaint begins with a thorough history. This includes delineating the exact nature and chronicity of the problem, specifying exacerbating and relieving factors, and assessing for red flag symptoms. Individuals should be questioned about the location, quality, and radiation of any pain as well as the relationship of symptoms to food ingestion. Symptoms related to the upper GI tract include nausea, vomiting, bloating, and excessive belching. Lower tract symptoms include crampy/spasmodic abdominal pain, constipation, and diarrhea. Individuals should be questioned about the location, quality, and radiation of any dietary history to assess pretraining and precompetition in food, fluid, and supplement intake. Any dietary changes that predate the onset of symptoms could identify the culprit. It is also important to inquire about the relationship of symptoms to transitions in training, especially any escalation in training volume and intensity.

Clinical Pearl

A comprehensive history correlates symptoms to sporting activities. Special attention should be given to the time course of symptoms and their relation to any escalation in training volume and intensity as well as changes in food, fluid, and supplement intake.

The presence of red flag symptoms should prompt a gastroenterology referral. Upper tract alarm symptoms include dysphagia, odynophagia, hematemesis, melena, and early satiety. For the lower GI tract, a diminution of stool caliber and hematochezia should cause concern. Unremitting pain, especially pain that awakens an individual from sleep, as well as any systemic symptoms such as fevers, night sweats, and unplanned weight loss, is especially concerning. Additionally, even moderate symptoms that are failing maximal conservative management should trigger further evaluation.

The review of systems should key on symptoms that indicate involvement of a specific portion of the digestive system or involvement of organ systems masquerading as a GI condition. The middle-aged athlete with apparent exertional GI complaints such as heartburn, epigastric pain, and nausea may actually be having angina. Providers need to have a high index of suspicion for coronary artery disease in these individuals and should thoroughly explore their cardiac risk factors. The athlete with chronic constipation or diarrhea should be asked about environmental temperature intolerance, palpitations, tremor, skin and hair changes, and menstrual irregularities that could point to hyper- or hypothyroidism. The presence of right upper quadrant or epigastric pain that is specifically triggered by fatty foods could indicate symptomatic cholelithiasis or recurrent pancreatitis. If the athlete is having flank or lower quadrant abdominal pain associated with gross or microscopic hematuria, then nephrolithiasis or other urinary tract pathology should be considered. Female athletes with abdominal complaints should be questioned about the relationship of their symptoms to their menstrual cycle, looking for ovarian and uterine pathology or pregnancy. Orthopedic issues such as sacral, pelvic, and femoral neck stress fractures can also present with lower abdominal symptoms. If a stress fracture is in the differential, providers should assess for risk factors such as rapid progression in training, poor nutritional status, and the presence of the female athlete triad.

56.3.2 Physical Examination

The physical exam, while fairly insensitive, should be used to provide evidence to corroborate or refute what is found in the history. While the physical is often tailored to upper versus lower tract complaints, it should be kept in mind that some conditions, such as inflammatory bowel disease, may affect anywhere from the mouth to the anus. Working top to bottom, the oral cavity should be assessed for signs of ulceration or posterior pharyngeal inflammation. The tooth enamel should be examined for deterioration that can occur with chronic acid reflux or forced vomiting in conjunction with an eating disorder. It is important to examine the neck for lymphadenopathy, thyroid nodules, and thyromegaly.

The abdominal exam should start with inspection, focusing on distension or overt organomegaly. To avoid altering the bowel sound pattern, auscultation for hypo- or hyperactive bowel sounds should be accomplished prior to percussion or palpation. Percussion is useful in evaluating for hyperresonance, which would indicate bowel distension or obstruction. Dullness to percussion can be seen focally when hepatosplenomegaly or a mass lesion is present. Shifting dullness with positional changes is seen with accumulation of ascitic fluid. Palpation should start in areas remote from symptoms and then conclude by focusing over the area of concern. The provider should note any rigidity, organomegaly, involuntary guarding, or rebound tenderness. In the acute setting, special tests can also be helpful. A positive Murphy's sign is suggestive of acute cholecystitis. Classically, focal pain over McBurney's point indicates an acute appendicitis. Obturator, psoas, and "heel tap" signs are all tests that can be performed to document peritoneal irritation.

The exam should conclude with at least a visual inspection of the anus, looking for perianal disease. When lower GI symptoms are present, however, providers should perform a digital rectal exam and assess for occult blood. In the female athlete with lower quadrant tenderness, no exam would be complete without performing a bimanual pelvic exam to assess the uterus and adnexa.

56.4 UPPER GASTROINTESTINAL DISEASES

56.4.1 Gastroesophageal Reflux Disease

56.4.1.1 Presentation

As in the nonathletic population, the most common presenting complaints in athletes with gastroesophageal reflux disease (GERD) are heartburn and acid regurgitation. When an individual describes the classic presentation of retrosternal burning, exacerbated by meals, intense workouts, and recumbency with resolution on antacids, the diagnosis is clear; however, many athletes present with more atypical symptoms, including hoarseness, cough, sore throat, bronchitis, asthma, recurrent pneumonia, intermittent choking, or chest pain.[45] Still others may present only with extraintestinal complaints, such as sore throat, exertional dyspnea, cough, or wheezing (see Table 56.2).

TABLE 56.2
GERD Symptom Patterns

Classic symptoms
- Heartburn
- Acid regurgitation

Nonspecific symptoms
- Nausea
- Dyspepsia
- Bloating
- Belching
- Indigestion
- Hypersalivation/water brash

Atypical symptoms/signs
- Pulmonary
  - Asthma/wheezing
  - Chronic cough
- Ear, nose, and throat
  - Dental erosions
  - Halitosis
  - Lingual sensitivity
  - Chronic pharyngitis
  - Hoarseness
  - Rhinitis/sinusitis
  - Globus
- Cardiac
  - Atypical chest pain

Red flags
- Chronic untreated symptoms
- Dysphagia
- Weight loss
- Hematemesis
- Melena
- Odynophagia
- Vomiting
- Early satiety

56.4.1.2 Pathophysiology

To understand the pathophysiology of acid reflux, one must first be familiar with the tiered defense system of the esophagus. The primary mechanical barriers to reflux are the lower esophageal sphincter (LES) and the diaphragm. The tonic contraction of the LES, when not swallowing, prevents the free reflux of gastric contents. The diaphragm encircles the LES and acts as a mechanical support, especially during physical exertion. This mechanical barrier is reinforced by luminal acid clearance. Large bolus clearance is accomplished by gravity and swallow-induced peristalsis. Salivary and esophageal gland secretions, rich in bicarbonate, clear the residual acidity. The final barrier is the esophageal epithelium itself. Intercellular junctions limit hydrochloric acid diffusion between cells. Intracellular buffering is reinforced by transmembrane channels that exchange hydrogen ions for sodium and chloride for bicarbonate. The esophageal blood supply delivers bicarbonate and removes H^+ and CO_2 to restore cellular buffering capacity and maintain normal tissue acid balance.[29]

Clinical Pearl

High-intensity exercise directly increases the duration of exposure to acid reflux worsening GERD symptomatology.

The pathophysiology of GERD involves the movement of gastric contents from the stomach into the esophagus. Symptoms develop when substances in the refluxate, including hydrochloric acid and the proteolytic enzyme pepsin, cause irritation of the esophageal epithelium. Reflux alone is insufficient to explain why individuals become symptomatic because healthy individuals have a physiologic amount of acid reflux. In fact, GERD patients have rates of gastric acid and pepsin reflux similar to healthy individuals.[16] The critical factor in symptom development appears to be that the contact time between refluxed material and the epithelium is so excessive that the normal gastric contents overwhelm the epithelial protective mechanisms. Alternatively, symptoms may develop when normal contact time occurs in the face of insufficient protective mechanisms.

Symptomatic reflux episodes during exercise are likely multifactorial but appear to involve transient LES relaxations (TLESRs), increased pressure gradient between the stomach and esophagus, and decreased esophageal clearance.[15] When reflux events coincide with TLESRs, the decrease in LES tone lasts longer and is not accompanied by a swallow-induced peristaltic sweep, leading to prolonged acid exposure. Prolonged acid exposure may also occur due to delayed acid clearance from body positioning. Supine or forward-flexed posture during particular modes of exercise increases intra-abdominal pressure and overcomes the mechanical protection of the LES; this posture also negates the bolus acid clearance achieved by gravity. Impaired esophageal motility during exercise also contributes to delayed acid clearance. GERD worsens with higher intensity of exercise and postprandial exercise and is more common with endurance sports. Increasing exercise intensity correlates with a rise in the duration of acid exposure and reflux episodes.[39] More specifically, both the number and the duration of esophageal reflux episodes increase when exercise intensity is greater than or equal to 90% VO_{2max}.[11,43] High-intensity exercise also reduces splanchnic blood flow, which may inhibit restoration of acid base balance and deprive the epithelium of the oxygen and nutrients needed for damage repair. It may also play a role in delayed gastric emptying, thereby promoting GERD.[32]

56.4.1.3 Evaluation and Management

If the history and physical exam raise red flags, the athlete should be referred for evaluation by a gastroenterologist (see Figure 56.1). Likewise, if an individual's symptoms are particularly severe or if the diagnosis is unclear, a GI referral is warranted. For patients with extraintestinal manifestations or atypical GERD symptoms, providers can consider an initial therapeutic trial; however, if empiric therapy fails, it is important to consult not only a gastroenterologist but also a specialist that would evaluate for any extraintestinal complications. In the face of a classic history and normal physical exam, it is reasonable to institute empiric therapy in a stepwise fashion (see Figure 56.2), starting with addressing any modifiable risk factors such as food and medication triggers, exercising immediately after meals, and wearing tight-fitting workout apparel.

Persistent symptoms despite behavioral interventions warrant medical therapy. If an athlete's complaints are episodic, over-the-counter (OTC) antacids or an H-2 receptor antagonist (H2RA) can be employed on an as-needed basis. This can be advanced to prescription-strength H2RA therapy if control is insufficient. The OTC H2RAs are particularly useful when taken prior to an activity that may result in reflux symptoms (heavy meal or exercise). The peak potencies of OTC H2RAs and antacids are similar, but the former have a longer duration of action (up to 10 hours). Should symptoms continue after 6 weeks of H2RA therapy, neither continuing therapy nor increasing the

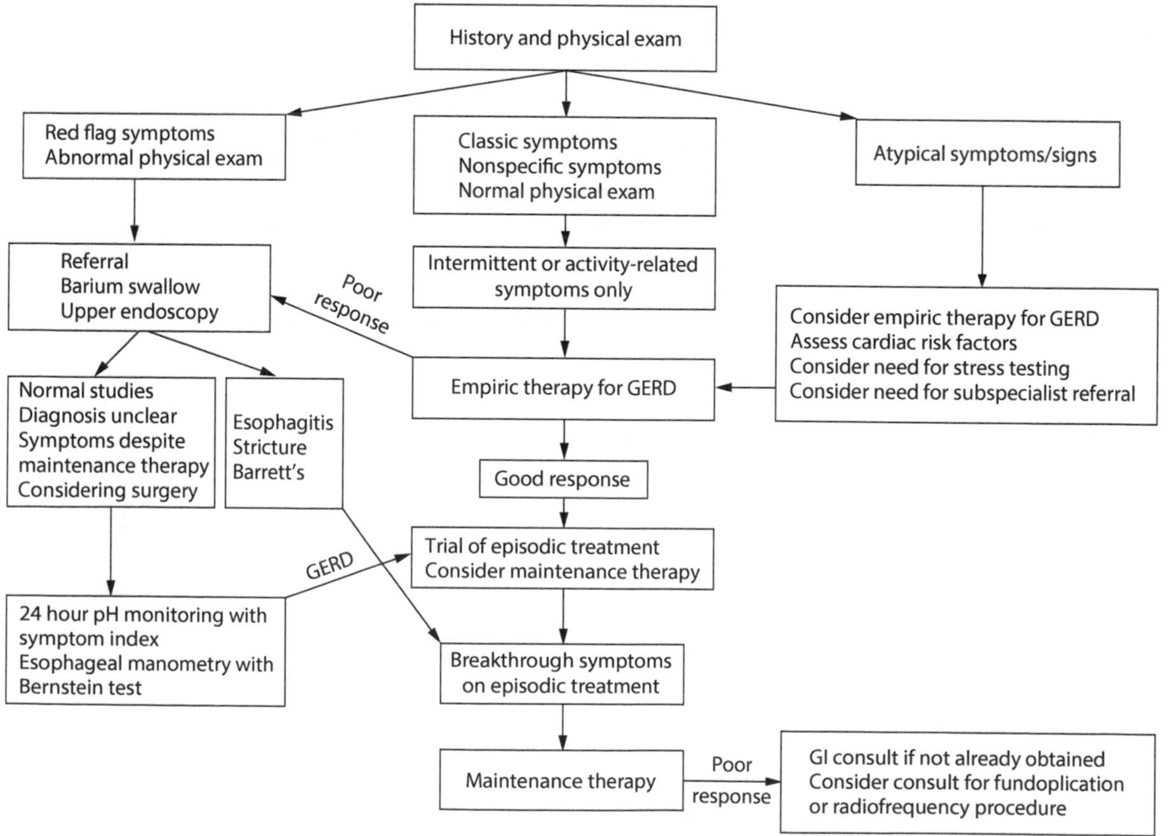

FIGURE 56.1 Evaluation of GERD. (Adapted from O'Connor, F.G., *Textbook of Running Medicine*, 1st edn., McGraw-Hill, New York, 2001. With permission.)

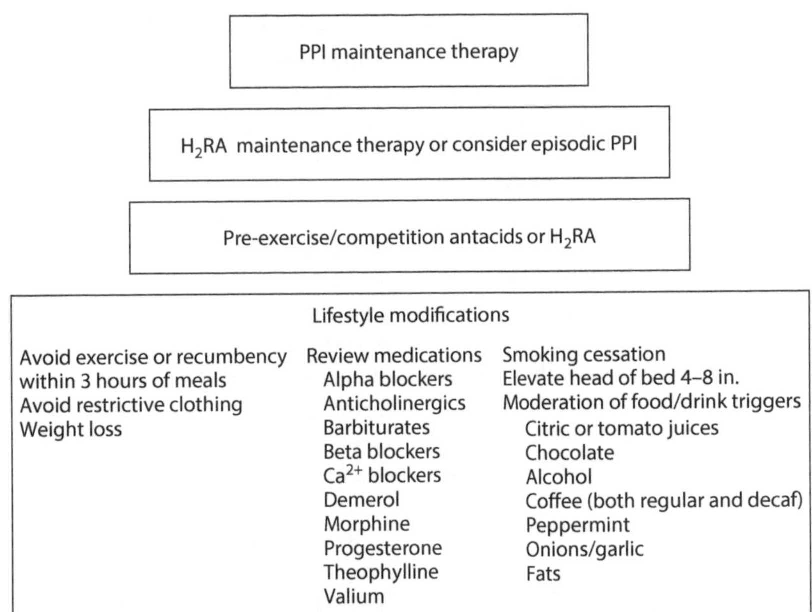

FIGURE 56.2 Therapeutic pyramid for exercise-related GERD. (Adapted from O'Connor, F.G., *Textbook of Running Medicine*, 1st edn., McGraw-Hill, New York, 2001.)

dose is likely to achieve control (level II evidence).[13] At this point, it was previously common practice to consider add-on therapy with a prokinetic agent to improve LES tone, gastric emptying, and peristalsis. These agents all have side effects that make them undesirable for use in athletes. Bethanechol has generalized cholinergic effects. Metoclopramide has a high incidence of fatigue, restlessness, tremor, and tardive dyskinesia, making it a poor choice for anything more than sporadic use. Cisapride, formerly the prokinetic agent of choice, was found to be associated with arrhythmia development, especially with concomitant use of agents metabolized by the cytochrome P-450 system, to include macrolides, imidazoles, or protease inhibitors.[6] This discovery led to severe prescribing restrictions in the United States, and it is currently available only by directly petitioning the manufacturer.

Thus, in individuals who fail to respond to H2RAs, standard-dose proton pump inhibitors (PPIs) are the treatment of choice. PPIs have been shown to provide more rapid relief of symptoms and are more likely than H2RAs to heal erosive esophagitis compared to higher and more frequent dosing of H2RAs.[6] The results of a systematic review of PPI therapy show that the agents in this class are equally efficacious in controlling heartburn and had similar healing and relapse rates.[19] If the response to episodic treatment is generally favorable but symptoms are occurring on a more chronic basis, maintenance therapy is beneficial. Because their efficacy is dose dependent, PPI therapy can be stepped up to control symptoms. Insufficient response to standard dosing can be reasonably treated with higher than approved PPI dosing.[1] Failure to respond to high-dose PPI therapy requires gastroenterologist evaluation to rule out complications of GERD. In the absence of findings consistent with reflux disease, a gastroenterologist can help confirm GERD or assess for other esophageal disorders.

More invasive treatments are available for patients with an established diagnosis of GERD who respond poorly to PPIs, who are intolerant of medical therapy, or who desire a permanent solution to potentially eliminate their need for medication. Laparoscopic antireflux surgery has been shown to provide a 96% improvement in primary symptoms and 96% long-term satisfaction rate; however, 2% of patients were worse after surgery and 14% still required medication.[46] Four trials with a total of 1232 randomized participants revealed that laparoscopic fundoplication surgery is more effective than medical management in the treatment of GERD in adults, at least in the short-to-medium term.[17,47] While the potential exists for excellent results, the best outcomes occur in carefully selected patients under the care of an experienced surgeon. It is advisable to have the surgery performed by an experienced surgeon, since more complications and poorer outcomes occur in low-volume centers. In a study of 100 patients, the best predictors of a good surgical outcome were age less than 50 years old and reflux symptoms that had completely resolved on medical therapy.[37] A fundoplication for severely obese patients (BMI between 25 and 30 or over 30) is presumably not the best strategy to control GERD. Of all surgical techniques, the Roux-en-Y gastric bypass having both restrictive and malabsorptive properties seems to be most promising. Adjustable gastric banding is known to have antireflux properties, especially in the short term.[26]

56.4.2 Peptic Ulcer Disease

56.4.2.1 Presentation

Epigastric pain is the hallmark of PUD. Both gastric and duodenal ulcers typically present with deep burning or gnawing pain, sometimes with radiation to the back. With duodenal ulceration, symptoms usually develop 2–3 hours after meals and are relieved with food or antacid ingestion. The symptoms of gastric ulcers develop sooner after meals and are less consistently relieved with food or antacids. In fact, food ingestion can actually precipitate gastric ulcer pain in some individuals. Most PUD patients have associated anorexia and weight loss. Some patients, particularly with duodenal ulcers, experience hyperphagia and weight gain, presumably due to the mitigating effects of food. Not uncommonly, the initial presentation of PUD can be life-threatening upper GI hemorrhage or perforation.[28]

Peptic ulcers are erosions in the surface of the stomach or duodenum that extend down to the muscularis mucosa. *H. pylori* induces ulcers by both direct and indirect mechanisms. *H. pylori* infection impairs negative feedback regulation of gastrin release through its high urease activity and alkaline ammonia production, leading to inappropriate secretion of somatostatin and gastrin. The inhibitory antral-fundic neural connections that downregulate acid production are also impaired.[28] Bacterial phospholipases weaken the protective mucus barrier, allowing toxic compounds from their breakdown of urea to damage the epithelium directly. The same urease enzyme that promotes this direct cell damage acts as a potent antigenic stimulator of immune cells. By inciting an exuberant host inflammatory response, *H. pylori* produces indirect epithelial damage.[44]

PUD secondary to NSAIDs occurs from postabsorptive inhibition of GI COX. By inhibiting gastric COX-1, NSAIDs may reduce mucosal blood flow, causing local ischemic injury. NSAIDs may also impair specific prostaglandin-dependent defenses, which protect the gastric mucosa, such as the thick bicarbonate-containing mucous layer lining the interior of the stomach, which buffers luminal gastric acid and thus protects the stomach wall. When these defenses have been weakened by NSAID inhibition of GI COX-1, a second wave of injury caused by luminal gastric acid may facilitate deeper ulceration, bleeding, and even perforation of the stomach wall.[24]

NSAID prostaglandin inhibition affects multiple layers of the protective barrier of the GI tract. As organic acids (except nabumetone), they easily penetrate the hydrophobic mucous layer and by decreasing mucosal surface nitric oxide production degrade the ability of the stomach to elaborate its protective mucous layer. NSAIDs inhibit bicarbonate synthesis and thereby decrease acid buffering capacity. They also inhibit glutathione, a superoxide radical scavenger, and consequently facilitate free radical damage. As NSAID concentrations rise, there is increased penetration of the epithelial cells and diminished mucosal blood flow, which leads to mitochondrial oxidative uncoupling and cell death.[12] No studies have directly related NSAID use to upper GI symptoms or bleeding specifically in athletes; nevertheless, the increased mucosal permeability and decreased splanchnic blood flow that occurs with prolonged exercise may serve as a pathophysiologic foundation on which the effects of *H. pylori* and the NSAIDs can build.

56.4.2.2 Evaluation and Management

Athletes should be questioned regarding any relationship of symptom onset with NSAID use. Laboratory analysis should assess for occult GI bleeding and anemia. If any alarm signs or symptoms are present or if an individual has new onset dyspepsia after the age of 45 or has a family history of gastric cancer, early gastroenterology referral is recommended.

Initially, NSAID use should be discontinued if possible. If analgesic therapy is crucial, replacing a nonselective NSAID with acetaminophen or a COX-2 inhibitor would be prudent. A systematic review of the upper GI safety and tolerability of one of the COX-2 inhibitors found a 46% lower rate of medication withdrawal for adverse events, a 71% lower risk of ulcers on endoscopy, and a 39% lower incidence of symptoms due to ulcers, perforations, bleeding, or obstruction compared to nonselective NSAIDs (level I evidence).[20]

Regardless of their risk status, all who are about to start long-term traditional NSAID therapy should be considered for testing for *H. pylori* and treated accordingly if *H. pylori* positive (LOE: 2, SOR: A).[27] These patients should have a noninvasive test for *H. pylori* infection. Urea breath test (UBT) is the favored test, with the stool antigen assay as an alternative. The use of PPIs within 2 weeks of testing can interfere with the results.[9] It is currently recommended that bismuth and antibiotics be withheld for at least 28 days and a PPI for 7–14 days prior to the UBT. Individuals who are *H. pylori* negative should receive short-term H2RA or PPI therapy (4–6 weeks). If they fail empiric antisecretory therapy or if symptoms recur upon cessation of treatment, they should be referred for endoscopy. Endoscopy should also be considered for all patients age 50 or older as well as patients with persistent symptoms, anorexia, weight loss, vomiting or signs of GI bleeding.[7,28] Symptomatic *H. pylori* positive individuals should have eradication therapy. The recommended primary therapies for *H. pylori* infection include the following: a PPI, clarithromycin, and amoxicillin or metronidazole (clarithromycin-based triple therapy) for 14 days or a PPI or H_2RA, bismuth, metronidazole, and tetracycline (bismuth quadruple therapy) for 10–14 days.[7] All patients should be retested for evidence of cure after a minimum of 4 weeks of therapy. The athlete should be off any antisecretory medication, especially PPIs, for a minimum of 2 weeks prior to retesting. Urea breath analysis is the posttreatment diagnostic test of choice, with stool antigen testing as the alternative if the former is unavailable. Individuals who fail second-line therapy and those with persistent dyspepsia should be referred to gastroenterology for further evaluation. See Table 56.3.

Clinical Pearl

All patients being started on long-term traditional NSAID therapy should be considered for noninvasive *H. pylori* testing and treated if positive.

TABLE 56.3
Regimens for the Treatment of *H. pylori* Infection

Regimen	Eradication Rate (%)[a]
Omeprazole 20 mg BID Amoxicillin 1000 mg BID Clarithromycin 500 mg BID	96.4
Omeprazole 20 mg BID Metronidazole 500 mg BID Clarithromycin 500 mg BID	89.8
Omeprazole 20 mg BID Bismuth subsalicylate 525 mg QID Tetracycline 500 mg QID Metronidazole 250 mg QID	85–90
Omeprazole 20 mg BID Amoxicillin 1000 mg BID Metronidazole 500 mg BID	79.0

Source: Adapted from O'Connor, F.G., *Textbook of Running Medicine*, 1st edn., McGraw-Hill, New York, 2001. With permission.

[a] All eradication rates are based on a 7-day regimen. Although European data suggest that 7 days are adequate, this has not been confirmed by U.S. studies; thus, a full 14-day treatment course is recommended.

56.5 LOWER GASTROINTESTINAL DISEASES

56.5.1 Runner's Diarrhea

56.5.1.1 Presentation

Athletes with runner's diarrhea suffer from a syndrome encompassing a spectrum of exertional or immediately postexertional lower GI symptoms. Their presentation ranges from abdominal cramping and fecal urgency to diarrhea and frank incontinence. Often, runner's diarrhea occurs in association with increases in training mileage or with particularly strenuous training sessions and competitions. An individual may be able to endure an episode by transiently reducing their pace; however, when symptoms are more severe, it may be necessary to completely suspend the workout and quickly seek relief.

56.5.1.2 Pathophysiology

While the true etiology of runner's diarrhea remains unknown, several possible physiologic mechanisms have been proposed. Body position and movement appear to play a role; for example, the forward positioning of cyclists appears to protect them from lower GI tract issues compared to the higher impact, jostling abdominal movements of runners.[35] Suggested mechanisms for runner's diarrhea include increased catecholamines and increased GI peptides including gastrin, motilin, secretin, peptide histidine–methionine, and vasoactive intestinal peptide that negatively affect GI homeostasis and cause more rapid gut transit time.[2,10,42,47] Alternatively, strenuous exercise may lead to rapid shifts in intestinal fluid and electrolytes, causing colonic irritability.[35] Another hypothesis is that the 70%–80% reduction in splanchnic blood flow that occurs with vigorous exercise may lead to an ischemic enteropathy. The resulting poor tissue perfusion maintained over the length of the exercise session could cause mucosal ischemia, leading to fluid shifts and diarrhea. This may explain the high prevalence of GI bleeding in marathon runners. The prolonged ischemia could result in mucosal necrosis, superficial erosions, and hemorrhage.[41] Another theory suggests that enteric ischemia results from reperfusion injury. According to this theory, after exercise has ceased, various chemical and vascular changes compromise the GI tract's protective barrier. When the bowel partially loses its ability to protect against irritating intraluminal substances such as endotoxins, food antigens, digestive enzymes, and bile, it results in a *leaky mucosa*.[4]

56.5.1.3 Evaluation and Management

The history should thoroughly detail the onset, severity, and chronicity of symptoms. Documenting any recent travel, unusual food ingestion, or exposure to sick contacts can help distinguish a potential infectious etiology. It is important to inquire about diarrhea not associated with training as well as melena and hematochezia. If available, reviewing the athlete's training log is a crucial part of the evaluation. A detailed diary can help correlate symptoms with changes in exercise mode, frequency, duration, and intensity. A dietary journal, if not already included in the training log, can be helpful in identifying particular replacement fluids, nutritional supplements, or food products that may be triggering the athlete's symptoms. The past medical history should be reviewed, looking for any history of inflammatory bowel disease or previous GI hemorrhage. Other comorbid diseases should be looked at carefully as several conditions, and potentially the medicine used to treat them, can lead to diarrhea. The individual's family history should be scrutinized for any inflammatory bowel disease or other chronic bowel conditions. A focused lab assessment includes fecal occult blood testing and a complete blood count to look for anemia. In the presence of severe diarrhea, serum electrolytes should be drawn. Liver enzymes and pancreatic enzymes can also be considered. If the history is suggestive of an infectious process, stool cultures should be obtained and the stool examined for leukocytes and ova and parasites.

For classic runner's diarrhea, reduction of training intensity, duration, and distance for 1–2 weeks may lead to resolution of symptoms.[47] During this time, cross-training with low or non-impact activities can be used to maintain the athlete's aerobic capacity. Any dietary or fluid replacement triggers should be eliminated. If a specific trigger is not identified, individuals with ongoing symptoms may benefit from dietary manipulation. A diet low in fiber can be helpful.[31] Ingestion of a lower carbohydrate liquid meal before exercise may help maintain GI tract perfusion and may prevent gut ischemia related to decreased splanchnic blood flow.[14] While not an adequate regimen for the control of chronic symptoms, some individuals may benefit from a complete liquid diet on the day prior to competition or a scheduled intense exercise session. When the diarrhea is under control, a full return to high-intensity exercise can be achieved by gradually increasing training as symptoms tolerate. Antidiarrheal medication should be used sparingly and with great caution. Antispasmodics, such as loperamide, are generally safe; however, anticholinergic medications such as diphenoxylate with atropine (Lomotil®) are to be avoided due to the potential for increased heat injury risk secondary to their effect on sweating. Consulting gastroenterology is necessary should an individual have difficult-to-control symptoms or if any red flags are found during the history, physical, or laboratory evaluation.

Clinical Pearl

The management of classic runner's diarrhea starts with a temporary reduction in training intensity and duration. Once symptoms are controlled, training can be gradually escalated as symptoms allow.

56.5.2 Abdominal Pain (Side Stitch)

56.5.2.1 Presentation and Proposed Etiology

In the young, active population, abdominal pain with exertion is a common symptom. The previously discussed conditions notwithstanding, the so-called side stitch is the most common cause o abdominal pain in athletes. Typically seen in runners, it presents as a somewhat pleuritic aching sensation, usually in the right upper abdominal quadrant. It is often seen in deconditioned individuals starting an exercise program but can also be observed in athletes intensifying their training. Exercise in the postprandial period is a frequent exacerbating factor. Side stitches usually stop immediately upon ceasing exercise. As an individual gains aerobic fitness, the frequency and severity of attacks tend to subside. While their true etiology remains elusive, they are most likely caused by hypoxia-induced diaphragmatic muscle spasm. Other theories note the stress placed on peritoneal ligaments (such as the gastrophrenic, lienophrenic, and coronary ligaments) that extend from the diaphragm to the abdominal viscera and irritation of the parietal peritoneum (which has been called an *exertional peritonitis*) as potential etiologies.[38] The pain may also be referred to the shoulder, possibly implicating hepatic, splenic, or phrenic nerve involvement.[21] Other potential causes include pleural irritation, hepatic capsule irritation, symptomatic abdominal adhesions, and right colonic gas pain.[14]

The management of side stitches involves using the history to rule out not only the other GI diseases discussed in this chapter but also other exertional pain syndromes, especially angina. Fortunately, other serious causes of abdominal pain with exercise, such as mesenteric ischemia, bowel infarction, omental infarction, and hepatic vein thrombosis, are rare. However, in the setting of unremitting pain, especially with signs of systemic illness or shock, these conditions need to be considered in the differential and patients referred for potential surgical evaluation.

Athletes with the typical features of a side stitch should be reassured that it is a benign process and will get better as their conditioning improves. They should be advised against exercise immediately after eating and to avoid large meals or drinks shortly before a workout. While running, athletes are advised to sip small amounts of fluid regularly. If an episode of pain does occur, slowing the pace, bending forward, pushing a hand inward and upward on the area of pain, tightening the abdominal muscles, and breathing out through pursed lips are recommended for immediate pain alleviation. Changing the footstrike-to-breathing cadence can also work. For example, if the stitch pain is on the right and the athlete normally exhales when the right foot hits the ground, the athlete can try exhaling instead when the left foot hits the ground. If the stitch becomes unbearable, stopping the exercise, walking slowly with arms raised above the head to stretch, or lying supine with hips elevated can relieve side stitch pain within a few minutes.[25]

56.6 ELEVATED LIVER ENZYMES

5.6.1 Etiology

Liver enzyme elevations have been described in otherwise asymptomatic long-distance runners as well as other athletes. They are usually found as incidental findings in lab studies obtained for reasons other than evaluating for liver disease. The suspected etiology is an ischemic insult secondary to reduced splanchnic blood flow and oxygen tension during vigorous exercise.[22] Both aspartate aminotransferase (AST) and alanine aminotransferase (ALT) are expressed in skeletal muscles, and conditions associated with myocyte damage, including primary muscle diseases and strenuous exercise, may lead to transaminitis.[8] Increases in ALT, AST, alkaline phosphatase, creatinine phosphatase, and lactate dehydrogenase have been observed in response to musculoskeletal injury. However, elevated measurements of glutamate dehydrogenase and gamma-glutamyl-transferase, which are more specific to the liver, confirm hepatocellular injury.[5]

5.6.2 Management

Because these asymptomatic enzyme abnormalities are often discovered in the convalescent setting, the history and physical should focus on recent training sessions and environmental exposure, evaluating for evidence of a missed heat injury or episode of exertional rhabdomyolysis. The athlete should be questioned regarding any history of chronic liver disease or alcohol dependence and their medication list reviewed for any potentially hepatotoxic agents. With the nearly ubiquitous use of nutritional supplements, it is crucial to investigate this often-overlooked area.

The majority of athletes can be reassured that this appears to be a benign process and the enzyme abnormalities usually revert to normal within just 1 week after abstaining from exercise. Thus, the first step in the laboratory evaluation is to obtain a repeat liver enzyme panel after abstaining from NSAIDs, alcohol, and exercise for 1 week. If the liver enzymes have not reached normal levels in that time, the athlete can be rechecked in 3 months. If the liver enzymes remain elevated on serial examinations, the athlete needs further evaluation, starting with an iron panel, total iron-binding capacity, and hepatitis serologies. If these are unrevealing, antinuclear antibody titer, anti-smooth-muscle antibody, ceruloplasmin, alpha-1-antitrypsin, and serum protein electrophoresis should be obtained as second-line tests. It is prudent to obtain a right upper quadrant ultrasound to evaluate for fatty liver, cholelithiasis, or other obstruction.[22] If testing is abnormal, if the liver enzymes have been mildly elevated for over 6 moths with a negative evaluation, if there are signs of evolving hepatic insufficiency, or if the ultrasound reveals evidence of dilated bile ducts or a liver mass, it is reasonable to refer the athlete to a gastroenterologist for consideration of MRI cholangiopancreatography, endoscopic ultrasound, endoscopic retrograde cholangiopancreatography and liver biopsy.

Clinical Pearl

The first step in evaluating the athlete with an incidental finding of elevated liver enzymes is to repeat testing after abstaining from NSAIDs, alcohol, and exercise for 1 week.

TABLE 56.4
SORT: Key Recommendations for Practice

Clinical Recommendation	Evidence Rating	References
Should GERD symptoms continue after 6 weeks of H2RA therapy (first-line treatment), neither continuing therapy nor increasing the dose is likely to achieve control. Transitioning to PPI therapy is indicated.	C	[20,22]
Patients with GERD who respond poorly to PPIs are intolerant of medical therapy, or patients who desire a permanent solution are candidates for surgical intervention. Optimal results from laparoscopic antireflux surgery require careful patient selection and an experienced surgeon.	C	[24–27]
For patients with PUD, NSAID use should be discontinued if possible. If analgesic therapy is crucial, replacing a nonselective NSAID with acetaminophen or a COX-2 inhibitor would be prudent.	C	[33]
For patients with PUD, evaluation with EGD should be considered for all patients 50 years of age or older, with persistent symptoms, anorexia, weight loss, and vomiting, and in the presence of signs of GI bleeding.	C	[29,36]
For classic runner's diarrhea, reduction of training intensity, duration, and distance for 1–2 weeks and transitioning to a diet low in fiber are recommended.	C	[40,44]

56.7 SUMMARY

Both upper and lower GI problems affect the exercising population. Primary care physicians should be ever cognizant that athletes can fall prey to conditions that affect the general population. By being aware of red flag symptoms, the sports physician can expedite the evaluation and treatment of potentially serious conditions. By following an organized evaluation and management process, clinicians can accurately diagnose and offer prompt treatment for GI conditions, thereby minimizing their impact on the active lifestyles of our athletes (Table 56.4).

REFERENCES

1. Bammer T, Hinder RA, Klaus A et al. Five- to eight-year outcome of the first laparoscopic nissen fundoplications. *Journal of Gastrointestinal Surgery: Official Journal of the Society for Surgery of the Alimentary Tract.* January–February 2001;5(1):42–48.
2. Bounous G, McArdle AH. Marathon runners: The intestinal handicap. *Medical Hypotheses.* December 1990;33(4): 261–264.
3. Brouns F, Beckers E. Is the gut an athletic organ? Digestion, absorption and exercise. *Sports Medicine (Auckland, N.Z.).* April 1993;15(4):242–257.
4. Brouns F, Saris WH, Rehrer NJ. Abdominal complaints and gastrointestinal function during long-lasting exercise. *International Journal of Sports Medicine.* June 1987; 8(3):175–189.
5. Bunch TW. Blood test abnormalities in runners. *Mayo Clinic Proceedings.* February 1980;55(2):113–117.
6. Caro JJ, Salas M, Ward A. Healing and relapse rates in gastroesophageal reflux disease treated with the newer proton-pump inhibitors lansoprazole, rabeprazole, and pantoprazole compared with omeprazole, ranitidine, and placebo: Evidence from randomized clinical trials. *Clinical Therapeutics.* 2001;23(7):998–1012.
7. Chey WD, Wong BCY, Practice Parameters Committee of the American College of Gastroenterology. American College of Gastroenterology guideline on the management of *Helicobacter pylori* infection. *American Journal of Gastroenterology.* August 2007;102(8):1808–1025.
8. Chiorean MV, Locke GR 3rd, Zinsmeister AR et al. Changing rates of *Helicobacter pylori* testing and treatment in patients with peptic ulcer disease. *American Journal of Gastroenterology.* December 2002;97(12):3015–3022.
9. Ciociola AA, McSorley DJ, Turner K et al. *Helicobacter pylori* infection rates in duodenal ulcer patients in the United States may be lower than previously estimated. *American Journal of Gastroenterology.* July 1999;94(7):1834–1840.
10. Collings KL, Pratt FP, Rodriguez-Stanley S et al. Esophageal reflux in conditioned runners, cyclists, and weightlifters. *Medicine & Science in Sports & Exercise.* May 2003; 35(5):730–735.
11. De Oliveira EP, Burini RC. The impact of physical exercise on the gastrointestinal tract. *Current Opinion in Clinical Nutrition and Metabolic Care.* September 2009;12(5):533–538.
12. Deeks JJ, Smith LA, Bradley MD. Efficacy, tolerability, and upper gastrointestinal safety of celecoxib for treatment of osteoarthritis and rheumatoid arthritis: Systematic review of randomised controlled trials. *BMJ (Clinical Research Ed.).* September 2002;325(7365):619.

13. DeVault KR, Castell DO, American College of Gastroenterology. Updated guidelines for the diagnosis and treatment of gastroesophageal reflux disease. *American Journal of Gastroenterology*. January 2005;100(1):190–200.
14. Eichner ER. Stitch in the side: Causes, workup, and solutions. *Current Sports Medicine Reports*. December 2006; 5(6):289–292.
15. Green GA. Gastrointestinal disorders in the athlete. *Clinics in Sports Medicine*. April 1992;11(2):453–470.
16. Hirschowitz BI. A critical analysis, with appropriate controls, of gastric acid and pepsin secretion in clinical esophagitis. *Gastroenterology*. November 1991;101(5):1149–1158.
17. Jackson PG, Gleiber MA, Askari R et al. Predictors of outcome in 100 consecutive laparoscopic antireflux procedures. *American Journal of Surgery*. March 2001;181(3):231–235.
18. Jyotheeswaran S, Shah AN, Jin HO et al. Prevalence of *Helicobacter pylori* in peptic ulcer patients in greater Rochester, NY: Is empirical triple therapy justified? *American Journal of Gastroenterology*. April 1998;93(4):574–578.
19. Katzka DA, Paoletti V, Leite L et al. Prolonged ambulatory pH monitoring in patients with persistent gastroesophageal reflux disease symptoms: Testing while on therapy identifies the need for more aggressive anti-reflux therapy. *American Journal of Gastroenterology*. October 1996;91(10):2110–2113.
20. Lanza FL, Chan FKL, Quigley EMM et al. Guidelines for prevention of NSAID-related ulcer complications. *American Journal of Gastroenterology*. March 2009;104(3):728–738.
21. Lauder TD, Moses FM. Recurrent abdominal pain from abdominal adhesions in an endurance triathlete. *Medicine & Science in Sports & Exercise*. May 1995;27(5):623–625.
22. Lee TH, Kim WR, Poterucha JJ. Evaluation of elevated liver enzymes. *Clinics in Liver Disease*. May 2012;16(2):183–198.
23. Li Z, Zou D, Ma X et al. Epidemiology of peptic ulcer disease: Endoscopic results of the systematic investigation of gastrointestinal disease in china. *American Journal of Gastroenterology*. December 2010;105(12):2570–2577.
24. Lichtenstein DR, Syngal S, Wolfe MM. Nonsteroidal antiinflammatory drugs and the gastrointestinal tract. The double-edged sword. *Arthritis and Rheumatism*. January 1995;38(1):5–18.
25. Lijnen P, Hespel P, Fagard R et al. Indicators of cell breakdown in plasma of men during and after a marathon race. *International Journal of Sports Medicine*. April 1988;9(2): 108–113.
26. Malfertheiner P, Chan FKL, McColl KEL. Peptic ulcer disease. *Lancet*. October 2009;374(9699):1449–1461.
27. Najm WI. Peptic ulcer disease. *Primary Care*. September 2011;38(3):383–394.
28. Nilius M, Malfertheiner P. *Helicobacter pylori* enzymes. *Alimentary Pharmacology & Therapeutics*. April 1996; 10(Suppl 1): 65–71.
29. Orlando RC. Pathogenesis of gastroesophageal reflux disease. *Gastroenterology Clinics of North America*. December 2002;31(4 Suppl):S35–S44.
30. Papatheodoridis GV, Sougioultzis S, Archimandritis AJ. Effects of helicobacter pylori and nonsteroidal anti-inflammatory drugs on peptic ulcer disease: A systematic review. *Clinical Gastroenterology and Hepatology: The Official Clinical Practice Journal of the American Gastroenterological Association*. February 2006;4(2):130–142.
31. Perko MJ, Nielsen HB, Skak C et al. Mesenteric, coeliac and splanchnic blood flow in humans during exercise. *Journal of Physiology*. December 1998;513(Pt 3):907–913.
32. Peters HP, Wiersma JW, Koerselman J et al. The effect of a sports drink on gastroesophageal reflux during a run-bike-run test. *International Journal of Sports Medicine* 21(1) (January 2000): 65–70; Kahrilas PJ, Fennerty MB, Joelsson B. High-versus standard-dose ranitidine for control of heartburn in poorly responsive acid reflux disease: A prospective, controlled trial. *American Journal of Gastroenterology*. January 1999;94(1):92–97.
33. Peters HP, Bos M, Seebregts L et al. Gastrointestinal symptoms in long-distance runners, cyclists, and triathletes: Prevalence, medication, and etiology. *American Journal of Gastroenterology*. June 1999;94(6):1570–1581.
34. Peters HP, Zweers M, Backx FJ et al. Gastrointestinal symptoms during long-distance walking. *Medicine & Science in Sports & Exercise*. June 1999;31(6):767–773.
35. Peters HP, De Vries WR, Vanberge-Henegouwen GP et al. Potential benefits and hazards of physical activity and exercise on the gastrointestinal tract. *Gut*. March 2001;48(3):435–439.
36. Rehrer NJ, Janssen GM, Brouns F, Saris WH. Fluid intake and gastrointestinal problems in runners competing in a 25-km race and a marathon. *International Journal of Sports Medicine*. May 1989;10(Suppl 1):S22–S25.
37. Schijven MP, Gisbertz SS, van Berge Henegouwen MI. Laparoscopic surgery for gastro-esophageal acid reflux disease. *Best Practice & Research: Clinical Gastroenterology*. February 2014;28(1):97–109.
38. Simons SM, Kennedy RG. Gastrointestinal problems in runners. *Current Sports Medicine Reports*, April 2004; 3(2):112–116.
39. Simrén M. Physical activity and the gastrointestinal tract. *European Journal of Gastroenterology & Hepatology*. October 2002;14(10):1053–1556.
40. Talalwah NAl, Woodward S. Gastro-oesophageal reflux. Part 3: Medical and surgical treatment. *British Journal of Nursing*. April 2013;22(7):409–415.
41. Ter Steege RWF, Van der Palen J, Kolkman JJ. Prevalence of gastrointestinal complaints in runners competing in a long-distance run: An internet-based observational study in 1281 subjects. *Scandinavian Journal of Gastroenterology*. 2008;43(12):1477–1482.
42. Van Nieuwenhoven MA, Brouns F, Brummer R-JM. Gastrointestinal profile of symptomatic athletes at rest and during physical exercise. *European Journal of Applied Physiology*. April 2004;91(4):429–434.
43. Viola TA. Evaluation of the athlete with exertional abdominal pain. *Current Sports Medicine Reports*. March–April 2010;9(2):106–110.
44. Vonkeman HE, van de Laar MAFJ. Nonsteroidal anti-inflammatory drugs: Adverse effects and their prevention. *Seminars in Arthritis and Rheumatism*. February 2010;39(4):294–312.
45. Waterman JJ, Kapur R. Upper gastrointestinal issues in athletes. *Current Sports Medicine Reports*. March–April 2012;11(2):99–104.
46. Wileman SM, McCann S, Grant AM et al. Medical versus surgical management for gastro-oesophageal reflux disease (GORD) in adults. *Cochrane Database of Systematic Reviews*. 2010;3:CD003243.
47. Worobetz LJ, Gerrard DF. Effect of moderate exercise on esophageal function in asymptomatic athletes. *American Journal of Gastroenterology*. November 1986;81(11):1048–1051.
48. O'Connor FG. *Textbook of Running Medicine*, 1st edn. New York: McGraw-Hill; 2001.

57 Genitourinary Considerations in the Athlete

Nicholas A. Piantanida

CONTENTS

TABLE 57.1
Key Clinical Considerations

1. Physiologic changes in renal function can occur during exercise that can lead to proteinuria and hematuria in the absence of trauma or injury and, in most cases, follow a benign course of resolution following 72 hours of relative rest.
2. With renal associated abdominal trauma, a decision on further work-up, including imaging, is based on the age of the athlete (child versus adult), the mechanism of injury, and the presence of hypotension or the length of symptoms, including microscopic hematuria.
3. Primary care providers evaluating patients with genitourinary concerns must become astute in recognizing contributing factors and then intervene to modify risk through patient education, particularly in conditions such as STDs, pudendal neuropathy, and recommendations regarding sports participation with a solitary kidney.

57.1 INTRODUCTION

The athlete's genitourinary system responds dynamically to the physiologic demands of exercise and demonstrates compensatory changes to sustain function. Although genitourinary injuries will occur infrequently in traditional sports, the growth and popularity of extreme sports and ultraendurance events has increasingly tasked the genitourinary system to function under higher levels of stress. Genitourinary considerations in the athlete require knowledge of the genitourinary system and the mechanism of sports-specific injury that occurred. Diagnosis and return-to-play decisions must follow a careful history and physical exam with specific algorithmic guidance to assist the treating primary care provider in arriving at a quality management plan (Table 57.1).

57.2 GENITOURINARY ANATOMY

The kidneys are retroperitoneal organs that lie obliquely along the borders of the psoas muscles. The position of the liver slightly displaces the right kidney so that it is lower than the left kidney. The kidneys are partially mobile creating displacement of 4–5 cm with the extremes of inspiration. The kidneys are supported by the perirenal fat (surrounded by perirenal fascia), the renal vascular pedicle, abdominal muscle tone, and the expansive effects of the abdominal viscera. A shared autonomic innervation with intraperitoneal organs explains, in part, some of the gastrointestinal symptoms that accompany genitourinary disease.[27]

The plasma filters through several segments of the kidney starting with the glomerular capillary tuft and then arrives into the tubular portions. At the glomerular capillary tuft, 20% of the plasma water is filtered and 80% of plasma, along with larger solutes, travels along an efferent capillary network surrounding the tubular network of the nephron. The efferent arteriole, in the tubular portions, will capture reabsorbed water and solutes and transition substances to be secreted.[31]

The remainder of the genitourinary system is comprised of the ureters, bladder, and genital organs. These segments are located in the lower abdominal and pelvis region. The bladder is a hollow and flaccid organ, which despite its anterior pelvis location is rarely injured. The genital organs in both males and females are tethered with the potential for injury by torsional rotation or direct trauma. In the male, the testes embryonically settle into the scrotum surrounded anteriorly by the tunica vaginalis and posteriorly by the epididymis.[27]

57.3 RENAL PHYSIOLOGY

The kidneys require more blood flow per unit weight than any other organ. At rest, 20%–25% of cardiac output goes to the kidneys. The majority of this blood flow passes into the renal cortex, with the glomerular portion of the nephron filtering an average of 180 L of plasma each day. The tubular portion of the nephron reabsorbs 99.5% of the filtered water and essential solutes.[31]

Renal blood flow (RBF) and glomerular filtration rate (GFR) are renal perfusion indices. RBF is regulated, similar to blood flow in any organ, by the net arteriovenous pressure difference across the vascular bed. GFR is the volume of plasma per minute filtered at the level of the glomerulus. RBF and GFR are linked in differing degrees to intrinsic and extrinsic mechanisms of profusion modulation.[31]

A process known as autoregulation is an intrinsic renal mechanism to maintain relatively constant GFR. Neural and hormonal influences represent extrinsic mechanisms for modulating RBF and GFR. These extrinsic mechanisms are capable of overriding autoregulation. Therefore, in the event of physical or emotional stress, the patient's neural inputs, through systemic sympathetic vasoconstriction, will decrease RBF; however, renal autoregulation will maintain GFR as high as possible.[31]

With moderate exercise (50% VO_{2max}), RBF diminishes from the resting volume by 25%–30%, whereas with heavy exercise (65% VO_{2max}), RBF diminishes by 75%. This reduced rate of profusion translates to altered renal function to include changes in electrolyte, protein, and cellular excretion. Although both exercise intensity and duration have a role in establishing changes in renal function, renal autoregulation is augmented by neural and hormonal inputs to preserve the GFR.[5,10] Above all, the rise in filtration fraction is blunted by prudent hydration measures in the athlete.

During exercise, the kidneys protect body hydration levels by increasing the secretion of antidiuretic hormone (ADH). ADH is produced in the hypothalamus and stored in the posterior pituitary. ADH is released under conditions of high plasma osmolality and/or low plasma volume. Osmoreceptors are the most sensitive measure for increased secretion of ADH, but the plasma volume receptors, once activated, elicit the strongest response. Thirst is triggered by low plasma volume and is the most recognized symptom in an exercising athlete to guide oral hydration.[31]

57.4 UROLOGIC LABORATORY EXAMINATION

Patients with urinary tract symptoms or signs should undergo a screening urine test. Macroscopic urinalysis (dip strip) is a useful preliminary clinic-based screening tool for symptomatic patients. A normal dip strip is sensitive enough to make the microscopic analysis of the urine unnecessary. Abnormalities on dip strip require further investigation by complete microscopic urinalysis to include sediment examination.[27]

Specimen collection is a critical step in urinalysis. A properly obtained midstream urine specimen is vital to accurate urinalysis. Refer to Table 57.2 for a review of the dip strip indices and sensitivities, as well as confounders to dip strip interpretation.

TABLE 57.2
Dip Strip Indices

	Description	Modifying Agents
Color and appearance	Assess gross hematuria and pyuria	Drugs, foods, dyes
Specific gravity	Measure of urinary concentration	ADH, glucose, protein
pH	Degree of urine acidity	Uric acid stones or *Proteus* sp.
Protein	Measures urine albumin Trace = 15–29 mg/dL 1+ = 30–99 mg/dL 2+ = 100–299 mg/dL 3+ = 300–999 mg/dL 4+ > 1000 mg/dL	Fever, exercise, dehydration, highly concentrated urine, or orthostatic factors
Glucose	Accurate for urinary glucose	Ascorbic acid, cephalosporins
Hemoglobin	Screen for erythrocytes	Myoglobin, ascorbic acid
Nitrite	Positive when # of bacteria >100 k	Coagulase-splitting sp., PM void
Leukocytes	Indicator of pyuria	Glucosuria, ascorbic acid, drugs

The microscopic exam of urinary sediment allows the provider to accurately define the complete picture of renal or bladder pathology. The morphology and the quantity of various elements of urinary sediment can assist the provider with a diagnosis. For example, red blood cell (RBC) casts are pathognomonic of intrinsic renal disease in the form of glomerulitis or vasculitis.

The routine practice of screening urine dip strips as a component of the preparticipation physical examination on healthy athletes is not recommended.[21]

57.5 PROTEINURIA

The average person has a 24 hours urinary protein excretion of approximately 80–150 mg/day and the albumin excretion rate for healthy adults is <30 mg/24 hours. In normal ratios, urine protein is comprised of 30% albumin, 30% serum globulins, and 40% tissue proteins. Although proteinuria can be a common finding on dip strip within 48 hours of exercise, fewer than 2% of all cases screened will have a serious and treatable urinary tract disorder. Proteinuria is defined as grade > 1+ on dip strip, >30 mg/g creatinine on albumin-to-creatinine ratio, or a 24 hour urinary protein excretion >150 mg/day.[5]

Common causes of benign proteinuria include dehydration, orthostasis, fever, heat or cold injury, emotional stress, vigorous exercise, and acute illnesses. Pathologic causes of proteinuria include chronic disease states, such as hypertension, diabetes, or collagen vascular diseases, which produce end organ renal disease. Also, processes that involve cancer, infection, or autoimmune disease can directly invade or injure the renal structure to cause proteinuria.[30]

Clinical Pearl

In the presence of contributing disease, the rate of proteinuria change is a predictor of renal decline.

Transient or episodic proteinuria is seen with exercise. The reported prevalence of exercise-induced proteinuria ranges from 18% to 100% depending on the type of exercise and its intensity. An increased incidence of proteinuria is reported in higher-intensity sports such as boxing, wrestling, sprinting, football, and gymnastics. These athletes experience proteinuria from the increased glomerular permeability coupled with impaired tubular resorption of plasma proteins. Athletic effort at brief maximal intensity produces a macromolecule load and solute demand that overwhelm the ability of the renal tube to reabsorb protein.[6]

Proteinuria is usually detected qualitatively with the use of a screening urine dip strip (Table 57.2). A correlation with urine specific gravity is important to avoid a false-positive result due to a high urine concentration (specific gravity levels over 1.025). In cases where urine dip strip for protein is 2+ or greater, urine specific gravity is less important.[10]

Urinalysis, in an athlete with proteinuria, should be repeated after a period of 48–72 hours free from exercise. A more generous period of 1 week should be considered in your athlete recovering from a febrile illness. If this second dip strip is positive, then a detailed evaluation should be pursued. See the proteinuria algorithm in Figure 57.1 and the diagnostic tests in Table 57.3 for a stepwise approach to the athlete with proteinuria.[6]

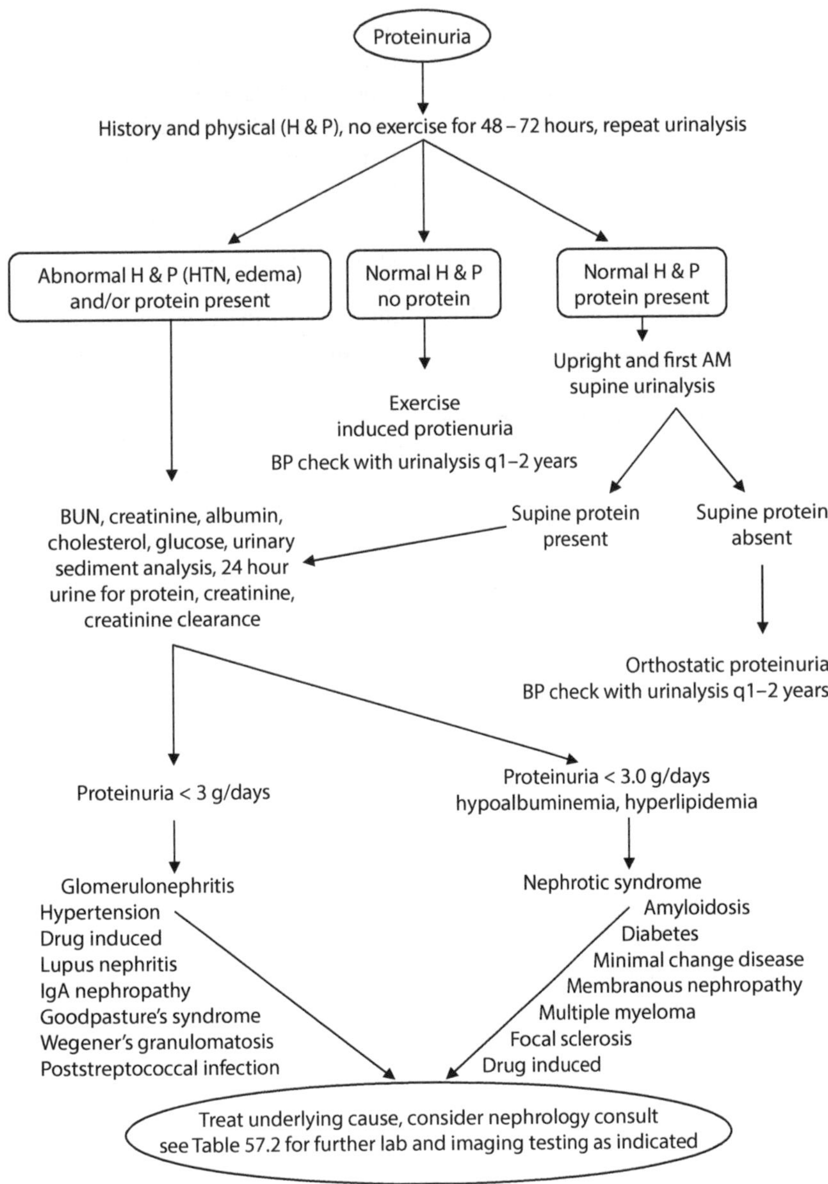

FIGURE 57.1 Proteinuria algorithm.

TABLE 57.3
Diagnostic Testing in Proteinuria and Hematuria

Test	Interpretation of Finding
Blood chemistries	Identify any abnormalities following renal disease
Complete blood count	Demonstrate any renal impairment on hematopoiesis
Antinuclear antibody	Elevated in systemic lupus erythematosus
C-reactive protein	Normal, rules out an inflammatory cause
Serum and urine electrophoresis	Abnormal in multiple myeloma
HIV, antistrep O titer, hepatitis	Defines infectious causes for glomerular proteinuria
Cryoglobulins	Present in myeloma, lupus, and other autoimmune dz
Complement C3 and C4	Decreased, with increased immune complexes
Renal ultrasound or MRI	Alternative anatomic survey of renal anatomy
Chest x-ray	Rule out evidence of systemic disease (*Strep. pneumoniae*, amyloidosis, sarcoidosis)

Clinical Pearl

Dip strip positive color change for proteinuria (tan to green) always merits clinical correlation.

A medical history taken from a proteinuric athlete should focus on drug exposure, voiding history, metabolic disease, and recent illnesses. Family and personal history of developmental anomalies should be defined including hereditary nephritis and polycystic kidney disease. Review of systems should include a discussion of fever, weight loss, renal colic pain, and other urinary symptoms. Physical exam should include vital signs, BMI, and a focused assessment searching for hypertension, an infectious source, and edema in the extremities.

The differential diagnosis includes orthostatic proteinuria, which is seen in 2%–5% of adolescents. Furthermore, orthostatic proteinuria is rarely seen in age > 30. Orthostatic proteinuria is seen with upright void, which then resolves with a morning supine urine collection. There is no therapy required and this clinical entity often resolves with time.[5]

Treatment for benign proteinuria in the athlete involves correcting the underlying cause, whether it is poor hydration, acclimatization, stress management, or avoiding exercise during periods of temperature stress or physical illness. Exercise-induced proteinuria will recur at a specific level of individual exertion. Athletes with exercise-induced proteinuria have no increased risk for chronic renal disease. They should participate in the full capacity of their sport and obtain a medical checkup with urinalysis yearly.[5,6]

57.6 HEMATURIA

Several medical conditions can produce blood in the urine or microscopic hematuria. Asymptomatic microscopic hematuria (AMH) in athletes is known by several names, including "sports hematuria," "stress hematuria," and "10,000-m hematuria." The incidence of exercise-induced hematuria is variable and ranges from 13% to 38% depending on the population studied. This broad variability follows in the order of exercise intensity, type of exercise, and degrees of dehydration. Fortunately, the incidence of serious disease in men and women is low and episodes of microscopic or gross exercise-induced hematuria resolve following 72 hours of rest.[6,11]

The etiology of AMH or sports hematuria is multifactorial and varies from physiologic to traumatic sources. As previously mentioned, exercise physiologic stress to the kidney diminishes blood flow and GFR is preserved with a compensatory renal vasoconstriction. In this configuration, two forces are at play that cause hematuria. First, vasoconstriction of the efferent glomerular arteriole creates stasis in the glomerular capillaries favoring passage of RBCs into the urine. Second, hypoxic injury occurs in the nephron with subsequent increased glomerular permeability leading to RBC loss into the urine. Direct trauma at any site along the genitourinary system can precipitate bleeding. Bladder irritation or microtrauma, also known as "bladder slap," can result in a runner with a bladder nearly empty of urine causing hematuria. Under these circumstances, hematuria results from the multiple times the anterior and posterior bladder wall impact each other. Heel strike or "march" hemoglobinuria appears in runners with mechanical destruction of RBCs in the heels that exceed the binding capacity of haptoglobin in the blood and are directly excreted as free hemoglobin.[6,11,18]

The "other" causes of hematuria are diverse and a broad differential ranges from causes to include neoplasm, autoimmune disease, infection, nephrolithiasis, hematologic disorders, polycystic kidney disease, and drug induced. The algorithm in Figure 57.2 and the diagnostic tests in Table 57.3 provide a sequential approach to hematuria in the athlete and should facilitate a simplified approach to testing, diagnosis, and treatment. In cases where history and physical exam demonstrates unstable vital signs, new-onset hypertension, edema, and/or gross hematuria in a patient over 35, an expedited assessment must follow to find a treatable cause for glomerular disease or an evaluation plan for a possible urologic neoplasm.[11,23]

Clinical Pearl

A positive dip strip does not define AMH; a microscopic urine exam is required in all potential cases.

The medical history should define any traumatic or atraumatic mechanisms. Events of a recent illness or medication profiles should be reviewed. A genitourinary history should define any associated urologic symptoms and search for

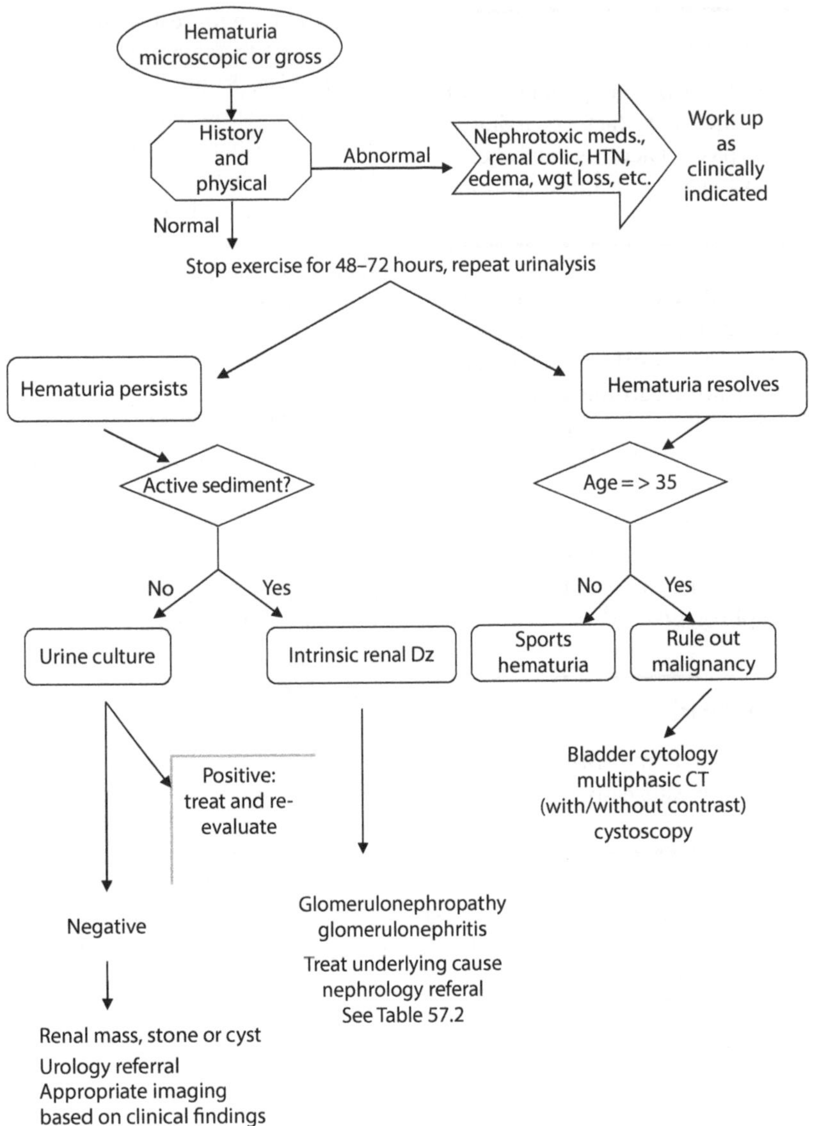

FIGURE 57.2 Hematuria algorithm.

evidence of genitourinary tenderness, swelling, or voiding abnormalities. Review of systems should include fever, weight loss, fatigue, menstrual dating, sickle cell status, nephrolithiasis, and connective tissue disease. Family history should be reviewed for bleeding disorders, polycystic kidney disease, and renal disease. Microscopic urinary exam will further assist with RBC morphology and other urinary sediment findings than can suggest the level of genitourinary injury or irritation.[5]

Clinical Pearl

Dysmorphic RBCs, proteinuria, cellular casts, and/or renal insufficiency warrants concurrent nephrology work-up as well as the potential need for urologic evaluation.

The 2002 American Urology Association (AUA) AMH guideline stipulated 2 of 3 urines and 3 or greater RBCs per high power field (HPF) as criteria for obtaining intravenous pyelography (IVP) or multiphasic CT. The new 2012 AUA AMH guideline recommends work-up for patients 35 years or older with a positive urinalysis following 72 hours of exercise rest with 3 or more RBCs/HPF using multiphasic renal CT scan and cystoscopy[23] (Level of Evidence C: consensus opinion). The following circumstances are rarely consistent with benign exercise-induced hematuria and other causes for the hematuria should be pursued[11,23]:

1. Microscopic hematuria does not resolve with an exercise rest for 72 hours.
2. Episodes of hematuria are associated with exertional renal colic pain[15] or hypertension and edema.
3. Gross hematuria is present on more than one occasion and not associated with a genitourinary infection or drug interaction.
4. The athlete is a man over the age of 35 years and has recurrent episodes of hematuria.

Clinical Pearl

Cystoscopy should be performed on patients with exercise-induced hematuria and risk factors: irritative voiding symptoms, current or past tobacco use and chemical exposures, and recurrent episodes in those with age over 35 years.

In these instances where the athlete presents with hematuria not consistent with exercise-induced hematuria, the patient should have a preliminary work-up to include a 24 hour urine collection to measure creatinine clearance and urine cytology, urine culture, serum creatinine, blood urea nitrogen (BUN), diagnostic imaging in the form of a multiphasic CT scan or renal ultrasound, and a referral to urology for cystoscopy. Recommendations for renal ultrasonography (US) instead of CT exist for nonsmoking women age < 40. A renal biopsy to rule out glomerular or renal tubular disorders is best deferred to the nephrologist.[11,23]

Clinical Pearl

Combining magnetic resonance imaging (MRI) with retrograde pyelograms provides an alternative to patients with CT contraindications.

Treatment for exercise-induced hematuria is based on the suspected pathophysiology of the condition. There is no evidence that exercise-induced hematuria causes permanent renal damage. The common medical practice is to return these athletes back to play after the hematuria resolves in 24–72 hours with rest. Athletes resuming exercise should be encouraged to maintain adequate hydration before and during exercise. Runners should avoid emptying their bladder completely before exercise to prevent "bladder slap" hematuria and further ensure adequate shoe cushioning to prevent "heel strike" hematuria. Therefore, in the presence of normal renal function and no changes in medical history, an athlete who has recurrent bouts of hematuria that clear with rest may proceed to enjoy the benefits of sports with no limitations. Annual monitoring measures should include a microscopic urinary exam and serum creatinine.[1]

57.7 ATRAUMATIC RENAL INJURY

Nephrotoxicity: Drug-induced renal dysfunction is seen with many common medications and rare supplements. During exercise, the renal endothelial surface is a vulnerable target for drugs and their metabolites. As described earlier, exercise couples diminished renal profusion with a concentrated filtrate that can be further impaired by drug-associated injury to tubular or glomerular structures, allergic interstitial inflammation, and/or vascular compromise. Since the clinicopathologic presentation of a drug-induced nephropathy is variable, its true incidence is difficult to describe.[9,13] Drugs and complementary and alternative substances that are associated with nephrotoxic effects on the kidney are listed in Table 57.4.

Rhabdomyolysis: Exercise-induced rhabdomyolysis is a relatively common complication of strenuous exercise, as evidenced by military recruit data. Acute renal failure, in the setting of exertional rhabdomyolysis, has a variable incidence ranging from 17% to 40%.[24] Sinert et al. explained, from their investigation, that several nephrotoxic cofactors (significant hypovolemia and/or aciduria) are required to precipitate acute

TABLE 57.4
Nephrotoxic Medications and Complimentary/Alternative Substances

Renal Disease	Pathophysiology	Medications
Acute renal failure	Prerenal failure due to decreased renal profusion	Diuretics, NSAIDs, ACE inhibitors, cyclosporine, radiocontrast agents
Renal toxic effect	Acute tubular injury due to a direct toxic effect	Quinolones, aminoglycosides, carbamazepine, tacrolimus
Immune-mediated interstitial nephritis	Acute interstitial nephritis due to immune-mediated inflammation of the interstitium	Penicillins, rifampin, sulfonamides, thiazide, cimetidine, furosemide, NSAIDs, ciprofloxacin.
Chronic interstitial fibrosis	Toxic to proximal tubule with lifelong risk for uroepithelial cancers	Aristolochic acid found in the Chinese herb *Aristolochia clematitis*
Renal vascular injury	Vascular endothelial injury manifested as hemolytic-uremic syndrome	Conjugated estrogens, tacrolimus, cocaine, quinine
Immune-mediated glomerulopathy	Acute immune mediated inflammation of the glomerulus	Gold, captopril, NSAIDs, penicillamine
Postrenal obstruction—intratubular	Intratubular obstruction due to medication precipitation	Acyclovir, sulfonamides, methotrexate
Postrenal obstruction—ureteral	Ureteral obstruction due to retroperitoneal fibrosis	Atenolol, ergotamine, dihydroergotamine, methyldopa
Chronic renal failure	Chronic interstitial fibrosis with or without papillary necrosis	NSAIDs, acetaminophen, aspirin, lithium

Source: Modified from Choudhury, D. and Ahmed, Z., *Med. Clin. North Am.*, 81, 705, 1997.
Note: NSAIDs, nonsteroidal anti-inflammatory drugs; ACE, angiotensin-converting enzyme.

renal failure with exertional rhabdomyolysis. In the presence of acidic urine (pH below 5.6), myoglobin dissociates into globulin and hematin. Hematin produces free hydroxy radicals that render a toxic effect on the cellular tubular level. Furthermore, in urine below pH 5.0, myoglobin forms casts that occlude the renal tubules and precipitate acute renal failure.[26]

Management of rhabdomyolysis starts with a strong measure of prevention with attention to factors of acclimatization, rest/work cycles under conditions of heat exposure, and hydration. Illness, aggravating medications, and specific substances such as ephedra and stimulant-based products are potentially contributing factors. In the presence of rhabdomyolysis, vigorous IV hydration, careful monitoring of urinary production, and tracking metabolic serum indices such as liver function tests and creatine kinase (CK) will assist with decisions on duration of hydration of the athlete and need to alkinalyze the urine. Metabolic indices peak 72–96 hours after the physical insult causing rhabdomyolysis. Return-to-play decisions follow several weeks of recovery where CK values are trending toward normal and a graded gradual reexposure to heat stress is observed after other contributing elements mentioned earlier are eliminated or treated.[20,24] Exertional rhabdomyolysis is further discussed in the hematology chapter.

57.8 TRAUMATIC RENAL INJURY

The kidney is the most common urologic organ injured. Reviews of pediatric sports trauma data registries characterize the kidney-related injuries as associated with blunt trauma to the flank or abdomen and commonly associated with a rapid deceleration. The overall incidence of genitourinary injury from blunt trauma is approximately 10%. The National Pediatric Trauma Registry (1990–1999) characterizes 62% of kidney injuries as related to football with cycling, baseball, basketball, hockey, and soccer comprising lower percentages. Children are more likely than adults to incur renal injury due to higher fall risk and less renal protection (less perirenal fat, less abdominal muscular stability, and larger kidney size to body surface area).[29]

Measures to clinically decide which athletes with blunt abdominal trauma require a work-up are the presence of hematuria (including microscopic RBCs 50/HPF), rapid deceleration event, and/or other symptoms to include hypotension. A focused evaluation adds a complete urinalysis, complete blood count (CBC), electrolytes, liver function tests, creatinine, glucose, amylase, lipase, and HCG in females.[29]

Clinical Pearl

Renal trauma, in the right clinical setting, should be suspected with hematuria, flank hematoma, abdominal ecchymosis or tenderness, rib fractures/pain, and/or peritoneal signs.

The imaging gold standard is a multiphase contrast-enhanced renal CT. It is important to note that most blunt renal injuries are managed successfully without operative intervention with CT grading and staging. See Table 57.5

TABLE 57.5
Renal Injury Management Based on AAST Staging

AAST Grade	Injury Description	Immediate Treatment	CT Imaging?
I	Nonexpanding subcapsular hematoma or renal contusion without parenchymal lesion	No gross hematuria: outpatient management, no routine imaging*	*Unless SBP < 90 or in child with >50 RBC/HPF
		Gross hematuria.	Multiphasic CT
		Bed rest until gross hematuria resolves, observation, routine imaging.	
II	Nonexpanding retroperitoneal perirenal hematoma, *or* cortical renal laceration less than 1 cm without urinary extravasation	Admit for observation, no routine imaging unless gross hematuria or.*	N/A
III	Laceration >1 cm without extravasation or collecting system rupture	Admit for observation, no routine imaging unless gross hematuria or.*	N/A
IV	Laceration extending through the collecting system with extravasation, *or*	Urinary extravasation: repeat CT at 48 hours.	CT stable: monitor Arterial: angiography Uro stent vs. drain
	Vascular injury with contained hematoma	No urinary extravasation. No repeat imaging.	N/A
V	Fractured kidney with multiple lacerations, *or*	93% will require surgical treatment and 86% will require a nephrectomy.	Multiphasic CT
	Devascularized kidney with hilar avulsion		

Source: Modified from Santucci, R.A. et al., *BJU*, 93(7), 937, 2004.
Note: AAST, American Association for the Surgery of Trauma; SBP, systolic blood pressure; N/A, not applicable.

for the renal injury management based on staging by the American Association for the Surgery of Trauma (AAST). In the absence of gross hematuria or hypotension (systolic blood pressure less than 90 mmHg), Grade I–II can be managed conservatively with observation and supportive care. Grade III–V are best comanaged with a surgeon[25] (Level of Evidence C: consensus/expert opinion).

Clinical Pearl

Hemodynamic instability in a child is a late sign of collapse and should therefore cause the examiner to proceed cautiously with serial examinations.

Athletes should not return to sports participation until all hematuria has resolved. This time frame is variable and ranges from 2 to 6 weeks with pediatric-age athletes requiring more time to allow a complete recovery. Renal injuries involving laceration with diastasis generally follow a longer time frame to heal with a period of 6–12 months of no contact sports to avoid relapse.[29]

57.9 SCROTAL MASS AND PAIN

Scrotal pain in an athlete accounts for many diagnostic possibilities and can be challenging, especially given the serious nature of a misdiagnosis. The primary etiologies for acute traumatic scrotal pain include testicular contusion, testicular rupture, testicular torsion, and scrotal hematoma. Common causes of insidious scrotal pain include epididymitis, testicular appendage torsion, inguinal hernia, and testicular tumor.[7]

The medical history should focus on the mechanism and time course of presentation. The physical exam should follow a focused inspection and palpation of the scrotal anatomy. Scrotal masses should be further described by transillumination as cystic or solid. Examination of the abdomen and groin should rule out referred pain. One useful examination technique[16] is described where three fingers are applied to the posterosuperior neck of the scrotum and the thumb is placed anteriorly. The examiner finding swelling below the thumb suggests testicular injury, epididymal injury, or hydrocele, while swelling above the thumb suggests incarcerated hernia or spermatocord injury. Regardless, a urinalysis should be performed in all cases of scrotal trauma. Adjunctive imaging evaluation should follow with an ultrasound. In the interim period, these injuries are acutely treated by support, ice, elevation, and analgesics. If there is evidence of an expanding scrotal hematoma, then immediate surgical consultation is indicated.[16]

Testicular torsion has its own diagnostic challenges and represents a surgical urgency. The incidence of testicular torsion is highest during early puberty through the teenage years with only 4%–8% resulting from trauma. When trauma has an association with this injury, it is more often minor. Pain onset is acute and tenderness is diffuse, affecting a single testicle. Pain is aggravated with testicular elevation above the symphysis pubis. Focal tenderness at the testicular upper pole is more suggestive of an appendiceal torsion. Imaging should not delay definitive treatment for a suspected testicular torsion.[16]

Clinical Pearl

Two reliable clinical signs of testicular torsion are absent cremasteric reflex and high/horizontal testicular lie.

Prompt surgical exploration and correction are the treatment of choice. Manually untwisting the torsed testicle is successful in 26%–80% of patients. Typically, the testicle twists toward the midline; the examiner may attempt to rotate the testis manually lateral toward the thigh (as if opening a book). If the testicular torsion cannot be reduced, then immediate surgical intervention is indicated. Greatest testicular salvage exists with manual or surgical reduction under 4–6 hours from onset. At 12 hours, the rate of salvage decreases to 50% and at 24 hours the success rate is 10%. Torsion of a testicular appendage is managed over several weeks of scrotal elevation, rest, and nonsteroidal anti-inflammatory drugs (NSAIDs).[7]

Epididymitis has an occasional association with trauma with more frequent causes being attributed to sexually transmitted diseases (STDs) and urinary tract infections. Epididymitis is not uncommonly seen from adolescent years into adulthood. Pain is insidious and localizes to the epididymis; the testis is not tender. Epididymitis that accompanies a urinary tract infection should have a renal/bladder sonogram and a voiding cystourethrogram to rule out structural abnormalities. Epididymitis treatment includes NSAIDs, scrotal elevation, and empiric antibiotic therapy, fluoroquinolone, until the urine culture yields an infected organism. If no organism is identified, epididymitis treatment duration is extended 1 week beyond the period of scrotal tenderness resolution, typically totaling 2–4 weeks.[7]

A testicular tumor presents as a firm testicular mass. The patient or a medical provider on routine physical exam may find it, and occasionally it is associated with a dull scrotal ache. Testicular cancer represents only 1% of all cancers in males, but one of the bimodal incidence peaks during a common age group for athletes, 15 years to 35 years old. Ninety-seven percent of testicular tumors are germinal in origin. See Table 57.6

TABLE 57.6
Testicular Cancers

Germinal Cell[a]	Nongerminal Cell
Seminoma	Leydig cell tumors
Embryonal cell carcinoma	Sertoli's cell tumors
Teratoma	Gonadoblastoma
Choriocarcinoma	

[a] 97% of testicular cancers.

for a listing of testicular tumors. A testicular ultrasound is a reliable means to initially evaluate a testicular tumor. A urologic consult should be placed in a timely fashion.[7]

57.10 GENITOURINARY INFECTIONS

The incidence of urinary tract infections has not been demonstrated in any study to have a higher prevalence rate among athletes. However, athletes may, by virtue of physiologic factors, experience a decrease in natural barriers such as thinner urethral tissues in amenorrheic or postmenstrual women. Poor hydration practices and voluntary urinary retention in athletes can lead to urinary stasis and/or urinary reflux that can form the nidus of infection. Finally, some sports, such as bicycling, generate recurrent incidental injury to the urethra, prostate, and bladder that can establish an inflammatory process that may be difficult to differentiate from infection.[14]

STDs in a 2010 Centers for Disease Control (CDC) report continue to reflect a major impact on society with 19 million new STDs per year, costing U.S. healthcare $16.4 million annually. Athletes are among the young, risk takers of the sexually active population. Indiscriminate sexual behavior puts them at greater risk to contract STDs.[12] The 3 most prevalent STDs among the young athletic population are chlamydia, gonorrhea, and human papillomavirus (HPV).[17] All 3 merit education, and where clinically appropriate (age less than 25 or genital urinary [GU] symptoms), screening is indicated. The concern regarding the burden of asymptomatic *Chlamydia trachomatis* and *Neisseria gonorrhoeae* infections in women less than 25 supports recommendations for universal screening in this age group during annual Papanicolaou/gynecological (PAP/GYN) exams.[28] See Table 57.7 for treatment selections for the previously mentioned STDs in accordance with the latest CDC guidelines.[8] Return-to-play guidelines depend on the cause of the infection and whether any complication exists. As a general rule, athletes should be held from competition until treatment is started for 72 hours and symptoms resolved.

57.11 PUDENDAL NERVE INJURY

The pudendal nerve is formed from the sacral plexuses (S2, S3, and S4) innervating the external genitalia and providing both bladder and rectal sphincter motor control. Sports with increased risk for prolonged compression along the perineum, such as cycling, are prime suspects for pudendal neuropathy. The incidence of pudendal nerve injury in cyclists increases with advancing age, increased BMI, and advancing duration of riding. The prevalence of pudendal nerve injury is variable among cyclists, 50%–90% as reported in several studies. Symptoms range across a spectrum of compression location and severity. Genital numbness is probably the most common and recognizable symptoms. Advancing symptoms include erectile dysfunction, difficulty obtaining an orgasm, and reduced sensation of rectal function. Management starts with rest from cycling until the saddle numbness resolves. Return to sports must include making changes in riding style and riding duration. There are benefits in selecting a seat structure (V-groove saddle, split saddle design, or seat with a central cutout) that reduces pressure on the perineum.[4,19]

TABLE 57.7
CDC 2010 Sexually Transmitted Disease Treatment Guidelines

STD	Primary	Alternative	Recurrent
Gonococcal urethritis/cervicitis	Ceftriaxone 250 mg IM Cefixime 400 mg po single dose	Any single-dose injectable cephalosporin *plus* doxycycline 100 mg bid × 7 days or Azithromycin 1 gm po single dose	N/A
Nongonococcal urethritis/cervicitis or chlamydia	Doxycycline 100 mg bid × 7 days Azithromycin 1 gm po single dose	Erythromycin Base 500 mg PO qid × 7 days Levofloxacin 500 mg po qd × 7 days	Metronidazole 2 gm po single dose Erythromycin base 500 mg qid × 7 days
Genital herpes virus	Acyclovir 400 mg po tid × 7–10 days	Famciclovir 250 mg po tid × 7–10 days Valacyclovir 1 gm po bid × 7–10 days	Acyclovir 400 mg po tid or 800 mg po bid × 5 days Famciclovir 125 mg po bid × 5 days Valacyclovir 1 gm po qd × 5 days
Herpes virus suppression	Acyclovir 400 mg po bid	Famciclovir 250 mg po bid Valacyclovir 500 mg–1 g po bid	N/A
Genital warts	Imiquimod or podofilox 0.5% solution or gel Apply 3 days a week for 30 days	Office-based treatments include cryotherapy each week or podophyllin resin 10%–25%	N/A

Source: Centers for Disease Control (CDC) and Prevention, *2010 Guidelines for Treatment of Sexually Transmitted Diseases*, Public Health Agency of Canada, Ottawa, Ontario, Canada, MMWR 60(No. RR-12) 2011.

Note: po, denotes by mouth; IM, denotes intramuscular; N/A, denotes nothing applies. Use these regimens in nonpregnant adult patients.

57.12 SOLITARY KIDNEY

Physicians may be asked to clear an athlete for sports participation with a solitary kidney. Special considerations exist in making this assessment, but automatic disqualification is not always necessary. The incidence of a solitary kidney (congenital or acquired) is estimated in the American population to be one in 1100– 1800. The results of a questionnaire sent to the membership of the American Medical Society for Sports Medicine in 1994 reported 237 of the 438 respondents (54.1%) indicating that they would allow full participation in sports for an athlete with a solitary kidney after discussion of the possible risks.[3]

In May 2001, the American Academy of Pediatrics published a policy statement regarding "Medical Conditions Affecting Sports Participation." In this policy statement, an athlete with a solitary kidney was a qualified "yes" for sports participation after completing an individual assessment for contact, collision, and limited contact sports. Even for contact sports, the literature has continued to demonstrate a very small risk of kidney injury. The 2010 Preparticipation Physical Evaluation monograph 4th edition, endorsed by the leading sports medicine societies, the American Academy of Family Physicians and the American Academy of Pediatrics, published a consensus opinion: "If the athlete chooses to play in a sport that may place a solitary kidney at increased risk for damage, a full explanation should be given to the athlete, his or her parent(s) or guardian(s) and the coaches. The explanation should include available protection (i.e. flak vest), potential serious long term consequences, and treatment of injuries if they occur."[2] As with all conditions of athletic genitourinary consideration, a knowledgeable primary care physician is best able to inform the athlete and advocate for measures that preserve and protect the health of the athlete. Guidelines on performing this type of counseling are available in the literature (Table 57.8).[22]

TABLE 57.8
SORT: Key Recommendations for Practice

Clinical Recommendation	Evidence Rating	References
The new 2012 AUA AMH guideline recommends work-up for patients 35 years or older with a positive urinalysis following 72 hours of exercise rest with 3 or more RBCs/HPF using multiphasic renal CT scan and cystoscopy.	C	[23]
Renal injury management based on staging by the American Association for the Surgery of Trauma (AAST). In the absence of gross hematuria or hypotension (systolic blood pressure less than 90 mmHg), Grade I–II can be managed conservatively with observation and supportive care. Grade III–V are best comanaged with a surgeon.	C	[25]
A solitary kidney is a qualified "yes" for all sports participation after completing an individual assessment for contact and collision and ensuring consultation with a physician versed in describing the risks, to include applying mitigating measures for protection.	C	[2]

REFERENCES

1. Abarbanel J, Benet AE, Lask D, Kimche D. Sports hematuria. *Journal of Urology.* 1990;143:887–890; Blair SN, Kohl HW 3rd, Barlow CE, Paffenbarger RS Jr, Gibbons LW, Macera CA. Changes in physical fitness and all-cause mortality. A prospective study of healthy and unhealthy men. *Journal of the American Medical Association.* April 1995;273(14):1093–1098.
2. American Academy of Family Physicians, American Academy of Pediatrics, American College of Sports Medicine, American Medical Society for Sports Medicine, American Orthopedic Society for Sports Medicine, American Osteopathic Academy of Sports Medicine. *Preparticipation Physical Exam Evaluation*, 4th edn. The McGraw-Hill Companies; 2010.
3. Anderson CR. Solitary kidney and sports participation. *Archives of Family Medicine.* 1995;4:885–888.
4. Asplund C, Barkdull T, Weiss B. Genitourinary problems in bicyclists. *Current Sports Medicine Reports.* 2007; 6:333–339.
5. Bellinghieri G, Savica V, Santoro D. Renal alterations during exercise. *Journal of Renal Nutrition.* January 2008;18(1):158–164.
6. Bernard J. Renal trauma: Evaluation, management, and return to play. *Current Sports Medicine Reports.* March/April 2009;8(2):98–103.
7. Bradley S, Hartmann B, Berkson D, Hong E. Testicular conditions in athletes: Torsion, tumors, and epididymitis. *Current Sports Medicine Reports.* March/April 2012;11(7):92–95.
8. Centers for Disease Control and prevention. 2010 STD treatment guidelines. 2010. Available at http://www.cdc.gov/sTD/treatment/2010/default.htm. Accessed May 29, 2014.
9. Choudhury D, Ahmed Z. Drug-induced nephrotoxicity. *Medical Clinics of North America.* 1997;81:705–717.
10. Cianflocco AJ. Renal complications of exercise. *Current Sports Medicine Reports.* 1992;11:437.
11. Gambrell RC, Blount BW. Exercise-induced hematuria. *American Family Physician.* 1996;53:905–911.
12. Habel MA, Dittus PJ, De Rosa CJ, Chung EQ, Kerrndt PR. Daily participation in sports and students' sexual activity. *Perspectives on Sexual and Reproductive Health.* December 2010;42(4):244–250.
13. Harirforoosh S, Jamali F. Renal adverse effects of nonsteroidal anti-inflammatory drugs. *Expert Opinion on Drug Safety.* November 2009;8(6):669–681.
14. Harris MD. Infectious disease in athletes. *Current Sports Medicine Reports.* March/April 2011;10(2):84–89.
15. Hebert LA, Betts JA, Sedmak DD, Cosio FG, Bay WH, Carlton S. Lion pain-hematuria syndrome associated with thin glomerular basement membrane disease and hemorrhage into renal tubules. *Kidney International.* 1996;49:168–173.
16. Hunter SR, Lishnak TS, Powers AM, Lisle DK. Male genital trauma in sports. *Clinics in Sports Medicine.* 2013;32:247–254.
17. Jaworski CA, Donohue B, Kluetz J. Infectious disease. *Clinics in Sports Medicine.* 2011;30:575–590.
18. Jones GR, Newhouse I. Sport-related hematuria: A review. *Clinical Journal of Sport Medicine.* 1997;7:119–125.

19. Leibovitch I, Mor Y. The vicious cycling: Bicycling related urogenital disorders. *European Urology*. 2005;47:277–287.
20. O'Connor FG, Brennan FH, Campbell W, Heled Y, Deuster P. Return to physical activity after exertional rhabdomyolysis. *Current Sports Medicine Reports*. 2008;7(6):328–331.
21. Peggs JF, Reinhardt RW, O'Brien JM. Proteinuria in adolescent sports physical examinations. *Journal of Family Practice*. 1986;22:80–81.
22. Psooy K. Sports and the solitary kidney: How to counsel parents. *Canadian Journal of Urology*. June 2006;13(3):3120–3126.
23. Rodney D, Jones JS, Barocas DA et al. Diagnosis, evaluation and follow-up of asymptomatic microhematuria (AMH) in adults: AUA guideline. *Journal of Urology*. December 2012;188:2473–2481.
24. Rosenberg J. Exertional rhabdomyolysis: Risk factors, presentation, and management. *Athletic Therapy Today*. 2008;13(3):11–12.
25. Santucci RA, Wessells H, Bartsch G et al. Evaluation and management of renal injuries: Consensus statement of the renal subcommittee. *BJU International*. 2004;93(7):937–954.
26. Sinert S, Kohl L, Rainone T, Scalea T. Exercise-induced rhabdomyolysis. *Annals of Emergency Medicine*. 1994;23:1301–1306.
27. Tansgho EA, McAninch JW (eds.). *Smith's General Urology*, 18th edn. Los Altos, CA: Lange Medical Publications/McGraw-Hill; 2013.
28. Turner CF, Rogers SM, Miller HG, Miller WC, Gribble JN, Chromy JR, Leone PA, Cooley PC, Quinn TC, Zenilman JM. Untreated gonococcal and chlamydial infection in a probability sample of adults. *Journal of the American Medical Association*. 2002;287(6):726–733.
29. Viola TA. Closed kidney injury. *Clinics in Sports Medicine*. 2013;32:219–227.
30. Viswanathan G, Upadhyay A. Assessment of proteinuria. *Advances in Chronic Kidney Disease*. July 2011;18(4):385–394.
31. West JB (ed.). *Best and Taylor's Physiologic Basis of Medical Practice*, 11th edn. Baltimore, MD: Williams & Wilkins; 1985.
32. Centers for Disease Control (CDC) and Prevention. *2010 Guidelines for Treatment of Sexually Transmitted Diseases*. Ottawa, Ontario, Canada: Public Health Agency of Canada, MMWR 60(No. RR-12); 2011.

58 Hematologic Concerns in the Athlete

William B. Adams

CONTENTS

TABLE 58.1
Key Clinical Considerations

1. While exercise does not predispose to hematologic disturbances, impaired physical performance is a frequent presentation for unmasking a hematologic disorder.
   Despite the fact that exercising adults tend to be more health conscious with regard to exercise and nutrition, exercise can cause a dilutional pseudoanemia and iron deficiency is the most common cause of a true anemia in athletes.
2. Athletes with anemia warrant the same diagnostic evaluation for anemia as do nonathletes.
3. Exertional rhabdomyolysis is a potentially limb- and life-threatening illness that is a not infrequent consequence of overexertion in both recreational and elite athletes, with the clinical hallmarks being myalgia, weakness, and myoglobinuria.
4. Sickle-cell trait, while generally a benign disorder that does not interfere with exercise participation, has been associated on rare occasion with severe exertional rhabdomyolysis and sudden death.

58.1 INTRODUCTION

Exercise per se does not predispose to hematologic disease states. Although athletes as a group tend to be healthier, they are still susceptible to the same hematologic diseases as nonathletes; however, symptoms from hematologic disturbances may present earlier and at lower severity often manifesting as impaired physical performance.[7,8] Maximal or prolonged exertion efforts typically cause transient changes in several hematologic indices. Regular endurance and altitude training generally result in more sustained alterations of hematologic parameters.[24] Dietary inadequacies, not uncommon in athletes, may cause hematologic problems due to a deficit of calories or critical nutrients.[11] This chapter discusses the evaluation, diagnosis, and management of common hematologic disorders identified in the recreational and elite athlete (Table 58.1).

58.2 HEMATOLOGIC DISORDERS IN ATHLETES

58.2.1 Evaluation for Hematologic Disorders in Athletes

The search for hematologic disorders in an athlete should be prompted by symptoms, history, or other clinical indications from physical evaluation. If there are no clinical concerns and no particular risk factors for hematologic disorders, routine blood testing for "screening" in a healthy athlete is not warranted. Hematologic testing in athletes without clinical indication may lead to additional unnecessary testing as well as erroneous diagnoses and possibly inappropriate, even hazardous, treatment. In situations where there is an incidental finding of a hematologic test abnormality in the absence of pathologic indicators, it may be prudent to initially repeat the test (e.g., complete blood count [CBC]) after the athlete has rested for several days to eliminate acute transient hematologic perturbations as cited in the following.[12,17] Ideally, blood drawn for hematologic study should be collected when the patient is normally hydrated and in a calm, well-rested state with no recent food intake or use of caffeine, nicotine, or other stimulants. Stress, emotional disturbance, and stimulants may artifactually increase the white blood cell (WBC) and platelet counts. Dehydration and overhydration may alter all parameters through hemoconcentration or dilutional effects. The possible influence of these factors should be considered in analyzing results of blood collected under these conditions.[12,17]

Clinical Pearl

In the absence of pathologic indicators, hematologic abnormalities incidentally found on an athlete's CBC are often physiologic. Repeating test with the athlete in a resting state after abstaining from exercise for several days may resolve the abnormalities precluding the need for further testing.

58.2.2 Anemia

Anemia is the reduction of total red blood cell (RBC) volume concentration (hematocrit [Hct]) or hemoglobin (Hgb) below normal values. It is a common clinical condition with a multitude of causes.[17] The prevalence of anemia for males in the United States ranges from 6/1000 below age 45 to 18.5/1000 males ages 75 and above. For women of all ages, the prevalence is 30/1000.[20] While athletes tend to be healthier than the general population, they may have a slightly higher prevalence of anemia from certain nutritional deficiencies, particularly those trying to restrict weight or those following special diets that are deficient in iron, vitamins, or calories.[3,24] Anemia arises from either excessive loss or inadequate production of RBCs or a combination of both. Symptoms and physical manifestations depend upon decrements in RBC volume and oxygen delivered to tissues, the rate at which these changes occur, and the cardiopulmonary compensatory capacity.[16,17]

58.2.2.1 Athletic Pseudoanemia (Sports Anemia)

Sweat losses and intravascular fluid shifts during sustained aerobic exercise may decrease plasma volume in 5%–20%. Trained endurance athletes tend to have a greater reduction in plasma volume during exercise due to greater sweat losses, which is offset by a physiologic plasma volume expansion in the resting or preexercise state. RBC production is increased with regular endurance training; however, this increased RBC mass is offset by a greater expansion of plasma volume. Consequently, a slight reduction in Hgb and Hct levels occurs in the resting state. This is not a true anemia but rather a physiologic adaptation that promotes increased cardiac output and enhanced oxygen delivery to tissues and protects against hyperviscosity. Hence, it is termed *athletic pseudoanemia* or is sometimes called *sports anemia*.[4,5,24] Hgb values typically run 0.5 g/dL lower for athletes pursuing moderate-intensity training and 1.0 g/dL lower for elite-level athletes.[4] This hemodilution from conditioning is temporary, however, and may resolve within days of terminating endurance-level training.[24] Diagnosis may be confirmed by testing the athlete after several days of rest from training or can be inferred from CBC testing revealing normal RBC indices and RBC distribution width (RDW) with a normal reticulocyte count and normal serum ferritin level. In athletes, normal ferritin levels may be as low as 12 μg/L, particularly with high-intensity training.[3] If iron-deficiency anemia is in question, a brief trial of oral iron supplementation with a repeat reticulocyte count at 1–2 weeks may provide the answer. A rise in the reticulocyte count confirms iron deficiency as the etiology of the anemia.[23]

58.2.2.2 Iron-Deficiency Anemia

Iron-deficiency anemia is the most common cause of true anemia in the athlete as in the nonathlete.[4,5] It occurs more often in female athletes mostly due to menstrual losses coupled with inadequate consumption of meat or other sources of iron.[3,5] Laboratory testing reveals a low Hgb and Hct with low mean corpuscular volume (MCV) and mean corpuscular hemoglobin (MCH). RDW is increased unless iron deficiency is chronic. Peripheral smear reveals hypochromic microcytic cells with a low to normal reticulocyte count. Serum ferritin levels that are low (≤ 12 μg/L) better reflect total body iron content, as serum iron levels are unreliable. Total iron binding capacity (TIBC) and transferrin saturation (serum iron × 100/TIBC) more accurately reflect iron status. In isolated iron deficiency, TIBC tends to be elevated, while transferrin saturation tends to be low (particularly <16%).[3,16,17] In the evaluation of iron-deficiency anemia, it is imperative to determine the cause of the deficiency in order to best effect the therapy and avoid overlooking potentially serious conditions. Iron replacement should continue until 6–12 months after anemia has resolved.[23]

Clinical Pearl

Athletic pseudoanemia is differentiated from true iron-deficiency anemia by normal RBC indices and a normal RDW.

58.2.2.3 Anemia due to Blood Loss

Acute heavy bleeding may cause anemia before the onset of iron deficiency. Typically, the diagnosis is obvious from history or exam findings of gross blood, melena, or hypovolemia. Bleeding contained within tissues or body cavity may be less obvious, particularly in the retroperitoneal space. In the absence of fluid administration, Hgb and Hct (both concentration values) are initially normal. Platelet counts transiently drop but become elevated within an hour if no ongoing hemorrhage is present. Over the ensuing days, Hgb and Hct values decline with plasma expansion from endogenous reservoirs. RBC indices remain normal until 3–5 days later when a reticulocytosis occurs, increasing MCV and RDW. Bilirubin levels are normal unless internal bleeding is present. With internal bleeding, unconjugated bilirubin and lactate dehydrogenase (LDH) rise as in hemolysis; however, no indicators of hemolysis can be found on peripheral smear.[15,17] If blood loss is slow and insidious, anemia may not manifest until iron stores are depleted. Often, this occurs with gastrointestinal (GI) bleeding and with menstrual blood loss in women; however, this situation may be revealed by a reticulocytosis with concomitant increase in RDW before iron stores are depleted.

58.2.2.3.1 Gastrointestinal Losses

GI bleeding is a very common and often serious cause of anemia. Accordingly, a stool occult blood test is indicated in initial assessment of any anemia workup.[20] GI bleeding may arise from the mucosa due to peptic ulcer disease or medication use (e.g., nonsteroidal anti-inflammatory drugs [NSAIDs]), vascular anomalies, inflammatory bowel diseases, ischemic syndromes, infection, diverticula, or tumors. In prolonged endurance events, low-grade GI bleeding is tremendously common. The source of this bleeding is seldom detectable and is theorized to arise from acute transient ischemia or mechanical contusion (e.g., cecal slap syndrome).[3,11,23,24] Athletes frequently pursuing long-distance running and those using NSAIDs may accrue enough cumulative blood loss to impact RBC mass.[4,23,24] However, in the absence of this or other pathology, exercise-associated GI bleeding is seldom significant enough to cause anemia.[8] Regardless of this, any GI bleeding warrants thorough investigation to rule out serious conditions.

58.2.2.3.2 *Menstrual Losses*

Blood loss from menstruation may be significant, particularly if a woman is prone to heavy or frequent menses or her diet is inadequate to compensate for cumulative menstrual losses. Characteristics of excessive flow are a requirement for 12 or more pads throughout menses, passage of clots beyond the first day, or duration of flow greater than 7 days.[17] Quantitation of menstrual flow and assessment of adequacy of iron replacement for chronic menstrual losses should be considered in the evaluation of all women athletes with anemia. Treatment focus is on reduction of menstrual flow if excessive and on iron replacement.

58.2.2.3.3 *Hematuria/Hemoglobinuria*

Bleeding from the urologic system is not typically of a volume to produce anemia. Some runners experience hematuria that is thought to arise either from increased filtration of RBCs into the urine (as a result of vascular shunting) or from bladder wall contusion during prolonged running. Any gross or microscopic hematuria, however, requires evaluation with particular concern to rule out urologic tumors.[24] Hemoglobinuria secondary to hemolysis is occasionally seen in long-distance running. It has been attributed to foot-strike hemolysis but typically is not a significant source of blood or iron loss (see the following section).[3,23]

58.2.2.3.4 *Exertional Hemolysis (Foot-Strike Hemolysis)*

Exertional hemolysis is a condition of intravascular destruction of RBCs in association with various exertional activities. Originally described as march hemoglobinuria in foot soldiers in the late 1800s, it was thought to arise from the foot strike causing compression of capillaries and rupturing RBCs; however, it is also seen in swimmers, rowers, and weight lifters, although usually to a much lesser degree.[5,23,24] It is now hypothesized that intravascular turbulence, acidosis, and elevated temperature in muscle tissues may be causative factors as well.[4] Typically, hemolysis is not significant enough to affect CBC parameters; however, if enough cumulative hemolysis occurs, the reticulocyte count RDW and MCV may be elevated and haptoglobin levels reduced. Transient hemoglobinuria may occur if hemolysis exceeds the capacity of serum haptoglobin to bind up released Hgb (approximately 20 cc of blood).[4,5,24] Generally, no treatment is necessary. Reducing impact forces to the feet (e.g., improved shoe cushioning, softer running terrain) may benefit some, particularly elite-level, runners.[4]

58.2.2.3.5 *Other Disorders Causing Anemia*

Anemia may result from other several other conditions or as a consequence of various disease processes. These may manifest in the form of accelerated RBC destruction or hemolysis or through impaired erythropoiesis. Details regarding diagnosis and evaluation of these may be found in standard hematology texts.[16]

58.2.2.3.6 *Evaluation of Anemia*

58.2.2.3.6.1 History The evaluation of anemia in the athlete should start with a search for historical clues, symptoms, and physical signs that point toward a specific etiology. Historical factors to solicit include character and duration of symptoms and whether onset was abrupt or insidious. Prior history of hematologic problems, malignancy, chronic diseases, or any family history of blood disorders is important as well. Assessment of calorie intake versus expenditure, endeavors at weight control, and use of exclusionary diets may reveal problems of caloric inadequacy or deficiency of critical nutrients. The use of nutritional aids, supplements, ergogenic agents, medications (particularly NSAIDs and inhibitors of DNA synthesis or folic acid), tobacco, or alcohol may be contributory as well.[12,17] Anemia classically presents with fatigue or malaise, but athletes often complain of decline in performance or endurance or an elevated heart rate.[8] Reports of petechiae, bruising, or bleeding problems, abdominal discomfort, jaundice, alteration of bowel patterns, dyspnea, fever, or pica may suggest particular etiologies. It is important to seek out indicators of GI bleeding as this is a common and oftentimes serious cause of anemia. Menstrual blood loss commonly contributes to anemia in women and should be quantified. Chemical exposure through work or hobbies may have hemolytic or hematopoietic effects as well.[17]

Clinical Pearl

A decrease in athletic performance may be the earliest manifestation of anemia in an athlete.

58.2.2.3.6.2 Examination The physical examination should assess overall health and nutrition as well as hemodynamic status, particularly orthostasis. Pallor and relative or absolute resting tachycardia indicate significant anemia. Findings of scleral icterus, jaundice, and splenomegaly suggest a hemolytic process. Bruising and petechiae may indicate a coagulation or platelet disorder. Certain integument changes may characterize dietary deficiencies or hypothyroidism. Findings of adenopathy, foci of skeletal tenderness in the limbs or sternum, and abdominal or pelvic masses may suggest underlying malignancy. Signs of chronic diseases (particularly renal and hepatic), infection, endocrinopathies, and malignancies particularly should be sought out along with stool testing for occult blood.[16,17]

58.2.2.3.6.3 Studies Evidence of heavy bleeding, severe hemolysis, malignancy, or profound deficiency in one or more hematologic cell lines necessitates specialized testing and specialist referral early on; otherwise, if the history, physical examination, and testing for occult bleeding do not point toward a specific etiology, a systematic laboratory evaluation should ensue.[17] In analyzing laboratory studies, verify that blood was not collected under conditions that spuriously alter hematologic parameters, as noted earlier. Repeating studies after several days of rest may preclude much unnecessary workup and anxiety.[12,17] Stool occult blood testing is indicated early as GI bleeding is a common cause of anemia[1]; otherwise, initial workup should start with a CBC, differential count, peripheral smear review, and reticulocyte count. Adult males and postmenopausal women with iron-deficiency anemia should be considered for screening for a GI malignancy. These studies allow classification of anemia according to conditions of excessive loss (bleeding or hemolysis) or inadequate production (ineffective erythropoiesis). Using this scheme with subsequent subcategorization according to RBC size (MCV) and Hgb content (MCH) allows for a more focused approach to determine the etiology of the anemia. If initial assessment reveals gross or occult bleeding, the evaluation is directed toward identification of the source and implementation of corrective measures (to include iron and blood replacement as indicated).

The first step in assessing anemia is to determine if the condition is one of excess blood loss or inadequate RBC production. This requires determination of the reticulocyte count and calculation of the reticulocyte production index (RPI). The RPI accounts for expected variance in reticulocyte percentage for different Hct values; hence, it is a more reliable parameter. The formula for determination of the RPI is

$$\text{Reticulocyte index} = \text{Reticulocyte count} \times \text{Hematocrit}/\text{Normal hematocrit}$$

RPI values of 3 or more indicate increased erythrocyte production as seen with blood loss (see Figure 58.1).[17]

Elevations of serum bilirubin (particularly unconjugated), LDH, and urobilinogen with decreased haptoglobin indicate hemolysis.[17] In this setting, determine the cause of hemolysis and implement corrective measures. Normal values for these tests indicate bleeding and should be followed with investigations to identify and treat the bleeding source. Internal bleeding, however, may mimic hemolysis, yielding the same chemistry disturbances as RBCs are broken down and reabsorbed. The difference is distinguished by history, examination findings, and a paucity of fragmented cells on peripheral smear.[15–18]

Anemia with RPI values less than 2 indicates impaired erythropoiesis (see Figure 58.2). In this setting, the next step involves using CBC results to subcategorize anemia according to erythrocyte indices of MCV and MCH. The MCV allows classification of the anemia as normocytic (normal MCV), microcytic (low MCV), or macrocytic (elevated MCV). Decreased MCH indicates hypochromia as seen in prolonged iron deficiency. It is important to realize that these parameters are averages and may not adequately reflect the clinical state early on when morphologic variation within the RBC population is averaged out. This situation, however, is revealed by an increase in the RDW, which reflects size variance in the RBC population and can identify acute alterations in RBC morphology long before the MCV is affected (e.g., early iron-deficiency anemia). The peripheral smear also may reveal morphologic characteristics in RBCs or other cell lines indicative of certain pathologic processes (e.g., hematologic malignancies, hemolysis, hemoglobinopathies).[12,16,17]

Another useful study at this stage, particularly in evaluating microcytic anemia, is the serum ferritin level (see Figure 58.3).

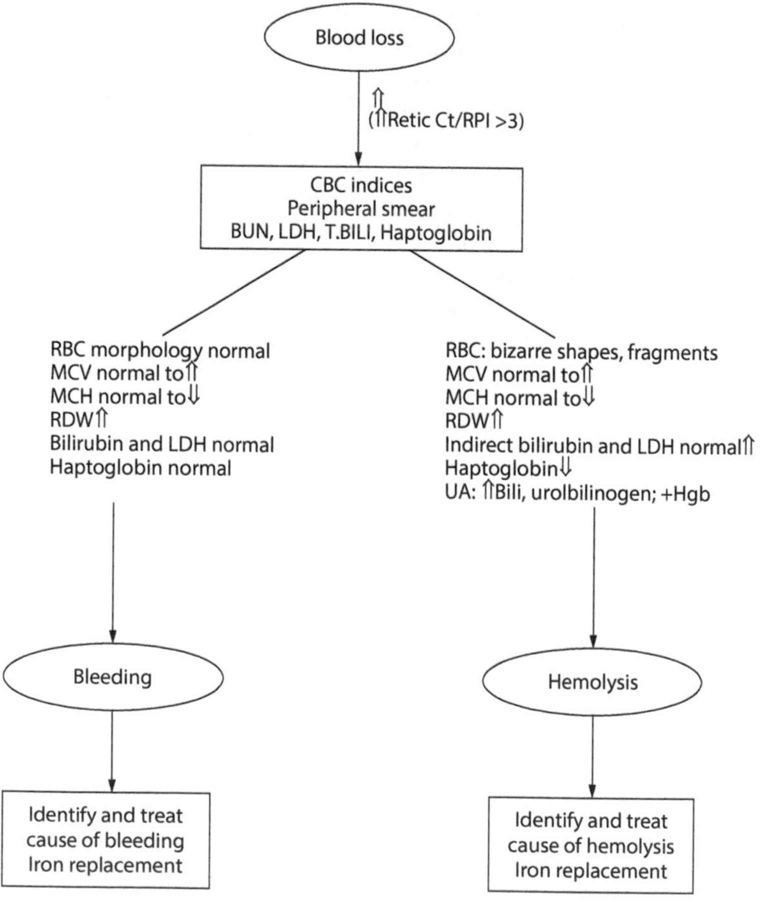

FIGURE 58.1 Evaluation of anemia secondary to blood loss (third edition).

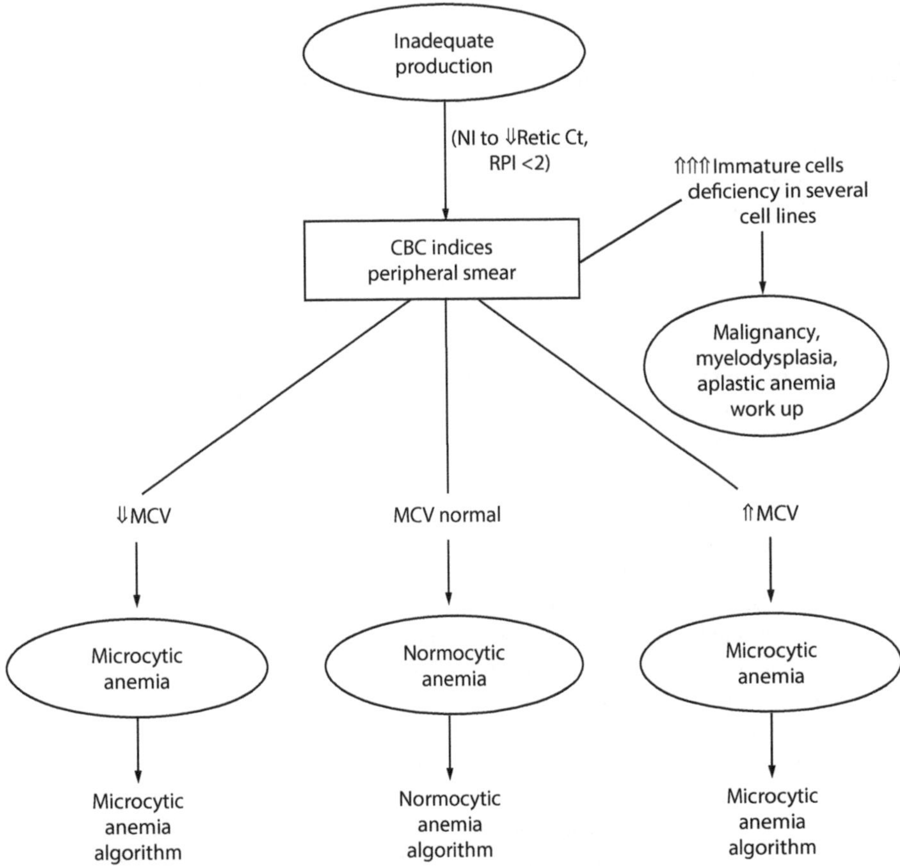

FIGURE 58.2 Evaluation of anemia secondary to inadequate production (third edition).

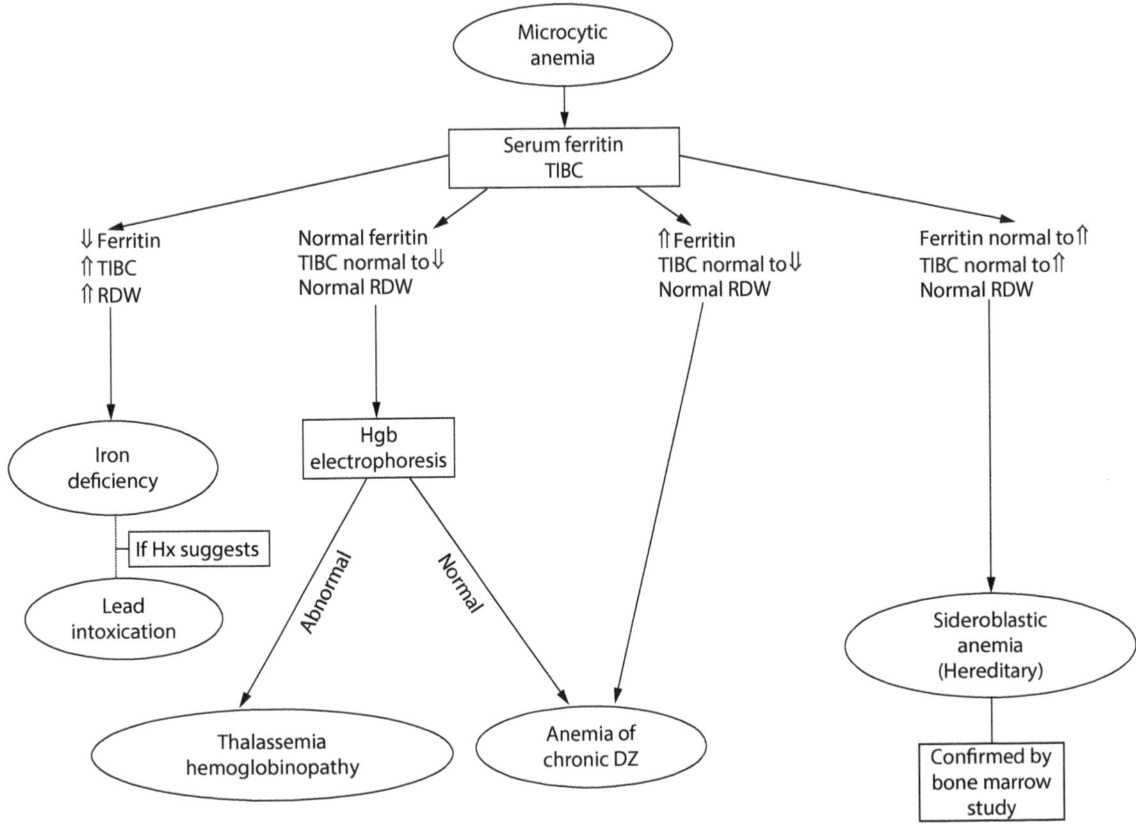

FIGURE 58.3 Evaluation of microcytic anemia (third edition).

TABLE 58.2
Common Causes of Microcytic Anemia

Iron-deficiency anemia
Anemia of chronic disease
Disorders of iron metabolism
Disorders of globulin synthesis (thalassemias)
Disorders of porphyrin and heme synthesis
Sideroblastic anemia
Lead toxicity

In the absence of concomitant disease processes, serum ferritin reflects total body iron stores. Serum ferritin tends to be low in iron deficiency (typically, <12 μg/L); however, inflammatory disease processes may elevate ferritin levels into the normal range, masking diagnosis of iron deficiency.[16] Ferritin levels tend to be elevated in thalassemia, anemia of chronic disease, liver disease, and various malignancies. Determination of TIBC and transferrin saturation (serum iron × 100/TIBC) may further aid in the determination of etiology. TIBC tends to be elevated in iron deficiency and decreased in anemia of chronic disease. Transferrin saturation tends to be lower in iron deficiency than anemia of chronic disease, particularly for values <16%.[16] Various etiologies of microcytic anemia are listed in Table 58.2.

Macrocytic anemia may be either a megaloblastic or nonmegaloblastic anemia (see Figure 58.4). The former typically results from deficiency of vitamin B12 or folate, although intrinsic defects in DNA synthesis and use of drugs that inhibit folate or DNA synthesis may be at fault as well. Nonmegaloblastic anemias typically result from alcoholism, liver disease, or hemolytic anemia. Megaloblastic anemia tends to manifest higher MCV values and is often associated with pancytopenia and hypersegmentation of neutrophils and oval macrocytes on peripheral smear. LDH is significantly elevated as well. Serum or erythrocyte vitamin B12 or folate assays help differentiate between these diagnoses. In unclear situations, a bone marrow examination may be necessary.[16] Table 58.3 lists many etiologies of macrocytic anemia.

TABLE 58.3
Common Causes of Macrocytic Anemia

Vitamin B_{12} deficiency
Folate deficiency
Combined vitamin B_{12} and folate deficiency
Disorders of DNA synthesis (inherited)
Alcoholism
Drug or toxin inhibition of DNA synthesis
Erythroleukemia
Recent subacute blood loss (hemolysis or hemorrhage)
Liver disease
Hypothyroidism
COPD
Myelodysplastic anemia
Myelophthisic anemia
Acquired sideroblastic anemia

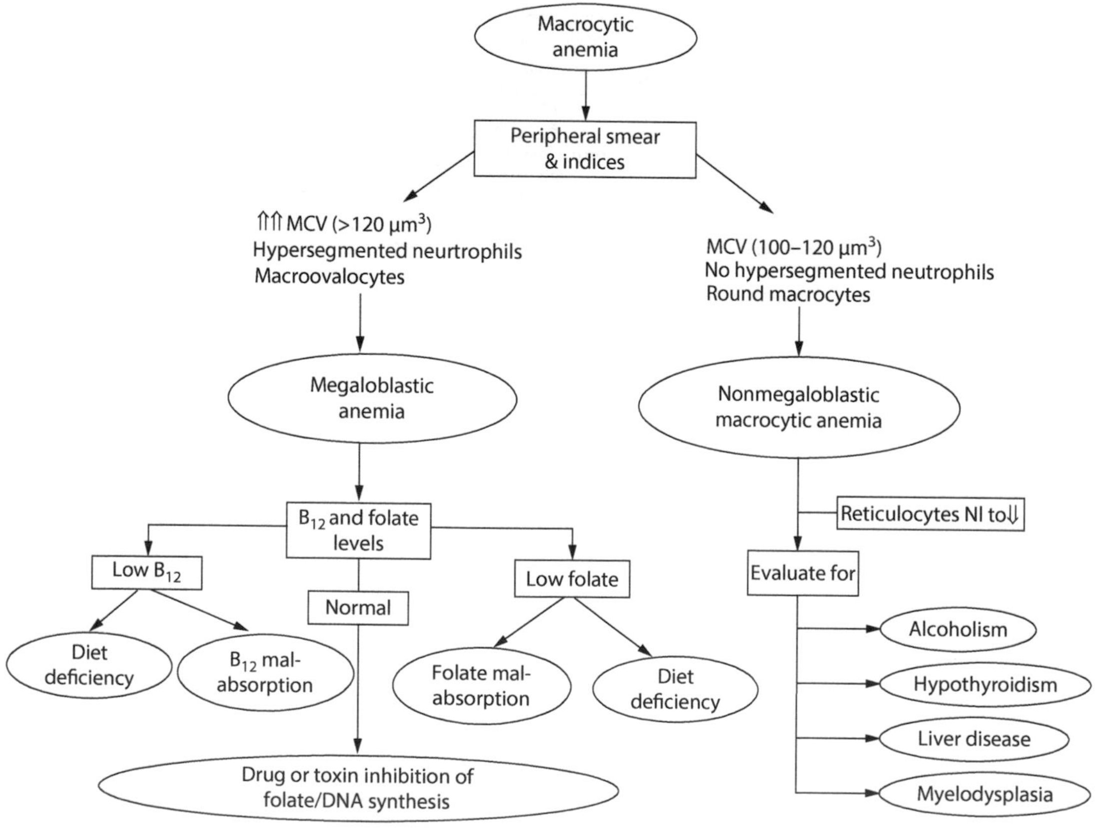

FIGURE 58.4 Evaluation of macrocytic anemia (third edition).

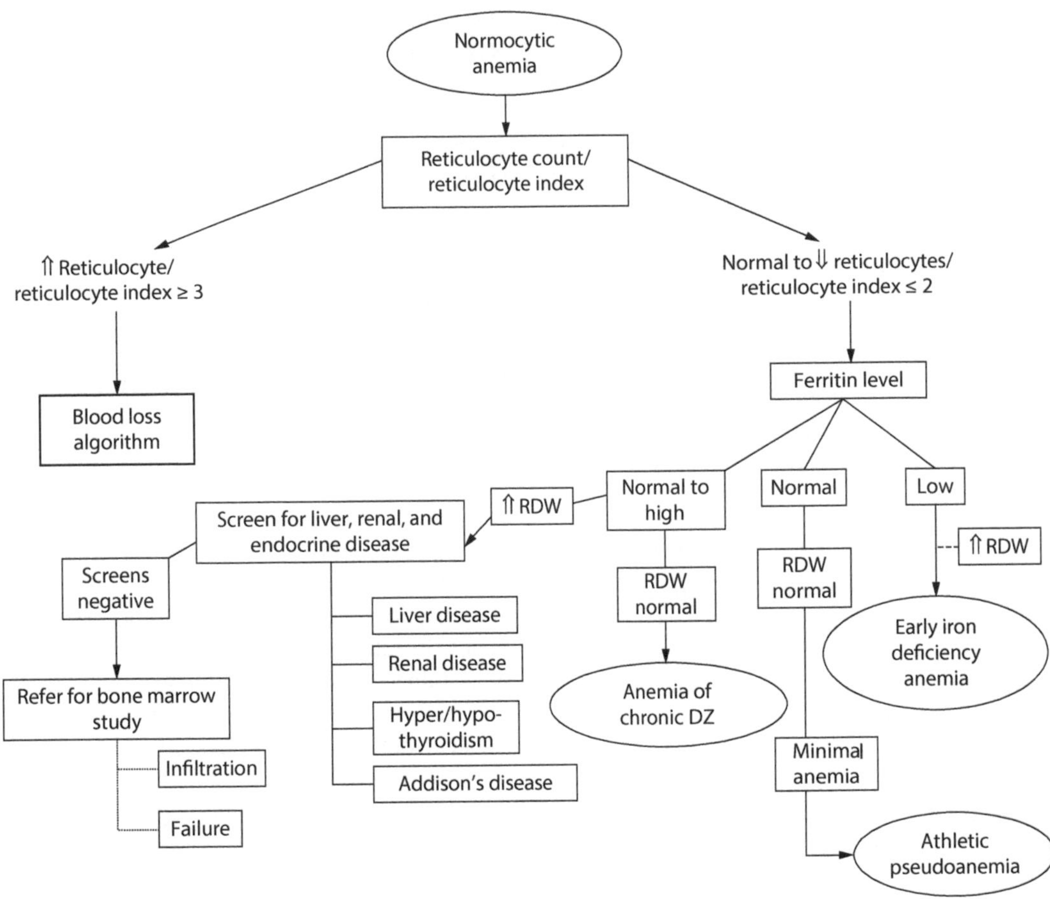

FIGURE 58.5 Evaluation of normocytic anemia (third edition).

A normocytic anemia may be a mild manifestation of systemic disease, an anemia in transition to becoming macrocytic or microcytic, or a state where concomitant conditions yield mixed microcytic and macrocytic erythrocyte populations with normal indices due to averaging. The latter situation would be apparent from evaluation of RDW and review of the peripheral smear. Normocytic anemia may represent early acute hemolysis or bleeding. These states should be distinguishable from clinical exam findings and laboratory results as detailed earlier; otherwise, the remaining etiologies fall into the category of impaired erythropoiesis arising from impaired marrow activity (hypoplastic or aplastic anemia, leukemia, and similar marrow infiltrative diseases) or decreased erythropoietin activity, as seen in renal and liver disease, endocrinopathies, and severe malnutrition. Also, anemia of chronic disease often manifests a normocytic anemia. This condition is characterized by elevated ferritin levels. Intrinsic marrow diseases are typically characterized by pancytopenia and immature or bizarre morphologies on peripheral smear. These are confirmed by bone marrow biopsy.[16] Renal, liver, and endocrine diseases should be identified in clinical evaluation but may be missed if symptoms are mild or more insidious in development. Figure 58.5 outlines an approach to evaluating normocytic anemia and Table 58.4 lists common etiologies.[16,17]

TABLE 58.4
Common Causes of Normocytic Anemia

Blood loss (initially after acute loss)
Hemolysis (initially after acute loss)
Anemia with impaired marrow response
Aplastic/hypoplastic anemia
Leukemia
Multiple myeloma
Myelodysplastic anemia
Early iron deficiency
Renal disease
Mixed anemia (iron-deficiency/thalassemia and megaloblastic anemia)
Anemia of chronic disease
Malnutrition

58.2.3 Erythrocythemia (Polycythemia) and Erythropoietin

RBC mass may be increased as a physiologic response to hypoxic stress or disease processes or may be induced by drug use. Smoking, carbon monoxide exposure (e.g., ice rinks), and training at altitude may also increase RBC mass in athletes. A spurious erythrocytosis may also arise from transient plasma volume contraction (e.g., exercise and dehydrated status).[21]

True polycythemia arises from conditions of excess RBC production, either as part of a hyperplastic marrow response (polycythemia vera) or as a secondary response to excess erythropoietin production (secondary polycythemia). Polycythemia vera is a myeloproliferative disorder involving trilineage marrow hyperplasia. Thus, the elevations of RBC mass are often with concomitant leukocytosis and thrombocytosis. It is typically characterized by low erythropoietin levels in the presence of markedly elevated Hct. These patients require regular phlebotomy to prevent a hyperviscosity state.[19] Secondary polycythemia results from elevated erythropoietin. This occurs as a response to hypoxia or reduced oxygen delivery to tissues in cases of Hgb variants with excessively high oxygen affinity. This is characterized by elevated RBC and erythropoietin levels with normal WBC and platelet counts.

58.2.4 White Blood Cell Line Abnormalities

Strenuous or prolonged vigorous exercise may produce acute profound perturbations of WBC populations. This effect, however, resolves with rest and is not typically associated with persistent abnormalities of WBC lines. Various drugs may either elevate or depress WBC production, as may infection. Persistent leukopenia may be indicative of human immunodeficiency virus infection or marrow disorders. Some populations (e.g., black males) may manifest a mild neutropenia that is nonpathologic.[12] If blood work indicates a pathologic alteration of the WBC population, examination should include a thorough assessment of lymphatic and hematologic systems with investigation for infectious, toxic, or oncologic causes. Readily treatable etiologies such as infection are addressed as indicated; otherwise, early referral to a hematologist for bone marrow assessment may be necessary, particularly if the etiology is unclear or profound leukopenia, leukocytosis, or disturbances of other cell lines are present suggestive of hematologic malignancy.[26]

58.2.5 Abnormalities of Platelets and Coagulation

Exercise, particularly endurance activities, seems to have a net neutral effect on platelets and coagulation. Certain drugs, toxins, autoimmune disorders, infections, malignancies, and other conditions that trigger disseminated intravascular coagulation (DIC) may produce thrombocytopenia ranging from mild to severe.[26] Acute development of petechiae, bruising, and bleeding problems should prompt investigation for etiologies in these areas. Long-standing history of mild bleeding or bruising problems may indicate von Willebrand's disease or mild factor VIII or IX deficiency. Also, diets deficient in green vegetables may manifest coagulopathy due to impairment of vitamin-K-dependent factors.[26] Evaluation of platelet and coagulation disorders focuses on identification of causative conditions as listed earlier. Laboratory assessment should start with a CBC with peripheral smear looking for abnormalities in all hematologic cell lines. Coagulation studies (prothrombin time [PT], partial thromboplastin time [PTT], and international normalized ratio) should be conducted as well. If the clinical picture suggests DIC (low platelets, fragmented RBCs, prolonged coagulation times), confirmatory testing to include fibrinogen, fibrin split products, and D-dimer should be added.[26] Thrombocytosis is often a transient condition, typically a manifestation of an acute response to physiologic stress. Transient isolated thrombocytosis is rarely of significance. Persistent thrombocytosis should prompt investigation for infection, inflammatory disorders, malignancies, or other hyperproliferative disorders (e.g., polycythemia vera and myeloproliferative diseases).[19]

58.3 SPECIAL CONSIDERATIONS

58.3.1 Sickle-Cell Trait

Sickle-cell trait (SCT) is a common condition present in 8% of blacks in the United States. It typically does not cause anemia and seems to have little impairment of athletic performance[6,8]; however, SCT may confer heightened risk of complications with exercise at altitude, in heat stress environments, in settings of rapid conditioning, or under conditions of sustained maximal exertion efforts. Individuals with SCT may also manifest mild microscopic hematuria that appears to occur independent of physical exertion.[6,13] This hematuria is rarely significant, but should be attributed as hematuria from SCT only after other etiologies are ruled out.[6,13] Hypoxic environments, particularly altitudes above 10,000 ft, may provoke sickling and cause a clinical picture similar to sickle-cell anemia. Exertion at altitudes of 5000 ft or more may produce enough hypoxic and metabolic stress to induce sickling and its sequelae.[6,13]

Individuals with SCT may be at higher risk of exertion-related rhabdomyolysis, particularly in heat stress conditions. Retrospective studies of recruit training populations indicate that SCT may confer increased risk of sudden death and exertional rhabdomyolysis. Although the total incidence is low, the occurrence of sudden death and exertional rhabdomyolysis in blacks with SCT was 30 times higher than in those without and 100 times higher than nonblack recruits without sickle trait.[13] While causative factors are difficult to discern, it is suggested that rapidly advanced conditioning training and sustained maximal exertion efforts increase the risk.[6,13]

Clinical Pearl

While SCT is largely a benign hemoglobinopathy and does not preclude athletic participation, it has rarely been associated with exercise collapse and sudden death.

In light of exertion-related risks, it may be prudent to screen individuals for SCT who are in higher prevalence groups or those with a family history of sickle-cell disease or trait. With known SCT, avoidance of hypoxic environments and strict adherence to heat illness prevention are crucial. Also, avoidance of rapid accelerated training and maximal sustained exertion in unconditioned individuals with SCT may be warranted.

58.3.2 Exertional Rhabdomyolysis

Rhabdomyolysis is a condition of skeletal muscle breakdown with release of myocyte contents into the circulation. Biochemically, muscle injury causes a release of myoglobin and muscle enzymes (creatine phosphokinase [CPK], LDH, transaminases). Severe states with a large volume of muscle damage typically cause electrolyte disturbances (potassium, phosphate, and calcium) plus extracellular fluid shifts into injured tissues.[22,27] Rhabdomyolysis may arise from a variety of insults (e.g., drug or toxin exposure, infection, ischemia, direct trauma such as crush injury or electrical shock, and heat stroke).[22,27] Excessive overload as in weight lifting can produce rhabdomyolysis of an isolated muscle or muscle group. Typically, this is self-limited, rarely manifesting systemic effects beyond the involved muscle. *Exertional rhabdomyolysis* is the term applied to rhabdomyolysis associated with vigorous exercise; it is most frequently seen in running or prolonged exertion activity and often associated with exertional heat illness[2,9,13,22] Certain individuals have higher susceptibility to exertional rhabdomyolysis, particularly those with underlying muscle enzyme deficiencies or metabolic diseases such as diabetes or thyroid disease.[2,22,25] An increased risk of severe rhabdomyolysis is associated with SCT as well. Often, this occurs in conjunction with exertional heat illness (particularly heat stroke) but occasionally manifests in settings of rapidly accelerated physical training and events involving sustained maximal exertion (see Section 58.3.1).[6,9,13] Alcohol consumption, infection, dehydration, preexisting electrolyte disturbances, and chronic acidosis also enhance susceptibility to exertional rhabdomyolysis.[22,27]

The spectrum of exertional rhabdomyolysis ranges from mild muscle injury with negligible symptoms and systemic effects to fulminate cases with large muscle mass injury, severe metabolic derangements, DIC, and death.[9,13,27] Many cases fall between these extremes, with symptoms and laboratory studies indicative of mild-to-moderate injury. While not at imminent risk, these individuals may incur renal injury from myoglobin release and be susceptible to severe rhabdomyolysis if injured muscles are overtaxed prior to completion of healing. The renal toxicity from myoglobin may correlate with both total myoglobin load and duration of renal tubule exposure[27]; therefore, patients with myoglobinuria or myoglobinemia must be treated with aggressive hydration to maintain high urine output until the myoglobin has cleared.[2,22]

Management of rhabdomyolysis focuses on recognizing the occurrence of significant myocyte injury, determining the magnitude of injury, and initiating interventions appropriate to the degree of injury. Clinical indicators of concern are severe muscle pain or weakness much greater than expected. Symptoms may start off being relatively mild but progress in intensity in subsequent hours. Concomitant occurrence of dark urine indicates myoglobinuria. Initial laboratory studies should include basic electrolyte panel ("Chem 7"), CPK, transaminases, LDH, uric acid, CBC, and urinalysis with microscopy. In more severe cases, calcium, phosphate, PT, PTT, fibrinogen, and fibrin split products should be added. It is important to note that muscle enzyme abnormalities often peak 1–2 days after the injury. Urinalysis findings of positive Hgb with no RBCs are used as indicators of myoglobinuria, as myoglobin studies are not quickly available in most settings.[2,10] Muddy casts indicate heavy myoglobin load and likely renal toxicity.[27]

Severity of rhabdomyolysis is gauged initially by magnitude of symptoms and perturbations of blood chemistries. Extreme pain, collapse during exertion, and early electrolyte shifts with acidosis are ominous indicators. In the presence of heat stroke, mental status alterations are typical, with multisystem toxicity manifesting early.[9,10,27] Assessment for the presence and resolution of myoglobinuria is important, as myoglobin-associated renal failure may occur even with mild symptoms.[2,22,27] Initial treatment in all cases of rhabdomyolysis is hydration.[2,22]

Mild cases manifest minimal symptoms that quickly resolve. CPK levels remain low (typically, ≤ 3000 IU/L) with no other laboratory abnormality. If these individuals remain asymptomatic, they may be treated with oral rehydration and rest with return to activity the next day. With more prominent symptoms, rapid IV hydration with 2 L isotonic fluids is indicated. If heat illness is present, rapid cooling measures must be implemented. The patient should be reassessed as fluid bolus is completed and laboratory studies become available. The patient with near or complete resolution of symptoms, modest muscle enzyme elevations (e.g., CPK, 3,000–10,000; transaminases less than twice normal), and otherwise normal studies may be released with continued oral hydration and restricted activity but must be reevaluated within 12–24 hours to assess for persistent or worsening symptoms or significant rise in muscle enzymes (e.g., CPK rise, >1000 mg/dL; transaminase values greater than thrice normal). Serial evaluations should continue until all parameters return to normal. Any case with severe or inadequately improving symptoms, continually rising muscle enzymes, early metabolic derangement, or persistent myoglobinuria requires more aggressive fluid treatment that is optimally done in the hospital.[10] Hospitalization is also warranted if the clinical picture is unclear, other features of concern are present, or compliance with rest is suspect.

Occasionally, patients present with fulminate rhabdomyolysis with massive muscle necrosis. These individuals manifest early severe metabolic derangements with acidosis often accompanied by shock. Many cases of noncardiac exertional sudden death are believed to arise from this condition due to electrolyte-induced dysrhythmias.[2,13] These cases require treatment according to advanced life support protocols for the dysrhythmias and transfer to an intensive-care facility for management of the metabolic derangements. Muscle necrosis in these cases is often perpetuated by increased compartment pressures, even with low elevations, and improves with early fasciotomy of involved muscle areas.[14,28]

Experience with marine recruits demonstrates that healthy individuals with uncomplicated mild to moderate rhabdomyolysis may return to activity immediately after all enzymes have returned to normal. It may be prudent, though, to resume exercise in a graduated manner, particularly if restricted from activity for more than a few days. Recurrent bouts of rhabdomyolysis or any severe episodes warrant investigation for an underlying disease process.[13]

58.4 CONCLUSION

With the exception of athletic pseudoanemia, it is uncommon to encounter significant persistent hematologic alterations from running. While high-intensity and prolonged endurance training may result in alterations of several hematologic parameters and occasionally lysis of RBCs, rarely are these of pathologic significance; however, signs and symptoms of hematologic disease may manifest at an earlier state in athletes due to physiologic demands that require maximal hematologic system performance. The condition of exertional rhabdomyolysis may occasionally manifest in athletes advancing training too rapidly but may also appear in a conditioned athlete in association with underlying disease states or as a consequence of severe overexertion or exertional heat illness. Identification and early treatment of those with myoglobin release or severe myocyte injury is crucial to preclude serious complications (Table 58.5).

TABLE 58.5
SORT: Key Recommendations for Practice

Clinical Recommendation	Evidence Rating	References
In situations where there is an incidental finding of a hematologic test abnormality in the absence of pathologic indicators, it may be prudent to initially repeat the test (e.g., CBC) after the athlete has rested for several days to eliminate acute transient hematologic perturbations.	C	[12,17]
Iron replacement should continue until 6–12 months after anemia has resolved.	C	[23]
All adult men and postmenopausal women with iron-deficiency anemia should be screened for gastrointestinal malignancy.	C	[16]
Initial treatment in all cases of rhabdomyolysis is hydration.	A	[2,22]
Recurrent bouts of rhabdomyolysis or any severe episodes warrant investigation for an underlying disease process.	C	[13]

REFERENCES

1. Abramson SD, Abramson N. "Common" uncommon anemias. *American Family Physician.* 1999;59(4):851–861.
2. Baggaley PA, *Rhabdomyolysis.* http://members.tripod.com/~baggas/rhabdo.html#pathogenesis; 1997. Accessed July 30, 2015.
3. Cook JD, The effect of endurance training on iron metabolism. *Seminars in Hematology.* 1994;31(3):146–154.
4. Eichner ER, Anemia and blood doping. In: Sallis RE, Massimino F (eds.). *Essentials of Sports Medicine.* St. Louis, MO: Mosby; 1997: pp. 35–38.
5. Eichner ER, Sports anemia, iron supplements and blood doping. *Medicine & Science in Sports & Exercise.* 1992; 24(9, Suppl):315–318.
6. Eichner ER. Sickle cell trait, heroic exercise and fatal collapse. *Physician and Sportsmedicine.* 1993;21(7):51–64.
7. Eichner ER, Scott WA. Exercise as disease detector. *Physician and Sportsmedicine.* 1998;26(3):41–52.
8. Fields KB. The athlete with anemia. In: Fields KB, Fricker PA (eds.). *Medical Problems in Athletes.* Malden, MA: Blackwell Scientific; 1997: pp. 259–265.
9. Gardner JW, Kark JA. Clinical diagnosis, management, and surveillance of exertional heat illness. In: *Textbooks of Military Medicine: Medical Aspects of Harsh Environments,* Vol. 1. Washington, D.C.: U.S. Government Printing Office; 2002: pp. 231–181.
10. Gardner JW, Kark JA. Heat-associated illness. In: Srickland GT (ed.). *Hunter's Tropical Medicine,* 8th edn. Philadelphia, PA: Saunders; 2000: pp. 140–147.
11. Harris SS. Helping active women avoid anemia. *Physician and Sportsmedicine.* 1995;23(5):35–48.
12. Jandl JH. Blood cell formation. In: Jandl JH (ed.). *Blood Textbook of Hematology.* New York: Little Brown & Co.; 1996: pp. 53–55.
13. Kark JA, Ward FT. Exercise and hemoglobin S. *Seminars in Hematology.* 1994;31(3):181–225.
14. Kuklo TR et al. Fatal rhabdomyolysis with bilateral gluteal, thigh, and leg compartment syndrome after the army physical fitness test. *American Journal of Sports Medicine.* 2000;28(1):112–116.
15. Lee GR. Acute posthemorrhagic anemia. In: Nique TA (ed.). *Wintrobe's Clinical Hematology,* 10th edn. Baltimore, MD: Lippincott Williams & Wilkins; 1999: pp. 1485–1488.
16. Lee GR. Anemia: A diagnostic strategy. In: Nique TA (ed.). *Wintrobe's Clinical Hematology,* 10th edn. Baltimore, MD: Lippincott Williams & Wilkins; 1999: pp. 908–940.
17. Lee GR. Anemia: General aspects. In: Nique TA (ed.). *Wintrobe's Clinical Hematology,* 10th edn. Baltimore, MD: Lippincott Williams & Wilkins; 1999: pp. 897–907.
18. Lee GR. Hemolytic disorders: General considerations. In: Nique TA (ed.). *Wintrobe's Clinical Hematology,* 10th edn. Baltimore, MD: Lippincott Williams & Wilkins; 1999: pp. 1109–1131.
19. Levine SP. Thrombocytosis. In: Nique TA (ed.). *Wintrobe's Clinical Hematology,* 10th edn. Baltimore, MD: Lippincott Williams & Wilkins; 1999: pp. 897–940, 1109–1131, 1485–1488, 1648–1660.
20. Little DR. Ambulatory management of common forms of anemia. *American Family Physician.* 1999;59:1598–1604.
21. Means RT. Polycythemia: Erythrocytosis. In: Nique TA (ed.). *Wintrobe's Clinical Hematology,* 10th edn. Baltimore, MD: Lippincott Williams & Wilkins; 1999: pp. 1538–1554.

22. O'Connor FG, Deuster PA. Rhabdomyolysis. In Goldman L, Schafer A (eds.) *Goldman-Cecil Medicine, 25th Edition.* Philadelphia, PA: Saunders Elsevier, pp. 723–726.
23. Selby G. When does an athlete need iron? *Physician and Sportsmedicine.* 1991;19(4):96–102.
24. Selby GB, Eichner ER. Hematocrit and performance: The effect of endurance training on blood volume. *Seminars in Hematology.* 1994;31(2):122–127.
25. Simon TL. Induced erythrocythemia and athletic performance. *Seminars in Hematology.* 1994;31(2):128–133.
26. Tenglin R. Hematologic abnormalities. In: Lillegard WA, Butcher JD, Rucker KS (eds.). *Handbook of Sports Medicine: A Symptom-Oriented Approach*, 2nd edn. Boston, MA: Butterworth-Heinemann; 1999: pp. 331–335.
27. Vivweswaran P, Guntupalli J. Environmental emergencies: Rhabdomyolysis, *Critical Care Clinics.* 1999;15(2):415–428.
28. Wise JJ, Fortin PT. Bilateral exercise induced thigh compartment syndrome diagnosed as exertional rhabdomyolysis: A case report and review of the literature. *American Journal of Sports Medicine.* 1997;25(1):126–129.

59 Allergic Diseases in Athletes

David L. Brown, Linda L. Brown, and Alain Michael P. Abellada

CONTENTS

TABLE 59.1
Key Clinical Considerations

1. Athletes have to be especially careful as medication use may affect their eligibility for competition. Because restrictions on over-the-counter and prescription medications can change, athletes should discuss the status of medications with the governing body for their particular sport or level of competition prior to use.
2. Oral decongestants and antihistamines can potentially interfere with heat dissipation and should be avoided during athletic training or competition in the heat.
3. Consultation with an allergy specialist is indicated when considering immunotherapy for allergic rhinitis and/or drastic environmental interventions.
4. For effective AIT, athletes need to commit to 3–5 years of treatment in order to sustain remission of their symptoms. Any individual who is unable to fully commit to treatment, has poorly controlled asthma, or is on a beta-blocker should not receive AIT.
5. For urticaria/angioedema, referral to an allergist is recommended for persistent symptoms poorly controlled on the usual medical therapy, suspected allergic component precipitating symptoms, severe angioedema, or a history of respiratory distress or hypotension.
6. Athletes presenting with anaphylaxis should be observed a minimum of 3 hours after symptoms have resolved following a mild reaction. An individual should be observed at least 6 hours after a more severe reaction, and hospitalization should be strongly considered to monitor for late-phase reactions.

59.1 INTRODUCTION

While allergic symptoms may at first appear to be a minor nuisance affecting athletes, medical providers should not underestimate their prevalence and impact. Allergic rhinitis alone affects approximately 58 million people in the United States annually.[30] Worldwide, allergic rhinitis affects 400 million people.[13] It is the fifth most common chronic disease and the most prevalent in patients under 18 years of age. Compared to patients without allergic rhinitis, the average number of annual prescriptions for patient with allergic rhinitis is almost double (10 prescriptions vs. 19 prescriptions).[29] The cost to treat allergic rhinitis almost doubled from 6.1 billion dollars in 2000 to 11.2 billion dollars in 2005.[11] Other allergic conditions can beset athletes as well. Overall, 12%–22% of the general population will suffer from at least one subtype of urticaria at some time in their lives, with a prevalence of 0.11%–0.6%.[27] The incidence of anaphylaxis is 50–2000 episodes per 100,000 person-years, with a possible *lifetime* prevalence of 0.05%–2%[4] with a mortality rate of 1%.[18,37] More important to the individual athlete is that these conditions can affect not only their physical capacity but also their psychological motivation to train and compete. Allergic rhinitis, in particular, may also be a harbinger of other atopic conditions such as eczema and asthma (Table 59.1).

59.2 RHINITIS

59.2.1 Pathophysiology

Allergic rhinitis occurs when an individual develops immunoglobulin E (IgE) sensitization to aeroallergens. Subsequent inhalation of these aeroallergens cross-links IgE receptors on mast cells in the respiratory epithelium, leading to the release of histamine and other chemical mediators of inflammation. The etiology of nonallergic rhinitis, which can be difficult to distinguish clinically from allergic rhinitis, is unknown.

59.2.2 Evaluation

A detailed history is of utmost importance in differentiating allergic and nonallergic rhinitis. Allergic rhinitis is typically associated with rhinorrhea, postnasal drip, and congestion. Other common symptoms include sneezing and cough as well as nasal and soft palate pruritus. Eye pruritus, injection, irritation, and watery discharge may indicate coexisting allergic conjunctivitis. Patients may also complain of generalized irritability and fatigue. Symptoms will occur upon reexposure to any aeroallergen to which a patient is sensitized; therefore, asking about seasonal exacerbations as well as indoor versus outdoor predominance of symptoms is crucial. Seasonal symptoms will often be due to pollen exposure. Spring and early summer exacerbations will occur with tree and grass pollination, while late summer and fall symptoms are usually due to weeds and mold. Perennial symptoms may be a sequential combination of these allergens. Alternatively, especially if symptom flares are mainly indoors, the athlete may be sensitive to cockroaches, dust mites, pet dander, or molds.

Allergic and nonallergic rhinitis presentations can be nearly identical, but nonallergic rhinitis patients complain about prominent nasal congestion, while nasal, eye, and soft palate pruritus are usually absent. Nonallergic rhinitis symptoms are often perennial and triggered by strong odors or smoke. However, fluctuations in air temperature, humidity, and barometric pressure occurring with the change in seasons may lead to exacerbations, making it difficult to differentiate from allergic rhinitis. After questioning the athlete regarding the symptoms and precipitants listed, the physician should also conduct a thorough review of the athlete's past medical and family history looking for asthma, allergies, and eczema that would lead to a higher index of suspicion for allergic rhinitis.

Clinical Pearl

Though allergic and nonallergic rhinitis presentations can be nearly identical, nonallergic rhinitis patients complain about prominent nasal congestion, while nasal, eye, and soft palate pruritus are usually absent.

The utility of physical examination in distinguishing allergic and nonallergic rhinitis is poor; however, some pertinent clues can be helpful. The nasal mucosa in allergic rhinitis is classically described as pale or bluish; however, as in nonallergic rhinitis, the mucosa can be red and edematous or may appear normal. Posterior pharyngeal cobblestoning is associated with postnasal drip of any etiology. Likewise, the so-called allergic shiners from infraorbital venous congestion are also nonspecific. Findings that are more suggestive of allergic rhinitis include an accentuated transverse nasal crease seen in children who repeatedly rub their nose due to pruritus, atopic stigmata such as eczema, and wheezing on auscultation.

59.2.3 Management

Treatment for allergic rhinitis is multifaceted but typically starts with avoidance measures. If these are ineffective, medical therapy can be initiated in a stepwise fashion (Figure 59.1). Ultimately, immunotherapy may be necessary if symptoms remain uncontrolled.[12]

59.2.3.1 Allergen Avoidance

Allergen avoidance, especially for allergies triggered by pollen or irritants (i.e., tobacco smoke and formaldehyde), is a very important treatment modality in managing allergic rhinitis. For patients allergic to animal dander, avoidance is always best.[8] However, consistent exclusion of the pet from the bedroom and the use of an HEPA filter may provide some benefit. For dust mite allergy, occlusive covers on the pillows, mattress, and box springs are essential. Frequent washing of bed linens and blankets in hot water is helpful. Dehumidifiers and removing carpet may also be required for highly sensitive patients. There is increasing evidence that HEPA filters are effective for reducing dust mite exposure.[31] Mold allergen

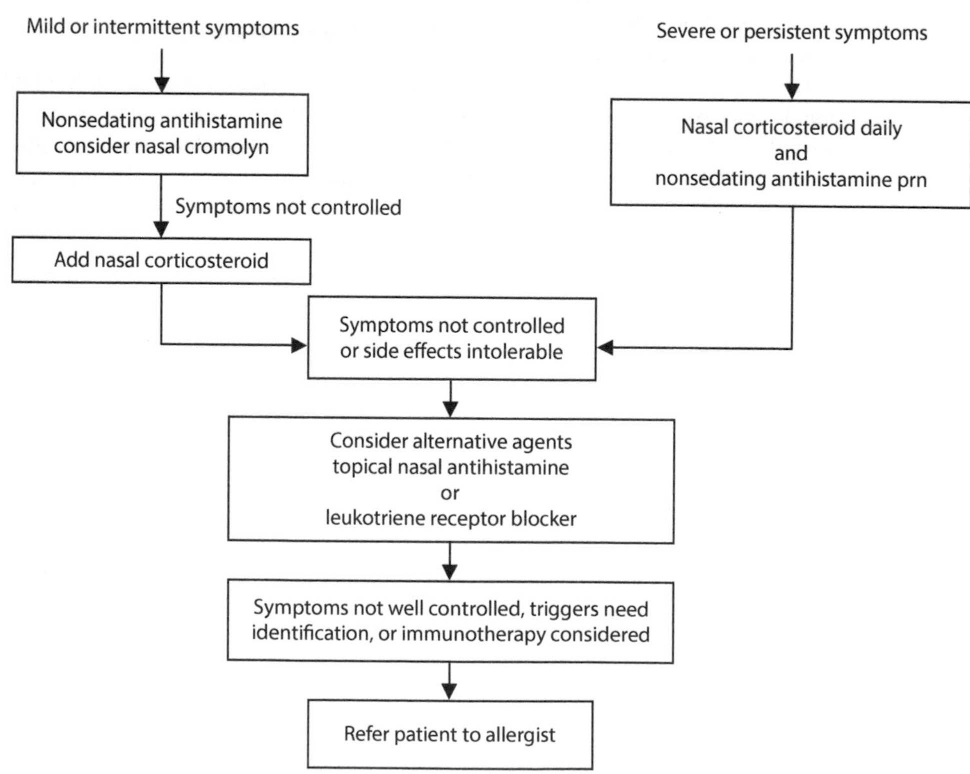

FIGURE 59.1 Stepwise therapy for allergic rhinitis.

can be difficult to control, but dehumidifiers and scrupulous cleaning can be beneficial.

59.2.3.2 Medical Therapy

Several medication classes are available for the control of rhinitis, including decongestants, oral and topical antihistamines, cromolyn, corticosteroids, and leukotriene (LT) receptor blockers. Oral decongestants, such as pseudoephedrine, are effective at relieving nasal congestion in patients with allergic rhinitis. However, there is insufficient evidence that combining an oral decongestant with an antihistamine increases the efficacy for treatment of allergic rhinitis compared to either drug alone.[8] The side effects of oral decongestants include insomnia, loss of appetite, irritability, and palpitations, and thus athletes should exercise caution in using them.[11] Because of peripheral vasoconstriction, they also interfere with heat dissipation and should be avoided during training or competition in the heat. Topical nasal decongestants such as oxymetazoline should be reserved for short-term control of severe congestion. Their use should be limited to no more than 3 days. If used longer than 5–7 days, they can cause severe rebound congestion and rhinorrhea known as rhinitis medicamentosa. Antihistamines act as competitive binders to the H1 receptor and are proven effective in relieving sneezing, itching, and watery rhinorrhea in allergic rhinitis. Their efficacy is roughly equivalent to nasal cromolyn but less than nasal steroids. They provide little relief of nasal obstruction and are generally ineffective in the treatment of nonallergic rhinitis. First-generation antihistamines can cause significant sedation, decreased alertness, and performance impairment, making them undesirable for most competitive athletes. These effects can exist even without an individual being aware of them. Dosing sedating antihistamines only at night may still cause daytime impairment. When compared to first-generation antihistamines, second-generation antihistamines are generally preferred. Second-generation antihistamines have less tendency to cause sedation, performance impairment, and/or anticholinergic adverse effects[6,36,39] (see Table 59.2). The other caveat to antihistamine use is that they have the potential to decrease heat dissipation by their anticholinergic effects on sweat glands. Thus, as is true for sympathomimetics, athletes should use them with caution during high-intensity training or competition and when ambient temperatures are high. Intranasal corticosteroids are the most effective medications for treating allergic rhinitis. They are more effective than the combined use of an antihistamine and an LT antagonist.[9,25,40] Intranasal corticosteroids act by inhibiting gene expression of inflammatory mediators. Several days of treatment are usually necessary for maximal effectiveness. Nasal steroids can be used periodically during the year, depending on the athlete's allergy season. However, when such treatment is initiated, the steroid must be administered regularly for consistent efficacy (see Table 59.3). Topical steroids have a low rate of side effects, which include irritation, burning, sneezing, and bloody nasal discharge.

Some providers may be concerned about starting nasal steroids for fear of side effects from chronic use or growth disturbance in a skeletally immature athlete; however, when taken appropriately, even chronic nasal steroid use is not associated with any significant adrenal suppression, nasal or pharyngeal candidiasis, cataracts, or glaucoma.[3,19] Intranasal fluticasone propionate, mometasone furoate, and budesonide have no effect on growth at recommended doses compared with placebo[1,22,33] and even when used at reference values (at as much as two times the recommended doses).[33] Although growth studies on beclomethasone dosed at 168 μg twice daily for 1 year in children aged 6–9 years showed a mean decrease in height compared to placebo of 0.9 cm ($p < 0.01$), growth studies for mometasone furoate (Nasonex®) dosed at 100 μg daily for 1 year in children aged 3–9 years and for fluticasone (Flonase®) dosed at two sprays daily in children aged 4–11 years showed no difference in growth compared to placebo.[1,32,33]

Cromolyn, a topical mast cell stabilizer, has a low potential for toxicity and provides modest improvement in the sneezing, itching, and rhinorrhea associated with allergic rhinitis. It is

TABLE 59.2
Second-Generation Oral Antihistamines

	Dose	Sedation
Cetirizine (Zyrtec®)	Age ≥ 6, 5–10 mg qd Age 2–5, 2.5–5 mg qd (syrup)	Slightly higher than placebo but less than first generation
Desloratadine (Clarinex®)	Age ≥ 12, 5 mg qd	No different than placebo[a]
Fexofenadine (Allegra®)	Age ≥ 12, 180 mg qd or 60 mg bid Age 6–11, 30 mg bid	No different than placebo
Levocetirizine (Xyzal®)	Age ≥ 12, 5 mg qd Age 6–11, 2.5 mg qd (syrup)	Slightly higher than placebo but less than first generation
Loratadine (Claritin®)	Age > 6, 10 mg qd	No different than placebo at 10 mg; sedating at higher doses

[a] Note that 7% of population may have sedation due to decreased metabolism of the drug.

TABLE 59.3
Topical Nasal Corticosteroids

	Dose (Sprays per Nostril)
Beclomethasone (Beconase AQ®, Vancenase AQ DS®)	Age ≥ 12, 1–2 bid; ages 6–11, 1 bid
Budesonide (Nasonex)	Age ≥ 12, 1–4 qd; ages 6–11, 1–2 qd
Ciclesonide (Omnaris®)	Age ≥, 2 qd
Fluticasone (Flonase)	Age ≥ 12, 2 qd; ages 4–11, same, but start at 1 qd
Flunisolide (Nasarel®)	Age > 14, 2 bid to qid; ages 6–11, 1–2 qd
Mometasone furoate (Nasonex)	Age ≥ 12, 2 qd; ages 3–11, 1 qd
Triamcinolone (Nasacort AQ®)	Age ≥ 12, 2 qd; ages 6–11, 1–2 qd

useful when administered prophylactically prior to allergen exposure; however, it often requires dosing up to 4–6 times daily to be effective, which may affect compliance and therefore symptom control.

LT receptor antagonists such as montelukast (Singulair®) provide mild improvement in symptoms of seasonal allergic rhinitis with efficacy similar to second-generation antihistamines.[24] These agents are well tolerated with a side effect profile no different than placebo. LT receptor antagonist therapy should be considered when nasal steroids and/or antihistamines fail or side effects are intolerable. They can also be considered for use in an athlete who may benefit from this therapy for treatment of concomitant asthma. Dosing is 4 mg for ages 2–5, 5 mg for ages 6–11, and 10 mg for ages 12 and above.

Topical nasal antihistamines such as azelastine (Astelin®, Astepro®) and olopatadine (Patanase®) are effective in providing short-term relief of symptoms due to both allergic and nonallergic rhinitis. Intranasal antihistamines are efficacious and have been shown to be equal to oral second-generation antihistamines for treatment of seasonal allergic rhinitis.[2] Side effects include drowsiness and an unpleasant aftertaste. Intranasal antihistamines may be considered as a first-line treatment for allergic rhinitis or as part of combination therapy with intranasal corticosteroids.[26] Dosing for patients aged 5–11 years is one spray twice daily; for those 12 years or older, the dose is two sprays twice daily. Ipratropium bromide (Atrovent®) 0.03% nasal spray is effective for treating rhinorrhea, particularly vasomotor-induced rhinorrhea triggered by cold air or exercise. It has no effect on pruritus or congestion. Side effects include occasional epistaxis and nasal dryness but no systemic anticholinergic or rebound effects. The dose is two sprays 30 minutes prior to exercise or exposure, and it may be used two or three times daily for patients over 6 years of age. When these treatments fail, it is important to consider not only medication inadequacy or noncompliance but also the possibility of other diagnoses such as anatomical or physical obstruction and chronic sinusitis.

59.2.3.3 Athlete-Specific Medication Issues

Athletes, especially at the collegiate or elite levels, have to be especially careful as medication use may affect their eligibility for competition. Because restrictions on over-the-counter and prescription medications can change, athletes should discuss the status of medications with the governing body for their particular sport or level of competition prior to its use. This would include the National Collegiate Athletic Association (NCAA) and U.S. Olympic Committee (USOC). In general, the NCAA has no restrictions on any allergy-related products with the exception that any products containing ephedrine are banned. The USOC, however, is much more stringent. All sympathomimetic-containing medications are banned. All glucocorticosteroids are prohibited when administered by oral, intravenous, intramuscular, or rectal routes.[38]

59.2.3.4 Allergy Testing

Typically, referral to an allergy specialist for skin testing should be made when a patient's history is suggestive of allergic rhinitis and institution of immunotherapy is being considered for poor response to medical therapy. Allergy consultation is also recommended when drastic environmental interventions are being considered such as pet elimination, taking up carpets, or purchasing new mattresses, bedding, dust mite covers, etc. It is important to stop antihistamines for 1 week prior to testing so as not to blunt the cutaneous response to skin testing. Allergy testing is contraindicated in the setting of severe lung disease or poorly controlled asthma with a forced expiratory volume in 1 second of less than 70%. Skin testing is generally preferred over in vitro tests such as ImmunoCAP® or radioallergosorbent testing because it is considered more sensitive. In vitro testing is helpful for validating the diagnosis and supporting environmental controls. Although it is less sensitive than skin testing, it is a reasonable alternative when skin testing cannot be performed.

Clinical Pearl

Consultation with an allergy specialist is indicated when considering immunotherapy for allergic rhinitis and/or drastic environmental interventions.

59.2.3.5 Allergen Immunotherapy

Allergen immunotherapy (AIT) desensitizes the allergic individual to an allergen over an extended treatment period to diminish allergic symptoms. It is an effective treatment for allergic rhinitis and allergic asthma. AIT also has persistent benefits after immunotherapy is discontinued[10,16] and can reduce the risk for the future development of asthma in patients with allergic rhinitis.[14–16,23,31,34] Prior to starting any AIT, it is important to verify allergen sensitivities by skin or in vitro testing. Subcutaneous AIT starts with a buildup phase involving weekly injections. Upon completion of the buildup phase, patients receive monthly maintenance injections. Patients should be advised that notable symptom relief usually takes several months of treatment. Athletes also need to commit to 3–5 years of treatment in order to sustain remission of their symptoms. Any individual who is unable to fully commit to treatment, has poorly controlled asthma, or is on a beta-blocker should not receive AIT. There is a small risk of a systemic allergic reaction with each injection, so it is important that AIT be administered by a board-certified allergist who can engage in a thorough discussion with the athlete regarding the benefits and potential risks of therapy. Ongoing follow-up with the allergist is warranted to ensure appropriate dosing to achieve optimal benefit while avoiding systemic reactions.

Clinical Pearl

Athletes need to commit to 3–5 years of AIT treatment in order to sustain remission of their symptoms.

Sublingual immunotherapy (SLIT) involves placement of the allergen under the tongue for local absorption. This is a viable alternative to subcutaneous AIT and has garnered much attention due to its ease of administration and lower rate of systemic reactions. One systematic review involving 63 randomized controlled trials (n = 5131) showed strong evidence that SLIT use improves asthma symptoms, moderate evidence showing a decrease in rhinitis and rhinoconjunctivitis symptoms, and moderate evidence demonstrating a > 40% decrease in medication use for asthma and allergies. However, the authors concluded that high-quality studies are still needed to determine optimal dosing strategies.[20] SLIT is widely used in Europe but has been less available in the United States. Recently, the FDA approved sublingual tablets for allergies caused by grass (Grastek®, Oralair®) and ragweed (Ragwitek®) and more allergens are in development. The advantage of this form of immunotherapy is that after the first dose in the doctor's office, the daily administrations may be taken at home. This has obvious advantages for a busy athlete's schedule. Patients must be counseled on the risk of anaphylaxis and advised to carry an epinephrine autoinjector. Because therapy must be initiated at least 3–4 months prior to the start of the pollen season, patients should be referred to an allergist well before the patient's allergy season if they are interested in this form of treatment.

TABLE 59.4
Allergic Conjunctivitis Topical Medications

Topical Agent	Mechanism of Action	Dose
Azelastine (Optivar®)	Antihistamine	1 drop bid
Cromolyn (Crolom®)	Mast cell blocker	1–2 drops, 4–6 times/day
Emedastine (Emadine®)	Antihistamine	1 drop qid
Ketotifen (Zaditor®)	Mast cell blocker/ antihistamine	1 drop bid to tid
Levocabastine (Livostin®)	Antihistamine	1–2 drops qid
Lodoxamide (Alomide®)	Mast cell blocker	1–2 drops qid
Naphcon A®, Opcon A®, Vasocon A®, Visine A®	Antihistamine/ decongestants	Up to qid
Nedocromil (Alocril®)	Inhibits activation and mediator release from inflammatory cells	1–2 drops bid
Olopatadine (Patanol®)	Mast cell blocker/ antihistamine	1 drop bid; age >3
Pemirolast (Alamast®)	Mast cell blocker	2 drops qid

59.3 ALLERGIC CONJUNCTIVITIS

The etiology for acute allergic conjunctivitis is the same as for allergic rhinitis. In this particular case, symptoms occur upon inoculation of the allergen onto the mucosa of the eyes. Individuals with animal dander sensitivity are especially prone to ocular symptoms. Seasonal allergic conjunctivitis is most likely to be severe in pollen-sensitive patients during tree pollen season. The treatment of allergic conjunctivitis can be achieved with the same measures as discussed with allergic rhinitis; however, if ocular symptoms persist despite other therapies or occur in isolation, targeted use of medications specifically for the eye is warranted (see Table 59.4). Combination mast cell blocker and antihistamine topical therapy is very effective. Other options include topical mast cell blockers or antihistamine alone, topical decongestants, and topical mast cell stabilizers. Topical corticosteroids are associated with significant complications and should only be used after consultation with an ophthalmologist.

59.4 URTICARIA AND ANGIOEDEMA

59.4.1 Pathophysiology

Urticaria is a condition occurring secondary to mast cell degranulation in the superficial dermis. It is characterized by pruritic, erythematous, cutaneous elevations that blanch with pressure. These evanescent hives may occur anywhere on the body but more often occur on the trunk and extremities. Immunologically, a variety of potential mediators are involved in urticaria, but all lead to blood vessel dilation and edema. These mediators include histamine, prostaglandins, LTs, platelet-activating factor, anaphylatoxins, bradykinin, and Hageman factor. Acute urticaria is defined as new-onset symptoms of less than 6 weeks in duration. If symptoms persist longer than 6 weeks, it is considered chronic urticaria. In patients who go on to have chronic urticaria, 75% have symptoms over 1 year, 50% have symptoms over 5 years, and 20% have symptoms for decades. Angioedema is similar pathologically to urticaria but occurs in the deeper dermis and subcutaneous tissues. Unlike urticaria, angioedema is more painful and burning than it is pruritic and often involves the face. Urticaria can occur at any age but is most common in children and young adults. Approximately 50% of patients at presentation have both urticaria and angioedema, 40% have urticaria only, and 10% have angioedema only.[37]

In the vast majority of cases, the cause of urticaria is idiopathic. Over half of all cases of chronic idiopathic urticaria are thought to be caused by an autoimmune mechanism with either IgG autoantibody acting against the IgE receptor or against IgE itself causing mast cell and basophil activation. In the minority of urticaria cases caused by an inciting factor, potential triggers include medications, insect stings, foods and food additives, and infections. It is beyond the scope of this chapter to review all of these, but Table 59.5 lists the most common known triggers. In addition to these triggers, various physical exposures can lead to urticaria as well (see Table 59.6). These physical urticarias are especially important to consider in athletes because they can be triggered by conditions that occur during practice and competition.[5]

Cholinergic urticaria is caused by an elevation in core body temperature and is classically precipitated by exercise or use of hot tubs. Initially small, papular, pruritic papules will occur followed by wheals with flare. Symptom onset is usually within 2–30 minutes and lasts up to 90 minutes.

TABLE 59.5
Common Triggers for Urticaria

Medical Conditions
- Autoimmune-mediated urticaria
- Autoimmune thyroid disease

Medications
- Antibiotics (beta-lactams, sulfa compounds)
- Nonsteroidal anti-inflammatories
- Progesterone
- Local anesthetics
- Opioid analgesics

Physical Contacts
- Latex
- Nickel
- Plants and plant resins
- Fruits/vegetables
- Raw fish
- Animal saliva

Insect Stings

Foods and Food Additives
- Milk
- Egg
- Peanut
- Nuts
- Soy
- Wheat
- Fish/shellfish
- Sulfites

Infections
- Coxsackie A and B
- Hepatitis A, B, C
- HIV
- Epstein–Barr virus
- Herpes simplex
- Intestinal parasites
- Dermatophyte infections

Cold urticaria is precipitated by rewarming following contact with a cold object. Within 2–5 minutes, the area exposed to the cold develops swelling and pruritus. Symptoms generally worsen after the area is warmed and can last up to 2 hours. Placing an ice cube on the skin for 15 minutes and observing for presence of hive formation can confirm the diagnosis. A risk of anaphylaxis exists with this condition due to massive histamine release if patients have a significant drop in core body temperature, such as with swimming or diving; therefore, patients with cold urticaria should avoid these activities.

Aquagenic urticaria is extremely rare and is caused by contact with water. In athletes who participate in water sports, this condition could be confused with both cholinergic and cold urticaria. Unlike cholinergic urticaria, with aquagenic urticaria, symptoms still occur even when the water temperature is cool and even if the patient is not exercising in the water. It can be distinguished from cold urticaria because it will not be precipitated by application of a cold object that is not water based.

Solar urticaria is rare and is precipitated by exposure to ultraviolet light. Anaphylaxis could occur if large body areas are exposed. Avoidance of ultraviolet light exposure is the best therapy in addition to liberal sunscreen use.

Pressure urticaria (angioedema) accounts for less than 1% of all urticarias. It is precipitated by direct pressure on the skin. In this type of urticaria, skin pressure is followed 3–12 hours later by localized hives as well as fever, malaise, and leukocytosis. Symptoms can last up to 24 hours. It can be precipitated by running, clapping, sitting, or using hand equipment. The diagnosis can be confirmed by applying a 15 lb weight to an individual's skin for 20 minutes and then examining the patient 4–8 hours later for characteristic signs and symptoms.

Symptomatic dermatographism is another type of physical urticaria. It occurs in 2%–5% of the general population and is characterized by the development of linear, pruritic wheals 2–5 minutes after stroking or rubbing the skin.

TABLE 59.6
Physical Urticarias

Type	Precipitant	Evaluation	Treatment
Cholinergic urticaria	Elevation in core temperature; exercise	History.	Premedicate with nonsedating antihistamine.
Cold urticaria	Rewarming after contact with cold object	Place cold object on skin for 15 minutes and look for urticaria upon rewarming.	Use nonsedating antihistamines as needed; avoid swimming and diving sports due to risk of anaphylaxis.
Aquagenic urticaria	Water contact	History; expose skin to water and look for changes.	Use nonsedating antihistamines.
Solar urticaria	Ultraviolet light exposure	Expose small, unprotected patch of skin to sunlight.	Limit sun exposure; wear protective clothing; use sunscreen.
Pressure urticaria/ angioedema	Direct pressure on skin; running, prolonged sitting, clapping, etc.	Place 15 lb weight on patient for 20 minutes and look for skin changes; test for fever and leukocytosis 3–12 hours later.	Avoid precipitants; use nonsedating antihistamines and NSAIDs; consider steroid burst/taper if symptoms are severe.
Symptomatic dermatographism	Stroking or rubbing skin; areas where clothing or equipment abrades skin	Look for linear, pruritic wheal 2–5 minutes after rubbing the skin.	Wear loose-fitting clothing; treatment usually not necessary; nonsedating antihistamines can be used but only for severe symptoms.

59.4.2 Evaluation

The history is most important in helping to define the onset and time course of these conditions. In the acute setting, providers should also assess the existence of coexisting symptoms that could indicate anaphylaxis rather than isolated urticaria or angioedema (see section on anaphylaxis and anaphylactoid reactions). While in most cases the precipitant remains unknown, a detailed history may isolate a trigger. Searching for a trigger is more beneficial in acute urticaria as compared to chronic urticaria, where an etiology is found in less than 10% of cases.

When the cause is found, drug hypersensitivity is most common; thus, individuals should be asked about any recent prescription or over-the-counter medications. For athletes, in particular, it is important to inquire about supplement use. Food and food additives rarely cause isolated urticaria, but the relationship to food inhalation, contact, and consumption should be documented. It is also important to document the relationship to physical triggers (e.g., heat, cold, sunlight, water, and skin pressure), occupational exposures, recent insect envenomation, and any recent illnesses. A thorough review of systems is important to help rule out any disease associations such as an acute bacterial or viral illness, parasitic infection, autoimmune/collagen vascular disease, serum sickness, endocrine disease, and malignancy.[7] The physical examination is especially helpful in the acute setting when skin manifestations are present. This can help document whether urticaria and angioedema are occurring in isolation or together as well as any signs of an anaphylactic reaction. A thorough exam should also look for evidence of the other diseases that are more rarely associated with urticaria and angioedema.

The use of laboratory and imaging studies should be targeted by the history and physical assessment. Given the association of chronic autoimmune urticaria with autoimmune thyroid disease, a thyroid function panel and thyroid autoantibodies should be drawn. If enlargement or nodularity of the thyroid is present, a thyroid ultrasound and nuclear medicine thyroid studies should be considered. A monospot or Epstein–Barr virus antibody titers can be ordered if acute mononucleosis is suspected. Testing for hepatitis A, B, and C as well as acute human immunodeficiency virus (HIV) infection may be warranted. The association of urticaria with other viral infections remains unclear, and routine testing for other viral pathogens is not recommended. If a significant travel history is discovered and the complete blood count shows eosinophilia, stool studies should be obtained looking for intestinal parasites. Progressive weight loss and/or the presence of lymphadenopathy or hepatosplenomegaly on exam would warrant an evaluation for an underlying lymphoreticular malignancy. Testing for hereditary or acquired C1 esterase inhibitor deficiency should be considered in any athlete presenting with recurrent isolated angioedema. A skin biopsy looking for vasculitis is indicated when individual urticarial lesions last longer than 24 hours or are associated with purpura, pain, hyperpigmentation, or systemic symptoms.[28]

Clinical Pearl

A skin biopsy looking for vasculitis is indicated when individual urticarial lesions last longer than 24 hours or are associated with purpura, pain, hyperpigmentation, or systemic symptoms.

If the history and physical exam are unrevealing, conducting a limited laboratory evaluation consisting of a complete blood count with differential, C-reactive protein, erythrocyte sedimentation rate, thyroid function panel, liver panel, and urinalysis is reasonable to screen for occult conditions. See Table 59.6 for evaluation of the physical urticarias.

59.4.3 Management

After the initial evaluation, the management of urticaria and angioedema becomes primarily symptomatic. Because food and food additives are a rare cause of chronic urticaria and angioedema, elimination diets are usually unnecessary unless the patient gives a history pinpointing a specific food. Any known trigger, of course, should be avoided.

Mild symptoms can be controlled with a low sedating antihistamine (see Table 59.2). If symptoms are more moderate or poorly controlled, the antihistamine dose should be maximized prior to considering add-on therapy. Additive therapies include LT antagonists, H2 blockers, and nighttime doxepin. For periods of moderate to severe symptoms, prednisone therapy tapered over 6–12 days can be helpful.

Referral to an allergist is recommended when a suspected allergic component is precipitating symptoms, when symptoms are not well controlled with the therapies listed earlier, when the patient has a history of respiratory distress or hypotension suggesting anaphylaxis, or in cases of severe angioedema. The athlete should be referred to a dermatologist for skin biopsy if urticarial vasculitis is suspected. The management of the physical urticarias is detailed in Table 59.6.

The allergist may consider other immunomodulatory medication options to include cyclosporin, dapsone, and methotrexate. Most recently, omalizumab (Xolair), a humanized monoclonal antibody that binds IgE, has been approved by the FDA to treat chronic urticaria. Doses of 150–300 mg every 4 weeks have been shown to significantly improve symptoms in patients with chronic idiopathic urticaria whose symptoms cannot be adequately controlled on antihistamines.[21] Although more costly than other treatments, omalizumab's efficacy, more favorable side effect profile, and monthly dosing make it a preferred option.

59.5 ANAPHYLACTIC AND ANAPHYLACTOID REACTIONS

59.5.1 Pathophysiology

Anaphylaxis is an acute, life-threatening, systemic reaction mediated through IgE antibodies and their receptors. It requires previous sensitization and subsequent reexposure to an allergen.

Anaphylactoid reactions are clinically indistinguishable from true anaphylaxis because both are caused by massive release of potent chemical mediators from mast cells and basophils. As such, both are managed with the same treatment measures discussed here. The difference is that anaphylactoid reactions are not mediated by IgE antibodies, they do not require prior sensitization, and they are less commonly associated with severe hypotension and cardiovascular collapse.

A typical case of anaphylaxis includes cutaneous signs or symptoms accompanied by obstructive respiratory symptoms and/or hemodynamic changes. Additional features include gastrointestinal complaints and a sense of impending doom. The onset of symptoms typically begins seconds to minutes after the inciting cause. More rarely, symptoms may be delayed for up to 2 hours. Approximately half of cases have a uniphasic course with abrupt, severe onset and death within minutes despite treatment. Up to 20% of cases have a biphasic presentation with immediate symptoms followed by an asymptomatic period for 1–8 hours. A late-phase reaction subsequently ensues with recurrence of severe symptoms. These symptoms are protracted, persisting for several hours in 28% of individuals.[17,35]

59.5.2 Evaluation

Making the diagnosis of anaphylaxis can be affected by variability in the standard definition of a case. Obtaining as much information from the affected athlete and any witnesses is important to define the time course and severity of the reaction as well as the potential cause. Anaphylaxis has many triggers including food, medications, and insect stings (see Table 59.7). Thus, exposure to any of these causes needs to be documented in the history. Hymenoptera sensitivity should be suspected as a cause of anaphylaxis in any athlete with a reaction that occurs outdoors, even if the patient does not recall being stung. Any food exposure prior to the onset of symptoms should be documented. Of special concern would be exposure to the most common food allergens, which include eggs, peanut, cow's milk, nuts, fish, soy, shellfish, and wheat. Several medications have been known to cause anaphylaxis, with the most common being beta-lactam antibiotics. Documenting exposure to prescription medications as well as over-the-counter medications and supplements is also important.

Because this is a sports medicine text, the discussion would be incomplete without mentioning exercise-induced anaphylaxis (EIA). This rare condition is associated with exercising within 2–4 hours after food ingestion. It is characterized by the usual manifestations of anaphylaxis beginning within 5–30 minutes of exercise and lasting up to 3 hours. The medical history should explore the relationship of symptom onset to physical exercise to assess for this rare trigger.

The physical manifestations of anaphylaxis involve multiple sites including the skin, upper airway, lower airway, and cardiovascular system (see Table 59.8). The physical

TABLE 59.7
Causes of Anaphylaxis

Idiopathic
Medications
Antibiotics
Intravenous and local anesthetics
Aspirin/NSAIDs
Chemotherapeutic agents
Opiates
Vaccines
Allergy immunotherapy sera
Radiographic contrast media
Blood products
Latex
Hymenoptera envenomation
Foods
Eggs
Peanut
Cow's milk
Nuts
Seafood
Soy
Wheat
Exercise (EIA)

TABLE 59.8
Symptoms and Signs of Anaphylaxis

Psychological
Sense of impending doom
Cutaneous
Tingling/pruritus
Generalized erythema
Urticaria
Angioedema
Upper Airway
Nasal congestion
Rhinorrhea
Sneezing
Globus sensation
Throat tightness
Dysphonia
Dysphagia
Lower Airway
Dyspnea
Wheezing
Cough
Cardiovascular
Lightheadedness
Syncope
Palpitations
Shock
Gastrointestinal
Abdominal cramps
Bloating
Nausea/vomiting

examination should start by evaluating upper-airway patency by listening for inspiratory stridor and looking for oral or pharyngeal edema. The athlete's respiratory status should then be assessed by observing their work of breathing and accessory muscle use. Auscultation may reveal wheezing, indicating acute bronchospasm. A set of vital signs is critical to patient management, looking for any evidence of cardiovascular or respiratory compromise. Once the ABCs are assessed and secured, the skin can be examined for the presence of generalized erythema, urticaria, and angioedema.

59.5.3 Acute Management

Initial management of anaphylaxis should always include administration of epinephrine (0.2–0.5 mL IM or SQ of 1:1000), even if symptoms are mild. The IM route is preferred, especially in children, as SQ injection may delay absorption. The dose may be repeated every 10–15 minutes if symptoms are not resolving. Using intravenous epinephrine at 1 μg/min of 1:10,000 (10 μg/mL) can be considered for ongoing symptoms resistant to repeated SQ or IM administration. This dosage can be increased to 2–10 μg/min for severe reactions. Patients on beta-blockers may not respond to epinephrine. In these cases, glucagon (2–5 mg IM/SQ) is beneficial. Supportive therapy with oxygen for hypoxemia, recumbent positioning, and intravenous fluids for hypotension, as well as inhaled beta-agonists or racemic epinephrine for bronchospasm, are also important tools. Antihistamines such as diphenhydramine (1–2 mg/kg or 25–50 mg IV/PO) may provide additional benefit. Corticosteroids, such as prednisone (0.5–2.0 mg/kg up 125 mg), should also be considered to prevent late-phase reactions. However, it cannot be overemphasized that neither antihistamines nor steroids should be used as substitutes for epinephrine. Their onset of action is much slower and they are insufficient to prevent or treat more severe anaphylaxis with respiratory or cardiovascular involvement. Athletes presenting with anaphylaxis should be observed a minimum of 3 hours after symptoms have resolved following a mild reaction. An individual should be observed at least 6 hours after a more severe reaction, and hospitalization should be strongly considered to monitor for late-phase reactions.

Clinical Pearl

Antihistamines and steroids should never be used as substitutes for epinephrine. Their onset of action is much slower, and they are insufficient to prevent or treat more severe anaphylaxis with respiratory or cardiovascular involvement.

59.5.4 Long-Term Management

It is critical that all patients with anaphylaxis have an action plan. This should include not only identification of their particular allergens but also symptom recognition and appropriate treatment. All of these individuals should carry an epinephrine autoinjector on their person at all times. While remembering to carry the injector is important, it is equally crucial that they have good education on indications and proper technique for its use. A provider knowledgeable in allergic disease should offer education on allergen avoidance, hidden allergens, and cross-reacting substances. These athletes should wear medical alert bracelets at all times, indicating their condition and allergy if known.

Unfortunately, for the athlete with EIA, no proven preventive therapy exists for this condition. Strategies for prevention include strict avoidance of relevant cotriggers (such as food, medications, ethanol ingestion, cold air or cold water exposure), as well as awareness of other concomitant risk factors, such as acute infection, emotional stress, menses, temperature/humidity extremes, and high pollen counts.[23]

Premedication and warm-up are not effective in preventing EIA.[1,23] Occasionally, skin testing can identify a specific food that the patient can avoid, but often, the results are inconclusive. The individual must always have access to an epinephrine autoinjector during practice and competition. Athletes such as cross-country runners, cyclists, or skiers should carry the autoinjector on their person when they do not have immediate access to their gear bags. They should discontinue exercising at the first sign of symptoms and self-administer their epinephrine. Their trainers and coaches should also be familiar with the recognition of anaphylaxis and use of epinephrine. Affected athletes should be advised to wear a medical alert bracelet, never to exercise alone, and carry a cell (mobile) phone for calling emergency medical services.

Referral for an allergy specialist is indicated when further testing is necessary for an unclear diagnosis or when the inciting agent is unknown, when reactions are recurrent and difficult to control, or when desensitization is required such as for stinging insects or antibiotic administration. Allergists also serve as an important resource for athletes, parents, and coaches who need additional education on allergen avoidance as well as institution or reinforcement of an individual's action plan.

59.6 SUMMARY

Allergic diseases can be important causes of morbidity and potentially mortality in athletes. Management begins with an understanding of the pathophysiologic mechanisms involved and hinges on an appropriate history and physical assessment. In the majority of athletes, rhinitis and urticaria can be managed at the primary care level with allergen avoidance and medications. Special attention should be paid to the use of any restricted or banned medication as dictated by the athlete's level of competition. When symptoms are more significant or difficult to control and when advanced testing is required, appropriate subspecialist referral is necessary (Table 59.9).

TABLE 59.9
SORT: Key Recommendations for Practice

Clinical Recommendation	Evidence Rating	References
Chronic nasal steroid use is not associated with any significant adrenal suppression, nasal or pharyngeal candidiasis, cataracts, or glaucoma.	C	[3, 19]
For the treatment of allergic rhinitis, intranasal corticosteroids have no effect on growth at recommended doses compared with placebo.	B	[1, 23, 32, 33]
AIT is an effective treatment for allergic rhinitis and allergic asthma, reduces the risk for the future development of asthma in patients with allergic rhinitis, and may have persistent benefits after immunotherapy is discontinued.	A	[10, 14–16, 23, 31, 34]
There is strong evidence that SLIT use improves asthma symptoms, moderate evidence showing decrease in rhinitis and rhinoconjunctivitis symptoms, and moderate evidence demonstrating > 40% decrease in medication use for asthma and allergies.	B	[20]

REFERENCES

1. Allen DB, Meltzer EO, Lemanske RF et al. No growth suppression in children treated with the maximum recommended dose of fluticasone propionate aqueous nasal spray for one year. *Allergy and Asthma Proceedings: The Official Journal of Regional and State Allergy Societies*. December 2002;23(6):407–413.
2. Berger W, Hampel F, Bernstein J et al. Impact of azelastine nasal spray on symptoms and quality of life compared with cetirizine oral tablets in patients with seasonal allergic rhinitis. *Annals of Allergy, Asthma & Immunology: Official Publication of the American College of Allergy, Asthma, & Immunology*. September 2006;97(3):375–381.
3. Boner AL. Effects of intranasal corticosteroids on the hypothalamic-pituitary-adrenal axis in children. *Journal of Allergy and Clinical Immunology*. July 2001;108(1 Suppl):S32–S39.
4. Brown SG, Kemp SF, Lieberman PL. Anaphylaxis. In: Adkinson NF Jr, Bochner BS, Burks AW, Busse WW, Holgate ST, Lemanske RF, O'Hehir RE (eds.). *Middleton's Allergy: Principles and Practice*, 8th edn. Philadelphia, PA: Saunders; 2014: pp. 1237–1259.
5. Casale TB, Sampson HA, Hanifin J et al. Guide to physical urticarias. *Journal of Allergy and Clinical Immunology*. November 1988;82(5, Pt 1):758–763.
6. Casale TB, Blaiss MS, Gelfand E et al. First do no harm: Managing antihistamine impairment in patients with allergic rhinitis. *Journal of Allergy and Clinical Immunology*. May 2003;111(5):S835–S842.
7. Darlenski R, Kazandjieva J, Zuberbier T et al. Chronic urticaria as a systemic disease. *Clinics in Dermatology*. June 2014;32(3):420–423.
8. Wallace DV, Dykewicz MS, Bernstein DI et al. The diagnosis and management of rhinitis: An updated practice parameter. *Journal of Allergy and Clinical Immunology*. August 2008;122(2 Suppl):S1–S84.
9. Di Lorenzo G, Pacor ML, Pellitteri ME et al. Randomized placebo-controlled trial comparing fluticasone aqueous nasal spray in mono-therapy, fluticasone plus cetirizine, fluticasone plus montelukast and cetirizine plus montelukast for seasonal allergic rhinitis. *Clinical and Experimental Allergy: Journal of the British Society for Allergy and Clinical Immunology*. February 2004;34(2):259–267.
10. Eng PA, Borer-Reinhold M, Heijnen IaFM et al. Twelve-year follow-up after discontinuation of preseasonal grass pollen immunotherapy in childhood. *Allergy*. February 2006; 61(2):198–201.
11. Eng PA, Reinhold M, Gnehm HPE. Long-term efficacy of preseasonal grass pollen immunotherapy in children. *Allergy*. April 2002;57(4):306–312.
12. Greiner AN, Meltzer EO. Pharmacologic rationale for treating allergic and nonallergic rhinitis. *Journal of Allergy and Clinical Immunology*. November 2006;118(5):985–998.
13. Greiner AN, Hellings PW, Rotiroti G et al. Allergic rhinitis. *Lancet*. December 2011;378(9809):2112–2122.
14. Jacobsen L. Preventive aspects of immunotherapy: Prevention for children at risk of developing asthma. *Annals of Allergy, Asthma & Immunology: Official Publication of the American College of Allergy, Asthma, & Immunology*. July 2001;87 (1 Suppl 1):43–46.
15. Jacobsen L, Niggemann B, Dreborg S et al. Specific immunotherapy has long-term preventive effect of seasonal and perennial asthma: 10-year follow-up on the PAT study. *Allergy*. August 2007;62(8):943–948.
16. Jacobsen L, Petersen BN, Wihl JA et al. Immunotherapy with partially purified and standardized tree pollen extracts. IV. Results from long-term (6-year) follow-up. *Allergy*. September 1997;52(9):914–920.
17. Kemp SF. Currents concepts in the pathophysiology, diagnosis, and management of anaphylaxis. *Immunology and Allergy Clinics of North America*. 2001;21(4):611–634.
18. Kemp SF. Navigating the updated anaphylaxis parameters. *Allergy, Asthma, and Clinical Immunology: Official Journal of the Canadian Society of Allergy and Clinical Immunology*. June 2007;3(2):40–49.
19. Krahnke J, Skoner D. Benefit and risk management for steroid treatment in upper airway diseases. *Current Allergy and Asthma Reports*. November 2002;2(6):507–512.
20. Lin SY, Erekosima N, Kim JM et al. Sublingual immunotherapy for the treatment of allergic rhinoconjunctivitis and asthma: A systematic review. *Journal of the American Medical Association*. March 2013;309(12):1278–1288.
21. Maurer M, Rosén K, Hsieh H-J et al. Omalizumab for the treatment of chronic idiopathic or spontaneous urticaria. *New England Journal of Medicine*. March 2013;368:924–935.
22. Möller C, Ahlström H, Henricson K-A et al. Safety of nasal budesonide in the long-term treatment of children with perennial rhinitis. *Clinical and Experimental Allergy: Journal of the British Society for Allergy and Clinical Immunology*. June 2003;33(6):816–822.
23. Möller C, Dreborg S, Ferdousi HA et al. Pollen immunotherapy reduces the development of asthma in children with seasonal rhinoconjunctivitis (the PAT-study). *Journal of Allergy and Clinical Immunology*. February 2002;109(2):251–256.
24. Nathan RA. Pharmacotherapy for allergic rhinitis: A critical review of leukotriene receptor antagonists compared with other treatments. *Annals of Allergy, Asthma & Immunology: Official Publication of the American College of Allergy, Asthma, & Immunology*. February 2003;90(2): 182–190.

25. Pullerits T, Praks L, Ristioja V et al. Comparison of a nasal glucocorticoid, antileukotriene, and a combination of antileukotriene and antihistamine in the treatment of seasonal allergic rhinitis. *Journal of Allergy and Clinical Immunology*. June 2002;109(6):949–955.
26. Ratner PH, Hampel F, Van Bavel J et al. Combination therapy with azelastine hydrochloride nasal spray and fluticasone propionate nasal spray in the treatment of patients with seasonal allergic rhinitis. *Annals of Allergy, Asthma & Immunology: Official Publication of the American College of Allergy, Asthma, & Immunology*. January 2008;100(1):74–81.
27. Sabroe RA. Acute urticaria. *Immunology and Allergy Clinics of North America*. February 2014;34(1):11–21.
28. Saini SS. Urticaria and angioedema. In: Adkinson NF Jr, Bochner BS, Burks AW, Busse WW, Holgate ST, Lemanske RF, O'Hehir RE (eds.). *Middleton's Allergy: Principles and Practice*, 8th edn. Philadelphia, PA: Saunders; 2014: pp. 575–587.
29. Schatz M, Zeiger RS, Chen W, Yang S-J, Corrao MA, Quinn VP. The burden of rhinitis in a managed care organization. *Annals of Allergy, Asthma & Immunology: Official Publication of the American College of Allergy, Asthma, & Immunology*. September 2008;101(3):240–247.
30. Settipane RA. Rhinitis: A dose of epidemiological reality. *Allergy and Asthma Proceedings: The Official Journal of Regional and State Allergy Societies*. June 2003;24(3):147–154.
31. Sheikh A, Hurwitz B. House dust mite avoidance measures for perennial allergic rhinitis. *Cochrane Database of Systematic Reviews*. 2001;4.
32. Schenkel EJ, Skoner DP, Bronsky EA et al. Absence of growth retardation in children with perennial allergic rhinitis after one year of treatment with mometasone furoate aqueous nasal spray. *Pediatrics*. February 2000;105(2):E22.
33. Skoner DP, Rachelefsky GS, Meltzer EO et al. Detection of growth suppression in children during treatment with intranasal beclomethasone dipropionate. *Pediatrics*. February 2000;105(2):E23.
34. Soni A. *Allergic Rhinitis: Trends in Use and Expenditures, 2000 to 2005*. Statistical Brief #204, Bethesda, MD: Agency for Healthcare Research and Quality; 2008.
35. Tang MLK, Osborne N, Allen K. Epidemiology of anaphylaxis. *Current Opinion in Allergy and Clinical Immunology*. August 2009;9(4):351–356.
36. Tashiro M, Horikawa E, Mochizuki H et al. Effects of fexofenadine and hydroxyzine on brake reaction time during car-driving with cellular phone use. *Human Psychopharmacology*. October 2005;20(7):501–509.
37. Tharp MD. Chronic urticaria: Pathophysiology and treatment approaches. *Journal of Allergy and Clinical Immunology*. December 1996;98(6, Pt 3):S325–S330.
38. The World Anti-Doping Code. The 2014 prohibited list international standard. Accessed June 24, 2014. http://www.wada-ama.org/Documents/World_Anti-Doping_Program/WADP-Prohibited-list/2014/WADA-prohibited-list-2014-EN.pdf.
39. Weiler JM, Bloomfield JR, Woodworth GG et al. Effects of fexofenadine, diphenhydramine, and alcohol on driving performance. A randomized, placebo-controlled trial in the Iowa driving simulator. *Annals of Internal Medicine*. March 2000;132(5):354–363.
40. Wilson AM, O'Byrne PM, Parameswaran K. Leukotriene receptor antagonists for allergic rhinitis: A systematic review and meta-analysis. *American Journal of Medicine*. March 2004;116(5):338–344.

60 Infectious Disease and Athletes

Mark D. Harris

CONTENTS

TABLE 60.1
Key Clinical Considerations

1. Infectious diseases are the most common illnesses that prompt athletes to seek medical care. This is true of athletes at all levels, from recreational to Olympic.
2. Moderate exercise helps boost the immune system and improves resistance to infectious disease, but lack of exercise and excessively vigorous and prolonged exercise probably lead to poorer immune function.
3. Diagnosis, treatment, and prevention of infectious disease in athletes are usually the same as for less athletic patients. However, sports medicine providers must also keep in mind effects on performance, restricted substances, and return to play concerns.
4. Given the communal activities of many sports teams, team doctors must educate coaches, players, and other team staff on good public health and hygiene practices, must enforce their use, and must be a good example.
5. As athletic events are held in increasingly underdeveloped and exotic locations, travel medicine issues such as immunizations and chemoprophylaxis have become more important.

60.1 INTRODUCTION

Though athletes and the public think of musculoskeletal injuries when they consider the discipline of sports medicine, an important part of taking care of athletes at every level is addressing their medical concerns, the most common of which are infectious diseases. During the 13th International Association of Athletics Federations World Championships in Athletics (2011) in Daegu, Korea, which lasted only nine days, 60 time-loss injuries and 68 illnesses occurred per 1000 athletes.[3] The most common diagnoses were upper respiratory tract infection (URTI), dehydration, and gastroenteritis/diarrheal disease. What is true for elite athletes is also true for others; infectious diseases cause as many as 50% of visits to high school and college training rooms.[27] Mass gatherings of people for events increase the risk for infectious diseases among participants and spectators.[40] Therefore, primary care providers must understand the most common infectious diseases and their sports-specific implications including prevention, disqualifying medications, and when athletes can safely return to play. The diagnosis and management of skin infections are detailed in Chapter 55 (Table 60.1).

60.2 EXERCISE AND THE IMMUNE SYSTEM

Much has been studied and written, and much is still unknown, about how exercise affects immune function. Overall, it appears from the literature that moderate exercise improves immune function, and prolonged or intense exercise

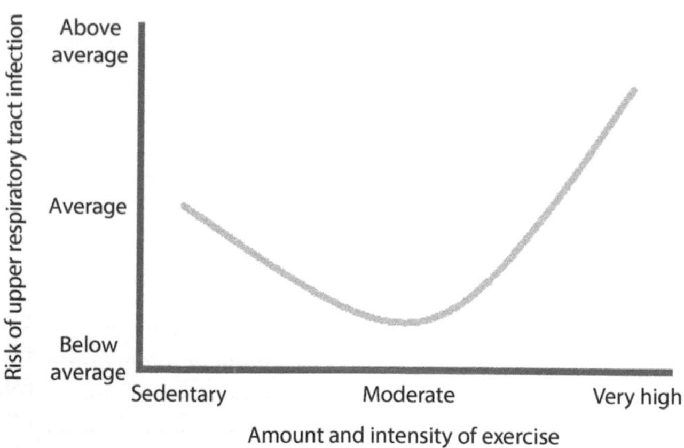

FIGURE 60.1 The "J" hypothesis.

impairs it. Neiman described the relationship between URTI incidence and exercise as a J-shaped curve, with sedentary individuals at greater risk for a URTI than moderate exercisers, but strenuous exercisers at the greatest risk of all[49] (see Figure 60.1). The negative effects of exercise on immune function are greatest when exercise lasts greater than 1.5 hours, is done at 55%–75% of VO_{2max}, and is without food intake during exercise.[32]

The human immune system comprises two parts: the innate immune system and the acquired or adaptive immune system. The innate immune system is constantly on guard, repelling invaders and responding instantly to threats whether or not it has encountered the threat before. It includes mechanical barriers such as the skin, hair, mucosal epithelial barriers, and nasal hairs. It also includes functional barriers such as areas of turbulent airflow that help keep particles laden with pathogens out of the lungs, elevated body temperatures that augment immune function and decrease pathogen replication, and stomach acids that protect the gastrointestinal (GI) tract. Other mechanisms serve to remove harmful invaders, such as the mucociliary elevator and the GI tract.[1,9] The innate immune system includes infection-fighting cells such as phagocytes and natural killer (NK) cells and infection-fighting proteins including complement and cytokines.[1,10] Finally, salivary antimicrobial polypeptides (such as human cathelicidin and lysozyme) and antimicrobial lipids provide frontline defense.[36]

The acquired or adaptive immune response includes B and T lymphocytes and immunoglobulins (Ig's).[1] IgA secreted from mucosa defends the body against invaders at the body surface, while IgM is present in the blood about seven days and IgG about 14 days after infection. While delayed, the acquired immune system provides powerful and enduring protection against pathogens.

Moderate exercise, defined as exercise from 5 to 60 minutes at 40%–60% of VO_{2max},[9] improves salivary IgA concentrations.[37] Levels of neutrophils and NK cells increase.[10,49,50] Proinflammatory cytokines such as interleukin (IL)-1, IL-6, and tumor necrosis factor, and anti-inflammatory cytokines such as IL-10 and IL-1 receptor antagonist increase with exercise.[10] Some studies suggest that URTIs are less common in moderate exercisers than in sedentary individuals[13] by as much as 20%–30% 11. Nonetheless, few studies have shown a direct association between an increased incidence of clinically confirmed infection and any specific measure of exercise-induced immune function.[23]

Vigorous exercise lasts 5–60 minutes at 70%–80% of VO_{2max}, and prolonged exercise lasts over 1 hour.[9] Both vigorous and prolonged exercises have been demonstrated to have a detrimental effect on the immune system, beginning at the end of the exercise session and lasting up to 24 hours.[9,50] Increased levels of cortisol, prolactin, growth hormone, and adrenaline suppress immune function.[11] T and B lymphocyte function diminishes, as do neutrophil levels,[66] and the normal ratio of CD4/CD8 cells of 1.5:1 reverses.[10] Lactoferrin and lysozyme concentrations transiently rise during and then fall after acute exercise,[62] and Kimata found that moderate–vigorous exercise decreased antimicrobial lipid levels in sedentary but not in active subjects.[36] Serum IgG and IgE concentrations decline,[45] as do nasal and salivary IgA levels.[51] Short, high-intensity exercise disrupts the mitochondria of leukocytes, decreasing function and increasing the risk of apoptosis.[60]

Vigorous exercise impairs the immune system in other ways as well. As oxygen demand increases, athletes shift to mouth breathing to increase their respiratory rate and tidal volume, bringing more air into the lungs faster and with less opportunity for warming, humidifying, and capturing airborne pathogens in the nose. The cooler, drier air disrupts the mucociliary elevator's ability to capture and remove harmful particles.[10] Airway inflammation increases.[6] More intense exercise increases the likelihood of small abrasions and lacerations that can admit invaders. Extreme exercisers may be at the greatest risk.[23,49] Thus, at baseline, the immune function of moderate and vigorous exercisers is the same, but the period from 3 to 24 hours after intense exercise may be an immunologic "open window" in which infections such as URTI are more likely.

Clinical Pearl

Overtraining not only impairs performance but also increases the athlete's risk for infectious disease. Primary care providers should be alert for this and intervene with players and coaches when it occurs.

60.3 INFECTIONS AND EXERCISE

Infections can impact an athlete's ability to perform in sports and exercise, but studies suggest that the effect is small.[10] Fever impairs temperature regulation and endurance. Infections can impact muscle strength, aerobic power, coordination, and concentration.[27] Drugs used to treat infectious diseases can also be problematic. Acetaminophen can be dangerous in patients who consume high levels of alcohol and those with underlying liver disease. Antibiotics can cause diarrhea, and quinolones are associated with an increased risk for tendon rupture. Antihistamines can be sedating and directly impact performance. Stimulants such as ephedrine-containing medications may disqualify the athlete from competition.[48] The World Anti-Doping Agency (WADA) regularly updates a list of prohibited substances (www.wada-ama.org).

Clinical Pearl

Some medications that are used for symptomatic treatment for infectious diseases, such as inhaled beta-agonists and ephedrine-containing compounds, may be disqualifying for competition. Primary care providers must be aware of what their athletes are taking, whether they prescribed them or not, and warn athletes of the potential repercussions.

60.4 UPPER RESPIRATORY TRACT INFECTION

In the general population, adults typically get 1–6 URTIs per year; accordingly, URTIs are the most common illnesses for which athletes seek care.[3,30] URTI is typically viral, with rhinovirus (10%–40%), coronavirus (20%), and respiratory syncytial virus (10%) being the most common.[53] Adenovirus, influenza virus, and echovirus are other frequent causes.[10] Secondary attack rates can be 25%–70% in closed communities.[53]

URTI is transmitted primarily by direct contact of contaminated hands with the hands, nose, eyes, or mouth of an uninfected person. Symptoms and signs include nasal congestion, boggy nasal mucosa, fatigue, cough (generally nonproductive), sore throat, and occasionally fever ($T_{max} > 100.4$). After an incubation period of 1–3 days, symptoms last for 3–7 days and resolve without treatment. Asthma exacerbations, bacterial sinusitis, and even pneumonia are occasional complications.[53] Viral myocarditis is a rare but potentially serious complication.[30]

Primary care providers can provide symptomatic treatment, including fluids, nonnarcotic pain medications, antitussives, antihistamines, and decongestants. Saline nasal spray can improve symptoms.[57] Antibiotics are not indicated unless the evaluation suggests a bacterial complication of URTI. If a specific virus such as influenza can be confirmed, antivirals such as oseltamivir can be useful.[19]

Handwashing and alcohol-based hand sanitizer use minimizes the risk of transmission. Adequate sleep and hydration, a healthful diet, and regular exercise can decrease the risk of developing clinical disease. People with URTI symptoms should cough onto their sleeve, not their hands, should wash their hands frequently, and should avoid crowded places. Since influenza is prevalent during the fall, winter, and spring, athletes should receive the vaccine annually.[41]

The "neck check" is a good rule of thumb to decide when an athlete can be cleared to return to play. If symptoms are only above the neck, such as nasal congestion, or sore throat, the athlete should exercise at moderate intensity (less than 70% of VO_{2max}) for 10 minutes. If symptoms worsen, he or she should stop exercising until symptoms improve. If they do not worsen, the athlete should exercise at 50% intensity until symptoms resolve. If any are below the neck, such as cough, myalgias, malaise, diarrhea, or fever, the athlete should not exercise until all below the neck symptoms improve.[18]

Clinical Pearl

The "neck check" is a useful guideline for most infectious disease respiratory tract return to play decisions.

60.5 RHINOSINUSITIS

Rhinosinusitis, inflammation of the mucosa of the nose and paranasal sinuses, is a common complication of URTI, affecting 1 in 7 American adults annually.[4] It is generally caused by the same viruses that cause URTI, the symptoms are similar to those of URTI, and treatment is the same. A small percentage of cases of rhinosinusitis are caused by bacteria, with *Haemophilus influenza, Moraxella catarrhalis, Streptococcus pneumoniae*, and *Staphylococcus aureus* being the most common pathogens.[4] Fever, purulent nasal discharge, and sinus tenderness on exam suggest a bacterial cause, as does worsening after 5–7 days or lasting more than 10 days.[4] Uncomplicated bacterial rhinosinusitis will resolve spontaneously in one month in 75% of cases.[53] Athletes who participate in water sports such as surfing, water polo, swimming, and diving seem to be at greater risk.

Antibiotics may be considered for patients with acute bacterial rhinosinusitis and are indicated for patients with complications such as high fever, intense facial pain, and periorbital swelling or erythema.[4] Amoxicillin (875 mg every 12 hours for 10 days) or trimethoprim–sulfamethoxazole (800 mg/160 mg twice per day for 10 days) is appropriate for first-line therapy. Other possibilities include amoxicillin/clavulanate, azithromycin, or clarithromycin. A shorter course of 3–5 days may be equally effective.[4] The "neck check" is a useful guideline for return to play.

60.6 PHARYNGITIS

Pharyngitis, inflammation of the oral and nasal pharynx, frequently accompanies URTI but can occur independently. It is most often caused by the same viruses that cause URTI, but additional causes include Epstein–Barr virus (EBV), herpes simplex virus (HSV), Coxsackie virus, group A beta-hemolytic streptococci (GABHS), and rarely *Neisseria gonorrhea*.[30,35] Sore throat, pain with swallowing, and fever are common. The presence of common URTI symptoms suggests a viral etiology, while fever >100.9, palatal petechiae, tonsilar exudates, and cervical adenopathy suggest a bacterial etiology.[12] GABHS is the cause in 5%–15% of cases of pharyngitis.[35] The modified Centor score is a clinical decision rule that can aid in diagnosis.[12]

Treatment for viral pharyngitis as part of a URTI is the same as for URTI without pharyngitis. Treatment for pharyngitis as part of infectious mononucleosis (IM) will be covered in that section. Treatment for GABHS includes penicillin 500 mg twice per day for 10 days. Erythromycin (800 mg two times per day for 10 days) is a good choice in penicillin allergic patients.[12] GABHS pharyngitis resolves in a few days even without treatment; however, antibiotic therapy shortens symptom duration and reduces complications such as suppurative peritonsillar abscesses, retropharyngeal abscesses, and acute rheumatic fever.[12] Rheumatic fever historically occurs in 0.1%–3.0% of untreated patients, typically children, with GABHS.[7] The "neck check" is a useful guideline for return to play.

60.7 INFECTIOUS MONONUCLEOSIS

Adolescents and young adults are often competitive athletes, and those same age groups often get mononucleosis. IM is self-limited, caused the EBV, secreted in saliva, and spread by direct contact. The peak incidence of infection is from 15 to 25 years of age, decreasing substantially by age 35, with 95% of adults eventually becoming immune.[31]

The clinical course for IM begins with an incubation period of 30–50 days, a 1–2 week prodrome, and several weeks of clinical disease.[10,56] The classic triad of symptoms and signs includes sore throat, fever, and cervical lymphadenopathy (often posterior). Other clinical manifestations include palpable splenomegaly, palatal petechiae, headache, poor appetite, myalgias, and fatigue. Maculopapular, urticarial, or petechial rash can occur, especially if the patient receives a beta-lactam or other antibiotic.[56] While IM is usually self-limited, clinical disease can last longer than 4 weeks, and symptoms are often worse in immunocompromised patients.

Lymphocytosis with greater than 10% atypical lymphocytes and a positive heterophile antibody absorption test (monospot) are consistent with a diagnosis of IM. The Monospot test has a 25% false-negative rate in the first week of symptoms, but this decreases to 5% by week 3.[56] Liver transaminase levels are commonly elevated and jaundice can occur. Viral capsid antigen titers (IgM and IgG), as well as Epstein–Barr nuclear antigen, can be helpful in challenging cases.

Treatment of uncomplicated IM includes maintaining good hydration, rest, and pain and fever control. Salt water gargles and throat lozenges can improve throat pain, but aspirin is contraindicated in adolescents because of the risk of Reye's syndrome.[56] Corticosteroids may be considered in patients with potential airway compromise, severe splenomegaly, myocarditis, or hemolytic anemia. Other rare complications include Guillain–Barre syndrome, encephalitis, disseminated intravascular coagulation, and aplastic anemia.[31,56]

One of the most feared complications is splenic rupture, which occurs in 0.1%–0.2% of patients, typically in the first 3 weeks of clinical disease.[31] Rupture can occur with trauma, without trauma, and even without exertion. While ultrasound and abdominal computed tomography are reliable in detecting splenomegaly, normal spleen sizes vary dramatically, and most athletes do not receive baseline measurements. As a result, imaging is generally not helpful in diagnosing splenomegaly, guiding return to play decisions, or in predicting rupture.[56]

Athletes with IM should avoid exercise entirely for at least 3 weeks after the onset of symptoms.[56] If they are afebrile and clinically improving, they can begin light, noncontact exercise and increase duration and intensity by about 10% per week. Recovery can take 2–3 months or more. The appropriate time for a safe return to contact activity is unclear, given the risk for splenic rupture; however, most authorities recommend no sooner than 3 weeks from the time of illness, and that the patient is asymptomatic.

60.8 OTITIS MEDIA AND EXTERNA

Over 20 million cases of otitis media (OM) are diagnosed in the United States per year, many of which are adult cases.[30] OM is caused by many of the same bacteria that cause rhinosinusitis, including *H. influenza, M. Catarrhalis,* and *S. Pneumoniae*.[26] Viral pathogens cause 30% of cases of OM.[30] In addition to URTI symptoms, clinical presentation includes mild, moderate, or severe TM bulging with ear pain and erythema, and otorrhea not associated with otitis externa (OE).[26] OM is usually self-limited and treatment is symptomatic, including analgesics, fever control, and interventions for URTI symptoms. Observation is appropriate in uncomplicated OM as antibiotics frequently do not change the course of the infection, but follow-up should be available in 48–72 hours.[26] Antibiotics should be used in diabetics or immunocompromised patients and in patients who develop complications such as mastoiditis.

OE, a typically bacterial or fungal infection involving the external auditory canal, is often associated with inadequate cerumen, preexisting allergies, or repetitive water exposure.[30] *S. aureus* and *Pseudomonas aeruginosa* are common bacterial causes and *Aspergillus* is a common fungal cause. Clinical manifestations include ear pain and itching, tragal tenderness, purulent discharge, and lymphadenopathy (pre- or postauricular or cervical).[10] Treatment includes cleaning the debris from the ear canal. If the tympanic membrane is intact, topical steroids and antibiotics can be used. Athletes can decrease their risk of OE by not placing objects into their ears and by using drying/acidifying drops such as isopropyl alcohol and acetic acid.[30] Ear plugs are controversial.

Athletes with OM can return to water sports when their TMs are intact and have normal mobility. However, because changes in barometric pressure can rupture the TM, air travel and underwater activities should be avoided while symptomatic.[30] Athletes with OE can return to water sports when they are asymptomatic. Athletes not in water sports have no limitations to participation.

60.9 CONJUNCTIVITIS

The conjunctiva, the superficial layer of tissue overlying the white sclera of the eye, can become irritated and red from many causes common in sports, such as dust, bright light, allergens, irritants, other foreign bodies, rubbing, and infectious agents. Organisms associated with infectious conjunctivitis include adenovirus, HSV, *H. influenza, S. pneumoniae, S. aureus,* chlamydia, and rarely *N. gonorrhea.*[16] Spread is usually via direct contact but fomites such as personal items can be involved.

Clinical manifestations of infectious conjunctivitis include eye redness, watering, and discharge. Viral conjunctivitis is self-limiting, lasting no more than 1–2 weeks. Treatment for viral conjunctivitis is symptomatic, including ocular decongestants, cold compresses, and artificial tears.[16] Bacterial conjunctivitis is more likely to present with purulent than watery discharge, and while symptoms often resolve over several days, they can persist for up to 3 weeks. Bacterial conjunctivitis is self-limiting and can be treated expectantly, but it is frequently treated with antibiotics to speed recovery, diminish transmission, and accelerate return to activity.[16] Topical azithromycin, ciprofloxacin, erythromycin, gentamycin, and trimethoprim/polymyxin B are effective. Treatment for chlamydial conjunctivitis includes topical erythromycin and oral azithromycin, and sexual partners must be treated.[16]

More serious causes of conjunctivitis include HSV and *N. gonorrhea.* Hyperacute bacterial conjunctivitis is associated with *N. Gonorrhea* in sexually active adults and has sudden onset with rapid progression. Eyes have a copious purulent discharge, pain, and some vision loss.[16] Rapid corneal perforation is a threat. HSV conjunctivitis can also follow a rapid course. Topical corticosteroids should only be used under the supervision of an ophthalmologist because they exacerbate HSV conjunctivitis.[16] Patients with either of these conditions should be immediately referred to an ophthalmologist for aggressive treatment.

Because causative agents for conjunctivitis are transmitted via direct contact and even pool water, athletes in high-contact sports such as wrestling and those in water sports should be restricted from competition or even training with others until the infection has completely cleared.

60.10 MENINGITIS

Meningitis, an infection of the tissue layers covering the central nervous system, usually occurs after local infection (recent OM or sinusitis) or hematogenous spread (recent pneumonia).[5] Aseptic meningitis is typically caused by enterovirus, HSV, *Borrelia burgdorferi*, and varicella zoster. Human immunodeficiency virus (HIV), *Treponema pallidum*, *Mycoplasma pneumoniae*, Rocky Mountain spotted fever, ehrlichiosis, mumps, tuberculosis, HIV, and arboviruses are less common causes of aseptic meningitis.[5] Septic meningitis, primarily caused by such bacteria as *H. influenza, S. pneumoniae,* and *Neisseria meningitidis*, is universally fatal if untreated. Even with treatment, mortality in septic meningitis is 21%.[5] Those who survive face neurological sequela such as hearing loss (14%) and hemiparesis (4%). In one study, 74.7% of patients with pneumococcal meningitis developed intracranial complications such as seizures, cerebrovascular events, and diffuse brain swelling.[34]

Aseptic meningitis is diagnosed when clinical and laboratory evidence of meningitis are present but bacterial cultures are negative. It is most prevalent from July to December.[30] Enterovirus infections, transmitted by the fecal–oral route, cause 55%–70% of cases of aseptic meningitis.[30] Patients with an identified cause such as HSV or *Mycobacterium tuberculosis* should receive specific therapies, but treatment otherwise is supportive.

The classic triad of symptoms of meningitis is nuchal rigidity, fever, and headache, but this is evident in only 44% of patients with meningitis.[5] Other clinical manifestations include altered mental status, the Kernig's and Brudzinski's signs, petechial rash, and occasionally seizures.[5] Diagnosis is made by analysis of the cerebrospinal fluid. Athletes with evidence of meningitis should receive immediate emergency care.

Immunization against *H. influenza, S. pneumoniae,* and *N. meningitidis* can help prevent septic meningitis. Hand washing and not sharing personal items, including protective gear and water bottles, are also important. Team members should be considered for antibiotic prophylaxis as clinically indicated.

60.11 ACUTE BRONCHITIS

Acute bronchitis, inflammation of the lining of the bronchial tree, is the most common diagnosis in adults who present with cough.[2] It is caused by viruses in 90% of cases, including adenovirus, coronavirus, rhinovirus, influenza and parainfluenza, and other viruses commonly associated with URTI. Bacterial causes include *Bordetella pertussis*, *M. pneumoniae*, and *Chlamydia pneumoniae*.[35] In addition to cough, patients present with URTI symptoms, and acute bronchitis generally resolves within 3 weeks. Fever, tachypnea, tachycardia, decreased O_2 saturation, and abnormalities on lung exam suggest pneumonia, but neither color nor consistency of sputum reliably distinguishes bronchitis from pneumonia.[2]

Treatment is symptomatic, similar to that for URTI, and antibiotics rarely change the disease course unless a specific bacterial cause such as pertussis is suspected.[2] Pertussis should be suspected in young athletes where the cough persists over two weeks; consideration should be given for prophylaxis of teammates after discussion with infectious disease or preventive medicine specialists. Oseltamivir is useful if influenza is confirmed. Antitussives and expectorants are not effective in treating bronchitis. Bronchodilators are helpful if the patient has concomitant wheezing and may be continued in such patients to mitigate postbronchitic airway inflammation. Oral corticosteroids confer no benefit in acute bronchitis, but inhaled steroids may have a small benefit.[2] Pelargonium (South African geranium) has shown some promise in helping patients return to activity.[2] The neck check is a good guide for return to play decisions.

60.12 PNEUMONIA

Community acquired pneumonia (CAP) is an infection of lung parenchyma and is the most common cause of infectious mortality in the United States. Bacterial causes include *S. pneumoniae, C. pneumoniae, M. pneumoniae,* and *Legionella*, although viruses cause about 30% of cases.[61] Five to eleven people per 1000 population develop CAP every year, especially in the winter months.[61] Symptoms include fever, chills, pleuritic chest pain, productive cough, and dyspnea.[35] Signs include asymmetric breath sounds, egophony, fremitus, pleural rub, rales, tachypnea, tachycardia, and dullness to percussion. Radiographs should be ordered in patients with two or more of these findings and considered in patients with at least one.[61] Chest radiographs (CXRs) sometimes show infiltrates, and a complete blood count may show leukocytosis with a left shift.[39] Blood and sputum cultures are useful, and urine antigen tests for *Legionella* and *Pneumococcus* are available.

The CURB-65 helps clinicians decide whether a patient should be admitted or treated as an outpatient. It evaluates prognostic variables such as mental status, blood urea nitrogen, blood pressure, respiratory rate, and age. The SMART COP score predicts the need for intensive respiratory or vasopressor support.[61] It adds multilobar involvement on CXR, albumin level, tachycardia, oxygen level, and arterial pH.

In previously healthy patients without antibiotic use in the past 3 months, macrolides or doxycyclines are first-line therapy. Outpatients with comorbidities or those with recent antibiotic use should receive a fluoroquinolone or a beta-lactam plus a macrolide.[61] The standard duration is 10–14 days but 7 days may be adequate. Influenza and pneumococcal vaccines can help prevent disease. Athletes should rest while symptomatic and gradually return to play afterward; primary care providers can estimate one to two reduced training days for every day of acute illness when guiding return to play.

60.13 MYOCARDITIS

Myocarditis is an inflammation of the heart muscle, which rarely follows systemic infections. Viral causes include adenovirus, Coxsackie B, cytomegalovirus, echovirus, EBV, hepatitis C, and influenza.[39] Other causes include mycoplasma, chlamydia, or drugs.[11,39] Men aged 20–40 years are at the highest risk. Patients typically have symptoms of a nonspecific viral infection and over time develop chest pain, palpitations, fever, and fatigue. Severe symptoms include dependent edema, orthopnea, paroxysmal nocturnal dyspnea, muffled heart sounds, and mitral regurgitation.[39] The electrocardiogram can show nonspecific ST and T wave abnormalities, and the echocardiogram can show globally decreased function with a low ejection fraction. Patients with associated pericarditis may have a friction rub.[59]

Myocarditis is usually self-limiting, even in the minority of patients who develop heart failure, but rarely can result in dysrhythmias and sudden cardiac death.[42] Athletes with myocarditis should immediately withdraw from competitive sports and convalesce for 6 months from the onset of clinical symptoms. They may return to play once their electrocardiogram and echocardiogram are completely normal, they have no serum markers of cardiac inflammation or heart failure, and they have no arrhythmias.[42]

60.14 ACUTE GASTROENTERITIS

Competitive athletes, especially adolescents and young adults, frequent congregate settings, such as team buses and locker rooms, and share food, water, and personal items. It is no surprise, therefore, that acute gastroenteritis (AGE) is the second most common infection in this population.[3,47] Viruses are most frequent, including rotavirus and norovirus. Other common organisms include *Giardia*, *Entamoeba histolytica*, *campylobacter*, *Escherichia coli*, *Salmonella,* and *Shigella*.[33] Transmission is usually fecal–oral and the peak incidence is in the warmer months of late spring, summer, and early fall.

Patients present with diarrhea, abdominal pain, cramping, nausea, vomiting, and dehydration. Bloody diarrhea and fever are more common with bacterial causes.[33] Fluid deficits in exercise are calculated by change in body weight. With a fluid deficit (weight decrease) of 2%, work capacity decreases by 15%–20%. With a decrease over 3%–5%, sweat production and blood flow to the skin decrease. Patients should be rehydrated orally if tolerated and intravenously if not.[17] Cool water is preferred in most cases and isotonic sports drinks are useful. Other symptoms can be treated empirically with analgesics, antiemetics, and antidiarrheals.

Antibiotics are generally not useful for uncomplicated viral, *Campylobacter*, or *Salmonella* AGE and may increase the risk of hemolytic uremic syndrome in *E. coli* infection.[33] Antimicrobials such as trimethoprim–sulfamethoxazole and quinolones can shorten the disease course in *Shigella* infection, and metronidazole effectively treats *Giardia* and *Entamoeba histolytica*.[33] Antibiotics such as fluoroquinolones can be used for prophylaxis against traveler's diarrhea,[10] and bismuth subsalicylate provides 60% protection.[67] Probiotics containing lactobacillus may also be effective.

Gastroenteritis is highly communicable. In 1998, a foodborne outbreak of AGE occurred among the University of North Carolina football team. Twenty-nine players developed symptoms shortly before playing the University of Florida, and after the game, 11 Florida players, who had not eaten the food, developed the same symptoms.[33] Therefore, athletes must be well hydrated and asymptomatic before returning to play.

Hepatitis A is generally found in areas with poor sanitation. It presents with nausea, vomiting, diarrhea, and sometimes jaundice.[43] It is transmitted through fecal–oral contact and is usually self-limited, though rarely it can progress to fulminant hepatitis and death. Hepatitis A can be prevented through vaccination and good sanitation and hygiene practices. Vaccination and hepatitis A Ig are useful for postexposure prophylaxis.[43]

60.15 BLOOD-BORNE INFECTIONS

The HIV, hepatitis C virus (HCV), and hepatitis B virus (HBV) are infections transmitted by blood or other body fluids that are of concern in sports. Over one million Americans are currently infected with HIV, 3.5 million Americans are infected with HCV, and 60,000 people in the United States are infected with HBV every year.[11] Sexual contact, needle sharing, tattooing, and body piercing are common ways to transmit these infections.

There is evidence that HIV has been transmitted in household contacts without needle sharing or sexual contact, probably from unrecognized wound or mucous membrane exposure. There was one possible case of HIV transmission during a soccer match and a few reports of transmission during bloody street fights.[10] However, there has never been a validated case of HIV transmission in an athletic setting.[48] The NCAA does not recommend routine mandatory testing but does encourage voluntary testing for athletes engaged in high-risk activities. Fourteen percent of all new cases of HIV occur in people between 12 and 24 years of age.[48] Asymptomatic HIV infection does not disqualify the infected athlete from play.

HIV-infected patients respond like non-HIV-infected people to moderate exercise. Aerobic exercise (AE) and progressive resistance exercise (PRE) improve VO_{2max} and CD4 count and decrease viral load.[52] AE decreases adiposity and enhances lipid profiles, and PRE increases limb girth and improves body weight.[21] Both improve quality of life.[15]

HCV is the most common blood-borne disease in the United States. One case report exists of HCV being transmitted via a bloody rag during a fist fight, but no cases of transmission during sport are known.[11] Three players on an amateur soccer club were infected with HCV because they shared needles to inject vitamin complexes.[55] Clinical manifestations include nausea and vomiting, abdominal pain, dark urine, light stools, fever, and jaundice. Liver failure can occur, with ascites and hepatic encephalopathy. Treatment includes interferon, ribavirin, and supportive care.[64] Up to 85% of patients infected will develop chronic HCV.[55]

HBV is a sturdy virus, surviving up to 7 days in the environment, and risk of transmission is 100 times greater than for HIV.[24] Transmission during sports competition has been documented. In 1982, 5 of 10 members of a sumo wrestling club at a Japanese high school were infected in a single year, and in 2000, 11 of 65 members of an American football team acquired HBV in 19 months. In both instances, infection was related to exposure to an open wound of an HBV carrier.[55] Symptoms and signs are similar to those for HCV. Only 5% of adults infected will develop chronic HBV, of which 20% will develop hepatic failure.[63] Treatment includes interferon, nucleotide reverse transcriptase inhibitor, and supportive care.

There is no vaccine for HIV or HCV, but the HBV vaccine is 95% effective. All athletes in a contact or collision sport should receive the HBV vaccine.[10] Universal precautions such as handwashing; wearing mask, gloves, and eyewear when exposed to body fluids; and covering open wounds are essential to decreasing transmission. Athletes with acute hepatitis should be allowed to play or not based on their clinical signs and symptoms. Patients with persistent hepatomegaly or splenomegaly should avoid contact and collision sports.[10]

60.16 SEXUALLY TRANSMITTED INFECTIONS

In 2010, over 1.3 million cases of chlamydia were reported to the U.S. Centers for Disease Control (CDC), but the CDC estimates that there were actually 2.8 million new cases.[46] Women aged 15–24 years carry the highest burden of disease, and the rates increased from 2006 to 2009. Women are usually asymptomatic but can present with vaginal discharge or bleeding, dysuria, and abdominal pain. Men are almost always asymptomatic. Azithromycin (1 g single dose) or doxycycline (100 mg twice daily for 7 days) is the preferred treatment, but erythromycin and quinolones can be used.[46] The sexual partner must be treated, and chlamydia can be prevented by abstinence, mutually monogamous sexual activity, and condom use. All sexually active women 24 years old and younger should be screened annually, and those 25 years old and older should be screened if they acquire a new partner or have multiple partners.[46] There is insufficient evidence to recommend screening men.

The CDC estimates that there are over 700,000 new cases of gonorrhea in the United States per year, and rates are highest in women from ages 15 to 19.[44] More than 95% of women are asymptomatic, but a few present with cervicitis, vaginal bleeding, and discharge. Complications include pelvic inflammatory disease, infertility, and disseminated gonococcal infection. The first-line treatment for uncomplicated gonorrhea infection is ceftriaxone 250 mg intramuscularly followed by azithromycin 1 g orally in a single dose.[44] Cefixime plus doxycycline and other regimens can be used as well. Screening and prevention are the same as for chlamydia. Infection with chlamydia, gonorrhea, or both can increase the risk of HIV infection.[44] Because the rate of reinfection is high with all sexually transmitted infections (STIs), providers should retest patients 3–6 months after treatment.

60.17 REPORTABLE DISEASE

The blood-borne and STIs noted earlier are reportable to county and state health departments and the CDC. Meningitis and outbreaks of any kind are also reportable, although specific guidelines vary somewhat by state. Every medical practice should have a mechanism for reporting communicable diseases.

Clinical Pearl

All athletes should be up to date on all immunizations recommended by the CDC, and all team medical personnel should teach and enforce good hygiene practices.

60.18 EXERCISE IN UNUSUAL PLACES

In the past decades, athletes have done more unusual things and gone to more unusual places, and infectious disease risks have increased. Five of 507 athletes participating in a triathlon in Heidelberg, Germany, in 2006 were infected with leptospirosis from the Neckar River.[8] Forty-two percent of athletes in a triathlon in Copenhagen, Denmark, in 2010 developed AGE after a storm contaminated the water a few days before.[25] Three runners racing in Martinique in 2009 were infected with leptospirosis, which infected wounds that participants received in the jungle.[29]

Diseases such as malaria, cholera, and dengue, rarely seen in the developed world, are genuine threats in the developing world, and pretrip vaccinations, chemoprophylaxis, and other interventions are vital. Clinicians must be well versed in travel medicine to care for their athletes both before and after the trip.

Clinical Pearl

Because of communal traveling (such as team buses), communal living, competing in underdeveloped areas, and high-risk behaviors, sports teams may be at higher risk for respiratory, food- and waterborne, and sexually transmitted diseases. Team medical personnel should evaluate the hazards likely to be present at future venues and intervene with players, coaches, administrators, sponsors, and the host facility personnel to decrease risks.

60.19 IMMUNOMODULATORS

The threat of infectious diseases of all types is high, and athletes, coaches, and clinicians alike have long sought ways to enhance the immune system and decrease risk. In 2005, a military study of a novel nutritional immune formula (NNIF) containing vitamins A, C, D, E, and K, zinc, B complex, folic acid, and trace metals improved phagocytosis, enhanced the activation of B cells, and increased the proportion of helper T cells. NNIF also attenuated the decrease in leukocytes and the increase in neutrophils that occurred after intense exercise.[65]

Zinc has been shown to improve diarrheal symptoms by 18% and decrease diarrheal disease by 14% in children in the developing world.[58] It is also associated with reduced URTI symptoms in these children. Neither benefit has been demonstrated in the developed world, suggesting that an underlying zinc deficiency may be present.[58] Carbohydrates are fuel for the muscles and athletes must have adequate stocks to compete effectively. Carbohydrates are also essential for immune system function.[50] However, there is no evidence that increasing consumption enhances immune function.

Vitamin C has been evaluated as prevention and treatment for respiratory diseases since the 1930s. One study in South Africa suggested that supplementation led to fewer reports of URTI.[54] However, a Cochrane review in May 2013 found the evidence insufficient to recommend vitamin C for URTI.[28] Echinacea, derived from the Midwestern purple coneflower, was marketed as a blood purifier and dizziness treatment in the nineteenth century and as a cold and flu remedy in the twentieth century.[38] Though echinacea was the third top-selling herbal supplement in the United States, existing studies suggest that it is not effective for URTI prophylaxis and of limited use for URTI treatment.[20,38]

Glutamine, a nucleoside precursor, has been suggested as an immune system booster. It is ingested in meats and greens and produced in the intestines, muscle, and lungs. Glutamine helps in B and T cell proliferation and in antibody and IL-2 syntheses. Hard, prolonged exercise tends to decrease glutamine levels, but there is no evidence that supplementation to increase levels provides any immunological benefit.[22]

Endurance athletes such as long-distance runners, cross-country skiers, and swimmers often have chronic inflammation in their upper airways. Throat sprays such as Difflam Forte have been studied, and it has shown an improvement in severity but not the frequency of upper respiratory symptoms.[14] IgA is an important mucosal immune defense and IgA levels decrease with hard exercise. As a result, some have posited that lactobacillus supplements, which may stimulate mucosal immune function, may decrease the incidence of URTI. A 2007 report suggested that prophylactic lactobacillus administration may decrease the duration and severity of URTI.[14] Further study is needed.

60.20 CONCLUSION

Infectious diseases are the most common illnesses that affect athletes. They are a significant threat to athletes at home and abroad, causing missed practices, missed games, lost tournaments, lost careers, and rarely even lost lives. Sports medicine practitioners must be well aware of these threats, how to diagnose and treat them, and how to prevent them. Diagnosis and treatment are similar to that for nonathletes, but performance, prevention, public health, and return to play issues are especially acute in the athletic population. Athletes should be vaccinated with all indicated vaccines against all relevant threats, and teams should establish and enforce solid public health practices (Table 60.2).

TABLE 60.2
SORT: Key Recommendations for Practice

Clinical Recommendation	Evidence Rating	References
Treatment for mild URTI symptoms includes supportive care such as saline nasal irrigation, decongestants, and antihistamines.	B	[20,57]
Antibiotics should not be used for the treatment of cold symptoms.	A	[20]
Using clinical decision rules improves care and decreases cost in patients with GABHS.	A	[12]
Beta-agonists and high-dose inhaled steroids can be useful in patients with wheezing in acute bronchitis.	B	[2]
The USPSTF recommends against screening low-risk patients for gonorrheal infection.	A	[44]

REFERENCES

1. Abbas AK, Lichtman AH. *Basic Immunology*. Philadelphia, PA: Saunders Elsevier; 2010: p. 312.
2. Albert RH. Diagnosis and treatment of acute bronchitis. *American Family Physician*. December 2010;82(11):1345–1350.
3. Alonso J, Eduard P, Fischetto G, Adams B, Depiesse F, Mountjoy M. Determination of future prevention strategies in elite track and field: Analysis of Daegu 2011 IAAF Championships injuries and illness surveillance. *British Journal of Sports Medicine*. 2012;46:505–514.
4. Aring AM, Chan MM. Acute rhinosinusitis in adults. *American Family Physician*. May 2011;83(9):1057–1063.
5. Bamberger DM. Diagnosis, initial management, and prevention of meningitis. *American Family Physician*. December 2010;82(12):1491–1498.
6. Belda J, Ricart S, Casan P et al. Airway inflammation in the elite athlete and type of sports. *British Journal of Sports Medicine*. 2008;42:244–248.
7. Benedek TJ. Rheumatic fever and rheumatic heat disease. In: Kiple KF (ed). *The Cambridge World History of Human Disease*. Cambridge, UK: Cambridge University Press; 1993: p. 970.
8. Brockman S, Piechotowski O, Bock-Hensley O, Winter C, Oehme R, Zimmerman S, Hartelt K, Luge E, Nockler K, Schneider T, Stark K, Jansen A. Outbreak of leptospirosis among triathlon participants in Germany, 2006. *BMC Infectious Diseases*. 2010;10:91.
9. Brolinson PG, Elliott D. Exercise and the immune system. *Clinics in Sports Medicine*. 2007;26:311–319.
10. Brukner P, Khan K. Common sports related infections. In: *Clinical Sports Medicine*. New York: McGraw Hill; 2012: pp. 1102–1117.
11. Callahan LR, Giugliano DN. Infections in athlete. In: Madden CC, Putukian M, Young CC, McCarty EC (eds.). *Netter's Sports Medicine*. Philadelphia, PA: Saunders Elsevier; 2010; pp. 197–203.
12. Choby BA. Diagnosis and treatment of streptococcal pharyngitis. *American Family Physician*. 2009;79(5):383–390.
13. Chubak J, McTiernan A, Sorensen B et al. Moderate-intensity exercise reduces the incidence of colds among postmenopausal women. *American Journal of Medicine*. 2006;119(11):937–942.
14. Cox AJ, Gleeson M, Pyne DB, Saunders PU, Fricker PA. Oral administration of the probiotic lactobacillus fermentum VRI-003 and mucosal immunity in endurance athletes. *British Journal of Sports Medicine*. 2010;44(2):127–133.
15. Clem KL, Borchers JR. HIV and the athlete. *Clinics in Sports Medicine*. 2007;26:413–424.
16. Cronau H, Kankanala RR, Mauger T. Diagnosis and management of red eye in primary care. *American Family Physician*. January 2010;81(2):137–144.
17. Divine J, Takagishi J. Exercise in the heat and heat illness. In: Maden CC, Putukian M, Young CC, McCarty EC (eds.). *Netter's Sports Medicine*. Philadelphia, PA: Saunder Elsevier; 2010: pp. 136–148.
18. Eichner R. Infection, immunity and exercise: What to tell patients. *Physician and Sportsmedicine: Home*. 1993;21:125.
19. Erlikh IV, Abraham S, Kondamudi VK. Management of influenza. *American Family Physician*. November 2010;82(9): 1087–1095.
20. Fashner J, Ericson K, Werner S. Treatment of the common cold in children and adults. *American Family Physician*. July 2012;86(2):153–159.
21. Fillipas S, Cherry CL, Cicuttini F et al. The effects of exercise training on metabolic and morphological outcomes for people living with HIV: A systematic review of randomized controlled trials. *HIV Clinical Trials*. 2010;11(5):270–282.
22. Gleeson M. Dosing and effectiveness of glutamine supplementation in human exercise and sport training. *Journal of Nutrition*. 2008;138(10):2045S–2049S.
23. Gleeson M. Immune function in sport and exercise. *Journal of Applied Physiolog*. 2007;103:693–699.
24. Gutierez RL, Decker CF. Blood borne infections and the athlete. *Disease-a-Month*. 2010;56:436–442.
25. Harder-Lauridsen NM, Kuhn KG, Erichsen AC, Molbak K, Ethelberg S. Gastrointestinal illness among triathletes swimming in non-polluted versus polluted seawater affected by heavy rainfall, Denmark 2010–2011. *PLoS One*. 2013;8(11):e78371.
26. Harmes KM, Blackwood RA, Burrows HL, Cooke JM, Harrison RV, Passamani PP. Otitis media: Diagnosis and treatment. *American Family Physician*. October 2013; 88(7):435–440.
27. Harris M. Infectious disease in athletes. *CSMR*. March/April 2011;12(2):84–89.
28. Hemilä H, Chalker E. Vitamin C for preventing and treating the common cold, http://summaries.cochrane.org/CD000980/vitamin-c-for-preventing-and-treating-the-common-cold#sthash.rcGdjsvr.dpuf. Accessed April 23, 2014.
29. Hochedez P, Rosine J, Theodose R, Abel S, Bourhy P, Picardeau M, Quenel P, Cabie A. Outbreak of Leptospirosis after a race in the tropical forest of Martinique. *American Journal of Tropical Medicine and Hygiene*. 2011;84(4):621–626.
30. Hosey RG, Rodenberg RE. Training room management of medical conditions: Infectious diseases. *Clinics in Sports Medicine*. 2005;24:477–506.
31. Hosey RG, Rodenberg RE. Infectious disease and the college athlete. *Clinics in Sports Medicine*. 2007;26:451.
32. Jaworski C, Donohue B, Kluetz J. Infectious disease. *Clinics in Sports Medicine*. 2011;30:575–590.
33. Karagenanes SJ. Gastrointestinal infections in the athlete. *Clinics in Sports Medicine*. 2007;26:434.
34. Kastenbauer S, Pfister HW. Pneumococcal meningitis in adults. *Brain*. 2003;126(5):1015–1025.
35. King OS. Infectious disease and boxing. *Clinics in Sports Medicine*. 2009;28:545–560.

36. Kiwata J, Anouseyan R, Desharnais R, Cornwell A, Khodiguian N, Porter E. Effect of aerobic exercise on lipid effector molecules of the innate immune response. *Medicine & Science in Sports & Exercise*. 2014;46(3):506–512.
37. Klentrou P, Cieslak T, MacNeil M et al. Effect of moderate exercise on salivary IgA. *European Journal of Applied Physiology*. 2002;87:153–158.
38. Kligler B. Echinacea. *American Family Physician*. January 2003;67(1):77–80.
39. Kruse RJ, Cantor CL. Pulmonary and cardiac infections in athletes. *Clinics in Sports Medicine*. 2007;26:321–344.
40. Kupferschmidt K. Do sports events give microbes a chance to score? *Science*. June 2012;336:1224–1225.
41. Luke A, D'Hemecourt P. Prevention of infectious diseases in athletes. *Clinics in Sports Medicine*. 2007;26:321–344.
42. Maron BJ, Ackerman MJ, Nishimura RA et al. Task force 4: HCM and other cardiomyopathies, mitral valve prolapse, myocarditis, and Marfan syndrome. *Journal of the American College of Cardiology*. 2005;45:1340–1345.
43. Matheny SC, Kingery JE. Hepatitis A. *American Family Physician*. December 2012;86(11):1027–1034.
44. Mayor MT, Roett MA, Uduhiri KA. Diagnosis and management of Gonococcal infections. *American Family Physician*. November 2012;86(10):931–938.
45. McCune AJ, Smith LL, Semple SJ et al. Immunoglobulin responses to a repeated bout of downhill running. *British Journal of Sports Medicine*. 2006;40:844–849.
46. Mishori R, McClaskey EL, Winkleprins VJ. *Chlamydia Trachomatis* infections: Screening, diagnosis, and management. *American Family Physician*. December 2012; 86(12):1127–1132.
47. Natarajan B. Gastrointestinal problems. In: Madden CC, Putukian M, Young CC, McCarty EC (eds.). *Netter's Sports Medicine*. Philadelphia, PA: Saunders Elsevier; 2010: pp. 204–208.
48. NCAA. *2014–2015 NCAA Sports Medicine Handbook*, Indianapolis, August 2014.
49. Neiman D. Is infection risk linked to exercise workload? *Medicine & Science in Sports & Exercise*. 2000; 32(7):S406–S411.
50. Neiman D. Nutrition, exercise and immune system function. *Clinics in Sports Medicine*. 1999;18(3):537.
51. Novas AD, Rowbotton DG, Jenkins DG. Tennis, incidence of URTI and salivary IgA. *International Journal of Sports Medicine*. 2003;24(3):223–229.
52. O'Brien K, Nixon S, Tynam AM, Glazier RH. Effectiveness of aerobic exercises in adults living with HIV/AIDs: Systematic review. *Medicine & Science in Sports & Exercise*. 2004;38(10):1659–1666.
53. Page CL, Diehl JJ. Upper respiratory tract infections in athletes. *Clinics in Sports Medicine*. 2007;26:345–359.
54. Peters EM, Goetzchee JM, Grobbelaar B, Noakes TD. Vitamin C supplementation reduces the incidence of postrace symptoms of upper respiratory tract infection in ultramarathon runners. *American Journal of Clinical Nutrition*. 1993;57(2):170–174.
55. Pirizzolo JJ, LeMay DG. Blood borne infections. *Clinics in Sports Medicine*. 2007;26:425–431.
56. Putukian M, O'Connor FG, Sticker PR et al. Mononucleosis and athletic participation: An evidence based review. *Clinical Journal of Sport Medicine*. 2008;18(4):309–315.
57. Rabago D, Zgierska A. Saline nasal irritation for upper respiratory conditions. *American Family Physician*. 2009; 80(10):1117–1119.
58. Saper RB, Rash R. Zinc: An essential micronutrient. *American Family Physician*. May 2009;79(9):768–772.
59. Synder MJ, Bepko J, White M. Acute pericarditis: Diagnosis and management. *American Family Physician*. April 2014;89(7):553–560.
60. Tuan TC, Hsu TG, Fong MC, Hsu CF, Tsai KKC, Lee CY, Kong CW. Deleterious effects of short term, high intensity exercise on immune function: Evidence from leukocyte mitochondrial alterations and apoptosis. *British Journal of Sports Medicine*. 2008;42:11–15.
61. Watkins RR, Lemonovich TL. Diagnosis and management of community-acquired pneumonia in adults. *American Family Physician*. June 2011;83(11):1299–1306.
62. West NP, Pyne DB, Kyd JM et al. The effect of exercise on innate mucosal immunity. *British Journal of Sports Medicine*. 2010;44:227–231.
63. Wilkins T, Zimmerman D, Schade RR. Hepatitis B: Diagnosis and treatment. *American Family Physician*. April 2010;81(8):965–972.
64. Wilkins T, Malcolm JK, Raina D, Schade RR. Hepatitis C: Diagnosis and treatment. *American Family Physician*. June 2010;81(11):1351–1357.
65. Wood SM, Kennedy JS, Arsenault JE, Thomas DL, Buck RH, Shippee RL, DeMichele SJ, Winship TR, Schaller JP, Montain S, Cordle CT. Novel nutritional immune formula maintains host defense mechanisms. *Military Medicine*. November 2005;170(11):975–985.
66. Yamamoto Y, Nakaji S, Umeda T et al. Effects of long term training on neutrophil function in male university judoists. *British Journal of Sports Medicine*. 2008;42:255–259.
67. Yates J. Traveler's Diarrhea. *American Family Physician*. June 2005;71(11):2095–2100.

61 Neurological Disorders in the Athlete

Gayan P. Poovendran and Joel L. Shaw

CONTENTS

TABLE 61.1
Key Clinical Considerations

1. Exertional headaches in athletes, while generally benign, require a careful history and physical examination, as well as careful risk stratification for ruling out serious intracranial pathology.
2. Epilepsy, in and of itself, should not be a contraindication to athletic activity, and clinicians should work with the patients to encourage safe sport and recreational activity.
3. Severe and atypical pain presentations should alert the astute clinician to the potential diagnosis of chronic regional pain syndrome to afford timely intervention with a multidisciplinary approach.

61.1 INTRODUCTION

Neurological conditions not uncommonly affect recreational and elite athletes, while exercise can assist in most cases in minimizing morbidity and medications utilized as treatments can complicate performance. When considering neurological disorders in an active patient population, participating in both recreational and sports activities, a physician may generally divide these disorders into (1) headaches, (2) epilepsy and other seizure-type disorders, (3) concussions and postconcussion syndromes, and (4) chronic pain disorders and nerve entrapments. This chapter focuses on headache, seizure-type disorders, and chronic pain conditions, whereas concussions and sequelae are discussed in Chapter 40 (Table 61.1).

61.2 HEADACHE

The literature has demonstrated that up to 35% of people who participate in physical exercise experience some form of headache.[63] While active patients suffer from the same types of headaches as the general population, there are several types of headache that may be more closely linked to physical activity. The most common form of headache experienced by sportspersons is effort related, while traumatic headaches are limited to participants in contact sports.[12]

61.2.1 Classification

Classification[21,64] of exercise-induced headaches is problematic due to limited studies that directly address exercise-associated headaches. Exercise-associated headaches are typically classified under a subset of *other primary headache disorders*, as opposed to their own category (see Table 61.2).

When evaluating an athlete in order to diagnose and classify the headache, in particular on the sideline, it is most important to initially triage the patient to facilitate an appropriate treatment plan. When evaluating a sportsperson with headaches, the first responsibility is to determine the severity and urgency of the headache.

61.2.1.1 Serious

Serious headaches require immediate and in-depth evaluation and treatment. There are some *red flags* regarding headache that should cue the physician to a more serious headache (see Table 61.3).

Headache *red flags* include association with any neurological changes, mental status changes, nausea or vomiting, increasing neck stiffness, focal neurological signs, and description as "thunderclap" or "the worst headache of my life." The aforementioned signs and symptoms should warrant immediate evaluation. These signs and symptoms could indicate a hemorrhagic etiology, both within and outside of the brain parenchyma. It is important to remember that not every patient with subarachnoid hemorrhage will declare a *thunderclap* or *the worst headache of my life.*

61.2.1.2 Concerning

Concerning headaches can be associated with traumatic injury. When considering concerning headache, the patient may meet criteria for concussion (displaying confusion,

TABLE 61.2
International Headache Society, Classification of Headache, Third Edition Beta

1. Migraine
2. Tension-type headache
3. Trigeminal autonomic cephalalgias
4. Other primary headache disorders
5. Headache attributed to trauma or injury to the head and/or neck
6. Headache attributed to cranial or cervical vascular disorder
7. Headache attributed to nonvascular intracranial disorder
8. Headache attributed to a substance or its withdrawal
9. Headache attributed to infection
10. Headache attributed to disorder of homoeostasis
11. Headache or facial pain attributed to disorder of the cranium, neck, eyes, ears, nose, sinuses, teeth, mouth, or other facial or cervical structure
12. Headache attributed to psychiatric disorder
13. Painful cranial neuropathies and other facial pains[13]
14. Other headache disorders

TABLE 61.3
Headache Red Flags

Headache associated with any neurological changes
Headache with mental status changes
Headache with nausea or vomiting
Headache with increasing neck stiffness
Headache with focal neurological signs
Description as *thunderclap* or *the worst headache of my life*

delayed motor response, amnesia, incoordination), but does not meet criteria of serious headache discussed earlier. Both serious and concerning headache may also be related to barotrauma from high altitude of diving.

61.2.1.3 Benign

Benign headache should be a diagnosis of exclusion. They may be either vascular or tension type in origin. Typically, they lack the aforementioned associated signs and symptoms of serious or concerning headache. Though immediate treatment is not required in cases of benign headache, the consequences and impact of headache during training and competition are significant.

61.2.2 Primary Headache Disorders

61.2.2.1 Migraine with Aura (IHS 1.2)

61.2.2.1.1 Definition

Migraine is a common and, sometimes, debilitating disorder. It is subdivided into types based on the presence or absence of aura. Migraine without aura is discussed in Tables 61.2 and 61.4. Migraine with aura is primarily characterized by the focal neurological symptoms that usually precede or sometimes accompany the headache. Some patients also experience a premonitory phase, occurring hours or days before the headache, and a headache resolution phase. Premonitory

TABLE 61.4
International Headache Society Criteria for Migraine without Aura

A. At least five attacks fulfilling criteria B–D
B. Headache attacks lasting 4–72 hours (untreated or unsuccessfully treated)
C. Headache has at least two of the following characteristics:
  1. Unilateral location
  2. Pulsating quality
  3. Moderate or severe pain intensity
  4. Aggravation by or causing avoidance of routine physical activity (e.g., walking or climbing stairs)
D. During headache at least one of the following:
  1. Nausea and/or vomiting
  2. Photophobia and phonophobia
E. Not attributed to another disorder

and resolution symptoms include hyperactivity, hypoactivity, depression, craving for particular foods, repetitive yawning, and other less typical symptoms reported by some patients.

61.2.2.1.2 Aggravating Factors

Migraine may be aggravated by a number of factors. These factors are associated with a long-term (weeks to months) increase frequency or severity of headaches. Some commonly reported aggravating factors include psychological stress and frequent intake of alcoholic beverages.

61.2.2.1.3 Precipitating Factors

Trigger factors increase the probability of a migraine attack in the short term (usually <48 hours) in a person with migraine. These include

- Endocrine changes (premenstrual or menstrual, oral contraceptive pills, thyroid disease)
- Metabolic changes (fever, anemia)
- Altitude or temperature change
- Alcohol (particularly red wine)
- Foods (particularly foods high in tyramine such as chocolates, aged cheese, nuts, hot dogs)

61.2.2.1.4 Premonitory Symptoms

Premonitory symptoms may occur hours to a day or 2 before a migraine attack (with or without aura). They include various combinations of fatigue, difficulty in concentrating, neck stiffness, sensitivity to light or sound, nausea, blurred vision, yawning, and pallor. It is best to avoid the previous term, prodromal, because it is mistakenly used to include aura.

61.2.2.1.5 Aura

Aura is the complex of neurological symptoms that occurs just before or at the onset of migraine headache. Symptoms of aura include the following:

- Blind spots (scotomas), which are sometimes outlined by simple geometric designs
- Zigzag lines that gradually float across your field of vision

TABLE 61.5
International Headache Society Criteria for Tension-Type Headache

A. At least 10 episodes occurring and fulfilling criteria B–D
B. Headache lasting from 30 minutes to 7 days
C. Headache has at least two of the following characteristics:
D. Bilateral location
E. Pressing/tightening (nonpulsating) quality
F. Mild or moderate intensity
G. Not aggravated by routine physical activity such as walking or climbing stairs
H. Both of the following:
  1. Absence of nausea or vomiting (anorexia may occur)
  2. No more than one of photophobia or phonophobia
I. Not attributed to another disorder

- Shimmering spots or stars
- Changes in vision
- Flashes of light
- Paresthesias
- Dysarthria

Treatment and management of migraine with aura is similar to treatment of migraine without aura, which is discussed in Table 16.5. A summary of common medications used in the management of headache is found in Table 61.6.

61.2.3 Tension (IHS 2)

Tension-type headaches (TTHs) are the most common type of primary headache: its lifetime prevalence in the general population ranges in different studies from 30% to 78%. The ICHD-IIR1 has specific diagnostic criteria for TTH (see Table 61.5),

TABLE 61.6
Medications for Use in Athletes with Headache Disorder

Class/Drug	Trade Name	Dosing	Maximum Daily Dosing
Analgesic			
Acetaminophen	Tylenol	325–1000 mg PO Q4–6 hours as needed	3000 mg
Nonsteroidal anti-inflammatories			
Aspirin	Ecotrin	325–650 PO Q4–6 hours as needed	4000 mg
Ibuprofen	Advil, Motrin	400–800 mg PO Q8 hours as needed	2400 mg
Naproxen	Aleve, Naprosyn, Anaprox	220–500 mg PO Q12 hours as needed	1500 mg
Muscle relaxants			
Cyclobenzaprine	Flexeril	10 mg PO Q12 hours as needed	30 mg
Methocarbamol	Robaxin	500–1500 mg PO Q6 hours as needed	8000 mg
Tizanidine	Zanaflex	4–8 mg PO Q6–8 hours as needed	36 mg
Migraine sedatives			
Butalbital + acetaminophen + caffeine	Fioricet	1 tab PO Q6 hours as needed	6 caplets
Butalbital + aspirin + caffeine	Fiorinal	1 tab PO Q6 hours as needed	6 tablets
Isometheptene + dichloralphenazone + acetaminophen	Midrin	2 tabs at headache onset, then one per hour until headache relieved	8 capsules
Ergotamines			
Ergotamine tartrate + caffeine	Cafergot	2 tabs at headache onset, then one per hour until headache relieved	6 tablets a day; 10 tablets a week
Dihydroergotamine mesylate	Migranal nasal	One spray in each nostril, repeat in 15 minutes if needed	6 sprays a day; 8 sprays a week
Dihydroergotamine	D.H.E. 45	1 mg IV/IM ×1, may repeat in 1 hour	3 mg per attack; 6 mg per week
Triptans			
Sumatriptan	Imitrex	One tablet at onset, repeat every 2 hours as needed One spray in each nostril at onset, may repeat once in 2 hours One injection SQ at onset, may repeat once after 1 hour	200 mg orally 40 mg nasally 12 mg subcutaneously
Migraine prophylaxis			
Topiramate	Topamax	50 mg PO BID	200 mg
Amitriptyline	Elavil	10–100 mg PO QHS	150 mg
Propranolol	Inderal	160–240 PO daily	
Verapamil	Calan	80 mg PO TID	480 mg
Divalproex	Depakote	250–500 mg PO BID	

subdividing it into episodic (ETTH) and chronic (CTTH), with a further subdivision of ETTH into frequent and infrequent.

61.2.3.1 Description

In patients presenting with TTH, pain is typically bilateral, pressing, or tightening in quality and of mild-to-moderate intensity, and it does not worsen with routine physical activity. There is no nausea but photophobia or phonophobia may be present.

61.2.3.1.1 Treatment

Treatment varies on chronicity and frequency of TTH. Infrequent TTH, with symptoms once a month or less, rarely has a significant impact on the patient's life. These patients respond well to analgesics on an as-needed basis. Patients with frequent TTH and CTTH can suffer from severe functional impairment. In either case, treatment goals should be limiting analgesic use to less than twice a week. More frequent use necessitates a prophylactic regimen, in which amitriptyline is the agent of choice. Relaxation techniques, biofeedback training, and cognitive behavior therapy are empirically validated behavioral treatments for TTH, with meta-analyses indicating that they produce similar results to amitriptyline prophylaxis.[33,51]

Clinical Pearl

The treatment goal of TTH is to limit analgesic and abortive agent use to less than twice a week.

61.2.4 Cluster (IHS 3.1)

Cluster headache presents as attacks of severe, strictly unilateral pain that is orbital, supraorbital, and temporal or in any combination of these sites. Pain lasts 15–180 minutes and occurs from once every other day to eight times a day. The attacks are associated with one or more of the following, all of which are ipsilateral: conjunctival injection, lacrimation, nasal congestion, rhinorrhea, forehead and facial sweating, miosis, ptosis, and eyelid edema. Most patients are restless or agitated during an attack. Cluster headaches are reportedly five times more common in men.

61.2.4.1 Treatment

Treatment of cluster headache is dependent on the age and health of patient and is aimed at cluster prevention. Drugs known to be effective prophylactic agents include verapamil, ergotamine, lithium, and prednisolone. Evidence for antiepileptic medications is limited. Acute attacks may be aborted with 100% oxygen and a rate of 7 L/min, though the mechanism of this is unclear. Additional abortive options include 5-hydroxytryptamine agonists such as sumatriptan and zolmitriptan.

61.3 Sports and Exercise-Related Primary Headache Disorders[33,51]

61.3.1 Exercise-Induced Migraine/Migraine without Aura (IHS 1.1)

Approximately 20% of individuals who experience migraine have their symptoms precipitated by physical activity and exercise, and effort induced migraine is seen in approximately 9% of sports-related headache. Headaches may be brought on in sports such as hockey, weight training, cycling, and rowing, among others. Exercise in extremes of temperature or altitude may also precipitate exercise-induced migraine. It is estimated that 10% of athletic migraines have an organic cause.[37]

According to the International Headache Society (IHS), migraine is a recurrent headache disorder manifesting in attacks lasting 4–72 hours. Typical characteristics of the headache are unilateral location, pulsating quality, moderate or severe intensity, aggravation by routine physical activity, and association with nausea and/or photophobia and phonophobia (see Table 61.4).

61.3.1.1 Treatment

In order to effectively treat migraines, it is important to have an accurate diagnosis, and treatment should be multifactorial. There are three main stages of treatment: (1) preventive treatment, (2) abortive treatment, and in some cases (3) prophylactic treatment.

Clinical Pearl

Use caution when prescribing beta-blockers in an athletic population, as the decrease in heart rate may cause these patients to experience decrease in exercise tolerance.

61.3.1.2 Preventive Treatment

Prevention is the most effective form of treatment. A healthy lifestyle is essential to limit headaches, including a healthy, well-balanced diet, adequate sleep (8 h/day), and adequate hydration. According to several studies, the use of riboflavin 200 mg twice a day and magnesium citrate 200 mg twice a day is beneficial.[36,51] Riboflavin improves mitochondrial energy and the magnesium decreases neurological hyperexcitability. Proper warm-up and breathing techniques will help to limit the effects of breath holding and Valsalva maneuver.

61.3.1.3 Abortive Treatment

During a migrainous attack, most patients will initially choose to lie quietly in a dark room and attempt to sleep. Sleep often terminates the attack. In other cases, more active treatment is necessitated. Active treatment of acute headaches is most commonly treated with nonsteroidal anti-inflammatory drugs

(NSAIDs), including ibuprofen and naproxen. When the pattern is more typical of migraines, 5-hydroxytryptamine blockers, such as sumatriptan or ergotamines, are effective as second-line therapy.

61.3.1.4 Prophylactic Treatment

Prophylactic treatment may include medications such as indomethacin or other NSAIDs, amitriptyline, SSRIs, beta-blockers, and calcium channel blockers. Caution should be used when using beta-blockers, narcotics, and caffeine in more competitive athletes, as they may be subject to substance screening. Similarly, side effects of these medications may adversely affect athletic performance. For difficult-to-manage patients, several alternative treatments have been shown to be effective. Botulinum toxin type A is effective and safe as prophylaxis for chronic headaches, exhibiting a 56% decrease in the number of headaches per month.[5] A randomized control trial demonstrated that acupuncture improves quality of life and decreases headache pain.[8]

61.3.2 Primary Exertional Headache (IHS 4.3)[27]

Primary exertional headache is the most common type of sports-related headache, having an incidence of 74% in one study. It is more frequently precipitated by aerobic activity, though any physical activity can be a factor. Patients will describe a mild-to-moderate headache that is either generalized or located in the frontal area. The etiology of this disorder is unknown. One theory regarded impaired vascular flow, but this has not been supported.

61.3.2.1 Definition

Per IHS, primary exertional headache is classified under *other primary headache disorders* (see Table 61.7). It is defined as headache precipitated by any form of exercise.

Subforms such as *weight lifter's headache* are recognized.[46] Weight lifter's headache has been proposed to be categorized under primary cough headache disorder, due to its proposed mechanism related to straining and Valsalva maneuvers in the absence of an intracranial abnormality.[10]

Clinical Pearl

You must investigate the first occurrence of exertional headache with MRI or CT scan to rule out subarachnoid hemorrhage or arterial dissection.

61.3.2.1.1 Management and Treatment

On first occurrence of this headache type, it is mandatory to exclude subarachnoid hemorrhage and arterial dissection. In one study, 43% of exertional headaches were associated with underlying pathology, though this was more prevalent in the middle-aged (average age of 42) as opposed to the younger (average age of 24) of the study population.[57]

TABLE 61.7
International Headache Society Criteria for Primary Exertional Headache

Pulsating headache fulfilling criteria 2 and 3
Lasting from 5 minutes to 48 hours
Brought on by and occurring only during or after physical activity
Cannot be attributed to another disorder

Diagnostic modalities include CT and MRI, depending on acuity and severity of symptoms. Other organic causes associated with primary exertional headache include Arnold–Chiari malformation, cerebral aneurysm, and intracranial neoplasm. Management and treatment revolve around either avoiding the precipitating activity, careful attention to breathing techniques, or prophylaxis with nonsteroidal anti-inflammatory medications.[46] Headaches tend to recur over weeks to months and then slowly resolve. In some cases, they may be lifelong.

Clinical Pearl

In cases of exertional headache, younger participants tend to have benign causes, whereas older participants tend to have underlying pathology.

61.4 SPORTS AND EXERCISE-RELATED SECONDARY HEADACHE DISORDERS

61.4.1 Acute and Chronic Posttraumatic Headache (IHS 5.1 and IHS 5.2)[12]

Headache is a symptom that may occur after injury to the head, neck, or brain. In cases of moderate-to-severe head trauma, imaging is required to rule out a traumatic brain lesion. In acute posttraumatic headache, symptoms generally develop within a week of trauma and resolve within 3 months. This temporal relationship helps establish trauma as cause for headache. There are case reports of symptoms developing months after inciting event, but these are rare and limited to case reports.

Chronic posttraumatic headache is often part of the posttraumatic syndrome that includes a variety of symptoms such as equilibrium disturbance, poor concentration, decreased work ability, irritability, depressive mood, and sleep disturbances. These patients present similarly to acute posttraumatic headache, but their symptoms have persisted beyond 3 months.

61.4.2 Cervicogenic Headache (IHS 11.2.1)

Cervicogenic, or cervical, headache is the term used to describe a headache that is caused by an abnormality of the joints, musculature, or neural structure of the neck. Physical exam and imaging studies lead to acceptance of cervical pathology causing headache. Treatment of cervicogenic headache requires correction of the abnormalities precipitating symptoms. A comprehensive exercise program includes motor control exercises of the neck. This may or may not be used in conjunction with soft tissue therapy. Postural retraining is an essential part of treatment, and stress reduction techniques may also be helpful.

61.4.3 High-Altitude Headache (IHS 10.1.1)

Headache is frequent sequelae to ascent to altitude, occurring in up to 80% of people traveling from lower elevations. Patients presenting with high-altitude headache will complain of bilateral frontal or frontotemporal headache that is dull or pressing quality. They are generally of mild or moderate intensity and aggravated by exertion, movement, straining, coughing, or bending.

These headache disorders occur within 24 hours of ascent to 2500 m and typically resolve within 8 hours of descent. High-altitude headache is a well-recognized accompaniment of acute mountain sickness. Prevention of this complication of altitude can be achieved through a slow ascent with acclimatization, with or without prophylactic acetazolamide 24 hours prior to ascent (see Chapter 63).

Clinical Pearl

Acetazolamide can be used for prevention and adjuvant treatment of high-altitude headache, but the cornerstone of treatment should always be safe descent.

High-altitude cerebral edema is a medical emergency and the sportsperson should receive prompt treatment, with descent to below 2500 m, to prevent permanent neurological damage. Adjuvant treatment options include dexamethasone and acetazolamide, though descent should be the mainstay of treatment.

61.4.4 Diving Headache (IHS 10.1.2)

Diver's headache is a nonspecific headache that is thought to be related to hypercapnia and vascular relaxation. The headache develops while diving to depths below 10 m and is accompanied by at least one symptom of CO_2 intoxication (light-headedness, mental confusion, dyspnea, flushed feeling of the face, motor incoordination) in the absence of decompression sickness. This headache resolves within 1 hour with treatment of 100% oxygen.

61.5 EPILEPSY

There has long been a controversy involving epileptic patients and their safety to participate in athletics and exercise. For the past several decades, the concerns of parents, administrators, and coaches have led to restrictions on athletic involvement for epileptic patients. Medical recommendations for a long period supported the exclusion of these patients and have only recently made some progress in allowing participation. Until 1974, organizations such as the American Medical Association (AMA) and the American Academy of Pediatrics (AAP) recommended significant restrictions in activity due to fear of injury and induction of seizure activity. Articles published in 1973 argued both for and against participation for epileptic patients.[30,34] This discussion led to a change in the change in the recommendations of the AMA in 1974 allowing participation in contact sports in some cases to assist in adjustment to school, social interactions, and the diagnosis of seizure disorder. In 1983, the AAP adjusted their recommendation to allow participation in most sports, including contact sports, as long as seizures were adequately controlled and supervision was available.

Clinical Pearl

Patients with well-controlled epilepsy may participate in most sports, including contact sports, as long as there is adequate supervision.

Epilepsy, defined as more than two seizures more than 24 hours apart in an individual greater than 1 month of age, is present in 1%–2% of the population.[9,25] Seventy-five percent of these patients have their first seizure by the age of 20, and thirty to forty percent of patients who have an initial seizure will have a recurrent episode and then are likely to have repetitive episodes in the future [9]. Despite this frequency, based on a study in 1997, 80% of patients are well controlled on two or fewer antiepileptic medications.[3] This should reassure patients and physicians that these would benefit from exercise. Multiple studies confirm the connection of decreased exercise and activity in epileptic patients with decreased self-esteem, increased anxiety and depression, and diseases associated with poor physical fitness, such as obesity, heart disease, and diabetes.[4,20,25] For this reason, the psychosocial and psychological benefits of physical activity should be used to encourage patients with well-controlled epilepsy to be involved frequently in physical activity, athletics, and exercise.

61.5.1 Classification

Seizures are generally classified based upon clinical presentation and the degree of involvement of the central nervous system, as well as their relationship to trauma (see Table 61.8). Seizures generally have unique etiologies based upon age (see Table 61.9) and have well-described precipitating risk factors (see Table 61.10).

Partial seizures are localized to one area of the brain with the activation of a smaller number of neurons. Partial seizures are further classified as simple or complex in reference

TABLE 61.8
Classification of Seizures

Focal
Simple
Complex
General
Tonic–clonic
Absence
Status epilepticus
Posttraumatic
Immediate
Early
Late

TABLE 61.9
Seizure Causes

Pediatrics	Neonatal injury, CNS infection, head trauma, metabolic disorder, tumor
Adults	Vascular insult, infection, tumor

TABLE 61.10
Precipitating Factors of Seizure

Idiopathic
New onset epilepsy
Stress
Sleep deprivation
Hyperthermia
Metabolic: hypoglycemia, hyponatremia, dehydration
Infections: meningitis, encephalitis
Trauma
Intracranial lesions: hematoma, tumor
Drugs/alcohol: intoxication or withdrawal

to the effect on consciousness. Seizures with no loss of consciousness are termed partial seizures but may include motor, sensory, or autonomic symptoms. Seizures associated with altered consciousness, which may include diminished responsiveness, staring, lip smacking, and repetitive swallowing, are termed complex seizures.

Generalized seizures are seizures associated with bilateral discharges on electroencephalography (EEG) and involve the entire cortex. Generalized seizures can be either convulsive or nonconvulsive. Nonconvulsive generalized seizures include absence and myoclonic seizures.

61.5.2 Benefits of Exercise

As stated before, epileptic patients have a higher rate of obesity, body mass index, and body fat ratio. Inactivity, in addition to the side effects of antiepileptic drugs, is a principal contributing factor. The effects of commonly used AEDs on weight are displayed in Table 61.11.[3]

TABLE 61.11
Effect of Antiepileptic Drugs on Weight

Weight Gain	Weight Loss	Weight Neutral
Gabapentin	*Topiramate*	*Lamotrigine*
Pregabalin	Zonisamide	*Phenytoin*
Valproate		Levetiracetam
Carbamazepine		

To counteract this medical risk, an active exercise program has been demonstrated to decrease cholesterol levels and increase aerobic performance. This same study showed that a regular exercise program reduces sleep problems and fatigue, improves psychosocial functioning, and increases sense of well-being. There are multiple studies that show decreased seizure risk in patients who follow a regular exercise program. Two studies showed improved EEG results, including a decrease in occurrence of epileptiform discharge, a normalization of EEG changes, and an increase of seizure threshold.[18,46]

In general, people with epilepsy report better seizure control when exercising regularly. A minority (up to 10%) of patients will provoke seizure with exercise. In one study, up to 36% of patients reported that regular exercise led to better seizure control and decreased epileptiform activity on EEG [38]. Also, sport participation does not appear to affect serum drug levels.

Clinical Pearl

For the large majority of patients (>90%), regular physical activity improves or has no effect on seizure threshold.

61.5.3 Epilepsy and Sports

61.5.3.1 Risk of Participation

It is important for patients and physicians to understand the things that may make participation in sports dangerous or unsafe. First, we need to understand the factors that may precipitate seizures. These include fatigue, emotional stress, fever, hormonal changes of the menstrual cycle, alcohol, caffeine, heat, humidity, and sleep deprivation (see Table 61.10). These vary depending on the patient and should be individualized.

Patients with epilepsy do not have a higher injury rate than those without epilepsy. In one study, exercise provoked seizure in 10% of participants,[30] though the risk of sustaining serious seizure-related injury was modest. In two separate studies, only 1%–2% of patients had identified exercise as a trigger for seizure activity.[15,37] Hypoglycemia and hyponatremia are also common abnormalities that may lower the seizure threshold, though there is no evidence to support that patients with epilepsy have more seizures related to these abnormalities compared with the general population. The concern for an increased risk of injury with sports participation is unfounded in most sports, although there are certain activities connected with a high risk.[1,22,52]

61.5.3.2 Specific Sports Guidelines

61.5.3.2.1 *Contact Sports: No Restrictions unless New Diagnosis or Unclear Course*

There are no recommendations or studies to support restricting the participation of epileptic patients in contact or collision sports.[35] Any current restrictions in sports should be based only on risk to the athlete or other participants if a seizure occurs during the sporting activity. According to the AMA and AAP, there should be no restriction for well-controlled epileptics to participate in football, hockey, rugby, soccer, basketball, or baseball. Boxing is the only collision sport without specific recommendations by the AMA, AAP, or American Association of Neurology. In the case of boxing, because there are no studies or consensus statements to restrict or allow participation, the decision to all participation should be done on an individual basis with full disclosure of potential risk to the patient.

61.5.3.2.2 *Water Sports: Permitted with Proper Precautions (No Open Water, Appropriate Flotation Devices, and Qualified Personnel)*

The main concern with swimming is the risk of drowning if a seizure occurs while in the water. One study showed a fourfold increase in the risk of drowning or near drowning from submersion in epileptic patients.[20] The general consensus is that epileptic patients with good control of seizure activity may participate in water competition and swimming if there is direct visual supervision by someone adequately trained in rescue and resuscitation techniques. This should only be permitted in events with clear water.

61.5.3.2.2.1 Not Permitted: Scuba, Competitive Underwater Swimming, and Diving Scuba diving is restricted due to the risk of dislodging the regulator, the poor airway protection during an emergency rapid ascent increasing the risk of aspiration or *the bends*, and the potential for injury to the rescue partner. Diving may be permitted after prolonged antiseizure period but is discouraged in patients with poor seizure control.

61.5.3.2.3 *Motor Sports: Discouraged*

The risk of injury to the driver, other drivers, or spectators in motor sports due to the high speed and force of collision is severe. For this reason, any effort to reduce the frequency of accidents and the risk of severe injury is essential. The general recommendation is that all epileptic patients should avoid participation in motor sports.

61.5.3.2.4 *Aerobic Sports: No Restrictions*

61.5.3.2.4.1 Sports at Heights Discouraged: Equestrian Sports, Free Climbing, and Gymnastics (High Bar and Rings) Sports in which a fall could cause serious injury require more serious consideration of seizure control and the benefit of participation for the athlete. Gymnastics requires appropriate planning and preparation for each individual. When seizures are well controlled, close observation and assistance by coaches and trainers are essential. In some cases, the use of safety harnesses is beneficial. Horseback riding and harnessed climbing may be possible with good seizure control and the assistance of a partner who can provide first aid and has the ability to contact emergency personnel, as long as the patient understands fully the risk.

Prohibited: Pilot Sports, Free Climbing, Skydiving, and Hang Gliding. Because of the potential risk of injury to the participant or others involved in these events, the risks outweigh the benefits of epileptic patients participating in these high-risk activities.

Shooting Sports: Permitted with Consideration of Type, Frequency, Pattern of Seizure, and Type of Weapon Fired.

TABLE 61.12
Antiepileptic Drugs and Their Common Side Effects

Drug Name	Common Side Effects
Gabapentin	Well tolerated compared to most antiepileptic medications, with minimal side effects or drug interaction.
Lamotrigine	Potential to cause dizziness, movement disorders, sedation, and headaches.
Valproate	Known to cause increased appetite, resulting in weight gain and tremors.
	Sedation and cognitive impairment are much less common.
Carbamazepine	May cause sedation, ataxia, nausea, and dizziness.
Phenytoin	Known to result in sedation, depressed cognitive function, and depressed activity.

61.5.4 Medication Guidelines for Sports

Medical treatment of epilepsy is difficult in the athletic population due to the frequent side effects from the medications that may affect the performance of the sportsperson. Discussed in Table 61.12 are side effects of several medications that may impact athletic performance, but the main point is that each patient must be treated individually for better seizure control with reduction of side effects (see Table 61.12).

61.6 COMPLEX REGIONAL PAIN SYNDROME

Complex regional pain syndrome (CRPS) is a disorder that typically affects the extremities and includes pain, swelling, decreased range of motion, vasomotor instability, skin changes, and, at the more advanced stages, bone demineralization. The development of this condition is often preceded by injury, surgery, or a vascular event. The commonly accepted definition involves regional pain with associated sensory changes following a noxious event.[54] Typically, the pain is described as more severe than would be expected based on the preceding injury. Typical associated skin changes include skin color changes, temperature changes, edema, allodia, loss of typical hair, and atypical sweat pattern.

Cases are categorized into two general types simply termed Type I and Type II. Type I, which has also been called reflex sympathetic dystrophy in the past, is defined by the symptoms listed earlier with no specific nerve lesion or no specific nerve involved. Type II, also referred to as causalgia, involves a case with a definitive and specific nerve lesion.

61.6.1 Etiology and Pathophysiology

One study that reviewed 140 cases of CRPS found the breakdown of the inciting event to be soft tissue injury (40%), fractures (25%), myocardial infarction (12%), and cerebrovascular events (3%).[43] Another study showed 35% of cases reviewed had no known precipitating event.[59] A study of 60 cases of knee CRPS showed the most common precipitating event being a knee arthroscopy.[39] One recurrent theme is the potential connection of current emotional stress as a common precipitating risk for the development of CRPS after an inciting event.[16,43]

The variety of causes coincides with the unclear understanding of the detailed pathogenesis of CRPS. The most common theory is the inciting event leads to development of a reflex arc. The arc is believed to follow along the sympathetic nervous system leading to peripheral vascular disturbances, cortical center dysfunction, increased sensitivity of injured axons to epinephrine, and abnormal response of local sympathetic nerves. The persistent pain and allodynia that develop in CRPS appear to be related to the peripheral nerves releasing inflammatory mediators and pain-producing peptides including substance P, neuropeptide Y, IL-6, TNF alpha, and IL-1 beta.[2,48] There also appears to be a central nervous system component based on improvement in symptoms after unilateral sympathetic nerve blocks and central changes found on functional MRI imaging of patients with CRPS.[14,45] Based on all of these studies, it appears the cause of CRPS is multifactorial and highly individual.

61.6.2 Clinical Presentation

CRPS is described as three clinical stages. Stage 1 involves burning pain, aching, increased sensitivity to touch and cold, edema, and vasomotor disturbances (altered color and temperature). Stage 2 may show increased edema, thickening of soft tissues such as skin, muscle wasting, and swollen, thicker skin. Stage 3 is associated with decreased range of motion, digit contractures, and brittle nails. This can also be associated with shoulder–hand syndrome where the patient may develop capsular retraction leading to frozen shoulder. CRPS is also typically associated with autonomic changes that may include cyanosis, mottling, abnormal sweating, loss of hair, diffuse soft tissue swelling, and coldness.[50]

Radiologic changes are common but sometimes difficult to interpret. Bone scans often show changes in CRPS. Early in the course of disease, there will be decreased perfusion of the affected area in early uptake.[38] Between 6 weeks and 6 months, the affected area will show increased uptake in the involved extremity during delayed perfusion.[29] After 6 months, bone scan changes are not very helpful. Plain film radiographs may show osteopenia in cases of CRPS. This is most evident in stage 3 disease.[27] MRI has the ability to differentiate soft tissue changes associated with CRPS including skin thickening, soft tissue edema, tissue enhancement of contrast material, and muscle atrophy. Based on these changes, MRI is most helpful in stages 1 and 3.[49] Based on expert opinion, the best recommendations at this point are to use bone scan in evaluation of apparent stage 1 and 2 disease and x-rays in stage 3 disease.

Other helpful diagnostic tools may include autonomic testing and response to therapy. Autonomic tests may include resting sweat output, resting skin temperature, and the quantitative sudomotor axon reflex test. These tests, although they can provide additional information, have not been well studied in comparison to typical response and recovery after a severe injury. Another diagnostic tool is response to sympatholysis. In the past, response to IV regional anesthesia or sympathetic nerve block was considered necessary for the diagnosis of CRPS. A Cochrane review in 2005[7] showed the evidence for this test is inconclusive, although the test is still helpful in demonstrating pain related to the sympathetic nervous system.

It is important to remember that the diagnosis of CRPS is a clinical diagnosis. There is no clinical test that it is the gold standard, and any laboratory or radiologic test should only be used as additional information to confirm diagnosis or assist with treatment.

61.6.3 Treatment

The best treatment for CRPS is prevention. The standard of prevention is early mobilization. This has been demonstrated especially in stroke patients,[6,44] although it appears clinically to be effective after trauma, prolonged IV use, and after myocardial infarction. Another potential preventive measure after fractures is the supplemental vitamin C. There are multiple studies demonstrating effectiveness after distal radius fractures,[56,66] although this has not been studied after any other fractures.

Further treatment requires a multidisciplinary approach. The first step is to educate the patient on the process, causes, and foundation for treatment. There have been limited studies on the use of psychological assessment and counseling, but the consensus is that this treatment would be beneficial, especially in later stage disease, based on the response in other chronic pain conditions. Physical therapy and occupational therapy are mainstay treatments, although the evidence is inconclusive regarding the effectiveness of these treatments.[40,41]

Multiple medications are used for treatment, with differing levels of evidence. The consensus guidelines[53] recommend as first choices tricyclic antidepressants, anticonvulsants (such as gabapentin and pregabalin), NSAIDs, and opioids for more severe pain. The most important concept of these treatments is to reduce pain in order to allow more aggressive physical therapy. Bisphosphonates were initially used to prevent bone resorption in CRPS, but further studies have shown benefits in pain relief.[32,60] Studies of short courses of glucocorticoids have demonstrated more benefit than NSAIDs and significant improvement compared to placebo. Due to the potential side effects, the expert consensus appears to be using glucocorticoids when the patient has not responded well to NSAIDs.[6,28] Calcitonin has been used due to its ability to slow bone resorption and its analgesic effect, similar to its benefit in the treatment of osteoporotic fractures. Studies have shown it to be effective, although the studies have not yet identified an optimal dose or duration.[17] Other medications that are sometimes suggested but have not been proven to be effective clinically include sympatholytics (propranolol, reserpine, or guanethidine), alpha-1 adrenoreceptor antagonists (terazosin or phenoxybenzamine), or clonidine patches.

If the oral therapies and physical therapy are not effective, the next step is to start one of several types of invasive therapy. The initial treatment would be a trigger point injection, most commonly used in the trapezius and suprascapular muscles. Nerve stimulation through transcutaneous electrical nerve stimulation (units) has shown some benefit.[19] Limited studies have shown some benefit with epidural clonidine although the side effects, such as hypotension and sedation, have been limiting factors.[24] Regional sympathetic nerve blocks may include ganglion blocks, stellate ganglion blocks, and intravenous regional blocks (Bier blocks). The results have been inconsistent but potentially beneficial.[7] Spinal cord stimulators may be an option if typical therapeutic measures have failed. Studies have shown decrease in pain but no significant improvement in function.[23] The last, most invasive choice is sympathectomy, which can be chemical or surgical treatment. Although a surgical clinic study showed significant decrease in pain,[42] other studies have shown adverse effects to include increased pain, new neuropathic pain, and uncontrolled sweating.[31] The concern for adverse effects and the significant invasiveness should leave this treatment as a last resort only for patients with stage 3 disease.

61.6.4 Prognosis

CRPS Type I, estimated to be the cause of 90% of cases, has a favorable prognosis, with 74% of cases resulting in complete resolution of symptoms.[47] The rate of recurrence ranges from 10% to 30% over multiple studies. A study of 1183 patients with CRPS showed a recurrence rate of 10%.[61] In this study, recurrences were more common in a different limb (76 patients) compared with the originally affected limb (34 patients). Recurrences may develop spontaneously or as a result of trauma, cold exposure, new surgery, or emotional trauma. In this same study, recurrences most commonly occurred spontaneously (53%) and the measured incidence of recurrence was less than 2% per patient per year.

61.6.5 Recurrence of CRPS

There are reported cases of recurrence of CRPS, although the cases are poorly understood. One of the factors that can predispose to a recurrence is surgery on a previously affected extremity. The general consensus is to avoid surgery during an exacerbation of CRPS and wait to perform elective surgeries until these episodes have improved. Based on a study of 47 patients with CRPS undergoing surgery of a previously affected extremity, the use of aggressive perfusion, avoidance of tourniquets, and perioperative mannitol infusions decreased the recurrence rate to 13%.[62] Also, in this study, the recurrence was mild and temporary in all but one recurrence. Proposed measures for prevention, although not proven to be effective, include aggressive rehabilitation, preoperative sympathetic blocks, postsurgery neuromodulation, and perioperative calcitonin prophylaxis. Exacerbations and recurrences are often treated with tricyclic antidepressants and anticonvulsants.

61.7 PARSONAGE–TURNER SYNDROME

Parsonage–Turner syndrome is a nontraumatic, idiopathic brachial plexopathy caused by an inflammatory disorder of the brachial plexus. The pathology of this condition is speculative but suggested based on clinical and electrophysiologic changes. It appears to have a multifactorial etiology that tends to affect motor nerves more significantly than sensory nerves.[11] The most common hypothesis is some relation to an atypical or exaggerated autoimmune response. Approximately half of patients describe a preceding event or condition including infection, exercise, surgery, or recent vaccination.[58]

61.7.1 Pathophysiology

The initial clinical symptom is sudden onset of severe pain in the shoulder. The pain is most often unilateral involving the shoulder girdle and the lateral arm. The severe pain often lasts up to 4 weeks before slowly decreasing.[60] There are frequently related sensory symptoms, most often of which is hypesthesia or paresthesia of the lateral shoulder and arm. Weakness develops after the pain, though the timing varies from the first 24 hours or up to several weeks later. The weakness may be associated with atrophy. These neurological changes can involve an isolated nerve or several nerves. The most commonly involved nerves are the suprascapular, long thoracic, musculocutaneous, radial, or axillary nerves. Resolution of weakness does not begin for several months, and complete recovery may require several years.[56]

61.7.2 Diagnosis

Diagnosis is typically made clinically, and diagnostic testing is used to confirm the clinical suspicion. Clinical diagnosis is made based on a pattern of sudden onset of severe pain progressing to weakness and atrophy that resolves slowly. When this pattern is present, the diagnosis can be confirmed by nerve conduction and electromyography. These studies may confirm specific nerve pathology or a more extensive distribution of damage. Laboratory and radiologic testing will be normal.

TABLE 61.13
SORT: Key Recommendations for Practice

Clinical Recommendation	Evidence Rating	References
Headache *red flags* and first episode of exertional headache warrant radiologic investigation.	C	[33,36]
Epileptic patients should be encouraged to be physically active.	B	[18,20,25]
Sympathectomy for patients with CRPS should be used with caution, in carefully selected patients, after thorough assessment, and probably only after failure of other treatment options or in palliative cases.	C	[31,42]
In patients requiring medications for headache, attention to adverse effects can help avoid time away from physical activity.	C	[33,36,46]

61.7.3 Treatment

There are no treatments proven to be effective for Parsonage–Turner syndrome. The main form of management is conservative to include pain medications as needed for the acute severe pain. Physical therapy is often used to assist with range of motion although there is no evidence that it will accelerate recovery. Although steroids are sometimes prescribed, again there is no evidence of benefit. The estimated time for recovery ranges from 1 to 3 years. Recurrence rate is around 5%.[56] It is not uncommon to have chronic residual weakness after recovery, although the percentages in the studies range from single digits to 60%[10] (Table 61.13).

REFERENCES

1. Aisonson MR. Accidental injuries in epileptic children. *Pediatrics.* 1948;2(1):85–88.
2. Alexander GM, van Rijn MA, van Hilten JJ et al. Changes in cerebrospinal fluid levels of pro-inflammatory cytokines in CRPS. *Pain.* 2005;116:213.
3. Baker GA, Jacoby A, Buck D, Staglis C, Monnet D. Quality of life of people with epilepsy: A European study. *Epilepsia.* 1997;38(3):353–362.
4. Ben-Menachem E. Weight issues for people with epilepsy—A review. *Epilepsia.* 2007;48(5):42–45.
5. Blumenfield A. Botulinum toxin type A as an effective prophylactic treatment in primary headache disorders. *Headache.* 2003;43(8):853–860.
6. Braus DF, Krauss JK, Strobel J. The shoulder-hand syndrome after stroke: A prospective clinical trial. *Annals of Neurology.* 1994;36:728.
7. Cepeda MS, Carr DB, Lau J. Local anesthetic sympathetic blockade for complex regional pain syndrome. *Cochrane Database of Systematic Reviews.* 2005;(4):CD004598.
8. Coeytaux RR, Kaufman JS, Kaptchuk TJ et al. A randomized controlled trial of acupuncture for chronic daily headache. *Headache.* 2005;45(9):1113–1123.
9. Corbitt RW, Cooped DL, Erickson DJ, Kriss FC, Thornton ML, Craig TT. American Medical Association Committee on Medical Aspects of Sports: Epileptics and contact sports. *Journal of the American Medical Association.* 1975;229(7):820–821.
10. Cup EH, Ijspeert J, Janssen RJ et al. Residual complaints after neuralgic amyotrophy. *Archives of Physical Medicine and Rehabi.* 2013;94:67.
11. Daniel JC, Nassiri JD, Wilckens J, Land BC. The implementation and use of the standardized assessment of concussion at the U.S. Naval Academy. *Military Medicine.* 2002;167(10):L873–L876.
11. England JD, Sumner AJ. Neuralgic amyotrophy: An increasingly diverse entity. *Muscle Nerve.* 1987;10:60.
12. Evans RW. Posttraumatic headaches in civilians, soldiers, and athletes. *Neurologic Clinics.* May 2014;32(2):283–303.
13. Farooq K, Williams P. Headaches and chronic facial pain. *Continuing Education in Anaesthesia, Critical Care & Pain.* 2008;8(4):138–142.
14. Freund W, Wunderlich AP, Stuber G et al. Different activation of opercular and posterior cingulate cortex (PCC) in patients with complex regional pain syndrome (CRPS I) compared with healthy controls during perception of electrically induced pain: A functional MRI study. *Clinical Journal of Pain.* 2010;26:339.
15. Frucht MM, Quigg M, Schwaner C, Fountain NB. Distribution of seizure precipitants among epilepsy syndromes. *Epilepsia.* 2000;41(12):1534–1539.
16. Geertzen JH, de Bruijn H, de Bruijn-Kofman AT, Arendzen JH. Reflex sympathetic dystrophy: Early treatment and psychological aspects. *Archives of Physical Medicine and Rehabilitation.* 1994;75:442.
17. Gobelet C, Waldburger M, Meier JL. The effect of adding calcitonin to physical treatment on reflex sympathetic dystrophy. *Pain.* 1992;48:171.
18. Gotze W, Kubicki S, Munter M, Teichman J. Effect of physical exercise on seizure threshold. *Diseases of the Nervous System.* 1967;28:664–667.
19. Hassenbusch SJ, Stanton-Hicks M, Schoppa D et al. Long-term results of peripheral nerve stimulation for reflex sympathetic dystrophy. *Journal of Neurosurgery.* 1996;84:415.
20. Howard GM, Radloff M, Sevier TL. Epilepsy and sports participation. *Current Sports Medicine Reports.* 2004;3:15–19.
21. International Headache Society. *International Headache Classification*, 2nd edn. April 24, 2013. http://www.ihs-classification.org/en/02_klassifikation/01_inhalt/.
22. ILAE Commission report. Restrictions for children with epilepsy. Commission of Pediatrics of the International League Against Epilepsy. *Epilepsia.* 1997;38(9):1054–1056.
23. Kemler MA, de Vet HC, Barendse GA et al. Spinal cord stimulation for chronic reflex sympathetic dystrophy—Five-year follow-up. *New England Journal of Medicine.* 2006;354:2394.
24. Kirkpatrick AF, Derasari M. Transdermal clonidine: Treating reflex sympathetic dystrophy. *Regional Anesthesia.* 1993;18:140.
25. Knowles BD, Pleacher MD. Athletes with seizure disorders. *Current Sports Medicine Reports.* 2012;11(1):16–20.
26. Kordi R, Mazaheri R, Rostami M et al. Hemodynamic changes after static and dynamic exercises and treadmill stress test; different patterns in patients with primary benign exertional headache? *Acta Medica Iranica.* 2012;50(6):399–403.
27. Kozin F, Genant HK, Bekerman C, McCarty DJ. The reflex sympathetic dystrophy syndrome. II. Roentgenographic and scintigraphic evidence of bilaterality and of periarticular accentuation. *American Journal of Medicine.* 1976;60:332.
28. Kozin F, McCarty DJ, Sims J, Genant H. The reflex sympathetic dystrophy syndrome. I. Clinical and histologic studies: Evidence for bilaterality, response to corticosteroids and articular involvement. *American Journal of Medicine.* 1976;60:321.

29. Lee GW, Weeks PM. The role of bone scintigraphy in diagnosing reflex sympathetic dystrophy. *Journal of Hand Surgery (American Volume).* 1995;20:458.
30. Livingston S, Berman W. Participation of epileptic patients in sports. *Journal of the American Medical Association.* 1973;224(2):236–238.
31. Mailis A, Furlan A. Sympathectomy for neuropathic pain. *Cochrane Database of Systematic Review.* 2003;(2): CD002918.
32. Manicourt DH, Brasseur JP, Boutsen Y et al. Role of alendronate in therapy for posttraumatic complex regional pain syndrome type I of the lower extremity. *Arthritis & Rheumatology.* 2004;50:3690.
33. McCrory P. Headaches and exercise. *Sports Medicine.* 2000;30:221–229.
34. McLaurin RL. Epilepsy and contact sports: Factors contraindicating participation. *Journal of the American Medical Association.* 1973;224(2):236–238.
35. Miele VJ, Bailes JE, Martin NA. Participation in contact or collision sports in athletes with epilepsy, genetic risk factors, structural brain lesions, or history of craniotomy. *Neurosurgical Focus.* 2006;21(4):E9.
36. Nadelson C. Sport and exercise-induced migraines. *Current Sports Medicine Reports.* 2006;5(1):29–33.
37. Nakken KO. Physical exercise in outpatients with epilepsy. *Epilepsia.* 1999;40(5):643–651.
38. Nickeson R, Brewer E, Person D. Early histologic and radionuclide scan changes in children with reflex sympathetic dystrophy syndrome (abstract). *Arthritis & Rheumatology.* 1995;28:S72.
39. O'Brien SJ, Ngeow J, Gibney MA et al. Reflex sympathetic dystrophy of the knee. Causes, diagnosis, and treatment. *American Journal of Sports Medicine.* 1995;23:655.
40. Oerlemans HM, Goris JA, de Boo T, Oostendorp RA. Do physical therapy and occupational therapy reduce the impairment percentage in reflex sympathetic dystrophy? *American Journal of Physical Medicine & Rehabilitation.* 1999;78:533.
41. Oerlemans HM, Oostendorp RA, de Boo T, Goris RJ. Pain and reduced mobility in complex regional pain syndrome I: Outcome of a prospective randomized controlled clinical trial of adjuvant physical therapy versus occupational therapy. *Pain.* 1999;83:77.
42. Olcott C 4th, Eltherington LG, Wilcosky BR et al. Reflex sympathetic dystrophy—The surgeon's role in management. *Journal of Vascular Surgery.* 1991;14:488.
43. Pak TJ, Martin GM, Magness JL, Kavanaugh GJ. Reflex sympathetic dystrophy. Review of 140 cases. *Minnesota Medicine.* 1970;53:507.
44. Petchkrua W, Weiss DJ, Patel RR. Reassessment of the incidence of complex regional pain syndrome type 1 following stroke. *Neurorehabilitation and Neural Repair.* 2000;14:59.
45. Pleger B, Tegenthoff M, Ragert P et al. Sensorimotor retuning in complex regional pain syndrome parallels pain reduction. *Annals of Neurology.* 2005;57:425.
46. Rifat, Sami F, Moeller JL. Diagnosis and management of headache in the weight-lifting athlete. *Current Sports Medicine Reports.* 2003;2(5):272–275.
47. Sandroni P, Benrud-Larson LM, McClelland RL, Low PA. Complex regional pain syndrome type I: Incidence and prevalence in Olmsted county, a population-based study. *Pain.* 2003;103:199.
48. Schinkel C, Gaertner A, Zaspel J et al. Inflammatory mediators are altered in the acute phase of posttraumatic complex regional pain syndrome. *Clinical Journal of Pain.* 2006;22:235.
49. Schweitzer ME, Mandel S, Schwartzman RJ et al. Reflex sympathetic dystrophy revisited: MR imaging findings before and after infusion of contrast material. *Radiology.* 1995; 195:211.
50. Sheon RP, Moskowitz RW, Goldberg VM. *Soft Tissue Rheumatic Pain: Recognition, Management, Prevention*, 3rd edn., Williams & Wilkins, Baltimore, MD, 1996. p. 116.
51. Smith ED, Swartzon M, McGrew AC. Headaches in athletes. *Current Sports Medicine Reports.* 2014;13(1):27–32.
52. Committee on Children with Handicaps, Committee on Sports Medicine. Sports and the child with epilepsy. *Pediatrics.* 1983;72:884.
53. Stanton-Hicks M, Burton AW, Bruehl SP et al. An updated interdisciplinary clinical pathway for CRPS: Report of an expert panel. *Pain Practice.* 2002;2:1.
54. Stanton-Hicks M, Janig W, Hassenbusch S et al. Reflex sympathetic dystrophy: Changing concepts and taxonomy. *Pain.* 1995;63:127.
55. Stevermer JJ, Ewigman B. Give vitamin C to avert lingering pain after fracture. *Journal of Family Practice.* 2008;57:86.
56. Tsairis P, Dyck PJ, Mulder DW. Natural history of brachial plexus neuropathy. Report on 99 patients. *Archives of Neurology.* 1972;27:109.
57. Turner J. Exercise-related headache. *Current Sports Medicine Reports.* 2003;2:15–17.
58. Van Alfen N, van Engelen BG. The clinical spectrum of neuralgic amyotrophy in 246 cases. *Brain.* 2006;129:438.
59. Van Laere M, Claessens M. The treatment of reflex sympathetic dystrophy syndrome: Current concepts. *Acta orthopaedica Belgica.* 1992;58(Suppl 1):259.
60. Varenna M, Zucchi F, Ghiringhelli D et al. Intravenous clodronate in the treatment of reflex sympathetic dystrophy syndrome. A randomized, double blind, placebo controlled study. *Journal of Rheumatology.* 2000;27:1477.
61. Veldman PH, Goris RJ. Multiple reflex sympathetic dystrophy. Which patients are at risk for developing a recurrence of reflex sympathetic dystrophy in the same or another limb. *Pain.* 1996;64:463.
62. Veldman PH, Goris RJ. Surgery on extremities with reflex sympathetic dystrophy. *Unfallchirurg.* 1995;98:45.
63. Williams SJ, Nakuda H. Sport and exercise headache: Part 1. Prevalence among university students. *British Journal of Sports Medicine.* 1994;28(2):90–93.
64. Williams SJ, Nakuda H. Sport and exercise headache: Part 2: Diagnosis and classification. *British Journal of Sports Medicin.* 1994;28(2):96–100.
65. Zollinger PE, Tuinebreijer WE, Breederveld RS, Kreis RW. Can vitamin C prevent complex regional pain syndrome in patients with wrist fractures? A randomized, controlled, multicenter dose-response study. *Journal of Bone and Joint Surgery.* 2007;89:1424.

62 Rheumatology

Kevin deWeber and Brian C. Lowell

CONTENTS

TABLE 62.1
Key Clinical Considerations

1. OA is a condition of joint degeneration involving cartilage, synovium, bone, tendon, and ligament, with a distinct inflammatory component.
2. Acute injury and repetitive occupational and sporting stresses to joints increase the risk of developing OA. Obesity as a risk factor has both mechanical and biochemical causes. Family history and female gender also increase risk.
3. NSAIDs provide significant pain reduction in OA. Opiates should be limited to severe cases in which joint replacement is not an option. Injectable corticosteroids provide moderate pain reduction for about 6 weeks, and injectable hyaluronate provides modest pain reduction for about 6 months.
4. RA is a chronic inflammatory disease associated with early mortality, of which cardiovascular disease is significant. Significant efforts should be made at ensuring adequate blood pressure and cholesterol control in the outpatient setting.
5. Regular exercise is extremely important. It improves the quality of life and strength in patients with RA. Additionally, exercise has no effect on exacerbating joint disease.
6. RA has a strong association with smoking. Efforts at smoking cessation should be a priority in smokers with RA.

62.1 INTRODUCTION

Arthritis is one of the most common musculoskeletal presentations that confront the primary care provider. Generally occurring in the form of either osteoarthritis (OA) or rheumatoid arthritis (RA), these conditions can be functionally disabling to the individual patient and have second-order effects on family members and coworkers. In addition to considerable individual morbidity, these disorders have considerable burden on society. Arthritis management is relevant to sedentary patients, those who seek to exercise for health, and many elite athletes because it can adversely affect both athletic performance and activities of daily living. This chapter reviews the clinical presentation and diagnosis of these disorders and equips providers with evidence-based strategies to effectively manage those who are affected (Table 62.1).

62.2 OA

62.2.1 Incidence and Prevalence of OA

The incidence rate of OA is relatively low before age 50 but rises sharply and continues to increase steadily with advancing age. The age- and sex-standardized incident rates for symptomatic knee OA is estimated to be 240 cases per 100,000 person years. For hand OA, the rate is 100 per 100,000 and for hip 88.[34]

OA affects about 13.9% of adults age 25 and older and 33.6% of those over 65.[24] Radiographic (RG) prevalence is higher than symptomatic prevalence. Symptomatic prevalence of knee OA is 16% in adults over 45 years. The prevalence of hand OA is 8% in those over 60. Hip OA prevalence is 4.4% in adults over 55. Foot OA prevalence is 2.0% in those aged 15–74 years. The prevalence of ankle OA is about 1%.[52] Glenohumeral OA is much less common, but prevalence data are limited; in a general orthopedic patient population, the RG prevalence was 0.4%.[31] Acromioclavicular (AC) joint osteophytes have been found to be present on 28.9% of skeletons of persons over 15 years of age, but the prevalence of symptomatic AC joint OA is unclear.[27] Isolated OA of the elbows and wrists is very uncommon.

62.2.2 Pathophysiology of OA

Though OA is often referred to as a degenerative condition in which articular cartilage (see Chapter 9) is mechanically worn away through either repetitive forces and/or acute injuries, it is actually a far more complex condition with significant inflammation, involving several different joint structures. Pathologic changes seen in OA include thinning of the articular cartilage, thickening of subchondral bone, inflammation of the synovium to varying degrees, ligament and knee meniscal degeneration, and joint capsule hypertrophy. In OA, the normally quiescent chondrocytes become activated, leading to proliferation, cluster formation, and increased production of cartilage matrix proteins and matrix-degrading enzymes. These result in matrix remodeling, inappropriate hypertrophy-like maturation, and cartilage calcification. Agents causing chondrocyte activation include mechanical stresses, inflammatory mediators, and possibly systemic humoral mediators. Cell death that is associated with aging likely also leads to diminished reparative ability and increased matrix remodeling response.[25] Over time, the net loss of chondrocytes and the abnormal response of remaining cells lead to thinning, fibrillation, fissuring, and fragmentation of the articular cartilage.

Clinical Pearl

OA involves changes in not just cartilage but synovium, bone, adjacent tendons, and ligaments. Inflammation is also a significant contributor to the pathophysiology and should not be underestimated.

Joint ligaments (and in the knee, menisci) also suffer pathologic changes in OA. While ligament and meniscal traumas are risk factors for OA, as discussed in Section 62.2.3, the late pathologic changes within these structures closely resemble those seen in articular cartilage as well, including reduced cellularity, matrix disruption, fibrillation, calcification, and cell death. Increased vascular penetration and increased nerve densities in ligaments and menisci also serve as sources of pain in OA.[25]

Bone also responds to the mechanical and inflammatory stimuli in OA. At joint margins, new bone is added by endochondral ossification, resulting in osteophytes, which likely serve a joint stabilizing function rather than causing progression of OA. As deep articular cartilage becomes more calcified, the subchondral bone becomes thicker, more infiltrated with neovascularization, and more sensitive to painful stimuli.

Inflammation of the synovium is a key component of OA. Though synovitis seen in OA is far less vigorous than that in RA, OA should still be viewed as a disease with significant inflammation. The synovium becomes thicker, more infiltrated by macrophages and lymphocytes, and increasingly vascular, leading to villous hyperplasia and a significant source of pain. Synovitis can be seen even very early in the disease process before RG changes appear, and its presence is correlated with accelerated subsequent cartilage erosion. There is also a relationship between synovitis and knee symptoms. How synovitis is triggered, however, is still uncertain.[4]

62.2.3 Risk Factors

OA has a multifactorial etiology, with several factors increasing risk and acting together—often through a series of different pathways—to arrive at a common end-stage pathology. See Figure 62.1.

Clinical Pearl

Risk factors for OA include age, genetics, obesity, prior injury, and sports or occupations that place great demand on joints.

Risk factors can be broadly categorized as joint level and person level. Joint-level risk factors are specific to each particular joint and include occupation, physical activity, injury, muscle weakness, joint malalignment, bone/joint dysmorphology, and leg-length inequality. Person-level risk factors act more on a systemic level and include advancing age, female sex, obesity, genetics, low bone mineral density, and malnutrition.

Age and sex. One of the strongest risk factors for OA is advancing age. The exact mechanism is not known and may include loss of reparative capacity and/or the accumulation of other risk factors over time. Women have a higher prevalence and severity of all types of OA, but the mechanisms are not understood.[33]

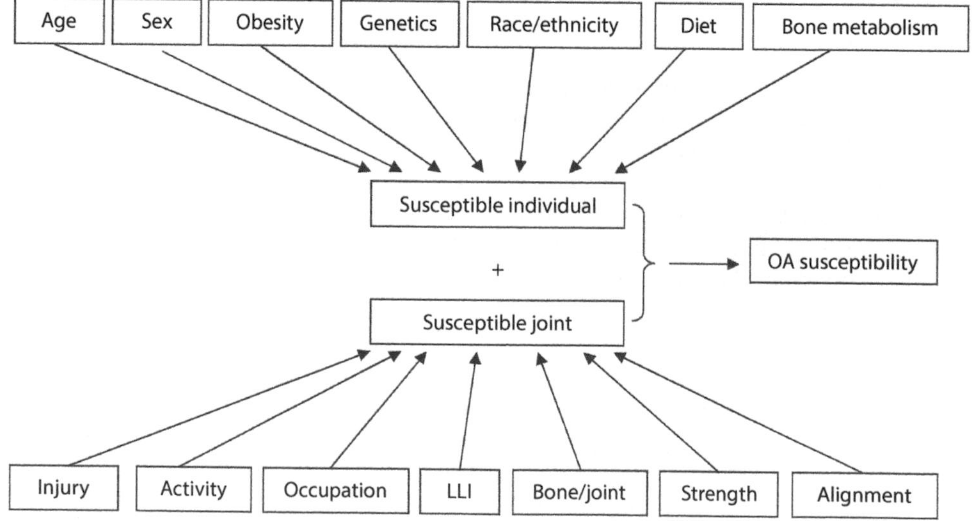

FIGURE 62.1 Potential risk factors for susceptibility of osteoarthritis. (From Neogi, T. and Zhang, Y., *Rheum. Dis. Clin. North Am.*, 39(1), 1, 2013.)

Obesity. Overweight and obesity are very strong risk factors, with a relative risk of 2.96 for knee OA compared to normal weight persons. About 29% of the population's attributable risk percent of OA is from obesity, assuming a prevalence of obesity of 25%. Furthermore, the risk of incident knee OA increases with increasing BMI. Conversely, weight loss—specifically decreasing BMI by 2 or more units over 10 years—is associated with a 50% lower risk of developing symptomatic knee OA in women. Weight loss has also been shown to improve symptoms of knee OA.[33]

While the added mechanical stress that obesity places on weight-bearing joints is a mechanism by which obesity increases the risk of OA, there may also be systemic factors that somehow affect cartilage. Hand OA is also more prevalent in obese persons, suggesting a possible metabolic or inflammatory effect of obesity on joints. Adipose tissue is known to be metabolically active, but its role in OA is not understood. However, total body fat is associated with decreased cartilage thickness, and lean mass is associated with increased cartilage thickness.[33]

Genetics. Approximately 40%–65% of OA is estimated to come from genetic factors. The associations are stronger for hand and hip OA than for knee OA. Pain severity from OA is also influenced by genetics.

Miscellaneous. Higher systemic bone mineral density is associated with an increased risk of incident OA, but this association is poorly understood. There may be some nutritional deficiencies that increase risk of OA, but studies are conflicting and inconclusive on the roles of vitamins C, D, E and K, selenium, and iodine.

Joint-level risk factors presumably exert their effect by alterations in the mechanical loading of joints, such as frank acute injuries to cartilage, unequal distribution of compressive or shearing forces, and high-volume repetitive forces.

Occupation. Jobs requiring kneeling or squatting are associated with increased risk of knee OA, especially in overweight persons and those whose jobs require carrying or lifting. These occupational activities confer about a 1.6 times increased risk of knee OA. While standing does not increase risk for knee OA, occupational standing and lifting are associated with hip OA. Risk of hand OA is increased in occupations requiring manual dexterity such as repeated pincer grip.

Physical activity and sports. Cartilage tissue needs physical stimulation and moderate stresses to maintain homeostasis and health, so physical activity has clear benefits for joints. Habitual, moderate levels of physical activity have not been found to increase risk of OA. A systematic review showed that whereas physical activity was associated with presence of RG tibial osteophytes, it was also associated with greater MRI-calculated cartilage volume and was not associated with RG joint space narrowing. This suggests that knee structures are affected differently by physical activity.[51] Running has not been proven to be associated with lower extremity OA. A few studies have suggested a link between high-mileage running (>20 miles a week) and hip OA, but the preponderance of studies has found no association, especially in knee OA.[56] A systematic review showed that elite soccer players have much higher prevalence rates of knee OA (between 40% and 80%) and ankle OA (12%–17%) than in the general population.[22] However, how much of this risk is attributable to repetitive increased joint load versus injury is unknown.

Injury. Joint trauma, including ligamentous injury, is a known risk factor for OA. Two meta-analyses have determined knee injury to confer a fourfold increase of developing knee OA.[5,30] In particular, 50% of persons who have tears of the anterior cruciate ligament or meniscus will develop knee OA in 10–20 years. This risk is not mitigated by ACL reconstructive surgery. It is therefore believed that the damage to the cartilage from the acute injury, not the resulting joint instability, is the greatest risk factor for future OA.[26] Injury is felt to be a significant contributor to a link between early OA and youth sports injuries, particularly acute injury of the knee and ankle.[7]

Other possible risk factors. Muscle weakness or strength, static joint malalignment, and leg-length inequality have not been conclusively shown to be risk factors for incident OA. However, knee malalignment is a strong risk factor for progressive knee OA, indicating a probable role of joint contact stresses in progression. Leg-length inequality of ≥2 cm was also shown to have double the prevalence of RG knee OA. Bone and joint shapes may play a role in developing OA. For example, cam-type femoral neck deformity and pincer-type acetabular shape have been associated with hip OA.[33]

62.2.4 Diagnosis and Severity Assessment

OA is diagnosed when either clinical findings or RG abnormalities suggest the pathologic changes characteristic of the disease. Clinical historical features include pain in the affected joint, joint stiffness lasting less than an hour, increased joint pain with increased activity, intermittent effusions, and occasional inflammatory exacerbations. Physical examination findings that suggest OA include joint line tenderness without marked synovial thickening, prominence of the joint lines due to osteophytes, and decreased range of motion in advanced disease. Enlarged distal interphalangeal (DIP) joints from OA are called Heberden's nodes, and enlarged proximal interphalangeal (PIP) joints are Bouchard's nodes (Figure 62.2).

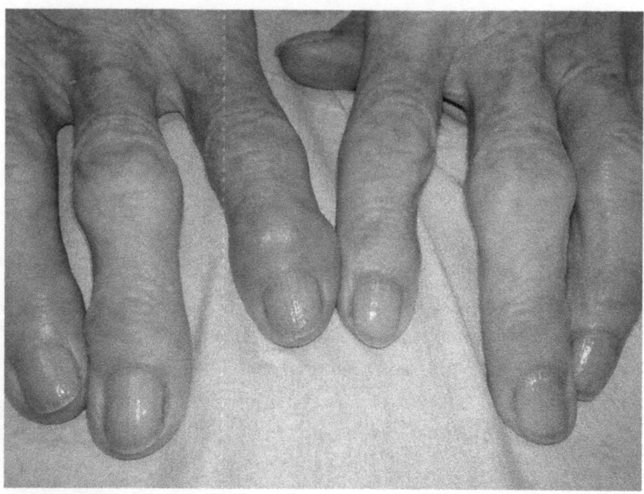

FIGURE 62.2 Hand osteoarthritis with Heberden's nodes (enlarged distal interphalangeal joints) and Bouchard's nodes (enlarged proximal interphalangeal joints). (From Heberden's node, http://en.wikipedia.org/wiki/Heberden%27s_node, accessed October 17, 2015.)

Joint effusion can be present in inflammatory exacerbations, but increased warmth will usually be very mild, and erythema is usually absent. In mild disease, examination may be normal in the office.

OA is radiographically defined by the presence of marginal osteophytes. Other features include joint space narrowing, subchondral sclerosis, and cystic changes (Figure 62.3).

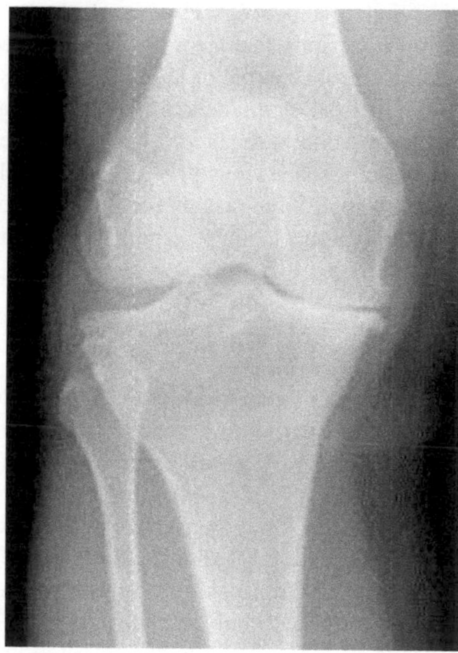

FIGURE 62.3 Osteoarthritis of knee. AP radiograph shows mild joint space narrowing laterally and total joint space loss medially, with medial osteophytes on femur and tibia and subchondral sclerosis of medial tibia.

Clinical Pearl

The Rosenberg view (AP weight bearing in 45° of knee flexion) is the most sensitive radiograph view for detecting early knee OA.

However, RG findings correlate poorly with joint symptoms; many persons with RG OA are asymptomatic; conversely, symptomatic joints may have an early absence of RG findings. Weight-bearing antero-posterior (AP) view of the knee in 45° of flexion—the Rosenberg view—is more sensitive than AP weight bearing in extension for detecting early joint space narrowing and should be the film of choice for initial detection of suspected knee OA. Progression of joint space narrowing over time can be used to monitor progression, and total lack of joint space ("bone on bone") is often used as an indicator for joint replacement if symptoms are also marked. The Kellgren–Lawrence grading system is widely accepted for assessing RG severity. Limitations of radiographs include lack of sensitivity and specificity for articular tissue damage and poor sensitivity to change at follow-up imaging (see Table 62.2).

Despite this, radiographs remain the gold standard for imaging-based diagnosis of OA in most clinical realms.[17]

Other imaging modalities may also be useful. Magnetic resonance (MR) imaging can detect pathologic changes of OA much earlier than radiography and can detect changes that radiographs cannot. Subchondral bone edema, meniscal damage, chondral damage (fraying, fissuring, thinning), synovitis, bony erosions (in hand OA), and effusion are all detectible on MR and usually occur prior to findings on radiographs. However, because of the high cost and lower availability of MR, it is not routinely used in diagnosis and clinical management of patients with OA.[17] Ultrasonography (US) can be used to diagnose OA. It has the advantage of real-time, multiplanar imaging at low cost and without ionizing radiation. The use of US for the assessment of hand OA is increasing. It can visualize cortical erosive changes, synovial hypertrophy, increased vascularity, marginal osteophytes, and effusion. Its limitations include inability to visualize deep structures and subchondral bone, and it is operator skill dependent. Nuclear medicine imaging, through its detection of increased bone turnover,

TABLE 62.2
Kellgren and Lawrence Classification of Radiographic Osteoarthritis Severity

Grade	Criteria
0	No RG features of OA
I	Doubtful narrowing of joint space; possible osteophytes
II	Small osteophytes; possible joint space narrowing
III	Multiple moderate-size osteophytes; definite joint space narrowing; some sclerosis; possible bony deformity
IV	Multiple large osteophytes; marked joint space narrowing; severe sclerosis; definite bony deformity

can detect osteophytes, subchondral sclerosis and cysts, bone marrow lesions, and synovitis. It can relatively easily provide a whole-body survey to help discriminate between soft tissues and bone origin of pain in patients with complex symptoms. Its limitations include poor anatomic resolution, lack of specificity, and use of ionizing radiation. Computed tomography is the method of choice for imaging cortical bone and soft tissue calcifications but does not detect soft tissue changes in OA. It is rarely used for initial diagnosis of nonaxial OA due to its lower sensitivity and high levels of ionizing radiation.[17]

62.2.5 Management

Patients with OA can and should be treated using a wide array of options. First and foremost, a biopsychosocial approach should be utilized, including assessment of mood, health education needs, health beliefs, motivation to self-manage, and participation in occupational and leisure activities, in addition to an assessment of physical status (pain, joint symptoms, sleep quality, mobility, strength, joint alignment, posture, comorbidities, and weight). Treatment plans should be individualized and are best managed by a multidisciplinary professional team that may include health-care providers, physical and/or occupational therapists, nutritional counselors, behavioral health specialists, and nursing staff.

Clinical Pearl

Patients with OA should be managed by a team consisting of not just the primary care provider but also professionals in the areas of nursing education, nutrition, physical therapy, behavioral health, and others as needed.

Education of patients with OA is critical. They must understand the disease, its natural course, treatments available, importance of personal behaviors in treatment success, and reasonable expectations. Cure is not possible for OA, but increased daily functional ability and reduced pain should be the universal goals. They must understand that maintenance of physical activity—even on affected joints—is necessary, but that pacing themselves and adjusting their routine based on how their joints respond are necessary. Information provided to patients should be individualized and included in every aspect of management. It should specifically address the nature of OA and its causes, consequences, and prognosis, should be reinforced and developed at subsequent clinical encounters, and should be supported by written and/or other types of information (DVD, website, group meetings, etc.). Patients undergoing surgery for OA will also benefit from preoperative education.[14]

Exercise management of OA in weight-bearing joints is paramount and strongly recommended by high-quality research. Aerobic, stretching, and strength exercises are all beneficial in OA, and patients should be instructed to incorporate them into their daily routines. Low-impact aerobic activities such as walking, biking, and aquatic activities should be the foundation of a good exercise regimen; national guidelines on activity levels can be used in OA patients. A balance should be sought where activity does not markedly increase pain in the long term, but is of sufficient intensity and duration to keep joints mobile and increase cardiovascular fitness. Strength exercise of the muscle groups surrounding affected joints is also highly beneficial since strong muscles assist in load bearing and increasing functional abilities. Yoga is also beneficial as it increases strength and flexibility.[23]

Weight loss is also critical for management of OA in weight-bearing joints. Patients should be educated and encouraged to regularly self-monitor their weight, to attend regular support group meetings and/or referred for nutritional counseling, to follow a structured meal plan, to reduce fat intake and increase intake of fruit and vegetables, and to address eating behaviors and triggers. A multidisciplinary management team is important for successful weight loss.[14]

Assistive devices and home/work adaptations should be considered and are generally recommended. The use of appropriate and comfortable shoes (highly cushioned, no high heels) should be advised; however, lateral wedge insoles for isolated medial knee OA are not effective. A walking stick may reduce pain for the contralateral side with hip, knee, or ankle OA. Walking frames or wheeled "walkers" may also be useful, but they have a risk of leading to spinal muscle contracture and back pain. Increasing the height of chairs, beds, and toilet seats can make sitting/standing less painful. Using hand rails for stairs and replacing baths with walk-in showers should be considered for safety purposes when OA is severe enough to limit mobility and balance.[14]

Many other therapies are effective for OA and can be recommended on an individual basis, as appropriate. Manual therapy with supervised exercise and manipulation with stretching are beneficial. Transcutaneous electrical nerve stimulation (TENS) may be tried and, if effective, can be prescribed for home use. Other treatments that have evidence to support recommendation include acupuncture, taping, and thermal-based therapy. Interventions for which there is scant evidence but may be tried include ultrasound and hand splints for hand OA. Interventions that are unsupported by evidence include laser therapy, magnetic bracelets, Chinese acupuncture, massage therapy, and cognitive behavior therapy.[23]

Pharmacologic treatments for symptomatic OA include topical, oral, and injectable medications. Nonsteroidal anti-inflammatory drugs (NSAIDs) are widely considered effective for analgesia for all types of OA and should be strongly considered. The use of the lowest effective dose, and intermittent use if possible, is advised to minimize risks. Acetaminophen is marginally effective and can be tried in patients with contraindications to NSAIDs or in addition to them. Tramadol is also effective for analgesia. Other opioids are not recommended unless patients with severe OA have failed other medical therapies and have contraindications for surgery or are unwilling to undergo surgery. Topical NSAIDs are effective and have a better safety profile than oral NSAIDs but require prolonged dosing to be effective. Topical capsaicin is also effective.[18] Glucosamine sulfate, when examined critically in meta-analyses, has been found to be ineffective for pain reduction in OA even when used for 6 months, but it may have marginal function-modifying effects.[57] Glucosamine combined with chondroitin also has no benefit over placebo in reducing pain or impacting joint space narrowing over time.[54]

Viscosupplementation with intra-articular injection of hyaluronate (IAHA) is FDA approved for knee OA in the United States but has also been used for OA in the shoulder, hip, ankle, first carpometacarpal (CMC), temporomandibular, and sacroiliac joints. Recent meta-analyses have concluded that IAHA for knee OA has a small but clinically irrelevant benefit compared to placebo. Of the many products available, none seems to be more effective than others.[12,13,41] Recommendations for this treatment vary across national organizations. IAHA can significantly reduce pain in ankle OA according to a recent meta-analysis[10] and in hip OA per a systematic review.[58] It is also likely to be beneficial in glenohumeral OA.[12]

Intra-articular injection of corticosteroid (IACS) has long been used for OA of various joints, with widely accepted efficacy in the short term, with most patients reporting reduced pain for 1–4 weeks and some longer. However, it has no proven long-term benefits. A Cochrane review concluded that IACS for knee OA has short-term benefits and few side effects.[3] Compared to IAHA, IACS for knee OA is more effective at 2 weeks, equally effective at 4 weeks, but less effective at 8, 12, and 26 weeks.[2]

Biologic therapies such as growth factor, stem cell, and platelet-rich plasma injections are currently being used by select practitioners who claim potential disease-modifying properties with these treatments. One pilot study on stem cells injected into knee OA claims long-term symptom improvement and increased cartilage quality by MRI at 1 year.[36] A systematic review and a meta-analysis of platelet-rich plasma injection for knee OA showed beneficial effects in 6–12 months compared with IAHA or saline injection.[9,20] Based on relatively scant evidence, these treatments cannot yet be widely recommended but may be considered in select patients.

Surgery. Knee arthroscopy with lavage and/or debridement for knee OA is not recommended since several studies have shown no benefit over placebo.[40] However, when OA is severe, with complete loss of articular cartilage and pain and dysfunction that significantly affect quality of life and activities of daily living, surgical management should be considered. Numerous commercial devices for total or partial joint replacement of joints such as shoulder, elbow, wrist, finger/thumb, hip, knee, and ankle are available and may be of benefit. Comparative efficacy is lacking, but surgical treatment of severe OA is widely considered to have a high patient satisfaction rate and to produce large increases in quality of life. Consultation with an experienced orthopedic surgeon is recommended when conservative treatments are inadequate in patients with severe OA.

62.3 RA

62.3.1 Incidence and Prevalence of RA

RA is a chronic autoimmune disease characterized by inflammation and destruction of the joint. The incidence of RA is estimated to be between 20 and 50 cases per 100,000 individuals in North America and Northern Europe with a prevalence of between 0.5% and 1.1%. Higher incidences and prevalence have been reported in closed American Indian tribes or Eskimos, while lower incidences and prevalence have been reported in southern Europeans, rural Africans, Asians, Latin Americans, and countries of the Middle East.[8,21] However, these disparities may be attributed to age distribution differences recognized in different geographic areas. RA is more common in the female population with a female-to-male ratio between 2 and 3:1. The peak age of onset is between the fifth and sixth decades of life.[44]

62.3.2 Pathophysiology of RA

RA is a chronic inflammatory arthritis with a largely unknown etiology. However, both genetic and environmental risk factors contribute to its development. It is assumed that the initiation and progression of RA occur when genetically predisposed individuals are exposed to environmental risk factors.[44]

RA is an extremely complex disease that involves both the innate and adaptive immune responses. Disease initiation likely occurs with activation of antigen-presenting cells (APCs), which include macrophages, dendritic cells and B cells, and autologous antigen to T cells. These activated T cells then produce an array of cytokines, importantly TNF, IL-6 and IL-1, which are ultimately responsible for recruiting and maintaining the inflammatory immune response.[11]

Rheumatoid factor (RF) and anticitrullinated protein antibody (ACPA) are two prevalent autoantibodies in RA. They are not only markers for disease but if present are associated with poor prognosis. Interestingly, only 50%–80% of individuals with RA have one or both of these autoantibodies. Thus, 30%–50% of the RA population have no identifiable autoantibodies and are considered to have seronegative disease.[43,48] Though ACPA has improved the diagnosis of RA, new biomarkers are being investigated for diagnosis of early and seronegative disease.[48]

Though RA is a systemic disease, it is thought to not only likely originate but also concentrate within the synovial membranes of individuals with active disease. This has been confirmed with identification of higher concentrations of ACPAs within the synovial membranes when compared to serum concentrations in individuals with rheumatic disease.[42]

Joint damage begins at the synovial membrane. Inflammation of the synovial membrane occurs with an influx of immune-mediated cell lines in addition to angiogenesis, resulting in synovial hyperplasia. The result of ongoing synovial hyperplasia is pannus formation at the boundary between cartilage and bone. This osteoclast (monocyte)-rich pannus destroys bone, while cellular enzyme secretion from polymorphonuclear, synoviocyte, and chondrocyte cell lines destroys cartilaginous tissue.[11]

62.3.3 Risk Factors for RA

62.3.3.1 Genetics

Familial disease clustering was the first indication for genetic susceptibility to RA. The prevalence of RA ranges 2%–12% in first-degree relatives of those affected with disease. There is a dramatic increase to 5%–10% in same sex dizygotic twins and further increases to 12%–30% in monozygotic twins. From such twin studies, it is estimated that genetic factors contribute up to 65% of the risk for developing RA.[38]

Clinical Pearl

The two greatest risk factors for RA are genetic and environmental. Genetic factors include age, female sex, and HLA-DRB1 gene positivity. The greatest environmental factor is smoking.

The HLA-DRB1 gene has the strongest association with developing RA and is the only gene ubiquitously seen amongst all studied populations. These alleles are derived from the major histocompatibility complex and are responsible for antigen binding and presentation to CD4+ T cells.[44] It is currently hypothesized that antigens are citrullinated, via posttranslational modification, resulting in better binding to these HLA alleles. These alleles then present these autologous antigens to T cells and antibody development ensues.[6,38,47]

With recent advancements in technology, and genome-wide association studies, approximately 60 additional non-HLA risk alleles associated with RA have been described. Interestingly, a large subset of these markers are related to immune function, although the risks are weak with very few of the alleles having odd risk ratios greater than 1.5.[6,29,38,53]

62.3.3.2 Environment

Environmental risk factors are more ill defined. Far and away, the greatest environmental risk associated with RA is smoking. Smoking not only increases susceptibility but also has a dose-dependent effect on risk. Smoking is likely associated with genetic predisposition, as it is associated with serologic positive disease.[8] Other environmental factors that may contribute to RA include aging, obesity, large birth weight, infectious trigger, pollutants, and lower socioeconomic status. Factors that may protect against disease include alcohol consumption, vitamin D intake, dietary factors (potentially Mediterranean diet), oral contraception use, and breastfeeding.[44,47]

62.3.4 Classification of RA

Typical features of RA include symmetric joint pain and/or tenderness, morning joint stiffness that lasts greater than 30 minutes, and joint swelling. RA most often is a disease of the small joints, including the metacarpophalangeal (MCP), PIP, and wrists. Joints not affected include the CMC, first metatarsophalangeal (MTP), and DIP joints.[19,21]

Clinical Pearl

Classifying RA in the patient population is dependent on the number of involved joints, serologic assessment, acute-phase reactant assessment, and symptom duration.

In 2010, the American College of Rheumatology (ACR) in collaboration with the European League Against Rheumatism (EULAR) updated the 1987 classification criteria for RA due to lack of sensitivity in early disease. The criteria were reassessed with the goal of early disease discovery and preventing individuals from reaching chronic, erosive disease. It is recognized that early intervention improves clinical outcomes with respect to joint preservation and reducing systemic complications. The change in criteria resulted in a definition of "definite RA" based on the presence of synovitis in at least one joint and achievement of a total score of 6 or greater from the individual scores in four domains: number of joints involved, serologic assessment, acute-phase reactant assessment, and symptom duration.[1,19,28]

The reclassification occurred in three phases. The aim of the first phase was to define both clinical and laboratory variables that practitioners deemed "RA-like" prior to initiating therapy to best control symptoms. The second phase derived the relative contributions of both clinical and laboratory factors that influenced developing the disease. Thus, each of the domains was weighted according to the probability each was associated with RA. The objective of the third phase was to refine the scoring criteria to define "definite RA" (≥6/10 points) and identify new patients with a high probability of developing destructive joint disease. According to the new criteria, a patient can be classified as either having or not having "definite RA" with a thorough symptom history, joint evaluation, serologic assessment (RF or ACPA), and acute-phase reactant assessment (ESR or CRP).[1,19,21,28]

It should be noted that other than the current ACR/EULAR classification criteria, there is no *gold standard* for definitive RA diagnosis. The diagnosis is made on signs and symptoms associated with RA phenotype.[28] The criteria were designed with the goal of classifying individuals with newfound disease so they may be appropriately enrolled into clinical trials and studies via uniform criteria. It is recognized, however, that these criteria will likely be used as a diagnostic aid. Further, recent scrutiny of the criteria deemed the measures a useful aid in making diagnoses when combined with clinical judgment. Additionally, when inflammatory arthritis is considered, it is absolutely necessary to refer to a rheumatologist for further evaluation, diagnosis, and appropriate management going forward.[1,28] See Table 62.3.

TABLE 62.3
Scoring Criteria for Rheumatoid Arthritis

The 2010 ACR-EULAR Classification Criteria for Rheumatoid Arthritis	Score
Specifies that patient present with at least one joint with clinical synovitis (swelling) that is not explained by another disease.	
A cumulative score of ≥6 from the following criteria receives classification of "definite RA."	
Patient with scores <6 should be periodically reassessed to evaluate for criteria fulfillment.	
Joint involvement: Swollen or tender joints on examination.	
1 large joint	0
2–10 large joints	1
1–3 small joints	2
4–10 small joints	3
>10 joints (at least 1 small joint)	5
Serology: RF and ACPA.	
Negative RF and negative ACPA	0
Low-positive RF or low-positive ACPA titers	2
High-positive RF or high-positive ACPA titers	3
Acute-phase reactants: C-reactive protein and erythrocyte sedimentation rate by laboratory standards.	
Normal CRP and normal ESR	0
Abnormal	1
Symptom duration: Patient reported symptoms of joint involvement.	
<6 weeks	0
≥6 weeks	1

Large joints: Shoulders, elbows, hips, knees or ankles.
Small joints: MCP, PIP, MTP joints (2–5), thumb, interphalangeal joints, and wrist.
Serology: Negative refers to normal limits. Low positivity refers to values ≤3 times the upper limit of normal. High positivity refers to values >3 times the upper limit of normal.

Source: Aletaha, D. et al., *Arthritis. Rheum.*, 62(9), 2569, 2010.

62.3.5 Management of RA

Early detection and treatment are the goals of care in managing RA. Treatment is aimed at preventing joint pain and swelling, minimizing joint damage (RG erosion), and maintaining quality of life by targeting low disease activity or remission.[55] Treatment initiation at disease onset is crucial since approximately 50% of individuals with RA develop joint abnormalities during the first year of disease.[39]

Clinical Pearl

Patients should swiftly be referred to a rheumatologist if RA is suspected. Minimizing joint damage is the primary goal of disease management.

62.3.5.1 Pharmacologic Treatment

Treatment currently includes the use of disease-modifying antirheumatic drugs (DMARDs) or biologics. In 2012, the ACR provided recommendations for the treatment of RA. Treatment of RA with either DMARD monotherapy, combination therapy, or biologic should continue for 3 months prior to reassessment and alteration of medication regimen.[50] Therapy is dictated by disease activity and the presence of poor prognostic factors. Poor prognostic factors include functional limitation, extra-articular disease, RF or ACPA positivity, or bony erosions by radiograph. Therapy should be guided by individual patient response, and although recommendations are in place, goals should be patient directed and should not substitute clinical judgment. See Table 62.4.

TABLE 62.4
Disease-Modifying Antirheumatic Drugs for Rheumatoid Arthritis

2012 ACR Medications
DMARDs
Hydroxychloroquine
Leflunomide
Methotrexate
Minocycline
Sulfasalazine
Biologic Agents
Anti-TNF:
Adalimumab
Etanercept
Infliximab
Certolizumab pegol
Golimumab
Non-TNF:
Abatacept (T cell costimulation with APCs)
Rituximab (CD20)
Tocilizumab (IL-6R)

The ACR recommendations for the treatment of RA are as follows:

Early RA (<6 months): Initiating therapy:

- Target low disease or remission.
- DMARD monotherapy for both low and moderate disease activities without poor prognostic factors. Methotrexate is the first-line therapy.
- DMARD combination therapy in patients with moderate or high disease activity with poor prognostic factors.
- Anti-TNF biologic agent use (± methotrexate) for high disease activity with poor prognostic factors.

Established RA (>6 months): Initiating and changing therapy:

- If after 3 months of DMARD monotherapy disease progressively worsens from low to moderate/high disease activity, in the absence of poor prognostic factors, DMARD combination therapy is warranted.
- If after 3 months of DMARD combination therapy disease progressively worsens, additional DMARD or changing DMARDs is warranted.
- If patient has moderate/high disease activity after 3 months of DMARD mono- or combination therapy, changing to biologic is recommended.
- If after 3 months of anti-TNF biologic use moderate/high disease activity is present, recommend changing ant-TNF biologic or initiating non-TNF biologic (abatacept, rituximab, or tocilizumab).
- If after additional 3 months still no benefit is seen, recommend again switching anti-TNF biologic or non-TNF biologic agent.[45,50]

As mentioned previously, RA is a chronic inflammatory disease associated with early mortality (3–10 years), and as time with the disease lengthens, so does mortality.[8,47] Despite current therapy with DMARDs or biologics, the mortality benefit has lagged behind that of the general public. Mortality is greatly associated with cardiovascular, pulmonary, and infectious disease entities. Armed with this information, it is appropriate to treat the RA population not only with pharmacologic intervention but also with appropriate screening tools associated with these conditions.[32] Specifically, efforts should be made with cardiovascular risk stratification, managing blood pressure and cholesterol, and smoking cessation.[55] Depression is an additional significant comorbidity associated with RA that should be appropriately monitored.[43]

62.3.5.2 Nonpharmacologic Treatment

The goals of such forms of therapy are to reduce pain, prevent loss of function, and improve quality of life.[15] Despite the severity of disease, strengthening and dynamic exercises should regularly be performed on patients with RA. This includes aerobic exercises for cardiopulmonary protection and weight-bearing exercises with moderate joint impact. Research demonstrates that exercise improves quality of life and strength but has no effect on exacerbating joint disease.[37] Despite the aforementioned attributes to exercise, it has not been shown to improve disease activity or joint damage.[46] There are conflicting data for relief of pain associated with RA. Other forms of nonpharmacologic intervention such as dietary change, acupuncture, tai chi, and yoga have been investigated, without significant evidence of benefit or lack of quality evidence.[49,55]

62.3.6 Severity Assessment

Treatment is directed toward minimizing end-stage disease, mainly through prevention of articular damage, minimizing functional loss, and maintaining quality of life. Thus, remission is the goal of RA therapy. Defining remission is difficult, but nonetheless numerous groups have put forth assessment tools to ensure that disease is being adequately treated. To date, many remission tools have been developed, but the most reliable criteria for assessing disease activity are with guidance from the ACR (ACR) and the EULAR.

Most remission indices are directed toward both qualitative and quantitative measures of disease activity. Most severity assessment tools combine joint evaluation for swelling and tenderness, physician and patient global assessments, and serologic marker measurement (ESR or CRP). The aforementioned variables ultimately lead to a score that indicates disease severity. The severity scores correlate with remission, low activity, moderate activity, or high activity.

RA assessment tools such as the DAS, DAS28, SDAI, and CDAI can be found at the following sites:

- http://www.das-score.nl
- http://wwwrheumatology.org/Practice/Clinical/Forms/Clinical_Forms/

All of the aforementioned criteria have been used in the clinical setting to assess RA disease severity (remission, low/moderate/high activity). There are numerous other indices besides the ones mentioned that are also applicable. Research suggests that all adequately measure disease activity severity. The fact remains that despite these tools, remission rates in both clinical trials and practice remain low. The relevance of these tools is to ensure rheumatic disease is appropriately treated and disease activity is routinely assessed to minimize progression of this chronic inflammatory disease (Table 62.5).[16,19,35,39]

TABLE 62.5
SORT: Key Recommendations for Practice

Clinical Recommendation	Evidence Rating	References
Education of patients with OA should include nature of OA, its natural course, treatments available, importance of personal behaviors in treatment success, and reasonable expectations.	A	[14,23]
Aerobic, stretching, and strength exercises are all beneficial in OA, and patients should incorporate them into their daily routines, using national guidelines for activity levels and adjusting exercises as needed based on joints affected.	A	[12,23]
Weight loss is beneficial for managing OA in weight-bearing joints. A multidisciplinary management approach should be utilized.	A	[14]
Aquatic exercise and hydrotherapy are beneficial for OA.	A	[23]
Yoga is beneficial for managing OA.	A	[23]
TENS is beneficial for reducing pain from OA.	B	[23]
Unloader knee bracing is beneficial for isolated medial or lateral compartment knee OA.	B	[23]
Wedged insoles are not recommended for isolated medial or lateral compartment knee OA.	B	[23]
Manual therapy with supervised exercise is beneficial for OA.	B	[23]
Balneotherapy (passive relaxation in mineral or thermal water) is beneficial for reducing pain from OA.	B	[23]
Tai chi is beneficial for OA.	C	[23]
Walking aids are beneficial for reducing pain from OA in weight-bearing joints.	C	[23]
Acupuncture is beneficial for reducing pain from OA.	C	[23]
For hand OA, recommended pharmacologic choices include topical or oral NSAIDs, topical capsaicin, or oral tramadol.	A	[18]
For hip and knee OA, recommended pharmacologic choices include acetaminophen, oral or topical NSAIDs, tramadol, and intra-articular corticosteroid injections.	A	[18]
Glucosamine and chondroitin sulfate are no longer recommended for hip or knee OA.	B	[18,54]
Intra-articular hyaluronate injection for knee OA leads to a small but clinically irrelevant benefit compared to placebo.	A	[12,41]
Knee arthroscopy with lavage/debridement for knee OA is not recommended.	A	[40]
Low-target disease or remission is the goal of therapy in all patients with RA.	C	[45]
Methotrexate is the recommended first-line therapy for treatment of RA unless it is not tolerated.	B	[43,45,55]
RA classification criteria are based on a combination of history, physical examination of the joints, and serology.	C	[1]
Exercise programs for PA patients can improve quality of life and muscle strength, while having no effect on exacerbating joint disease.	B	[37]

REFERENCES

1. Aletaha D, Tuhina N, Silman AJ et al. Rheumatoid arthritis classification criteria. *Arthritis & Rheumatology*. 2010;62(9): 2569–2581.
2. Bannuru RR, Natov NS, Obadan IE et al. Therapeutic trajectory of hyaluronic acid versus corticosteroids in the treatment of knee osteoarthritis: A systematic review and meta-analysis. *Arthritis & Rheumatology*. 2009;61(12):1704–1711.
3. Bellamy N, Campbell J, Robinson V et al. Intraarticular corticosteroid for treatment of osteoarthritis of the knee. *Cochrane Database of Systematic Reviews*. 2006;19(2):CD005328.
4. Berenbaum F. Osteoarthritis as an inflammatory disease (osteoarthritis is not osteoarthrosis!). *Osteoarthritis and Cartilage*. 2013;21:16–21.
5. Blegojevic M, Jinks C, Jeffery A et al. Risk factors for onset of osteoarthritis of the knee in older adults: A systematic review and meta-analysis. *Osteoarthritis and Cartilage*. 2010;18:24–33.
6. Bowes J, Barton A. Recent advances in the genetics of RH susceptibility. *Rheumatology (Oxford)*. 2008;47(4):399–402.
7. Caine DJ, Golightly YM. Osteoarthritis as an outcome of paediatric sport: An epidemiological perspective. *British Journal of Sports Medicine*. 2011;45(4):298–303.
8. Carmona L, Cross M, Williams B et al. Rheumatoid arthritis. *Best Practice & Research Clinical Rheumatology*. 2010;24(6):733–745.
9. Chang KV, Hung CY, Aliwarga F et al. Comparative effectiveness of platelet-rich plasma injections for treating knee joint cartilage degenerative pathology: A systematic review and meta-analysis. *Archives of Physical Medicine and Rehabilitation*. 2014;95(3):562–575.
10. Chang KV, Hsiao MY, Chen WS et al. Effectiveness in infra-articular hyaluronic acid for ankle osteoarthritis treatment: A systematic review and meta-analysis. *Archives of Physical Medicine and Rehabilitation*. 2013;94(5):951–960.
11. Choy E. Understanding the dynamics: Pathways involved in the pathogenesis of rheumatoid arthritis. *Rheumatology*. 2012;51(Suppl 5):v3–v11.
12. Colen S, Haverkamp D, Mulier M, van den Bekerom MP. Hyaluronic acid for the treatment of osteoarthritis in all joints except the knee: What is the current evidence? *BioDrugs*. 2012;26(2):101–112.
13. Colen S, van den Bekerom MP, Mulier M, Haverkamp D. Hyaluronic acid in the treatment of knee osteoarthritis: A systematic review and meta-analysis with emphasis on the efficacy of different products. *BioDrugs*. 2012;26(4):257–268.
14. Fernandes L, Hagen KB, Bijlsma JW et al. EULAR recommendations for the non-pharmacological core management of hip and knee osteoarthritis. *Annals of the Rheumatic Diseases*. 2013;72(7):1125–1135.
15. Forestier R, Andre-Vert J, Guillez P et al. Non-drug treatment (excluding surgery) in rheumatoid arthritis: Clinical practice guidelines. *Joint Bone Spine*. 2009;76(6):691–698.

16. Fransen J, Stucki G, van Riel PLCM. Rheumatoid arthritis measures: Disease Activity Score (DAS), Disease Activity Score-28 (DAS28), Rapid Assessment of Disease Activity in Rheumatology (RADAR), and Rheumatoid Arthritis Disease Activity Index (RADAI). *Arthritis & Rheumatology.* 2003;49(5):214–224.
17. Guermazi A, Hayashi D, Foemer FW, Felson DT. Osteoarthritis: A review of strengths and weaknesses of different imaging options. *Rheumatic Disease Clinics of North America.* 2013;39(3):567–591.
18. Hochberg MC, Altman RD, April KT et al. American College of Rheumatology 2012 recommendations for the use of nonpharmacologic and pharmacologic therapies in osteoarthritis of the hand, hip, and knee. *Arthritis Care & Research (Hoboken).* 2012;64(4):465–474.
19. Jeffery RC. Clinical features of rheumatoid arthritis. *Medicine.* 2014;42(5):231–236.
20. Khoshbin A, Leroux T, Wasserstein D. The efficacy of platelet-rich plasma in the treatment of symptomatic knee osteoarthritis: A systematic review with quantitative synthesis. *Arthroscopy.* 2013;29(12):2037–2048.
21. Kourilovitch M, Galarza-Maldonado C, Ortiz-Prado E. Diagnosis and classification of rheumatoid arthritis. *Journal of Autoimmunity.* 2014;48–49:26–30.
22. Kuijt MT, Inklaar J, Gouttebarge V, Frings-Dresen MH. Knee and ankle osteoarthritis in former elite soccer players: A systematic review of the recent literature. *Journal of Science and Medicine in Sport.* 2012;15(6):480–487.
23. Larmer PJ, Reay ND, Aubert ER, Kersten P. Systematic review of guidelines for the physical management of osteoarthritis. *Archives of Physical Medicine and Rehabilitation.* 2014;95(2):375–389.
24. Lawrence RC, Felson DT, Helmick CG et al. Estimates of the prevalence of arthritis and other rheumatic conditions in the United States. Part II. *Arthritis & Rheumatology.* 2008;58(1):26–35.
25. Loeser RF, Goldring ST, Scanzello CR, Goldring MB. Osteoarthritis. A disease of the joint as an organ. *Arthritis & Rheumatology.* 2012;64(6):1697–1707.
26. Lohmander LS, Englund PM, Dahl LL, Roos EM. The long-term consequence of anterior cruciate ligament and meniscus injuries: Osteoarthritis. *American Journal of Sports Medicine.* 2007;35(10):1756–1769.
27. Mahakkanukrauh P, Surin P. Prevalence of osteophytes associated with the acromion and acromioclavicular joint. *Clinical Anatomy.* 2003;16(6):506–510.
28. Mjaavatten MD, Bykerk VP. Early rheumatoid arthritis: The performance of the 2010 ACR/EULAR criteria for diagnosing RA. *Best Practice & Research Clinical Rheumatology.* 2013;27(4):451–466.
29. Morgan AW, Robinson JI, Conaghan PG. Evaluation of the rheumatoid arthritis susceptibility loci HLA-DRB1, PTPN22, OLIG3/TNFAIP3, STAT4 and TRAF1/C5 in an inception cohort. *Arthritis Research & Therapy.* 2010;12(2):R57.
30. Muthuri SG, McWilliams DF, Doherty M, Zhang W. History of knee injuries and knee osteoarthritis: A meta-analysis of observational studies. *Osteoarthritis and Cartilage.* 2011;19:1286–1293.
31. Nakagawa Y, Hyakuna K, Otani S et al. Epidemiologic study of glenohumeral osteoarthritis with plain radiography. *Journal of Shoulder and Elbow Surgery.* 1999;8(6):580–584.
32. Naz SM. Mortality in establishing rheumatoid arthritis. *Best Practice & Research Clinical Rheumatology.* 2007; 21(5):871–883.
33. Neogi T, Zhang Y. Epidemiology of OA. *Rheumatic Disease Clinics of North America.* 2013;39(1):1–19.
34. Oliveria SA, Felson DT, Reed JI et al. Incidence of symptomatic hand, hip, and knee osteoarthritis among patients in a health maintenance organization. *Arthritis & Rheumatology.* 1995;38(8):1134–1141.
35. Ometto F, Botsios C, Raffeiner B et al. Methods used to assess remission and low disease activity in rheumatoid arthritis. *Autoimmunity Reviews.* 2010;9(3):161–164.
36. Orozco L, Munar A, Soler R et al. Treatment of knee osteoarthritis with autologous mesenchymal stem cells: A pilot study. *Transplantation.* 2013;95(12):1535–1541.
37. Perandini LA, de Sa-Pinto AL, Roschel H et al. Exercise as a therapeutic tool to counteract inflammation and clinical symptoms in autoimmune rheumatic diseases. *Autoimmunity Reviews.* 2012;12(2):218–224.
38. Perricone C, Ceccarelli F, Valesini G. An overview on the genetic of rheumatoid arthritis: A never-ending story. *Autoimmunity Reviews.* 2011;10(10):599–608.
39. Polido-Pereira J, Vieira-Sousa S, Fonseca JE. Rheumatoid arthritis: What is refractory disease and how to manage it? *Autoimmunity Reviews.* 2011;10(11):707–713.
40. Reichenbach S, Rutjes AW, Nuesch E et al. Joint lavage for osteoarthritis of the knee. *Cochrane Database of Systematic Reviews.* 2010;12(5):CD007320.
41. Rutjes AW, Juni P, da Costa BR et al. Viscosupplementation for osteoarthritis of the knee: A systematic review and meta-analysis. *Annals of Internal Medicine.* 2012;157(3):180–191.
42. Schaeverbeke T, Truchetet M, Richez C. When and where does rheumatoid arthritis begin? *Joint Bone Spine.* 2012;79(6): 550–554.
43. Scott DL, Wolfe F, Huizinga TWJ. Rheumatoid arthritis. *Lancet.* 2010;376(9746):1094–1108.
44. Scott IC, Steer S, Lewis CM et al. Precipitating and perpetuating factors of rheumatoid arthritis immunopathology—Linking the triad of genetic predisposition, environmental risk factors and autoimmunity to disease pathogenesis. *Best Practice & Research Clinical Rheumatology.* 2011;25(4):447–468.
45. Singh JA, Furst DE, Bharat A et al. 2012 Update of the 2008 American College of Rheumatology recommendations for the use of disease-modifying antirheumatic drugs and biologic agents in the treatment of rheumatoid arthritis. *Arthritis Care & Research.* 2012;65(5):625–639.
46. Theodora PM, Vlieland V, Pattison D et al. Non-drug therapies in early rheumatoid arthritis. *Best Practice & Research Clinical Rheumatology.* 2009;23(1):103–116.
47. Tobon GJ, Youinou P, Saraux A. The environment, geo-epidemiology, and autoimmune disease: Rheumatoid arthritis. *Journal of Autoimmunity.* 2010;35(1):10–14.
48. Trouw LA, Mahler M. Closing the serological gap: Promising novel biomarkers for the early diagnosis of rheumatoid arthritis. *Autoimmunity Reviews.* 2012;12(2):318–322.
49. Uhlig T. Tai Chi and yoga as complementary therapies in rheumatologic conditions. *Best Practice & Research Clinical Rheumatology.* 2012;26(3):387–398.
50. Upchurch KS, Kay J. Evolution of treatment for rheumatoid arthritis. *Rheumatology.* 2012;51(Suppl 6):vi28–vi36.
51. Urquhart DM, Tobling JF, Hanna FS et al. What is the effect of physical activity on the knee joint: A systematic review. *Medicine & Science in Sports & Exercise.* 2011;43(3):432–442.
52. Valderrabano V, Horisberger M, Russell I et al. Etiology of ankle osteoarthritis. *Clinical Orthopaedics and Related Research.* 2009;467(7):1800–1806.

53. Viatte S, Plant D, Raychaudhuri S. Genetics and epigenetics of rheumatoid arthritis. *Nature Reviews Rheumatology.* 2013;9(3):141–153.
54. Wandel S, Juni P, Tendal B et al. Effects of glucosamine, chondroitin, or placebo in patients with osteoarthritis of hip or knee: Network meta-analysis. *BMJ: British Medical Journal.* 2010;341:c4675.
55. Wasserman AM. Diagnosis and management of rheumatoid arthritis. *American Family Physician.* 2011;84(11):1245–1252.
56. Willick SE, Hansen PA. Running and osteoarthritis. *Clinics in Sports Medicine.* 2010;29(3):417–428.
57. Wu D, Huang Y, Gu Y, Fan W. Efficacies of different preparations of glucosamine for the treatment of osteoarthritis: A meta-analysis of randomized, double-blind, placebo-controlled trials. *International Journal of Clinical Practice.* 2013;67(6):585–594.
58. Zhang W, Nuki G, Moskowitz RW et al. OARSI recommendations for the management of hip and knee osteoarthritis: Part III: Changes in evidence following systematic cumulative update of research published through January 2009. *Osteoarthritis and Cartilage.* 2010;18(4):476–499.

63 Environmental Injuries and Illness

Brian V. Reamy and Douglas J. Casa

CONTENTS

TABLE 63.1
Key Clinical Considerations

1. Individuals at the extremes of age are most at risk for hypothermia, and subtle, nonspecific clinical presentations are common. An accurate core temperature is key to diagnosis.
2. The severity of frostbite injury can be lessened by avoiding cycles of recurrent rewarming and refreezing.
3. The two key diagnostic criteria for exertional heatstroke are extreme hyperthermia at the time of collapse (>40.5°C) and central nervous system dysfunction (coma, altered consciousness, aggression, confusion).
4. Initial field treatment for possible symptoms of altitude illness involves stopping the ascent and rest. A lack of improvement in 12 hours should lead to a descent in altitude.

63.1 INTRODUCTION

The environment in which we compete and play can pose many significant challenges to the trained athlete or outdoor adventurer. An awareness and understanding of heat-, cold-, and altitude-related injuries will help the physician and other medical professionals prevent, recognize, and treat these injuries and facilitate enjoyment of sports in the outdoors (Table 63.1).

63.2 HYPOTHERMIA

Hypothermia occurs when the body's core temperature drops below 35°C (95°F). It is the primary cause of death of more than 1500 patients per year just in the United States and a contributing cause of significant morbidity and mortality.[4] Increasing homelessness and sports activities in inclement environments have contributed to an increased incidence of hypothermia in the past decade.

63.2.1 Epidemiology

Individuals at the extremes of age, younger than 2 and older than 60 years, are most at risk of accidental hypothermia. Risk factors include the use of intoxicants, psychiatric illness, medical illnesses, sleep deprivation, dehydration, malnutrition, and trauma. The impaired judgment resulting from psychiatric illness or the use of ethanol are the most common predisposing factors in leading individuals to ignore the early symptoms of hypothermia.

63.2.2 Pathophysiology

The body combats the fall in core temperature through shivering thermogenesis, by shunting of blood from the periphery to the core, and by increased gluconeogenesis. When the core temperature drops below 35°C, the victim becomes poikilothermic and cools to the ambient temperature.[2] Central nervous system (CNS) function is directly depressed by the cold. The electroencephalogram becomes abnormal below a temperature of 33.5°C (92.5°F) and silent at 19°C (66°F).[2] Initial reflex tachypnea continues until core temperature falls below 30°C (86°F). Failure of brainstem control of respiratory drive and the freezing of the thoracic musculature eventually lead to a cessation of breathing.[2]

Cold triggers peripheral vasoconstriction and tachycardia. Below 34°C (93°F), bradycardia, hypotension, decreased cardiac output, and a lengthening of cardiac electrical conduction ensue. A J-wave (Osborn hypothermic hump) may be noted at the QRS–ST junction. The myocardium becomes increasingly irritable, and spontaneous atrial and ventricular dysrhythmias can occur.[2]

Below 28°C (82°F), ventricular fibrillation can develop with minor stimuli such as removing a patient's wet clothing or ambulance transport.[2]

63.2.3 Clinical Features

Nonspecific symptoms and signs predominate and mimic the effects of mild dementia or ethanol intoxication. The CNS effects of cold lead to impaired memory, judgment, slurred speech, and decreased alertness. Paradoxic bradycardia and hypoventilation occur despite hypotension. Multiple cardiac dysrhythmias develop as the core temperature falls. A cold-induced ileus, abdominal spasm, and rigidity can mimic an acute abdomen.

63.2.4 Diagnosis

An accurate core temperature is crucial and is ideally obtained with a rectal thermistor probe. At a minimum, a rectal temperature obtained with a thermometer scaled for hypothermia is required. Oral and ear temperatures are grossly inaccurate. A core temperature above 35°C can rapidly exclude hypothermia. Hypothermia is classified as mild, moderate, or severe based on the core temperature.

Hypothermia can also be staged clinically on the basis of vital signs and the use of the Swiss staging system of hypothermia with stages I–IV.

Common laboratory findings include a falsely elevated hematocrit caused by dehydration, a low leukocyte count caused by sequestration, hyperamylasemia resulting from pancreatic injury, an aberrant coagulation profile, hypokalemia, and hypoglycemia caused by glycogen depletion. Below 30°C, insulin is rendered inactive, and a paradoxic hyperglycemia can ensue.

63.2.5 Treatment

Field treatment should focus on *gentle handling* of the victim so as to not cause cardiac dysrhythmias. Wet clothing should be removed and dry clothing or a blanket applied. Massage of cold-injured limbs should be avoided; it can damage fragile, frozen parts and trigger dysrhythmias. Traumatic injuries to the spine or limbs should be stabilized. An airway should be maintained and cardiac monitoring begun if available. If the skin is frozen, needle electrodes should be used or fashioned by passing a 20-gauge needle through an electrode pad into the frozen skin. If the patient is alert, warm, noncaffeinated beverages can be provided. Fluid resuscitation with IV D5NS should be started. Lactated Ringers should be avoided because of potential problems with the metabolism of lactate by a cold-injured liver. Emergency room treatment should focus on rewarming of the patient. Defibrillation is generally limited to one countershock until the core temperature is raised above 30°C (86°F) (Level of Evidence B: nonrandomized clinical trials (ECC Guidelines of the American Heart Association [AHA], 2010).[28] It may also be reasonable to perform defibrillation attempts concurrent with rewarming regardless of core temperature (ECC guidelines of AHA, 2010).[28] Medications may be less effective with severe hypothermia, but it is not unreasonable to consider the use of vasopressors according to standard ACLS algorithms.

Clinical Pearl

Except for mild hypothermia, rewarming should include a combination of passive external rewarming, active core rewarming, and active external rewarming.

There are three techniques of rewarming. In all but the mildest of cases, a combination of techniques that include active core rewarming (ACR) should be utilized. Passive external rewarming by covering the victim with a blanket or wrap is ideal in an alert patient whose core temperature is greater than 32°C (90°F). Below 90°F, rewarming should proceed with ACR concurrent with active external rewarming (AER). ACR can be accomplished with IV D5NS warmed to 40°C–42°C (104°F–108°F) or the inhalation of humidified oxygen warmed to 104°F–108°F. More invasive techniques include peritoneal lavage with dialysate warmed to 104°F–108°F, thoracic lavage with normal saline at 104°F–108°F, or warming of the gastrointestinal tract with gastric/colonic lavage.[2] These invasive techniques can trigger cardiac irritability and should be used sparingly. If cardiopulmonary bypass is available, it is now preferred in cases of severe hypothermia.[4]

AER (fires, hot water bottles, and heating pads) should be employed when ACR has already begun to avoid the life-threatening risk of core temperature afterdrop. This devastating process occurs when sudden exposure of vasoconstricted cool extremities to AER, causes peripheral vasodilatation, a drop in central blood pressure, and a sudden influx of cool blood from the periphery to the core that can trigger dysrhythmias and shock.[2] Tables 63.2 and 63.3 provide overviews of hypothermia severity and ideal treatment modalities.[2,4]

63.2.6 Prevention

Good conditioning, proper nutrition, experienced leadership in backcountry environments, normal hydration, avoidance of ethanol or tobacco, habituation to the cold environment (both physiologic and behavioral), and the use of proper clothing help prevent hypothermia.[9] Clothing choice centers on the three Ls: layered, loose, and lightweight. A waterproof outer layer is key.[25] If exercise is occurring in a temperature of <0°F, three-layered hand and footwear are optimal for the prevention of frostbite.

TABLE 63.2
Hypothermia Severity and Treatment

Temperature	Clinical Features	Treatment
Mild		
35°C/95°F	Maximum shivering	Passive external rewarming
33°C/91°F	Ataxia, apathy, tachypnea	Passive external warming
Moderate		
32°C/90°F	Stupor, shivering stops	Active core rewarming (± active external rewarming)
Severe		
28°C/82°F	Decreased v-fibrillation threshold, hypoventilation	Active core rewarming
14°C/57°F	Lowest adult accidental hypothermia survival	Active core rewarming
9°C/48°F	Lowest therapeutic survival	Active core rewarming

TABLE 63.3
Swiss Staging System and Management of Hypothermia

Stage	Symptoms	Treatment
HT I	Awake and shivering	Passive external rewarming
HT II	Impaired alertness and not shivering	Cardiac monitoring; active core rewarming with warm oxygen and warm IV fluids and active external rewarming
HT III	Unconscious, not shivering, vital signs present	As with HT II and usage of cardiopulmonary bypass if available or patient is refractory to medical management
HT IV	Unconscious, no vital signs present	As with HT III plus CPR, ACLS guidelines with epinephrine and defibrillation and cardiopulmonary bypass

Source: Brown, J.A. et al., *N. Engl. J. Med.*, 367, 1930, 2012.

63.3 FROSTBITE

Frostbite is freezing of tissues leading to damage. Frostnip is the formation of superficial ice crystals and causes *no tissue damage.* Chilblains is an *autoimmune* lymphocytic vasculitis, common in women, that leads to localized nodules or ulcers on the extremities 12 hours after cold exposure.

63.3.1 Epidemiology

Frostbite is most common in active individuals from 30 to 49 years of age. High-risk outdoor activities in inclement environments account for a large percentage of injuries. Risk factors for frostbite are shown in Table 63.4.

Ethanol and psychiatric problems underlie up to 70% of most cases of frostbite. The need for amputation correlates more with the *duration* of cold exposure rather than the *lowness* of the temperature. This explains why the impaired judgment resulting from ethanol use and psychiatric illness account for such a large percentage of injuries.[26] Anatomic sites of injury are in order: feet and hands (90% of all frostbite), ears, nose, cheeks, and the penis (a particular concern for runners).

TABLE 63.4
Risk Factors for Frostbite

Predisposing Factors	
Behavioral	**Organic**
Ethanol use	Prior cold injury
Psychiatric illness	Wound infection
Motor vehicle problems	Atherosclerosis
Homelessness	Diabetes mellitus
Smoking	Fatigue
Improper clothing	
High-risk outdoor activities (back-country skiing/ mountaineering)	

63.3.2 Pathophysiology

There are three synchronous pathways that lead to tissue damage in frostbite: tissue freezing, hypoxia, and the release of inflammatory mediators. Each pathway multiplies and catalyzes the damage caused by the other pathways. Freezing leads to denaturation of the membrane lipid–protein matrix and cellular disruption. Hypoxia occurs from cold-induced vasoconstriction that triggers acidosis, increased viscosity, microthrombosis, and vessel endothelial damage. Inflammatory mediators (PGF2α, thromboxane A2) are released from damaged endothelium, which triggers more vasoconstriction, platelet aggregation, thrombosis, hypoxia, and cell death. The same prostaglandins are found in the blister fluid of heat and frostbite damaged skin.[26] The release of these prostaglandins peaks during rewarming; *therefore, cycles of recurrent freezing and rewarming must be avoided to lessen the extent of injury.*

63.3.3 Clinical Features

Symptoms include numbness, clumsiness, tingling, and throbbing pain after rewarming. The signs of frostbite were classically divided into first through fourth degrees. This scheme is not prognostically useful. It is better to distinguish between two types of injury: superficial and deep frostbite. Superficial injury is characterized by normal skin color, large blisters filled with clear or milky fluid, intact pinprick sensation, and skin that will indent with pressure. Deep frostbite shows small blood-filled dark blisters, nonblanching cyanosis, skin that is wooden to the touch and will not indent with pressure.

63.3.4 Diagnosis

Tissue viability is not ultimately determined until 22–45 days postinjury. The primary utility of diagnostic tests is to help define tissue viability at an earlier time. Doppler flow studies and angiography can determine tissue viability and predict the need for surgical intervention as early as 7 days postinjury. Technetium 99 m scintigraphy can be employed as soon as 72 hours from injury to assess tissue viability with a *positive predictive value* (ppv) of 0.84. A scan on day 7 raises the ppv to 0.92 (Level of Evidence A: randomized clinical trial).[10] Magnetic resonance imaging or magnetic resonance angiography may emerge as the optimal modality for early tissue assessment.

63.3.5 Treatment

Field warming should not be instituted until refreezing can be prevented. The injured part should be protected with a loose bulky splint during transport for definitive care. Hypothermia should be treated, and smoking, ethanol, and massage of the frozen part should be avoided. Definitive emergency department care is outlined in Table 63.5. It is based on the work of Heggars and McCauley and guidelines from the Wilderness Medicine Society.[16,19–22]

TABLE 63.5
Stepwise Treatment of Frostbite

Treat hypothermia and any concomitant injuries.
Rapidly rewarm the affected parts in water at 40°C–42°C (104°F–108°F) until thawing is complete and the skin is pliable in texture (typically 15–30 minutes of rewarming).
Debride blisters filled with clear or milky fluid. Apply aloe vera (at least 70%; Dermaide Aloe); cover with a bulky dressing; and leave hemorrhagic blisters intact.
Splint and elevate the extremity.
Administer ibuprofen orally at standard doses. (Avoid aspirin or steroids, but consider the use of pentoxifylline 400 mg po tid.)
Give tetanus toxoid and tetanus immune globulin if >10 years since last booster.
Administer IV penicillin 500,000 units q. 6 hours for 72 hours. (Clindamycin is the recommended alternative for penicillin-allergic patients.)
Treat pain with parenteral narcotics as needed.
Begin daily hydrotherapy with hexachlorophene at 40°C for 30–60 minutes daily.
No smoking.

Clinical Pearl

Frostbite maims, but hypothermia kills. It is critical to treat hypothermia as the first priority before managing frostbite injuries.

Adjuvant therapies with heparin, warfarin, steroids, vitamin C, and hyperbaric oxygen have not been proven to be helpful. Pentoxifylline (Trental) has been shown to be useful in pedal frostbite.[15,21]

63.4 HEAT ILLNESS

Heat illness is best thought of as a continuum of severity along a spectrum from the mild (heat cramps), through the moderate (heat exhaustion), to the life threatening (exertional heatstroke [EHS]).[5] Heat cramps are involuntary, painful contractions of skeletal muscle typically occurring during or after prolonged exercise. Heat exhaustion is a sign of systemic vascular strain in the body's attempt to maintain normothermia—*untreated it may progress to heatstroke.* Heatstroke occurs when heat generation exceeds heat loss leading to a rise in core temperature and thermoregulatory failure. Classical heatstroke is confined to individuals without access to cool environments or debilitated by medical illness. EHS is the form most common in athletes and is defined by a rectal temperature >40.5°C with CNS changes.[1,5,23]

63.4.1 Epidemiology

Frequency correlates with the *wet bulb globe temperature* (WBGT). WBGT = (wet bulb temp × 0.7) + (dry bulb × 0.1) + (black globe × 0.2) where the wet bulb represents the humidity, the dry bulb the air temperature, and the black globe the radiant heat. Risk factors for EHS include obesity, low physical fitness, improper intensity based on physical fitness, improper work-to-rest ratio based on WBGT, dehydration, fatigue, recent episode of heat illness, concomitant febrile illness, sleep deprivation, wear of impermeable garments, the lack of heat acclimatization, the use of medicines or supplements that decrease sweating, and increased thermogenesis (antihistamines, ephedra, caffeine, diuretics).[5,17]

63.4.2 Pathophysiology

The cause of heat cramps is unclear.[1,5] EHS occurs when heat storage outpaces heat loss that leads to deleterious changes at the cellular level. Core temperature >41°C leads to a release of many inflammatory mediators to include *interleukin 1* (IL-1), *interleukin 6* (IL-6), and *tumor necrosis factor.* These cytokines amplify cellular and endothelial damage that triggers systemic vascular collapse and multiorgan failure.

63.4.3 Clinical Features

Symptoms of heat exhaustion and EHS overlap. The diagnosis of EHS rests not on absolute temperature criteria—rather it is due to the presence of an altered mental status and the progression of disease despite first-line treatments. Initial symptoms include headache, dizziness, fatigue, irritability, anxiety, chills, nausea, vomiting, and heat cramps. Seizures and disordered thoughts are evidence of heatstroke. Signs include a core temperature greater than 40.5°C, tachycardia, hyperventilation, hypotension, and syncope. It is important to remember that most cases of EHS are still sweating profusely at the time of collapse. The two key diagnostic criteria for EHS are extreme hyperthermia at the time of collapse (>40.5°C) and CNS dysfunction (coma, altered consciousness, aggression, confusion, inappropriate comments and actions, etc.).[5,23] Please note that a lucid interval may be present surrounding the occurrence of EHS; if the individual collapsed during intense exercise in the heat and cardiac condition has been ruled out, assume EHS until proven otherwise.[23]

Clinical Pearl

Field temperature assessment in the collapsed athlete requires a rectal temperature; auricular and oral temperatures have not been found to be valid when assessing the athlete at risk for heat stroke.

63.4.4 Diagnosis

The diagnosis hinges on an elevated core temperature *combined* with the presence of the symptoms and signs noted earlier. Ideally, this temperature should be rectal; no other expedient field measure to assess core body temperature has been proven valid for individuals who have been doing intense exercise in the heat.[6] Any collapse during exertion should include heat illness in the differential and early core temperature measurement is crucial. Of note, healthy athletes can raise their core temperature to 39°C–41°C simply from exertion alone and be asymptomatic. Laboratory tests are normal until EHS is present. Lab alterations such as increased liver function tests, disordered coagulation profile, leukocytosis, electrolyte disturbances, and evidence of acute renal failure are nonspecific and similar to other shock states.

63.4.5 Treatment

The key is to not delay treatment while trying to determine where on the continuum of heat illness a particular patient is located. Immediate treatment increases the likelihood of the body's return to normal thermoregulation and prevents progression to heatstroke. Field treatment should involve cessation of activity, removal to a shaded, cool environment, fluid replacement beverages, and fanning after spraying the patient with a cool mist. Heat cramps can be treated with passive stretching of the affected muscles.[17,19,27] In case of altered mental status, seizures, or a core temperature greater than 40.5°C, EHS should be presumed, and the patient should be evacuated for definitive emergency care. If the patient responds to field treatment, they should avoid exertion for at least 24–48 hours to avoid a transient but increased risk of recurrent heat illness. EHS treatment involves the nine steps shown in Table 63.6.

Immediate whole body cooling with cold water immersion is the key to a successful outcome.[5,7,8,23] The evidence strongly indicates that the key to surviving EHS without long-term sequelae is getting the patient's body temperature under 40°C within 30 minutes of onset of condition. Emergency action plans need to be able to realize this goal and have appropriate strategies in place for transport and cooling modalities for the specific venue in which they are training or competing.[7,8,23] Concerns that ice water immersion would increase seizures or trigger shivering thermogenesis have been allayed by recent studies (Level of Evidence A: ACSM, 2007 Position Stand Exertional Heat Illness).[1,12]

TABLE 63.6
Treatment of Heatstroke

Immediate cooling. If available, ice water immersion is best. If not, fanning after misting the patient should be undertaken. Cool until rectal temp reaches 39°C (102.2°F).
Avoid antipyretics. The hypothalamic set point is normal. They can aggravate hepatic or renal injury.
Avoid alcohol baths. Vasodilated skin can lead to systemic absorption.
Monitor core temperature until it is <38°C (100.5°F).
Consider diazepam (5 mg) or lorazepam (2 mg) to control shivering and as prophylaxis against seizures.
Monitor renal function closely. Early dialysis is indicated.
Correct *persistent* electrolyte abnormalities.
Check coagulation profile at admission and serially until 72 hours have passed.
Use fresh frozen plasma and/or platelets as needed.
Rehydrate vigorously; monitor for fluid overload and hyponatremia.

63.4.6 Five Keys to Prevention

Acclimatization to high heat and humidity for 10–14 days prior to competition is ideal. The first 4–5 days are when two key physiologic changes occur: changes in sweat composition and an increase in the ability of the body to rapidly dissipate heat. *Clothing* should be light colored, lightweight, and offer sun protection. *Medications* that impair heat loss should be stopped or changed, e.g., change antihistamines to nasal steroids to treat allergic rhinitis and stop ephedra compounds. *Activity planning or reduction* should be based on the WGBT scale: <65 low risk for heat illness, 65–72 high-risk individuals should be monitored or told not to compete, 72–78 risk rises for all, 78–82 high-risk individuals should not exercise, 82–86 unacclimated or unfit athletes should stop, 86–90 exercise should be limited for even fit and acclimated individuals, >90 all activities should stop (ACSM, 2007).[1,17] *Prehydration and hydration per ACSM* recommendations. These can be summarized for patients as follows: drink 16 oz of water or sports beverages several hours before exercise. The goal of drinking is to prevent a greater than 2% body weight loss and should be customized to the activity and the athlete. Approximately 400–800 mL (13–27 oz) per hour is a reasonable amount of fluid consumption to recommend. After exercise, replace each kilogram of weight lost with approximately 1.5 L of fluids (ASCM, 2007).[1]

63.5 ALTITUDE ILLNESS

Rapid ascent past 8000 ft. leads to the onset of the physiologic effects of decreased oxygen concentration at altitude. These effects are most pronounced for those attempting exercise at altitude. Several clinical syndromes exist:

- *High altitude headache* (HAH) is the first symptom of altitude exposure. It may or may not progress to acute mountain sickness (AMS).
- AMS is a syndrome that includes HAH and at least one of four symptoms: nausea/vomiting, fatigue/lassitude, dizziness, or insomnia.
- *High altitude cerebral edema* (HACE) is the clinical progression of AMS so that severe CNS symptoms develop, such as ataxia, altered consciousness, confusion, drowsiness, stupor, or coma.
- *High altitude pulmonary edema* (HAPE) is the most common cause of altitude-related death. It is characterized by classic signs of pulmonary edema: wet cough, dyspnea at rest, weakness, and orthopnea.

63.5.1 Epidemiology

Altitude illness is most common in the unacclimatized, regardless of fitness level, which ascend rapidly past 8000 ft. The severity is linked to the rate of ascent, altitude attained, sleeping altitude, length of altitude exposure, level of exertion, and an individual's inherent physiologic susceptibility that remains static despite reexposure.[11]

63.5.2 Pathophysiology

A rapid rate of ascent, an inappropriately slowed hypoxic ventilatory response to ambient hypoxia and hypercarbia, fluid retention, and vasogenic edema are the initial pathologic changes. Days later, cerebral edema, pulmonary hypertension, and alveolar leakage lead to death if untreated.[13,14] *Maximal oxygen uptake* (VO_{2max}) falls 10% for each 3281 ft. of altitude gained over 5000 ft. VO_{2max} at sea level is *not* predictive of performance at altitude. Many of the world's elite mountaineers have average sea level VO_{2max} values. Past performance and personal problems with altitude illness are the best predictors of future performance and the need for aggressive preventive interventions.

63.5.3 Differential Diagnosis

Any of the symptoms of AMS on ascent past 8000 ft. should trigger suspicion for altitude illness. Key differential diagnostic considerations include dehydration, hypothermia, and a viral infection. Dehydration can be differentiated by response to a fluid challenge. Hypothermia can be distinguished by a low core temperature and improvement with exertion/increased body temperature. Altitude illness worsens with exertion. Although viral syndromes have similar symptoms, they are typically accompanied by fever, myalgia, or diarrhea and are more subacute in onset than AMS. Dyspnea at rest, worsening of symptoms after sleeping, and gait disturbance point toward altitude illness. Abnormal tandem gait is a sensitive examination finding for severe AMS progressing to HACE. Improvement with descent confirms the diagnosis.[14]

63.5.4 Treatment

Initial field treatment involves stopping the ascent and rest. A lack of improvement in 12 hours should lead to a descent in altitude. Typically, descending 1000–3000 ft. is sufficient. Acetazolamide (125–250 mg bid) should be given. If available, low flow oxygen and portable hyperbaric bags are helpful. Additional useful medications are ibuprofen or aspirin for headache and promethazine (25–50 mg) or prochlorperazine (5–10 mg) for nausea and vomiting. Treatment of HACE or HAPE should include *immediate* descent and evacuation. Dexamethasone (4 mg po/IM q. 6 hours) for HACE and nifedipine (10 mg po once followed by 30 mg of the extended release tablet bid) should be instituted for HAPE.[3,18] Tadalafil 10 mg twice daily has growing evidence for usefulness in the prevention of HAPE.[18] Hospital treatment will also include high flow oxygen or hyperbaric oxygen to obtain an arterial saturation of greater than 90%, and loop diuretics for pulmonary edema.[18,24] Mechanical ventilation is only required in cases of coma.

63.5.5 Prevention

Altitude illness can be prevented by proper acclimatization.[18,25] Physiologic changes of hyperventilation, tachycardia, erythropoiesis, and a variety of cellular changes take from minutes to months to reach their peak. Recommendations for the prevention of altitude illness are provided in Table 63.7.

Key recommendations for practice are provided in Table 63.8.

Clinical Pearl

Acclimatization is the key to altitude illness prevention. Begin exertion below 8,000 ft. and spend two to three nights sleeping between 8,000 and 10,000 ft. before ascending above 10,000 ft.

TABLE 63.7
Prevention of Altitude Illness

1. Begin exertion below 8,000 ft. Spend two to three nights sleeping between 8,000 and 10,000 ft. before ascending above 10,000 ft.
2. Sleep no more than 1,500 ft. higher each day above 10,000 ft.
3. Avoid alcohol or sedatives.
4. Avoid dehydration or hypothermia.
5. Consider acetazolamide 125–250 mg po bid beginning the day before ascent: for any individual with a prior history of AMS, when climbing above 11,400 ft., or when acclimatization is not possible. (Continue until after 48 hours at maximum altitude.)
6. In the face of symptoms of AMS, do not go higher. Descend if symptoms do not improve in 12 hours.
7. Reserve dexamethasone (4 mg q. 6 hours) for the treatment of severe AMS or HACE.
8. Nifedipine 30 mg twice per day of the sustained release preparation can be used for HAPE prevention or treatment.
9. Tadalafil (10 mg twice per day) or sildenafil (50 mg three times per day) can be used for HAPE prevention.

TABLE 63.8
SORT: Key Recommendations for Practice

Clinical Recommendation	Evidence Rating	References
Defibrillation is generally limited to one countershock until the core temperature is raised above 30°C (86°F).	B	[28]
It may be reasonable to perform defibrillation attempts concurrent with rewarming regardless of core temperature.	C	[28]
Technetium 99 m scintigraphy can be employed as soon as 72 hours from injury to assess tissue viability with a *positive predictive value* (ppv) of 0.84. A scan on day 7 raises the ppv to 0.92.	A	[10]
Refreezing of thawed tissue needs to be avoided to lessen the extent of frostbite injury.	B	[21,26]
Immediate whole body cooling with cold water immersion to get the patient's body temperature under 40°C within 30 minutes of onset is the key to a successful outcome in EHS.	A, B	[5,7,8,12,23]
Descent of 300–1000 m is the single best treatment for AMC and HACE.	A	[18]
Nifedipine SR 30 mg bid is effective for the prevention of HAPE.	A	[18]

REFERENCES

1. Armstrong LE, Casa DJ, Millard-Stafford M et al. Exertional heat illness during training and competition. *Medicine & Science in Sports & Exercise*. 2007;39(3):556–572.
2. Auerbach PS (ed.). *Wilderness Medicine*, 5th edn. Chapters 1, 5, 8 and 11. St Louis, MO: Mosby; 2007.
3. Bartsch P, Maggiorini M, Ritter M et al. Prevention of high-altitude pulmonary edema by Nifedipine. *New England Journal of Medicine*. 1991;325:1284.
4. Brown JA, Brugger H, Boyd J et al. Accidental hypothermia. *New England Journal of Medicine*. 2012;367:1930–1938.
5. Casa DJ, Armstrong LE, Kenny GP et al. Exertional heat stroke: New concepts regarding cause and care. *Current Sports Medicine Reports*. 2012;11(3):115–123.
6. Casa DJ, Becker SM, Ganio MS et al. Validity of devices that assess body temperature during outdoor exercise in the heat. *Journal of Athletic Training*. 2007;42(3):333–342.
7. Casa DJ, McDermott BP, Lee EC et al. Cold water immersion: The gold standard for exertional heat stroke treatment. *Exercise and Sport Sciences Reviews*. 2007;35(3):141–149.
8. Casa DJ, Kenny GP, Taylor AS. Immersion treatment for exertional hyperthermia: Cold or temperate water. *Medicine & Science in Sports & Exercise*. 2010;42(7):1245–1252.
9. Castellani JW, Young AJ, Ducharme MB et al. Prevention of cold injuries during exercise. *Medicine & Science in Sports & Exercise*. 2006;38(11):2012–2029.
10. Cauchy E, Marsigny B, Allamel G et al. The value of technetium 99 scintigraphy in the prognosis of amputation in severe frost-bite injuries of the extremities. *Journal of Hand Surgery*. 2000;25(5):969–978.
11. Fiore DC, Hall S, Shoja P. Altitude illness: Risk factors, prevention, presentation and treatment. *American Family Physician*. 2010;82(9):1103–1110.
12. Gaffin SL, Gardner J, Flinn S. Current cooling method for exertional heatstroke. *Annals of Internal Medicine*. 2000;132:678.
13. Graham CA, McNaughton GW, Wyatt JP. *Wilderness & Environmental Medicine*. 2001;12(4):232–235.
14. Hackett PH, Roach RC. High-altitude illness. *New England Journal of Medicine*. 2001;345:107–114.
15. Hayes DW, Mandracchia VJ, Considine C et al. Pentoxifylline adjunctive therapy in the treatment of pedal frostbite. *Clinics in Podiatric Medicine and Surgery*. 2000;17(4):715–722.
16. Heggers JP, Robson MC, Manavalen K et al. Experimental and clinical observations on frost-bite. *Annals of Emergency Medicine*. 1987;16:1056.
17. Herring SA, Bernhardt DT, Boyajian-O'Neil L et al. Selected issues in injury and illness prevention and the team physician: A consensus statement. *Medicine & Science in Sports & Exercise*. 2007;39(11):2058–2068.
18. Luks AM, McIntosh SE, Grissom CK et al. Wilderness Medical Society consensus guidelines for the prevention and treatment of acute altitude illness. *Wilderness & Environmental Medicine*. 2010;21:146–155.
19. Markenson D, Ferguson JD, Chameides L et al. First aid: 2010 American Heart Association and American Red Cross guidelines for first aid. *Circulation*. 2010;122(Suppl 3):S934–S946.
20. McCauley RL, Hing DN, Robson MC et al. Frostbite injuries: A rational approach based on pathophysiology. *Journal of Trauma*. 1983;23:143.
21. McIntosh SE, Hamonko M, Freer L et al. Wilderness Medical Society consensus guidelines for the prevention and treatment of frostbite. *Wilderness & Environmental Medicine*. 2011;22(2):156–166.
22. Murphy JV, Banwell PE, Roberts AHN et al. Frostbite: Pathogenesis and treatment. *Journal of Trauma*. 2000;48: 171–181.
23. O'Connor FG, Casa DJ, Bergeron MF et al. American College of Sports Medicine roundtable on exertional heat stroke—Return to duty/return to play: Conference proceedings. *Current Sports Medicine Reports*. 2010;9(5):314–321.
24. Pennardt A. High altitude pulmonary edema: Diagnosis, prevention and treatment. *Current Sports Medicine Reports*. 2013;12(2):115–119.
25. Pescatello LS, Arena R, Riebe D, Thompson P. Chapter 8: Exercise prescription for healthy populations. In: *ACSM's Guidelines for Exercise Testing and Prescription*, 9th edn. Lippincott Williams &Wilkins; 2014: pp. 216–235.
26. Reamy BV. Frostbite: Review and current concepts. *J Am Board Fam Pract*. 1998;11:34–40.
27. Sawka MN, Burke LM, Eichner R et al. Exercise and fluid replacement. *Medicine & Science in Sports & Exercise*. 2007;39(2):377–390.
28. Vanden Hoek TL, Morrison LJ, Shuster M et al. Cardiac arrest in special situations: 2010 American Heart Association guidelines for cardiopulmonary resuscitation and emergency cardiovascular care. *Circulation*. 2010;122(Suppl 3):S829–S861.

64 The Young Athlete

Sally S. Harris and Andrew J.M. Gregory

CONTENTS

TABLE 64.1
Key Clinical Considerations

1. Increasing levels of obesity in children are in part due to declining levels of physical activity.
2. Children in sports and exercise programs are less likely to be overweight and children who watch more television are more overweight.
3. Physical activity in childhood is an important determinant of physical activity in adulthood.
4. Strength training can be beneficial in prepubescent children if it is supervised and appropriate weights/ machines are used.
5. Children do not appear to be more at risk for heat illness than adults; however, the same precautions that are in place for adults should be in place for children.
6. ACL injury prevention programs should be utilized in young female athletes to reduce ACL injury incidence.
7. Physeal injuries should be considered in any young athlete who may still be skeletally immature (sometimes in the early 20s in certain bones).

64.1 INTRODUCTION

Pediatric and adolescent sports medicine is a relatively new and rapidly growing field. It has developed in response to the explosion of organized sports participation for children that has occurred over the past several decades. The participation of girls in sports has increased dramatically since the passage of Title IX in 1972, raising specific concerns with regard to the health consequences of sports participation for young girls. In certain sports, such as gymnastics, figure skating, swimming, and tennis, young girls in particular manifest a unique ability to excel on an international level during the pubertal years. We have also witnessed the emergence of the elite child athlete. Children are specializing at younger ages in one specific sport and training exclusively in that sport year-round. In addition, training programs are becoming increasingly rigorous, and it is quite common to find children training multiple hours each day, with regimens of intensity equivalent to those formerly demanded only of adult athletes (Table 64.1).

The trend toward greater participation by children in organized sports and their involvement in intensive training has raised a number of concerns with regard to the appropriateness and health consequences of these activities. This is offset by the opposite end of the spectrum where decreased activity is associated with increasing rates of pediatric obesity and lack of fitness. Concurrent with the rise of organized sports has been a dramatic increase in musculoskeletal injuries, particularly overuse injuries, which were previously encountered almost exclusively in adults. Other concerns include the risk of injury to the growth centers of the immature skeleton, as well as the effects on overall growth, maturation, and psychological well-being. Optimal care of young athletes requires an understanding of the fact that young athletes are not merely small adults but have distinct musculoskeletal, physiologic, psychologic, and developmental responses and needs with regard to sports training and participation.

64.2 GENERAL ISSUES

64.2.1 Youth Fitness

Concern is growing that children are becoming more overweight and less physically fit. Studies suggest that increasing levels of obesity among children are due in part to declining levels of physical activity over the past several decades.[42] Measures of physical fitness and endurance among children have also declined, and measures of body fatness, such as skinfold thickness and body mass index, have increased.[42,63,64] Children spend less time in physical education classes in school and more time in sedentary activities such as watching television and playing computer games. Low levels of physical activity are associated with several negative health behaviors such as cigarette smoking, marijuana use, lower consumption of fruit and vegetables, greater television watching, failure to wear seat belts, and low perception of academic performance.[55] Studies show that participants in sports and exercise programs are less likely to be overweight and that children who watch more television are more overweight.[26,16] The prevalence of obesity is lowest among children watching one or fewer hours of television daily and highest among those watching four or more hours of television per day.[19] One randomized controlled trial provides evidence that television viewing is a cause of increased body fatness and that reducing television watching reduces childhood obesity.[62]

Physical activity is an important factor for preventing obesity in children.[14] Overweight children are more likely to become overweight adults. As the prevalence of obesity increases, the need to reduce sedentary behaviors and to promote a more active lifestyle becomes essential. Studies suggest that physical activity in childhood is an important determinant of physical activity in adulthood.[3] It is estimated that at least 50% of today's youth do not engage in appropriate levels of physical activity.[64,68] Unfortunately, participation in regular physical activity declines consistently from ages 12 to 21, particularly declining from ages 15 to 18 and continues into young adulthood.[15] Adolescent females are less active than their male counterparts. Early and ongoing intervention is necessary to offset these declines in physical activity throughout adolescence and young adulthood. Three factors have been identified as important in promoting physical activity in young people: utilizing afternoon time for sports and physical activity, enjoyment of physical education, and family support for physical activity.[68]

The long-term health benefits of physical activity during childhood are unclear; however, the benefits of physical activity in adulthood are well documented and include prevention of coronary artery disease, stroke, hypertension, obesity, non-insulin-dependent diabetes mellitus, osteoporosis, mental illness, and some cancers.[29] Studies show a modest relationship between physical fitness in adolescence and favorable lipid profiles and body fatness in young adulthood.[6] Physical activity during childhood and adolescence may also be important in maximizing bone density.[51] Sixty percent of children exhibit at least one modifiable adult risk factor for coronary heart disease by age 12.[63] Promotion of physical activity in adolescence may reduce exposure to other risk factors lasting into early adulthood. Establishment of regular physical activity during childhood is an important foundation for continued physical activity in adulthood and the associated health benefits.[57]

It may seem ironic that, despite the growth of organized sports participation, children in general are more overweight and less fit. In part, the selective competitive structure of organized sports limits opportunities for large numbers of children who are not talented, or competitive athletes or do not have the means to participate. Informal, recreational physical activities available to such children in the past are increasingly limited by urbanization and safety concerns.[52]

It is important to make the distinction between sports performance and health-related measures of physical fitness. The emphasis in organized sports is typically on acquisition of sports-specific skills and other attributes related to performance, such as power, agility, and speed. Health-related physical fitness, on the other hand, refers to those components of fitness required for optimal health and disease prevention, such as cardiorespiratory endurance, muscle strength and flexibility, and body composition. Although optimal physical fitness can improve performance in sports and certain sports activities do enhance physical fitness, many children involved in organized sports may not be achieving adequate fitness levels. Children should be encouraged to participate in activities that will develop both sports skills and physical fitness (see Table 64.2).

TABLE 64.2
Strategies to Increase Physical Activity among Youth at School

Provide enhanced physical education that increases lesson time, is delivered by well-trained specialists, and emphasizes instructional practices that provide substantial moderate-to-vigorous physical activity.
Provide classroom activity breaks.
Develop activity sessions before and/or after school, including active transportation.
Build behavioral skills.
Provide after-school activity space and equipment.
Develop and implement a well-designed PE curriculum.
Enhance instructional practices to provide substantial moderate-to-vigorous physical activity.
Provide teachers with appropriate training.
Involve school personnel in intervention efforts.
Educate and encourage parents to participate with their children in active transportation to school.
Add short bouts of physical activity to existing classroom activities.
Encourage activity during recess, lunch, and other break periods.
Promote environmental or systems change approaches, such as providing physical activity and game equipment, teacher training, and organized physical activity during breaks before and after school.

Source: U.S. Department of Health and Human Services, *Physical Activity Guidelines for Americans Midcourse Report: Strategies to Increase Physical Activity among Youth*, Washington, DC, 2012.

Clinical Pearl

Children and adolescents should do 60 minutes (1 hour) or more of physical activity each day.

64.2.1.1 Sports Readiness and Selection of Developmentally Appropriate Sports Activities

A child's readiness to participate in organized sports or structured training sessions depends on a combination of factors: (1) neurodevelopmental level (motor skills acquisition), (2) social development (interaction with coaches and teammates), and (3) cognitive level (ability to understand instructions).[28,50] No evidence indicates that a child's motor development can be accelerated or their subsequent sports ability maximized by physical training at very young ages,[8] for example, we have no proof that special training can groom a preschooler to become a future champion. The acquisition of motor skills appears to be an innate process that follows the same sequence in all children; however, the rate at which children master motor skills is highly variable and cannot be predicted on the basis of age, size, weight, or strength of the child on an individual basis.[71] Specific skills can be refined through repetitive practice only after the relevant level of motor development has been reached.

At what age is a child ready to begin participation in a specific activity? Although this is a commonly asked question, it has no scientific answer from a neurodevelopmental standpoint. The best answer is that sports activities should match, or be modified to match, the developmental capabilities of the individual child. Sports activities requiring skills beyond the developmental level of the participants are unlikely to be successful. When given the opportunity, children naturally select and modify activities so that they can participate successfully and have fun. Therefore, modification of equipment and rules should be made to suit the developmental level of the participants, such as smaller equipment, smaller fields, shorter duration of games and practices, reduced number of participants playing at the same time, frequent changing of positions, and less emphasis on score keeping. An example of such an adaptation is the game of T-ball, in which children hit a stationary baseball mounted on a stand rather than a pitched ball that requires more advanced visual tracking skills.

Prior to age 6, most children do not have the basic skills required to participate in organized sports. Balance and attention span are limited, and vision and ability to track moving objects are not fully mature. Emphasis in this age group should be on development of fundamental motor skills, such as running, tumbling, swimming, kicking, throwing, and catching, in an environment emphasizing fun and experimentation, limited instruction, and avoidance of competition.

By age 6, most children have acquired the fundamental motor skills to begin participation in simple organized sports activities. They still lack the hand–eye coordination necessary to perform complex motor skills and the cognitive ability to understand and remember concepts of teamwork and strategies. Organized sports that can be played without complex motor skills and strategies, such as entry-level baseball and soccer, are more appropriate than sports such as football that do not lend themselves as easily to adaptation to a more basic level. Emphasis should be on skill acquisition rather than winning. By age 10–12 years, most children have acquired the motor skills and cognitive ability to begin participation in sports at a more sophisticated level, requiring complex motor skills, teamwork, and strategies.

Is it all right for young children, such as 9-year olds, to participate in a contact sport, such as football, hockey, lacrosse, and rugby? When parents ask this question, their main concern is risk of injury. They can be reassured that young children actually have a lower risk of injury in contact sports than do older children, because they do not have the size and strength to generate forces great enough to cause more serious injuries. In addition, significant physical mismatches that could put a smaller child at increased risk of injury do not occur until puberty. A more relevant concern is whether the physical contact and associated aggressiveness and competition are developmentally appropriate or enhancing the value of the experience at this age. The child's enjoyment and eagerness to participate are some of the best indicators of the appropriateness of the activity.

Motivational factors for children's participation in sports include fun, success, skill development, variety, freedom, family participation, participation with friends, and enthusiastic leadership, whereas failure, embarrassment, competition, boredom, and regimentation discourage participation.[65,81] In general, children are much more interested in personal involvement and lots of action than in winning and scores. Attrition in children's sports occurs to a large extent because of lack of playing time, feelings of failure, and overemphasis on competition.[69] Sports programs for children should be designed with these factors in mind in order to promote long-term participation.

Clinical Pearl

In order to keep kids participating in youth sports, the emphasis should be placed on fun, not winning or losing.

64.3 EXERCISE PHYSIOLOGY

64.3.1 Aerobic Training

An increase in maximal oxygen uptake (VO_{2max}), a measure of aerobic fitness, occurs in part as a function of growth alone. Absolute VO_{2max} increases with age during childhood and adolescence as a function of increasing body size.[80] In this regard, growth mimics the effects of training, as even untrained children will show an increase in VO_{2max} over time due to growth; however, maximal oxygen uptake relative to body mass (VO_{2max}/kg) remains essentially stable during childhood and adolescence then slowly declines with age in adulthood.[79] Throughout childhood, boys have a slightly higher VO_{2max}/kg than girls. Gender differences become most apparent at puberty, when VO_{2max} rises dramatically in boys, reflecting increased muscle mass, and declines somewhat in girls, owing to an increase in body fat.

Some evidence suggests that children do experience a training response from aerobic activities, although less dramatic than that seen in adults. Cardiorespiratory profiles of child athletes are superior to those of unathletic children, although the difference is smaller than that seen between sedentary and athletic adults (Figure 64.1). When training programs meet adult standards (in terms of the intensity,

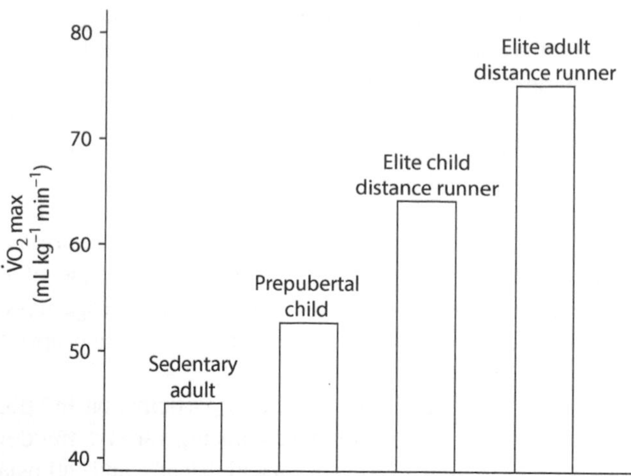

FIGURE 64.1 Typical values of maximal oxygen uptake in trained and athletic children and adults (males). (From Rowland, T.W., *Exercise and Children's Health*, Human Kinetics, Champaign, IL, 1990, p. 57. With permission.)

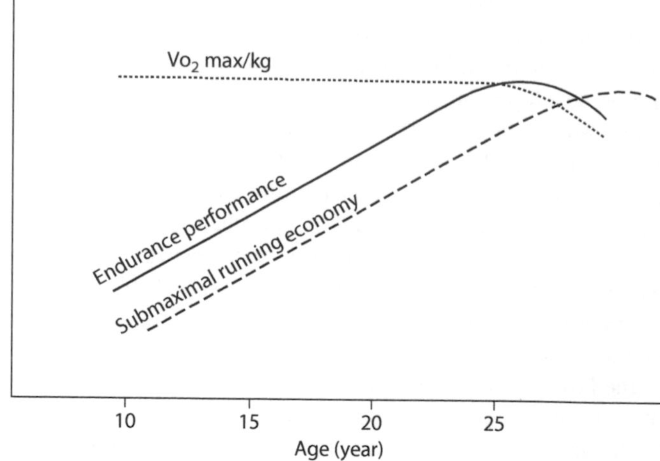

FIGURE 64.2 Changes in maximal oxygen uptake, running economy, and endurance performance with age. (From Rowland, T.W., *Exercise and Children's Health*, Human Kinetics, Champaign, IL, 1990, p. 56. With permission.)

frequency, and duration of the training stimulus), most studies in children show improvements in VO_{2max}.[74] The magnitude of improvement in VO_{2max} is equal to that observed in adults (7%–26%) (Level of Evidence B: systematic review).[74] Children show other adaptations to training similar to those seen in adults, such as lower resting heart rate, decreased submaximal heart rate, increased left ventricular mass, and higher stroke volume with exercise. However, children's response to aerobic training is limited due to several factors. Children are metabolically less efficient than adults and therefore require more oxygen per kilogram of body weight to perform the same level of exercise. Children work at a higher heart rate and lower stroke volume to achieve the same cardiac output as adults. Ventilation rates are also higher, reflecting a less efficient ventilatory system.

The yield of additional aerobic training in child athletes who are already relatively fit appears to be very low. Studies have consistently failed to show a training response in child athletes as opposed to unathletic children. The difficulty in demonstrating a training response in athletic children is probably due to several factors: (1) it is difficult to separate the effects of training from those of growth alone, (2) the magnitude of the training response in children is limited by certain physiologic factors, and (3) significant gains are more difficult to detect in individuals who are already highly fit.

It is interesting to note that in children, significant improvements in endurance performance can occur even though VO_{2max} does not change. For instance, although VO_{2max}/kg remains essentially unchanged during childhood, progressive improvement in endurance performance is observed with age (see Figure 64.2). This apparent discrepancy can be explained by the fact that in children, improvements in economy of motion (metabolic cost of the activity) contribute substantially to gains in endurance performance, irrespective of improvements in VO_{2max}.

64.3.2 Strength Training

Development of muscle strength during childhood is in part a function of the cross-sectional area of muscles; therefore, strength gains parallel growth. An individual is born with a fixed number of muscle fibers, and growth occurs as a result of hypertrophy and increase in fiber diameter. Prior to puberty, females and males have similar muscle mass and strength. At puberty, boys show marked acceleration in development of strength secondary to increased muscle mass, while in girls, strength and muscle mass do not change appreciably.

Traditional dogma held that prepubertal children were incapable of improving muscle strength, a belief based on the fallacy that improvement in strength is dependent on the presence of androgens and associated increase in muscle mass; however, significant strength gains can occur independently of increases in muscle size. This is particularly true for children and women and is even seen in adult males during the early phases of a strength-training program, before any change in muscle size occurs. Neurologic factors, such as increased muscle fiber recruitment, synchronization of motor unit fibers, and improved motor skill coordination, appear to be important mechanisms for strength gains in these instances. Studies of strength training in children show that both boys and girls demonstrate significant gains in strength.[72] Prepubescent children make similar relative strength gains (percent improvement) compared to older children and adults but demonstrate smaller absolute strength increases.

Clinical Pearl

Prepubescent children can make gains in strength with training via neuromuscular recruitment instead of increased muscle mass.

From a practical standpoint, the value of strength training in children is of low yield. Prior to puberty, the gains in strength due to strength training are relatively small and unlikely to confer any significant performance advantages. No compelling evidence suggests that strength gains translate to improved athletic performance. Although strength training has been shown to improve performance on selected motor fitness tests, the improvement is less than that gained by practicing the skill itself. For instance, knee extension weight training improves performance of the vertical jump, but not as much as practicing the vertical jump itself.[78] Children are more likely to improve sports performance by practicing and perfecting the skills of the sport itself, rather than from strength training.

Although the efficacy of strength training in children has been confirmed, concern has been raised about the safety of this activity with regard to risk of injury to the immature skeleton. Although numerous case reports of epiphyseal fracture due to weight training in children have been reported, the majority appear preventable and occur as a result of improper technique, excessive loading, and ballistic movements.[67] The majority of such injuries occur in the home setting, where supervision may be inadequate. Supervised, prospective studies of resistance training in prepubescent children have not reported epiphyseal injury.[2,5,61,72] The majority of injuries are neither epiphyseal nor acute but rather are soft-tissue injuries, such as sprains and strains, especially of the low back.[7,10] No evidence suggests that weight training is more risky in this regard than participation in other sports and recreational activities. Concerns that weight training might lead to muscle boundness and decreased flexibility, which could predispose to injury, appear unwarranted; numerous prospective studies show no change or show slight improvements in flexibility.[5,61,72,73] In addition, some evidence suggests that strength training in adolescents may result in a decreased rate of injuries and rehabilitation time during other sports activities.[11,34]

The term "strength training" should be distinguished from "weight lifting" and "power lifting." Strength training refers to a variety of resistance training modalities (free weights, kettle bells, body weight, elastic bands, and weight machines) designed to increase muscle strength and endurance by performing multiple repetitions and sets of each exercise. Weight lifting and power lifting, on the other hand, are competitive sports emphasizing maximal lifts, such as the clean and jerk and the snatch (weight lifting), and the squat, dead lift, and bench press (power lifting). These activities are not recommended for children and adolescents[75] Weight training is thought to be safe when closely supervised and appropriately designed. This would include emphasis on sets of low resistance and high repetitions, no maximal lifts (although there is some evidence that this may be safe), and no Olympic-style lifts. A sample weight training program for children and adolescents is listed in Tables 64.3 and 64.4.

TABLE 64.3
Sample Strength-Training Program

2–3 sets of 8–15 repetitions per set
Frequency of 2–3 sessions per week with rest day in between
Duration of 30–60 minutes
At least 8 weeks in length
Progressive resistance
Start at no resistance/weights until proper form is achieved
Initiate resistance at the 8-repetition level; advance to 15 repetitions
Add weight in increments of 1–3 lbs until child can do just 8 repetitions
Advance again to 15 repetitions before increasing weights

64.3.3 Thermoregulation

Again, traditional dogma has held that children were at increased risk for heat stress due to a multitude of predisposing factors.[4] However, more recent studies have demonstrated that children tolerate the heat much the same way that adults do.[18] Recent investigations have failed to indicate group differences in heat dispersal when adult–child comparisons are considered in respect to relative exercise intensity. Children rely more on dry heat dissipation by their larger relative skin surface area than on evaporative heat loss. This also enables them to evaporate sweat more efficiently with the added bonus of conserving water better than adults. These findings imply that no differences exist in thermal balance or endurance performance during exercise in the heat nor that child athletes are more vulnerable to heat injury.[18]

Children may take longer than adults to acclimatize to new environments. Often, children are less aware of early signs of heat stress and may fail to decrease their activity level. Voluntary hypohydration occurs frequently in children, and for a given level of dehydration, children experience a faster rise in core temperature than adults. Obese children and very young children may be at particular risk, due to the insulating effect of increased layers of adipose tissue. The most common cause of heat-related illness in healthy children is insufficient acclimatization. In this regard, heat-related illness is entirely preventable by taking appropriate precautions and providing unrestricted access to fluids. Although water is adequate for fluid replacement, children voluntarily drink more of flavored beverages. The additional carbohydrate in sports drinks is helpful only for sustained activities of over 60 minute duration.

Clinical Pearl

Children tolerate heat stress the same as adults, but utilize more nonevaporative mechanisms to facilitate thermoregulation.

Less is known with regard to cold tolerance of children. Like adults, most children generate adequate metabolic heat to maintain and usually increase body core temperature during

TABLE 64.4
Strength-Training Recommendations

Proper resistance techniques and safety precautions should be followed so that programs are safe and effective. Whether it is necessary or appropriate to start such a program and which level of proficiency the youngster already has attained in his or her sport activity should be determined before a strength-training program is started.

Power lifting, body building, and maximal lifts should be avoided until physical and skeletal maturity is reached.

Athletes should not use performance-enhancing substances or anabolic steroids and should be educated about the risks associated with the use of such substances.

Before beginning, a medical evaluation should be performed by a pediatrician or family physician. Youth with uncontrolled hypertension, seizure disorders, or a history of childhood cancer and chemotherapy should be withheld from participation until additional treatment or evaluation.

Children with complex congenital cardiac disease (cardiomyopathy, pulmonary artery hypertension, or Marfan syndrome) should have a consultation with a pediatric cardiologist before beginning a strength-training program.

Aerobic conditioning should be coupled with resistance training if general health benefits are the goal.

Strength-training programs should include a 10–15 minute warm-up and cooldown.

Athletes should have adequate intake of fluids and proper nutrition, because both are vital in maintenance of muscle energy stores, recovery, and performance.

Specific strength-training exercises should be learned initially with no load (no resistance). Once the exercise technique has been mastered, incremental loads can be added using either body weight or other forms of resistance. Strength training should involve 2–3 sets of higher repetitions (8–15) 2–3 times per week and be at least 8 weeks in duration.

A general strengthening program should address all major muscle groups, including the core, and exercise through the complete range of motion. More sports-specific areas may be addressed subsequently.

Any sign of illness or injury from strength training should be evaluated fully before allowing resumption of the exercise program.

Instructors or personal trainers should have certification reflecting specific qualifications in pediatric strength training.

Proper technique and strict supervision by a qualified instructor are critical safety components in any strength-training program involving preadolescents and adolescents.

Source: Adapted from the AAP COSMF, Policy Statement: Strength Training by Children and Adolescents.

moderate and intense exercise in cold weather. Children do not appear to be at greater risk of hypothermia than adults except with regard to exercise in water. In this situation, the child's larger ratio of surface area to mass allows for greater conductive heat loss: the smaller and leaner the child, the faster the cooling rate and the greater the risk of hypothermia.

64.3.4 Intensive Training, Growth, and Maturation

Does intensive training have adverse effects on growth and pubertal maturation? Children performing heavy physical labor have been noted to have decreased stature.[38] Nutritional deprivation is often a confounding factor. Cause for concern is also raised by studies in animals showing shortened long bones due to prolonged training. It is reassuring that studies of child athletes show no apparent adverse effect of intensive training on growth or skeletal maturation.[21,22] However, proper nutrition may be particularly important in growing children involved in intensive training.

It is well recognized that athletic girls experience menarche at least 1–2 years later than other girls. This has raised the concern that training may adversely affect sexual development and reproductive function. Frisch reported a statistical association of a 0.4-year delay in menarche per year of prepubertal training.[30] It remains controversial whether delayed menarche is a direct consequence of athletic activity. More likely, the relationship is a result of selectivity. Girls with delayed menarche are perhaps more likely to engage and succeed in sports, as a prepubertal body habitus (i.e., slender physique, narrow hips, long legs, and low body fat) may be advantageous in sports such as track, gymnastics, ballet, and swimming.[45] However, some athletes have experienced extreme delays in menarche, beyond age 16 or until after cessation of their high school or college athletic careers. In these cases, it is believed that the associated long-standing caloric deprivation and extreme weight restrictions, rather than the intensive training of the sport itself, are significant contributing factors. Evidence also suggests that intense training combined with insufficient caloric intake may restrict development of height during adolescence; however, in most cases, catch-up growth occurs when training is reduced or ceases, and final adult height is not affected.[21,22] In extreme cases, though, catch-up growth may be incomplete. Children participating in intensive training programs over many years should have their growth parameters monitored closely so that reductions in training intensity and increases in caloric intake can be implemented if growth problems are detected.[46]

In boys, on the other hand, evidence of delay of secondary sexual characteristics associated with sports participation is lacking. Sports such as football, baseball, and basketball seem to favor early maturers, who are initially stronger, heavier, and taller than their later maturing peers.

Delayed menarche has no effect on ultimate fertility; however, concern exists with regard to the effects on bone density. It is certainly well recognized that athletes with secondary amenorrhea experience progressive and irreversible loss of bone density, probably due to hypoestrogenism.[27] Amenorrhea and osteoporosis often occur in conjunction with disordered eating and comprise a condition referred to as the female athlete triad.[32,80] Premature osteoporosis is associated with increased risk of stress fractures.[49] It is unclear whether delayed menarche has similar effects on bone density; however, studies in young ballet dancers have found that delayed menarche is associated with a delay in bone density development.[77,78] It remains to be seen whether the delay in bone density development is merely temporary, with catch-up bone development after menarche occurs, or whether the reduction of bone density is permanent.

Gender differences in both aerobic capacity and muscle strength become apparent at puberty, due to the increase in muscle mass in boys and the rise in body fat in girls. Prior to puberty, no appreciable differences between boys and girls in endurance, strength, height, or body mass are observed; therefore, coeducational participation prior to puberty is not thought to place girls at a competitive disadvantage or at increased risk of injury. After puberty, however, most girls are unlikely to compete on an equal basis with boys their age and may be at increased risk of injury due to the discrepancy in strength and size.

There may be dramatic physical differences between individuals of the same gender, particularly boys, as children experience puberty across a wide age spectrum. For this reason, many authorities feel that children's participation in contact sports would be more appropriately matched on the basis of size and maturational stage than on the basis of chronologic age.[60] Skeletally immature athletes should be counseled with regard to the potential risks of injury in competing in contact sports against athletes who are physically more mature.

64.4 INJURIES IN THE IMMATURE SKELETON

Musculoskeletal injuries in sports typically fall into two categories: (1) acute traumatic injuries (macrotrauma), which generally occur as a result of a single event such as a fall, direct blow, or a twist, and (2) overuse injuries (microtrauma), which occur insidiously as a result of repetitive musculoskeletal stress, such as with rigorous training and/or biomechanically incorrect activity. Although overuse injuries were once considered rare in children, they now account for approximately half of all sports injuries seen in children.[24,25] The rise in overuse injuries is thought to be a direct consequence of the rise in organized sports and the repetitive training programs often associated with these activities. Risk factors are outlined in Table 64.5.

TABLE 64.5
Risk Factors for Overuse Injury in Children

Training error
Incorrect biomechanics
Anatomic malalignment
Improper environment
Muscle–tendon imbalance
Vulnerability of growth cartilage
Growth process
Associated disease states
Nutritional factors
Cultural deconditioning

Children differ from adults with regard to susceptibility and patterns of sports injuries. Both the presence of growth cartilage and the growth process itself are thought to place children at increased risk for injury. Growth cartilage occurs at three sites in the immature skeleton: (1) the epiphysis (growth plates), (2) the joint surface (articular cartilage), and (3) the apophysis (secondary growth centers around joints that are the attachment sites of ligaments and tendons) (Figure 64.3). Both acute injury (macrotrauma) and overuse injury (microtrauma) can occur at all three sites (Table 64.3). The musculoskeletal system appears to be most vulnerable to injury during the period of peak height velocity during adolescence,[20] perhaps due to biochemical changes that occur during rapid growth. In addition, rapid bone growth that occurs during the adolescent growth spurt results in relative tightness of muscle–tendon units spanning the joints. The resulting diminished flexibility places the adolescent at increased risk of overuse injury. For these reasons, it may be prudent to decrease the intensity of training during the periods of rapid growth and to place increased emphasis on stretching exercises to improve flexibility (see Table 64.6).[53]

Surveys of high school sports injuries show that 70%–80% are considered minor, causing the athlete to miss less than a week of participation. Most are sprains, strains, and contusions. Highest rates of injury occur in the sports of wrestling, football, gymnastics, cross-country, and soccer. Girls sustain a higher proportion of injuries to the lower extremities than boys. Younger athletes (prepubertal) are more likely to sustain injuries to the upper extremity, such as fractures of the wrist,

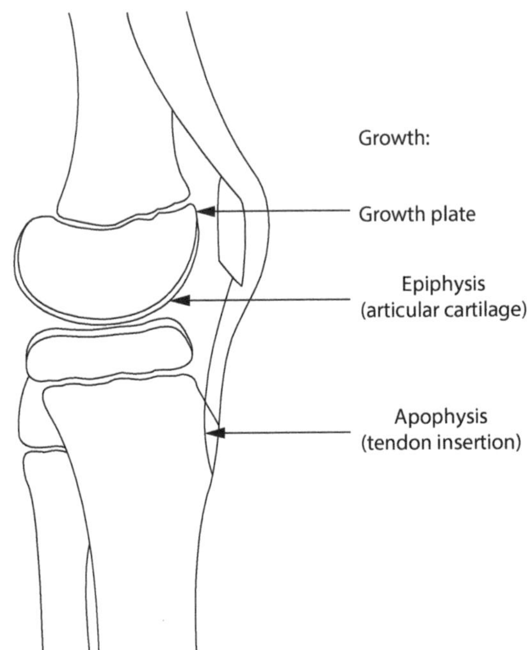

FIGURE 64.3 Growth cartilage is present at three sites: the growth plate, the articular surface, and the apophyses, and is susceptible to overuse injury at each of these sites. (From O'Neill, D.B. et al., *Injuries in the Young Athlete*; Micheli, L.J., ed., *Clin. Sports Med.*, 7(3), 591, 1988, p. 596. With permission.)

TABLE 64.6
Prevention of Overuse Injuries, Overtraining, and Burnout in Young Athletes

Encourage athletes to have at least 1–2 days off per week from competitive athletics, sport-specific training, and practice to allow both physical and psychological recovery.

Advice athletes that the weekly training time, repetitions, or total distance should not increase by more than 10%/week (e.g., increase 2 miles/week if running 20 miles/week).

Encourage the athlete to take at least 2–3 months away from a specific sport during one year.

Emphasize that the focus of sports should be on fun, skills, safety, and sportsmanship.

Encourage the athlete to participate on only 1 team per season. If the athlete is a member of multiple teams, then total participation time should be considered in the limits.

If the athlete complains of nonspecific muscle or joint problems, fatigue, or poor academic performance, be alert for burnout. Questions pertaining to sport motivation are appropriate.

Advocate for the development of a medical advisory board for weekend athletic tournaments to educate athletes about heat illness, overparticipation, overuse injuries, and/or burnout.

Encourage the development of educational opportunities for athletes, parents, and coaches to provide information about appropriate nutrition and fluids, sport safety, and the avoidance of overtraining to achieve optimal performance and good health.

Convey a special caution to parents with younger athletes who participate in multigame tournaments in short periods of time.

forearm, and clavicle, due to falls on the outstretched arm. These injuries occur more commonly from accidents during recreational activities such as skating, cycling, and playing on playground equipment than during organized sports. Lower extremity injuries predominate in older children and adolescents, particularly in girls (shown in Table 64.7).

64.4.1 Injury Patterns in Girls

In 1970, 1 out of 27 girls played sports as opposed to 1 out of 2.5 today. Between 1972 and 2001, the number of girls participating in high school sports exploded from 294,000 to 2.8 million. The increased participation of girls has raised concerns whether girls are at higher risk of injury than boys. Evidence suggests that injury rates for girls are different from those for boys, especially with regard to anterior cruciate ligament (ACL) tears of the knee.[59] Adolescent female athletes are at two and a half to six times greater risk for ACL tears than males, especially in the sports of basketball, soccer, and volleyball.[41] Possible risk factors include deficiencies in training or skill level, lower extremity malalignment, smaller femoral notch size, hormonal factors, muscle firing and strength imbalances, and suboptimal biomechanics (knee valgus, hip adduction) during jumping, landing, cutting, and pivoting. Evidence suggests that training girls to land, cut, jump, and pivot more like boys may reduce ACL injuries.[33,35] A cohort study done in adolescent female soccer players found an 88% reduction in ACL tears in the group participating in a preventive training program including stretching, strengthening, plyometrics, agility drills, and avoidance techniques.[44]

TABLE 64.7
Common Injuries of Growth Centers of the Immature Skeleton

Site	Macrotrauma (Acute)	Microtrauma (Overuse)
Epiphysis	**Acute epiphyseal fracture**	**Epiphysitis**
	Distal femur	Distal femur (swimming, tennis)
	Distal tibia/fibula	
	Proximal humerus	Proximal humerus (little league shoulder)
	Distal radius/ulna	Distal radius (gymnast's wrist)
	Proximal femur	
	Metacarpal/metatarsal Epiphysis	
	Phalanges	
Articular cartilage	**Osteochondral fracture**	**Osteochondritis dissecans**
	Knee	Knee: femoral condyles
	Talar dome	Talar dome
	Elbow: lateral condyle	Elbow: capitellum
Apophysis	**Apophyseal avulsion fracture**	**Apophysitis**
	Anterior superior iliac spine: sartorius origin	Apophyses about the hip and pelvis (see left column)
	Anterior inferior iliac spine: rectus femoris origin	
	Iliac crest–iliotibial band origin and abdominal muscles insertion	
	Ischial tuberosity: hamstring origin	
	Greater trochanter: gluteus medius insertion	
	Lesser trochanter: iliopsoas insertion	
	Medial humeral epicondyle: ulnar collateral ligament origin	Medial humeral epicondyle (little league elbow)
	Tibial tubercle: patellar tendon insertion	Tibial tubercle (Osgood–Schlatter's disease)
	Posterior calcaneus: Achilles tendon insertion	Posterior calcaneus (Sever's disease)
	Base of the fifth metatarsal	Base of the fifth metatarsal (Iselin's disease)

A systematic review and meta-analysis of eight cohort (observational) studies and six randomized trials of various types of neuromuscular and educational interventions appear to reduce the incidence rate of ACL injuries in adolescents and adults by approximately 50%.[31]

Clinical Pearl

ACL prevention programs should be utilized as they reduce the incidence of ACL tears in adolescent females.

After puberty, girls seem more prone to overuse injuries, particularly of the lower extremities. This is thought to be due to lower extremity malalignment (femoral anteversion, genu valgum, external tibial torsion, foot pronation) that is more prevalent in girls than boys and becomes more pronounced with the body changes of puberty in girls. An additional contributing factor is the increase in body fat that girls experience at puberty, in contrast to the increased muscle mass that occurs in boys. Increased body fat may also contribute to decreased performance and a less fit appearance, triggering extreme weight control behaviors and eating disorders.

64.4.2 Epiphyseal Injury

Children are at unique risk of injury to the epiphysis. It is estimated that 10% of all skeletal trauma in childhood involve epiphyseal injury.[43] Epiphyseal injury can lead to major skeletal growth disturbances such as limb length discrepancies and joint angle deformities; however, epiphyseal injuries associated with sports are usually not severe, and less than 5% of epiphyseal injuries result in subsequent growth disturbance.[55]

The epiphyseal plate is two- to five-fold weaker than the surrounding ligamentous structures.[54] The epiphysis is particularly vulnerable during the period of rapid growth at puberty. For this reason, the incidence of epiphyseal injuries peaks during puberty in conjunction with the adolescent growth spurt. In the skeletally immature, acute physeal fractures rather than ligament injuries usually occur. As the skeleton matures, ligament injury is more likely. Therefore, injuries that would result in ligamentous damage in adults may cause epiphyseal fracture in children and adolescents with open epiphyseal plates. A common example is a valgus injury to the knee, which would result in a sprain of the medial collateral ligament in an adult but may cause epiphyseal fracture of the distal femoral epiphysis in adolescents. Similarly, inversion injury at the ankle, which results in the typical sprain of lateral ankle ligaments in adults, may cause a fracture of the distal fibular epiphysis in children. Similarly, injury to the wrist in children often results in distal radial epiphyseal fracture rather than the wrist sprains seen in adults. A slipped capital femoral epiphysis is a variant of epiphyseal fracture that presents as hip pain at the onset of the adolescent growth spurt, particularly in children who are obese or of large build.

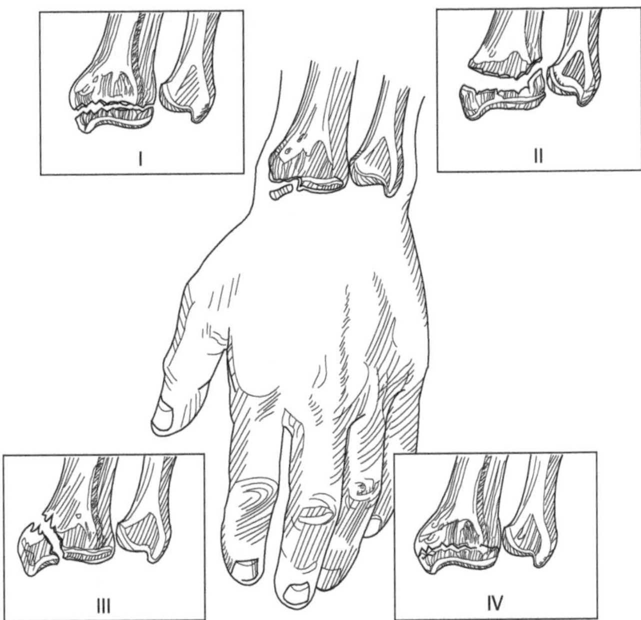

FIGURE 64.4 The Salter–Harris classification of epiphyseal fractures. A Salter V typically is not visualized radiographically. The epiphysis usually fuses in whole or in part with the metaphysis within 1 year.

Epiphyseal fractures are usually categorized according to the Salter and Harris classification scheme (Figure 64.4).[70] The majority of epiphyseal injuries in athletes are type I and type II injuries. If good reduction and adequate immobilization are achieved, type I and type II injuries rarely result in growth disturbances. Orthopedic consultation is advisable. Type III, IV, and V injuries have a higher likelihood of subsequent growth disturbance due to bone bridge formation across the physeal plate and often require surgical intervention to obtain appropriate alignment. These types of injuries occur infrequently in sports and are usually associated with trauma from falls or motor vehicle accidents. The possibility of epiphyseal injury should be suspected in any joint injury in a child with open epiphyses, particularly during the time of the adolescent growth spurt. The diagnosis of "sprain," implying ligamentous injury only, should be made with caution in the immature skeleton.

The epiphysis is not only vulnerable to fractures as a result of macrotrauma but is also susceptible to overuse injury as a result of repetitive stress to the region. This is most likely to occur in children involved in intensive training programs with emphasis on a single sport and presents as persistent pain at the location of the physis. Common sites include the distal femoral epiphysis associated with breaststroke swimming or tennis and the proximal humeral epiphysis in baseball ("little league shoulder") and tennis. These conditions usually respond well to temporary activity modification and lead to no long-term sequelae. Epiphyseal growth arrest and associated degenerative changes secondary to sustained repetitive microtrauma are observed at two sites: the distal radius in gymnasts,[12,66] and the proximal humerus in baseball pitchers.[37] Studies of weight lifting in children have found no evidence of even subclinical epiphyseal microtrauma on the basis of bone scan[61] or evidence of cartilage or connective tissue injury on the basis of various serum and urinary markers.[5] However, caution should be exercised with regard to the skeletal consequences of intensive training during childhood[36] and participation in endurance events such as marathons and triathlons[9] because long-term studies are lacking.

64.4.3 Apophyseal Injury

The apophysis is a center of ossification similar to an epiphysis, but it does not contribute to the long growth of bones. It is the site of attachment of muscle–tendon units on bone and often is associated with a prominence of the bone at the site, such as the tibial tubercle at the knee or the medial epicondyles of the elbow. In children, the junction between the apophysis and the underlying bone has not completely ossified and is weaker than the muscle or tendon attached to it; therefore, tensile forces at this site result in injury to the apophysis rather than to the muscle–tendon unit (as would present as muscle strains in adults). Injury from both macrotrauma and microtrauma can occur at these apophyseal sites.[76]

Sudden contractile forces during sports can result in avulsion fracture of the apophysis, in which a portion of the apophysis is pulled off the underlying bone with the muscle–tendon unit still attached. Typically, such injuries are associated with a sudden, painful popping sensation. Most commonly, they occur around the hip and pelvis at the following sites: the iliopsoas insertion into the lesser trochanter, the sartorius origin at the anterior superior iliac spine, the rectus femoris origin at the anterior inferior iliac spine, the hamstring origin at the ischium,[40] the abdominal muscles attachment along the iliac crest, and the hip adductors attachment at the pubic ramus. Although associated with marked pain and disability, such injuries generally respond to rest and rehabilitation and rarely require surgical intervention, unless the avulsed fragment is large or significantly displaced.

In addition to acute avulsion fractures, overuse injuries of the apophysis also occur. They are often referred to as apophysitis and represent chronic repetitive traction at the site. These injuries can occur at all the aforementioned apophyses about the hip and pelvis, in addition to several other sites. Perhaps, the four most common sites are at the calcaneus (Sever's disease), the tibia (Osgood–Schlatter disease), medial epicondyle of the elbow, and the iliac crest. Iliac crest apophysitis occurs as a result of traction of the abdominal muscles at their site of insertion along the iliac crest. Fusion of the iliac crest apophysis occurs at about age 16 in boys and age 14 in girls. The condition presents as tenderness over the iliac crest and is exacerbated by activity requiring extension of the hip or extension and rotation of the back. It is frequently seen in association with hill running, throwing, rowing, and hurdling.

64.4.4 Articular Cartilage Injury: Osteochondritis Dissecans

Osteochondritis dissecans (OCD) refers to the development of an osteochondral fragment of articular cartilage at a joint surface. The fragment may be composed entirely of cartilage or have an osseous component of various sizes. The fragment may be *in situ*, partially detached, or completely detached. Although the etiology of OCD is most likely multifactorial,[13,17] it is thought that trauma may play a role.[17] OCD can occur as a result of acute macrotrauma to the joint surface, leading to fragment formation and chronic nonunion secondary to avascular osteonecrosis. In addition, growing evidence suggests that repetitive microtrauma to the joint surface may also contribute to the development of OCD. OCD usually presents during the second decade of life. The vast majority of cases occur at the distal femur, classically on the lateral aspect of the medial femoral condyle. The patella, the talus, and the capitellum of the humerus are other common sites. Initial symptoms are often vague and consist of pain, often related to activity level. If the fragment becomes detached, mechanical symptoms such as catching, locking, and joint effusion may develop. Because history and physical findings are usually nonspecific, the diagnosis is usually made on the basis of x-rays. Often, special x-ray views, such as a tunnel view of the knee, or advanced imaging techniques such as magnetic resonance imaging (MRI) are required to visualize the lesion. Prognosis and treatment depend on the age of the patient, skeletal maturity, degree of symptoms, and stability and location of the lesion. The goal is to achieve union of the fragment and restore the integrity of the joint surface. Nonoperative treatment is often successful in patients with open epiphyses, and spontaneous healing can occur with activity modification, protection, and physical therapy for range of motion and strength. Surgical treatment is usually indicated for those who fail conservative treatment, have detached fragments, or are skeletally mature. Surgery involves either debridement to the fragment or internal fixation with drilling or bone grafting of the base.

64.4.5 Osteochondroses

The osteochondroses represent a group of developmental abnormalities of ossification that can occur at any epiphysis and can involve the articular surface, secondary ossification center of the epiphysis, or the physeal plate. The most common of these are listed in Table 64.8. It is often difficult to distinguish osteochondrosis from normal variations in ossification on radiographs. Some osteochondroses, such as Legg–Calve–Perthes disease and Kienbock's disease, are thought to be due to avascular osteonecrosis. For other osteochondroses, such as Panner's disease of the elbow, the etiology is unclear but is thought to be due in part to stress applied to bone in which ossification

TABLE 64.8
Osteochondroses

Femoral head (Legg–Calve–Perthes disease)
Capitellum (Panner's disease)
Vertebral endplates (Scheuermann's disease)
Tarsal navicular (Kohler's disease)
Metatarsal head (Freiberg's disease)
Lunate (Kienbock's disease)

is delayed, resulting in disordered endochondral ossification of the epiphysis.[58] In most cases, the condition is self-limited, and reconstitution of the ossification center will occur with evidence of radiographic healing and relief of symptoms.

64.4.6 Discoid Lateral Meniscus

The lateral meniscus may develop as a discoid-shaped variant in approximately 3% of people.[39] Normally, the meniscus is crescent shaped, but in this case, it is more circular and thicker. This can present as a snapping knee (asymptomatic popping) in the younger child or with a meniscus tear (lateral pain and swelling) in the adolescent. In a snapping knee, a palpable pop is felt in the lateral joint line with McMurray's maneuver whereas in a meniscus tear, lateral joint line tenderness, and an effusion are present. Widening of the lateral joint space may appear on an AP x-ray, but MRI is the gold standard for diagnosis. No treatment is necessary for asymptomatic popping but arthroscopic meniscectomy is recommended for discoid meniscus tears.

64.4.7 Tarsal Coalition

Tarsal coalition refers to congenital fusion of two or more of the tarsal bones of the foot. True incidence is unknown but is seen in families and can be bilateral. Most (90%) occur between either the calcaneus and navicular or the calcaneus and talus and are often bilateral. The connection may be bony or fibrous but ossification increases with time. Patients usually present with medial or lateral ankle pain with activity during the adolescent time period. On exam, patients have decreased inversion of the subtalar joint with reproduction of the pain. Diagnosis can be made with oblique x-ray of the foot in the case of calcaneonavicular coalition, but CT is required to see a talocalcaneal coalition and is the gold standard for any coalition. Surgery for resection of the coalition is usually necessary for relief of pain but conservative treatment with orthotics, bracing or casting, may be attempted first.[23]

Clinical Pearl

If tarsal coalition is suspected, order an oblique radiograph or CT scan of the foot not the ankle.

64.4.8 Stress Fractures of the Spine

Stress fracture of the spine is the most common cause of back pain in activity adolescents. These stress fractures occur commonly at the pars interarticularis portion of the posterior elements and are considered high risk for nonunion. A stress fracture should be suspected in any adolescent athlete complaining of back pain. On exam, patients have tenderness of the lumbar spinous processes and pain with single leg hyperextension. X-rays may be negative early in the process and so MRI with fluid-sensitive sequences of the pars is recommended if the plain films are not diagnostic. The mainstay of treatment is rest from activity and physical therapy concentrating on core strengthening and hamstring flexibility. Bracing is controversial and is not necessary for treatment of most of these stress fractures.[1]

Clinical Pearl

If stress fracture of the spine is suspected, order an MRI that includes sagittal and axial STIR sequences of the lumbar spine.

64.5 SUMMARY

Recreational and sporting activities for children are generally safe. Most injuries are minor and self-limiting; catastrophic injuries are rare. While youth are capable of high levels of training intensity and competition, enjoyment with acquisition of sport-specific skills is the appropriate goal for children's physical activities. Sound coaching, careful preparticipation assessment, regular preventive strategies, and effective injury management will maintain children's already high levels of health and reinforce a lifelong habit of fitness through exercise (Table 64.9).

TABLE 64.9
SORT: Key Recommendations for Practice

Clinical Recommendation	Evidence Rating	References
To encourage long-term participation, sports programs for children should emphasize fun, personal involvement, variety, and success rather than competition, regimentation, and winning.	B, C	[68,69,57,65]
Prior to puberty, no appreciable differences exist between boys and girls in endurance, strength, height, or body mass, and they can compete in a coeducational setting on an equal basis.	B	[34,73]
Children are at risk for heat stress the same as adults; appropriate precautions should be taken to ensure adequate hydration and acclimatization.	B	[18]
For optimal physical matching of children in contact sports, consideration should be given to body size and maturational stage in addition to chronological age.	C	[60]
Early specialization in a single sport, intensive training, and year-round training should be undertaken with caution with regard to increased risk of overuse injury, psychological stress, and burnout.	C	[9,36]
Supervised strength training is safe and can be recommended for prepubertal children as they can gain strength but will not gain muscle mass.	B	[34,73,75]

REFERENCES

1. Anderson SJ, Harris S (eds.). *Care of the Young Athlete*, 2nd edn. American Academy of Orthopaedic Surgeons and American Academy of Pediatrics. Rosemont, IL; 2009.
2. Bale P. The functional performance of children in relation to growth, maturation, and exercise. *Sports Medicine.* 13(3);1992;151–159.
3. Baranowski T, Bouchard C, Bar-Or O et al. Assessment, prevalence, and cardiovascular benefits of physical activity and fitness in youth. *Medicine & Science in Sports & Exercise.* 1992;24(65):237–247.
4. Bar-Or O. Temperature regulation during exercise in children and adolescents. In: Gisolfi C, Lamb DR (eds.). *Perspectives in Exercise and Sport Medicine, Vol. 2, Youth, Exercise, and Sport.* Indianapolis, IN: Benchmark Press; 1989: pp. 335–362.
5. Blimkie CJR, MacDougall D, Sale D et al. Soft-tissue trauma and resistance training in boys. *Medicine & Science in Sports & Exercise.* 1989;21(Suppl 533):S89.
6. Boreham C, Twisk J, Neville C et al. Associations between physical fitness and activity patterns during adolescence and cardiovascular risk factors in young adulthood: The Northern Ireland Young Hearts Project. *International Journal of Sports Medicine.* 2002;23(Suppl 1):S22–S26.
7. Brady TA, Cahill B, Bodnar L. Weight training-related injuries in the high school athlete. *American Journal of Sports Medicine.* 1982;10:1–5.
8. Brant C, Hanbenstricker J, Seefeldt V. Age changes in motor skills during childhood and adolescence. *Exercise and Sport Sciences Reviews.* 1984;12:467–520.
9. Brenner J. Overuse injuries, overtraining, and burnout in child and adolescent athletes. *Pediatrics.* 2007;1242:119.
10. Brown EW, Kimball RG. Medical history associated with adolescent powerlifting. *Pediatrics.* 1983;72:636–644.
11. Cahill BR, Griffith EH. Effect of preseason conditioning on the incidence and severity of high school football knee injuries. *American Journal of Sports Medicine.* 1978;6:180–184.
12. Caine DJ. Growth plate injury and bone growth: An update. *Pediatric Exercise Science.* 1990:2;209–229.
13. Cambell CJ, Ranawat CS. Osteochondritis dissecans: The question of etiology. *Journal of Trauma.* 1966:6;210–221.
14. Cambell K, Waters E, O'Meara S et al. Interventions for preventing obesity in children. *Cochrane Database of Systematic Reviews.* 2003;1:CD001872.
15. Caspersen CJ, Pereira MA, Curran KM. Changes in physical activity patterns in the United States, by sex and cross-sectional age. *Medicine & Science in Sports & Exercise.* 2000:32(9):1601–1609.
16. Children, adolescents, and television, American Academy of Pediatrics, Committee on Public Education. *Pediatrics.* 2001;107(2):423–426.
17. Clanton TO, DeLee JC. Osteochondritis dissecans: History, pathophysiology and current treatment concepts. *Clinical Orthopaedics.* 1982;62:50–64.
18. Climatic heat stress and exercising children and adolescents, Council On Sports Medicine and Fitness and Council on School Health. *Pediatrics.* 2011;128:e741.
19. Crespo CJ, Smit E, Troiano RP et al. Television watching, energy intake, and obesity in U.S. children: Results from the third National Health and Nutrition Examination Survey, 1988–1994. *Archives of Pediatrics and Adolescent Medicine.* 2001;155(3):360–365.
20. Dalton SE. Overuse injuries in preadolescent athletes. *Sports Medicine.* 1992;13(1):58–70.
21. Daly RM, Bass S, Caine D et al. Does training affect growth? Answers to common questions. *Physician and Sportsmedicine.* 2002;30(10):21–29.
22. Damsgaard R, Bencke J, Matthiessen G et al. Is prepubertal growth adversely affected by sport? *Medicine & Science in Sports & Exercise.* 2000;32(10):1698–1703.
23. Dare DM, Dodwell ER. Pediatric flatfoot: Cause, epidemiology, assessment, and treatment. *Current Opinion in Pediatrics.* February 2014;26(1):93–100.
24. DiFiori J. Overuse injuries in children and adolescents. *Physician and Sportsmedicine.* 1999;27:75.
25. DiFiori JP, Benjamin HJ, Brenner J et al. overuse injuries and burnout in youth sports: A position statement from the American Medical Society for Sports Medicine. *Clinical Journal of Sport Medicine.* 2014;24(1):3–20.
26. Dowda M, Ainsworth BE, Addy CL et al. Environmental influences, physical activity, and weight status in 8 to 16 year olds. *Archives of Pediatrics and Adolescent Medicine.* 2001;155(6):711–717.
27. Drinkwater BL, Bruemner B, Chestnut III, CH. Menstrual history as a determinant of current bone density in young athletes. *Journal of the American Medical Association.* 1990;263:545–548.
28. Dyment PG. Neurodevelopmental milestones, when is a child ready for sports participation? In: Sullivan JA, Grana WA (eds.). *The Pediatric Athlete.* Baltimore, MD: Port City Press; 1990: pp. 27–29.
29. Foster C, Murphy M. Does physical activity reduce the risk of vascular events in asymptomatic people? *Clinical Evidence.* 2002:8;99–100.
30. Frisch RE. Body fat, menarche, fitness, and fertility. *Human Reproduction.* 1987:2;521–533.
31. Gagnier J, Morgenstern H, Chess L. Interventions designed to prevent anterior cruciate ligament injuries in adolescents and adults: A systematic review and meta-analysis. *American Journal of Sports Medicine.* August 2013;41(8): 1952–1962.
32. Harris SS. Developmental and maturational issues. In: Puffer JC (ed.). *Twenty Common Problems in Sports Medicine.* New York: McGraw-Hill; 2000: pp. 337–352.
33. Heidt RS Jr, Sweeterman LM, Carlonas RL et al. Avoidance of soccer injuries with preseason conditioning. *American Journal of Sports Medicine.* 2000;28:659–662.
34. Henja WF, Rosenberg A, Buturusis DJ et al. The prevention of sports injuries in high school students through strength training. *National Strength and Conditioning Association.* 1982;4:28–31.
35. Hewett TE, Lindenfeld TN, Riccobene JV et al. The effects of neuromuscular training on the incidence of knee injury in female athletes: A prospective study. *American Journal of Sports Medicine.* 1999;27:699–706.
36. Intensive training and sports specialization in young athletes. American Academy of Pediatrics, Committee on Sports Medicine and Fitness. *Pediatrics.* 2000;106(1):154–157.
37. Jobe FW, Nuber G. Throwing injuries of the elbow. *Clinics in Sports Medicine.* 1986;5:621–636.
38. Kato S, Ishiko T. Obstructed growth of children's bones due to excessive labor in remote corners, in *Proceedings of the International Congress of Sports Sciences*, Kato K, Ed. Tokyo, Japan: Japanese Union of Sports Sciences; 1966: pp. 479–486.
39. Kouteres C, Wonj V. *Pediatric Sports Medicine.* Slack Inc.; 2014.
40. Kujala UM, Orava S. Ischial apophysis injuries in athletes, *Sports Medicine.* 1993;16(4):290–294.

41. LaBella CR, Hennrikus W, Hewett TE. Anterior cruciate ligament injuries: Diagnosis, treatment, and prevention. *Pediatrics.* 2014;133:e1437.
42. Luepker RV. How physically active are American children and what can we do about it? *International Journal of Obesity and Related Metabolic Disorders.* 1999;23(Suppl 2):S12–S17.
43. Mafful N. Intensive training in young athletes. *Sports Medicine.* 1990;9(4):229–243.
44. Mandelbaum BR, Silvers HJ, Watanabe DS, Knarr JF, Thomas SD, Griffin LY, Kirkendall DT, Garrett W Jr. Effectiveness of a neuromuscular and proprioceptive training program in preventing anterior cruciate ligament injuries in female athletes: 2-year follow-up. *American Journal of Sports Medicine.* July 2005;33(7):1003–1010.
45. Malina RM. Menarche in athletes, a synthesis and hypothesis. *Annals of Human Biology.* 1983;10:1–24.
46. Medical concerns in the female athlete, American Academy of Pediatrics, Committee on Sports Medicine and Fitness, *Pediatrics.* 2000;106(3):610–613.
47. Medical conditions affecting sports participation. American Academy of Pediatrics, Committee on Sports Medicine and Fitness. *Pediatrics.* 2008;121:841–848.
48. Micheli LJ (ed.). Pediatric and adolescent sports injuries. *Clinics in Sports Medicine.* 2000;19(4):593–619.
49. Myburgh KH, Hutchins J, Fataar AB et al. Low bone density as an etiologic factor for stress fractures in athletes. *Annals of Internal Medicine.* 1990;113:754–759.
50. Nelson MA. Developmental skills and children's sports. *Physician and Sportsmedicine.* 1991;19(2):67–79.
51. Neville CE, Murray LJ, Boreham CA et al. Relationship between physical activity and bone mineral status in young adults: The Northern Ireland Young Hearts Project. *Bone.* 2002;30(5):792–798.
52. Organized sports for children and preadolescents, American Academy of Pediatrics, Committee on Sports Medicine and Fitness. *Pediatrics.* 2001;107(6):1459–1462.
53. Outerbridge AR, Michele LJ. Overuse injuries in the young athlete. *Clinics in Sports Medicine.* 1995;14(3):503–516.
54. Pappas AM. Epiphyseal injuries in sports. *Physician and Sportsmedicine.* 1983;11(6):140–148.
55. Pate RR, Heath GW, Dowda M et al. Associations between physical activity and other health behaviors in a representative sample of U.S. adolescents. *American Journal of Public Health.* 1996;86(11):1577–1581.
56. U.S. Department of Health and Human Services, *Physical Activity Guidelines for Americans Midcourse Report: Strategies to Increase Physical Activity among Youth*, Washington, DC, 2012.
57. Physical fitness and activity in schools, American Academy of Pediatrics, Committee on Sports Medicine and Fitness. *Pediatrics.* 2000;105(5):1156–1157.
58. Pizzutillo PD. Osteochondroses. In: Sullivan JA, Grana WA (eds.). *The Pediatric Athlete.* Baltimore, MD: Port City Press; 1990: pp. 211–234.
59. Powell JW, Barber–Foss KD. Sex-related injury patterns among selected high school sports. *American Journal of Sports Medicine.* 2000;28(3):385–391.
60. Reducing injury risk from body checking in boys youth ice hockey. *Pediatrics.* June 2014;133(6):1151–1157.
61. Rians CB, Weltman A, Cahill BR et al. Strength training for prepubescent males: Is it safe? *American Journal of Sports Medicine.* 1987;15:483–489.
62. Robinson TN. Reducing children's television viewing to prevent obesity: A randomized controlled trial. *Journal of the American Medical Association.* 1999;282(16):1561–1567.
63. Ross JG, Gilbert GG. The National Children and Youth Fitness Study: A summary of findings. *JOPERD.* 1985;56(1):45–50.
64. Ross JG, Gilbert GG. The National Children and Youth Fitness Study II: a summary of findings. *JOPERD.* 1987;58(9):51–56.
65. Rowland TW. Clinical approaches to the sedentary child. In: Rowland TW (ed.). *Exercise and Children's Health.* Champaign, IL: Human Kinetics; 1990: pp. 259–274.
66. Roy S, Caine D, Singer KM. Stress changes of the distal radial epiphysis in young gymnasts: A report of 21 cases and a review of the literature. *American Journal of Sports Medicine.* 1985;13:301–308.
67. Sale DG. Strength training in children. In: Gisolfi C, Lamb DR (eds.). *Perspectives in Exercise and Sport Medicine, Vol. 2, Youth, Exercise, and Sport.* Indianapolis, IN: Benchmark Press; 1989: pp. 165–222.
68. Sallis JE, Prochaska JJ, Taylor WC et al. Correlates of physical activity in a national sample of girls and boys in grades 4 through 12. *Health Psychology.* 1999;18(4):410–415.
69. Sallis JF, Simons–Morton BG, Stone EJ et al. Determinants of physical activity and interventions in youth. *Medicine & Science in Sports & Exercise.* 1992;24(65):248–257.
70. Salter RB, Harris WR. Injuries involving the epiphyseal plate. *Journal of Bone and Joint Surgery.* 1963;45:587–622.
71. Seefeldt V, Haubenstricker J. Patterns, phases or stages: An analytical model for the study of developmental movement. In: Kelso JAS, Clark JE (eds.). *The Development of Movement Control and Coordination.* New York: John Wiley & Sons; 1982: pp. 309–318.
72. Servidio FJ, Bartels RL, Hamlin RL et al. The effects of weight training using Olympic style lifts on various physiological variables in pre-pubescent boys. *Medicine & Science in Sports & Exercise.* 1985;17:288.
73. Sewall L, Micheli LJ. Strength training for children. *Journal of Pediatric Orthopaedics.* 1986;6:143–146.
74. Shephard RJ. Effectiveness of training programs for prepubescent children. *Sports Medicine.* 1992;13(3):194–213.
75. Strength training by children and adolescents, American Academy of Pediatrics, Committee on Sports Medicine and Fitness. *Pediatrics.* 2008;121:835.
76. Stricker PR, Wasilewski C. Apophysis. In: Puffer JC (ed.). *Twenty Common Problems in Sports Medicine.* New York: McGraw-Hill; 2000: pp. 353–357.
77. Warren MP. The effects of exercise on pubertal progression and reproductive function in girls. *Journal of Clinical Endocrinology and Metabolism.* 1980;51:1150–1157.
78. Warren MP, Brooks–Gunn J, Hamilton LH et al. Scoliosis and fractures in young ballet dancers: Relation to delayed menarche and secondary amenorrhea. *New England Journal of Medicine.* 1986;314:1348–1353.
79. Weltman A. Janney C. Rians CB et al. The effects of hydraulic resistance strength training in prepubertal males. *Medicine & Science in Sports & Exercise.* 1986;18(6):629–638.
80. Yeager KK, Agostine R, Nattiv A et al. The female athlete triad. *Medicine & Science in Sports & Exercise.* 1993;25:775–777.
81. Zauner CW, Maksud MG, Melichna J. Physiological considerations in training young athletes. *Sports Medicine.* 1989;8(1):15–31.
82. O'Neill, D.B., Micheli, L.J. Overuse injuries in the young athlete, *Clinics in Sports Medicine*, 7, 591–610, 1988.

65 The Female Athlete

Rochelle M. Nolte and Jacqueline S. Lamme

CONTENTS

TABLE 65.1
Key Clinical Considerations

1. The female athlete triad refers to the interrelationship among energy availability, menstrual function, and bone health.
2. Physicians should perform a full history and physical and appropriate laboratory tests on any athlete with primary or secondary amenorrhea.
3. Healthy pregnant women with no contraindications should get at least 150 minutes of moderate intensity exercise per week.
4. Exercise during pregnancy has many benefits, including improved cardiovascular fitness, prevention and control of gestational diabetes, control of maternal weight gain, reduced back pain and musculoskeletal discomfort, improved body image, and improved sense of well-being.
5. Athletes can use combination oral contraceptives in an extended cycle manner to regulate their menstrual cycle and avoid having their menses during competitions.

65.1 INTRODUCTION

As the number of girls and women participating in sports grows, the amount of information available about female athletes continues to increase. However, as with any other relatively new area of medicine, the initial information being gathered points out how much more there is to learn. While many of the benefits (physical, psychological, and social) and risks (injury) of sports and exercise are the same for women and men, some issues are specific to women. This chapter addresses issues for adolescent, reproductive-aged, and postmenopausal women (Table 65.1).

65.2 EXERCISE IN ADOLESCENTS

65.2.1 Primary Amenorrhea

Primary amenorrhea is defined as delayed menarche or the absence of menses by the age of 15.[3] Athletes who begin intensive training before puberty are at risk, especially gymnasts and ballet dancers. The athlete presenting with primary amenorrhea should have a thorough history documented, including pubertal milestones. A lack of any pubertal development can indicate hypothalamic, pituitary, or gonadal failure. An interruption of normal pubertal development can indicate ovarian failure or pituitary failure, as happens with a pituitary neoplasm. Normal breast and pubic development in the absence of menstrual periods can indicate an abnormality of the reproductive organs.[17]

Clinical Pearl

Pregnancy is the most common cause of amenorrhea in sexually active women and should always be ruled out.

A training history should include a dietary history, including a history of weight gain or loss, and a detailed history of the type, frequency, duration, and intensity of exercise. A history of the athlete's perception of stress associated with her sport, school, work, home, and peers should be elicited, as well as the support system available to her and an assessment of her coping methods. Athletes who associate more stress with their sport and competition are more likely to be amenorrheic.[17]

A full review of systems should be done, including a history of sexual activity. A thorough history of past medical problems and treatments, especially chemotherapy or radiation therapy, is also important. The athlete should be questioned about medications, illicit drug use, and anabolic steroid use, which can result in amenorrhea. A family history of age at menarche or any family history of endocrinopathies, hirsutism, amenorrhea, or congenital anomalies may be important.[17]

The physical exam should include vital signs, height, weight, body mass index (BMI), arm span, Tanner stage, any characteristics of chromosomal anomalies, any traits of androgen excess such as hirsutism or acne, fundoscopic exam and visual field confrontation, evaluation for galactorrhea, palpation of the thyroid, and a pelvic exam to assess for normal anatomy.[17]

Laboratory testing for amenorrhea is shown in Figure 65.1. The progestin challenge is done by giving medroxyprogesterone as a 10 mg daily dose for 5–10 days.[12] A karyotype should

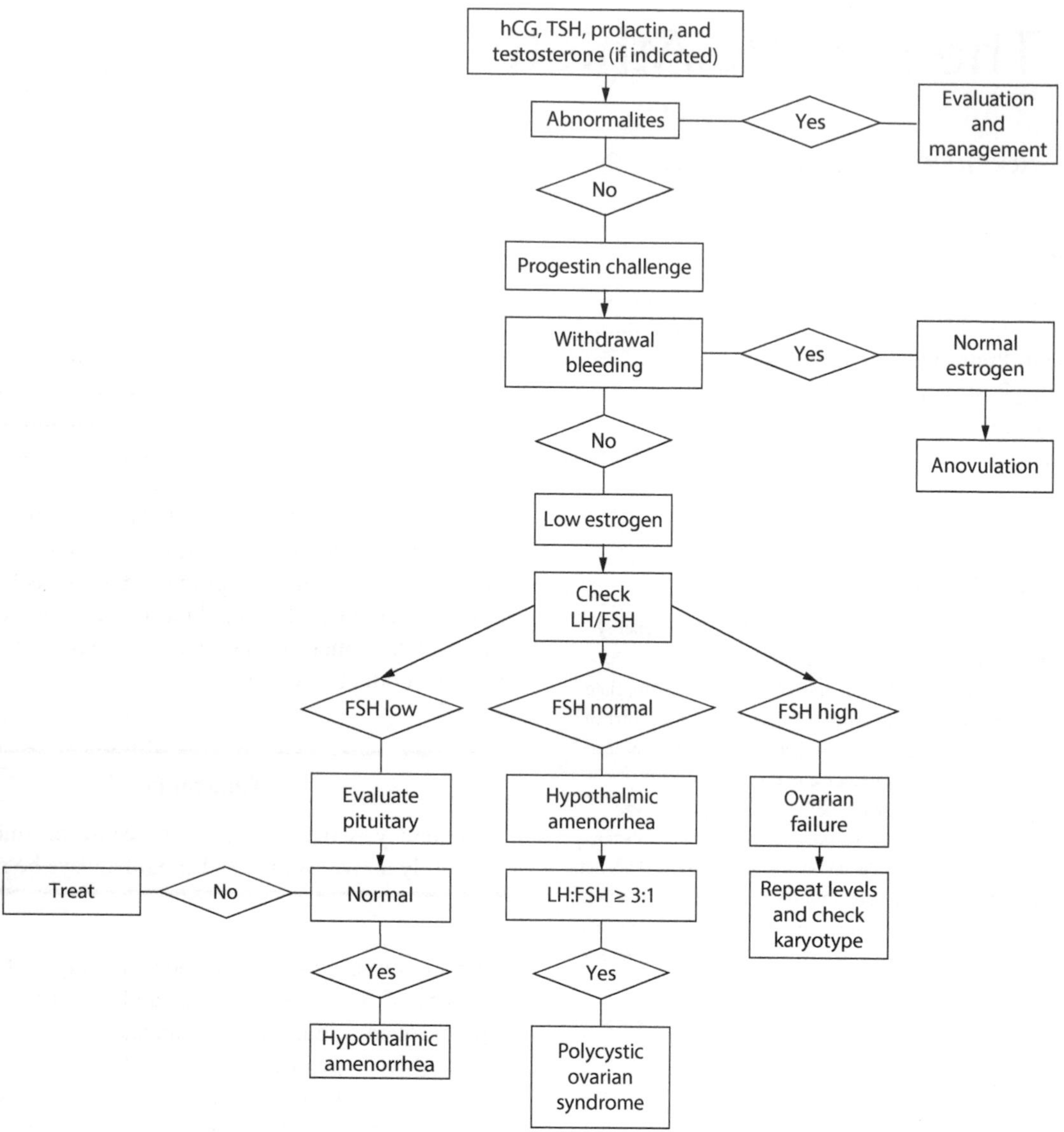

FIGURE 65.1 Special considerations for the female runner. (Adapted from Fieseler, C.M., *J. Back Musculoskel. Rehab.*, 6, 37, 1996.)

be done in any patient who is found to have no uterus on pelvic exam or pelvic ultrasound, as well as any patient under the age of 30 years found to have ovarian failure.

Hypothalamic amenorrhea can be a cause of secondary or primary amenorrhea. In hypothalamic amenorrhea, the pulsatile gonadotropin-releasing hormone (GnRH) is abnormal. Rarely, this can be caused by a tumor or trauma to the hypothalamus. A developmental defect in the hypothalamus can result in an isolated gonadotropin deficiency characterized by a lack of sexual development, primary amenorrhea, low luteinizing hormone and follicle-stimulating hormone levels, normal female karyotype, and sometimes an undeveloped sense of smell.[17] Psychological stress (such as moving away to college, divorce, death in the family, stressful social situations, or stress associated with scholastic or athletic performance) and physical stress (such as weight loss or gain or increase in training) are thought to affect neurohormones that regulate GnRH, leading to hypothalamic amenorrhea.[17] It is also thought that all women must reach a critical body weight and body fat percentage before reproductive function spontaneously starts. Exercise-associated or athletic amenorrhea is considered to be a subset of hypothalamic amenorrhea.[17]

Amenorrhea is a chronically estrogen-deficient state. Because estrogen facilitates calcium uptake into bone, athletes with amenorrhea are at risk of osteoporosis and stress fractures, much like postmenopausal women. If exercise-associated amenorrhea is suspected, the patient should be counseled on the risk of having decreased bone mass. Because women reach their peak bone mass by the end of the second decade and then bone mass starts to decline, the concern is that not only will these athletes be at an increased risk of stress fractures now, but they will also be at risk of osteoporosis in the future secondary to never achieving their peak bone mass. Recent studies have also indicated that hypothalamic amenorrhea is an independent risk factor for coronary artery disease in premenopausal women.[19] The weight-bearing exercise done by athletes can help protect them but may not be enough to overcome long periods of estrogen deficiency. Prevention of this loss of bone mass is one of the main goals of treating amenorrhea.

65.2.2 Secondary Amenorrhea

Secondary amenorrhea is the absence of menstrual bleeding in a woman who has previously had menstrual cycles.[17] Exercise-related amenorrhea is a diagnosis of exclusion. Pregnancy is the most common cause of amenorrhea in sexually active women and must be excluded. Other diagnoses to rule out include endocrine disorders such as polycystic ovarian syndrome, diabetes mellitus, Cushing's syndrome, and thyroid disorders. Anatomic abnormalities such as Asherman's syndrome should also be considered. If a woman aged over 30 years is presenting with secondary amenorrhea, other etiologies to be considered are premature ovarian failure, endometrial hyperplasia, and carcinoma. Exercise-related amenorrhea can be considered a subset of hypothalamic amenorrhea, which also includes amenorrhea related to anorexia nervosa and weight loss, as well as psychological stress, such as moving away to college, divorce, or death in the family. The evaluation and management of secondary amenorrhea is similar to that of primary amenorrhea discussed earlier.

65.2.3 Female Athlete Triad

As the name implies, the female athlete triad has three components: (1) low-energy availability with or without disordered eating, (2) amenorrhea or oligomenorrhea, and (3) osteoporosis or osteopenia.[10] Given the central role of energy availability in the female athlete triad, and the fact that other physiological functions in addition to menstrual function and bone health can be affected, the International Olympic Committee expert panel has proposed the term "Relative Energy Deficiency in Sport" to replace the term "female athlete triad."[20] At this time, the term female athlete triad is more commonly used, but the term refers to the same syndrome of lack of energy availability in the athlete. The prevalence of the female athlete triad is unknown given the secretive nature of eating disorders and underreporting by female athletes. Risk factors include chronic dieting, low self-esteem, family dysfunction, physical abuse, biologic factors, perfectionism, and a lack of nutrition knowledge.[25] Trigger factors include an emphasis on body weight for performance or appearance; pressure to lose weight from parents, coaches, judges, and peers; a drive to win at any cost; self-identity as an athlete only (no identity outside of sports); a sudden increase in training; exercising through injury; overtraining (especially when undernourished); a traumatic event, such as an injury or loss of a coach; and vulnerable times such as an adolescent growth spurt, entering college, retiring from athletics, and postpartum depression.[25]

While we do not know the prevalence, we do know that adolescent girls and young adult women are at risk for developing eating disorders. Whether or not the prevalence of anorexia or bulimia is higher in the athletic population is unknown, but disordered eating does seem to be a problem for female athletes, especially those who participate in sports where leanness is encouraged (runners) or where appearance is judged (dancers, gymnasts). Female athletes with disordered eating and decreased energy intake can develop amenorrhea. As noted previously, the athlete with amenorrhea is at an increased risk of cardiovascular disease as well as low bone mass secondary to either inadequate bone formation or premature bone loss. This leads to an increased risk of fractures, including stress fractures.[19,25]

When taking the history from a female athlete, the physician should be aware of the characteristics of an eating disorder, such as severe self-imposed weight loss, altered body image, an intense fear of becoming fat, lightheadedness, syncopal episodes, weakness, palpitations, overuse injuries, and decreased school and sport performance. They may also complain of fatigue, chest pain, abdominal pain, bloating, diarrhea, constipation, or recurrent pharyngitis. Other history to obtain is a family history of disordered eating, obesity, depression, anxiety, or substance abuse. Psychological history should include smoking, alcohol, and other substance abuse, life stresses, self-esteem and control issues, and symptoms of depression.[25] The 2014 Female Athlete Triad Coalition Consensus provides a list of screening questions for physicians to screen female athletes at risk for the triad and to address the previously discussed risk factors.[10] Important historical questions related to amenorrhea were discussed in the previous sections.

When examining the female athlete, the physician should be aware of physical characteristics of eating disorders, including fat and muscle loss, dry hair and skin, lanugo (particularly on the trunk), cold and discolored hands and feet, decreased body temperature, hypotension, bradycardia, swollen parotid glands, conjunctival petechiae, periodontal disease and caries, pharyngeal erythema, face and extremity edema, knuckle scars, and rectal fissures.[25] Laboratory and EKG studies should be ordered as indicated by the history and physical. Dual-energy x-ray absorptiometry (DEXA) can be used to evaluate bone density.[18] There is now reference data for pediatric DEXA studies.[4] The patient's values should be compared to healthy youth matched for gender, age, ethnicity, and height to generate a Z-score.[4] As there are systemic differences among manufacturers, pediatric patients should be evaluated on equipment for which there are pediatric norms available as values cannot be reliably compared on different equipment and software. The T-score, which is used to compare postmenopausal women to females at peak bone mass, should never be used in the pediatric, adolescent, and young adult population. A Z-score that is more than two standard deviations below expected should be labeled as "low for age."[4]

Management of the female athlete triad is multidisciplinary and requires involvement by the primary care physician, a mental health professional, and a nutritionist with the goal of increasing their energy availability. These patients need guidance and education about their condition, their diet, their training, their stress, and other issues in their life.

They may also be candidates for hormone replacement therapy (HRT), as well as additional calcium and vitamin D. It is recommended that calcium intake be 1000–1300 mg/day.[2] Current vitamin D recommendations are 600–800 IU daily or supplementation as needed to maintain vitamin D levels greater than 32 ng/mL. While bisphosphonates are indicated in the treatment of postmenopausal osteoporosis, their use in young amenorrheic athletes is not recommended, and they should be used with extreme caution in women of childbearing age given the risk of teratogenicity.[10] Combined oral contraceptives (COCs) may be used to provide contraception in amenorrheic athletes; however, most studies indicate that this is not adequate to increase BMD and reduce the risk of stress fracture in these women. In young athletes between 16 and 21 years of age with BMD Z-scores <2.0 or Z-scores <1.0 and a significant fracture history, HRT may be initiated with 100 ug transdermal estrogen and cyclic progesterone (either 200 mg micronized progesterone or 5–10 mg of medroxyprogesterone) for 12 days every month.

It is the job of the team physician to determine if an athlete is healthy enough to participate in her sport. At this time, there are no standardized guidelines for clearance and return to play for girls and women with the female athlete triad. The 2014 Female Athlete Triad Coalition Consensus statement proposes a risk stratification module that assists physicians in making this determination. The consensus panel recommends that athletes diagnosed with anorexia nervosa with a BMI<16 or bulimia nervosa with more than four purging episodes a week be categorically restricted from returning to play until resolution of their eating disorder.[10]

65.3 EXERCISE IN REPRODUCTIVE-AGED WOMEN

65.3.1 Exercise in Pregnant Women

Pregnancy is a normal condition. In the absence of medical or obstetric complications, pregnant women should follow the recommendations of the Centers for Disease Control and Prevention and the American College of Sports Medicine on exercise. The guidelines are accumulation of 30 minutes or more of moderate exercise per day on most, if not all, days of the week.[1] Guidelines for physical activity in pregnant women were addressed by the U.S. Department of Health and Human Services in 2008, recommending that healthy women should begin or continue a minimum of 150 min/week of moderate-intensity exercise while pregnant. Additionally, they specified that women who engaged in vigorous physical activity prior to pregnancy could continue their activity as long as their pregnancy remained uncomplicated.[24] The specific exercise prescription will have to be tailored for each woman based on her baseline level of fitness, her preferred activities, and her gestational age. However, there is no evidence of adverse fetal effects from maternal participation in moderate level activity, whether she was active or inactive prior to pregnancy.[6]

Clinical Pearl

There is no evidence that moderate exercise has a detrimental effect on pregnancy, labor, or fetal well-being.

Exercise during pregnancy has many benefits. Exercise helps maintain or improve cardiovascular fitness. Exercise also helps control maternal weight gain. The American Diabetes Association endorses exercise in the management of gestational diabetes when euglycemia is not achieved by diet alone.[1] Exercise can help reduce low back pain and other musculoskeletal discomforts during pregnancy, as well as assisting with the prevention of urinary incontinence.[21,28] Exercise is also associated with improved body image and sense of well-being, much as it is in nonpregnant patients.

No evidence indicates that moderate exercise has a detrimental effect on pregnancy, labor, or fetal well-being.[8] The babies of regularly exercising women appear to tolerate labor well. They also have been shown to have a similar head circumference and length, but lower body fat, than babies born to nonexercising mothers. However, there have been recent studies of elite, Olympic level athletes demonstrating transient fetal bradycardia after maternal exercise in excess of 90% of maximum maternal heart rate (MHR).[26] The long-term effect of these transient bradycardic events is unknown, and fetal heart rate tracings were reassuring within 20 minutes of these episodes in the studies done to date. There appeared to be no bradycardic events in these women if exercise intensity remained below 90% of MHR. Definitions of exercise intensity vary. However, moderate activity can be described as 40%–59% of MHR and vigorous activity as 60%–84% of MHR with strenuous activity being >90% MHR. Studies on long-term impact of strenuous activity are still underway, but most research to date appears to agree that moderate physical activity should be recommended for all healthy pregnant women and vigorous physical activity can be continued in those women who exercised at this level prior to pregnancy.[21,24,28]

An exercise program should be safe and comfortable and allow the mother to maintain her fitness while minimizing risk to the fetus. The highest risk to mother and fetus with exercise is trauma, and this can be minimized by avoiding sports with a high risk of contact or falling, especially as the woman's balance changes in the later stages of pregnancy.

Environmental conditions should be taken into account when exercising. Pregnant women should dress appropriately and drink appropriate amounts of fluids during exercise and avoid exercising in extreme heat or on uneven terrain. Exertion at altitudes of up to 6000 ft appears to be safe,[8] but engaging in physical activities at higher altitudes carries various risks, and women who travel to higher altitudes should be aware of the signs and symptoms of altitude sickness, for which they should cease activity and descend to a lower altitude. Additionally, it is recommended that the pregnant patient allow 2–3 days for acclimatization prior to moderate exercise at high altitudes and allow two weeks

TABLE 65.2
Contraindications to Exercise during Pregnancy

Absolute Contraindications to Exercise during Pregnancy	Relative Contraindications to Exercise during Pregnancy	Warning Signs to Terminate Exercise while Pregnant
Hemodynamically significant heart disease	Severe anemia	Dyspnea prior to exertion
Incompetent cervix/cerclage	Unevaluated maternal cardiac arrhythmia	Amniotic fluid leakage
Multiple gestation at risk for premature labor	Chronic bronchitis	Preterm labor
Persistent second- or third-trimester bleeding	Poorly controlled type 1 diabetes	Vaginal bleeding
Restrictive lung disease	Poorly controlled hyperthyroidism	Decreased fetal movement
Placenta previa after 26 weeks of gestation	Extreme underweight (BMI < 12)	Dizziness
Premature labor during the current pregnancy	History of extremely sedentary lifestyle	Headache
Ruptured membranes	Intrauterine growth restriction in current pregnancy	Chest pain
Preeclampsia/pregnancy-induced hypertension	Poorly controlled hypertension	Muscle weakness
	Heavy smoker	Calf pain or swelling (rule out thrombophlebitis)
	Orthopedic limitations	
	Poorly controlled seizure disorder	
	Extreme morbid obesity	

Source: Adapted from ACOG Committee Opinion No 267, *Obstet. Gynecol.*, 99(1), 171, 2002, reaffirmed 2009.

for full acclimatization prior to vigorous activity at these altitudes given the increased risk of acute mountain sickness (AMS). While medications commonly used to treat AMS (nifedipine, dexamethasone, and acetazolamide) are not contraindicated in pregnancy, the recommendation is to instead prevent AMS through proper acclimatization.[16] Scuba diving should be avoided throughout pregnancy as the fetus is at increased risk for decompression sickness secondary to the inability of the fetal pulmonary circulation to filter bubble formation (see Table 65.2).

No definitive guidelines have been agreed upon for elite or endurance athletes during pregnancy. There is no well-defined upper limit of safety for strenuous exercise in pregnancy.[21] Elite athletes have to deal with the changing physiology of pregnancy, which may necessitate changing their exercise regimen. After the first trimester, the uterus can cause obstruction of venous return in the supine position, so athletes will have to adjust resistance training and floor exercises appropriately. Motionless standing also causes a significant decrease in cardiac output and should be avoided as much as possible. Athletes should stop exercising when they feel fatigued; they should not try to "train through" fatigue during pregnancy. The increased oxygen consumption of pregnancy will lead to most women experiencing a decline in their exercise tolerance. The goal of exercise during pregnancy is to maintain fitness while avoiding fetal risk. Common sense about the environment, and the type, frequency, duration, and intensity of exercise should be recommended.

65.3.2 Contraception

COCs that contain both an estrogen and progesterone may have potential benefits for female athletes that extend beyond pregnancy prevention. They can help with cycle control, premenstrual syndrome, dysmenorrhea, menorrhagia, and iron deficiency secondary to excessive menstrual blood loss. For athletes who prefer to avoid menses during competition (adventure race participants, triathletes, swimmers, distance runners, and potentially dancers and gymnasts), monophasic pills can be taken in an extended cycle manner. Regimens ranging from taking placebo pills every 3 months to continuous hormonal therapy without placebo are commonly prescribed. There is no evidence at this time that there are any increased safety concerns with extended use of contraceptive pills above the standard precautions for any COC.[22]

Intrauterine devices (IUDs) may be a good option for athletes who are looking for long-term contraception who want to avoid hormonal manipulation, but the athlete should be counseled on the possibility of heavier menstrual bleeding and increased uterine cramping with use of the copper IUD. The Mirena intrauterine system (IUS) (levonorgestrel-containing IUS, also known as the LNG-IUS) is indicated for heavy menstrual bleeding and may lead to amenorrhea in up to 60% of users. This may be a beneficial side effect in the female athlete who would prefer to not experience menses. The Skyla IUS is a LNG-IUS that is indicated for nulliparous women. However, due to its lower progesterone content, it may not cause amenorrhea as found with the Mirena IUS and is not indicated for heavy menstrual bleeding.

Clinical Pearl

The Mirena IUS (levonorgestrel-containing IUS or LNG-IUS) is indicated for heavy menstrual bleeding and may lead to amenorrhea in up to 60% of users. This may be a beneficial side effect in female athletes who would prefer to not experience menses.

65.3.3 Fertility

All women who wish to conceive should be advised to get their health care up to date and ensure that they are eating a healthy diet and including adequate amounts of folic acid and avoiding tobacco and alcohol. They should also have their physicians evaluate any medications they are taking to ensure they are safe to be taken during pregnancy. If a woman is exercising heavily and not having regular menstrual cycles, she should be advised to decrease her exercise intensity in order to allow resumption of normal ovulatory cycles. It is thought that endorphins, cortisol, or other neurohormones such as melatonin or dopamine suppress the pulsatile GnRH[3,17] when they are released with extensive exercise, having an adverse effect on fertility. More research is needed on this hypothesis. If decreasing the exercise intensity does not work, other causes of infertility should be ruled out. If the woman is over the age of 35 and worried about age-related infertility, ovulation induction may be offered. Any effects of athletic amenorrhea on fertility and reproductive health appear to be reversible with treatment of the amenorrhea, after the athlete has decreased her activity level and increased her caloric intake and body fat percentage.

65.3.4 Mastalgia

Mastalgia is a common complaint of the general female population and may be something to consider in athletes. A survey of female registrants of the London Marathon in 2012 revealed that 32% of participants experienced mastalgia, with the prevalence increasing with cup size. A confirmed link between exercise and mastalgia has yet to be established, but it is hypothesized that the lack of intrinsic support in breast tissue, combined with excessive motion during high-impact activity can cause pain. Sports bras with appropriate support based on the athlete's breast size and her activity level should be recommended.[7]

65.4 EXERCISE IN POSTMENOPAUSAL WOMEN

The health benefits of exercise for postmenopausal women include decreased hypertension and diabetes, improved muscle strength and balance, weight control, and psychological benefits. In order for a woman to have an exercise program she is comfortable with and will continue, all of the barriers to exercise, including bone health, medical problems, incontinence, and social issues, need to be addressed.

65.4.1 Hormone Replacement Therapy

Whether or not to use HRT, and the duration of this therapy, is a decision each woman will have to make with the counseling and guidance of her physician. Benefits of HRT include control of perimenopausal vasomotor symptoms (hot flashes, flushes, night sweats), prevention of urogenital atrophy, and prevention of osteoporosis. The only absolute contraindications to HRT are known or suspected estrogen or progesterone receptor positive breast cancer, thromboembolic disease, undiagnosed uterine bleeding (which could indicate uterine cancer), and liver dysfunction.

65.4.2 Osteoporosis

Over 40 million Americans have osteoporosis or low bone mineral density (BMD). Osteoporosis is associated with about 600,000 vertebral fractures and over 200,000 hip fractures annually in the United States. Over 400,000 radial and other extremity fractures occur annually that are associated with osteoporosis. Women have an eightfold increase in their risk of vertebral fracture and a twofold increase in their risk of hip fracture compared to men. Women experience a fourfold increase in the risk of hip fracture with each decade after the age of 50. Over 25% of the patients who present with a hip fracture will be discharged to a nursing home. Over 35% will never walk normally again.[18]

Osteoporosis is diagnosed if BMD in a postmenopausal woman is >2.5 standard deviations below the BMD of a normal young woman (*T*-score) when measured by DEXA. Postmenopausal osteoporosis in women is the most common form with which people are familiar, but other groups are at risk of developing osteoporosis as well. Elderly men, people who have been taking steroids or high doses of levothyroxine for a long period of time, and young female athletes with eating disorders and amenorrhea are also at risk. Low bone mass is defined as a *T*-score of –1 to –2.5 in postmenopausal women.[2]

BMD screening by DEXA is indicated for women aged over 65 years. It may also be indicated before age 65 for women identified as being high risk for developing osteoporosis. Risk factors include weight low BMI, current smoker, excessive alcohol use, medical causes of bone loss, history of a fragility fracture, parental history of a hip fracture, and rheumatoid arthritis.[2] Determining who is at risk for osteoporotic fractures is based largely on history. Nonmodifiable risk factors such as age, sex, race, history of a low-trauma fracture, and family history of osteoporosis should all be noted. Modifiable risk factors include low body weight, low calcium intake, tobacco use, excessive alcohol use, deconditioning, low muscle mass, poor balance, poor vision, estrogen deficiency, and fall hazards in the environment, all of which can be addressed in the treatment and prevention of osteoporosis and fractures.

Nonpharmacologic measures used in the treatment and prevention of osteoporosis include decreasing tobacco and alcohol use and encouraging weight-bearing exercise, which helps increase bone density and muscle mass and improves balance. Nutritionally, postmenopausal women should be taking in 1000–1300 mg of calcium daily, divided into at least two to three doses, as more than 500 mg of calcium cannot be effectively absorbed at one time. Women should also be taking 600–800 IU of vitamin D daily.[2] The vitamin D should be taken with the calcium to aid in the absorption of the calcium. More research needs to be done on other nutrients to determine their effect on osteoporosis before specific recommendations can be made.

Pharmacologic treatment and prevention of osteoporosis includes estrogen, bisphosphonates, selective estrogen receptor modulators, and calcitonin.

Appropriate prevention and treatment of osteoporosis is something that can have a huge impact on the quality of life of patients by helping them remain active and independent. Osteoporosis is clinically silent until the very late stages. Thinking about screening for osteoporosis so treatment can be started early is one of the most important things we can do to help prevent fractures from osteoporosis.

65.4.3 Urogenital Symptoms

Urinary incontinence is defined by the International Continence Society as the "involuntary loss of urine which is objectively demonstrable and a social and hygienic problem."[11] Urinary incontinence affects up to 30% of community-dwelling postmenopausal women and can be a huge barrier to exercise.[23] It can also be an embarrassing topic that a patient may not bring up voluntarily. The most common types of incontinence include stress (stress urinary incontinence [SUI]), urge, or a mixed type that has symptoms of both stress and urge incontinence. Overflow incontinence resulting from urinary retention is less common in active community-dwelling individuals and is more specific to certain medical and neurological conditions. The World Health Organization Consultation on Incontinence concluded that while strenuous exercise is likely to unmask urinary incontinence in otherwise asymptomatic women, there is no evidence that it is the underlying cause of the incontinence. That being said, a higher prevalence of both SUI and urge urinary incontinence (UUI) is seen in athletes with coinciding eating disorders.[5] It is hypothesized that this increased risk is due to the low-estrogen state found in women with hypothalamic amenorrhea and the female athlete triad.

Stress urinary incontinence (SUI) is the loss of urine related to increased intra-abdominal pressure. This type of incontinence is common in premenopausal as well as postmenopausal women, especially after vaginal deliveries. It has also been reported in 28% of nulliparous elite athletes during exercise.[11] The primary complaint is a loss of urine with activities that increase intraabdominal pressure, such as sneezing or coughing, or exercises that include running or jumping. Athletes involved in high-impact activities such as gymnastics (dismount/tumbling) or basketball (jumping) are also at risk.[11,23] Management is directed at correcting the underlying pelvic relaxation using exercises that strengthen the muscles of the pelvic floor. Pelvic floor muscle training exercises can be taught by providing the patient with a Kegel exercises handout or having the patient see a clinic that has nursing or physical therapy staff instructed in biofeedback. Advantages of having the patient followed in a clinic include one-on-one instruction and ability to track progress with a manometer. Doing the exercises requires a motivated patient and there is no guarantee that pelvic floor muscle training will work for everyone. Some women have extreme pelvic floor relaxation and pelvic prolapse that cannot be overcome with strengthening and will require surgery as a final treatment or a pessary as a temporizing measure. The estrogen deficiency associated with menopause can cause vaginal and urethral atrophy, contributing to incontinence. Systemic or topical estrogen can be used to correct the deficiency.

UUI is the loss of urine associated with an uncontrollable sensation of having to void immediately. Patients complain of urgency, frequency, and dribbling on the way to the bathroom or spontaneous complete bladder emptying. They can also complain of feeling the urge to void with provocative stimuli such as running water. UUI can be secondary to detrusor instability or hyperreflexia and can be managed with bladder retraining through the use of a prompted voiding program or with medications that decrease detrusor activity by blocking muscarinic receptors on detrusor smooth muscle. Oxybutynin (Ditropan®), a commonly used antimuscarinic, has the side effects of dry mouth and constipation and occasionally sedation leading many women to discontinue this medication. Other antimuscarinics have been developed with improved side-effect profiles and dosing regimens, such as a sustained-release version of oxybutynin (Ditropan XL®) and tolterodine (Detrol®). These anticholinergic drugs must be used with caution in athletes as they may compromise the sweating mechanism, increasing the chances of heat injury. Other drugs used in the treatment of incontinence include imipramine (Tofranil®) and hyoscyamine (Levsin®), but neither of these medications has been studied in athletes. Duloxetine may possibly improve the quality of life in patients with SUI, but it is unclear whether or not it cures the symptoms.[14]

Postmenopausal women have a higher incidence of mixed incontinence, with traits of both stress and urge incontinence. Treatment should address the dominant symptom first and then address any secondary symptoms if they remain bothersome.

65.5 SUMMARY

Many of the risks and benefits of exercise are the same for men and women, but certain issues are gender specific. Female athletes of all ages have issues such as primary and secondary amenorrhea, fertility, HRT, pregnancy, incontinence, osteoporosis, eating disorders, and the female athlete triad that must be addressed. This is a relatively new area of medicine, and we should be able to make more specific recommendations in the future as we learn more about the physiology of the female athlete (Table 65.3).

TABLE 65.3
SORT: Key Recommendations for Practice

Clinical Recommendation	Evidence Rating	References
In the absence of medical or obstetric complications, pregnant women should get 30 minutes of exercise on most, if not all days of the week.	C	[1]
Exertion at altitudes of up to 6000 ft appears to be safe for pregnant women.	C	[1]
Scuba diving should be avoided throughout pregnancy as the fetus is at increased risk for decompression sickness secondary to the inability of the fetal pulmonary circulation to filter bubble formation.	C	[1]
Female athletes at risk of the female athlete triad should undergo a cumulative risk assessment prior to clearance for sports participation.	C	[10]
Women over the age of 65 and younger women who are at high risk for developing osteoporosis should be screened with DEXA.	C	[2]

REFERENCES

1. American College of Obstetricians and Gynecologists, ACOG Committee Opinion No 267, Exercise during pregnancy and the postpartum period. *Obstetrics & Gynecology.* 2002;99(1):171–173, reaffirmed 2009.
2. American College of Obstetricians and Gynecologists, Osteoporosis. Practice bulletin No 129. *Obstetrics & Gynecology.* 2012;120(3):718–734.
3. American Society of Reproductive Medicine Practice Committee, Current evaluation of amenorrhea. *Fertility and Sterility.* 2004;82(1):266–272.
4. Bachrach LK, Sills IN. Clinical report- bone densitometry in children and adolescents. *Pediatrics.* 2011;127(1):189–194.
5. Bo K, Borgen JS. Prevalence of stress and urge urinary incontinence in elite athletes and controls. *Medicine & Science in Sports & Exercise.* 2001;33(11):1797–1802.
6. Bredin SS et al. Risk assessment for physical activity and exercise clearance in pregnant women without contraindications. *Canadian Family Physician.* 2013;59:515–517.
7. Brown N et al. The experience of breast pain (mastalgia) in female runners of the 2012 London Marathon and its effect on exercise behavior. *British Journal of Sports Medicine.* 2014;48:320–325.
8. Clapp JF. Exercise during pregnancy: A clinical update. *Clinics in Sports Medicine.* 2000;19(2):2.
9. Clapp JF et al. Continuing regular exercise during pregnancy: Effect of exercise volume on fetoplacental growth. *American Journal of Obstetrics & Gynecology.* 2002;186(1):142–147.
10. DeSouza MJ et al. 2014 Female athlete triad coalition consensus statement on the treatment and return to play of the female athlete triad: *First International Conference* held in San Francisco, California, May 2012 and *Second International Conference* held in Indianapolis, Indiana, May 2013. *British Journal of Sports Medicine.* 2014;48(289):1–20.
11. Elia G. Stress urinary incontinence in women. *Physician and Sportsmedicine.* 1999;27(1):39–52.
12. Fieseler CM. Special considerations for the female runner. *Journal of Back and Musculoskeletal Rehabilitation.* 1996;6:37–47.
13. Frankovich RJ, Lebrun CM. Menstrual cycle, contraception, and performance. *Clinics in Sports Medicine.* 2000;19(2):253.
14. Goldstick O, Constantini N. Urinary incontinence in physically active women and athletes. *British Journal of Sports Medicine.* 2014;48:296–298.
15. http://nihseniorhealth.gov/osteoporosis/faq/faq3.html. Accessed March 2014.
16. Jean D, Moore L. Travel to high altitude during pregnancy: Frequently asked questions and recommendations for clinicians. *High Altitude Medicine & Biology.* 2012;13(2):73–81.
17. Marshall LA. Clinical evaluation of amenorrhea in active and athletic women. *Clinics in Sports Medicine.* 1994;13(2):2.
18. Meier DE. Chapter 29: Osteoporosis and other disorders of skeletal aging. In: Cassel CK et al. (eds.). *Geriatric Medicine,* 3rd edn. New York: Springer-Verlag; 1997.
19. Merz CNB et al. Hypoestrogenemia of hypothalamic origin and coronary artery disease in premenopausal women: A report from the NHLBI-sponsored WISE study. *Journal of the American College of Cardiology.* 2003;41:413–419.
20. Mountjoy M et al. The IOC consensus statement: Beyond the female athlete triad—Relative energy deficiency in sport (RED-S). *British Journal of Sports Medicine.* 2014; 48:491–497.
21. Nascimento SL et al. Physical exercise during pregnancy: A systemic review. *Current Opinion in Obstetrics and Gynecology.* 2012;24(6):387–394.
22. Panicker S et al. Evolution of extended use of the combined oral contraceptive pill. *Journal of Family Planning and Reproductive Health Care.* 2014;40(2):133–141.
23. Resnick NM. Chapter 48: Urinary incontinence. In: Cassel CK et al. (eds.). *Geriatric Medicine,* 3rd edn. New York: Springer-Verlag; 1997.
24. Salvesen KA et al. Fetal wellbeing may be compromised during strenuous exercise among pregnant elite athletes. *British Journal of Sports Medicine.* 2012;46:279–283.
25. Sanborn CF et al. Disordered eating and the female athlete triad. *Clinics in Sports Medicine.* 2000;19(2):2–5.
26. Szymanski LM, Satin AJ. Exercise during pregnancy: Fetal responses to current public health guidelines. *Obstetrics & Gynecology.* 2012;119(3):603–610.
27. Szymanski LM, Satin AJ. Strenuous exercise during pregnancy: Is there a limit? *American Journal of Obstetrics & Gynecology.* 2012;207:79e1–79e6.
28. Tanji JL. The benefits of exercise for women. *Clinics in Sports Medicine.* 2000;19(2):6.

66 The Older Athlete

Ted Epperly and Todd Palmer

CONTENTS

TABLE 66.1
Key Clinical Considerations

1. Muscle loss (sarcopenia) can be minimized by continual use and exercising of the body muscles.
2. The cardiovascular–pulmonary system is exceedingly responsive to conditioning with regular exercise.
3. Overuse injuries, especially of the lower extremities, account for 70%–85% of total injuries.
4. The majority of athletic injuries in the elderly athlete can be diagnosed with nothing more than a good history and physical exam.
5. The need for cardiac stress testing prior to developing an exercise program is controversial and often unnecessary.
6. There are four categories of the exercise prescription in the elderly: (1) aerobic exercise, (2) muscle strengthening, (3) flexibility, and (4) balance.
7. Dehydration is relatively more common in the elderly with as little as 2% reduction. Active hydration before, during, and after exercise is very important.

66.1 INTRODUCTION

As America grows older, it is also becoming progressively more health conscious and exercising more. These are good things! As these two processes overlap, an unprecedented number of elderly athletes (65 years of age or older) are lacing up their jogging or walking shoes, putting on their golf gloves, toning up, trimming down, and basically deciding to "use it or lose it" (Table 66.1).

That our society is aging is of little doubt. Demographers have relished pointing out that, in 1995, 34 million people were aged over 65 years (12.5% of the population) and that, in 2030, when all of the baby boomers have reached 65, the country will have 69 million elderly (20% of the total population). By 2050, it is projected that 80 million people in the United States will be over age 65.[10] The average life expectancy is increasing, in part through better exercise and nutrition, so that persons reaching age 65 will have a life expectancy of 81.4 years for men and 85 years for women. The older population is itself becoming older, with those in the 65–74 age group being three times more numerous than the population of that age in 1900, those in the 75–84 years age group being 13 times greater, and the 85 plus age group (the fastest growing segment of our population) being 24 times more numerous.[7]

That America and elderly Americans are being encouraged to exercise more is also undisputed. The American Heart Association (AHA); President's Council on Fitness, Sports, and Nutrition; American Association of Retired Persons; and U.S. Preventive Services Task Force are encouraging the elderly to become more physically active and to develop a program of physical activity tailored to their health status and lifestyle.[4,27]

Not only are the elderly responding to this call to athletic arms by becoming more active, but they are also becoming more competitive. The Senior Olympics and the Senior Professional Golf Tour are just two examples of this trend, and many more competitions for the elderly have emerged. Dramatic improvements have also occurred in most seniors- or masters-level world records in swimming and track and field.[35] The intensity and commitment to training and exercising that characterize many young adults is now being carried into the elderly years especially by the ultracompetitive baby boomers.

66.2 PHYSIOLOGIC CONSIDERATIONS/ BENEFITS

It is important to keep in mind that sometimes, it is very difficult to determine which bodily changes are due strictly to aging and which are due to disuse. These physiologic changes probably result from a combination of both factors.

66.2.1 Muscle

Sarcopenia is a decline in muscle mass and strength that occurs with the normal aging process. All humans lose muscle mass and function as they age, even master athletes who are very active into advanced age.[28] The loss of muscle tissue is both quantitative (decline in myocytes) and qualitative (decline in strength). Sarcopenia is no doubt multifactorial, with neurological, hormonal, nutritional, metabolic, and physical-activity-related changes and other disease comorbidities all playing key roles. As one ages from 30 to 80, muscle mass decreases in relation to body weight by about 30%–40%.[7]

Most studies indicate that maximal strength measures peak in the third decade of life and plateau until about age 50, with a steady decline after that.[30] Muscle size and mass appear to decrease with aging; by age 65–75 years, men show a 20%–25% decrease in quadriceps size by ultrasound scanning compared to men in their 20s.[30,35] Isometric strength of the quadriceps is also reduced by 39% in this elderly group.[35] Computed tomography (CT) scanning of arm and leg muscle size in young (25–38) and elderly (65–90) men demonstrated that the elderly men's muscles were smaller by 28% and 36%, respectively.[35] The lower extremity musculature declines at a faster rate than upper extremity musculature.[28] Other studies, however, have demonstrated little or no change in strength up to age 60.[35] An age-related decrease in muscle fibers and number of motor units has been observed, as well as a possible reduction in the number of Na–K pumps, which effect excitation–contraction coupling.[35]

Clinical Pearl

Muscle mass and strength are lost slowly with aging. How much of this loss is secondary to disuse and how much is strictly age related is unclear. This loss can be minimized or even negated by continual use and exercise of the body's musculature, and improvement in strength and size of "old muscle" can be achieved.

Nonetheless, isometric and isokinetic strength and muscle mass in an older athlete can improve with a training program, and the training response is similar to that seen in younger men.[2,30,35] Aerobic capacity has also been shown to decline with age in active runners and swimmers, reflecting a decline in muscle and aerobic capacity.[28]

Muscle mass and strength are lost slowly with aging. How much of this loss is secondary to disuse and how much is strictly age related is unclear, however. This loss can be minimized or even negated by continual use and exercise of the body's musculature, and improvement in strength and size of "old muscle" can be achieved.

66.2.2 Bone

Bone is a very dynamic tissue that is constantly undergoing deposition and reabsorption. The aging process slows the process of resorption and redeposition of the salts and protein in bone matrix, resulting in a weaker bone. Additionally, an age-related decrease in total body calcium occurs.[35] Bone increases in mass by radial deposition until about the age of 30 years. Bone mass then plateaus until about age 40 in both sexes, after which cortical bone loss occurs at approximately 0.3%–0.5% per year in both men and women.[32,35] At menopause, bone loss accelerates in women, with 2%–3% being lost per year for approximately 5 years after menopause.[30] Trabecular bone loss is more variable and independent of menopausal changes, with a loss of roughly 1.2% per year in men and women.[35] Trabecular bone loss precedes cortical bone loss by at least a decade in both sexes. At this rate, women may lose 30%–35% of their cortical bone mineral mass and 50% of their trabecular mass by age 70 years.[30,35] The corresponding loss in men is about 20% of cortical and 33% of trabecular bone.[35]

Bone loss can be diminished by regular activity and exercise of the skeleton, in combination with good nutrition. Cross-sectional studies of athletes have demonstrated a larger bone mass and density compared to age-matched sedentary controls.[35] Additionally, CT scans of the first lumbar vertebrae of runners with osteoarthritis and osteoporosis, when compared to age- and sex-matched controls who did not run, showed them to have maintained greater bone density than the nonrunners.[20]

66.2.3 Cartilage

Aging produces change in articular cartilage structure and function. Those changes primarily include smaller proteoglycan subunits and a loss of cartilage water content. These alterations decrease the elasticity of cartilage and may lead to an increased incidence of osteoarthritis. Joints postulated to be of greatest risk for this degenerative cartilaginous change include the knees, hips, ankles, and spinal facet joints.[32] Additionally, the small distal joints of the feet and hands are often involved. Multiple studies and papers have addressed the issue of degenerative arthritis or osteoarthritis and its association with running.[19,20,21,24,25] None of these studies has demonstrated evidence of premature osteoarthritis changes in patients studied, and it appears that running actually slows the rate of premature degenerative arthritis.[32] Clinically, if an older runner already has degenerative arthritic changes, the impact of running may accelerate the condition.[32] It is therefore prudent to suggest for these patients an alternative exercise regimen that does not have the same impact on the ankle, knee, and hip. Athletic endeavors that involve quick cutting, jarring, and impact motions, such as tennis, racquetball, and basketball, carry the most injurious forces to cartilage.

66.2.4 Ligaments and Tendons

Ligaments and tendons become less elastic secondary to a decrease in water content, predisposing the elderly to an increased risk of sprains and strains.[32] Decreased flexibility is common with both disuse and aging. A well-designed and regular stretching program before and after exercising is very important in the elderly and helps to maintain muscle flexibility, decreases the formation of excess collagen fiber cross-linkages, and helps to preserve full joint range of motion.[30] Lack of flexibility and decreased range of motion in the elderly increase the stress and force directly borne by the joint and predispose the musculature to tears.[30]

66.2.5 Nervous System

Aging produces a 37% decrease in the number of spinal cord axons and a 10% decline in nerve conduction velocity.[32] The sensory nerves are also more predisposed to neuromas and hypersensitivity secondary to weather changes. Vision and hearing also decrease, as do reaction time and quickness. In fact, quickness is lost long before flexibility and strength.

66.2.6 Cardiovascular System

As one ages, maximum oxygen uptake (VO_{2max}) declines steadily, and anaerobic endurance decreases by approximately 35% or 6.9% per decade.[12,32] Cardiac output similarly decreases by about 6%–8% per decade throughout adulthood, and maximum heart rate declines by 3.2% per decade. The reliability of heart rate based formulae in the older athlete is marginalized by concurrent medication, comorbid disease, exercise/activity history and basic physiology (see Chapters 7, 14, and 27).

Clinical Pearl

Cardiac output decreases by about 6%–8% per decade throughout adulthood, and maximum heart rate declines by 3.2% per decade.

Average 10 km run times slow by approximately 6% per decade.[35] The cardiovascular–pulmonary system, however, is exceedingly responsive to conditioning and with regular exercise, such as running, maximum heart rate decline can be slowed and VO_{2max} and endurance can be maintained.[15,26,32] Not surprisingly, it has also been demonstrated that a running or similar aerobic program is a better way to improve cardiovascular endurance, VO_{2max}, and physical capacity than is a weight-lifting program for trained, healthy elderly.[29] Cross-training in the elderly utilizing a combination of aerobic conditioning (such as running, swimming, elliptical training, cycling, or rowing) and weight lifting for potential additive results make intuitive sense.

Regularly performed endurance exercise favorably modifies the lipid and lipoprotein profile in elderly male runners (66 ± 5 years) by producing an increase in high-density lipoprotein cholesterol and thus may reduce the risk of coronary artery disease in the elderly.[13] Regular exercise, however, is not a panacea or vaccine against coronary artery disease, and the athlete's perception of risk reduction should be discussed.[31]

66.2.7 Kidneys

Glomeruli are lost as one ages, with a corresponding loss in kidney filtration, and a decrease in cellular and total body water predisposes the elderly to dehydration.[4] It is therefore recommended that the elderly move indoors in extremely hot weather and/or breakup workouts into alternating sequences of jogging or cycling for 10 minutes and walking for 5 minutes.[4] Because the elderly are often not aware of dehydration because of blunted thirst, it is advisable to have them drink fluids before, during, and after exercising.

66.2.8 Psychologic Benefits

The psychologic benefits of regular exercise cannot be overemphasized. Older athletes who run and walk regularly have been found to be less tense, depressed, fatigued, angry, and confused and to have greater vigor, a more positive attitude, and higher self-esteem with regard to themselves and their physical fitness.[11,33] When asked why they exercised, 93% of the population over 55 years of age reported exercising to feel better.[22]

66.3 COMMON INJURIES

Injuries seen in the exercising elderly are almost exclusively overuse injuries (Tables 66.2 and 66.3) accounting for 70%–85% of the total injuries.[8,14,18,22] The knee is by far the most common injury site in the elderly, similar to injuries in younger athletes. Most of these injuries are related to running or walking. The elderly tend to gravitate away from high-impact, contact, and team sports and settle on more individual sports that they can master and control. The reason for the increase in knee and foot problems in the older athlete is probably secondary to reduced strength and flexibility of the lower limb and thus decreased shock-absorbing capabilities of the knee and foot.[22] The clinician should examine the patient carefully to determine if the elderly athlete's symptoms are due to osteoarthritis or to an extra-articular soft-tissue syndrome occurring in conjunction with radiographic evidence of osteoarthritis.[22] The elderly often take a wait-and-see attitude toward their injuries, as many of the overuse injuries are slow to develop[18]; therefore, they tend to present late, may be more

TABLE 66.2
Sports Injuries in the Elderly

Diagnosis	Percent (%)
Tendinitis	23.0
Patellofemoral pain syndrome	10.0
Osteoarthritis	9.3
Muscle strain	8.8
Ligament sprain	8.1
Plantar fasciitis	6.0
Metatarsalgia	5.7
Meniscal injury	5.0
Degenerative disk disease	4.3
Stress fracture/periostitis	3.7
Unknown	3.3
Morton's neuroma	2.8
Inflammatory arthritis	2.5
Multiple diagnoses	2.0
Vascular compartment	1.3
Bursitis	1.3
Adhesive capsulitis	1.0
Rotator cuff tear	0.6
Subcromial impingement	0.5
Achilles tendon rupture	0.4
Spondyloarthritis of C-spine	0.25

Source: Data from Mathewson, G.O. et al., *Med. Sci. Sports Exerc.*, 21(4), 379, 1989; Kannus, P. et al., *Age Aging*, 18, 263, 1989; DeHaven, K. and Lintner, D.M., *Am. J. Sports Med.*, 14(3), 218, 1986.

TABLE 66.3
Sites of Sports Injuries in the Elderly

Sites of Sports Injuries in the Elderly [14,18,22]

Location	Percent (%)
Knee	31.0
Foot	18.0
Lower leg	10.1
Shoulder	8.8
Ankle	8.1
Lumbosacral spine	5.6
Multiple sites	5.6
Elbow	4.4
Hip/pelvis	4.0
Upper leg	2.6
Neck	1.4
Wrist/hand	0.9

Source: Data from Mathewson, G.O. et al., *Med. Sci. Sports Exerc.*, 21(4), 379, 1989; Kannus, P. et al., *Age Aging*, 18, 263, 1989; and Hogan, D.B. and Cape, R.D., *J. Am. Ger. Soc.*, 32, 121, 1984.

recalcitrant, and have been treating their injuries at home. Most of the older athlete's shoulder, tendon, and ligament problems are secondary to degenerative changes in combination with overuse.

Clinical Pearl

Injuries seen in the exercising elderly are almost exclusively overuse injuries accounting for 70%–85% of the total injuries.

66.4 DIAGNOSIS AND TREATMENT

Diagnosis can easily be made in 70%–84% of injured older athletes with nothing more than a good history and physical exam.[18,22] The following questions are helpful and necessary to ask these elderly athletes: Are your symptoms aggravated by activity? Exacerbated by a preexisting problem? Precipitated by a sudden change in intensity level, a single severe session, or trauma?[11] Further diagnostic aids such as a plain radiograph, CT scan, magnetic resonance imaging, or radionuclide scan are obtained when felt necessary. Consultation may be helpful in about 15% of cases.[22]

Clinical Pearl

Diagnosis can easily be made in 70%–84% of injured older athletes with nothing more than a good history and physical exam.

Because most of the elderly athlete's problems are overuse injuries, a conservative treatment policy is warranted. These problems, as in younger athletes, should respond well to PRICEMM (prevention/protection, rest, ice, compression, elevation, modalities, and medications). When necessary to treat elderly with medications, three caveats should be remembered. First, start low and go slow. Start any nonsteroidal anti-inflammatory drug or COX II inhibitor at a low dose and proceed slowly before raising the dose. Second, remember that the elderly are frequently on other medications, so check for potential drug–drug interactions. Third, remember that therapy of injuries in the elderly takes longer than it does for younger persons, so begin rehabilitation as soon as possible. A useful guideline is that treatment duration should be at least twice as long for an athlete 60 years or older than for a 20-year-old athlete, and three times as long for athletes older than 75.[4] A successful return to activity can be obtained if adequate treatment, rest, and rehabilitation are provided. One useful approach is to decrease activities by 15%–25% of usual activities until symptoms disappear. Similarly, an increase in activities can gradually be returned in increments of 15%–25% over 3–6 weeks, depending on the condition.

Physical therapy has much to offer the older athlete including ultrasound, diathermy, iontophoresis, and range of motion and stretching exercises. Simple, inexpensive items such as handheld free weights and elastic rubber tubing can be used at home following simply written, printed instructions to increase patient compliance and reduce patient cost for rehabilitation. Muscle strengthening, particularly quadriceps strengthening, is crucial for knee-related problems and can easily be taught to the elderly. Orthotics and braces may also play a role for such problems as Achilles tendinitis, ankle instability, posterior tibial tendinitis, plantar fasciitis, and Morton's neuroma. If the aforementioned measures do not work, then local steroid injections and/or surgery may be necessary. Local steroid injection was used in 10% of the elderly seen for their sport-related injuries in one study.[22] Most sport-related injuries in the elderly are easily managed with a common-sense and conservative approach, with only 2%–4% requiring surgery.[18,22]

Contributing factors and age-related changes that may contribute to athletic problems in the elderly include decreases in muscle mass, flexibility, reaction time, bone mass, and cartilage thickness and resilience, as well as impaired vision, hearing, proprioception, temperature regulation, and balance. A regular program of exercise and range of motion activities will help maintain muscle mass and flexibility. In return, muscle mass and flexibility will decrease musculoskeletal injuries. Problems with arthritis can subsequently be helped with reduced-weight-bearing activities such as swimming, stationary cycling, or elliptical training devices. Osteoporosis can be helped by a regular exercise program (full weight bearing). For elderly patients who suffer from poor vision, hearing, and balance problems, a stationary bicycle or elliptical training machine may provide good exercise while maintaining balance in a safe environment.

Exercise after myocardial infarction is in no way contraindicated; however, a program must be tailored to the individual's condition and should start with low-impact aerobic exercise (such as walking or stationary cycling) and should build up slowly in duration, frequency, and intensity as the patient demonstrates tolerance. Exercise after arthroplasty or joint replacement also is not contraindicated. However, limited-weight-bearing activity is preferred initially, such as water conditioning, stationary cycling, or elliptical training for endurance while decreasing joint stress.

66.5 PREPARTICIPATION SCREENING

The American College of Sport Medicine (ACSM) and the AHA recommend consultation with primary care providers when developing an activity/exercise plan for older adults.[9] Optimally, discussions between elderly patients and providers regarding physical activity and exercise should be occurring at least once a year regardless of whether or not there is a definite plan for increased physical activity. Because chronological age does not equate to physiologic function,[1] it is extremely important that the physician individualize exercise prescriptions to the needs and abilities of the particular older athletes being evaluated. The principles of exercise prescription are similar for people of all ages. The goal is to improve cardiovascular and muscle fitness. The physician's role is to understand these principles and suggest an exercise plan that is safe and takes into account an individual's goals and physical abilities and to keep the patient motivated and compliant. Many older patients, however, have some unique challenges and conditions that must be carefully considered and managed in order to achieve this.

A history and physical examination should be performed prior to initiating an exercise program in order to identify significant risk factors and conditions that could play a role in regard to the safety and efficacy of general and specific types of exercises. The history and physical examination should focus on conditions that may impede the success of exercise or affect the motivation of the individual if they are not considered. Medications also need to be carefully evaluated considering the fact that side effects and physiologic changes can be exaggerated in the elderly and be a significant factor during exercise.

There are very few absolute and relative contraindications for aerobic and resistance training for the older athlete. The absolute contraindications are fairly obvious and include recent electrocardiogram changes or myocardial infarction, unstable angina, third-degree heart block, acute heart failure, uncontrolled hypertension, and uncontrolled metabolic disease.

Other significant conditions would include current infections, recent surgeries, deep venous thrombosis, fevers with muscle aches, arthritis, osteoporosis, foot sores, arrhythmias, peripheral vascular disease, and cognitive dysfunction. Many conditions may be treatable prior to exercise and not recognizing some could lead to injury.

Muscle strength should always be assessed especially in the lower extremities as this is where most injuries occur. For the same reason, flexibility determination in the lower extremities is important.

The physician's knowledge of a patient's overall condition and specific problems is important in regard to identifying contraindications and limitations and leads to more successful exercise prescriptions and compliance.

Clinical Pearl

The physician's knowledge of a patient's overall condition and specific problems is important in regard to identifying contraindications and limitations and leads to more successful exercise prescriptions and compliance.

With regard to exercise stress testing prior to initiating an increased activity or exercise program, the evidence is conflicting and opinions are divergent leading to the U.S. Preventive Services Task Force not making a specific recommendation and some confusion for providers and trainers.[1] There are some principles that apply and should be carefully considered; both to prevent cardiac ischemia and also to unnecessarily prevent cardiac stress testing from becoming an obstacle to exercise. The first is related to gradual escalation of activity.[1] The rates of death and acute myocardial infarctions are highest in individuals who have a significant nongraduated change in their activity levels. The exact mechanism for this is not known, but there is some evidence pointing toward a phenomenon where increased heart rate, demand, and coronary artery excursion in a nonaccustomed or nonconditioned patient could cause bending and flexing of the coronary arteries to the point that atherosclerotic plaque cracking occurs followed by platelet aggregation and thrombosis. Another reason is simply that the coronary arteries cannot accommodate the required higher flow rates. For these reasons, and to improve adherence, guidelines from the AHA and ACSM emphasize gradual initiation of exercise. Both groups also endorse the statement that "exercise stress testing may be considered for previously sedentary older individuals who are planning to begin a vigorous exercise program." However, this is generally unnecessary because sedentary patients should not start out with a vigorous program, and they need to be given careful guidance consistent with this.

The second principle relates to risk factors and the existence of cardiovascular disease. These are well known to physicians with regard to medical decisions such as statin use, but they are also very significant here. Any patient with diabetes (especially if they also have accompanying macro vascular disease), symptomatic or known cardiovascular disease, pulmonary disease to include COPD, asthma, cystic fibrosis, or interstitial lung disease, or renal disease should have stress testing prior to initiating an exercise program. However, other than patients with known cardiovascular disease, most elderly patients should be able to initiate a light intensity program without significant risk. This would generally be defined as less than three metabolic equivalent units (METs). However, since METs can be misleading in the elderly, a better indication for light intensity activity would be that there is no noticeable change in their breathing or heart rate.[23]

Other risk factors to consider include, smoking, hypertension, age (male 45 or over and female 55 or over), dyslipidemia, family history, sedentary lifestyle, obesity, and prediabetes. Two or more of these risk factors put the patient in the moderate risk category, and although there are no definite recommendations to do cardiac stress testing, a careful physical exam should be done, and each patient should be considered individually as well as the intensity of the activity prescribed when determining the need for an exercise stress test. Often, a stress test is not needed if exercise is started out slowly using low-intensity exercises with continuing follow-up and assessment. In addition to providing information regarding cardiovascular safety, stress testing can also give the provider current information regarding fitness level and what an effective exercise prescription might consist of. However, in this regard, physical performance testing has largely replaced exercise stress testing and can help recognize functional limitations that can be targeted with exercise intervention.[1] Some useful physical performance tests include the senior fitness test, short physical performance battery, usual gait speed, 6 minute walk test, and the continuous-scale physical performance test.

Clinical Pearl

The need for cardiac stress testing prior to developing an exercise program is controversial. Risk factors need to be carefully assessed as well as the rate of escalation of physical activity. Rate of escalation should be kept slow.

The need for cardiac stress testing prior to developing an exercise program is controversial. Risk factors need to be carefully assessed as well as the rate of escalation of physical activity. Rate of escalation should be kept slow.

66.6 EXERCISE PRESCRIPTION

When prescribing exercise to the elderly, four categories should be addressed: aerobic exercise, muscle strengthening/endurance, flexibility, and balance.[1,6,23,34] Regarding intensity of exercise, because METs were largely derived from testing younger individuals and because of the great differences in fitness levels in the elderly, METs should not be used to measure or guide intensity. Rather, a 10-point scale should be used relative to a person's physical fitness and perceived exertion, with 0 representing complete rest like sitting and 10 representing an all-out effort. Using this scale, moderate activity would be defined as 5 or 6, coinciding with a noticeable increase in heart rate and breathing, and vigorous as 7 or 8, with a substantial increase in heart rate and breathing. During vigorous activity, they should be able to carry on a conversation, and if they cannot, they are exercising too hard.[23]

Clinical Pearl

When prescribing exercise to the elderly, four categories should be addressed: aerobic exercise, muscle strengthening/endurance, flexibility, and balance.

When prescribing exercise to the elderly, four categories should be addressed: aerobic exercise, muscle strengthening/endurance, flexibility, and balance.

METs should not be used to measure or guide intensity of exercise in the elderly. Heart rate, breathing, and speech are better indicators.

Clinical Pearl

METs should not be used to measure or guide intensity of exercise in the elderly. Heart rate, breathing, and speech are better indicators.

66.6.1 Aerobic

This is any activity that does not cause excessive orthopedic stress. Examples would be walking, swimming, cycling, jogging if able, tennis, and using cardio equipment. The AHA and ACSM suggests at least 30 minutes a day of moderate intensity exercise, 5 days a week, or 25 minutes a day of vigorous intensity exercise on 3 days a week, or a combination of the two. These are the minimum amounts, and exceeding them will lead to greater health benefits. This is especially true if weight loss is a goal as the minimum amount may be insufficient. The times do not have to be continuous and can represent a summation of activity throughout the day; for example, three periods of 10 minute moderate exercise would satisfy the minimum requirement.

Clinical Pearl

Older adults should get at least 150 minutes of moderate intensity exercise per week.

66.6.2 Muscle Strengthening

This is accomplished through weight training/lifting, weight-bearing calisthenics, or resistance training. It should be done at least 2 days a week and involve 8–10 of the major muscle groups (e.g., arms, legs, abdomen, shoulders, and hips). The goal is 10–15 repetitions for each exercise. Muscles strengthening and endurance is a gradual process and can be accomplished with progressively heavier weights. The individual should choose a weight size that he or she can lift about eight times and then work up to 10–15 repetitions. When this is achieved, they can try a heavier weight, which again they should be able to lift eight times followed by progression to 10–15 times. Muscle soreness is normal initially, but exacerbation of other chronic pain conditions should not occur.

Breathing should be normal when weight training avoiding valsalva, with exhalation occurring as the weight is lifted. Movements should be slow with good mechanics and position, taking 2–3 seconds to lift the weight, followed by hold for 1 second, and the return to starting position lasting 3–4 seconds.

With very frail individuals, especially ones with sarcopenia, muscle strengthening/endurance exercising may be necessary prior to aerobic conditioning.

66.6.3 Flexibility

This involves stretching each major muscle group slowly to the point of feeling tightness or slight discomfort (not pain) and holding for about 30 seconds with normal breathing the entire time. This should be done twice a week for at least 10 minutes. Stretching is best done after aerobic or strengthening exercises when the body is warmed up.

66.6.4 Balance (Neuromotor Exercises)

Balance and dizziness issues are not uncommon in the elderly, and neuromotor exercises and maneuvers combining balance, agility, and proprioception training, performed 2–3 times a week, can reduce and prevent falls. This can consists of a series of postures that gradually reduce the center of gravity (e.g., two-legged stand to semitandem to tandem to one-legged), standing with decreased sensory input like having eyes closed, dynamic movements that change the center of gravity (circle turns or tandem walks), or stressing postural muscles as one would do with heel-to-toe stands or walking. Tai chi classes have also been shown to decrease falls, and supervision during this as well as the other maneuvers described earlier may be needed.

In general, physical activity optimally should include a cooldown period, especially in patients with cardiovascular disease. This would include a gradual reduction in exercise volume and intensity and stretching.

66.7 PROMOTING EXERCISE

Motivating patients to exercise as with other lifestyle changes can be challenging.

The AHA and the American College of Preventive Medicine both endorse health-care providers advising elderly patients to exercise. Some potentially effective techniques include writing a prescription for exercise, modifications of stages of change, and the 5 As. The latter includes assessing physical activity, advising patient of benefits of exercise and guidelines, agreeing with patients' readiness to change based on their Prochaska's stage, assisting patient in developing an activity plan, and arranging for follow-up or referral.

Continuing praise and encouragement is key. Involving friends, family, and even pets, who in their own way will let you know when they want their daily walk, and getting patients into exercise groups like at senior centers or the YMCA can also help with compliance.

Cross-training with a variety of activities can make exercise more enjoyable as well as reduce overuse injuries. Striving for a safe and enjoyable exercise environment is also important and combining exercise with other enjoyable activities like a treadmill in front of the television can help.

A potentially effective technique for promoting exercise in the elderly is to write an exercise prescription.

Clinical Pearl

A potentially effective technique for promoting exercise in the elderly is to write an exercise prescription.

66.8 NUTRITION

Nutrition for the older adult is very important and should not be overlooked by the physician.[3] In fact, nutritional advice may have a greater impact on improving general health than on maintaining athletic performance. Of the eight most common causes of death in the United States in those aged 65 years and over, five of them have a known nutritional influence.[17] Nutrition for the exercising elderly can be broken down into four areas: (1) energy (calories), (2) macronutrients (protein, carbohydrates, fat), (3) micronutrients (vitamins and minerals), and (4) water.

66.8.1 Calories

Energy requirements decrease with age, and although this stems from many factors, it can be attributed in large part to a reduction in physical activity. In addition to the reduction in physical activity, there is also a reduction in basal metabolic rate due to decreased lean mass. The approximate reduction in average calories consumed goes from 1700 kcal/day for women to 1400 in women over 75 and from 2700 kcal/day to 1800 in men over 75.[5] With regard to athletes, there is also a reduction in caloric needs in the older athlete compared to the younger one, and this can be attributed to lower volumes of exercise in addition to the decreased metabolic rate. It has been seen that for older patients who maintain exercise volumes similar to younger athletes, they do not experience the decline in resting energy expenditure or caloric needs.

It is important for older athletes to monitor their energy expenditure and caloric intake to insure that they maintain their weight and proper body composition. Failure to do this may result in loss of muscle and bone mass and increase the risk for fatigue, weakness, and illness.

Clinical Pearl

Caloric requirements decrease with age, and in general, this applies to the older athlete. This general decrease in caloric intake can lead to inadequate ingestion of carbohydrates and protein in the older athlete, and in those who consumes less than 2000 kcal/day, protein and carbohydrate intake should be monitored.

Caloric requirements decrease with age, and in general, this applies to the older athlete. This general decrease in caloric intake can lead to inadequate ingestion of carbohydrates and protein in the older athlete, and in those who consumes less than 2000 kcal/day, protein and carbohydrate intake should be monitored.

66.8.2 Macronutrients

The energy requirements listed earlier are met by the ingestion of carbohydrates, fats, proteins, and alcohol. The ACMS and other groups recommend the following proportions for the older athlete: 55%–58% carbohydrate, 12%–15% protein, and 25%–30% fat. However, older athletes who consume less than 8380 kJ/day (2000 kcal/day) of energy may be at risk of not consuming adequate carbohydrate and protein to meet minimum requirements and are encouraged to monitor the intake of these macronutrients. For example, it is recommended that athletes consume 6–10 g/kg/day of carbohydrates depending on conditions like gender, amount of exercise, and environment. Carbohydrates are important macronutrients in that they provide energy to cells throughout the body (particularly the brain), maintain glucose levels during exercise, and restore glycogen stores to muscle during rest and recovery. An active elderly athlete, especially an endurance athlete, will likely need to consume a higher percentage of daily carbohydrates (around 65%).

66.8.3 Protein

The exact protein requirement of the older athlete is not known for sure, but it may be less than the younger athlete secondary to lower volumes of exercise and lower muscle mass.

The RDA for protein is 0.8 g/kg/day for all healthy adults, with no increase for persons who exercise regularly. However, the ACSM states that the need for highly active people may be greater, 1.2–1.4 g/kg/day, and this may even be higher for adults heavily into weight training. The discrepancy between the RDA and the ACSM may stem from the ACSM addressing the needs of highly trained athletes. Decrease in muscle mass has been seen in sedentary people consuming only the RDA recommended amount of protein. Atrophy in specific muscle groups can be halted by resistive training, but there can still be a loss of whole body fat free mass. Exercise and consuming more than the RDA for protein (125%) showed an increase in the whole body fat free mass.

As seen earlier, the data are somewhat mixed, but the very active adult athlete should consider consuming 1.2–1.4 g/kg of protein a day.

66.8.4 Fat

Intake is important in that it provides energy, fat-soluble vitamins, and essential fatty acids. As stated earlier, the ACMS recommends that 25% of 30% of calories be in the form of fat. It is not recommended that athletes have diets that are fat restrictive (less than 20% of calories) or fat abundant as they will not enhance athletic performance.

66.8.5 Micronutrients (Vitamins and Minerals)

A well-balanced diet should meet the micronutrient needs of athletes in general in most cases; however, intense training may increase the athlete's requirements to the aforementioned recommended levels, and inadequate intake of micronutrients may have a small impact on exercise capacity. Because the overall energy intake is lower in the elderly, one cannot always assume that micronutrient demands are being met, so diet, intensity of exercise, underlying medical conditions, and medications all need to be looked at carefully. A consultation with a dietitian in the very active older athlete can be helpful.

There are some special micronutrient considerations in the elderly. Older adults have a 12% prevalence of vitamin B12 deficiency, which can lead to neurologic, hematologic, or psychological disease. A daily intake of 2.4 μg/day is recommended from fortified foods or supplements in all people over 51 because decreased absorption from food bound B12 is more of an issue with older adults. Some groups advocate screening people over 65 years and since the sequelae mentioned earlier can occur even with low normal B12 levels, a methylmalonic acid and/or homocysteine level should be obtained when these levels are found, as they are more sensitive for diagnosing true deficiency.

Clinical Pearl

Older adults have a 12% prevalence of vitamin B12 deficiency, which can lead to neurologic, hematologic, or psychological disease.

Vitamin D deficiency increases with aging probably largely related to decreased sun exposure. Some studies have found an association between low levels and a number of medical problems. However, with supplementation, the only benefits that certain studies have shown relate to decreased falling and decreased fracture rates in patients with low bone mineral density. The RDA for vitamin D is 600 international units through age 70 and 800 in patients 71 and over, and checking levels in high-risk adults is recommended. The American Geriatrics Society recommends at least 1000 international units daily and the National Osteoporosis Foundation recommends 800 to 1000 int. units daily to older adults (≥65 years) to reduce the risk of fractures and falls. The US Preventative Task Force suggests 800.

There should be adequate daily calcium (1200 mg/day) intake in older athletes with osteopenia and osteoporosis, with as much as possible coming from food sources rather than supplements.

Riboflavin requirements have been found to be increased in endurance-trained older women.

66.8.6 Water

For athletes of all ages, performance can be affected even at less than 2% dehydration.[16,33] As we age, there are a myriad of physiologic reasons making us more prone to dehydration[34] as well as the deleterious effects of it during exercise, including impairment of cardiovascular function. Complicating this is the fact that the thirst mechanism becomes less sensitive as we age. These factors all support the statement that water intake in the active elderly needs to be well monitored and managed proactively. Older athletes should consume generous amounts of fluids 24 hours before activity including 400–600 mL (14–22 oz.) 2–3 hours before exercise. During exercise, they should consume 6–12 oz. every 15–20 minutes, and this should start early in the training session. Following exercise, they should replace fluid losses by drinking 450–675 mL (16–24 oz.) for every pound of body weight lost. Fluids should be cooled (40°F–50°F) to enhance palatability and promote gastric emptying.[6]

For many reasons, dehydration is more common in the elderly and can be dangerous as well as affect athletic performance with as little as a 2% reduction. Active hydration before, during, and after exercise is very important.

Clinical Pearl

For many reasons, dehydration is more common in the elderly and can be dangerous as well as affect athletic performance with as little as a 2% reduction. Active hydration before, during, and after exercise is very important.

66.9 ENVIRONMENT

The environment is often overlooked as a factor that can cause problems with exercise for the elderly. Heat, cold, high relative humidity, strong winds, and high altitudes can adversely affect exercise. In addition, the elderly often have risk factors that can make them less tolerant of environmental hazards. The use of diuretics or psychotropic medications, low-sodium diets, impaired thirst drive, and poor conditioning can cause the elderly to be more susceptible to the environment. For example, exercise in heat and high relative humidity along with the use of diuretics can easily lead to dehydration. It is important to educate patients about these risks and offer suggestions about alternative exercise plans. For example, walk inside a mall during extreme heat or cold or garden in the early morning hours rather than in the middle of the day. This will make the activity not only safer for the patient but also more enjoyable.

66.10 SUMMARY

That America is aging and that the level of exercise in the elderly is increasing is undisputed. This is good! For many years, society supported the myth that the elderly should not be active and athletic. Studies demonstrate that the elderly person's musculature and cardiovascular status can adapt to and improve performance with exercise. The physician's responsibility is to evaluate a potential older athlete thoroughly with a preexercise screen; appropriately prescribe and direct a slowly progressive, individualized program of training that includes conservative treatment and adequate rehabilitation for overuse injuries; and educate the patient with regard to preventive strategies (nutrition, safety, and special precautions) and to engage, encourage, and activate them to achieve more quality days through their excessive and participation programs (Table 66.4).

TABLE 66.4
SORT: Key Recommendations for Practice

Clinical Recommendations	Evidence Rating	References
Consultation with a primary care physician is advisable when developing an activity/exercise plan for the elderly to assess for contraindications, relative contraindications, and other conditions, which could impede the success or safety of the plan.	C	[1,23]
Exercise stress testing might be considered prior to initiation of a new exercise program, and this should be based on risk factors and rate of escalation of physical activity, although the rate should be kept slow.	C	[1]
Any exercise plan for the elderly should include components of aerobic exercise, muscle strengthening/endurance, flexibility, and balance, and include at least 150 minutes a week of moderate intensity exercise. If appropriate and safe, higher intensity exercise can be substituted and can shorten total minutes needed.	C	[1,6,23,34]
Because caloric needs and consumption are generally decreased, elderly athletes can be at risk for micro- and macronutrient deficiencies, and this should be assessed and monitored. This is especially true for carbohydrates, proteins, vitamin B12, and vitamin D.	C	[5]
Elderly patients are at increased risk for dehydration, so it is important to counsel patients on active hydration associated with exercise.	C	[5]

REFERENCES

1. American College of Sports Medicine, *ACSM's Guidelines for Exercise Testing and Prescriptions*, 9th edn. Baltimore, MD: Lippincott Williams & Williams; 2014.
2. Brown AB, McCartney N, Sale DG. Positive adaptations to weight lifting training in the elderly. *Journal of Applied Physiology*. 1990;69(5):1725–1733.
3. Benardot D. *Advanced Sports Nutrition*, 2nd edn., Paperback, Human Kinetics Inc., December 27, 2011.
4. Brown MB. Special considerations during rehabilitation of the aged athlete. *Clinics in Sports Medicine*. 1989;8(4):893–901.
5. Campbell WW, Geik RA. Nutritional considerations for the older athlete. *Nutrition*. July–August 2004;20(7–8):603–608.
6. Centers for Disease Control and Prevention, How much physical activity do older adults need? http://www.cdc.gov/physicalactivity/everyone/guidelines/olderadults.html. Last updated: June 17, 2014.
7. Cobbs EL, Duthie EH, Murphy JB (eds.). *Geriatrics Review Syllabus: A Core Curriculum in Geriatric Medicine*, 4th edn. Dubuque, IA: Kendall/Hunt Publishing (for the American Geriatrics Society); 1999.
8. DeHaven K, Lintner DM. Athletic injuries: Comparison by age, sport and gender. *American Journal of Sports Medicine*. 1986;14(3):218–224.
9. Durso SC, Sullivan GM. *Geriatrics Review Syllabus: A Core Curriculum in Geriatrics Medicine*, 8th edn. New York: American Geriatrics Society; 2013.
10. Federal Interagency Forum on Aging-Related Statistics, *Older Americans Update 2010: Key Indicators of Well-Being*. Washington, DC: U.S. Government Printing Office; 2010.
11. Frandin K, Grimby G, Mellstrom D. Walking habits and health related factors in a 70-year old population. *Gerontology*. 1991;37:281–288.
12. Fuchi T, Iwaoka K, Higuchi M et al. Cardiovascular changes associated with decreased aerobic capacity and aging in long distance runners. *European Journal of Applied Physiology*. 1989;58:884–889.
13. Higuchi M, Fuchi T, Iwaoka K et al. Plasmo-lipid and lipoprotein profile in elderly male long distance runners. *Clinical Physiology*. 1988;8:137–145.
14. Hogan DB, Cape RD. Marathoners over sixty years of age: Results of a survey. *Journal of the American Geriatrics Society*. 1984;32;121–123.
15. Iwaoka K, Fuchi T, Higuchi M et al. Blood lactate accumulation during exercise in older endurance runners. *International Journal of Sports Medicine*. 1988;9:253–256.
16. National Athletic Trainers', Association position statement: Fluid replacement for athletes. *Journal of Athletic Training*. 2000;35:212–224.
17. Position of the Academy of Nutrition and Dietetics, Food and nutrition for older adults: Promoting health and wellness. *Journal of the Academy of Nutrition and Dietetics*. 2012;112:1255–1277.
18. Kannus P, Niittymaki S, Jarvinen M et al. Sports injuries in elderly athletes: A three-year prospective, controlled study. *Age Aging*. 1989;18:263–270.
19. Konradsen L, Hansen EM, Sonder-gaard L. Long distance running and osteoarthrosis. *American Journal of Sports Medicine*. 1990;18(4):379–381.
20. Lane NE, Bloch DA, Hubert HB et al. Running, osteoarthritis, and bone density: Initial two-year longitudinal study. *American Journal of Medicine*. 1990;88:452–459.
21. Lane NE, Bloch DA, Wood PD et al. Aging, long distance running, and the development of musculoskeletal disability. *American Journal of Medicine*. 1987;82:772–780.
22. Mathewson GO, MacIntyre JG, Taunton JE. Musculoskeletal injuries associated with physical activity in older adults. *Medicine & Science in Sports & Exercise*. 1989;21(4):379–385.
23. Morey MC, Schmader KE, Sokol HN. Physical activity and exercise in older adults. UpToDate.com http://www.uptodate.com/contents/physical-activity-and-exercise-in-older-adults, April 2014.
24. Panush RS, Brown DG. Exercise and arthritis. *Sports Medicine*. 1987;4:54–64.
25. Panush RS, Schmidt C, Caldwell JR et al. Is running associated with degenerative joint disease? *Journal of the American Medical Association*. 1986;366(9):1152–1154.
26. Pollock ML, Foster C, Knapp D et al. Effect of age and training on aerobic capacity and body composition of master athletes. *Journal of Applied Physiology*. 1987;62(2):725–731.
27. Rock CL. Nutrition of the older athlete. *Clinics in Sports Medicine*. 1991;10(2):445–457.
28. Roubenoff R, Hughes VA. Sarcopenia: Current concepts. *Journals of Gerontology. Series A: Biological Sciences and Medical Science*. 2000;55A(12):M716–M724.
29. Sagiv M, Fisher N, Uaniv A et al. Effect of running versus isometric training programs on healthy elderly at rest, *Gerontology*. 1989;35:72–77.
30. Seto JL, Brewster CE. Musculoskeletal conditioning of the older athlete. *Clinics in Sports Medicine*. 1991;10(2):401–429.

31. Sperry L. Perceived cardiac risks and beliefs about health and running in elite older runners. *Perceptual and Motor Skills.* 1990;70:661–662.
32. Ting AJ. Running and the older athlete. *Clinics in Sports Medicine.* 1991;10(2):319–325.
33. Ungerleider S, Golding JM, Porter K. Mood profiles of masters track and field athletes. *Perceptual and Motor Skills.* 1989;68:607–617.
34. Physical Activity Guidelines for Americans, U.S. Department of Health and Human Services. Active older adults. ODPHP Publication No.U0036, October 2008, www.health.gove/paguidelines.
35. Wilmore JH. The aging of bone and muscle. *Clinics in Sports Medicine.* 1991;10(2):231–244.

67 The Disabled Athlete

James H. Lynch and Richard B. Birrer

CONTENTS

TABLE 67.1
Key Clinical Considerations

1. Physical and mental health is significantly improved with exercise, including competitive sports, in athletes with disabilities.
2. Injury rates for physically disabled athletes are approximately the same as those of athletes without a disability in similar sports.
3. Wheelchair athletes usually suffer from upper extremity injuries, and stump trauma is common in amputee athletes.
4. Preparticipation physical evaluation for the disabled athlete is similar to any athlete without physical or intellectual disability and should take into consideration common problems associated with different disabilities.

67.1 INTRODUCTION

Primary care providers in a multitude of professional settings encounter patients and athletes with physical and intellectual (ID) disabilities. It is our obligation to provide the same encouragement for participation and quality care that we do for able-bodied athletes. Summarizing the critical sports medicine information for disabled athletes is a complex task due to the wide range of disabilities and levels of competition. This chapter will address common issues while acknowledging that there are differences between recreational disabled athletes and highly competitive elite disabled athletes. Thus, this chapter will initially review terminology and common considerations for disabled athletes of all types. The chapter will then detail clinical considerations for specific populations according to different types of disabilities (Table 67.1).

67.2 TERMINOLOGY

Since some athletes have both physical disability and ID, a distinction between these two categories may not be universally applied. However, for our purposes in this context of sports medicine, we will separate the two for educational purposes. Thus, this chapter will differentiate "physical" from "intellectual" disabilities when appropriate. But when referring to issues common to any disability, the word "disabled" will be used.

The Americans with Disabilities Act (ADA) considers an individual disabled if he or she (1) has a physical or mental impairment that substantially limits one or more major life activities, or (2) has a record of such impairment, or (3) is regarded as having such impairment. A physical impairment is defined by the ADA as "any physiological disorder or condition, cosmetic disfigurement, or anatomical loss affecting one or more of the following body systems: neurological, musculoskeletal, special sense organs, respiratory (including speech organs), cardiovascular, reproductive, digestive, genitourinary, hemic and lymphatic, skin, and endocrine."[3]

The spectrum of physically disabled athletes covers any individual with a physical impairment that substantially limits one or more of the major activities of life. Sport for the disabled athlete can be therapeutic, recreational, and/or fiercely competitive. In general, the physical fitness profiles of physically disabled athletes improve with training and age but are lower than a normative sample. Regular training can increase the aerobic capacity, strength, and flexibility of a physically challenged athlete above that of able-bodied, active individuals.[9,26]

ID is defined by two expert organizations in similar ways with slight variations in terminology. According to the American Association on Intellectual and Developmental Disabilities (AAIDD), *ID* is defined as a disability characterized by significant limitations both in intellectual functioning (reasoning, learning, problem solving) and in adaptive behavior, which covers a range of everyday social and practical skills.[44] ID is a common developmental disorder that affects 7.5 million Americans. An individual is considered to have ID if they experience the following three criteria: (1) below-average intellectual functioning level (2 years or more behind peers or an IQ of 70 or less), (2) significant limitations in two or more adaptive skill areas, and (3) the condition manifesting itself before the age of 18. "Adaptive skill areas" refer to those daily living skills needed to live, work, and play in the community. They include communication, self-care, home living, social skills, leisure, health and safety, self-direction, functional academics, community use, and work. Adaptive skills are assessed in the person's typical environment across all aspects of an individual's life. A person with limits in intellectual functioning who does not have limits in adaptive skill areas may not be diagnosed as having ID.[44]

The American Psychiatric Association's (APA) diagnostic criteria for ID (formerly mental retardation) are found in the Diagnostic and Statistical Manual of Mental Disorders (DSM). According to the DSM-5, ID refers to (1) deficits in intellectual functioning (an IQ of approximately 70 or less), (2) concurrent deficits in adaptive functioning in skills required for daily living (such as communication, social skills, personal independence, or school/work functioning), and (3) these problems were evident during childhood or adolescence.[2] Mental retardation and intellectual disability are two names for the same thing, but ID has gained currency as the preferred term. In 2007, the American Association on Mental Retardation changed its name to the AAIDD. Despite this, the term "mental retardation" is still used today in some laws and public policy to determine eligibility for state and federal programs with regard to legal status, education, training, employment, income support, and health care.[44]

67.3 HISTORY

The first World Games for the Deaf were held in Paris during 1924, the same year that saw the formation of the International Committee on Silent Sports. Twenty years later, Sir Ludwig Guttmann introduced wheelchair sports as part of rehabilitation of war veterans in 1944. The next three decades were witness to the formation of a number of international and national organizations and competitions for disabled athletes. Among the more notable were the National Wheelchair Basketball Association (1949), National Wheelchair Games and Athletic Association (1957), International Stoke Mandeville Games Federation (1957), Paralympics (1960), International Special Olympics (1968), the Olympiad for the Physically Disabled (1976), and the International Paralympic Games (1996).[52] The latter hosted 3500 athletes from 120 countries and attracted over 500,000 spectators. In 1978 the Amateur Sports Act (PL95-606) renewed the commitment of the U.S. Olympic Committee to amateur athletes, particularly those with disabilities. Today, athletes with a disabilities have opportunities in sporting activities and physical education unknown to previous generations.[37,46] These include virtually every sport including the marathon, rock climbing, scuba diving, archery, kayaking, weight lifting, skydiving, golf, and the martial arts, and many have established world records.

Athletes with a wide range of individual physical disabilities have achieved recognition as elite performers in many sports.[21] Performance benchmarks include a 100 m dash by a blind athlete in 10.7 seconds, a 2.1 m (6′11″) high jump by a class 2 amputee (AMP), 1500 m in 3:57 using a wheelchair, a 291 kg (640 lb) bench press by a paraplegic weight lifter, a 2 hours 23 minutes Boston marathon by a blind competitor, and summiting Mt. Everest (29,028 ft) by AMPs, the blind, deaf, and those with epilepsy. Dong-Hyun, a blind Korean archer, has medaled in every Olympic since 2004, and the AMP George Eyser earned six gold medals in the 1904 Olympics in the sport of gymnastics.

67.4 DISABLED EVENTS: PARALYMPICS

The Paralympic Games are the equivalent of the Olympic Games for athletes with physical disabilities. First organized in 1960 in Rome for athletes with spinal cord injuries (SCIs), the Paralympic Games are held every 4 years and usually take place after the Olympic Games using the same venues. The International Paralympic Committee (IPC) is responsible for organizing the Paralympic Games, which now include athletes with four primary disability types: those with SCIs, developmental disabilities or cerebral palsy (CP), AMPs, and those who are blind or visually impaired (VI). At the Athens 2004 Paralympic Games, 3806 athletes from 136 nations competed in five categories: AMPs, wheelchair athletes, CP, VI, and "les autres" (French term for "others"—with physical disabilities not conforming to any of the aforementioned). There is not a category for athletes with IDs.[16,48]

67.5 SPORT CLASSIFICATIONS

Historically, a number of classification systems have arisen based on the particular disability.[7] Examples include those of the Special Olympics International, Paralympics, U.S. Les Autres Sports Association, U.S. Cerebral Palsy Athletic Association, U.S. Association of Blind Athletes, Wheelchair Sports USA, Disabled Sports USA, Dwarf Athletic Association of America, International Stoke Mandeville Games Federation, and the American Athletic Association

TABLE 67.2
Additional Preparticipation Evaluation Considerations

Examination	Notes
Vital signs	Blood pressure, respiratory rate, pulse, temperature
Skin	Bony prominences, prior breakdown site, insensate areas, catheter and ostomy sites in SCI, amputee, and neuromuscular disease
EENT	Correctible VA > 20/200 for non–visually impaired athlete HA > 55dB in the better ear in nonhearing impaired athlete Check visual fields
CVS	Check for congenital heart disease especially in developmentally disabled (Down and Turner's syndromes); cardiomyopathy in muscular dystrophy
Pulmonary	Diaphragmatic excursion as measured by percussion along posterior thorax >3 cm in females and >5 cm in males during respiratory cycle
	Consider PFTs for neuromuscular and scoliotic disabilities
GI/GU	Continence
	Bowel control
Neuro	Identification/confirmation of SCI level of muscle tone (Ashworth Scale) and primitive reflexes DEC cognitive ability, coordination and balance, both sitting and standing
Musculoskeletal	ROM (goniometer); ligamentous laxity
	Strength testing, structural deformities
	Orthotics usage; sitting posture evaluation—head position, thoracic kyphosis, pelvic tilt
Functional	Independence measures of transferring, ambulation/ mobility, and proficiency in using adaptive equipment
Neck	Atlantoaxial instability

Note: VA, visual acuity; HA, hearing acuity; PFT, pulmonary function testing; ROM, range of motion.

of the Deaf. The classification system of the International Paralympics Committee (IPC) recognizes six categories and ten eligible impairment types and is based on the WHO International Classification of Functioning, Disability and Health. It is sports specific, functionally based, determined by a panel of certified experts and may be modified as an individual's disability changes over time. A summary (Table 67.2) is provided as a guideline.

67.6 DISABLED EVENTS: SPECIAL OLYMPICS

Special Olympics International is a nonprofit, international program developed in the 1960s to provide athletic opportunities for people with IDs. The mission is "to provide year-round sports training and athletic competition in a variety of Olympic-type sports for children and adults with intellectual disabilities, giving them continuing opportunities to develop physical fitness, demonstrate courage, experience joy and participate in sharing of gifts, skills and friendship with their families, other Special Olympics athletes and the community."[19] Special Olympics provides opportunities for over two million athletes to develop physical fitness and to experience camaraderie in 30 different sports programs in almost 180 countries. Events in aquatics, gymnastics, bowling, figure and speed skating, alpine and cross-country skiing, soccer, softball, volleyball, floor and poly hockey, bowling, basketball, and track and field occur at thousands of local, area, chapter, and national settings. Contact sports are not allowed. Classification of athletes is based on gender, age, and prior sport performances and is commensurate with the official rules of national sport-governing organizations. To be eligible to participate, an individual must be at least 8 years old and be identified by a professional agency as having an ID.[39] The Special Olympics has established the motor activities training program to introduce the severely intellectually impaired to sports activities and physical fitness.[10] For many athletes, Special Olympics is a path to empowerment, competence, acceptance, joy, and friendship. The Special Olympics Athlete's Oath is "Let me win. But if I cannot win, let me be brave in the attempt."[19]

67.7 ROLE OF THE PRIMARY CARE PROVIDER

Some providers new to the sports world of the disabled may underestimate the level of rigor or risk undertaken by a disabled athlete. As a result, many athletes with disabilities do not have close relationships to sports medicine professionals and often do not seek medical assistance but rather choose to self-treat injuries.[8] The "medical home" concept has direct application to working with disabled patients. The primary care provider is in an ideal position to deal with the prejudice, stereotyping, and stigmatization of the physically or intellectually disabled athlete. The physician's role is one of evaluation, prescription, supervision, and support.[8,37] This requires careful coordination, creativity, and collaboration due to unique challenges and complex decision-making. Some areas deserve special mention to include preparticipation evaluation, exercise prescription, and event coverage as detailed in the following.

67.8 PREPARTICIPATION PHYSICAL EVALUATION

The goal in performing a preparticipation physical evaluation (PPE) is to promote the health and safety of the athlete in training and competition (see Chapter 3). The *PPE: Preparticipation Physical Evaluation*, fourth edition monograph was updated in 2010 by all major American sports medicine societies. The authors stress that PPE for the athlete with special needs should be similar to any athlete without physical disability or ID.[1] The PPE should address the particular concerns of the athlete with special needs (see Table 67.3).

TABLE 67.3
Sports and Recreation Options by Disability

	Individual Sports																						Team Sports																											
	Archery	Bicycling	Bowling	Canoeing\Kayaking	Cross Country	Diving	Fishing	Goal Ball	Golf	Gymnastics	Horseback Riding	Power Lifting	Rifle Shooting	Road Racing	Sailing	Scuba Diving	Skating: Roller and ice	Skiing: Cross	Skiing: Downhill	Speed Skating	Swimming	Tricycling	Baseball	Basketball	Basketball: Wheelchair	Bocce	Fencing	Floor Hockey	Football: Tackle	Football: Touch	Football: Wheelchair	Handball	Ice hockey	Poly Hockey	Racquetball	Slalom	Sledge Hockey	Soccer	Soccer: Wheelchair	Softball	Table Tennis	Team Handball	Tennis	Tennis: Wheelchair	Track	Track: Wheelchair	Volleyball	Weight Lifting	Wheelchair Poling	Wrestling
Amputation																																																		
Upper extremity	R	R	R	R		R	R		R		R	R	R	R	R	R	R	R	R		R	R	R	R			R		R	R			R		I	I		R		R	R		R		R		R	R		
	A			A					A				A																																					
Lower extremity AK	R	R	R	R		R	R		R		R	R	R	R	R	R	I	R	R		R	R	R		R		I		I	I	R				R	R	R	I	R	R	R		I	R	R	R	R	R	R	
																		A	A				a																	A					A					
Lower extremity BK	R	R	R	R	R	R	R		R		R	R	R	R	R	R	R	R	R	R	R	R	R	R	I		R		R	R	I		I		R	R	I	R	I	R	R		R	I	R	I	R	R		
Cerebral Palsy																																																		
Amputation	R	R	R	R	R	R	R		R		R	R	R	R	R	I	R	R	R		R	R	R	I		R	I		I	I			I		R	R		R		R	R	R	R		R		R	R		
																		A	A																															
Wheel chair	R	I	R	R	R	I	R		I		I	R	R	R	R						I	I	I		R	R	I	I			R		I			R	I		R	I	R	R		R		R	I	R	R	
																																										A								
Neuromuscular disorders																																																		
Muscular dystrophy	R	I	R	I			R		R		I		R		R	I	I	I	I		R	R	I	I	I	R					I		I			I	I	I	I	I	R		I	I	I	I	I		R	
	A												A																																					
Spinal muscular atrophy	R	I	R	I			R		R		I		R		R	I	I	I	I		R	R	I	I	I	R					I		I			I	I	I	I	I	R		I	I	I	I	I		R	
	A												A																																					
Charcot–Marie–Tooth synd.	R	R	R	R			R		R		R	R	R		R	R	R	R	R		R	R	R	R		R	R		R	R			I			R		R		R	R		R		R		R	R		
Ataxias	R	R	R	I			R		I		I	I	R		R	I	I	R	I		R	I	I	I	R	R				I	I		I			I	I	I	R	I	R		R	R	I	R	I	I	R	
Sensory impaired																																																		
Blind		R								R		R						R	R	R	R	R																							R			R		R
Deaf		R	R			R							R	R				R	R	R	R	R						R				R					R			R	R		R		R		R			R
Develop. disabled	R	R	R			R		R		R	R	R		R			R	R	R	R	R	R		R			R	R						R		R				R	R	R	R		R		R			

(Continued)

TABLE 67.3 (*Continued*)
Sports and Recreation Options by Disability

	Individual Sports																						Team Sports																											
	Archery	Bicycling	Bowling	Canoeing\Kayaking	Cross Country	Diving	Fishing	Goal Ball	Golf	Gymnastics	Horseback Riding	Power Lifting	Rifle Shooting	Road Racing	Sailing	Scuba Diving	Skating: Roller and ice	Skiing: Cross	Skiing: Downhill	Speed Skating	Swimming	Tricycling	Baseball	Basketball	Basketball: Wheelchair	Bocce	Fencing	Floor Hockey	Football: Tackle	Football: Touch	Football: Wheelchair	Handball	Ice hockey	Poly Hockey	Racquetball	Slalom	Sledge Hockey	Soccer	Soccer: Wheelchair	Softball	Table Tennis	Team Handball	Tennis	Tennis: Wheelchair	Track	Track: Wheelchair	Volleyball	Weight Lifting	Wheelchair Poling	Wrestling
Spinal cord injury																																																		
Cervical	R		R	I			R				X		R		R			I	I		R	R	R		I			I			I		I				I				R			I		R	I		I	
	A		A	A									A					A	A			A	A																		A			A			A			
High thoracic: T1–T5	R		R	R			R		R		I		R	R	R	R		I	I		R	R	R		R		R	R			R		R			R	I		R	R	R			R		R	R	R	R	
									A									A	A				A				A									A				A							A			
Lower thoracic: T6–L3	R		R	R			R		R		R	R	R	R	R	R		R	R		R	R	R		R		R	R			R		R			R	I		R	R	R			R		R	R	R	R	
									A									A	A								A									A				A							A			
Lumbosacral: L4 sacral	R	R	R	R		R	R		R		R	R	R	R	R	I	R	R	R		R	R		R	I		R		I	R	I		I			R		R		R	R		R		R		R	R		
Others																																																		
Osteogenesis imperfect	R	I	R	R			R		I		I	I	R		R	I	I	R	I		R	R	I	I	R		R		X	I	I		X				X	X	R	I	R		R	R	R	R	I	I	R	
Arthrogryposis	R	I	R	R			R		I		R	I	R		R	I	I	R	I		R	I	R	R			I		X	R	I		I					I		R	R		R		R	X	R	I	X	
Juvenile rheum atoid arthritis	R	I	R	R			R		I		I	I	R		R	I	I	I	I		R	I	I	I	I		I		I	I	I							I	I	I	R		I	I	I	I	I	I	I	
	A		A																																															
Hemophilia	R	R	R	R			R		R		R	I	R		R	R	I	R	I		R	R	I	R			R		X	I			X					I		R	R		I		R		R	I		
	A																																																	
Skeletal dysplasias	R	R	R	R			R		R		R	I	R		R	R	R	R	R		R	R	R	R		R	R		I	R			R					R		R	R		R		R		R	I		
																			A																															

The health care provider should be aware of common problems associated with different disabilities and be able to diagnose abnormalities that may endanger the athlete.[9,20] The preparticipation questionnaire has been shown to be helpful in detecting roughly three quarters of sports-significant abnormalities.[5] While the clearance is provided by the sports medicine physician, the assessment is made in the context of a multidisciplinary team—family, school officials, athletic staff, and medical consultants (e.g., neurology, surgery and rehabilitation).

A history of prior surgeries (gastrostomy, ventriculoperitoneal [VP] shunt) and injuries (brain trauma), comorbid conditions, adaptive equipment needs, fitness and training level, risk factors, and current medications is essential (evidence level C, consensus opinion).[53] Medication dosage schedules must be reviewed and individualized. Some prescription and over-the-counter (OTC) drugs (e.g., stimulants, antispasmodics, narcotic analgesics, steroids, diuretics, and beta blockers) may be restricted or prohibited by the appropriate governing body.[48]

67.9 EXERCISE PRESCRIPTION

Depending on the degree of disability and available resources, the exercise prescription may vary greatly per individual disabled athlete. For example, a competitive Paralympic skier's abilities and fitness level may differ greatly from an intellectually disabled recreational swimmer. Taking individual differences into account then, the primary care provider may find it useful to address activities of daily living, weight control, psychological well-being, and the fitness profile (i.e., range of motion, strength, and cardiopulmonary endurance).[20] For less conditioned athletes or those with more limiting disabilities, there are several other considerations. The training heart rate (THR), if not directly available from an exercise stress test (EST), may be lower than calculated by standard formula due to highly reduced vascularity and muscle mass (Chapter 7). The program should progress slowly (60%–80%) in order to improve compliance and minimize injuries. The prescription should be graded with respect to intensity since a vigorous program can cause early fatigue with secondary depressive affects. Flexibility, strengthening, and proprioceptive exercises based on the sport and physical impairment should be individualized in conjunction with the PPE. Neglected muscle groups should be emphasized. Appropriate warm-up and cooldown program elements as well as preventive taping and orthotics are important.[11]

The choice of a sport should reflect the preference of the patient, the type and degree of the disability, and his or her motivation and determination (see Table 67.2).[23,43] Horseback riding and ice-skating are two therapeutic modalities that have been shown to be very useful in the disabled population since they can participate in social or organized riding clubs. There also are carefully graded competitions for the disabled. Ice-skating helps disabled youngsters to gain confidence and self-control. Balance is essential, but less power and strength are required than for walking. A stable spine, good quadriceps, absence of knee flexion contractures, extension and abduction stability of the hips, and extension stability of the knee are required for participation. Additionally, relatively plantigrade feet, some dorsiflexion and plantar flexion stability of the ankle assisted by an orthosis, and motor power across the ankle joints are useful. Well-fitted, single-blade skates without toe picks are recommended. An outrigger skate aid of the Lofstrand type can be used to increase the support base. A Hein-A-Ken Skate aid is useful with children who cannot propel themselves with reciprocal action. Children with minimal brain dysfunction and attention deficit disorders benefit through precision movement, obstacle completion, and kinesthetic awareness.

67.10 EVENT COVERAGE

Providing sports medicine coverage at events for disabled athletes is similar to covering any athletic event. Systematic planning and an understanding of some issues specific to athletes with disabilities can help ensure success. Estimated crowd attendance must be factored into planning. Seizure precautions should be followed in all activities where there might be a risk of severe injury if a convulsion were to occur, such as in swimming, diving, skiing, or equestrian. Since many disabilities place athletes at increased risk of heat or cold injuries, environmental concerns such as adequate shelter, water, and restrooms must be addressed. Preparticipation screening results may assist in planning for unique issues and identifying specific athletes at increased risk. Medical records should be readily available to medical staff. Medical conditions, allergies, medications, and emergency contact information should be located in a central location or on identification badges or race bibs. For monocular athletes, eye protection with polycarbonate lenses should be worn, especially for missile-type sports. Supplies and equipment needed are comparable to other competitive sporting events. An automated external defibrillator (AED) as well as antiepileptic injectable medications is recommended.[27]

Coverage of events for intellectually disabled athletes, such as Special Olympics events, frequently relies on volunteers who may or may not have experience with past events. It is imperative to know the minimum medical facility requirements. Special Olympics requires the following for large competitions: A qualified emergency medical technician (EMT) must be in attendance or readily available at all times. A licensed medical professional must be on-site or on call at all times. First aid areas must be clearly identified, adequately equipped, and staffed by a qualified EMT for the entire event. An ambulance with advanced cardiac life support (ACLS) capabilities must be readily available at all times.[19] Most care will involve general first aid. Advanced emergency care by trained providers will usually involve initial stabilization and rapid transport to those who require more than basic first aid.[19,33]

67.11 SENSORY DISABILITIES: THE DEAF ATHLETE

Although the oldest international organization (1924) for disabled sport was developed for the deaf athlete (Comité International des Sports des Sourds [CISS]), public interest in and support for athletic programs for the deaf have never been strong. Deaf athletes appear normal and are capable of playing all sports that are open to people with normal hearing. Fitness levels and motor development do not appear to be significantly different from normal peers. Sensorineural defects (e.g., congenital rubella, infections, congenital malformations, Rh incompatibility, and drug therapy), rather than conduction problems, are the cause of significant deafness.[34] While the severity of the hearing deficit can be classified, a hearing loss of 55 dB or greater in the better ear (three-frequency pure tone average at 500, 1000, and 2000 Hz) is required for purposes of competition qualification (eligibility standard for World Games). Concomitant damage to the vestibular apparatus, although relatively uncommon, affects balance and coordination. Activities with sharp turns, spins, or cuts (i.e., skiing and skating), or those demanding balance (i.e., gymnastics and diving), may not be possible. Communication is the major problem for the deaf athlete, and its lack may prevent participation in some sports. Colored lights and flags and light dimmers are used to facilitate play. The athlete must maximize peripheral vision in order to recognize the field position of teammates. A full athletic program for deaf athletes is available at Gallaudet College, Washington, DC, the largest liberal arts institution for deaf people in the world. Many deaf people have excelled at the amateur, professional, and elite level.

67.12 SENSORY DISABILITIES: THE BLIND ATHLETE

Legal blindness is defined as 20/200 or 1/10 or less of normal vision in both eyes. Some blind athletes are legally blind; most (80%) have some useful vision, but others are completely blind. Certainly, the athlete with partial sight has the ability to perceive light, dark, and shadows. The International Blind Sports Federation in conjunction with the IPC governs worldwide sport competition among blind athletes and utilizes functional classification as assessed by usable vision rather than movement capability.

Unless there are other disabilities, the VI are generally fit, although their movements may not be as free (i.e., shuffling gait and stiffness of posture and movement) as those of the non-VI.[24] A wide range of sports activities are available to the blind athlete: swimming, track and field events, weight lifting, rowing, wrestling, golf, skiing, tandem bicycling, beep baseball, roller or goal ball, and even archery and skydiving. A sighted companion calls signals, uses clap sticks, counts steps or strokes, or touches the runner/skier in order to guide the athlete audibly. Blind bowlers utilize a portable, waist-high guide rail 12 feet (3.7 m) long. A battery emits a beep in a regulation softball used in beep baseball. Athletes should wear protective gear (face masks and chest and groin protectors) in this and other contact sports.

The Education Amendments to the Elementary and Secondary Act of 1965 (1972) (Section 904), Rehabilitation Act (1973) (Section 504), Education for All Handicapped Children Act (1975), and PL94-142 provide the opportunity for physical education instruction in the least restrictive environment for most blind children. Nonetheless, blind children and youth are not socialized into sport in the same ways and by the same significant factors as sighted youngsters. Learned dependence and stereotypic behaviors are problematic. Acute visual loss may be associated with an adverse psychological reaction and cognitive delays. While many blind people do compete in individual and team sports, it is estimated that for every blind individual who is given the opportunity to learn and engage in sport, two blind individuals are not. It is, therefore, a lack of experience rather than a lack of ability that is responsible for fitness and motor delays. The Lavelle School for the Blind in the Bronx, NY, is one example of a free school devoted to all blind individuals aged three through high school.

67.13 THE SPINAL CORD–INJURED ATHLETE

The wheelchair is the modus operandi for the SCI athlete. Track and field, swimming, table tennis, pentathlon, archery, weight lifting, fencing, snooker, marathon, bowling, pool/billiards, slalom, road running, precision javelin, basketball, and darchery (darts and archery) are some common activities for these athletes.[31,57] SCI persons are introduced to these activities at regional centers before joining park or recreation department programs or the national wheelchair organizations.

Classification of wheelchair athletes is intended to enable those with even the most severe disability to compete in a fair manner with others of similar degrees of disability. The system is anatomically based, and manual muscle testing of upper and lower extremities and trunk balance must be performed to determine classification. Training affects the cooperation, performance, and quality of life of the athlete.[49] Factors such as spasticity, sensation, deformities, orthoses and surgical procedures, the type of equipment, and certain pathologies (multiple sclerosis, polio, neuromuscular disease) mean that the two ends of the disability spectrum can present formidable classification problems.[50] One fair solution is split classification—classifying an athlete differently for each event. Thus, AMPs and individuals with such wide-ranging neurologic or paralyzing disorders as meningomyelocele, osteogenesis imperfecta, or brain injury can compete in the Paralympics with a wheelchair.

There are two basic types of wheelchair designs: medical/regular and sports. There are over 20 different sports chairs, which are built for performance rather than comfort. Acceleration, turning, and maneuverability are optimized by the use of a roll bar, antitip casters, rigid frame, lowered seat back, and adjustable axle plates. Additional wheelchair models include track and racing chairs and motorized chairs. The former utilize large cambered drive wheels, small hand rims, and a lowered seat position. Motorized chairs use two 12 V batteries and allow considerable independence for severely disabled persons for up to 8 hours (after an overnight charge) at speeds up to 5 mph and inclines of at least 10°.

Common problems include bowel and bladder dysfunction, urinary tract infection, osteoporosis, urinary calculi, muscle atrophy, decubitus ulcers, difficulties in temperature regulation, and respiratory compromise, especially for SCI < T6.

Autonomic dysreflexia (AD) has been observed in 80% of high-level athletes with paraplegia and is characterized by piloerection, paroxysmal hypertension and bradyarrhythmia, hyperhidrosis, and headache secondary to a noxious stimulus (e.g., pressure sore, distended bowel/bladder, infection, fracture, and tight clothes) below the SCI level (most problematic at or above T6).[8,35,53] Hyperthermia (50% of track competitors) and hypothermia (9% of swimmers) disorders have been noted in the quadriplegic population (secondary to AD) and in the Special Olympics (decreased perception of problem). Management of AD includes removal of the offending stimulus, if possible, and treatment of the hypertension. "Boosting" or self-induced AD by an SCI competitor to enhance performance has been reported in 15% and should be diligently screened for in the PPE.[20] Overdistention of the bladder and the use of sharp objects or tight lower extremity straps are commonly used.

Premature osteoporosis and osteopenia secondary to paraplegia can lead to fractures in the paralyzed extremities during contact sports. These should be suspected in the setting of AD, pain, angular deformity, and minimal mechanical force. Heterotopic ossification also occurs in SCI or traumatic brain-injured athletes, usually around major joints. While sports participation does not increase the risk of ectopic bone formation, it should be considered a stimulus to AD. Limitation of exercise capacity (decreased cardiac output), venous blood pooling, and the potential for deep venous thrombosis are additional problems in the SCI athlete. Management strategies include abdominal binders, positive pressure garments (stockings), and lower extremity functional electrical stimulation.

Bladder infections have been reported in 22% of pediatric SCI athletes.[20,24] Although overuse injuries occur with slightly more frequency than acute ones, functional deterioration, hypoactivity, and fear of accident cause most of the damage to these children. Preventive strategies emphasizing environmental control and strength and conditioning plus orthotics and similar devices to correct structural deformities and reduce biomechanical stress are important.[50]

SCI athletes participating in swimming, endurance races, and cold weather activities may experience hypothermia due to loss of muscle mass below the lesion level, loss of sweat, vasomotor and neural control, and decreased sensation. While preventive education is important, intra- and postcompetition monitoring is critical. Loss of sudomotor and vasomotor reflexes cut both ways and may also be responsible for hyperthermia—a condition potentially worse in the disabled athlete. In the 1990 U.S. Junior Wheelchair Games, 49% suffered from hyperthermia or heat-related illness.[4,50] The concomitant administration of anticholinergics or alpha blockers makes this even more likely. Both conditions require aggressive emergent treatment (see Chapter 35).

Clinical Pearl

Heat illness needs to be differentiated from boosting. The treatments are different, and timely, accurate diagnosis is critical.

Pressure sores afflict wheelchair athletes, AMPs, and all insensate athletes with improperly fitted prostheses and those sports involving high amounts of directional change and lateral movement (e.g., basketball and tennis). Anatomical areas that require attention are the greater trochanter of the hip, sacrum, and ischium. Pressure loads are further exaggerated by specially designed sports wheelchairs in which the athlete's knees are higher than the seat. Proper positioning, custom-fitted cushioning, the correct fit of prostheses and equipment, regular repositioning, and minimization of skin shear and moisture are important management strategies.

67.14 THE AMPUTEE ATHLETE

AMP sports are governed by the IPC for the Disabled (ISOD). AMP athletes can participate in practically any sport or recreational activity (see Table 67.2). AMP games include swimming, skiing, slalom, archery, riflery, football-kicking, table tennis, bowling, and a variety of track and field events. Amputations may be congenital or acquired, but this factor is irrelevant to the classification system, although congenital ones should suggest the possibility of other anomalies. There are nine general, five track, and seven field classifications for AMPs used by the IPC. The team physician should be familiar with the regulations and ethical issues concerning assistive devices, orthoses, and prostheses. For example, crutches and sticks are prohibited in all track events, while the wearing of a prosthesis is optional. Certainly as technology improves, the performance level gap between disabled and able-bodied athletes is closing. While a wheelchair may be utilized in basketball and marathons, most AMP athletes compete with a prosthesis. Some skiers "three track" with an outrigger that has a short ski tip and a swivel. Physical conditioning or training may decrease the metabolic cost of ambulation and the risk for heat-related illnesses for lower extremity AMPs.[51]

Most injuries occur in running sports and involve the stump, spine, and intact limbs. Uneven surfaces, misalignment of the prosthesis and/or pylon, and lack of cushioning cause impact and rotatory forces to be transmitted almost completely to the residual limb.[35] Loss of a heel strike necessitates greater quadriceps strength and may predispose to early fatigue following above-the-knee amputation (AKA). The hop–skip running pattern is associated with decreased pelvic rotation, exaggerated truncal, and asymmetric arm movements, and excessive vaulting off the sound limb occurs due to a prolonged swing phase of the prosthetic limb. Ischial bursitis and irritation of the ischial tuberosity are, therefore, common. Areas of minor irritation should be treated with protective dressings (e.g., DuoDERM) before a pressure ulcer develops. Socket alterations may be helpful in some cases. Strains and sprains of the sound limb, sacroiliac region, and lumbar spine are also secondary to increased mechanical stresses during running. Upper extremity and multiple coexisting amputations are more common in children, but complications such as phantom limb syndrome and skin breakdown are less frequent. Prostheses require repair and reconditioning more regularly in the younger AMP athlete due to increasing growth and expansion as well as the frequency of abuse and misuse.[38]

67.15 THE CEREBRAL PALSY ATHLETE

The degree of muscular involvement in CP can range from severe spasticity to slight speech impairment. Unlike spinal cord–injured athletes and competitors whose disabilities affect the range of motion, balance, and strength of lower extremities, the CP athlete usually has to cope with associated upper motor neuron dysfunction such as perceptual–motor problems (60%), learning disabilities (>50%), seizures (30%), visual dysfunction (75%), deafness (20%), abnormal reflex activity (startle and asymmetric tonic neck) and muscle tone (50%–85%), and other "soft signs" of neuron damage—impulsivity, hyperkinesis, and attention deficits. Of the general CP population, 85%–90% have three or more disabilities. In addition, 30%–70% of this population is intellectually impaired—a diagnosis that excludes the individual from sports events by the standards of the National Association of Sports for Cerebral Palsy (NASCP). The latter uses a functional classification system of eight categories that is sport- and disability-specific. About 50% of all CP athletes compete in wheelchairs (i.e., they are functionally nonambulatory), and about half are ambulatory. Seizures are best controlled with carbamazepine since it is the drug least likely to adversely affect athletic performance. Aerobic activity decreases seizure potential because the metabolic acidosis associated with lactic acid accumulation stabilizes neuromembranes.[6,22] If seizures occur with exercise, a stress test with an EEG is recommended. Vigilance for missed dosages due to travel and ataxia and nystagmus due to adjusted dosage schedules are paramount. Diazepam suppositories should be available at athletic events for intractable seizures.

67.16 LES AUTRES ATHLETE

A French term for "the others," les autres, includes athletes with locomotor disabilities exclusive of CP. Examples include muscular dystrophy, multiple sclerosis, organic brain syndrome, osteogenesis imperfecta, arthrogryposis, short stature, and ataxia. Some of these disabilities are static, others variable, and some progressive. Therefore, periodic medical reviews are appropriate. The IPC classification may not always be appropriate for the associated dysfunctions and tremendous individual differences of this group of athletes.

Spina bifida athletes generally tolerate sports well. A neurology or neurosurgical consultation is appropriate if there is a tethering concern. Damage to a VP shunt is uncommon. Athletes with an Arnold–Chiari malformation should be managed like a Down syndrome athlete with atlantoaxial instability (AAI). Because cognitive and learning disabilities are common, rule adaptation may be appropriate. Injury to the lower extremities is possible due to osteoporosis and sensorimotor problems. Wheelchair modification and orthotics should be considered. Bowel and bladder dysfunctions are usually not problematic but may be an inconvenience.

67.17 INTELLECTUAL DISABILITIES

The group of athletes with IDs includes those with Down syndrome, fragile X syndrome, autism, and certain degenerative metabolic disorders.

Athletes with IDs may have a variety of health-related issues that impact their participation in competitive athletics. With such a diverse population of athletes, there is no unifying list of diagnoses or conditions; however, there are some important points for the sports medicine team to consider. Epidemiologic studies of organized athletics for intellectually disabled athletes reveal some patterns and conditions that are more prevalent in this population. Generally speaking, intellectually disabled athletes as compared to general population athletes have a higher prevalence of hearing and visual impairment; decreased measures of strength and endurance; poorer agility, balance, speed, flexibility, and reaction time;

higher rates of obesity (half of all with ID); lower peak heart rate; and lower peak oxygen uptake.[14,25,29,36] Using preparticipation screening exam data for Special Olympics athletes, the incidence of sports-significant abnormalities detected is roughly 40%. The most common categories of problems detected among intellectually disabled athletes are neurologic (16%), ophthalmologic (15%), musculoskeletal (6%), and medical (5%). The most common diagnoses are seizures and vision loss.[27,28] As a comparison, the incidence of sports-significant abnormalities detected among nondisabled athletes is 1%–3% historically.

67.18 DOWN SYNDROME

The athlete with Down syndrome (trisomy 21) requires special consideration due to well-described conditions associated with increased risk in athletics. Down syndrome is the most common human malformation pattern with an estimated incidence at 1 in 600–800 live births. Up to 30% of Special Olympics athletes have Down syndrome. Phenotypically, Down syndrome can vary greatly, but frequent findings include ID, orthopedic issues, cardiac anomalies, vision problems, epilepsy, and obesity.[43] National health interview data of children with Down syndrome in the United States from 1997 to 2005 revealed the following general health information: children with Down syndrome were more than twice as likely as children in the general population to have seizures, recent food allergy, frequent diarrhea, or three or more ear infections.[45]

Cardiac anomalies are prevalent in about half of persons with Down syndrome as compared to about 1% in the general population. Atrioventricular septal defects make up the majority of these, most of which are surgically repaired at a young age. Ventricular septal defects, atrial septal defects, and patent ductus arteriosus comprise another 20% of the congenital heart disease associated with Down syndrome. Pulmonary hypertension is also more common in people with Down syndrome.[30] With or without cardiac malformations, athletes with Down syndrome have been found to have lower cardiovascular fitness levels than their peers.[43]

Persons with Down syndrome have a high prevalence of vision and eye health problems. Many eye problems are undetected secondary to infrequent examinations. Down syndrome is associated with an increased frequency of keratoconus, cataracts, high refractive error, glaucoma, strabismus, and macular disease. In studies screening Down syndrome athletes, about 20% were observed to have significant uncorrected refractive errors (greater than one diopter). About one third to one half of Down syndrome athletes screened prior to participation are observed to have pathology sufficient to affect vision.[17,56]

Due in part to inherent ligamentous laxity, the musculoskeletal system is a frequent cause of disability in Down syndrome athletes. The major areas of concern include the hips, patellofemoral joints, feet, and cervical spine. Acquired hip instability is seen in about 5% of persons with Down syndrome. The natural history of this condition is to progress from acute dislocation to recurrent dislocation, then eventually to fixed dislocation. If treated nonoperatively, caution should be used to modify sports participation to avoid complete hip dislocation.[12] Patellofemoral dislocation occurs in 4%–8% of persons with Down syndrome. Progression to fixed dislocations may occur but may do well with nonoperative management.

No restriction is necessary for asymptomatic instability. A patellar sleeve and activity restriction may be helpful for an athlete with symptoms. Foot deformities are very common in athletes with Down syndrome due to generalized ligamentous laxity. Athletes with Down syndrome are prone to pes planovalgus, metatarsus primus varus, and bunions. Surgery is rarely necessary as these conditions are well tolerated in athletes with Down syndrome with appropriately fitting shoes.[12,55]

Cervical spine instability is the most significant musculoskeletal issue for the athlete with Down syndrome. AAI, which affects 10%–30% of individuals with Down syndrome, denotes laxity of the articulation between C1 (atlas) and C2 (axis). While atlantoaxial dislocation can be a significant cause of cord compromise, approximately 98% of AAI cases are asymptomatic.[18] Symptoms of AAI include neck pain, fatigability, clumsiness, or altered sensation. Neurologic signs include abnormal gait, sensory deficits, spasticity, hyperreflexia, clonus, and extensor-plantar reflex. AAI is due to odontoid abnormalities or laxity of the transverse ligament that holds the odontoid process in place against the inner aspect of the arch of the atlas.[13] Radiographic evaluation is necessary to detect AAI. Lateral cervical spine radiographs in flexion, extension, and neutral will allow for examination of the atlantodens interval (ADI), which is measured from the anterior aspect of the odontoid to the posterior surface of the anterior arch of atlas. In the early 1980s, the Special Olympics and the American Academy of Pediatrics (AAP) began recommending cervical spine radiographic screening of Special Olympians with Down syndrome before participation in "high-risk" sports.[19] These recommendations remain in effect today. The high-risk sports include pentathlon, diving (either as a sport or in swimming starts), butterfly swimming stroke, high jump, gymnastics, soccer, judo, snowboarding, and alpine skiing. Currently, the AAP recommends obtaining screening x-rays between the ages 3 and 5 years for all children with Down syndrome, not just Special Olympians.[18,42] Using Special Olympics' guidelines, AAI is diagnosed when the ADI is more than 4.5 mm. Athletes with asymptomatic AAI should be restricted from high-risk activities that place undue stress on the neck, but no further intervention is warranted. For athletes with symptomatic AAI or an ADI greater than 5 mm, MRI evaluation is recommended. The guidelines do not recommend continued radiographic screening for children with an ADI less than

4.5 mm. Because some studies have shown AAI progresses over time, especially with young patients, it may be reasonable to obtain repeat evaluations until skeletal maturity is achieved, although there is no consensus on the proper interval.[47] Special Olympics does permit athletes with known AAI to play with a signed release only after they are evaluated and counseled in writing by two licensed physicians who determine that the athlete is not medically precluded from participation.[19]

Life expectancy for individuals with Down syndrome has increased from 12 years of age in 1949, to 35 years of age in 1982, to 55 years of age currently. Hence, there are many older persons with Down syndrome participating in athletics now.[5] Several health-related changes are associated with aging in athletes with Down syndrome. The following conditions apply to adults with Down syndrome: 40% will develop hypothyroidism; 46%–57% have mitral valve prolapse; 50% have sleep apnea; 70% have conductive hearing loss; 70% over the age of 65 years have visual impairments. Alzheimer disease increases with age from rates of 10% for ages 30–39 years up to 55% for ages 50–59 years.[5]

Clinical Pearl

Athletes with Down syndrome require cervical spine clearance clinically and radiographically. Persons with atlantoaxial subluxation or dislocation and neurologic signs should be restricted from *all strenuous activities.*

67.19 INJURY AND ILLNESS PATTERNS

Injury rates for *physically* disabled athletes are approximately the same as those of athletes without a disability in similar sports.[16] There are several comprehensive publications in the sports medicine literature that describe injury and illness patterns in the past few Paralympic Games.[32,41,54] Illnesses (25%–30%) were the most commonly reported problem. Injury patterns have been identified for certain groups, with wheelchair athletes typically sustaining upper extremity injuries, blind athletes sustaining lower extremity injuries, and CP athletes sustaining both. The most commonly injured body locations (with each representing roughly 10%–15% of all injuries) are (1) thorax/spine, (2) shoulder, and (3) lower leg/ankle/toes. The majority of these injuries were musculoskeletal soft tissue injuries to include strains 22%, sprains 6%, contusions 6%, and abrasions 5%.[15] There may be some variation between summer and winter sports with a trend for more fractures in winter sports such as alpine skiing and sledge hockey.[54]

Upper extremity soft tissue injuries (e.g., sprains, strains, bursitis, tendonitis) and skin problems (e.g., abrasions/wheelburns, pressure sores, blisters) occur in up to 97% of wheelchair athletes during training and competition in track events.[53] Shoulder pain is the most common complaint in wheelchair athletes.[49] The differential diagnosis should include biceps and rotator cuff pathology as well as osteonecrosis. Roughly 15% have elbow pain secondary to forearm extensor tendonitis, olecranon bursitis, triceps tendonitis, epicondylitis, and nerve entrapment. Nerve entrapment is quite common with site involvement varying as follows: carpal tunnel 50%–73%, ulnar 50%, and radial 16%. The point of hand–wheel contact at the proximal carpal tunnel is the site of impingement in carpal tunnel, whereas Guyon's canal is the ulnar entrapment site. Ganglion cysts of the long flexors or extensors are secondary to repetitive injury to the wrist joint capsule. Avascular necrosis of the lunate (Kienbock's disease), dorsal compartment tenosynovitis, and deQuervain's disease are additional repetitive use injuries. Track, road racing, and basketball also have the highest percentage of such injuries. Hand and wrist fractures are the most commonly encountered fractures in the wheelchair athlete, particularly during collision sports. Associated osteopenia may impair the healing process. In the childhood athlete, the epiphyseal plate is involved. Skiing by athletes with disabilities is relatively safe, but the knee and foot are injured more commonly in CP athletes due to problems with spasticity and foot deformities.[52]

Injury rates for individuals with IDs are less than those reported for physically disabled and general population athletes. Epidemiologic data have been reported for state, national, and international events.[6,28,33,40] Studies have shown that 3%–4% of all athletes are treated at Special Olympics events. Track and field, followed by softball, accounted for more sports injuries than other events. The most commonly injured site was the knee. Injury rates calculated per 1000 participant-hours are 0.4 for Special Olympics athletes and 2.0 for special education high school students in organized contact sports. These aforementioned rates can be compared to the following nondisabled adult athletes' injury rates (per 1000 participant-hours): 0.03 for swimming, 2.9 for badminton, 3.65 for soccer, 4.1 for football, and 4.7 for ice hockey. In a study of Special Olympics injuries in Texas, athletes with Down syndrome had a relative risk of injury or illness 3.2 times greater than the other athletes.[27]

67.20 SUMMARY

Regular physical activity for the disabled in the form of sports and recreational exercise improves fitness profile, increases muscular function, and builds courage and self-esteem. Sports participation advances disabled athletes beyond their specific disability, focuses on ability and achievement, and facilitates interaction with mainstream society. Disabled athletes face many challenges during training and competition. As the number of disabled athletes grows, sports medicine professionals must become proficient in dealing with some of the unique considerations in this population (Tables 67.4 and 67.5).

TABLE 67.4
Additional Resources for Disabled Athletes

National Sports Center for the Disabled
677 Winter Park Dr.
Winter Park, CO 80482
970-726-1540
www.nscd.org

Amputee Coalition
9303 Ctr. St. Suite 100
Manassas, VA 20110
888-267-5669
www.amputee-coalition.org

United States Association for Blind Athletes (USABA)
1 Olympic Plaza
Colorado Springs, CO 80909
719-866-3224
www.usaba.org

United States Deaf Sports Federation
PO Box 910338
Lexington, KY 40591
605-367-5761(TTY)
605-367-5760(Voice)
www.usdeafsports.org

Dwarf Athletic Association of America
708 Gravenstein Hwy
Sebastopol, CA 95472
888-598-3222
www.daaa.org

United Cerebral Palsy
1825 K St. NW Suite 600
Washington, DC 20006
800-872-5872
www.ucp.org

Special Olympics, Inc. (SO)
1133 19th St NW New York Avenue, N.W.
Suite 500
Washington, DC 20036
202-628-3630
800-700-8585
www.specialolympics.org

Disabled Sports USA
451 Hungerford Dr.
Suite 100
Rockville, MD 20850
301-217-0960
www.dsusa.org

National Disability Sports Alliance
25 West Independence Way
Kingston, RI 02881
401-792-7130
www.ndsaonline.org

National Center for the Disabled
Winter Park Resort
33 Parsenn Rd.
Winter Park, CO 80482
303-316-1518
www.nscd.org

Wheelchair and Ambulatory Sports USA
PO Box 5266
Kendall Park, NJ 08824
732-266-2634
www.wsusa.org

American Amputee Foundation Inc.
PO Box 94227
North Little Rock, AR 72190
501-835-9290
www.americanamputee.org

United States Olympic Committee
27 South Tejon
Colorado Springs, CO 80903
888-222-2313
www.teamusa.org

International Paralympics Committee
Adenauerallee 212-214
53113 Bonn, Germany
+49-228-2097-200
www.paralympic.org

Literature:
Pacwrek MJ, Jones JA. *Sports and Recreation for the Disabled: a Resource Manual.* Indianapolis, IN, Benchmark Press, 1989.
Batshaw MI(ed): *Children with disabilities.* 5th Ed. Baltimore: Paul Brookes Pub.Co. 2007.

TABLE 67.5
SORT: Key Recommendations for Practice

Clinical Recommendation	Evidence Rating	References
Cervical spine clearance should be performed for all athletes with Down syndrome. Screening x-rays should be obtained between ages 3 and 5 years for all children with Down syndrome to evaluate for atlantoaxial instability (AAI).	C	[13,18,42,47]
Injury rates for *physically* disabled athletes are approximately the same as those of athletes without a disability in similar sports	C	[16]
Injury rates for individuals with *intellectual* disabilities are less than those reported for physically disabled and general population athletes	C	[6,28,33,40]

REFERENCES

1. American Academy of Family Physicians et al. *PPE: Preparticipation Physical Evaluation*, 4th edn. Washington, DC: American Academy of Pediatrics; 2010: pp. 131–139.
2. American Psychiatric Association. *The Diagnostic and Statistical Manual of Mental Disorders: (Revised 5th edn.)*. Washington, DC: American Psychiatric Association; 2013.
3. Americans with Disabilities Act of 1990. Public Law 101-336. 108th Congress, 2nd session (July 26, 1990) [cited July 27, 2014]. Available from http://www.ada.gov/ada_fed_resources.htm. Accessed August 4, 2015.
4. Armstrong LE, Maresh CM, Riebe DH, Kenefick RW, Castellani JW, Senk JM, Echegaray MS, Foley MF. Local cooling in wheelchair athletes during exercise-heat stress. *Medicine & Science in Sports & Exercise*. 1995;27(2): 211–216.
5. Barnhart RC, Connolly B. Aging and Down syndrome: Implications for physical therapy. *Physical Therapy*. 2007;87(10):1399–1406.

6. Batts KB, Glorioso Jr, JE, Williams MS. The medical demands of the special athlete. *Clinical Journal of Sport Medicine.* 1998;8(1):22–25.
7. Bergeron JW. Athletes with disabilities. *Physical Medicine and Rehabilitation Clinics of North America.* 1999;10(1):213–228.
8. Bernardi M, Guerra E, Giacinto BD, Cesare AD, Castellano V, Bhambhani Y. Field evaluation of paralympic athletes in selected sports: Implications for training. *Medicine & Science in Sports & Exercise.* 2010;42(6):1200–1208.
9. Bhambhani Y. Physiology of wheelchair racing in athletes with spinal cord injury. *Sports Medicine.* 2002;32(1):23–51.
10. Birrer RB. The special olympics athlete: Evaluation and clearance for participation. *Clinical Pediatrics.* 2004;43(9):777–782.
11. Bluechardt MH, Wiener J, Shephard RJ. Exercise programmes in the treatment of children with learning disabilities. *Sports Medicine.* 1995;19(1):55–72.
12. Caird MS, Wills BPD, Dormans JP. Down syndrome in children: The role of the orthopaedic surgeon. *Journal of the American Academy of Orthopaedic Surgeons.* 2006; 14(11):610–619.
13. Cope R, Olson S. Abnormalities of the cervical spine in Down's syndrome: Diagnosis, risks, and review of the literature, with particular reference to the special olympics. *Southern Medical Journal.* 1987;80(1):33–36.
14. Durstine JL, Moore GE, Painter PL, Roberts SO. *ACSM's Exercise Management for Persons with Chronic Diseases and Disabilities*, 3rd edn. Champaign, IL: Human Kinetics; 2009: pp. 49–125.
15. Ferrara MS, Palutsis GR, Snouse S, Davis RW. A longitudinal study of injuries to athletes with disabilities. *International Journal of Sports Medicine.* 2000;21(3):221–224.
16. Ferrara MS, Peterson CL. Injuries to athletes with disabilities. *Sports Medicine.* 2000;30(2):137–143.
17. Gutstein W, Sinclair SH, North RV, Bekiroglu N. Screening athletes with Down syndrome for ocular disease. *Optometry—Journal of the American Optometric Association.* 2010; 81(2):94–99.
18. Hankinson TC, Anderson RCE. Craniovertebral junction abnormalities in Down syndrome. *Neurosurgery.* 2010; 66(3):A32–A38.
19. International Special Olympics Web site [Internet]. What we do: Special olympics mission. Washington, DC: Special Olympics International [cited July 27, 2014]. Available from http://www.specialolympics.org/mission.aspx?source=QL. Accessed August 4, 2015.
20. Jacob T, Hutzler Y. Sports-medical assessment for athletes with a disability. *Disability & Rehabilitation.* 1998;20(3):116–119.
21. Kavanagh E. Affirmation through disability: One athlete's personal journey to the London Paralympic Games. *Perspectives in Public Health.* 2012;132(2):68–74.
22. Klenck C, Gebke K. Practical management: Common medical problems in disabled athletes. *Clinical Journal of Sport Medicine.* 2007;17(1):55–60.
23. Kosel H. Various types of sports for the handicapped and their suitability for the disabled. *Zeitschrift fur Orthopadie und ihre Grenzgebiete.* 1975;113(4):599–605.
24. Lai AM, Stanish WD, Stanish HI. The young athlete with physical challenges. *Clinics in Sports Medicine.* 2000; 19(4):793–819.
25. Lynch James H. The athlete with intellectual disabilities. In: O'Connor FG (ed.). *ACSM's Sports Medicine: A Comprehensive Review.* Lippincott Williams & Wilkins; 2012.
26. Martin JJ, Whalen L. Self-concept and physical activity in athletes with physical disabilities. *Disability and Health Journal.* 2012;5(3):197–200.
27. McCormick DP, Ivey Jr, FM, Gold DM, Zimmerman DM, Gemma S, Owen MJ. The preparticipation sports examination in special olympics athletes. *Texas Medicine.* 1988;84(4):39–43.
28. McCormick DP, Niebuhr VN, Risser WL. Injury and illness surveillance at local special olympic games. *British Journal of Sports Medicine.* 1990;24(4):221–224.
29. Murphy NA, Carbone PS. Promoting the participation of children with disabilities in sports, recreation, and physical activities. *Pediatrics.* 2008;121(5):1057–1061.
30. National Association for Child Development Web Site [Internet]. Ogden, UT: Congenital heart disease in children with Down syndrome [cited July 27, 2014]. Available from http://downsyndrome.nacd.org/heart_disease.php. Accessed August 4, 2015.
31. Noreau L, Shephard RJ. Spinal cord injury, exercise and quality of life. *Sports Medicine.* 1995;20(4):226–250.
32. Nyland J, Snouse SL, Anderson M, Kelly T, Sterling JC. Soft tissue injuries to USA paralympians at the 1996 summer games. *Archives of Physical Medicine and Rehabilitation.* 2000;81(3):368–373.
33. O'Connor, Francis G (eds.). *Sports Medicine: Just the Facts.* New York: McGraw-Hill, Medical Publishing Division; 2005.
34. Palmer T, Weber KM. The deaf athlete. *Current Sports Medicine Reports.* 2006;5(6):323–326.
35. Patatoukas D, Farmakides A, Aggeli V, Fotaki S, Tsibidakis H, Mavrogenis A, Papathanasiou J, Papagelopoulos P. Disability-related injuries in athletes with disabilities. *Folia Medica.* 2011;53(1):40–46.
36. Patel DR, Greydanus DE. Sport participation by physically and cognitively challenged young athletes. *Pediatric Clinics of North America.* 2010;57(3):795–817.
37. Patel DR, Greydanus DE. The pediatric athlete with disabilities. *Pediatric Clinics of North America.* 2002;49(4): 803–827.
38. Pepper M, Willick S. Maximizing physical activity in athletes with amputations. *Current Sports Medicine Reports.* 2009;8(6):339–344.
39. Platt LS. Medical and orthopaedic conditions in special olympics athletes. *Journal of Athletic Training.* 2001;36(1):74.
40. Ramirez M, Yang J, Bourque L, Javien J, Kashani S, Limbos MA, Peek-Asa C. Sports injuries to high school athletes with disabilities. *Pediatrics.* 2009;123(2):690–696.
41. Reynolds J, Stirk A, Thomas A, Geary F. Paralympics—Barcelona 1992. *British Journal of Sports Medicine.* 1994;28(1):14–17.
42. Risser WL, Anderson SJ, Bolduc SP, Griesemer B, Harris SS, Mclain L, Tanner SM et al. Atlantoaxial instability in Down-syndrome: Subject review. *Pediatrics.* 1995; 96(1):151–154.
43. Sanyer ON. Down syndrome and sport participation. *Current Sports Medicine Reports.* 2006;5(6):315–318.
44. Schalock RL, Borthwick-Duffy SA, Bradley V, Buntix WHE, Coulter MD, Craig EM, Gomez SC et al. Intellectual disability. *Definition, Classification and Systems of Supports.* 2010;11:259.
45. Schieve LA, Boulet SL, Boyle C, Rasmussen SA, Schendel D. Health of children 3 to 17 years of age with Down syndrome in the 1997–2005 National Health Interview Survey. *Pediatrics.* 2009;123(2):e253–e260.
46. Shapiro DR, Martin JJ. Athletic identity, affect, and peer relations in youth athletes with physical disabilities. *Disability and Health Journal.* 2010;3(2):79–85.
47. Tassone JC, Duey-Holtz A. Spine concerns in the special olympian with Down syndrome. *Sports Medicine and Arthroscopy Review.* 2008;16(1):55–60.

48. Tsitsimpikou C, Jamurtas A, Fitch K, Papalexis P, Tsarouhas K. Medication use by athletes during the Athens 2004 Paralympic Games. *British Journal of Sports Medicine.* 2009;43(13):1062–1066.
49. Turbanski S, Schmidtbleicher D. Effects of heavy resistance training on strength and power in upper extremities in wheelchair athletes. *The Journal of Strength & Conditioning Research.* 2010;24(1):8–16.
50. Van de Vliet P. Paralympic athlete's health. *British Journal of Sports Medicine.* 2012;24(1):8–16.
51. Ward KH, Meyers MC. Exercise performance of lower-extremity amputees. *Sports Medicine.* 1995;20(4):207–214.
52. Webborn AD. Fifty years of competitive sport for athletes with disabilities: 1948–1998. *British Journal of Sports Medicine.* 1999;33(2):138.
53. Webborn N, Van de Vliet P. Paralympic medicine. *The Lancet.* 2012;380(9836):65–71.
54. Webborn N, Willick S, Reeser JC. Injuries among disabled athletes during the 2002 Winter Paralympic Games. *Medicine & Science in Sports & Exercise.* 2006;38(5):811–815.
55. Winell J, Burke SW. Sports participation of children with Down syndrome. *Orthopedic Clinics of North America.* 2003;34(3):439–443.
56. Woodhouse JM, Adler P, Duignan A. Vision in athletes with intellectual disabilities: The need for improved eyecare. *Journal of Intellectual Disability Research.* 2004; 48(8):736–745.
57. Wu SK, Williams T. Factors influencing sport participation among athletes with spinal cord injury. *Medicine & Science in Sports & Exercise.* 2001;33(2):177–182.

68 The Athlete with Chronic Illness*

Karl B. Fields, Timothy Ryan Draper, Zachary Smith, and Evan Corey

CONTENTS

TABLE 68.1
Key Clinical Considerations

1. Aerobic, isometric, and resistance exercise all offer potential benefits to hypertensive patients.
2. Hypertensive medication can be prescribed for athletes that will control their blood pressure without negatively affecting exercise capacity.
3. Coronary artery disease may occur in athletes without classic symptoms.
4. Weight management must begin in childhood to avoid adverse adult health outcomes.
5. Exercise has numerous beneficial effects for diabetes patients and is one of the cornerstones of successful management.
6. Symptoms of exercise-induced bronchospasm usually start 6–12 minutes after initiation of moderate or intense exercise.
7. Exercise-induced bronchospasm is common in all aerobically demanding sports and particularly in winter sports.
8. Expert opinion suggests that patients with epilepsy be allowed to participate in almost all sports.
9. For higher-risk sports, patients must have excellent epileptic control before participation.

68.1 INTRODUCTION

Medical problems are responsible for approximately 70% of the visits that athletes make to physicians. The majority of these are respiratory and other episodic infectious illnesses; however, a significant number of athletes have one or more chronic medical conditions. For individuals over age 35, the risk of known and occult disease increases substantially. Important to the care of these patients is an understanding of how sports activity affects their illness. The corollary to this concern is that the illness may also affect strength, endurance, coordination, or other parameters that can impact sports performance. The physician's ultimate goal becomes maximizing the athlete's ability to pursue sports safely and successfully (Table 68.1).

While athletes potentially experience any of the diseases seen in the nonathletic population, certain conditions occur frequently enough that physicians should have specific knowledge of the effect exercise has on disease management and participation risks. Individuals with obesity, hypertension, coronary artery disease, and diabetes mellitus benefit from physical activity, but sport poses risks for each condition. These disorders occur in a significant portion of the population, including athletes. Seizure disorders alter consciousness so that safe participation in water sports, vehicular activity, equestrian sport, and other special situations cannot be assured even with treatment. This chapter reviews these common medical conditions and how best to care for athletes affected.[31]

68.2 HYPERTENSION

The *JNC VII* and *VIII* define normal blood pressure (BP) in adults as less than 120/80 mmHg. Prehypertension is not a disease but a defined group of patients who have systolic BP of 120–139 or diastolic BP of 80–89. This group merits closer follow-up to be sure they do not develop hypertension. For an adult, a resting BP of 140/90 or above on a screening test followed by two office BP measurements at or above this level with an appropriate-sized cuff confirms the diagnosis of hypertension.[25] JNC VII further classified hypertension into stage 1, which are individuals with BPs between 140/90 and 159/99. Stage 2 hypertension includes individuals with BP of 160/100 or greater. Systolic or diastolic hypertension is a subcategory in which one of the two parameters exceeds normal values but not both.

In children and older adolescents, the diagnosis of hypertension is based on adjustment of BP levels for population demographics along with the level of physical maturity. In general, normal BP is defined as less than 90% for age and prehypertension as between the 90% and 95%. Stage 1 hypertension is defined as BP ranging from above 95% to 99% plus 5 mmHg and stage 2 as BP exceeding the 99% plus 5 mmHg.[26]

* In the second edition, this chapter was authored by Warren B. Howe.

Clinical Pearl

Strong evidence demonstrates that aerobic exercise lowers blood pressure. However, most trials also show that resistance exercise and even isometric exercise can help lower blood pressure as well.

Physical activity increases the heart rate and cardiac output. BP varies in relation to cardiac output and total peripheral resistance. Exercise generally causes some transient increase in pressure levels because peripheral resistance rarely decreases enough to counter the effect of tachycardia and greater blood flow. Resistance (isometric) and dynamic (isotonic) exercise trigger different pressor responses. Typically, heavy-resistance activities cause dramatic rises in BPs. Dynamic exercise leads to gradually higher BPs during activity, although a small subset of athletes show a marked hypertensive response to dynamic exercise. The overall effect of continuous training is to lower both systolic and diastolic pressures. Numerous trials of aerobic exercise have demonstrated drops in systolic BP of 5–15 mmHg and drops in diastolic BP of 3–6 mmHg. Recent data show similar drops with resistance training and, surprisingly, the drops with isometric exercise are somewhat larger. Studies of children and adolescents show a similar trend in BP reduction with exercise but a less dramatic drop in BP.[21]

Based on the positive effects of both resistance and dynamic exercise on BP, most hypertensive athletes do not have to substantially alter their training. If the hypertensive athlete is not in good control, exercise capacity drops substantially. Until control is reached, hypertensive patients should start with low-intensity warm-ups followed by moderate-intensity training. Once good control is established, periodic monitoring of BP response to intense workouts as well as periodic resting BP evaluations helps guide therapy. There is evidence that athletes with the greatest BP elevation during workouts have greater risk of left ventricular hypertrophy, and this is concerning for end organ damage. Thus athletes who have recurrent exaggerated BP responses may warrant tighter BP control.

A second concern for the hypertensive athlete is finding an effective medication with a side effect profile that will not hinder sports performance. Angiotensin-converting enzyme (ACE) inhibitors are the drug of choice for most athletes, as they effectively control pressures during exercise with minimal side effects. Calcium channel blockers are the preferred initial drug in African-American athletes.[17] Other options considered as primary therapy in JNC VIII include angiotensin-II receptor blockers (ARBs) and diuretics. While ARBs control exercise pressures equally well and also have limited adverse effects, diuretics often pose specific risks for athletes that limit their use. Diuretics may reduce maximal exercise capacity and increase risks of dehydration, cramps, and heat illness. Beta blockers, alpha blockers, central alpha agonists, and direct vasodilators are not primary choices for antihypertensive medications and rarely merit use in athletes. Concomitant nonsteroidal anti-inflammatory drug (NSAID) use may limit effectiveness of antihypertensive agents and also increase the risk of side effects.

Clinical Pearl

For patients with hypertension, ACE inhibitors, ARBs, and calcium channel blockers can be used without affecting exercise performance.

One area of research is whether certain sports actually increase the risk of hypertension. Studies show that American football athletes have a high prevalence of hypertension when compared to competitors in other sports and to nonathletic students.[4,18,22,39] In a study of a division 1 university football program, 19% of football athletes had hypertension when compared to only 7% of nonfootball athletes. In addition, over 60% of the football players had BP levels that fell into the prehypertension category. This association has also been seen in professional football athletes who have greater levels of hypertension than professional baseball athletes. In collegiate and professional football athletes, professional soccer athletes, and even elite endurance athletes, higher BP levels have an association with more left ventricular mass and true left ventricular hypertrophy. What is not known is the actual cause of this association. Is the type of training or diet of strength athletes more likely to lead to hypertension? Are these results affected by other variables including legal or illegal supplements? In any case, hypertension is a common chronic medical condition in this group of athletes, and more study of causes and long-term effects is warranted.[19]

A serious risk for hypertensive athletes or athletes who have any major cardiac risk factor is occult coronary artery disease. Coronary artery disease often occurs in conjunction with hypertension, diabetes mellitus, obesity, and/or hyperlipidemia. Silent myocardial ischemia and infarction occur in a significant portion of men and women with high BP. Because athletes place extreme physical demands on their cardiovascular systems, an exercise tolerance test (ETT) becomes an important test to determine the likelihood of coronary artery disease and can also measure the BP response to exertion.

68.3 CORONARY ARTERY DISEASE

Athletes with known coronary artery disease merit close monitoring for sports participation. While individuals have completed extreme exercise, including marathon runs, after a myocardial infarction, balloon angioplasty, or coronary artery bypass grafting (CABG), rarely would a physician recommend intense exercise. Because patients with known coronary syndromes can reduce their risks by maintaining high fitness levels, moderate exercise improves their prognosis. Patients with coronary artery disease who can achieve more than 10.7 MET of workload on standard exercise testing have a normal age-adjusted mortality. Under careful monitoring, a newer approach to athletes with coronary artery disease is to use high-intensity interval training. Athletes utilizing this make dramatic fitness gains, but the risk of triggering a cardiac event suggests that this approach be medically monitored.[24,40]

Clinical Pearl

Improved fitness can dramatically lower mortality risk in patients with known coronary artery disease. With careful monitoring, even higher-intensity exercise may be beneficial in these patients.

Careful adjustment of cardiac medications, including deciding when preexercise nitroglycerin should be utilized, improves the ability of these individuals to exercise safely. The current view of coronary artery disease is that this is a dynamic process. Research shows that plaque instability, platelet adhesiveness, epithelial responsiveness, and intravascular nitrous oxide levels all influence the likelihood that a specific lesion will lead to a myocardial infarction. With the myriad of possible triggers for acute coronary syndromes, specific research focuses on determining the effect of exercise on each of these parameters.

Physicians need to recognize that cardiac ischemia in well-conditioned athletes may cause vague symptoms or a drop in exercise tolerance with no additional symptoms. Thus any drop in exercise tolerance or more fatigue in either exercise or recovery may warrant more investigation. Currently, our best approach to secondary prevention of cardiac events centers around appropriate drug treatments, including aspirin, lipid-lowering agents, beta blockers, ace inhibitors, and other individualized medications.[12] Because we expect patients with coronary artery disease to exercise, the authors feel that yearly monitoring through the ETT seems reasonable. Additional testing and more frequent monitoring should follow if the athlete shows any signs of instability with his or her disease.[2,30]

68.4 OBESITY

In 2009–2010 more than 35% of men and women in the United States were obese.[27] Obesity contributes to excess morbidity from hypertension, type 2 diabetes, coronary artery disease, stroke, gallbladder disease, osteoarthritis, respiratory difficulty, and sleep apnea. In addition, multiple cancers have higher incidences in the obese, including endometrial, breast, prostate, and colon. Not surprisingly, higher body weights are associated with greater all-cause mortality. Centripetal obesity with a high waist-to-hip ratio indicates a subtype of obesity with an independently elevated level of risk, particularly for cardiovascular disease (CVD).[28]

Clinical Pearl

Centripetal obesity with a high waist-to-hip ratio indicates a high risk for cardiovascular disease.

Many obese athletes have achieved the highest pinnacles of athletic success. Some sports have such a focus on size that obesity has traditionally been considered advantageous, including football, weight throwing in track and field, heavyweight wrestling, and powerlifting. Rather than the athletic activity leading to a healthier lifestyle, sports with too much emphasis on size and strength have often encouraged dietary excess and other harmful practices such as using anabolic agents. Deaths from heat illness are more common in obese athletes. Fortunately, most athletic programs have redirected their focus to discourage obesity and to look more critically at lean body mass.

A more common problem confronting athletes is post-competition weight gain. An average professional football lineman weighing 300 pounds can rapidly develop to morbid obesity if he ceases activity and continues the same diet. Highly competitive athletes consume 1500–2000 excess calories a day to replace the expenditure from multiple training sessions. Considering that the body requires approximately 10 calories per pound to maintain body weight, an average male professional football lineman could be consuming an average intake of 4500–5000 calories daily. Even if this individual persists in exercising at a level considered vigorous by most Americans, without a marked reduction in calorie intake, he could stand to gain 30–50 pounds in his first year out of serious training.

With this in mind, sound nutritional practices must be implemented during the competitive life of most athletes. Focus should be toward ideal weight based on body fat, not on total pounds. Simple waist-to-hip ratios can identify individuals who have higher risk. Athletes need to be informed about the calorie demand of various training activities so they do not overestimate the impact on calorie need of a low-intensity workout. Strategies should teach healthy eating and avoidance of fast foods to establish patterns that lead to better postcompetition diet practices. Data from the Harvard Growth Study, with a follow-up period of 55 years, indicate that overweight adolescents have a higher risk of all-cause mortality and other adverse health effects independent of their adult weight.[23] This emphasizes the importance of sound weight management starting at the middle school and high school sports participation level.

Clinical Pearl

Overweight adolescents have higher risk of all-cause mortality and adverse health outcomes independent of adult weight.

68.5 DIABETES IN THE ATHLETE

Regular exercise has been shown to improve glycemic control, increase self-esteem, and decrease the incidence of cardiac disease in those with diabetes mellitus. Close monitoring of blood glucose and appropriate adjustments in medications and diet aid in optimizing performance and preventing complications associated with exercise. In 2010, 25.8 million people, or 8.3% of the U.S. population, have diabetes with approximately 5% having type 1 diabetes.[7] Type 1 is characterized by autoimmune destruction of insulin-producing beta cells in the pancreas, and these diabetics require a specialized diet along with exercise. In addition, exogenous insulin administration is needed to utilize glucose. Type 2 diabetes mellitus accounts for 95% of diabetes.[7] In addition to impaired production of insulin, type 2 diabetes is characterized by reduced sensitivity to insulin and excessive production of glucose by the liver. Fifty-seven percent of type 2 diabetics are obese.[8] Although they may be able to control their blood glucose by diet alone, type 2 diabetics often require oral medications or exogenous insulin.[5,10,11,38]

As in the general population, diabetics who exercise enjoy several benefits, including improved fitness levels, which correspond to longevity and decreased risk of cardiovascular death.[35] Exercise is considered a cornerstone in the control of diabetes, as exercise has been found to provide significant improvement in diabetes control.[33] Risks of exercise for the diabetic include hypoglycemia, hyperglycemia, and neuropathy. Hypoglycemia (defined as blood glucose <65 mg/dL) is most common in those requiring exogenous insulin and can lead to fatigue, confusion, and coma. Exercising with elevated blood glucose may cause a rapid rise in glucose and ketoacidosis, and fluid loss can ensue. Peripheral neuropathy can cause ulceration and infections in the feet of diabetics who lack adequate pain sensation.[20]

Clinical Pearl

Exercise provides significant improvement in control in both type 1 and type 2 diabetes.

Every athlete with diabetes may benefit from a thorough medical evaluation that includes history, physical exam, and appropriate laboratory tests. The history should elicit information about the degree of glycemic control, any diabetic complications, additional medical problems, and plans to change exercise regimens. This is also an excellent opportunity to gauge the patient's understanding of the disease and provide education.[32,36]

The physical exam should focus on the cardiovascular, ophthalmologic, and neurologic systems. There are no high-quality studies that show an ETT is absolutely required prior to exercise in otherwise healthy diabetics. However, many would suggest that diabetics should undergo exercise testing if they meet any of the following criteria: (1) age greater than 35 years, (2) type 1 diabetes for longer than 15 years or type 2 diabetes for longer than 10 years, or (3) presence of additional cardiac risk factors, autonomic neuropathy, or peripheral vascular or microvascular disease.[41] In addition to detecting coronary disease, an exercise test can aid in the diagnosis of hypertension or orthostatic hypotension and can establish a baseline fitness level.

Clinical Pearl

Higher-risk diabetic athletes should undergo exercise tolerance testing before beginning a vigorous exercise program.

The ophthalmologic examination should include a fundoscopic examination to assess for diabetic retinopathy. If proliferative retinopathy is present, isometric exercises should be avoided.[10] Other eye diseases to be assessed include cataracts and glaucoma.

A thorough neurologic and foot exam is important to assess for peripheral neuropathy and signs of infection. Blisters and abrasions can cause ulcerations and serious infections in diabetics with neuropathy. In addition, Charcot deformity may develop in patients with severe peripheral neuropathy. Appropriate footwear, evaluation of the need for orthoses, and frequent examination may help prevent complications.

Controlling glucose levels during exercise is optimized by adjusting the intensity of exercise, carbohydrate intake, and insulin or medication dosage. For type 1 diabetics, additional carbohydrate snacks may be all that is needed to supplement metabolic needs. A 15–30 g, readily absorbable carbohydrate snack should be consumed for every 30 minutes of exercise. For prolonged exercise, a reduction in insulin may be required. Decreasing short-acting insulin 30%–50% within 2–3 hours of exercise may help to prevent hypoglycemia. Short-acting insulin can be reduced by 30% for exercise less than 1 hour, 40% for 1–2 hours of activity, and 50% for more than 3 hours of activity. If the athlete uses an insulin pump, a reduction in the basal rate of 50% may be necessary, while a 50% decrease in the premeal bolus may be necessary for diabetics exercising after meals.[37]

Type 2 diabetics who are diet controlled rarely need any adjustments for exercise. Because of increased glucose utilization, the dose of oral hypoglycemic medication may have to be reduced by 50% or more on days of extended exercise. Type 2 diabetics, likewise, should have quick access to carbohydrate snacks to prevent hypoglycemia.

Prevention of hypoglycemia requires close monitoring of blood glucose before, during, and after exercise. Those at greatest risk for exercise-induced hypoglycemia are type 1 diabetics and type 2 diabetics who inject exogenous insulin. Carbohydrates should be given to a diabetic with a glucose level below 100 mg/dL at the start of activity.[41]

Athletes who exercise with hyperglycemia (blood glucose >240 mg/dL) are at risk of rapidly rising glucose levels, dehydration, and ketoacidosis. Exercise should be avoided if the blood glucose level is greater than 300 mg/dL or if greater than 250 mg/dL and ketones are present.[41]

Clinical Pearl

Diabetics with blood glucose greater than 300 mg/dL or greater than 250 mg/dL with ketones present should avoid exercise until control of blood glucose is improved.

The athlete with diabetes is able to compete at the highest levels. Close monitoring of glucose levels to establish glycemic patterns, adjustment in medication and food intake, and being familiar with potential complications will allow the diabetic athlete to compete effectively and safely.

68.6 SEIZURE DISORDERS

A seizure, defined as an abnormal electrical discharge of cortical neurons leading to sudden involuntary alterations in movement, perception, or behavior, affects up to 10% of the population at some point in one's lifetime. Epilepsy, a disorder of recurrent seizures, affects approximately 2%–3% of the population.[9] A number of athletes suffer from seizure disorders and caring for these individuals can add an element that can be challenging if the healthcare provider is not prepared.

To be prepared, healthcare providers should be familiar with classifying seizure disorders. Seizures are classified according to their characteristics and are separated into two major categories: partial and generalized. Partial seizures localize to a distinct section leading to a vast array of symptoms. Depending on where the electrical occurrence initiates, symptoms could include motor or sensation disturbances; disruption in smell, hearing, or vision; or psychological symptoms, to name a few. To further delineate, partial seizure can be categorized as simple or complex. Simple partial seizures produce no loss of consciousness, and the athlete may have repetitive actions such as lip smacking, involuntary muscle contractions, or be unresponsive to commands. Complex partial seizures, in contrast, do ultimately impair consciousness. Following seizure activity, which typically lasts less than 5 minutes, individual athletes typically have a brief state referred to as a postictal state indicated by headache, transient amnesia, and/or fatigue.[13] Both simple and complex partial seizures can evolve into secondary generalized seizures.

Generalized seizures involve cortical discharge from both cerebral hemispheres leading to bilateral symptoms and loss of consciousness. The most common type of generalized seizure is the tonic–clonic, or grand mal seizure. This type of seizure begins with abrupt loss of consciousness and stiffening of the axial musculature and extremities that subsequently turn to a more jerking motion, leading to potential injuries such as shoulder dislocation or clavicle, humeral, femoral, or ankle fractures.[14] Absence seizures are a subtype of generalized seizures consisting of blank staring spells with no associated memory of the seizure often seen in childhood. Other generalized seizure subtypes to be aware of are myoclonic, clonic, tonic, and atonic.

While the majority of epilepsy in children is idiopathic, known causes of childhood epilepsy include birth and neonatal injury (58%), central nervous system (CNS) infection (15%), head trauma (12%), and, rarely, metabolic disorders and tumors. In adults, epilepsy generally results from vascular insults (60%), tumors (10%), and CNS infection (9%) (9).

Regardless of the cause of epilepsy, certain inciting factors are known to predispose athletes to seizures. Depending on their action, they either decrease seizure threshold or increase seizure frequency. Triggers include fatigue, sleep deprivation, dehydration and overhydration, stress, hyperventilation, hypoxia, hyperthermia, electrolyte disturbances such as hypo- or hypernatremia, hypoglycemia, and certain illicit drugs. Although some of these factors occur with activity, exercise has not been shown to increase seizure frequency. Multiple studies have shown that seizures rarely occur during exercise and overall seizure control may improve with exercise. Current theories are based on B-endorphin release, lowered blood pH with lactic acid release, increased gamma-aminobutyric acid (GABA) concentration, and possibly increased mental alertness and attention. A few studies have shown that seizure activity can increase in the postexercise rest period.[16]

Although significant head trauma can lead to seizure activity, no data have shown that repetitive minor head injuries cause any deterioration of seizure control. In a study of 301 children including those with epilepsy, blunt head trauma was not shown to worsen seizure control in epileptics.[9]

Clinical Pearl

Exercise has not been shown to increase seizure frequency.

The treatment of epilepsy is limited to antiepileptic drugs (AEDs), such as phenytoin, carbamazepine, valproic acid, lamotrigine, gabapentin, and clonazepam. With AEDs, about 50% of epileptics remain seizure-free. AEDs unfortunately can have considerable side effects, such as fatigue, sedation, nystagmus, ataxia, confusion, and nausea.[13] Many of these side effects are undesirable, which potentially affect performance and can be dangerous for athletes.

If during activity an athlete experiences a seizure, a healthcare provider should follow standard first aid guidelines; management of airway, breathing, and circulation should be followed. If possible, help the athlete to the ground or a safe surrounding, removing any harmful objects from the surrounding area. Cushion the athlete's head but do not remove equipment during the seizure activity unless it is obstructing the airway. If the athlete is vomiting, then roll them into a lateral decubitus position to decrease the risk of aspiration but attempt to wait until the postictal phase due to risk of injury. If seizure activity occurs for longer than 3–5 minutes, then activate EMS and transport the athlete to the nearest medical facility. Avoid restraining the seizing athlete during convulsion secondary to risk of serious injury. Also, never put anything in the athlete's mouth, but safe removal of any mouth guard can be attempted if it is jeopardizing airway.

Overall, few guidelines for epileptic participation in sports exist. In 1968, the American Medical Association (AMA) advised that individuals with a "convulsive disorder not completely controlled by medications" be banned from collision sports, contact sports, and even some noncontact sports such as tennis. The discovery of the beneficial effects of exercise on epilepsy led to the AMA changing their stance by explaining that epileptics with reasonable control of seizures should be allowed to play any sport not proven to cause chronic head trauma. In 1983, the American Academy of Pediatrics (AAP) went a step further, declaring that "epilepsy *per se* should not exclude a child from hockey, baseball, football, basketball, and wrestling." (2) Exercise is currently recommended for most well-controlled epileptics to improve overall fitness and self-esteem. Some commonsense guidelines should be used to determine if participation is safe. Specific sports that involve heavy blows to the head, such as boxing and martial arts, are contraindicated. High-risk sports that may pose risk of injury or death to epileptics or others, such as archery and riflery, are considered by many to be too dangerous.

Aviation sports, mountain climbing, and water sports should be considered only for very-well-controlled epileptics under adequate supervision. There is concern for a greater risk of drowning in epileptics vs. the general population when water sports are unsupervised. Sports such as gymnastics and horseback riding, which have the potential for injury from a high fall, should also only be considered in well-controlled epileptics. If any of these activities are pursued by the epileptic, supervision must be present at all times.[3,34]

Clinical Pearl

Epileptic athletes should only participate in higher-risk sports if they are in good control and well supervised.

Motor sports are contraindicated in epileptics who have at least one to two seizures per year; however, epileptics who are well controlled and seizure-free for at least 2 years are eligible for a driver's license and can be considered eligible to participate in motor sports. Eligibility should be based on excellent seizure control, the safety of the driver, and the comfort level of the physician, driver, and other participants.[1,14,16,29]

To lessen the risk of participation, epileptics should be encouraged to use appropriate equipment and follow the rules of safe play. If, during the sport, major head trauma occurs or seizure frequency increases, the epileptic's participation should be discontinued. If a new seizure occurs in a participant involved in contact sports, that person should undergo a thorough work-up, observation period, and possibly treatment before returning to the sport. Ultimately, the decision on participation needs to be individualized based on athlete's type of seizure disorder, control, and specific sport. A summary can be seen in Table 68.2.

A more important issue may be that few epileptics actually participate in exercise. One survey of 3000 NCAA Division I athletes discovered only one athlete, a gymnast, with epilepsy. Estimates suggest less than 5% of epileptics participate in a regular exercise program. Often coaches, parents, physicians, and epileptics themselves limit involvement in sports out of fear of uncontrolled seizures, embarrassment, or ignorance about the disease. Exercise should be encouraged to improve the health of epileptics (15). Because epileptics have a five times higher risk of suicide, exercise may lessen the risk of depression and help boost self-esteem.

In summary, epileptics and healthcare providers who are familiar with understanding the types of seizures, precipitating factors, postictal recovery, and medications can follow commonsense guidelines and develop a plan to allow safe participation in sports (Table 68.3).

TABLE 68.2
Sports Participation in Athletes with Seizure Disorder

Type of Sport	Recommendations
Contact sports	No restrictions unless newly diagnosed or unclear course.
Water sports	Generally permitted with proper supervision. Scuba diving, competitive underwater swimming, and diving are prohibited or may participate if seizure-free for 5 years and off medications per U.K. Sport Diving Medical Committee.
Motor sports	Generally discouraged unless seizure-free for 2 years.
Aerobic sports	No restrictions and encouraged.
Sports from heights	Equestrian and certain gymnastic events are strongly discouraged. Skydiving, hang gliding, and free climbing also discouraged vs. prohibited by some.
Shooting sports	Depends on type of seizure, control, and weapons being fired. Generally discouraged.

Source: Adapted from Petron, D.J. and Crist, J.C., Neurologic problems in the athlete, in *Netter's Sports Medicine*, Putukian, M., Young, C.C., McCarty, E.C., and Madden, C.C. eds., Saunders, Philadelphia, PA, 2010, pp. 252–264.

TABLE 68.3
SORT: Key Recommendations for Practice

Clinical Recommendations	Evidence Rating	References
Strong evidence indicates that aerobic exercise lowers blood pressure. Moderate evidence indicates that resistance and isometric exercise lower blood pressure.	A	[17,21,22,25,26]
Fitness level dramatically lowers mortality risk in individuals with coronary artery disease.	A	[24,30,40]
Overweight adolescents have a higher risk of all-cause mortality.	A	[23]
Exercise benefits control in both type 1 and 2 diabetics.	A	[33,35,36]
Epilepsy should not preclude a child from participating in contact or collision sports.	C	[13,16,29]

REFERENCES

1. American Academy of Pediatrics. Medical conditions affecting sports participation. *Pediatrics*. 2001;107(5):1205–1209.
2. American College of Sports Medicine. *ACSM's Guidelines for Exercise Testing and Prescription*, 6th edn. Philadelphia, PA: Lippincott Williams & Wilkins; 2000.
3. Bartsokas T. The athlete with epilepsy. In: Garrett WE, Kirkendall DT, Squire DL (eds.). *Principles and Practice of Primary Care Medicine*. Philadelphia, PA: Lippincott Williams & Wilkins; 2001: pp. 265–271.
4. Berge HM, Gjerdalen GF, Andersen TE, Solberg EE, Steine K. Blood pressure in professional male football players in Norway. *Journal of Hypertension*. 2013;31(4):672–679.
5. Brukner P, Fricker P. Diabetes mellitus. In: Fields K, Fricker P (eds.). *Medical Problems in Athletes*. Boston, MA: Blackwell Science; 1997: pp. 216–220.
6. Cantu RC. Epilepsy and athletics. *Clinics in Sports Medicine*. 1998;61–69:17(1).
7. Centers for Disease Control and Prevention (CDC). National diabetes fact sheet: National estimates and general information on diabetes and prediabetes in the United States, 2011. U.S. Department of Health and Human Services, Centers for Disease Control and Prevention, Atlanta, GA, 2011.
8. Centers for Disease Control and Prevention (CDC). *Behavioral Risk Factor Surveillance System Survey Data*. U.S. Department of Health and Human Services, Centers for Disease Control and Prevention, Atlanta, GA, 2012.
9. Chang BS, Lowenstein DH. Epilepsy. *New England Journal of Medicine*. 2003;349:1257.
10. Christakos C, Fields K. Exercise in type 1 diabetes: Why benefits outweigh risks. *Sports Primary Care*. 2001;1(3):17–19.
11. Colberg S, Swain D. Exercise and diabetes control. *Physician and Sportsmedicine*. 2000;28:63–81.
12. De Lorgeril M, Renaud S, Mamelle N et al. Mediterranean alpha-linolenic acid-rich diet in secondary prevention of coronary heart disease. *Lancet*. 1994;343:1454–1459.
13. Dimberg EL, Burns TM. Management of common neurologic conditions. *Clinics in Sports Medicine*. 2005;24:637–662.
14. Dubow JS, Kelly JP. Epilepsy in sports and recreation. *Sports Medicine*. 2003;33(7):499–516.
15. Fallon KE. Neurology. In: Fields KB, Fricker PB (eds.). *Medical Problems in Athletes*. Boston, MA: Blackwell Science; 1997: pp. 186–208.
16. Fountain NB, May AC. Epilepsy and athletics. *Clinics in Sports Medicine*. 2003;22:605–616.
17. James PA, Oparil S, Carter BL, Cushman WC. Evidence-based guideline for the management of high blood pressure in adults: Report from the panel members appointed to the eighth Joint National Committee (JNC 8). *Journal of the American Medical Association*. 2014;311(5):507–520.
18. Karpinos AR, Roumie CL, Nian H, Diamond AB, Rothman RL. High prevalence of hypertension among collegiate football athletes. *Circulation: Cardiovascular Quality and Outcomes*. 2013;6(6):716–723.
19. Kim YJ, Goh CW, Byun YS, Lee YH, Lee JB, Shin YO. Left ventricular hypertrophy, diastolic dysfunction, pulse pressure, and plasma ET-1 in marathon runners with exaggerated blood pressure response. *International Heart Journal*. 2013;54(2):82–87.
20. LaPorte RE, Dorman JS, Tajima N et al. Pittsburgh insulin-dependent diabetes mellitus morbidity and mortality study: Physical activity and diabetic complications. *Pediatrics*. 1986;78:1027–1033.
21. Mark AE, Janssen I. Dose–response relation between physical activity and blood pressure in youth. *Medicine & Science in Sports & Exercise*. 2008;40(6):1007.
22. Millar PJ, McGowan CL, Cornelissen VA, Araujo CG, Swaine IL. Evidence for the role of isometric exercise training in reducing blood pressure: Potential mechanisms and future directions. *Sports Medicine*. 2014;44(3):345–356.
23. Must A, Jacques PF, Dallal GE et al. Long-term morbidity and mortality of overweight adolescents. *New England Journal of Medicine*. 1992;327:1350–1355.
24. Myers J, Prakash M, Froelicher V, Do D, Partington S, Atwood JE. Exercise capacity and mortality among men referred for exercise testing. *New England Journal of Medicine*. 2002;346(11):793–801.
25. National Heart, Lung, and Blood Institute. *JNC VII: The Seventh Report of the Joint National Committee on Prevention, Detection, Evaluation, and Treatment of High Blood Pressure*. NIH Publication No. 04-5230. Bethesda, MD: National Institutes of Health; 2004.
26. National Heart, Lung, and Blood Institute. The fourth report on the diagnosis, evaluation, and treatment of high blood pressure in children and adolescents. National High Blood Pressure Education Program Working Group on high blood pressure in children and adolescents. *Pediatrics*. 2004;114(2 Suppl, 4th report):555.
27. Ogden CL, Carroll MD, Kit BK, Flegal KM. Prevalence of obesity in the United States, 2009–2010. NCHS data brief, no 82. National Center for Health Statistics, Hyattsville, MD, 2012.
28. Perry AC, Miller PC, Allison MD et al. Clinical predictability of the waist-to-hip ratio in assessment of cardiovascular disease risk factors in overweight, premenopausal women. *American Journal of Clinical Nutrition*. 1998;68:1022–1027.
29. Petron DJ, Crist JC. Neurologic problems in the athlete. In: Putukian M, Young CC, McCarty EC, Madden CC (eds.). *Netter's Sports Medicine*. Philadelphia, PA: Saunders; 2010: pp. 252–264.
30. Reamy BV, Ledford CC. Cardiovascular considerations in middle-aged athletes at risk for coronary artery disease. *Current Sports Medicine Reports*. 2013;12(2):70–76.
31. Sachtleben TR, Mellion MB. The hypertensive athlete. In: Mellion MB, Walsh WM, Madden C, Putukian M, Shelton GL (eds.). *Team Physician's Handbook*, 3rd edn. Philadelphia, PA: Hanley & Belfus; 2002: pp. 277–287.
32. Schneider SH, Khachandurian AD, Amorosa LF et al. Ten-year experience with an exercise-based outpatient life-style modification program in the treatment of diabetes mellitus. *Diabetes Care*. 1992;15:1800–1810.
33. Sigal RJ, Kenny GP, Boulé NG et al. Effects of aerobic training, resistance training, or both on glycemic control in type 2 diabetes: A randomized trial. *Annals of Internal Medicine*. 2007;147(6):357.
34. Sirven JI, Varrato J. Physical activity and epilepsy; 1999. http://www.physsportsmed (accessed December 19, 2013).
35. Sluik D, Buijsse B, Muckelbauer R et al. Physical activity and mortality in individuals with diabetes mellitus: A prospective study and meta-analysis. *Archives of Internal Medicine*. 2012;172(17):1285.
36. Summerson JH, Koren JC, Dignan MB. Association between exercise and other preventive health behaviors among diabetics. *Public Health Reports*. 1991;106:543–547.
37. Tsiani E, Giacca A. Exercise and diabetes. *Canadian Journal of Diabetes*. 1999;22:39–46.

38. Wallberg-Henriksson H. Exercise and diabetes mellitus. *Exercise and Sport Sciences Reviews.* 1992;20:339–368.
39. Weiner RB, Wang F, Isaacs SK, Malhotra R, Berkstresser B, Kim JH, Hutter AM Jr, Picard MH, Wang TJ, Baggish AL. Blood pressure and left ventricular hypertrophy during American-style football participation. *Circulation.* 2013;128(5):524–531.
40. Weston KS, Wisløff U, Coombes JS. High-intensity interval training in patients with lifestyle-induced cardiometabolic disease: A systematic review and meta-analysis. *British Journal of Sports Medicine.* 2014;48(16):1227–1234.
41. White R, Sherman C. Exercise in diabetes management: Maximizing benefits, controlling risks. *Physician and Sportsmedicine.* 1999;27(4):63–76.

Appendix A: Sports Medicine Resource Guides

Richard B. Birrer, Francis G. O'Connor, and Shawn F. Kane

Position Statements and Guidelines
American College of Sports Medicine
Indianapolis, IN
www.acsm.org

American Medical Society for Sports Medicine
Leawood, Kansas
www.amssm.org

Appendix B: Types of Sports

Richard B. Birrer, Francis G. O'Connor, and Shawn F. Kane

Category I: Collision

Boxing
Football, tackle
Martial arts, full contact

Category II: Contact

Basketball
Baseball/softball
Wrestling
Soccer
Rugby
Lacrosse
Judo
Football, flag
Martial arts
Volleyball
Parachuting
Hockey
Cricket

Category III: Endurance

Trampolining
Track and field events
Jogging/walking
Sledding/tobogganing/luge
Racquet sports
Skateboarding
Cycling
Surfing
Swimming
Skating (roller/ice)
Rowing
Diving, scuba
Skiing
Water polo
Gymnastics
Handball
Climbing/hiking/mountaineering/orienteering
Ultimate Frisbee
Kayak
Dance
Cheerleading
Auto racing

Category IV: Nonendurance/sedentary

Golf
Bowling
Ballooning
Croquet
Gliding
Fishing
Flying
Yoga
Sailing
Diving
Shooting
Weightlifting
Horseshoe pitching
Caving
Camping
Billiards/snooker
Archery
Equestrian activities

Note: Classification represents a summary of average performance levels. Many sports could be placed in alternate categories under special circumstances. For example, the use of light weights numerous times during weightlifting would classify weightlifting as an endurance sport (i.e., circuit weight training), and the aerobic practice of a soft martial arts style such as Pakua would make it an endurance sport.

Appendix C: Sports and Sports Medicine Organizations

Richard B. Birrer, Francis G. O'Connor, and Shawn F. Kane

Academy for Sports Dentistry (ASD)
Farmersville, IL
www.academyforsportsdentistry.org

Amateur Athletic Union
AAU National Headquarters
Lake Buena Vista, FL
www.aauathletics.org
www.aausports.org

American Academy of Podiatric Sports Medicine (AAPSM)
Walkersville, MD
www.aapsm.org

Shape America (formerly American Alliance for Health, Physical Education, Recreation, and Dance)
Reston, VA
www.shapeamerica.org

American College of Sports Medicine (ACSM)
Indianapolis, IN
www.acsm.org

American Medical Athletic Association (formerly American Medical Joggers Association [AMJA])
Bethesda, MD

American Medical Society for Sports Medicine
Leawood, KS
www.amssm.org

American Orthopedic Society for Sports Medicine
Rosemont, IL
www.sportsmed.org

American Osteopathic Academy of Sports Medicine
Madison, WI
www.aoasm.org

American Physical Therapy Association (APTA)
Alexandria, VA
www.apta.org

Canadian Academy of Sport and Exercise Medicine (CASEM)
Ottawa, Ontario, Canada
www.Casem-acsme.org

International Federation of Sports Medicine
Lausanne, Switzerland
www.FIMS.org

International Olympic Committee
Lausanne, Switzerland
www.olympic.org

National Academy of Sports Medicine
Chandler, AZ
www.nasm.org

National Athletic Trainers Association (NATA)
Carrollton, TX
www.nata.org

National Collegiate Athletic Association
Indianapolis, IN
www.ncaa.org

National Federation of State High School Athletic Associations
Indianapolis, IN
www.nfhs.org

National High School Athletic Coaches Association
Easton, PA
www.nhsca.org

National Strength and Conditioning Association
Colorado Springs, CO
www.nsca.com

President's Council on Physical Fitness and Sports
Rockville, MD
www.fitness.gov
www.usa.gov

United States Olympic Committee
Colorado Springs, CO
www.teamusa.org

Appendix D: Medical Supplies and Equipment

Richard B. Birrer, Francis G. O'Connor, and Shawn F. Kane

First aid supplies

Examination gloves
Notebook and pencils
First aid manual
Various sizes of bandages
Gauze pads 2 × 2, 4 × 4 in.
Gauze rolls 2 and 4 in.
Adhesive tape: 1/2 × 2 in.
Scissors (surgical and 3 in. straight)
Elastic underwrap
Cotton
Razor and shaving cream
Finger splints: 1/2 and 2 in.
Tongue depressors
Wound irrigation materials:
  Povidone-iodine solution (Betadine®)/hydrogen peroxide
  Sterile normal saline
  10–50 cc syringes
Antibiotic ointment (Bacitracin® or Betadine®)
Alcohol swabs
Nail clippers
Tourniquet
Acetaminophen (Tylenol®)
Aspirin
NSAID of choice
Ammonia smelling salts
Saline in plastic squeeze bottle
Water in plastic squeeze bottle
Ethyl chloride spray
Petroleum jelly
Flashlight/penlight
Benzoin spray (firm grip)
Tape remover
Dental cotton rolls
Assorted felt/foam rubber
Container for sharps
List of contents

First aid equipment

Double-action bolt cutter (1)
Screwdrivers: Phillips, regular (2)
Stretcher (1)
Backboard (short aluminum recommended) (1)
Blankets, Army (2)
Blanket, Mylar space (1)
Sandbags, 4–5 lb (4)
Cervical collar, semi-rigid (1)
Crutches, adjustable lengths (2 pairs)
Slings, plus safety pins as required for muslin type (3)
Splints, upper and lower extremity (2 each)
Sling psychrometer or a device with humidity/temperature/activity risk chart (1)
Knee immobilizer
Elastic bandages: 3, 4, and 6 in. (12 each)
Ice, with small plastic bags to contain it
Styptic pencil
Weight scale
Chart for recording athletes' weights
Water containers, 5 gal (2)
Towels
Thomas 1/2 ring
Tables for examination, taping, treatments
Refrigerator
Whirlpool bath(s)
Telephone (coins available if pay phone)
Bulletin board for emergency phone numbers
List of phone numbers of each athlete's parents or guardian
Locked cabinet for medication
Sphygmomanometer (appropriate sizes)
Stethoscope
Goniometer
Stop watch
Skin staple application
Tape measure
Snellen chart
Thermometer
Skin calipers
Illness/injury patient care instructions
List of contents

Cardiopulmonary resuscitation crash kit

Equipment

1. Oral airways (small, medium, and large)
2. Mouth-to-mouth mask
3. Ambu bag with face mask (appropriate size) and adapter for endotracheal tubes
4. Endotracheal tubes, cuffed (small, medium, and large)
5. Disposable laryngoscope with light source
6. Cricothyrotomy kit
7. Syringe (50 mL) and large catheter for suction
8. 5 and 10 cc syringes with 22-gauge needles
9. 14-gauge angiocatheter
10. Automated external defibrillator

Drugs

1. Atropine sulfate, 2 mg in injectable prefilled syringe (10 mL)
2. Epinephrine, 1:10,000 in injectable prefilled syringe (10 mL)
3. Lidocaine hydrochloride, 100 mg in injectable prefilled syringe (5 mL)
4. Sodium bicarbonate, 50 mEq in injectable prefilled syringe (50 mL)
5. Lactated Ringer's (500 mL) and 5% dextrose (500 mL) with tubing and catheters
6. Nitroglycerin, 0.4 mg sublingual tablets
7. Morphine sulfate, 15 mg Tubex® with syringe
8. Meperidine, 100 mg in 2 mL ampoule
9. Furosemide, 40 mg IU ampoule
10. Diazepam (Valium®), 10 mg in prefilled syringe
11. 50% dextrose in water in a prefilled syringe
12. Dexamethasone (Decadron®), 24 mg/mL, 5 mL vial
13. Short-acting beta-agonist inhaler

The sports medicine bag

1. Tongue depressors
2. Padded tongue blade
3. Lidocaine 1% plain
4. Metaproterenol (Alupent®) inhaler
5. Ophthalmologic irrigating solution and eye cup
6. Fluorescein dye strips (3) for staining cornea
7. Tetracaine (Pontocaine®), 0.5%, 2 mL ampoule
8. Small eye spud
9. Sodium sulfacetamide (Sulamyd®) eye drops or ointment
10. Sterile suture set (1) with scalpel and #10 and #11 blades
11. Plastic suture material 5–0, 6–0 (2 each) with swaged PRE-2 needles
12. Ster-I-Strip, 1/4 and 1/2 in. (2 packages each)
13. Tape adherent, 1 can
14. Sterile gloves (2 pairs)
15. Sterile gauze pads, 2 × 2 in., 3 × 3 in., 4 × 4 in. (3 ea)
16. Povidone-iodine (Betadine®) solution
17. ABD pads (2)
18. Medicine cups (2)
19. Cotton-tipped applicators (Q-tips®), 1 package
20. Betadine® ointment
21. 8 in. heavy-duty bandage scissors
22. Swiss army knife with as many gadgets as possible
23. Disposable flashlight (1)
24. Elastic bandages: 3, 4, and 6 in. (1 each)
25. Prewrap foam bandage, 3 in. (1)
26. Elastic tape: 1 and 3 in. (2 each)
27. Cotton web roll, 4 in. (2)
28. Tufskin® (Cramer), 1 can
29. Skin lube® (Cramer), 1 tube
30. Plastic foam sheet, 3/4 in. thick
31. Felt padding, 3/8 in. (4 × 4 in. sheet)
32. Cyanoacrylate (Super Glue®) (1)
33. Stethoscope
34. Aneroid manometer
35. Reflex hammer
36. Ophthalmoscope-otoscope
37. Thermometer
38. Orthoplast® sheet (6 × 6 in.)
39. Band-Aids®, all sizes
40. Moleskin® (6 × 6 in.)
41. Rubber suction device for contact lens removal
42. Alcohol swabs
43. Nasostat®/tampons, regular (2)
44. Hemostat or tongue forceps
45. Two-way radio pager or mobile phone
46. Eye patches (2)
47. 3 and 5 cc syringe (1 each) with 22- and 25-gauge needles (2 each)
48. Antibiotics (penicillin, tetracycline, erythromycin, trimethoprim)
49. Topical antifungal
50. NSAID of choice
51. Ear drops
52. Cold medication of choice
53. Insect repellant
54. Sunscreen (SPF 15)
55. Scalpels (#11, 15) 1 each
56. Prescription blanks
57. 30% ferric subsulfate (Monsel's solution) for abrasions and cuts
58. Hank's balanced salt solution for dental avulsions
59. Small mirror
60. List of contents

REFERENCES

American Academy of Family Physicians (AAFP), American Academy of Orthopaedic Surgeons (AAOS), American College of Sports Medicine (ACSM), American Medical Society for Sports Medicine (AMSSM), American Orthopaedic Society for Sports Medicine (AOSSM), and the American Osteopathic Academy of Sports Medicine (AOASM), Sideline preparedness for the team physician: A consensus statement, 2000.

Ray, R.L. and Feld, F.X., The team physician's medical bag, *Clin. Sports Med.*, 8(1), 139–146, 1989.

Appendix E: Injury Surveillance and Prevention Organizations

Richard B. Birrer, Francis G. O'Connor, and Shawn F. Kane

Aerobics and Fitness Association of America (AFAA)
Sherman Oaks, CA
www.afaa.com
Joint survey of injuries incurred by 10,000 exercise instructors, including frequency, type, severity, and location of injuries.

American Aerobic Association International
New Hope, PA
www.aaai-ismafitness.com
Survey of 3,000 aerobics instructors and 30,000 participants, on injury severity, anatomic sites of injury, and equipment associated with specific injuries.

Cooper Institute for Aerobics Research (CIAR)
Dallas, TX
www.cooperinstitute.org
Survey of patients at Cooper Clinic regarding lifetime exercise patterns and orthopedic injury rates, plus planned study of relationship to baseline musculoskeletal fitness.

IDEA Health and Fitness Association (originally International Dance-Exercise Association)
San Diego, CA
www.ideafit.com
Multiple articles on training injuries and prevention

National Athletic Trainers Association (NATA)
Carrollton, TX
www.nata.org
Statistics, guidelines, and similar research on high school and collegiate sports

National Collegiate Athletic Association (NCAA) Injury Surveillance System
Indianapolis, IN
www.datalyscenter.org/programs/ncaa-injury-surveillance-program/
Tracks injuries in football, men's and women's soccer, lacrosse, gymnastics, women's volleyball, field hockey, ice hockey, wrestling, softball, and baseball from 10% of NCAA member schools that participate in a given sport. Includes type of injury, severity of injury, body part injured, cause of injury, field type, field condition, position played, special equipment worn, and time of season.

Nationwide Children's
Columbus, OH
www.nationwidechildrens.org/cirp-rio-study-reports
Captures high school athletic exposure (number of athlete practices and number of athlete competitions per week), injury (body site, diagnosis, severity, etc.), and injury event (mechanism, activity, position/event, field/court location, etc.) data weekly throughout the academic year using certified athletic trainers (ATCs) as data reporters.

The National Injury Information Clearinghouse/National Electronic Injury Surveillance System (NEISS)
Division of Hazard and Injury Data Systems
U.S. Consumer Product Safety Commission
Bethesda, MD
www.cpsc.gov
Collects, investigates, analyzes, and disseminates injury data (age, sex, diagnosis, body part injured, type of treatment, and location where accident occurred) and information relating to the causes and prevention of death, injury, and illness associated with consumer products.

National Safety Council (NSC)
Itasca, IL
Customer Service: customerservice@nsc.org
www.nsc.org
Data on number of participants, number and severity of injuries, and the number of facilities in 30 sports.

National Spinal Cord Injury Statistical Center (NSCISC)
Birmingham, AL
www.nscisc.uab.edu/sci-model-systems.aspx
Email: nscisc@uab.edu
A national network established to support and direct the collection, management, and analysis of the world's largest and longest spinal cord injury research database.

Prevent Blindness (formerly National Society to Prevent Blindness)
Chicago, IL
www.preventblindness.org
Collects and analyzes data on sports-related eye injuries.

Sport Safety International
Promotes injury prevention and safe participation in physical activity and sports by providing the highest quality educational programming to athletes, parents, coaches, and sports medicine professionals.
www.sportsafetyinternational.org

ThinkFirst (formerly National Injury Prevention Foundation)
Naperville, IL
www.ThinkFirst.org
Injury research in conjunction with other organizations.

Appendix F: Sports Classification

Richard B. Birrer, Francis G. O'Connor, and Shawn F. Kane

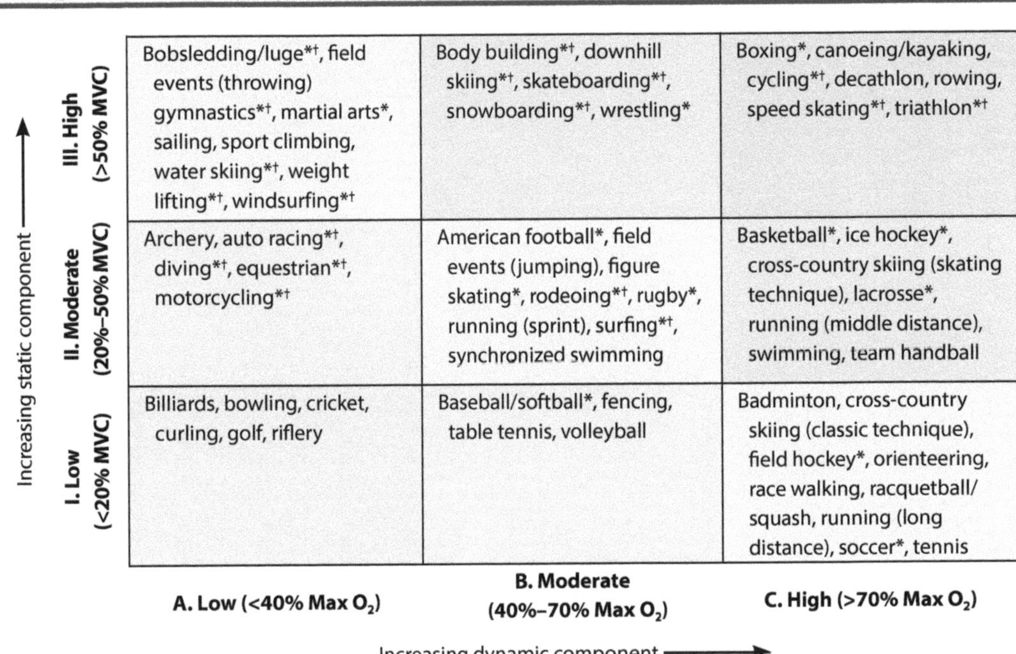

FIGURE F.1 Classification of sports. This classification is based on peak static and dynamic components achieved during competition. It should be noted, however, that higher values may be reached during training. The increasing dynamic component is defined in terms of the estimated percent of maximal oxygen uptake ($MaxO_2$) achieved and result in an increasing cardiac output. The increasing static component is related to the estimated percent of maximal voluntary contraction (MVC) reached and result in an increasing blood pressure load. The lowest total cardiovascular demands (cardiac output and blood pressure) are shown in green and the highest in red, blue, yellow, and orange depict low moderate, moderate, and high moderate total cardiovascular demands. *Danger of bodily collision. †Increased risk if syncope occurs. (From Task Force 8: Classification of sports, *J. Am. Coll. Cardiol.*, 45(8), 1364, 2005.)

Appendix G: Therapeutic Exercises for the Injured Athlete

Robert M. Barney Poole

Physical therapy in the rehabilitation of an injured athlete involves a variety of range-of-motion and strengthening exercises to restore the function of each injured body part.

G.1 SHOULDER RANGE OF MOTION

Active-assisted or passive-assisted range of motion in flexion for the shoulder, using a T-bar (Figures G.1 through G.3).

G.2 SHOULDER STRENGTHENING

High-repetition, low-weight, isotonic exercise incorporating eccentric and concentric contractions (Figures G.4 through G.8).

G.3 ELBOW

Stretching and strengthening using high-repetition, low-weight, isotonic exercise incorporating eccentric and concentric contractions (Figures G.9 through G.15).

G.4 KNEE

Strengthening and stretching, by means of isometric and isotonic exercise incorporating high-repetition, low-weight exercises (Figures G.16 through G.22).

G.5 ANKLE

Stretching and strengthening using high-repetition, low-weight exercises incorporating eccentric and concentric contractions (Figures G.23 through G.28).

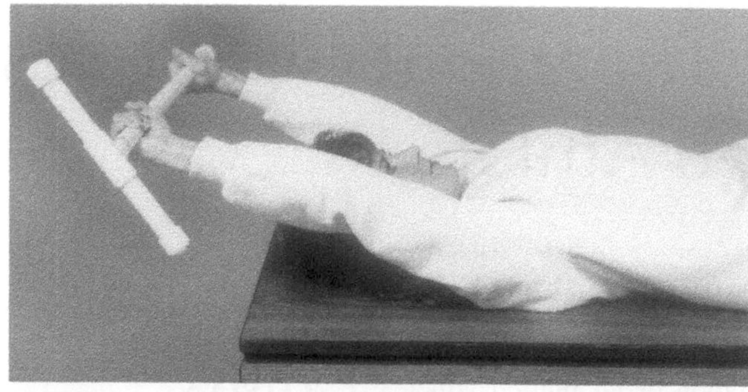

FIGURE G.1 *Shoulder flexion:* The athlete is positioned supine, gripping the stick with both hands, which are a shoulder-width apart. Move the arms over the head as far as possible and hold for 5 counts. Relax. Complete 5 sets of 10 repetitions, three times a day.

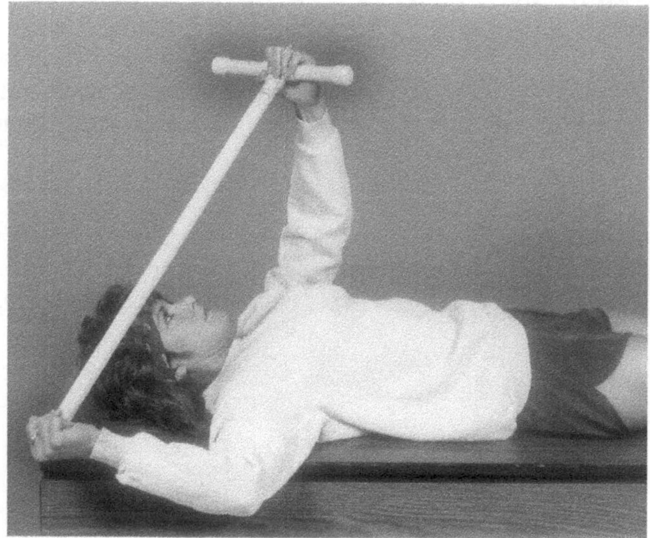

FIGURE G.2 *Shoulder external rotation:* The athlete is positioned supine with the arm abducted to 90°. Push the arm down toward the floor into external rotation and hold for 5 counts. Relax. Complete 5 sets of 10 repetitions, three times a day.

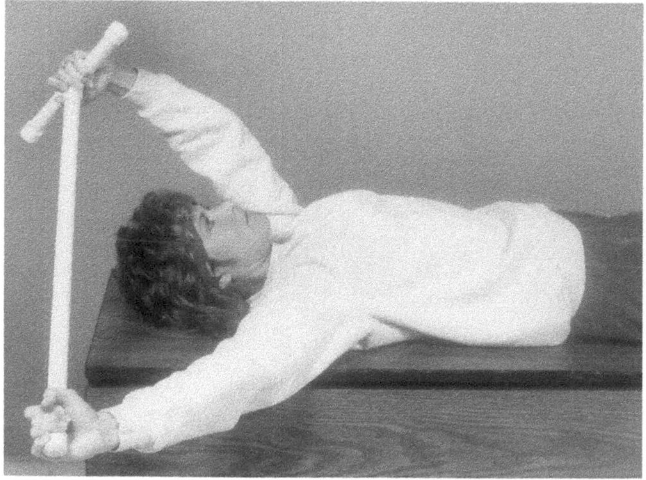

FIGURE G.3 *Shoulder abduction:* The athlete is positioned supine and uses the T-bar to push/pull the arm into abduction. (The arm must remain on the table to get the maximum benefit from this exercise.) Hold for 5 counts. Relax. Repeat 5 sets of 10 repetitions, three times a day.

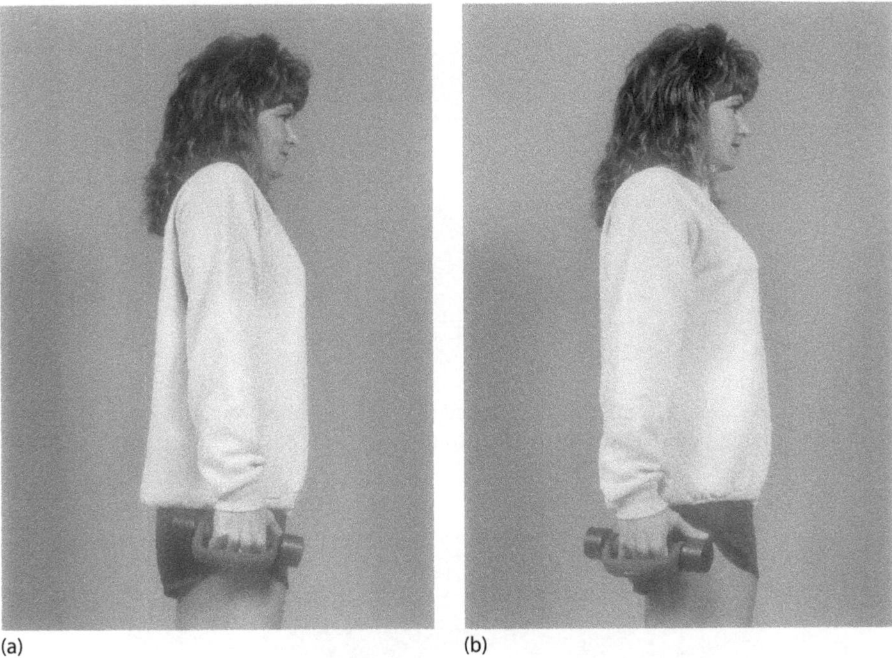

(a) (b)

FIGURE G.4 *Shoulder shrugs:* The athlete stands with the arms straight down at the sides and a 1 lb weight in each hand. (a) Lift the shoulders up toward the ears as far as possible and hold for 5 counts, then (b) pull them back, pinching the shoulder blades together. Again, hold for 5 counts. Relax the shoulders slowly. Repeat 5 sets of 10, gradually increasing the weight to 5 lbs.

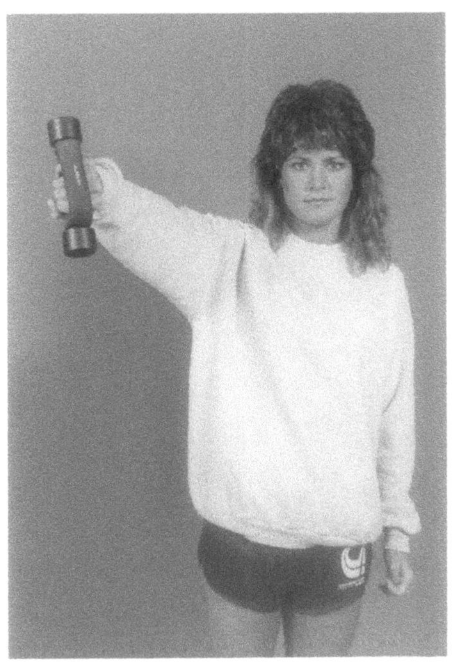

FIGURE G.5 *Supraspinatus strengthening:* The athlete stands with the affected arm straight at the side and the thumb joint pointed down. Raise the arm from this point to eye level, holding for 5 counts. Relax. Repeat 5 sets of 10, three times a day, gradually progressing from 1 to 5 lbs, as tolerated.

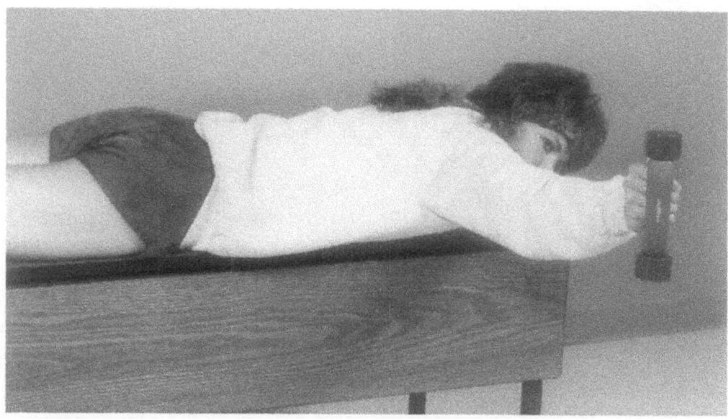

FIGURE G.6 *Prone horizontal abduction:* The athlete is positioned prone with the involved arm hanging straight toward the floor. Raise the arm to eye level, keeping the thumb pointed up toward the ceiling. Hold for 5 counts. Relax. Repeat 5 sets of 10, progressing from 1 to 5 lbs as tolerated.

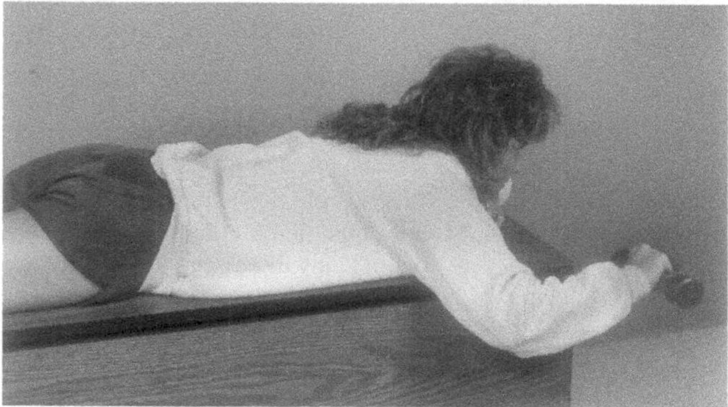

FIGURE G.7 *Prone external rotation:* The athlete lies prone with the arm at 90° of abduction, the elbow bent to 90°, and the forearm hanging straight down from the table. With the thumb pointed toward the body, lift the arm into external rotation to eye level. Hold for 5 counts. Relax. Repeat 5 sets of 10, progressing from 1 to 5 lbs as tolerated.

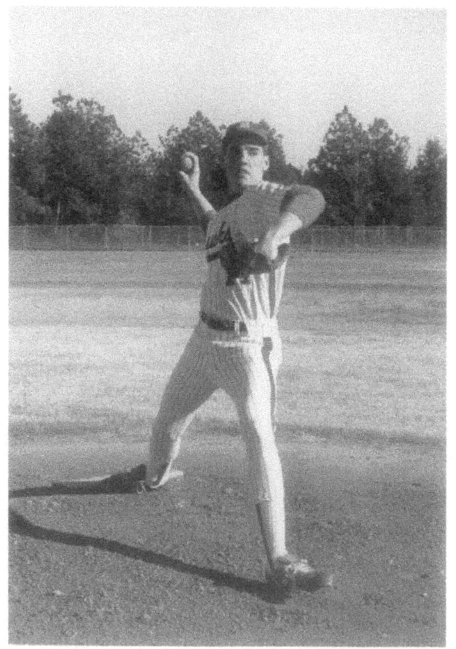

FIGURE G.8 A return-to-throwing program gradually progresses the throwing athlete back to competition. A program of short- and long-toss sessions is completed twice per day for two successive days, followed by a day of rest and then two more days of throwing.

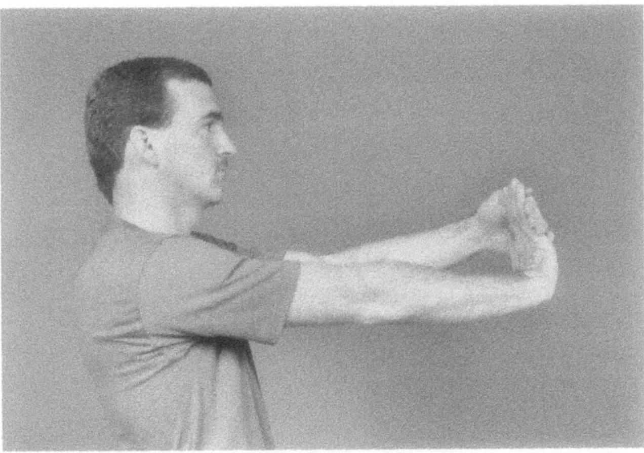

FIGURE G.9 *Stretching flexors:* With the elbow straightened, grasp the middle of the hand and thumb and pull the wrist back toward the elbow. Hold for 10 counts. Relax slowly. Repeat 3 sets of 10, three times a day.

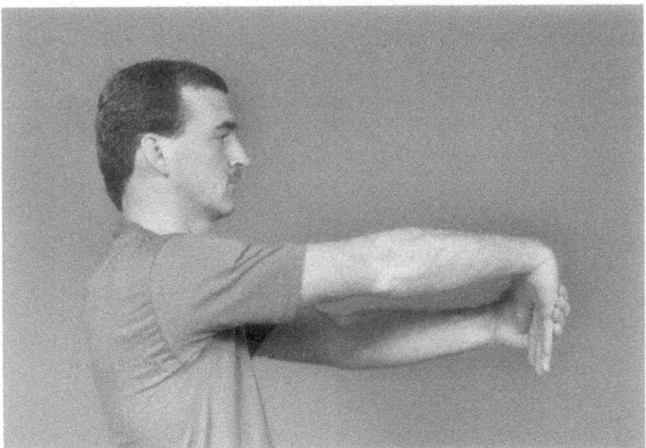

FIGURE G.10 *Stretching extensors:* With the elbow straightened, grasp the back of the hand and thumb and pull back toward the elbow. Hold for 10 counts. Relax slowly. Repeat 3 sets of 10, three times a day.

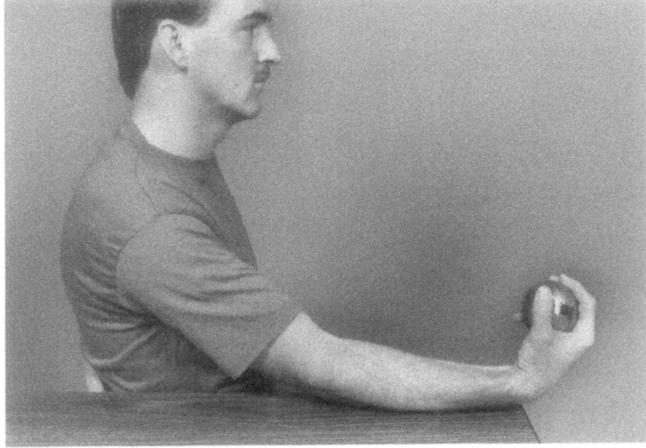

FIGURE G.11 *Wrist flexion curls:* The forearm is comfortably supported on a table with the hand over the edge, palm up. Using a 1 lb weight, curl the wrist up as far as possible and hold for 5 counts. Relax slowly. Repeat 5 sets of 10, three times a day, gradually progressing from 1 to 5 lbs, as tolerated.

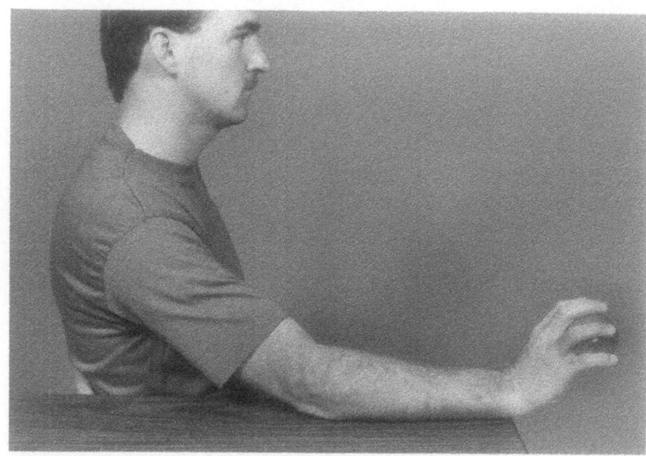

FIGURE G.12 *Wrist extension curls:* The forearm is supported comfortably on a table with the hand over the edge, palm down. Using a 1 lb weight, curl the wrist up as far as possible and hold for 5 counts. Relax slowly. Repeat 5 sets of 10, three times a day, gradually progressing from 1 to 5 lbs, as tolerated.

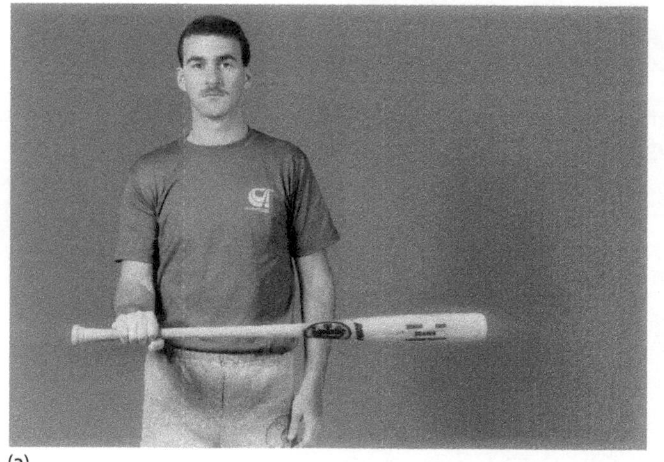

(a)

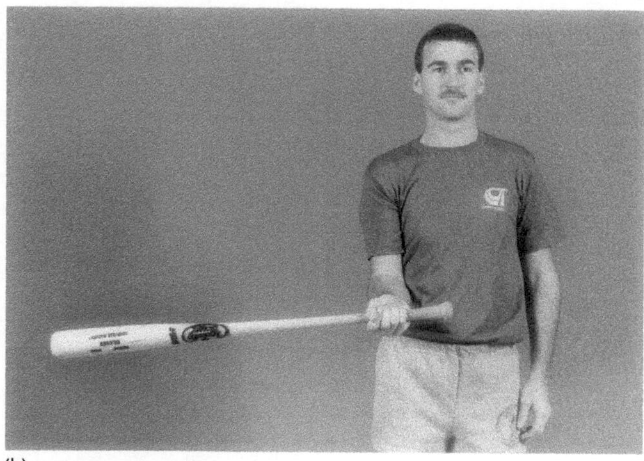

(b)

FIGURE G.13 *Pronation/supination using a baseball bat:* With the arm held at the side, bend the elbow to 90°, then grasp the middle of the bat with the arm in the neutral position. (a) Move the wrist and arm into pronation as far as possible and hold for 5 counts. (b) Move the arm slowly back to neutral and then into full supination, again holding for 5 counts. Relax briefly in neutral and repeat 3 sets of 10, three times a day. The resistance may be increased by moving the hand toward the end of the bat. *Note:* To make exercise more interesting, use objects with which the athlete is familiar.

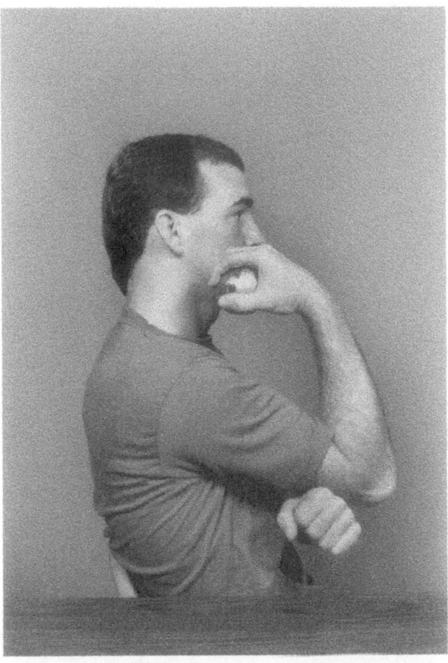

FIGURE G.14 *Biceps curl:* The straightened elbow is supported by the opposite arm, then bent as far as possible and slowly returned to full extension. Begin with a 2 lb weight and work up to 5 sets of 10 repetitions, five times a day, progressing to 10 lbs, as tolerated.

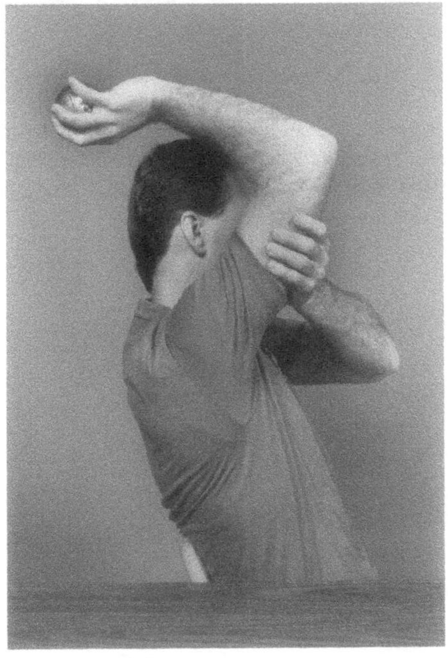

FIGURE G.15 *Triceps curl:* The straightened arm is supported by the opposite hand at the elbow with the arm raised overhead. Bend the elbow as far as possible and then slowly straighten it to full extension. Begin with a 2 lb weight and progress to 5 lbs as tolerated. Repeat 5 sets of 10 repetitions, three times a day. *Note:* Therapeutic putty is a good adjunct to an elbow program and is used to maintain strength and function.

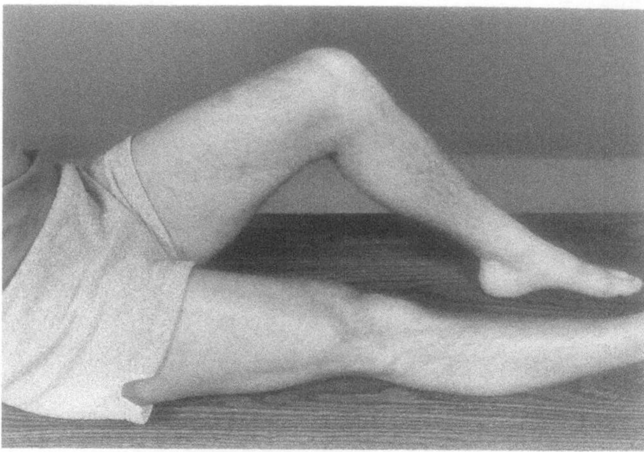

FIGURE G.16 *Quadriceps exercise:* A gradual isometric contraction of the quadriceps is performed by straightening the leg as much as possible. The patella should track proximally. Hold for 5 counts each and perform frequently during the day.

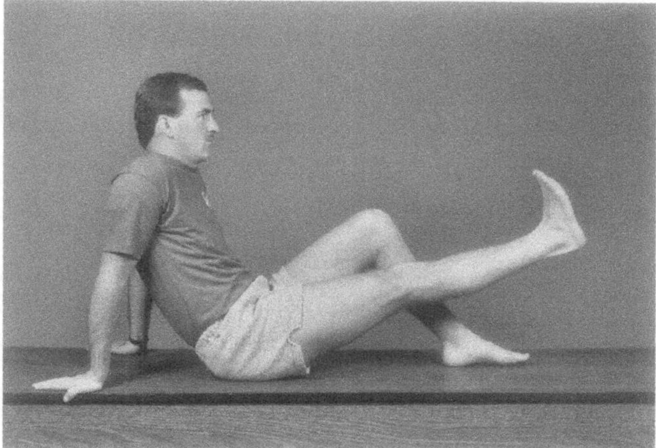

FIGURE G.17 *Straight leg raise:* The athlete is positioned semi-reclined or supine with the opposite leg flexed to 90° and the foot planted flat next to the involved knee. Contract the quadriceps and lift the left 45°. Hold this position for at least 5 counts, then slowly lower the leg to the floor. Relax and repeat. Lifts are done in sets of 10 with a 30 second rest between each set, three times a day. Weight is applied to the ankle for resistance. Gradually progress from 1 to 5 lbs, as tolerated.

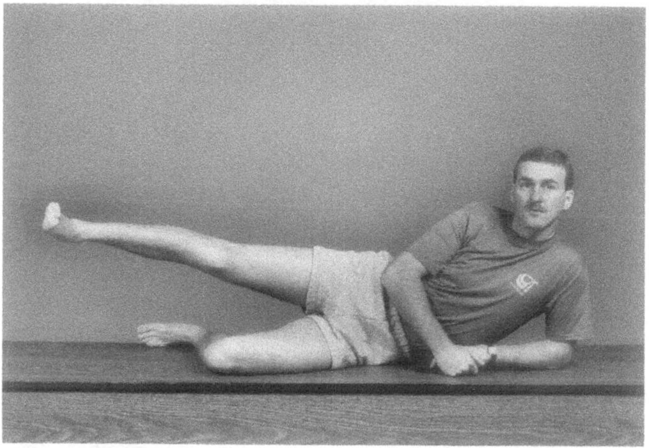

FIGURE G.18 *Hip abduction exercises:* The athlete is positioned side-lying with the unaffected knee flexed to 90° and the hip flexed at 45°. The affected leg is straight, and the body weight is shifted forward. Lift the leg and hold for 5 counts, then slowly lower it back to the starting position. Resistance can be added at the ankle, from 1 to 5 lbs, as tolerated. Repeat 5 sets of 10 repetitions, three times a day.

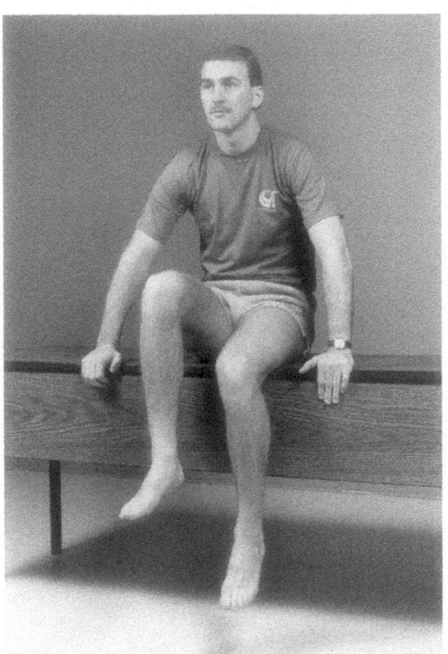

FIGURE G.19 *Hip flexion exercise:* The athlete is placed in a seated position. Lift the knee toward the chest at a 45° angle and hold for 5 counts. Slowly lower the knee and place the foot on the floor. Repeat 5 sets of 10 repetitions, three times a day. Resistance can be added gradually on top of the thigh, from 1 to 5 lbs, as tolerated.

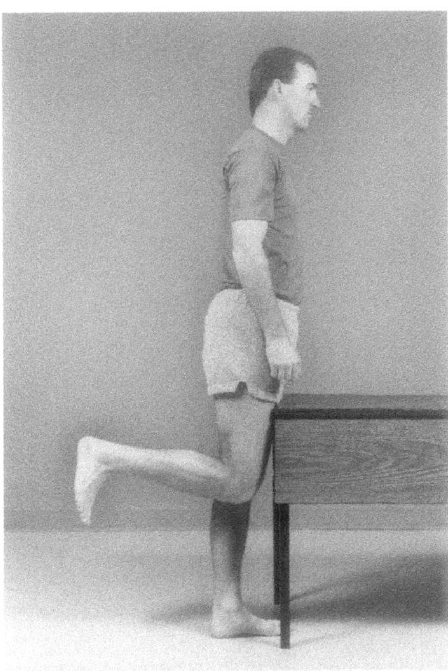

FIGURE G.20 *Hamstring curl:* The athlete stands with the thigh pressed against a wall or table to block hip flexion. Flex the knee as much as possible and hold for 5 counts. Slowly return to the starting position. Repeat 5 sets of 10, three times a day. Resistance can be added to the ankle, from 1 to 5 lbs, as tolerated.

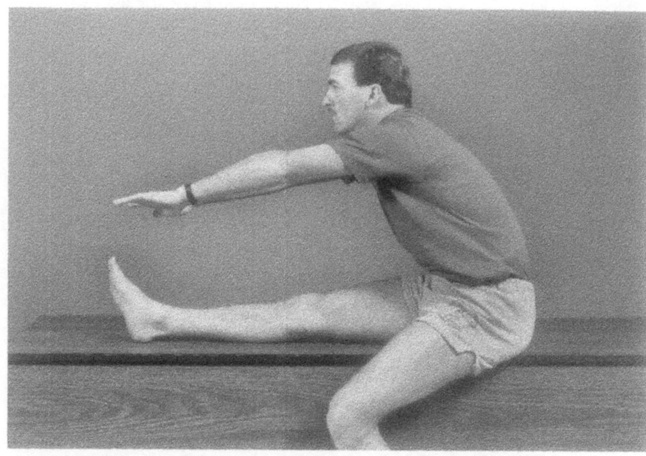

FIGURE G.21 *Hamstring stretch:* The athlete is in a sitting position with one leg off the exercise table. The back is straight, and the leg to be stretched is straight. Reach forward slowly and hold for 10 counts. Stretch for at least 5 minutes, three times a day. Do not bounce when stretching.

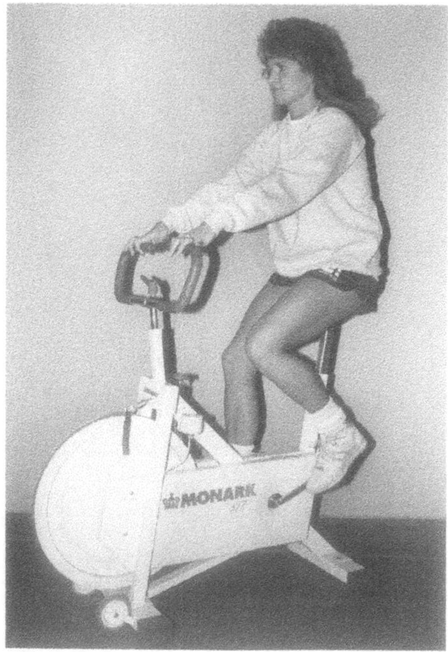

FIGURE G.22 *Exercise bike:* The exercise bicycle is a good way for athletes to increase endurance, strength, and range of motion. The bend in the knee should be 15° when the foot is at the bottom of the pedal stroke. Progress from 10 minutes at minimum resistance to 30 minutes, twice a day.

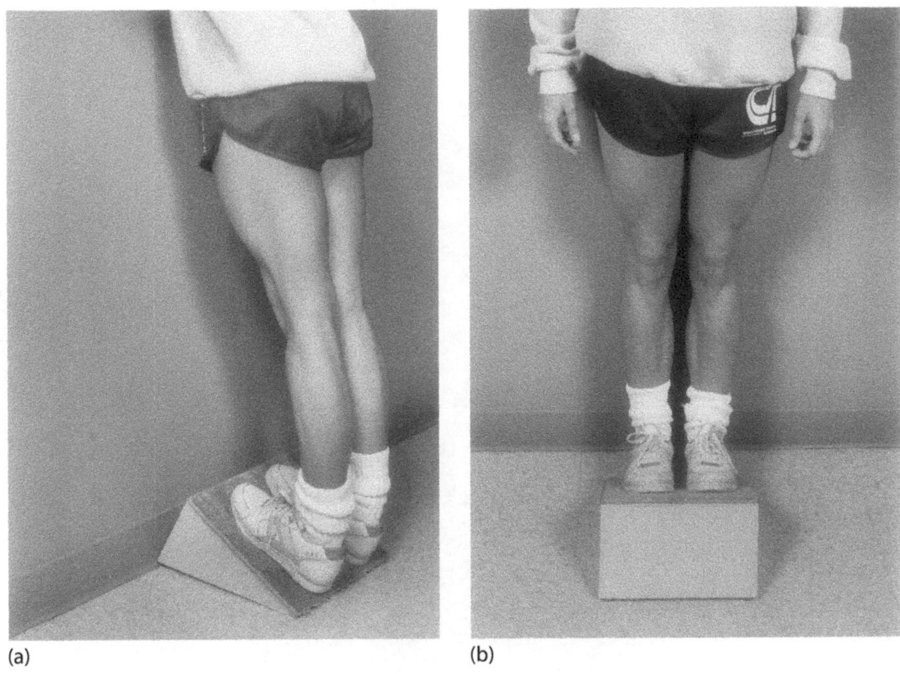

(a) (b)

FIGURE G.23 *Heelcord Stretching Using a Heelcord Box:* The feet should be positioned on the heelcord box for a comfortable, sustained stretch of about 5 minutes, three to five times daily. The box may be positioned with the higher edge (a) toward or (b) away from the wall. Heelcord stretching is especially important both *before* and *after* sports activities.

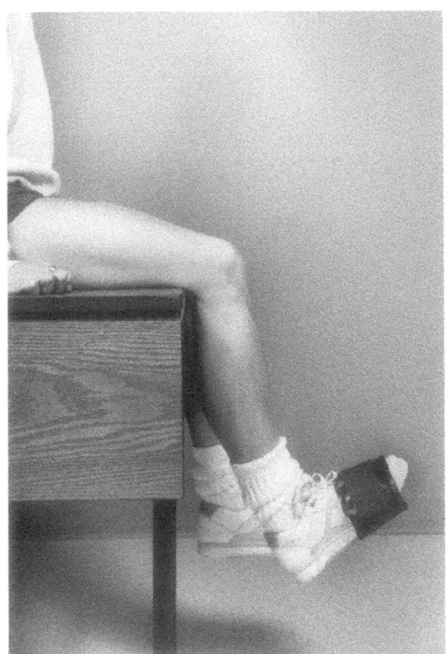

FIGURE G.24 *Anterior tibialis strengthening:* The athlete sits with the foot off the floor. With a 1 lb weight attached to the forefoot, pull the foot up as far as possible and hold for 5 counts. Relax slowly and repeat 5 sets of 10 repetitions, three times a day. Progress from 1 to 5 lbs, as tolerated.

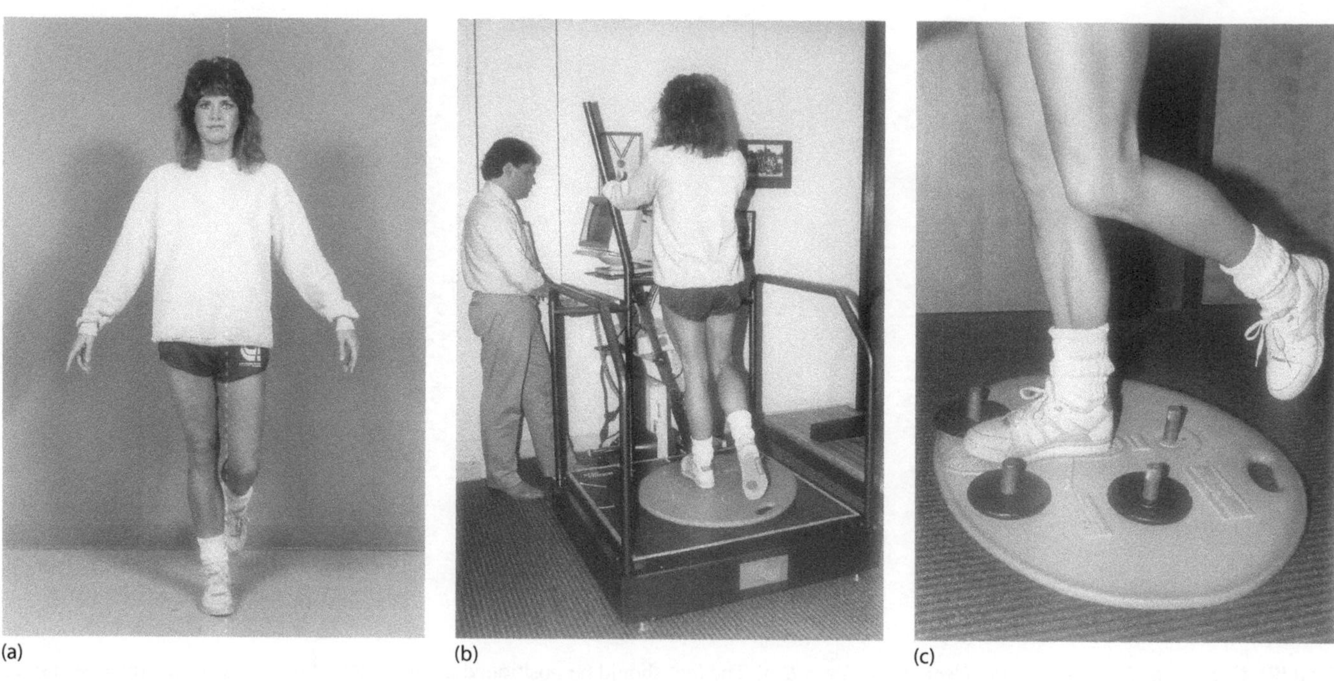

(a) (b) (c)

FIGURE G.25 *Proprioception exercises:* These may range from simple exercises, such as (a) balancing while standing on one foot, to more complex exercises. (b) The ankle balance board may be weighted to provide strengthening along with proprioception. (c) The new Star Station by Camp Corporation gives a computer-produced color printout of pressure monitored by a pressure-sensitive network beneath the balance board. This is possibly the most complex of all proprioception devices.

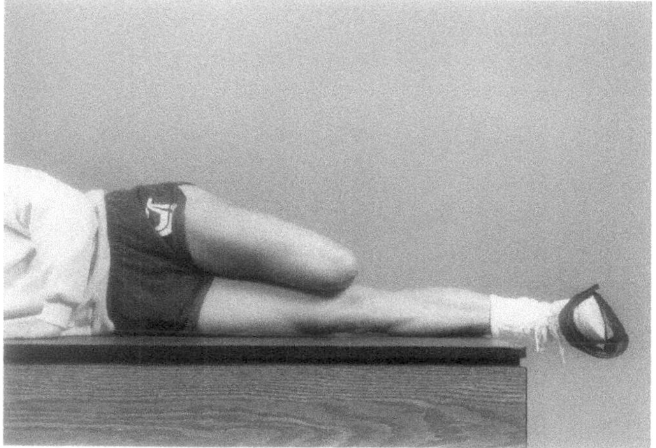

FIGURE G.26 *Peroneal strengthening:* The athlete lies on the involved side with the involved foot over the edge of the table. With a 1 lb weight placed on the forefoot, turn the lateral side of the foot up and hold for 5 counts. Relax slowly. Repeat 5 sets of 10 repetitions, progressing from 1 to 5 lbs, as tolerated.

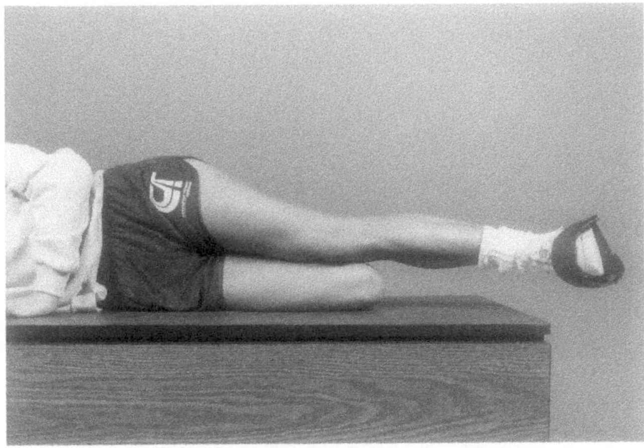

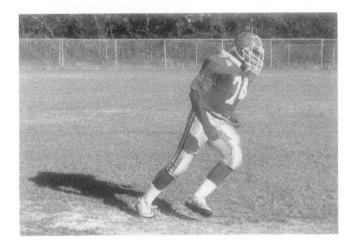

FIGURE G.27 *Posterior tibialis strengthening:* The athlete lies on the involved side with the involved foot over the edge of the table and a 1 lb weight on the forefoot. Turn the medial side of the foot up and hold for 5 counts. Relax slowly. Repeat 5 sets of 10 repetitions, progressing from 1 to 5 lbs, as tolerated.

FIGURE G.28 *Return to running program*: The running athlete is gradually progressed from walking to a slow jog to full-speed running and agility drills, as tolerated.

Appendix H: Glossary

Richard B. Birrer, Francis G. O'Connor, and Shawn F. Kane

With the marked growth of the field of sports medicine over the past 20 years, a new vocabulary has emerged; therefore, physicians interested in this subject may be inundated with many new terms with which they have no previous familiarity. It is well known that medical schools are trying to teach students not to use proper names or slang terms, but as the field of sports medicine grows, so does the use of this strange vocabulary. Along with the new terms, sports medicine has also incorporated many of the long-term standards of orthopedics (indicated by an asterisk). The intent of this glossary is to clarify some of the communication problems primary care physicians will face in the care of athletes.

Apprehension shoulder: Feeling of instability in a subluxed or dislocated shoulder than has been reduced.

Athlete's foot: *Tinea pedis (ringworm of the foot); characterized by itching, fissure formation, and inflammation.

Athlete's kidney: Upper calyceal scarring, usually in the right kidney, following multiple traumatic punches.

Athlete's pseudoanemia: Dilutional effect caused by a proportionately greater increase in plasma volume than in red blood cell mass and hemoglobin.

Athletic pseudonephritis: Abnormal urine analysis secondary to exercise-induced renal ischemia.

Backpack palsy: Compression of the upper trunk of the brachial plexus from a heavy backpack.

Baker's cyst: *Popliteal cyst.

Barked shin: Contusive abrasion of the anterior surface of the tibia.

Barton's fracture: *Marginal fracture of distal radial rim due to extreme fixed dorsiflexion of the wrist in association with a pronating force.

Baseball elbow: Worn-out elbow joint seen in veteran pitchers.

Baseball finger: Avulsion of the extensor tendon from its attachment to the dorsal surface of the base of the terminal phalanx; also called mallet finger.

Bends: Arthralgias in scuba diving due to joint air emboli.

Bennett's fracture: *Fracture/dislocation of the carpal metacarpal of the thumb, with fracture of some portion of the medial proximal margin of the base of the metacarpal.

Biker's knee: Occurs when saddle is too high or too low, resulting in excessive patellar pressure, inflammation, and pain.

Black dot heel: Calcaneal petechiae secondary to running.

Black eye: Periorbital hematoma.

Black heel: Calcaneal petechiae secondary to repeated microtrauma (e.g., sudden stops and starts); also called talon noir.

Bladder knock: Microtrauma to bladder wall in long-distance runners, frequently resulting in hematuria.

Blocker's exostosis: See Tackler's exostosis.

Blocker's node: See Tackler's exostosis.

Blowout fracture: Fracture of the orbital floor manifested by limited eye motion and diplopia if the extraocular muscles (i.e., inferior rectus) are entrapped.

Bonking: Seen in endurance athletes when they run out of liver glycogen, presumably due to low blood sugar, causing the patient to get dizzy, shaky, confused, have cold sweats, and experience lack of coordination.

Boot-top fracture: Comminuted fracture at the junction of the middle and lower third of the tibia secondary to high-speed forward fall, angling leg over high, rigid ski boot.

Boutonniére deformity: *See Buttonhole deformity.

Bowler's finger: Perineural fibrosis of the dorsal branch of the radial digital nerve of the ring finger due to repetitive microtrauma.

Bowler's thumb: Digital neuroma of the ulnar digital nerve due to repetitive microtrauma of the thumb base against the hard edge of ball's thumbhole during delivery.

Boxer's elbow: Chip fractures and loose bodies in the elbow joint, produced by repetitive microtrauma in hyperextension (e.g., jabs).

Boxer's fracture: *Fracture of the neck of the fourth or fifth metacarpal.

Boxer's knuckle: Chronically inflamed metacarpal phalangeal bursa due to repetitive trauma.

Breaststroker's knee: Grade 1 medial collateral sprain resulting from the "whip kick."

Buddy system: Alignment of an injured digit to an adjacent digit in order to immobilize it (also, pairing off partners for safety, as in swimming).

Bullrider's thumb: Sprain of the radial collateral ligament and avulsion fracture of the radial portion of proximal phalanx during mechanical bull riding.

Burner: See Stinger.

Button: Chin.

Buttonhole deformity: Disruption of the central slip of the extensor digitorum communis tendon over the PIPJ.

Catcher's hand: Repetitive trauma to the ulnar artery along its course through Guyon's canal, leading to thrombosis and aneurysm.

Cauliflower ear: Ear deformity due to repeated hemorrhage and fibrosis of the perichrondrium and cartilage of the ear. Also called scrum ear and wrestler's ear.

Charley horse: *Contusion of elements of the quadricep muscles.

Chokes: Pulmonary air embolism from rapid diving ascent.

Clarinetist's thumb: Carpometacarpal and metacarpophalangeal joint strain of the dominant thumb in clarinet players.

Clicking hip: *See Snapping hip.

Clipping injury: Valgus force to the knee.

Clothesline injury: Direct blow to the larynx, with pain and difficulty in swallowing and inspiration; acute laryngospasm may occur.

Clutched thumb: *See Trigger finger.

Coaches' finger: Dislocation of the proximal interphalangeal (PIP) joint of the finger, usually middle phalanx dislocated dorsal to the proximal phalanx, generally as a result of hyperextension.

Colles' fracture: *Distal forearm fracture resulting from a fall on the outstretched hand causing dorsal displacement of the distal radius (dinner fork deformity).

Crabs: Pediculosis pubis.

Crazy bone: Contusion of ulnar nerve in the ulnar groove.

Cuber's thumb: Repeated thenar contusions while working Rubik's Cube.

Cyclist's nipple: Cold, painful nipples following exposure to cold during cycling.

Cyclist's palsy: See Handle-bar neuropathy.

Dart thrower's elbow: Olecranon bursitis.

Dead arm syndrome: Sharp paralyzing pain during the cocking phase of throwing due to shoulder subluxation.

Ding: Also known as "getting your bell rung"—a first-degree head concussion with no loss of consciousness, but the athlete may be slightly confused and have dizziness and ringing in the ears.

Drummer boy's palsy: Rupture of the extensor pollicis longus in drummers from repetitive thumb motion.

Ear squeeze: Pressure differential during diving descent, causing otalgia, decreased hearing, tinnitus, and occasionally blood-tinged sputum due to transudation and blood vessel rupture.

Egyptian foot: Condition in which the first metatarsal ray is the longest.

Exercise addiction: Negative withdrawal symptoms (e.g., feelings of guilt, irritability, anxiety, constipation, sleep disturbance) that occur after stopping long-term, intense, regular exercise program; may be endorphin mediated.

Fartlek: "Speed play"—unstructured program incorporating a combination of techniques such that repetition, interval, and continuous training are used in a single session.

Fighter's fracture: See Boxer's fracture.

Foot drop: *Loss of motor function caused by contusion of the peroneal nerve by a direct blow with significant swelling or hemorrhage.

Football acne: Acne underneath a football tackler's chin strap.

Football finger: See Jersey finger.

Footballer's (English) ankle: Tenderness over the talar bone of the ankle due to talotibial exostoses from repeated explosive push-offs.

Footballer's migraine: Migraine headache secondary to unexpected head blows (e.g., soccer, wrestling) and thought to be due to trauma-induced vasospasm.

Fungo: Three- to four-weeks rehabilitation for injured pitchers utilizing long, easy throws that progress to short, strong throws.

Gamekeeper's thumb: *Rupture or chronic laxity of the ulnar collateral ligament of the first metacarpal-phalangeal joint (thumb).

Golden period: First 20–30 minutes after an injury, when it is easy to identify pathology before swelling sets in.

Golfer's elbow: Medial epicondylitis.

Greek foot: Condition in which the second metatarsal ray is longer than first.

Groin pull: Strain of hip flexors or adductors.

Guitarist's cramp: Spontaneous flexion of the third metacarpophalangeal joint of the right third finger in guitarists.

Gymnast's wrist: Acute or chronic osseous or soft-tissue injury to the wrist in association with compression dorsiflexion forces of gymnastics.

Hammer toe: *Permanent flexion of the mid-phalangeal joint.

Hamstring pull/tear: Strain of the posterior thigh muscles.

Handle-bar neuropathy: Overuse syndrome associated with cycling, appearing as weakness and loss of coordination in one or both hands due to compression entrapment of the ulnar nerve in Guyon's canal.

Heat cramps: Muscle cramps, twitching, and spasms in the legs, arms, or back, presumably due to electrolyte imbalance.

Heat exhaustion: Weakness, sweating, or dizziness with normal body temperature after prolonged heat exposure; may be associated with dehydration and tachycardia.

Heat fatigue: Inefficient muscle function due to lack of heat acclimatization.

Heatstroke: Extreme hyperthermia with thermoregulatory failure and profound CNS, electrolyte, and metabolic abnormalities.

Heel spur syndrome: *Plantar fasciitis. Inflammation reaction at insertion of the plantar fascia into the calcaneus.

Herpes gladiatorium: Herpes simplex infection; occurs in wrestlers.

Hip pointer: A contusion of the iliac crest.

Hitting the wall: Sudden onset of fatigue and depression usually seen in hot weather among long-distance runners, probably due to depletion of blood glucose and muscle glycogen.

Hooker's elbow: Lateral epicondylitis secondary to "hooking" in ice fishing—repeated jerking on a fishing line attached to a wooden stick.

Hot shot: See Stinger.

Hot spots: Trigger points.
Housemaid's knee: *Prepatellar bursitis.
Hurdler's injury: Avulsion of ischial tuberosity at the attachment of the long end of the biceps femoris and the semitendinosus, due to forcible flexion of hip with knee extended.
Hutchinson's fracture: Push-off fracture of the distal radial styloid.
Impact impotence: Loss of erectile capacity in association with groin paresthesias secondary to long-distance cycling (>100 miles/week).
Jammed finger: *Collateral ligament injury, volar plate injury, articular fracture, or dislocation following a jam injury.
Javelin throwers elbow: Repetitive valgus stress to medial collateral ligament, causing a sprain or avulsion fracture of the olecranon tip following forceful extension.
Jersey finger: A jam injury; rupture of the flexor digitorum profundus, usually of the second or third finger.
Jock itch: Tinea cruris (ringworm of groin); may also be caused by monilia.
Jogger's foot: See Runner's foot.
Jogger's heel: Nonspecific heel pain possibly due to a heel spur, bursitis, fat pad atrophy, stress fracture, fasciitis, or entrapment of the terminal branches of the posterior tibial nerve.
Jogger's itch: See Judo itch.
Jogger's nipple: Repeated irritation of the nipples from shirt during running.
Jogger's penis: See Penile frostbite.
Joint mice: *Small, opaque, loose bodies, unattached to bone, and interspersed between joint surfaces.
Jones's fracture: *Diaphyseal fatigue fracture of the fifth metatarsal due to repetitive microtrauma.
Judo itch: Intense itching around ankles and wrists, working up extremities to hips and shoulders; appears after judo workouts and sweating.
Jumper's ankle: See Footballer's ankle.
Jumper's knee: Inflammation of the patellar tendon at its attachment to the inferior pole of the patella.
Karate fracture: See Boxer's fracture.
Karate knuckle: See Boxer's knuckle.
Linebacker's arm: See Tackler's exostosis.
Little League shoulder: Injury of the proximal humeral epiphysis.
Little Leaguer's elbow: *Medial, lateral, and posterior elbow pathology secondary to repetitive throwing in youngsters.
Locked knee: See Trick knee.
Maisonneuve fracture: *Fracture of the proximal fibula with sprain of the deltoid and tibiofibular ligaments.
Malicious malalignment syndrome (Patellofemoral pain or stress syndrome): Most common etiology of patellofemoral pain, caused by a broad pelvis, femoral anteversion, genu varum and recurvatum, tibia varum, bilateral medial squinting of the patellae, and compensatory foot pronation.
Mallet finger: See Baseball finger.
Marathon foot: Subungual bleeding due to microtrauma of long-distance running.
March fracture: *Fatigue or stress fracture of the metatarsal shaft (Deutschländer's disease).
Mat burn: See Strawberry.
Miner's elbow: Olecranon bursitis.
Miserable malalignment syndrome: See Malicious malalignment syndrome.
Morton's foot: *Second metatarsal longer than the first, which causes weight and distribution problems and pain.
Morton's neuroma: *Interdigital mechanical neuritis that eventually leads to a fibrous reaction producing a neuroma usually between the third and fourth toes.
Musher's knee: *Iliotibial band irritation casing lateral knee pain while "mushing" dog team, secondary to sharp backward kicking of the leg.
Nun's knee: *Prepatellar bursitis.
Oarsman's wrist: Traumatic tenosynovitis of the wrist radial extensors seen in rowers, canoeists, and weightlifters.
Overreaching: Short-term overtraining.
Overtraining: Chronic imbalance between exercise and recover, resulting in severe and prolonged fatigue.
Overuse syndrome: A wide variety of muscle, tendon, ligament, and bone injury due to repetitive microtrauma.
Pac-Man wrist: See Space Invaders wrist.
Paddle soreness: Ischial bursitis and pruritus ani in novice cyclists.
Patellofemoral pain syndrome: See Malicious or Miserable malalignment syndrome.
Penile frostbite: Superficial penile frostbite seen in joggers training in cold weather (jogger's penis), particularly among those who wear training gear made of polyester.
Pianist's cramp: Spontaneous flexion of the metacarpophalangeal joint of the fourth and/or fifth fingers of the right hand in pianists.
Pitcher's elbow: See Baseball elbow.
Piriformis syndrome: Buttock pain secondary to compression of the sciatic nerve by the piriformis muscle.
Prepatellar bursitis: See Housemaid's knee, Nun's knee, Roofer's knee.
Pudendal neuropathy: Compression of dorsal branch of pudendal nerve between bicycle seat and pubic symphysis.
Pump bump: Inflamed nodule lateral to calcaneal attachment of Achilles tendons.
Punch drunk: Permanent dementia pugilistica—neurologic sequela secondary to multiple blows to the head (e.g., boxing, steeplechase jockeys); slurred monotonous speech, dull facies, irritability, slowness of mentality, and tremor are characteristics.
Punch fracture: See Boxer's fracture.
Racquet player's pisiform: Subluxation of the pisiform with subsequent chondromalacia of the piso-triquetral

joint and possible compression of the ulnar nerve in Guyon's canal; seen in tennis, badminton, and squash.

Raspberry: See Strawberry.

Reverse Colles' fracture: See Smith's fracture.

Reverse ear squeeze: Distension of the tympanic membrane due to overpressurization.

Rider's strain: Strain of adductor longus muscle of the thigh, seen in horseback riders.

Ringman's shoulder: Asymptomatic cortical irregularity of the proximal humerus, seen in all-around gymnasts.

Roofer's knee: Prepatellar bursitis.

Runner's ache: Stitch or catch in the side, thought to be from stretching of the large intestine by a gas pocket.

Runner's bump: Os calcis bone spur from repetitive microtrauma.

Runner's diarrhea: See Runner's trots.

Runner's foot: Tarsal tunnel syndrome or medial plantar nerve entrapment.

Runner's fracture: Stress fracture of the lower end of the fibula or tibia.

Runner's high: Euphoria associated with long-distance running.

Runner's knee: Patellofemoral dysfunction or stress syndrome.

Runner's nipple: See Jogger's nipple.

Runner's toe: See Tennis toe.

Runner's trots: Gastrointestinal cramping and/or diarrhea in long-distance runners.

Saddle soreness: Ischial bursitis and pruritus ani in novice cyclists.

Scrum ear: See Cauliflower ear.

Scrum herpes: See Herpes gladiatorum.

Second wind: Subjective feeling of less fatigue and ventilatory stress after first few minutes of continuous exercise. No definite physiological explanation; may be due to achievement of aerobic threshold.

Shin splints: *Pain of the anteromedial distal 2/3 of the tibial shaft due to muscle–tendon inflammation.

Shoulder pointer: Contusion of the clavicle or acromioclavicular joint.

Skier's douche: See Water skiing douche.

Skier's enema: See Water skiing douche.

Skier's fracture: Comminuted spiral fracture of the tibia in association with a fibular fracture.

Skier's nose: Cold-induced rhinorrhea commonly seen in winter sports (skiing, skating, sledding, etc.)

Skier's thumb: See Gamekeeper's thumb.

Skier's toe: See Tennis toe.

Smith's fracture: *Flexion fracture of distal radius with increased volar angulation (reverse Colles' fracture).

Snapping hip: Medial or lateral audible snap, pop, or click of the hip due to subluxation of the femoral tendon or ligament slipping over a bony prominence; associated pain is due to bursitis, synovitis, or tendinitis.

Snapping neck: *Snapping or popping neck (audible or palpable); may be due to either irregularity at articulation or forced snapping of a tendon over bony prominences.

Snapping shoulder: *Subluxation of the bicipital tendon.

Soccer ankle: Anterior capsule sprain with the development of a traction spur on the superior talar neck due to repetitive microtrauma of kicking a heavy soccer ball on a wet pitch with an extremely plantarflexed foot.

Space Invaders wrist: Overuse strain of the wrist secondary to playing video games.

Sports anemia: Mild anemia seen acutely from increased plasma volume during early adaptation to endurance exercise; chronically, from iron deficiency (inadequate dietary intake, gastrointestinal blood loss, and hemolysis).

Squat-jump syndrome: Myoglobinuria and rhabdomyolysis following vigorous squat jumping.

Staleness: See Overtraining.

Stinger: Stretch or impingement of the brachial plexus, cervical plexus, or supraclavicular nerves following improper blocking technique, inexperience, or poor conditioning in football players.

Stitch in side: Upper abdominal pain reported by endurance athletes; cause unknown, but may be due to diaphragm muscle spasm.

Stone bruise: Contusion of the bone (usually foot).

Strawberry: Severe abrasion of skin, usually with weeping, secondary to sliding or rubbing on a floor; also termed raspberry, mat or turf burn.

Student's elbow: Olecranon bursitis.

Surfer's knots: Painless hyperkeratotic skin nodules over the metatarsophalangeal joints and anterior tibial surface.

Swimmer's ear: Acute otitis externa.

Swimmer's knee: See Breaststroker's knee.

Swimmer's shoulder: Impingement of the rotator cuff under the coracoacromial ligament and the acromion (coracoacromial arch).

Tackler's exostosis: Calcified spur on midlateral humerus from repeated tackles/blocks with the arm in football; also called blocker's exostosis, blocker's node, and linebacker's arm.

Talon noir: See Black heel.

Tennis elbow: Lateral epicondylitis.

Tennis leg: Traditionally a tear of the plantaris muscle, actually a strain of gastrocnemius (medial head).

Tennis thumb: Tendinitis with calcification in the flexor pollicis longus, secondary to repeated friction.

Tennis toe: Subungual hematoma produced by pressure, usually of the second toe but also the first and third.

Tennis wrist: Strain/laxity of the radioulnar ligament or fracture of the hamate due to excessive wrist action or direct trauma from racquet butt.

Trick knee: *Medial or lateral cartilage damage causing the knee to pop, click, or lock.

Trigger finger: Stenosing tenosynovitis at metacarpophalangeal joint causing painful snapping, flexion, and extension.

Turf burn: See Strawberry.

Turf toe: Traumatic sprain of first metatarsophalangeal joint capsule secondary to hyperextension.

Unhappy triad: *Simultaneous tears of the anterior cruciate, medial collateral ligament, and medial meniscus, seen in football players (clipping tackle) or skiers.

Urban cowboy rhabdomyolysis: Cramps and tenderness in muscle that may be accompanied by a reddish urine secondary to myoglobinuria; all secondary to strenuous activity (in this particular case, riding a mechanical bull) and also seen with prolonged or excessive exertion (e.g., boxing, karate, and marathons).

Water skiing douche: Water under high pressure may enter body orifice—rectum (skier's enema), vagina (skier's douche), auditory canal, nose, etc.—resulting at times in significant trauma.

Water wart: Molluscum *contagiosum*.

Wind knocked out: Blow to the upper abdomen (solar plexus) causing an inability to catch one's breath.

Wrestler's ear: See Cauliflower ear.

Appendix I: SCAT3™—Sport Concussion Assessment Tool, 3rd Edition

Richard B. Birrer, Francis G. O'Connor, and Shawn F. Kane

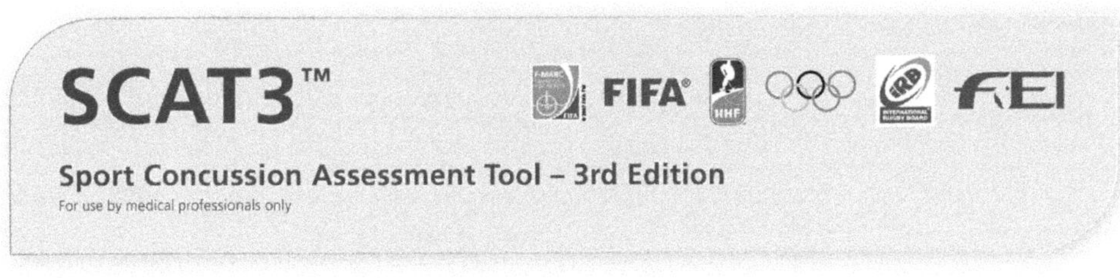

Name

Date/Time of Injury:
Date of Assessment:

Examiner:

What is the SCAT3?[1]

The SCAT3 is a standardized tool for evaluating injured athletes for concussion and can be used in athletes aged from 13 years and older. It supersedes the original SCAT and the SCAT2 published in 2005 and 2009, respectively[2]. For younger persons, ages 12 and under, please use the Child SCAT3. The SCAT3 is designed for use by medical professionals. If you are not qualified, please use the Sport Concussion Recognition Tool[1]. Preseason baseline testing with the SCAT3 can be helpful for interpreting post-injury test scores.

Specific instructions for use of the SCAT3 are provided on page 3. If you are not familiar with the SCAT3, please read through these instructions carefully. This tool may be freely copied in its current form for distribution to individuals, teams, groups and organizations. Any revision or any reproduction in a digital form requires approval by the Concussion in Sport Group.

NOTE: The diagnosis of a concussion is a clinical judgment, ideally made by a medical professional. The SCAT3 should not be used solely to make, or exclude, the diagnosis of concussion in the absence of clinical judgement. An athlete may have a concussion even if their SCAT3 is "normal".

What is a concussion?

A concussion is a disturbance in brain function caused by a direct or indirect force to the head. It results in a variety of non-specific signs and/or symptoms (some examples listed below) and most often does not involve loss of consciousness. Concussion should be suspected in the presence of **any one or more** of the following:

- Symptoms (e.g., headache), or
- Physical signs (e.g., unsteadiness), or
- Impaired brain function (e.g. confusion) or
- Abnormal behaviour (e.g., change in personality).

SIDELINE ASSESSMENT

Indications for Emergency Management

NOTE: A hit to the head can sometimes be associated with a more serious brain injury. Any of the following warrants consideration of activating emergency procedures and urgent transportation to the nearest hospital:

- Glasgow Coma score less than 15
- Deteriorating mental status
- Potential spinal injury
- Progressive, worsening symptoms or new neurologic signs

Potential signs of concussion?

If any of the following signs are observed after a direct or indirect blow to the head, the athlete should stop participation, be evaluated by a medical professional and **should not be permitted to return to sport the same day** if a concussion is suspected.

Any loss of consciousness?	Y	N
"If so, how long?"		
Balance or motor incoordination **(stumbles, slow/laboured movements, etc.)**?	Y	N
Disorientation or confusion **(inability to respond appropriately to questions)**?	Y	N
Loss of memory:	Y	N
"If so, how long?"		
"Before or after the injury?"		
Blank or vacant look:	Y	N
Visible facial injury in combination with any of the above:	Y	N

1 Glasgow coma scale (GCS)

Best eye response (E)	
No eye opening	1
Eye opening in response to pain	2
Eye opening to speech	3
Eyes opening spontaneously	4
Best verbal response (V)	
No verbal response	1
Incomprehensible sounds	2
Inappropriate words	3
Confused	4
Oriented	5
Best motor response (M)	
No motor response	1
Extension to pain	2
Abnormal flexion to pain	3
Flexion/Withdrawal to pain	4
Localizes to pain	5
Obeys commands	6
Glasgow Coma score (E + V + M)	of 15

GCS should be recorded for all athletes in case of subsequent deterioration.

2 Maddocks Score[3]

"I am going to ask you a few questions, please listen carefully and give your best effort."

Modified Maddocks questions (1 point for each correct answer)

What venue are we at today?	0	1
Which half is it now?	0	1
Who scored last in this match?	0	1
What team did you play last week/game?	0	1
Did your team win the last game?	0	1
Maddocks score		of 5

Maddocks score is validated for sideline diagnosis of concussion only and is not used for serial testing.

Notes: Mechanism of Injury (**"tell me what happened"**?):

Any athlete with a suspected concussion should be REMOVED FROM PLAY, medically assessed, monitored for deterioration (i.e., should not be left alone) and should not drive a motor vehicle until cleared to do so by a medical professional. No athlete diagnosed with concussion should be returned to sports participation on the day of Injury.

SCAT3 SPORT CONCUSSION ASSESMENT TOOL 3 | **PAGE 1**

259

BACKGROUND

Name: ______ Date: ______
Examiner: ______
Sport/team/school: ______ Date/time of injury: ______
Age: ______ Gender: M F
Years of education completed: ______
Dominant hand: right left neither
How many concussions do you think you have had in the past? ______
When was the most recent concussion? ______
How long was your recovery from the most recent concussion? ______

Have you ever been hospitalized or had medical imaging done for a head injury?	Y	N
Have you ever been diagnosed with headaches or migraines?	Y	N
Do you have a learning disability, dyslexia, ADD/ADHD?	Y	N
Have you ever been diagnosed with depression, anxiety or other psychiatric disorder?	Y	N
Has anyone in your family ever been diagnosed with any of these problems?	Y	N
Are you on any medications? If yes, please list:	Y	N

SCAT3 to be done in resting state. Best done 10 or more minutes post excercise.

SYMPTOM EVALUATION

3 How do you feel?

"You should score yourself on the following symptoms, based on how you feel now".

	none	mild		moderate		severe	
Headache	0	1	2	3	4	5	6
"Pressure in head"	0	1	2	3	4	5	6
Neck Pain	0	1	2	3	4	5	6
Nausea or vomiting	0	1	2	3	4	5	6
Dizziness	0	1	2	3	4	5	6
Blurred vision	0	1	2	3	4	5	6
Balance problems	0	1	2	3	4	5	6
Sensitivity to light	0	1	2	3	4	5	6
Sensitivity to noise	0	1	2	3	4	5	6
Feeling slowed down	0	1	2	3	4	5	6
Feeling like "in a fog"	0	1	2	3	4	5	6
"Don't feel right"	0	1	2	3	4	5	6
Difficulty concentrating	0	1	2	3	4	5	6
Difficulty remembering	0	1	2	3	4	5	6
Fatigue or low energy	0	1	2	3	4	5	6
Confusion	0	1	2	3	4	5	6
Drowsiness	0	1	2	3	4	5	6
Trouble falling asleep	0	1	2	3	4	5	6
More emotional	0	1	2	3	4	5	6
Irritability	0	1	2	3	4	5	6
Sadness	0	1	2	3	4	5	6
Nervous or Anxious	0	1	2	3	4	5	6

Total number of symptoms (Maximum possible 22)
Symptom severity score (Maximum possible 132)

Do the symptoms get worse with physical activity?	Y	N
Do the symptoms get worse with mental activity?	Y	N

self rated — self rated and clinician monitored
clinician interview — self rated with parent input

Overall rating: If you know the athlete well prior to the injury, how different is the athlete acting compared to his/her usual self?

Please circle one response:

no different	very different	unsure	N/A

Scoring on the SCAT3 should not be used as a stand-alone method to diagnose concussion, measure recovery or make decisions about an athlete's readiness to return to competition after concussion. Since signs and symptoms may evolve over time, it is important to consider repeat evaluation in the acute assessment of concussion.

COGNITIVE & PHYSICAL EVALUATION

4 Cognitive assessment

Standardized Assessment of Concussion (SAC)[4]

Orientation (1 point for each correct answer)

What month is it?	0	1
What is the date today?	0	1
What is the day of the week?	0	1
What year is it?	0	1
What time is it right now? (within 1 hour)	0	1
Orientation score		of 5

Immediate memory

List	Trial 1		Trial 2		Trial 3		Alternative word list		
elbow	0	1	0	1	0	1	candle	baby	finger
apple	0	1	0	1	0	1	paper	monkey	penny
carpet	0	1	0	1	0	1	sugar	perfume	blanket
saddle	0	1	0	1	0	1	sandwich	sunset	lemon
bubble	0	1	0	1	0	1	wagon	iron	insect
Total									

Immediate memory score total — of 15

Concentration: **Digits Backward**

List	Trial 1		Alternative digit list		
4-9-3	0	1	6-2-9	5-2-6	4-1-5
3-8-1-4	0	1	3-2-7-9	1-7-9-5	4-9-6-8
6-2-9-7-1	0	1	1-5-2-8-6	3-8-5-2-7	6-1-8-4-3
7-1-8-4-6-2	0	1	5-3-9-1-4-8	8-3-1-9-6-4	7-2-4-8-5-6
Total of 4					

Concentration: **Month in Reverse Order** (1 pt. for entire sequence correct)

Dec-Nov-Oct-Sept-Aug-Jul-Jun-May-Apr-Mar-Feb-Jan	0	1
Concentration score		of 5

5 Neck Examination:

Range of motion Tenderness Upper and lower limb sensation & strength

Findings: ______

6 Balance examination

Do one or both of the following tests.

Footwear (shoes, barefoot, braces, tape, etc.) ______

Modified Balance Error Scoring System (BESS) testing[5]

Which foot was tested (i.e. which is the **non-dominant** foot) Left Right

Testing surface (hard floor, field, etc.) ______

Condition

Double leg stance:	Errors
Single leg stance (non-dominant foot):	Errors
Tandem stance (non-dominant foot at back):	Errors

And/Or

Tandem gait[6,7]

Time (best of 4 trials): ______ seconds

7 Coordination examination

Upper limb coordination

Which arm was tested: Left Right

Coordination score — of 1

8 SAC Delayed Recall[4]

Delayed recall score — of 5

INSTRUCTIONS

Words in *Italics* throughout the SCAT3 are the instructions given to the athlete by the tester.

Symptom Scale

"You should score yourself on the following symptoms, based on how you feel now".

To be completed by the athlete. In situations where the symptom scale is being completed after exercise, it should still be done in a resting state, at least 10 minutes post exercise.

For total number of symptoms, maximum possible is 22.

For Symptom severity score, add all scores in table, maximum possible is 22 x 6 = 132.

SAC[4]

Immediate Memory

"I am going to test your memory. I will read you a list of words and when I am done, repeat back as many words as you can remember, in any order."

Trials 2 & 3:

"I am going to repeat the same list again. Repeat back as many words as you can remember in any order, even if you said the word before."

Complete all 3 trials regardless of score on trial 1 & 2. Read the words at a rate of one per second. **Score 1 pt. for each correct response.** Total score equals sum across all 3 trials. Do not inform the athlete that delayed recall will be tested.

Concentration

Digits backward

"I am going to read you a string of numbers and when I am done, you repeat them back to me backwards, in reverse order of how I read them to you. For example, if I say 7-1-9, you would say 9-1-7."

If correct, go to next string length. If incorrect, read trial 2. **One point possible for each string length.** Stop after incorrect on both trials. The digits should be read at the rate of one per second.

Months in reverse order

"Now tell me the months of the year in reverse order. Start with the last month and go backward. So you'll say December, November ... Go ahead"

1 pt. for entire sequence correct

Delayed Recall

The delayed recall should be performed after completion of the Balance and Coordination Examination.

"Do you remember that list of words I read a few times earlier? Tell me as many words from the list as you can remember in any order."

Score 1 pt. for each correct response

Balance Examination

Modified Balance Error Scoring System (BESS) testing[5]

This balance testing is based on a modified version of the Balance Error Scoring System (BESS)[5]. A stopwatch or watch with a second hand is required for this testing.

"I am now going to test your balance. Please take your shoes off, roll up your pant legs above ankle (if applicable), and remove any ankle taping (if applicable). This test will consist of three twenty second tests with different stances."

(a) Double leg stance:

"The first stance is standing with your feet together with your hands on your hips and with your eyes closed. You should try to maintain stability in that position for 20 seconds. I will be counting the number of times you move out of this position. I will start timing when you are set and have closed your eyes."

(b) Single leg stance:

"If you were to kick a ball, which foot would you use? [This will be the dominant foot] Now stand on your non-dominant foot. The dominant leg should be held in approximately 30 degrees of hip flexion and 45 degrees of knee flexion. Again, you should try to maintain stability for 20 seconds with your hands on your hips and your eyes closed. I will be counting the number of times you move out of this position. If you stumble out of this position, open your eyes and return to the start position and continue balancing. I will start timing when you are set and have closed your eyes."

(c) Tandem stance:

"Now stand heel-to-toe with your non-dominant foot in back. Your weight should be evenly distributed across both feet. Again, you should try to maintain stability for 20 seconds with your hands on your hips and your eyes closed. I will be counting the number of times you move out of this position. If you stumble out of this position, open your eyes and return to the start position and continue balancing. I will start timing when you are set and have closed your eyes."

Balance testing – types of errors

1. Hands lifted off iliac crest
2. Opening eyes
3. Step, stumble, or fall
4. Moving hip into > 30 degrees abduction
5. Lifting forefoot or heel
6. Remaining out of test position > 5 sec

Each of the 20-second trials is scored by counting the errors, or deviations from the proper stance, accumulated by the athlete. The examiner will begin counting errors only after the individual has assumed the proper start position. **The modified BESS is calculated by adding one error point for each error during the three 20-second tests. The maximum total number of errors for any single condition is 10.** If a athlete commits multiple errors simultaneously, only one error is recorded but the athlete should quickly return to the testing position, and counting should resume once subject is set. Subjects that are unable to maintain the testing procedure for a minimum of **five seconds** at the start are assigned the highest possible score, ten, for that testing condition.

OPTION: For further assessment, the same 3 stances can be performed on a surface of medium density foam (e.g., approximately 50 cm x 40 cm x 6 cm).

Tandem Gait[6,7]

Participants are instructed to stand with their feet together behind a starting line (the test is best done with footwear removed). Then, they walk in a forward direction as quickly and as accurately as possible along a 38mm wide (sports tape), 3 meter line with an alternate foot heel-to-toe gait ensuring that they approximate their heel and toe on each step. Once they cross the end of the 3m line, they turn 180 degrees and return to the starting point using the same gait. A total of 4 trials are done and the best time is retained. Athletes should complete the test in 14 seconds. Athletes fail the test if they step off the line, have a separation between their heel and toe, or if they touch or grab the examiner or an object. In this case, the time is not recorded and the trial repeated, if appropriate.

Coordination Examination

Upper limb coordination

Finger-to-nose (FTN) task:

"I am going to test your coordination now. Please sit comfortably on the chair with your eyes open and your arm (either right or left) outstretched (shoulder flexed to 90 degrees and elbow and fingers extended), pointing in front of you. When I give a start signal, I would like you to perform five successive finger to nose repetitions using your index finger to touch the tip of the nose, and then return to the starting position, as quickly and as accurately as possible."

Scoring: 5 correct repetitions in < 4 seconds = 1

Note for testers: Athletes fail the test if they do not touch their nose, do not fully extend their elbow or do not perform five repetitions. **Failure should be scored as 0.**

References & Footnotes

1. This tool has been developed by a group of international experts at the 4th International Consensus meeting on Concussion in Sport held in Zurich, Switzerland in November 2012. The full details of the conference outcomes and the authors of the tool are published in The BJSM Injury Prevention and Health Protection, 2013, Volume 47, Issue 5. The outcome paper will also be simultaneously co-published in other leading biomedical journals with the copyright held by the Concussion in Sport Group, to allow unrestricted distribution, providing no alterations are made.

2. McCrory P et al., Consensus Statement on Concussion in Sport – the 3rd International Conference on Concussion in Sport held in Zurich, November 2008. British Journal of Sports Medicine 2009; 43: i76-89.

3. Maddocks, DL; Dicker, GD; Saling, MM. The assessment of orientation following concussion in athletes. Clinical Journal of Sport Medicine. 1995; 5(1): 32–3.

4. McCrea M. Standardized mental status testing of acute concussion. Clinical Journal of Sport Medicine. 2001; 11: 176–181.

5. Guskiewicz KM. Assessment of postural stability following sport-related concussion. Current Sports Medicine Reports. 2003; 2: 24–30.

6. Schneiders, A.G., Sullivan, S.J., Gray, A., Hammond-Tooke, G. & McCrory, P. Normative values for 16-37 year old subjects for three clinical measures of motor performance used in the assessment of sports concussions. Journal of Science and Medicine in Sport. 2010; 13(2): 196–201.

7. Schneiders, A.G., Sullivan, S.J., Kvarnstrom. J.K., Olsson, M., Yden. T. & Marshall, S.W. The effect of footwear and sports-surface on dynamic neurological screening in sport-related concussion. Journal of Science and Medicine in Sport. 2010; 13(4): 382–386

ATHLETE INFORMATION

Any athlete suspected of having a concussion should be removed from play, and then seek medical evaluation.

Signs to watch for

Problems could arise over the first 24–48 hours. The athlete should not be left alone and must go to a hospital at once if they:

- Have a headache that gets worse
- Are very drowsy or can't be awakened
- Can't recognize people or places
- Have repeated vomiting
- Behave unusually or seem confused; are very irritable
- Have seizures (arms and legs jerk uncontrollably)
- Have weak or numb arms or legs
- Are unsteady on their feet; have slurred speech

Remember, it is better to be safe.
Consult your doctor after a suspected concussion.

Return to play

Athletes should not be returned to play the same day of injury.
When returning athletes to play, they should be **medically cleared and then follow a stepwise supervised program,** with stages of progression.

For example:

Rehabilitation stage	Functional exercise at each stage of rehabilitation	Objective of each stage
No activity	Physical and cognitive rest	Recovery
Light aerobic exercise	Walking, swimming or stationary cycling keeping intensity, 70% maximum predicted heart rate. No resistance training	Increase heart rate
Sport-specific exercise	Skating drills in ice hockey, running drills in soccer. No head impact activities	Add movement
Non-contact training drills	Progression to more complex training drills, eg passing drills in football and ice hockey. May start progressive resistance training	Exercise, coordination, and cognitive load
Full contact practice	Following medical clearance participate in normal training activities	Restore confidence and assess functional skills by coaching staff
Return to play	Normal game play	

There should be at least 24 hours (or longer) for each stage and if symptoms recur the athlete should rest until they resolve once again and then resume the program at the previous asymptomatic stage. Resistance training should only be added in the later stages.

If the athlete is symptomatic for more than 10 days, then consultation by a medical practitioner who is expert in the management of concussion, is recommended.

Medical clearance should be given before return to play.

Scoring Summary:

Test Domain	Score		
	Date:	Date:	Date:
Number of Symptoms of 22			
Symptom Severity Score of 132			
Orientation of 5			
Immediate Memory of 15			
Concentration of 5			
Delayed Recall of 5			
SAC Total			
BESS (total errors)			
Tandem Gait (seconds)			
Coordination of 1			

Notes:

CONCUSSION INJURY ADVICE

(To be given to the **person monitoring** the concussed athlete)

This patient has received an injury to the head. A careful medical examination has been carried out and no sign of any serious complications has been found. Recovery time is variable across individuals and the patient will need monitoring for a further period by a responsible adult. Your treating physician will provide guidance as to this timeframe.

If you notice any change in behaviour, vomiting, dizziness, worsening headache, double vision or excessive drowsiness, please contact your doctor or the nearest hospital emergency department immediately.

Other important points:

- Rest (physically and mentally), including training or playing sports until symptoms resolve and you are medically cleared
- No alcohol
- No prescription or non-prescription drugs without medical supervision. Specifically:
  - No sleeping tablets
  - Do not use aspirin, anti-inflammatory medication or sedating pain killers
- Do not drive until medically cleared
- Do not train or play sport until medically cleared

Clinic phone number

Patient's name

Date/time of injury

Date/time of medical review

Treatingphysician

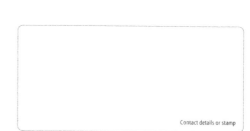

Index

B

C

F

G

H

I

J

N

P

T

U

V

W

Y

Z

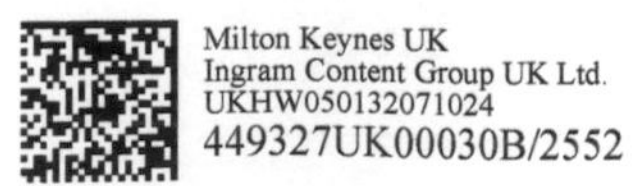

Milton Keynes UK
Ingram Content Group UK Ltd.
UKHW050132071024
449327UK00030B/2552